REFERENCE RANGE

DETERMINATION	Conventional	SI	NOTES
Leukocyte count	Newborn: 9000–30,000/μL 1 wk: 5000–21,000/μL 1 mo: 5000–19,500/μL 6–12 mo: 6000–17,500/μL 2 yr: 6200–17,000/μL	$9.0–30.0 \times 10^9$/L $5.0–21.0 \times 10^9$/L $5.0–19.5 \times 10^9$/L $6.0–17.5 \times 10^9$/L $6.2–17.0 \times 10^9$/L	Hemacytometer method
Erythrocyte count	Newborn: 4.4–5.8 million/μL Infant/child: 3.8–5.5 million/μL Adult male: 4.7–6.1 million/μL Adult female: 4.2–5.4 million/μL	$4.4–5.8 \times 10^{12}$/L $3.8–5.5 \times 10^{12}$/L $4.7–6.1 \times 10^{12}$/L $4.2–5.4 \times 10^{12}$/L	Hemacytometer method
Eosinophil count	50–400/μL	$0.05–0.4 \times 10^9$/L	Hemacytometer method
Reticulocyte count	Newborn: 2.5%–6.0% Adult: 0.5%–2.0%	2.5–6.0 g/L 0.5–2.0 g/L	New methylene blue
Absolute reticulocyte	24,000–84,000/μL	$24–84 \times 10^9$/L	Calculation: %Retic × RBC
Erythrocyte sedimentation rate (ESR)	Male: 0–15 mm/hr Female: 0–20 mm/hr		Westergren method EDTA (anticoagulant)
Osmotic fragility of erythrocytes	Initial hemolysis: 0.45% Complete hemolysis: 0.30%–0.35%		Heparin (anticoagulant)
Acidified serum test (Ham's test) for PNH	No hemolysis		
Sugar water test for PNH	< 5% hemolysis		
Autohemolysis test	Lysis at 48 hr: without added dextrose (0.2%–2.0%) Lysis at 48 hr: with added dextrose (0–1.0%) Lysis at 48 hr: with added ATP (0–0.8%)		
RBC enzymes			
G6PD	3.4–8.0 U/g Hgb	0.22–0.52 MU/mol Hgb	Bishop, modified method
Pyruvate kinase	13–17 U/g Hgb	0.84–1.1 MU/mol Hgb	ICSH method
Iron studies			
Serum iron	Adult male: 50–160 μg/dL Adult female: 40–150 μg/dL	8.95–28.64 μmol/L 7.16–26.85 μmol/L	Colorimetric
TIBC	250–400 μg/dL	44.75–71.60 μmol/L	Colorimetric
Transferrin saturation	20–50%		
Ferritin (serum)			

Iron deficiency
  Borderline
  Iron excess
	0–12 ng/mL
	13–20 ng/mL
	> 400 ng/L
		0–4.8 nmol/L
		5.2–8.0 nmol/L
		> 160 nmol/L
			RIA

Folic acid			
Normal Borderline	> 3.3 ng/L 2.5–3.2 ng/mL	> 7.3 nmol/L 5.75–7.39 nmol/L	RIA
Red cell folate	150–450 mg/mL	340–1020 nmol/L	Collect in EDTA
Haptoglobin	40–336 mg/dL	0.4–3.6 g/L	RID

SI = System of International Units; CV = coefficient of variation; SD = standard deviation; PNH = paroxysmal nocturnal hemoglobinuria; ATP = adenosine triphosphate; G6PD = glucose-6-phosphate dehydrogenase deficiency; TIBC = total iron-binding capacity; RIA = radioimmunoassay; RID = radioimmunodiffusion; ICSH = International Committee for Standardization of Hematology; EDTA = ethylenediamine tetra-acetic acid

Clinical Hematology and Fundamentals of Hemostasis

Clinical Hematology and Fundamentals of Hemostasis

Edition 4

DENISE M. HARMENING, PhD, MT(ASCP), CLS(NCA)
Chair and Professor
Department of Medical and Research Technology
University of Maryland School of Medicine
Baltimore, Maryland

F. A. Davis Company • Philadelphia

F. A. Davis Company
1915 Arch Street
Philadelphia, PA 19103
www.fadavis.com

Printed in the United States of America

Last digit indicates print number: 10 9 8 7 6 5 4

Acquisitions Editor: Christa Fratantoro
Developmental Editor: Peg Waltner
Production Editor: Jack Brandt
Cover Designer: Louis J. Forgione

As new scientific information becomes available through basic and clinical research, recommended treatments and drug therapies undergo changes. The author(s) and publisher have done everything possible to make this book accurate, up to date, and in accord with accepted standard at the time of publication. The authors, editors, and publisher are not responsible for errors or omissions or for consequences from application of the book, and make no warranty, expressed or implied, in regard to the contents of the book. Any practice described in this book should be applied by the reader in accordance with professional standards of care used in regard to the unique circumstances that may apply in each situation. The reader is advised always to check product information (package inserts) for changes and new information regarding dose and contraindications before administering any drug. Caution is especially urged when using new or infrequently ordered drugs.

Library of Congress Cataloging-in-Publication Data

Clinical hematology and fundamentals of hemostasis / Denise M. Harmening, editor. — 4th ed.
    p. ; cm.
  Includes bibliographical references and index.
  ISBN 0-8036-0783-0 (alk. paper)
   1. Hematology. 2. Blood—Diseases. 3. Homeostasis. I. Harmening, Denise.
  [DNLM: 1. Hematologic Diseases—Blood Cells. 2. Hemostasis—Blood Cells. WH 100
C6413 2001]
  RB145 .C536 2001
  616.1′5—dc21

               2001047699

To all students—full-time, part-time, past, present, and future—
who have touched and will continue to touch the lives of so many educators. . . .

It is to you this book is dedicated in the hope
of inspiring an unquenchable thirst for knowledge and love of mankind

PREFACE

The fourth edition of this text continues to set the standard for teaching and learning in clinical hematology and fundamentals of hemostasis. Thorough, yet concise, a total of 33 chapters serve as a combination of text, laboratory procedures manual, and atlas of cell morphology. This textbook is unique in its five-part format, featuring an introduction to clinical hematology and sections on the anemias, white blood cell disorders, hemostasis and thrombosis, and laboratory methods. Outlines, educational objectives, case histories, summary charts, and study guide questions support each chapter.

The new laboratory methods section includes chapters on routine hematology methods, automated differential analysis, flow cytometry, cytochemistry, coagulation, and molecular diagnostic techniques in hematopathology. The expanded color plate section of the cytochemistry chapter serves as a condensed atlas of cytochemistry. Numerous illustrations, including 293 color plates, aid in the process of learning. In addition, the fourth edition includes more than 950 figures (line drawings and black-and-white photographs) and 339 tables. The text has retained the popular listing of normal hematologic values on the inside covers for quick reference. In addition, an invaluable glossary provides easy access to definitions of medical terms unique to hematology and hemostasis. Summary charts have been added at the end of each chapter to identify for students the most important information to know for clinical rotations. An innovative instructor's guide emphasizing competency-based assessment accompanies the text, and an interactive test-generating question bank is also available, containing over 1800 questions with assigned taxonomy levels.

This new edition, like the first, second, and third, is a culmination of the dedicated efforts of many prominent laboratory professionals. Fifty-five contributors committed themselves to this project by donating their time and expertise out of concern for a common goal: improving patient care by providing a high-quality, practical, and usable textbook. To all of these contributors, thank you and congratulations on a wonderful book. A very special thank you and acknowledgment must also be given to Joanne Manning, my administrative assistant, for her superb organizational abilities and her tireless efforts and support. A special acknowledgment is also given to Virginia Hughes, who is currently enrolled in the SBB program at the National Institutes of Health (NIH)—her many hours of dedicated and meticulous review have ensured a more accurate and usable text—and to Angela Neale, a graduate of the medical technology program, for her countless hours of research and searching the Internet for references. In addition, I would like to acknowledge the contributions, throughout the book's preparation, of my dedicated coworkers and friends at the Department of Medical and Research Technology (DMRT), particularly Cynthia Stambach, Audrey Ford, Alicia Walters, and Tom Pennington.

Finally, my sincere appreciation is also extended to the following educators, clinicians and industry representatives for their thorough and thoughtful review of the manuscript:

- Paul Broden, MA, MT(ASCP)SH, RAC
  Vice President
  QARC, Sysmex Corporation
  Los Alamitos, California

- Donna Castellone, MS, MT(ASCP)SH
  Technical Supervisor, Special Coagulation
  Cornell University
  New York Presbyterian Hospital
  New York, New York

- Dan Holton
  Product Manager
  Abbott Laboratories
  Abbott Park, Illinois

- Nancy Lavon
  Marketing Manager
  Bayer Corporation
  Tarrytown, New York

- Janis Wyrick-Glatzel, MS, MT(ASCP)
  Associate Professor of
  Clinical Laboratory Science Program
  Program in Clinical Laboratory Science
  University of Nevada at Las Vegas
  Las Vegas, Nevada

In summary, this book has been designed to inspire an unquenchable thirst for knowledge in every medical technologist, hematologist, and practitioner whose knowledge, skills, and ongoing education provide the public with excellent health care.

D.M. Harmening, PhD, MT(ASCP), CLS(NCA)

CONTRIBUTORS

Ann Bell, MS, SH(ASCP), CLSpH(NCA)
Emeritus Professor, Clinical Laboratory
  Sciences
Emeritus Assistant Professor, Department
  of Medicine
University of Tennessee, Memphis
The Health Science Center, Department of
  Medicine
Division of Hematology Oncology
Memphis, Tennessee

Carlo Brugnara, MD
Director, Hematology Laboratory
Associate Professor of Pathology
Children's Hospital
Boston, Massachusetts

Carlos E. Bueso-Ramos, MD, PhD
Associate Professor
Department of Hematopathology
Division of Pathology and Laboratory
  Medicine
The University of Texas M.D. Anderson
  Cancer Center
Houston, Texas

Lambert Busque, MD, FRCP(C)
Associate Professor of Medicine,
  Universite de Montreal
Department of Hematology
Maisonneuve-Rosemont Hospital
Montreal, Quebec, Canada

Barbara Caldwell, MS, MT(ASCP)SH
Manager, Clinical Laboratory Services
Montgomery General Hospital
Olney, Maryland

Carol C. Caruana, H(ASCP)SH
Department of Laboratories
North Shore University Hospital
New York University School of Medicine
Manhasset, New York

Betty E. Ciesla, MS, MT(ASCP)SH
Morgan State University
Program in Medical Technology
Baltimore, Maryland

Theresa L. Coetzer, PhD
Department of Molecular Medicine and
  Haematology
South African Institute for Medical
  Research
School of Pathology
Department of Haematology
University of the Witwatersrand Medical
  School
Johannesburg, South Africa

Giovanni D'Angelo, FCMLS
Associate Director of Leukemic Cell Bank
Department of Hematology
Maisonneuve-Rosemont Hospital
Montreal, Quebec, Canada

Carmen Del Toro, MS, MT
Professor
Sacred Heart University
Medical Technology Program
Santruce, Puerto Rico

Aamir Ehsan, MD
Assistant Professor
Director of Flow Cytometry
Director of Hematology at Audie Murphy
  Veteran's Hospital
Department of Pathology
The University of Texas Health Science
  Center
San Antonio, Texas

Gordon E. Ens, MT(ASCP)
President, Colorado Coagulation
  Consultants, Inc.
Aurora, Colorado

Claudia E. Escobar, MT(ASCP)SH
Technical Service Specialist
Diagnostica Stago
Parsippany, New Jersey

Douglas Fish, MD, FRCP(C)
Assistant Professor of Medicine,
  Université de Montréal
Department of Hematology
Maisonneuve-Rosemont Hospital
Montreal, Quebec, Canada

Donna M. Gandour, PhD
Manager, Customer Education and
  Applications Support
BD Biosciences Immunocytometry
  Systems
San Jose, California

Armand B. Glassman, MD
Olla S. Stribling Distinguished Chair for
  Cancer Research
Professor
Division of Pathology and Laboratory
  Medicine
University of Texas M.D. Anderson
  Cancer Center
Houston, Texas

Ralph Green, BAppSci(MLS), FAIMLS
Associate Professor in Immunohematology
Acting Head
Department of Medical Laboratory Science
Faculty of Biomedical and Health Sciences
Royal Melbourne Institute of Technology
  University
Melbourne, Victoria, Australia

Margaret L. Gulley, MD
Associate Professor, Pathology
  Department
University of North Carolina at Chapel
  Hill
Chapel Hill, North Carolina

Sandra Gwaltney Krause, MA,
  MT(ASCP)
Former Instructor
Department of Medical Technology
University of South Alabama
Mobile, Alabama

Martin Gyger, MD, FRCP(C)
Director, Bone Marrow Transplant
  Program
King Faisal Specialist Hospital and
  Research Centre
Riyadh, Kingdom of Saudi Arabia

Walid Hamoudi, MD, PhD
Faculty Associate
Department of Hematopathology
Division of Pathology and Laboratory
  Medicine
The University of Texas M.D. Anderson
  Cancer Center
Houston, Texas

Denise M. Harmening, PhD, MT(ASCP), CLS(NCA)
Chair and Professor
Department of Medical and Research Technology
University of Maryland School of Medicine
Baltimore, Maryland

Chantal Ricaud Harrison MD
Professor of Pathology
University of Texas Health Sciences Center at San Antonio
San Antonio, Texas

Laurel D. Holmer, MEd, MT(ASCP)SH
Assistant Professor
Department of Clinical Laboratory Science
University of Nevada School of Medicine
Reno, Nevada

Ellen Hope Kearns, MS, SH(ASCP)H
Professor of Health Sciences
Division of Health Sciences
School of Health
California State University, Dominguez Hills
Carson, California

Virginia C. Hughes, MS, MT(ASCP), CLS(NCA)I
Specialist in Blood Banking Program
Department of Transfusion Medicine
Warren G. Magnuson Cinical Center
National Institutes of Health (NIH)
Bethesda, Maryland

Jerry W. Hussong, DDS, MD
Director of Hematopathology and Flow Cytometry
Laboratory Medicine Consultants
Department of Pathology
Sunrise Hospital
Las Vegas, Nevada

Dan M. Hyder, MD
Director, Department of Pathology and Laboratory Medicine
Southwest Washington Medical Center
Vancouver, Washington

Diane M. Joiner Maier, MLT(ASCP)
Technical Service Specialist
Diagnostica Stago
Parsippany, New Jersey

Cynthia S. Johns, MSA, MT(ASCP)SH
Laboratory Manager
Esoterix Coagulation
Aurora, Colorado

Carmen J. Julius, MD
Department of Pathology and Laboratory Medicine
The Ohio State University
Columbus, Ohio

Charles L. Knupp, MD
Professor of Medicine
Division of Hematology/Oncology
East Carolina University School of Medicine
Greenville, North Carolina

Lee A. LaMonica, BS, MT(ASCP), CLS(NCA)
Senior Medical Technologist
Endocrinology Department
Quest Diagnostics, Inc.
San Juan Capistrano, California

Teresa M. Launder, MD
Director of Hematology and Bone Marrow Lab
Assistant Professor, Pathology
Oregon Health Sciences University
Portland, Oregon

Lyle C. Lawnicki, MD
Resident in Pathology
Oregon Health Sciences University
Portland, Oregon

Louann W. Lawrence, DrPH, MT(ASCP)SH, CLS(NCA)
Professor and Department Head
Department of Clinical Laboratory Sciences
School of Allied Health Professions
Louisiana State University Health Science Center
New Orleans, Louisiana

John Lazarchick, MD
Professor, Director of Hematopathology and Hemostasis
Department of Pathology and Laboratory Medicine
Medical University of South Carolina
Charleston, South Carolina

Darla K. Liles, MD
Assistant Professor
Department of Medicine
Brody School of Medicine
East Carolina University
Greenville, North Carolina

James M. Long, MD, LtCol(sel), USAF
Department of Hematology and Oncology
David Grant Medical Center/SGOMO
Travis Air Force Base
Vacaville, California

Joe Marty, MS, MT(ASCP)
Assistant Professor (Clinical)
Department of Pathology
University of Utah Health Sciences Center
Salt Lake City, Utah

Deirdre DeSantis Parsons, MS, MT(ASCP)SBB
Assistant Professor
Department of Medical and Research Technology
University of Maryland School of Medicine
Baltimore, Maryland

Mary L. Perkins, MS, MT(ASCP)SH
Manager, Hematology, Medical Genetics
Legacy Laboratory Services
Portland, Oregon

Sherrie L. Perkins, MD, PhD
Medical Director of Hematopathology
University of Utah Health Sciences and ARUP Laboratories
Salt Lake City, Utah

Julie A. Plumbley, MD
Hematopathology Fellow
Department of Pathology
The University of Texas Health Science Center
San Antonio, Texas

Sharon L. Schwartz, MT(ASCP)SH, CLS(NCA)
Technical Specialist in Coagulation and Hematology
North Shore—Long Island Jewish Health System Laboratories
Lake Success, New York

Vickie L. Simmons, BS, MT(ASCP)SH
Field Technical Service Specialist Supervisor
Diagnostica Stago
Parsippany, New Jersey

Peggy Simpson, MS, MT(ASCP)
MLT Program Director
Alamance Community College
Graham, North Carolina

Kelly M. Smith-Moore, MT(ASCP)SH
Technical Service Specialist
Diagnostica Stago
Parsippany, New Jersey

Catherine M. Spier, MD
Associate Professor
University of Arizona
Department of Pathology
Health Science Center
Tucson, Arizona

Joan M. Steiner-Adler, EdD, MT(ASCP), CLS(NCA)
Program Director
School of Medical Technology
Eisenhower Medical Center
Rancho Mirage, California

Ronald Strauss, MD
Medical Director, DeGowin Blood Center
Professor of Pathology and Pediatrics
University of Iowa Hospitals and Clinics
Iowa City, Iowa

Mitra Taghizadeh, MS, MT(ASCP)
Clinical Assistant Professor
Department of Medical and Research Technology
University of Maryland School of Medicine
Baltimore, Maryland

Janis Wyrick-Glatzel, MS, MT(ASCP)
Associate Professor of Clinical Laboratory Science Program
Program in Clinical Laboratory Science
University of Nevada at Las Vegas
Las Vegas, Nevada

Stan Zail, MBBCh, MD, FCRPath
Department of Molecular Medicine and Haematology
South African Institute for Medical Research
School of Pathology
University of the Witwatersrand Medical School
Johannesburg, South Africa

Hallye Zeringer, BS, MT(ASCP)SH
Medical Technologist
Southern Baptist Hospital
New Orleans, Louisiana

CONTENTS

Clinical Hematology and Fundamentals of Hemostasis

COLOR PLATES

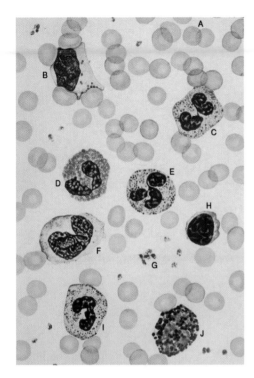

1. Peripheral blood (PB).
   A. RBC's, *B*. large lymphocyte
   C. neutrophil, *D*. eosinophil
   E. neutrophil, *F*. monocyte, *G*. platelets,
   H. small lymphocyte, *I*. neutrophilic
   band, *J*. basophil

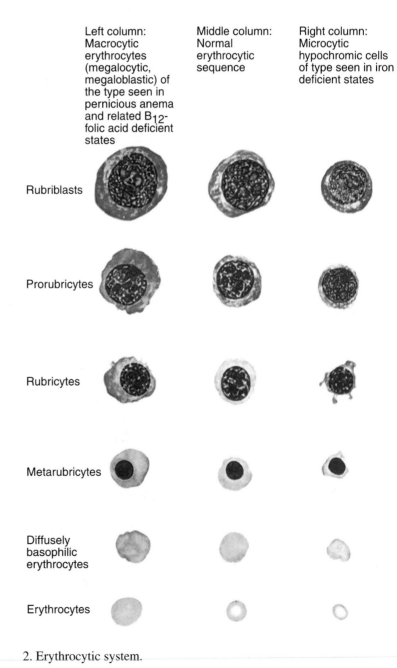

Left column: Macrocytic erythrocytes (megalocytic, megaloblastic) of the type seen in pernicious anema and related B$_{12}$-folic acid deficient states

Middle column: Normal erythrocytic sequence

Right column: Microcytic hypochromic cells of type seen in iron deficient states

Rubriblasts

Prorubricytes

Rubricytes

Metarubricytes

Diffusely basophilic erythrocytes

Erythrocytes

2. Erythrocytic system.

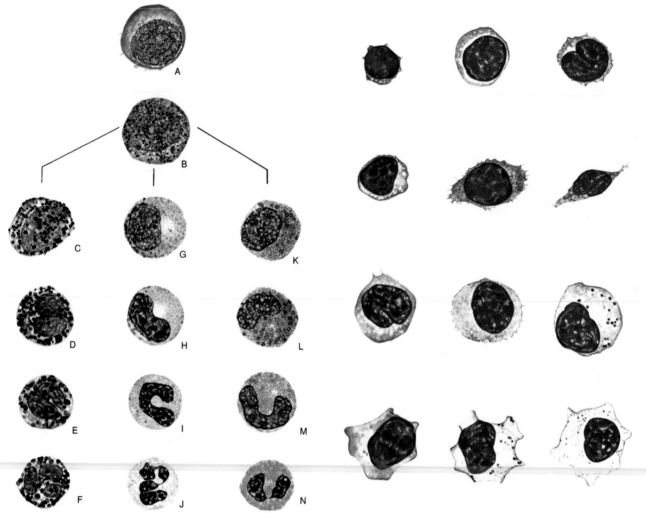

3. Granulocytopoiesis.

A. Myeloblast, B. Promyelocyte, C. Basophilic-Myelocytes,
D. Basophilic-Metamyelocytes, E. Basophilic-Bands,
F. Basophilic-Segmented, G. Neutrophilic-Myelocytes,
H. Neutrophilic-Metamyelocytes, I. Neutrophilic-Bands,
J. Neutrophilic-Segmented, K. Eosinophilic-Myelocytes,
L. Eosinophilic-Metamyelocytes, M. Eosinophilic-Bands,
N. Eosinophilic-Segmented.

4. Lymphocytes.

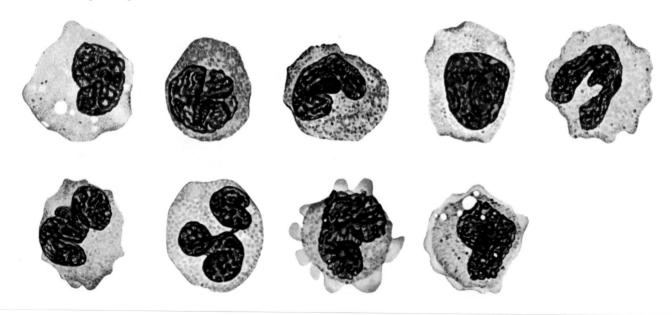

5. Monocytes.

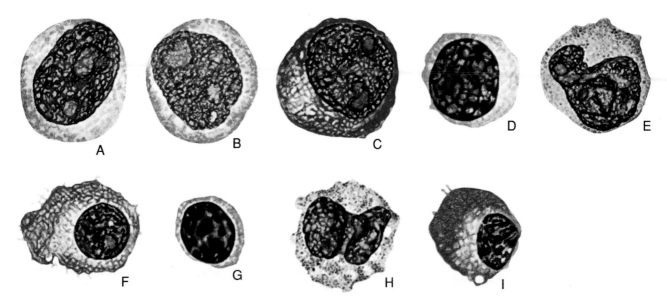

6. Lymphocytic, monocytic, and plasmacytic systems.
    A. Lymphoblast, *B*. Monoblast, *C*. Plasmablast, *D*. Prolymphocyte, *E*. Promonocyte,
    F. Proplasmacyte, *G*. Lymphocyte, *H*. Monocyte, *I*. Plasmacyte.

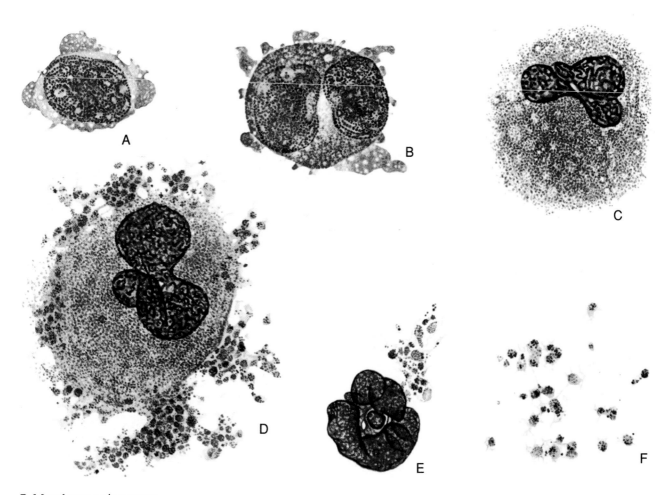

7. Megakaryocytic system.
    A. Megakaryoblast, *B*. Promegakaryocyte, *C*. Megakaryocyte, *D*. Metamegakaryocyte,
    E. Metamegakaryocyte Nucleous, *F*. Thrombocytes (platelets).

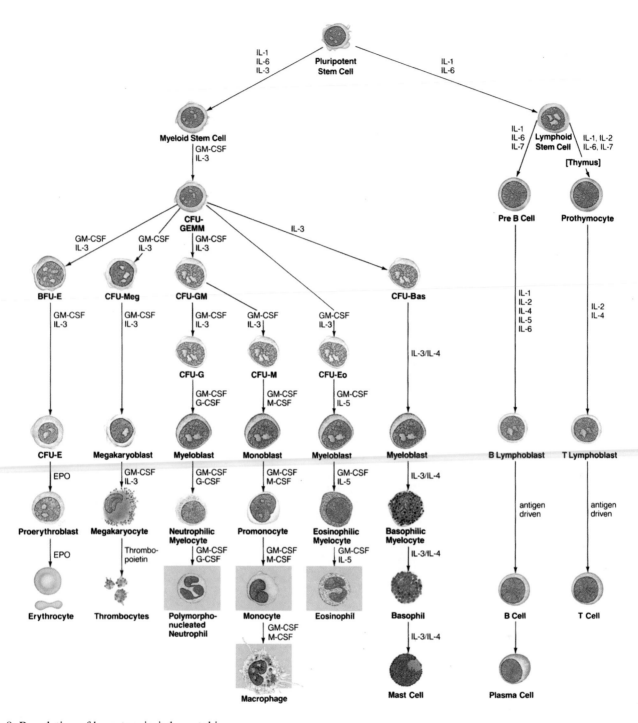

8. Regulation of hematopoiesis by cytokines.

9. PB: RBCs and platelets.   10. Neutrophils.

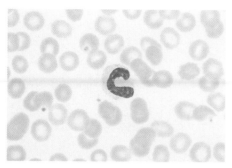

11. Neutrophil band.

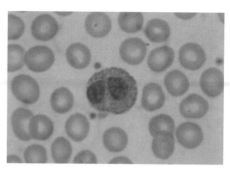

12. Eosinophil.

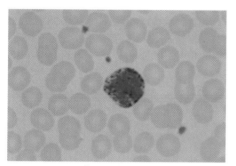

13. Basophil.

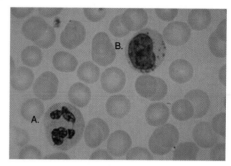

14. *A.* Neutrophil. *B.* Lymphocyte.

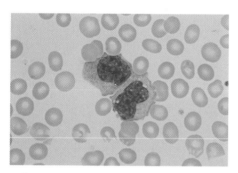

15. Monocytes.

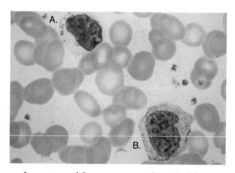

16. *A.* Lymphocytes with azure granules. *B.* Monocyte.

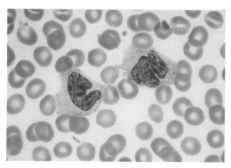

17. Monocytes.

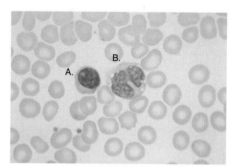

18. *A.* Lymphocyte. *B.* Monocyte.

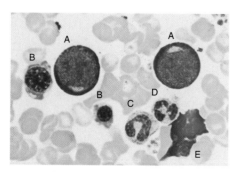

19. Bone marrow (BM). *A.* Rubriblasts. *B.* Rubricytes.
C. N. Band. *D.* Neutrophil. *E.* Smudge Cell.

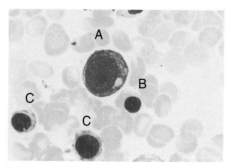

20. *A.* Rubriblast. *B.* Metarubricyte. *C.* Rubricytes.

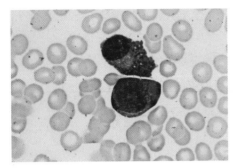

21. *Center:* Rubriblast; *upper center:* Plasmacyte.

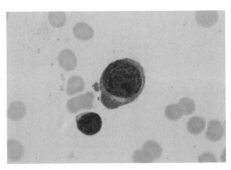

22. *Center:* Rubriblast; *lower center:* Lymphocyte.

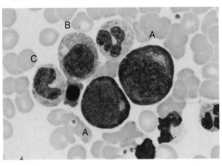

23. *A.* Rubriblasts. *B.* Myelocyte. *C.* Metamyelocyte.

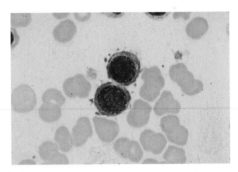

24. Prorubricytes.

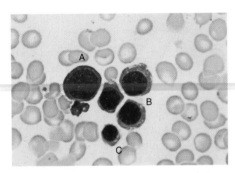

25. *A.* Prorubricyte. *B.* Rubricytes. *C.* Metarubricyte.

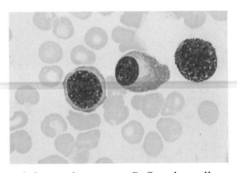

26. *L:* Prorubricyte, plasmacyte; *R:* Smudge cell.

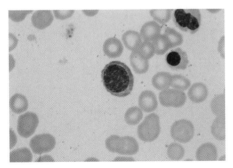

27. *Center:* Prorubricyte; *R:* Metarubricyte.

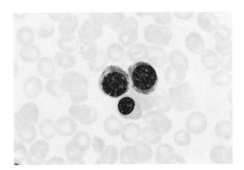

28. Rubricytes: Early and late stages.

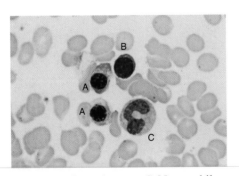

29. *A.* Rubricytes. *B.* Lymphocyte. *C.* Neutrophil.

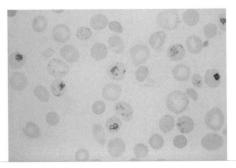

30. Reticulocytes.

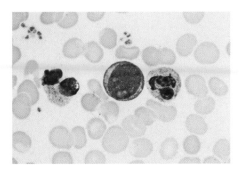

31. *Center:* Myeloblast; *R:* Neutrophil.

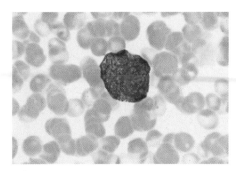

32. Promyelocyte.

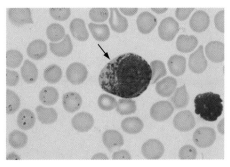

33. Promyelocyte *(center).*

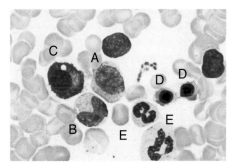

34. *A.* Myelocyte. *B.* Metamyelocyte. *C.* Plasmacyte. *D.* Metarubricytes. *E.* Neutrophils.

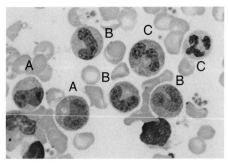

35. *A.* Myetamyelocytes. *B.* Bands. *C.* Neutrophils.

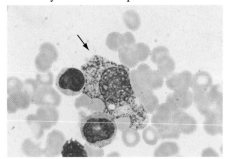

36. Tissue neutrophil *(large center cell).*

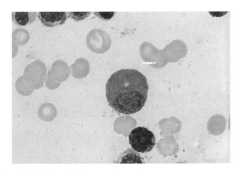

37. *Center:* Eosinophilic myelocyte.

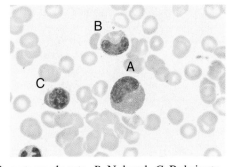

38. *A.* E. metamyelocyte. *B.* N. band. *C.* Rubricyte.

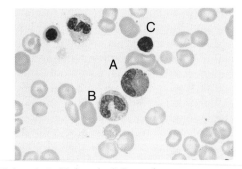

39. *A.* E. band. *B.* N. band. *C.* Lymphocyte.

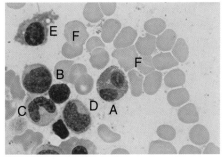

40. *A.* Eosinophil. *B.* Lymph. *C.* Band. *D.* Metamyelocyte. *E.* Plasmacyte. *F.* Polychromatophilic RBCs.

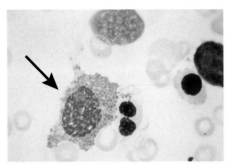

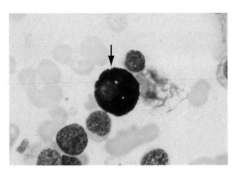

41. *L:* Tissue eosinophils; *R:* Binucleated metarubricyte.

42. Tissue basophil. *(arrow)*

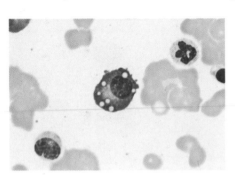

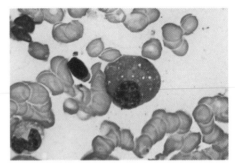

43. *Center:* Plasmacyte.

44. *Center:* Plasmacyte; *L:* small lymphocyte.

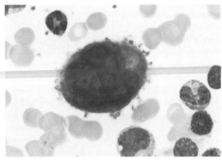

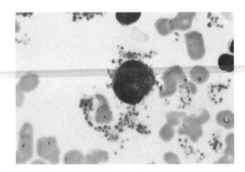

45. Early megakaryocyte (*center*).

46. Early megakaryocyte (*center*).

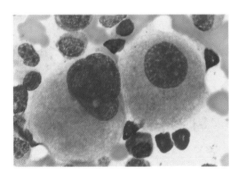

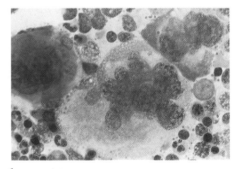

47. Megakaryocytes without platelets.

48. Megakaryocytes.

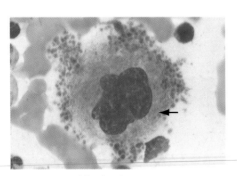

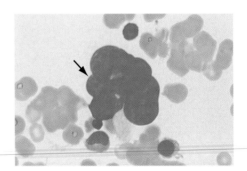

49. Megakaryocytes with platelets.

50. Naked nuclei, megakaryocyte.

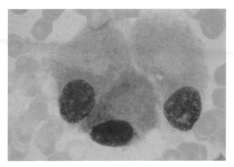

51. Three osteoblasts.

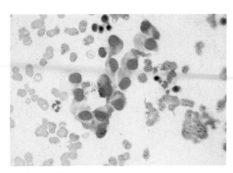

52. Group of osteoblasts *(center)*.

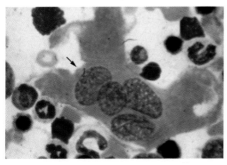

53. Osteoclasts.

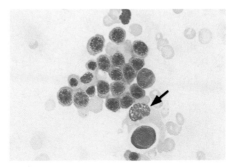

54. Polychromatophilic normoblasts; histiocyte *(arrow)*.

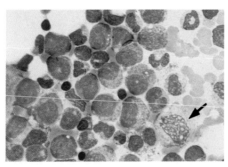

55. Granulopoiesis: with myelocytes; reticulum cell *(arrow)*.

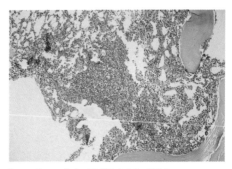

56. Lymphocytic nodule (follicle) in BM.

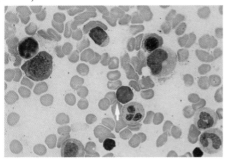

57. Hematogone *(arrow)*.

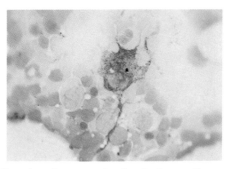

58. Alkaline phosphatase-stained reticulum cell.

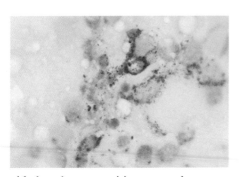

59. Two acid phosphatase-positive macrophages.

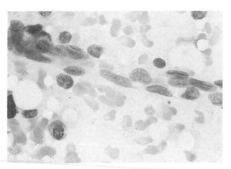

60. Endothelial cells aspirated from hypocellular BM.

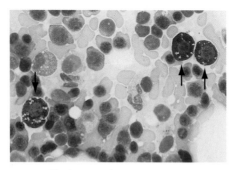

61. Three mast cells *(arrows)*.

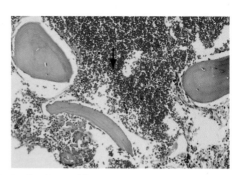

62. BM: Aspiration artifact.

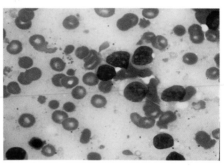

63. Hairy cell leukemia: with "dry-tap" BM.

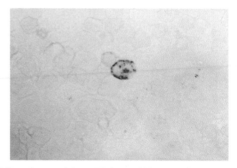

64. TRAP stain, positive: Hairy cell leukemia.

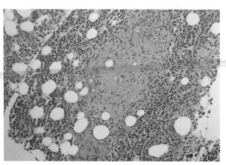

65. BM: HIV-positive patient with tuberculosis (TB).

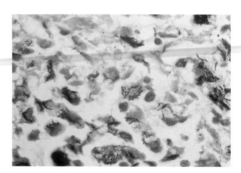

66. BM, acid-fast stain: TB.

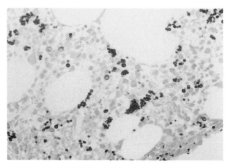

67. BM, GMS stain: HIV-positive patient, histoplasmosis.

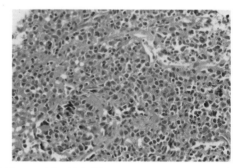

68. BM biopsy: T-cell ALL.

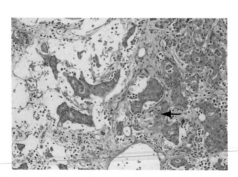

69. BM biopsy: Metastatic carcinoma.

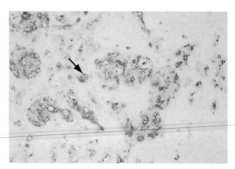

70. PSA (prostate-specific antigen) stain.

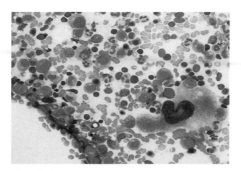

71. Normal cellular marrow.

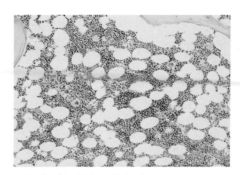

72. Normal BM with 50% cellularity.

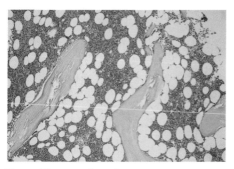

73. Severe aplastic anemia.

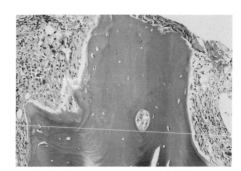

74. Hypercellular BM biopsy: 80% cellularity.

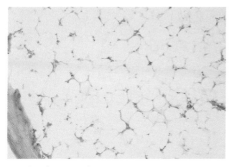

75. BM: Normal bony trabeculae.

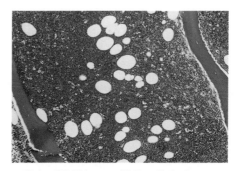

76. BM: Myelofibrosis in myeloid metaplasia.

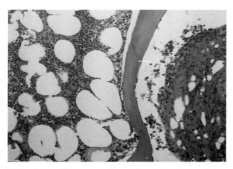

77. BM: Thinning of bony trabeculae (osteopenia).

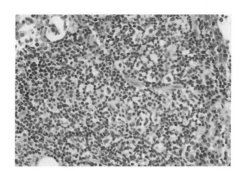

78. BM: Lymphoid aggregate.

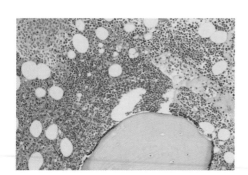

79. BM: Malignant lymphoma.

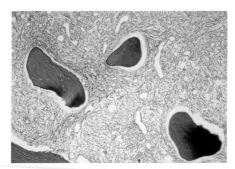

80. BM, reticulin stain: Hairy cell leukemia.

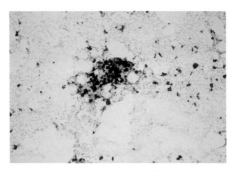

81. BM, iron stain: Increased storage iron.

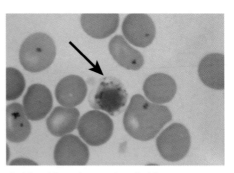

82. Ringed sideroblast *(center)* and siderocytes.

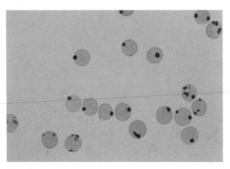

83. Heinz bodies.

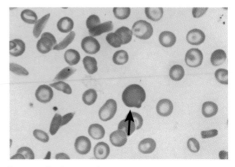

84. Polychromasia *(arrow)*.

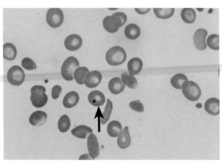

85. Howell-Jolly bodies.

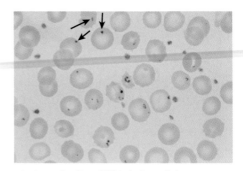

86. Pappenheimer bodies (Wright's stain)

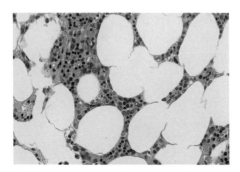

87. BM: Golden-brown hemosiderin granules.

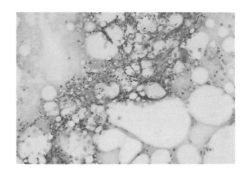

88. BM, Prussian blue stain: Iron-deficiency anemia (IDA).

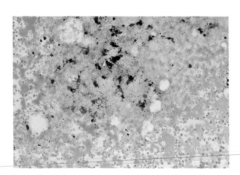

89. BM, Prussian blue stain: Anemia of chronic disease.

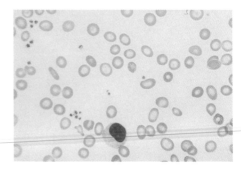

90. IDA: Microcytic, hypochromic RBCs.

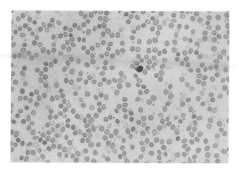

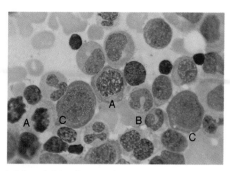

91. Dimorphic population of RBCs (sideroblastic anemia).

92. BM: *A.* Megaloblastic anemia. *B.* Band. *C.* Pronormoblast.

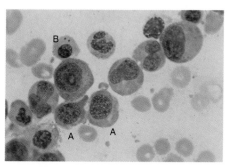

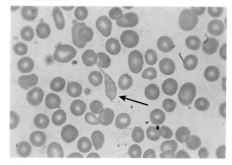

93. BM megaloblasts. *A.* Rubricyte. *B.* Metarubricyte.

94. Cabot ring, pernicious anemia (PA).

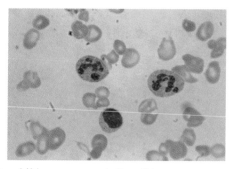

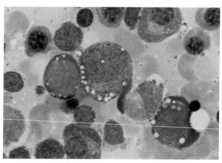

95. Neutrophil hypersegmentation, PA.

96. Vacuolization: BM cells; toxicity with chloramphenicol.

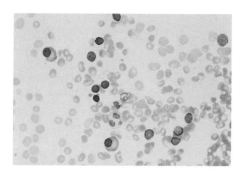

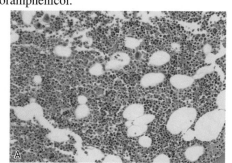

97. BM aplasia, hypocellular.

98. BM: *A.* Normocellular.

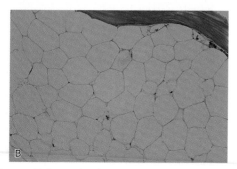

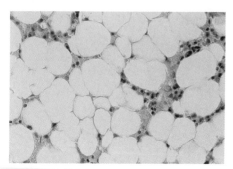

98. *B.* Hypocellular, aplastic anemia.

99. BM: Aplastic anemia.

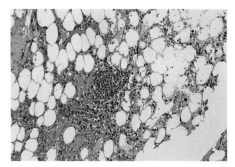

100. BM: Lymphoid aggregate, aplastic anemia.

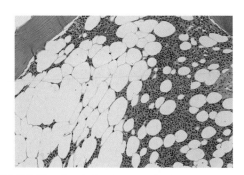

101. BM, H&E stain: Aplastic anemia.

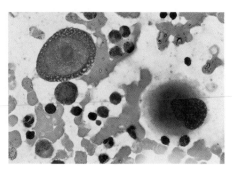

102. *L.* Rubriblast with parvovirus inclusions.

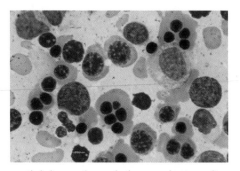

103. Congential dyserythropoietic anemia, type 2.

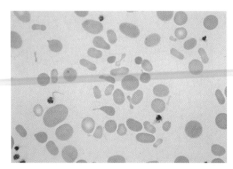

104. PB: Hereditary pyropoikilocytosis.

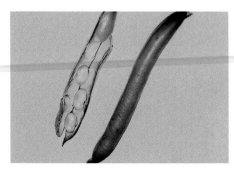

105. Fava beans.

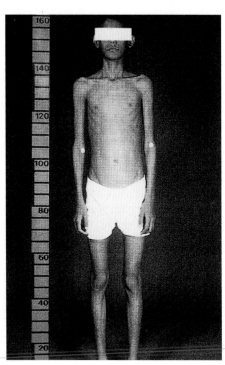

106. Asthenic physique with mild jaundice.

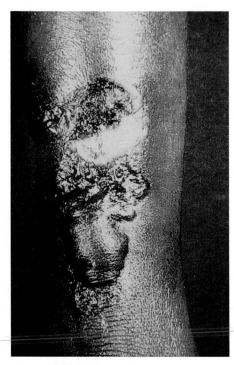

107. Leg ulcers, sickle cell anemia.

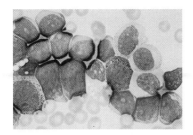

169. BM: AML, M2.

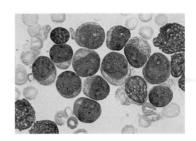

170. AML, M2.

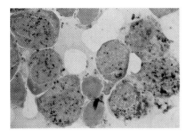

171. AML, M2 (myeloperoxidase stain).

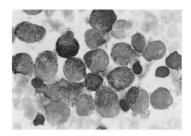

172. BM: Acute promyelocytic leukemia (APL), M3.

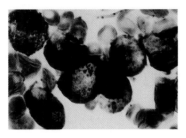

173. APL, M3 (Sudan black B stain).

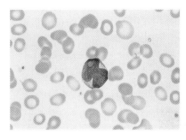

174. PB: "Microgranular" promyelocytic leukemia, M3m.

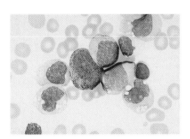

175. BM: Myelomonocytic leukemia (AMML), M4.

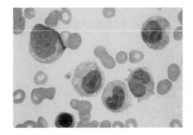

176. PB: AMML, M4.

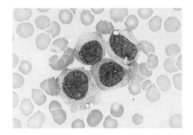

177. PB: Acute monocytic leukemia (AmoL), M5a.

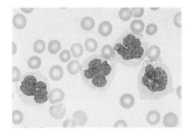

178. AmoL, well-differentiated (M5b).

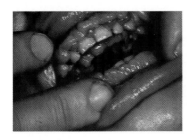

179. Gum hypertrophy.

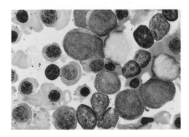

180. BM: Erythroleukemia, M6.

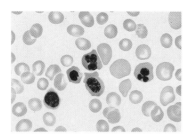

181. PB: Erythroleukemia, M6.

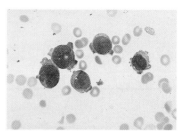

182. Acute megakaryoblastic leukemia (AmegL), M7.

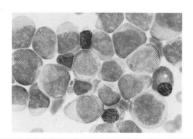

183. BM: AML.

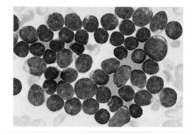

184. BM: Acute lymphoblastic leukemia (ALL), L1.

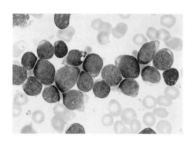

185. BM: ALL, L2.

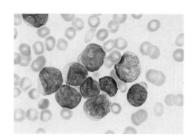

186. PB: ALL, L2.

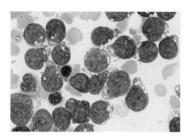

187. BM: ALL, L3.

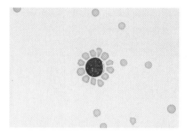

188. E-rosette formation in T-cell ALL.

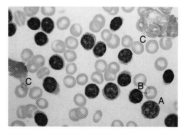

189. PB: Chronic lymphocytic leukemia (CLL).

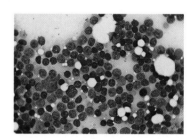

190. BM: CLL.

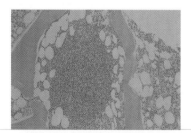

191. BM: CLL, nodular pattern.

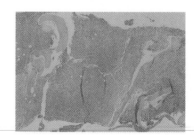

192. BM: CLL, diffuse pattern.

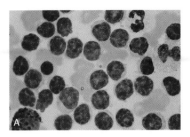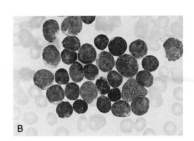

193. PB: Lymphoproliferative disorders. *A.* CLL.   *B.* ALL.

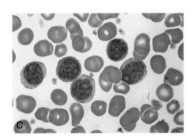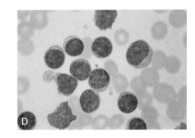

C. Prolymphocytic leukemia.   *D.* CLL, occasional prolymphocyte.

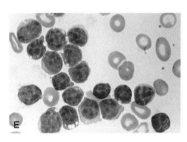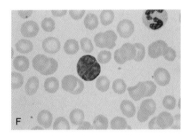

E. Small lymphocytic lymphoma (SLL), leukemic phase.   *F.* Small cleaved-cell leukemia (SCCL).

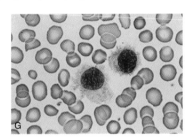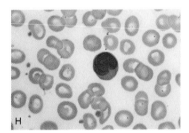

G. Hairy cell leukemia.   *H.* Sezary syndrome.

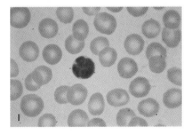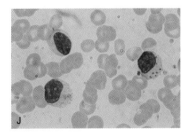

I. Adult T-cell leukemia/lymphoma.   *J.* T-γ lymphocytosis, large granular lymphocytes.

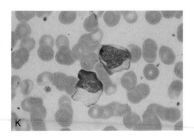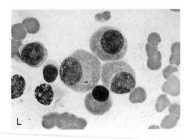

K. Infectious mononucleosis, atypical lymphocytes.   *L.* Plasma cell dyscrasia.

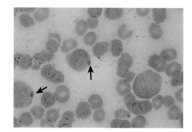

194. Naphthol acetate esterase (NAE)-positive T lymphocytes.

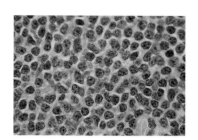

195. SLL.

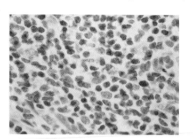

196. SCCL.

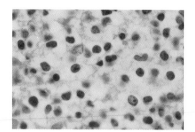

197. BM: Hairy cell leukemia (HCL).

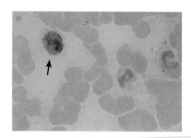

198. Tartate-resitant acid phosphatase (TRAP) stain, HCL.

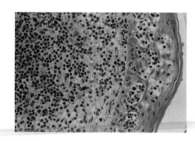

199. T-cell lymphoma mycosis fungoides (epidermis).

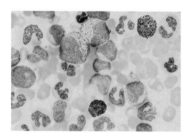

200. PB: CML.

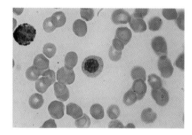

201. CML, pelgeroid granulocyte (pseudo-Pelger cell).

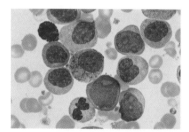

202. BM: CML, myeloid hyperplasia.

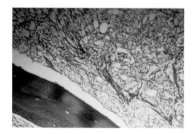

203. CML: Silver stain for reticulin and collagen fibers.

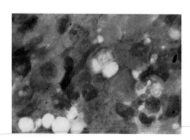

204. Sea-blue histiocytes, pseudo-Gaucher cells with CML.

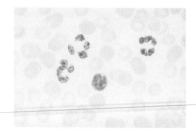

205. LAP-negative stain, CML.

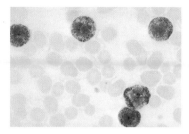

206. Leukemoid reaction; increased LAP.

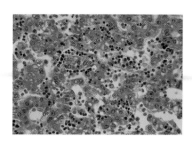

207. Extramedullary hematopoiesis (liver).

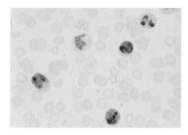

208. PB: Polycythemia vera (PV).

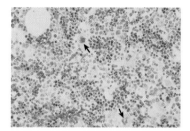

209. BM: Panhyperplasia in PV.

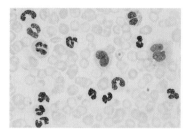

210. LAP-positive stain, PV.

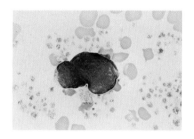

211. PB: Essential thrombocythemia; megakaryocyte.

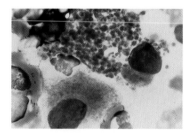

212. BM: Essential thrombocythemia.

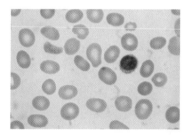

213. PB: Essential thrombocythemia; megakaryocyte.

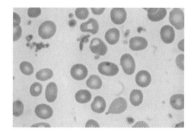

214. PB: 5q-Syndrome; anisomacrocytosis, ↑ Plt count.

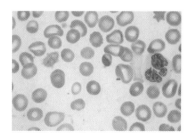

215. PB: RAEB anisomacrocytosis; platelet and Dohle body.

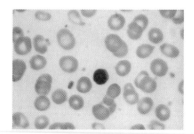

216. PB: RARS; dimorphic macrocytosis.

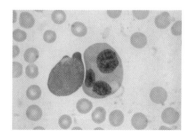

217. PB: RAEB-t (in transformation).

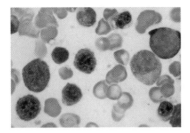

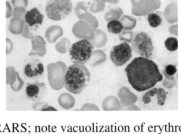

218. BM: RARS (refractory anemia with ringed sideroblasts).

219. BM: RARS; note vacuolization of erythroblasts.

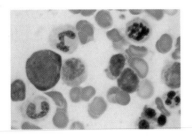

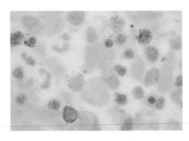

220. BM: RAEB (refractory anemia with excess blasts).

221. BM, Prussian blue stain: RARS.

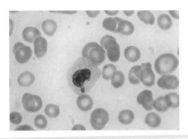

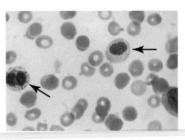

222. PB: RAEB; anisomacrocytosis, pelgeroid neutrophil.

223. PB: RAEB-t; mononucleated Pelger (Stodtmeister type).

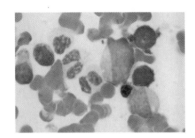

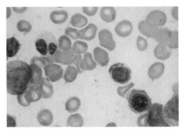

224. BM: RA; basophilic erythroblast with cytoplasm blebs.

225. BM: RAEB-t; pelgeroid neutrophil.

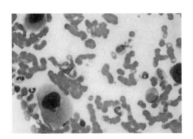

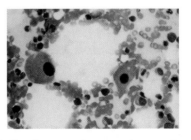

226. BM: 5q-Syndrome; monolobulated micromegakaryocytes.

227. BM: 5q Syndrome; micromegakaryocytes.

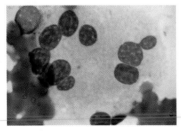

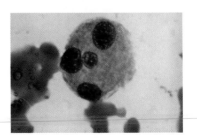

228. BM: RA; hypogranular megakaryocyte.

229. BM: RA; detached nuclei megakaryocyte.

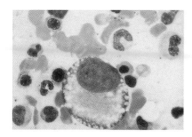

230. BM: RA; vacuolated immature megakarocyte.

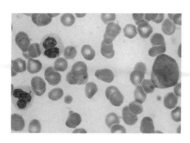

231. PB: RAEB-t; myeloblast, pelgeroid neutrophils.

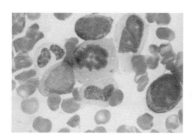

232. BM: RAEB; myeloblasts, mitosis, pelgeroid neutrophil.

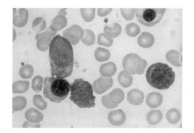

233. BM: RAEB-t; myeloblast with Auer rods.

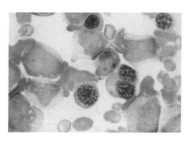

234. BM: RAEB-t; myeloblasts, megaloblastoid cell with HJB.

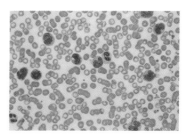

235. PB:CMML; promonocytes-monocytes, pelgeroid neutrophil.

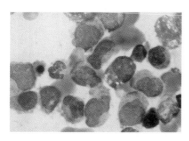

236. BM: CMML; myeloblasts, monocytes, promonocytes.

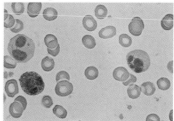

237. PB, peroxidase stain: RA; neutrophil, positive reaction.

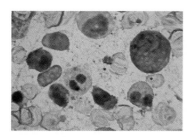

238. BM, peroxidase stain: RA; pseudo-Pelger-Huët-neg cells.

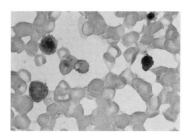

239. BM, PAS stain: RAEB; erythroblasts, positive granules.

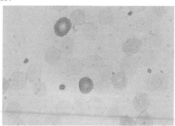

240. PB, Kleihauer-Betke stain: RA; positive RBCs, HbF.

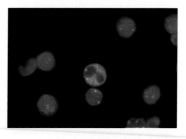

241. Fluorescence in situ hybridization (FISH), +8 in neutrophil.

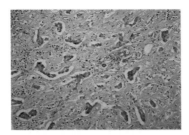

242. Amorphous amyloid deposits (liver).

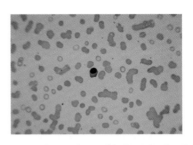

243. PB: rouleaux formation with "stacked coin" RBCs.

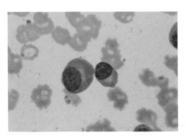

244. PB: Plasma cells with multiple myeloma.

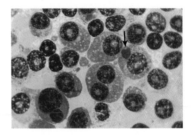

245. BM: Multiple myeloma.

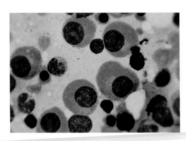

246. BM: Plasma cells.

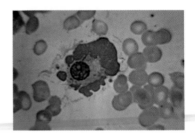

247. Flame cell, IgA myeloma.

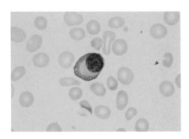

248. PB: Plasma cell leukemia.

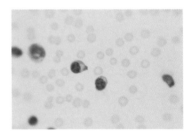

249. Plasmacytoid lymphocytes with red-staining Ig.

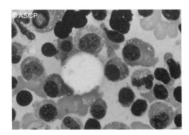

250. BM: Waldenstrom's plasmacytoid lymphocytes.

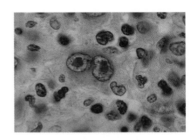

251. Classical Reed-Sternberg (RS) cell.

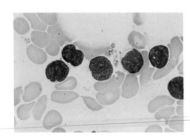

252. PB: Sézary cells in Sézary syndrome.

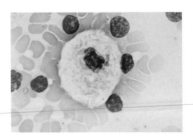

253. BM: Gaucher's cell.

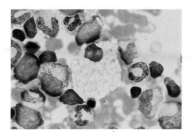

254. BM: Niemann-Pick cell.

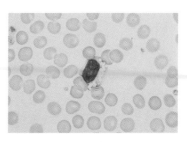

255. Tay-Sachs disease, vacuolated lymphocytes.

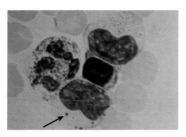

256. Hurler's anomaly.

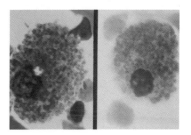

257. Sea-blue histiocytes.

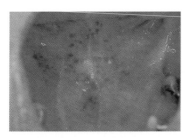

258. Oral cavity of a patient with ITP.

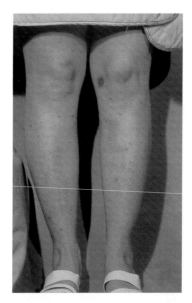

259. Petechial bleeding, ITP.

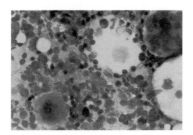

260. BM: Idiopathic thrombocytopenic purpura (ITP).

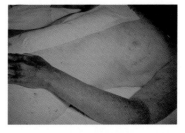

261. Post-transfusion purpura (PTP).

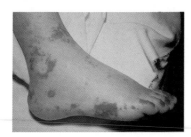

262. Anaphylactoid (Henoch-Schönlein) purpura (foot).

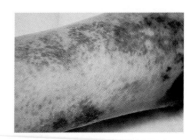

263. Steroid purpura (skin manifestations).

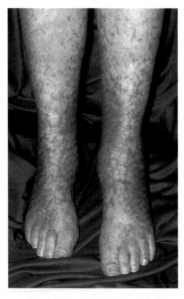

264. Legs, vascular lesion with Paraproteinemia.

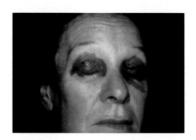

265. Amyloid purpura.

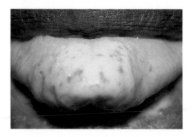

266. Tongue with hereditary hemorrhagic telangiectasias.

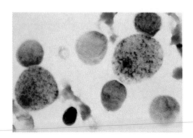

267. Diffuse hemorrhage in DIC.

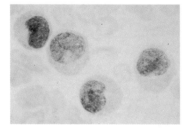

268. PB: DIC, schistocytes *(arrows)* and NRBCs.

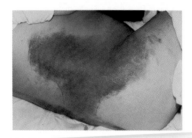

269. Myeloperoxidase-positive stain, AML, M2.

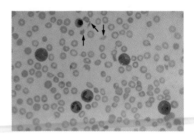

270. Alpha-naphtyl acetate-positive stain, AmoL, M5b.

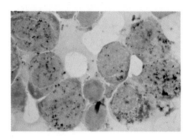

271. Nonspecific esterase with NaF inhibition, M5b.

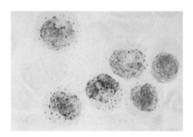

272. NCAE stain, acute promyelocytic leukemia, M3.

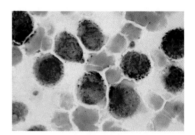

273. Combined esterase-positive stain, AMML, M4.

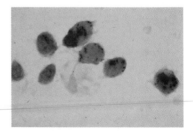

274. TRAP stain: Positive hairy cells.

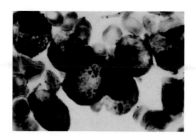

275. SBB stain: positive acute promyelocytic leukemia, M3.

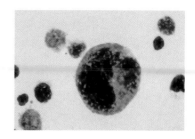

276. PAS-positive stain, erythroleukemia, M6.

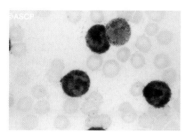

277. LAP test: Positive reaction.

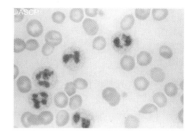

278. LAP test: Negative reaction.

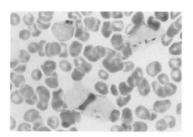

279. Peroxidase reaction in AML, M1.

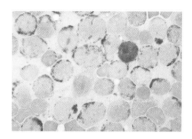

280. Cyanid-resistant peroxidase stain.

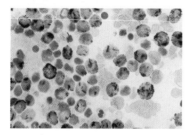

281. Sudan black B reaction in AML, M2.

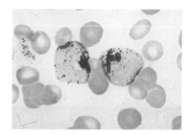

282. Sudan black B reaction in "myeloblast."

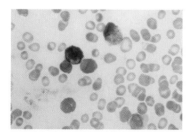

283. Napthol AS-D chloroacetate esterase, AML, M2.

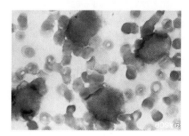

284. Nonspecific esterase reaction in monoblasts.

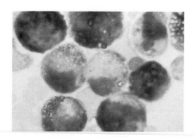

285. Naphthyl butyrate esterase, AmoL, M5b.

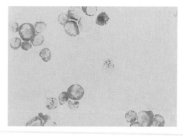

286. NCAE and α-Naphthyl acetate esterase, M4.

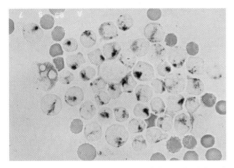

287. Acid phosphatase-positive T-cell lymphoblastic leukemia.

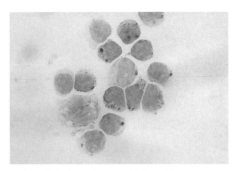

288. Cytospin acid phosphatase in lymphocytes.

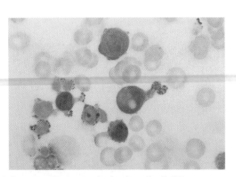

289. Cytospin tartrate-resistant acid phophatase "hairy cells."

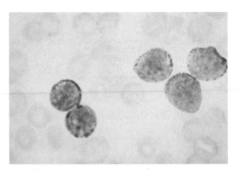

290. PAS in ALL.

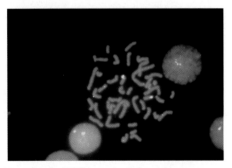

291. PAS in megakaryocytic leukemia, M7.

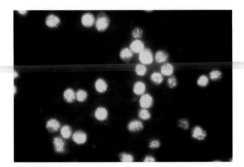

292. TdT in T-lymphoblast, ALL.

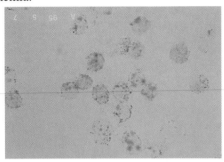

293. FISH analysis, DiGeorge syndrome.

1

Morphology of Human Blood and Marrow Cells:

Hematopoiesis

ANN BELL, MS, SH(ASCP), CLSpH(NCA)

BASIC MORPHOLOGY AND BASIC CONCEPTS

MORPHOLOGY OF CELLS ON THE NORMAL BLOOD SMEAR
Erythrocytes (Red Blood Cells)
Platelets (Thrombocytes)
Leukocytes (White Blood Cells)

HEMATOPOIESIS
Definition
Ontogeny (Origin) of Hematopoiesis

ERYTHROPOIESIS
Rubriblast (Pronormoblast, Proerythroblast)
Prorubricyte (Basophilic Normoblast, Basophilic Erythroblast)
Rubricyte (Polychromatophilic Normoblast, Polychromatophilic Erythroblast)
Metarubricyte (Orthochromatic Normoblast, Orthochromatic Erythroblast)
Diffusely Basophilic Erythrocyte (Polychromatophilic Erythrocyte)
Erythrocyte (Red Blood Cell, Discocyte)

MYELOPOIESIS (GRANULOCYTOPOIESIS)
Morphological Changes
Stages of Differentiation and Maturation (Granulocytes)

MONOPOIESIS
Monoblasts and Promonocytes
Monocytes and Macrophages

LYMPHOPOIESIS
Lymphoblasts and Prolymphocytes
Lymphocytes
Plasmablasts and Proplasmacytes
Plasmacytes (Plasma Cells)

MEGAKARYOCYTOPOIESIS

BONE-DERIVED CELLS
Osteoblasts
Osteoclasts

MOLECULAR HEMATOLOGY AND ADVANCED CONCEPTS
Introduction to the Cell Cycle
Specific Cell Line Ontogeny

TRENDS IN THERAPEUTIC MANIPULATION OF HEMATOPOIESIS
Recombinant Cytokines
Clinical Trials of Recombinant Cytokines
CD Nomenclature
Clinical Applications of Cell Surface Markers

OBJECTIVES

At the end of this chapter, the learner should be able to:

1. Describe two main differences between neutrophilic band and neutrophilic segmented cells.

2. Distinguish between eosinophils and basophils.

3. Describe four morphological features that are helpful in identifying monocytes.

4. List four characteristics of lymphocytes.

5. Compare a large lymphocyte with a monocyte.

6. Define *hematopoiesis*.

7. Name organs responsible for hematopoiesis in the fetus.

8. Define the term *erythropoiesis*.

9. List the proper cell maturation sequence of the erythroid series.

10. Recognize each cell in the erythrocytic series.

11. Give two or more characteristics of each nucleated red cell in the erythrocytic series.

12. List the proper cell sequence for myelopoiesis (granulocytopoiesis).

13. Recognize each cell in the myelocytic series.

14. Differentiate the morphological features of promyelocyte, neutrophilic myelocyte,

neutrophilic metamyelocyte, and neutrophilic band.

15. Describe the morphology of a myeloblast.

16. Describe three features of a mature plasmacyte.

17. State the mission of megakaryocytes.

18. Explain the process of platelet release from the bone marrow.

19. Distinguish between osteoblasts and osteoclasts.

20. Name two differences between a megakaryocyte and an osteoclast.

➤ BASIC MORPHOLOGY AND BASIC CONCEPTS

Hematology is the study of blood and its related disorders. Its birth can be traced to 1642, when Leeuwenhoek first noted cells in the blood. More than 200 years elapsed before other investigators expanded upon Leeuwenhoek's discovery. Table 1–1 outlines the significant milestones in the history of hematology.

The average blood volume in an adult is 4 to 6 L: women have 4 to 5 L, and men 5 to 6 L. This blood volume represents about 8% of the total body weight, and blood has a pH between 7.35 and 7.45. Blood is composed of 55% plasma (the fluid portion) and 45% formed elements or cells. Of the 45% cellular elements, approximately 44% of the cells are red blood cells (RBCs), whereas only 1% are white blood cells (WBCs) and platelets (PLTs) (Fig. 1–1).

Plasma is composed of about 91.5% water and 8.5% solutes. The solutes consist of three different kinds of proteins: albumins (55%), globulins (38%), and fibrinogen (7%); other solutes are electrolytes, hormones, nonprotein nitrogen compounds, nutrients, and respiratory gases.

The reference values for the cellular elements are as follows: RBCs (4.2 to 5.4 $\times$ 10^{12}/L for females and 4.7 to 6.1 $\times$ 10^{12}/L for males), WBCs (4.8 to 10.8 $\times$ 10^9/L) and PLTs (150 to 350 $\times$ 10^9/L) in adults. These reference values vary with age, gender, geographic location, and health or disease.

➤ MORPHOLOGY OF CELLS ON THE NORMAL BLOOD SMEAR

The primary step in assessing hematologic function and the presence of disease is an examination of the cellular elements in the blood. Examination of the blood frequently gives important information that aids in the diagnosis of hematologic disease and may suggest further testing.[1] A well-made and well-stained blood smear is vital, because the analysis of cell morphology may be greatly hindered by poorly made and poorly stained smears.[1] (See Chap. 28 for smear preparation.)

Careful examination of cell morphology on a blood smear and determination of the percentage of each type of blood cell present is an important skill to master. Blood cells normally present on a blood smear are RBCs (erythrocytes), white blood cells (leukocytes), and platelets (thrombocytes) (Fig. 1–2; see Color Plate 1). Morphological descriptions of each of these cellular elements in normal blood are presented in this chapter. After the description of normal blood cells, hematopoiesis and the morphological features of normal bone marrow cells are discussed (see Color Plates 2 through 8).

➤ Table 1-1
HISTORY OF HEMATOLOGY

1642	Leeuwenhoek first notes cells in blood
1842	Donne discovers platelets
1846	Gulliver differentiates lymphocytes from granulocytes by size
1874	Malassez counts white blood cells (WBCs) by hemocytometry
1875	Hayem defines methods for counting platelets
1879	Ehrlich uses aniline dyes to stain WBCs

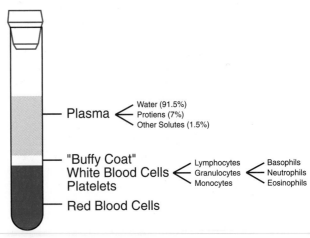

Plasma ⟵ Water (91.5%) / Proteins (7%) / Other Solutes (1.5%)

"Buffy Coat"
White Blood Cells ⟵ Lymphocytes / Granulocytes ⟵ Basophils / Neutrophils / Eosinophils
Platelets   Monocytes

Red Blood Cells

➤ FIGURE 1–1 Centrifuged whole blood depicting plasma, WBC, platelet, and RBC layers.

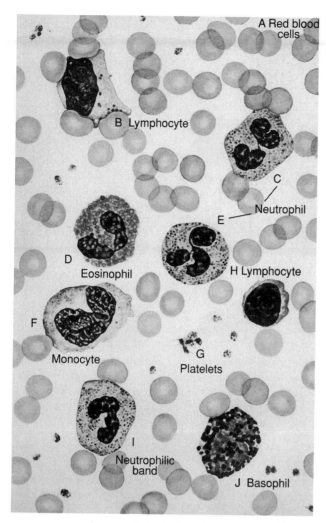

> ➤ **FIGURE 1–2** Cell types found in smears of peripheral blood from normal individuals. *A.* Red blood cells (RBCs). *B.* Large lymphocyte. *C.* Segmented neutrophil. *D.* Eosinophil. *E.* Segmented neutrophil. *F.* Monocyte. *G.* Platelets. *H.* Small lymphocyte. *I.* Neutrophilic band. *J.* Basophil.

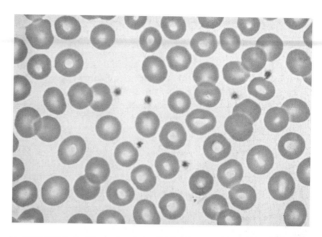

> ➤ **FIGURE 1–3**   Normal peripheral blood smear; normal erythrocytes and platelets.

Erythrocytes (Red Blood Cells)

Erythrocyte morphology is evaluated in an area of the stained smear where red cells are evenly distributed and do not overlap (Fig. 1–3 and Color Plate 9). Red cells consist of plasma membrane surrounding a solution of proteins (mainly hemoglobin) and electrolytes.[1] A normal mature erythrocyte is a biconcave disc that is 7 to 8 μm in mean diameter and 1.5 to 2.5 μm thick; it has a mean volume of 90 femtoliters (fL). After the smear is stained with Wright's stain, an erythrocyte appears as a circular cell with distinct and smooth margins and has a dull pinkish hue. In the central portion of the erythrocyte where the cell is thinnest, the intensity of the stain is less than at the marginal area, creating an area of central pallor. Red cells should be fairly uniform in size and relatively round in shape, with a small area of central pallor and no nucleus or inclusions (see Fig. 1–3 and Color Plate 9).[2–4]

Platelets (Thrombocytes)

In the same area where erythrocyte morphology is being studied, the number of platelets per oil immersion field and the morphology should be evaluated. Platelets are approximately 2 to 4 μm in diameter and vary in shape.[3] An average of 7 to 15 platelets per oil immersion field is normally observed. An estimate of the number of platelets in 10 oil immersion fields should be made. Platelets may be observed in small groups (see Fig. 1–2G and Color Plate 1–G). A count of individual platelets in a group should be made.[4]

In Wright's stain a platelet contains reddish-purple granules in a small amount of bluish cytoplasm, but there is no nucleus.[4] Platelets contain particular molecules needed for hemostasis and are able to adhere, aggregate, and supply a surface for coagulation reactions.[1,5]

Leukocytes (White Blood Cells)

The morphology and the distribution of leukocytes are evaluated. WBCs normally observed on a blood smear include neutrophils (neutrophil segmented and a few neutrophil bands), eosinophils, basophils, lymphocytes, and monocytes (see Fig. 1–2 and Color Plate 1). Immature cells of any type are abnormal. Cells should be examined for abnormalities in nucleus or cytoplasm.

Segmented Neutrophil (Filamented Neutrophil, Polymorphonuclear Neutrophil)

In normal peripheral blood of older children and adults, 50% to 70% of mature granulocytes called segmented neutrophils are found (Table 1–2). The nucleus of the segmented neutrophil is separated into two to five (usually three) lobes, with a narrow segment or filament connecting the lobes[4] (Fig. 1–4 and Color Plate 10). Approximately 6% of the neutrophils have one lobe (band neutrophil), 35% have two lobes, 41% have three lobes, 17% have four lobes, and 2% have five lobes.[4] Segmentation of the nucleus enables these motile cells to pass through an opening in endothelial lining cells of capillaries and to "home in" on selected prey (such as microorganisms causing infection).[6,7] Nuclear chromatin is heavily clumped, coarse, or pyknotic and stains purplish-red (see Figs. 1–2C, 1–2E, and 1–4; Color Plates 1 and 10). The cytoplasm is light pink when stained properly and the secondary granules (which are fine, numerous, and evenly distributed) stain either pink or a neutral color. Neutrophil secondary granules are lysosomes that contain alkaline phosphatase.[1]

➤ Table 1-2 PERIPHERAL BLOOD CELLS: NORMAL ADULT VALUES		
	Percent	**Absolute Values (per mm³)**
N. band	2–6	100–650
N. segmented	50–70	2400–7500
Eosinophil	0–4	0–450
Basophil	0–2	0–200
Lymphocyte	20–44	1000–4750
Monocyte	2–9	100–100

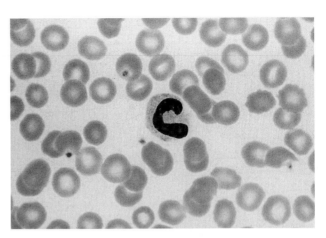

➤ FIGURE 1–5   Neutrophilic band.

Mature neutrophils are approximately twice the size of normal erythrocytes. Granulocytes, as well as monocytes, play a key role in inflammation and phagocytosis.[5] They migrate from the blood vessel into the tissues,[5] where they serve as the first line of defense against infections.

Band Neutrophil (Nonsegmented Neutrophil, Nonfilamented Neutrophil)

Peripheral blood of healthy individuals contains 2% to 6% of the band neutrophils (Table 1–2). Band neutrophils have a nucleus with a horseshoe shape in which the opposite edges of the nucleus become almost parallel for an appreciable distance.[4] These cells do *not* have a nucleus separated into lobes connected by a filament (Fig. 1–5 and Color Plate 11).

The nuclear chromatin is clumped, and there is usually a dark pyknotic mass at each pole where the lobe is destined to be.[4] The secondary neutrophil granules are small, evenly distributed, stain various shades of pink (on Wright's stain), and contain alkaline phosphatase.[1] There may be an occasional dark primary granule (see Fig. 1–2I and Color Plate 1).

Difficulty may arise in differentiating between band and segmented neutrophils and in deciding whether the link connecting the lobes is narrow enough to be called a filament or wide enough to be identified as a band. A filamented or segmented cell has a threadlike connection between two lobes, and there is no visible chromatin between the two sides of the filament. Lobes of nuclei often touch each other or overlap, and it may be impossible to see the

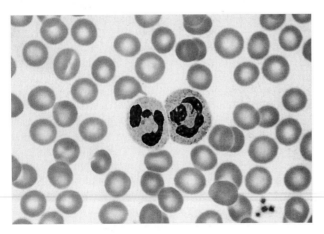

➤ FIGURE 1–4   Two segmented neutrophils.

connecting filaments. In a band neutrophil, there are two distinct margins with nuclear chromatin material visible between the margins. If the margin of a lobe can be traced as a definite and continuing line from one side of the nucleus across the isthmus to the other side, then it may be assumed that a filament is present even though it is not visible. In attempting to differentiate between a segmented and a band neutrophil, identification should not be made on a single morphological characteristic but on combined features. In case of doubt regarding a borderline cell, the questionable cell should be placed into the mature category.[4]

Eosinophil

Eosinophils are usually easily recognizable because of the large, round, secondary, refractile granules that have an affinity for the acid eosin stain (see Figs. 1–2D and 1–6, and Color Plates 1 and 12). With Wright's stain, normal eosinophilic granules become orange to reddish-orange. The granules are spherical, uniform in size, and evenly distributed. Because of the size and roundness of the granules, eosinophils may be recognized in unstained moist preparations of blood in light microscopy and using phase microscopy. The crystalloid core of the granule is composed mainly of major basic protein (MBP), which binds to acid aniline dyes and which may help to explain the staining qualities of the granule.[7–9]

Normal adult peripheral blood contains 0 to 4% eosinophils (Table 1–2). Normal blood eosinophils are about the size of or slightly larger than neutrophils and have a band or two-lobed nucleus with condensed chromatin; rarely does an eosinophil have three lobes.[4,8,9] There is a diurnal variation in the percentage of circulating eosinophils, with an increase at night and a decrease in the morning.[7]

Basophil

Although basophils constitute only 0 to 2% of normal blood cells (Table 1–2), the large, abundant, violet-blue (or purple-black) granules aid in the immediate recognition of this cell.[4,10] These granules are visible above the nucleus as well as lateral to it, and they obscure most of the nucleus. The granules vary in size from 0.2 to 1.0 μm.[4] They are coarse and unevenly distributed; vary in number, shape, and color; and are less numerous than eosinophil granules (see Figs. 1–2J and 1–7, and Color Plates 1 and 13). These granules have an affinity for blue or basic thiazine dyes.[10] Basophil granules are also water soluble. In cells that are poorly fixed

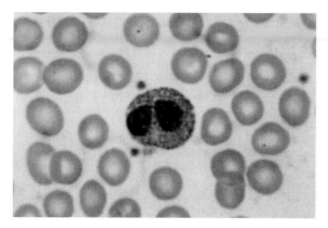

➤ FIGURE 1–6   Eosinophil (segmented).

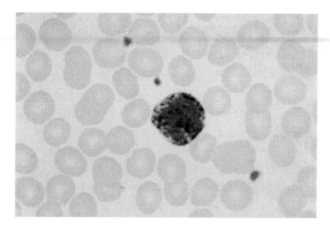

➤ FIGURE 1–7   Basophil.

during staining, the center of the granule may disappear or the entire granule may be washed away, leaving a small colorless cytoplasmic area.[4]

Basophils show a diurnal variation similar to that of eosinophils, increasing at night and decreasing in the morning.[7]

Lymphocyte

Lymphocytes are the second most numerous cells in the blood, comprising from 20% to 44% of the adult blood cells (Table 1–2). Most lymphocytes are small, varying from 7 to 10 μm. There are also intermediate sizes and some large lymphocytes (Fig. 1–8 and Color Plate 4). Size is not a reliable basis for determining the age of metabolic activity of

lymphocytes because their size varies with the thickness of the smear. Lymphocytes tend to become spherical and small in thick areas of the smear; in the thinnest end of the smear, lymphocytes may spread out and appear large.[4] Small lymphocytes are usually round with smooth margins (see Figs. 1–2*H* and 1–8*A,* and Color Plates 1 and 4). Rarely, a lymphocyte may have a spindle form with an oval nucleus and cytoplasmic filaments extending outward at each end (see Fig. 1–8*F* and Color Plate 4). The margin of large lymphocytes frequently is indented by neighboring erythrocytes, causing them to have a serrated (holly-leaf) shape[4] (see Figs. 1–8*J* through *L,* and Color Plate 4).

With Wright's stain, the color of the cytoplasm is blue, varying in intensity from light to dark in different cells. The

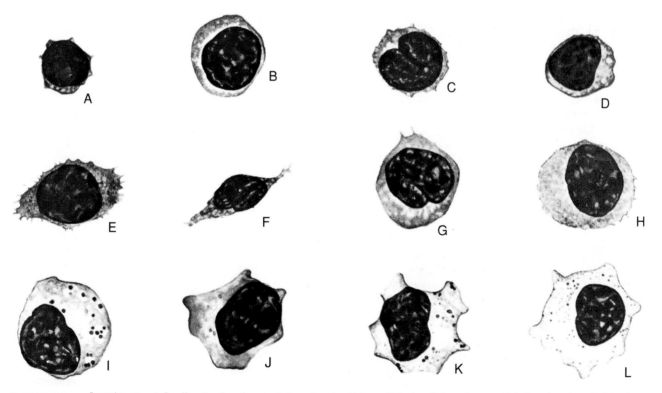

➤ FIGURE 1–8   Lymphocytes. *A.* Small mature lymphocyte. *B.* Lymphocyte of intermediate size. *C.* Lymphocyte with indented nucleus. *D.* Lymphocyte of intermediate size. *E.* Lymphocyte with pointed cytoplasmic projections (frayed cytoplasm); typical nucleus. *F.* Spindle-shaped and pointed cytoplasmic projections. *G.* Large lymphocyte with indented nucleus and pointed cytoplasmic projections. *H.* Large lymphocyte. *I.* Large lymphocyte with purplish-red (azurophilic) granules. *J.* Large lymphocyte with irregular cytoplasmic contours. *K.* Large lymphocyte with purplish-red (azurophilic) granules and with indentations caused by pressure of erythrocytes. *L.* Large lymphocyte with purplish-red (azurophilic) granules. (From Diggs, LW, et al: The Morphology of Human Blood Cells, ed 5. Abbott Laboratories, Abbott Park, IL, 1985, pp 1–18, 25–27, with permission.)

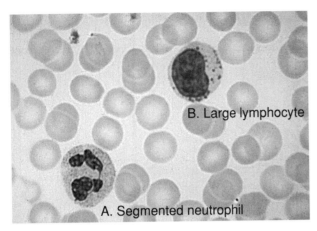

B. Large lymphocyte

A. Segmented neutrophil

➤ **FIGURE 1–9** *A*. Segmented neutrophil. *B*. Lymphocyte with azurophilic granules.

color is evenly distributed in some cells and uneven in other cells. The intensity of the blue stain is greater at the periphery of the cell than near the Golgi area adjacent to the nucleus.

Most lymphocytes do not have granules. In some large cells there may be a few well-defined granules that vary in size, are unevenly distributed, and can be easily counted. These granules are a purplish-red and have been called *azurophilic;* however, this term is misleading because these granules are predominantly red rather than blue[4] (see Figs. 1–8*I* and *K*, 1–9*B*, and Color Plates 4 and 14).

The diameter of the nucleus of a small lymphocyte in peripheral blood is slightly larger than, or the same size as, a normal erythrocyte in the same microscopic field. The lymphocyte's nucleus, in relation to its cytoplasm, is large (N:C ratio is 4:1); and the nuclei are round or slightly indented. Chromatin structure is lumpy or clumped and stains dark

purple with lighter bluish-purple areas between chromatin aggregates.[4,11]

Nucleoli are present in some lymphocytes but are not visible in light microscopy because they are obscured by the darkly stained chromatin masses. The fact that nucleoli may be present in small lymphocytes is evidence that these cells are capable of growth and replication.[11]

Monocyte

In the thin areas of the peripheral blood smear, a monocyte measures about 15 to 18 μm[12] and is larger than the mature neutrophil. Monocytes have abundant cytoplasm in relation to the nucleus (N:C ratio is 2:1 or 1:1). With Wright's stain the cytoplasm turns a dull gray-blue, in contrast to the pink cytoplasm of the neutrophils. Numerous fine, small, reddish- or purplish-stained, evenly distributed granules in the cytoplasm give the cell a ground-glass appearance (see Figs. 1–2*F* and 1–10, and Color Plates 1 and 5). There may be varying numbers of prominent granules in addition to the small granules. Some monocytes may appear nongranular, suggesting rapid turnover. Digestive vacuoles may be observed in the cytoplasm. In disease states, phagocytized erythrocytes, nuclei, cell fragments, bacteria, fungi, and pigment may be present.[12]

The nuclei of monocytes frequently may be kidney shaped, deeply folded or indented, or occasionally lobular. One of the distinctive features of the monocyte is the appearance of convolutions (like those in the brain) in the nucleus (Figs. 1–10 and 1–11, and Color Plates 5 and 15). Another characteristic is the lacy, often delicate chromatin network of intermingled fine strands with small chromatin clumps.[4,12]

The shape of the monocyte is variable. Many cells are round; other cells reveal blunt pseudopods that are manifestations of their slow mobility. These ameboid cells continue

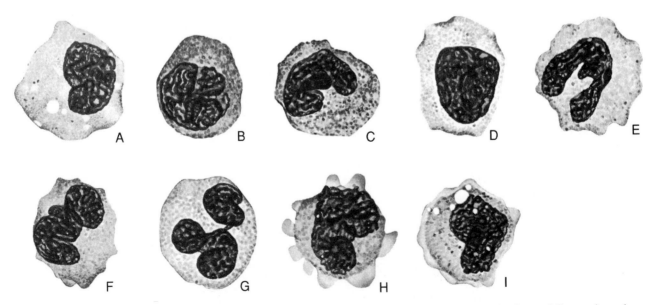

A   B   C   D   E

F   G   H   I

➤ **FIGURE 1–10** Monocytes. *A*. Monocyte with "ground-glass" appearance, evenly distributed fine granules, occasional azurophilic granules, and vacuoles in cytoplasm. *B*. Monocyte with opaque cytoplasm and granules and with lobulation of nucleus and linear chromatin. *C*. Monocyte with prominent granules and deeply indented nucleus. *D*. Monocyte without nuclear indentations. *E*. Monocyte with gray-blue color, band type of nucleus, linear chromatin, blunt pseudopods, and granules. *F*. Monocyte with gray-blue color, irregular shape, and multilobulated nucleus. *G*. Monocyte with segmented nucleus. *H*. Monocyte with multiple blunt nongranular pseudopods, nuclear indentations, and folds. *I*. Monocyte with vacuoles and with nongranular ectoplasm and granular endoplasm. (From Diggs, LW, et al: The Morphology of Human Blood Cells, ed 5. Abbott Laboratories, Abbott Park, IL, 1985, pp 1–18, 25–27, with permission.)

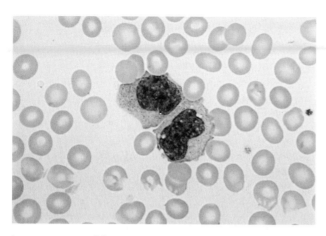

➤ FIGURE 1–11   Monocytes.

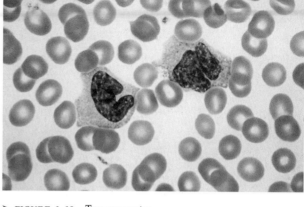

➤ FIGURE 1–13   Two monocytes.

to move while the blood film is drying and become fixed before the cytoplasmic extensions are retracted. Pseudopods vary in size and number; the outer portion of the outstretched cytoplasm may have a hyaline appearance without granules, in contrast to the inner granular cytoplasm.[4]

It is helpful to memorize four helpful characteristic features of the monocytes: nuclear convolutions; lacy, often delicate chromatin; dull gray-blue cytoplasm; and blunt pseudopods (see Fig. 1–10H and Color Plate 5). Kinetic studies have revealed that the half-life of monocytes in the circulation ranges from 8 hours to 3 days before these cells enter tissues and are transformed into macrophages.[1,2]

Monocytes account for 2% to 9% of normal blood leukocytes (Table 1–2).

Large Lymphocytes versus Monocytes

A monocyte (see Fig. 1–10D and Color Plate 5) is often mistaken for a large lymphocyte (see Fig. 1–8G through L, and Color Plate 4) because the monocytic cytoplasm may be blue, the granules may be indistinct, the nucleus is round, and the blunt pseudopods and digestive vacuoles are missing. To distinguish monocytes from large lymphocytes, it is useful to observe the nuclear chromatin structure, character of the cytoplasm, and shape of the cells. The nucleus of a lymphocyte tends to be clumped, rather than linear or lacy as it is in a monocyte (Fig. 1–12 and Color Plate 16). There is a greater tendency for the nuclear chromatin to be condensed at the periphery of the nucleus in the lymphocyte. The brain-like convolutions present in a monocyte (Fig. 1–13 and Color Plate 17) are *not* observed in a lymphocyte[4] (Fig. 1–14 and Color Plate 18).

Large lymphocytes and monocytes may have distinct bluish-red granules. In a monocyte the large bluish-red granules are interspersed with numerous fine granules in the cytoplasm and cannot be enumerated (see Figs. 1–10B and C, and Color Plate 5). In a lymphocyte these large granules are prominent (sometimes at the periphery of the cytoplasm) and can be counted easily because there are no other granules (see Figs. 1–8I and K, and Color Plate 4). Because of the finely granular cytoplasm the monocyte has a ground-glass appearance; the cytoplasm of the lymphocyte has a relatively clear, nongranular background. Large lymphocytes are often deeply indented by neighboring RBCs (see Fig. 1–8K). Monocytes tend to project blunt pseudopods between cells or to compress cells, rather than being indented by them.[4] Table 1–3 summarizes and compares the morphological characteristics of large lymphocytes versus monocytes.

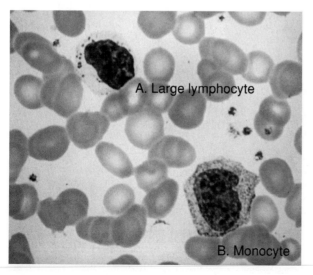

➤ FIGURE 1–12   A. Lymphocytes with azure granules. B. Monocyte.

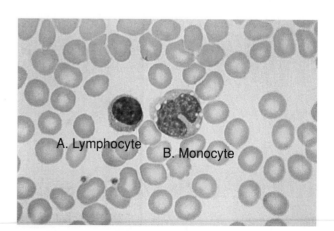

➤ FIGURE 1–14   A. Lymphocyte. B. Monocyte.

> ## Table 1-3
> ## MORPHOLOGICAL COMPARISON OF LARGE LYMPHOCYTES AND MONOCYTES

	Large Lymphocyte	Monocyte
Size, μm	12–15	15–18
Nucleus	Clumped, condensed at periphery	Lacy, brain-like convolutions
Cytoplasmic granules	Bluish-red, prominent granules, easily enumerated if present	Bluish-red, interdispersed with other granules, not easily enumerated
Cytoplasm	Clear, nongranular background	"Ground-glass" appearance
Cell interactions	Indented by erythrocytes	Projection of blunt pseudopodia

➤ HEMATOPOIESIS

Definition

Hematopoiesis is the name given to the dynamic processes of blood cell production and development of the various cells of the blood. Strong evidence exists that blood cells are the progeny of a hematopoietic stem cell.[5] Hematopoiesis is characterized by a constant turnover of cells. The normal hematopoietic system continuously maintains a cell population of erythrocytes, leukocytes, and platelets through a complex network of tissues, organs, stem cells, and regulatory factors.[1] This network is responsible for the maturation and division of hematopoietic stem cells into the lineage-committed stages that transport oxygen and excrete carbon

dioxide (RBCs), fight infection (granulocytes), perform immune functions (lymphocytes), and maintain hemostasis, a process in which blood clots and bleeding is halted (platelets)[5] (Table 1–4).

Hematopoietic stem cells duplicate themselves during division, as shown by the curved arrow in Figure 1–15.[13] The hematopoietic stem cell has the capacity for continuous self-replication and proliferation, together with the ability to differentiate into committed progenitor cells of lymphoid and myeloid lineages.[14] Under the influence of growth factors (cytokines) such as colony-stimulating factors and interleukins, progenitor cells divide and differentiate to form the mature cellular elements of the peripheral blood (see Fig. 1–15).[15]

The hematopoietic system consists of the bone marrow, liver, spleen, lymph nodes, and thymus. These tissues and organs are involved in the production, maturation, and destruction of blood cells. The entire process of hematopoiesis evolves from the stem cells that support hematopoiesis, the progenitor cells that are committed to particular cell lines, and the regulatory factors (growth factors) to which the hematopoietic system responds. These features enable the hematopoietic system to respond to stimuli such as infection, bleeding, or hypoxia by increasing hematopoiesis with emphasis on the cell type needed.[5]

> ## Table 1-4
> ## HEMATOPOIETIC CELL FUNCTION

Cell	Function
Granulocytes	Fight infection
Lymphocytes	Cellular and humoral immunity
Erythrocytes (red cells)	Transport oxygen and excrete carbon dioxide
Platelets	Maintain hemostasis

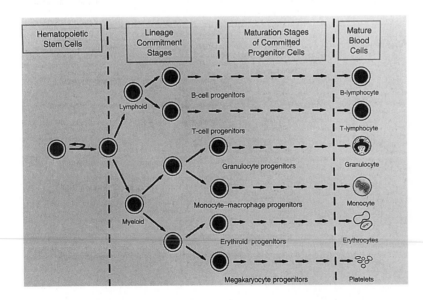

➤ FIGURE 1–15 Diagram of hematopoietic cell differentiation. Hematopoietic stem cells can duplicate themselves during cell division (self-replicate), as indicated by the curved arrow. Most descendants of the stem cells are committed to differentiate. This commitment process occurs through a series of steps or stages, each of which leads to further restriction of lineage choice, until finally the descendant cells are limited to a single lineage. After lineage commitment, the progenitor cells continue to differentiate and mature into the terminally differentiated cells found in the blood. The diagram shows only the steps of commitment and does not depict the proliferation of cells that occurs throughout the process. The amplification of cell numbers accompanying differentiation is very large. (From Koury, M, and Bondurant, M, News Physiol Sci 8:170–174, 1993, with permission.)

Ontogeny (Origin) of Hematopoiesis

During the first few weeks of embryonic life, hematopoiesis begins in the mesoderm of the yolk sac (Fig. 1–16) with mesenchymal stem cells forming large primitive nucleated erythroid cells. Yolk sac production of these nucleated erythroid cells begins to decline in about 6 weeks and ends in about 2 months.[5,14]

The fetal liver assumes responsibility for hematopoiesis during the second month, with the yolk sac nucleated RBCs migrating to the liver and remaining in the liver until the seventh month. From the third to the sixth month, splenic hematopoiesis also occurs. At approximately 7 months of fetal life, the responsibility for hematopoiesis shifts from the liver to the bone marrow, which then becomes the major site of blood cell development in the fetus. Fetal marrow becomes filled with RBCs during hematopoiesis. Bones of the toes, fingers, vertebrae, ribs, pelvis, long bones, and cranium are filled with erythroid cells; early

lymphocytic cells also may be formed during fetal life. A few megakaryocytes (precursors to platelets) first appear at approximately 3 months of fetal life, and granulocytes are observed at about 5 months.[5,15]

At birth, the liver and spleen have ceased hematopoietic cell development, and the active sites of hematopoiesis are in bone cavities (red marrow). Bone seems to provide a microenvironment most appropriate for proliferation and maturation of blood cells.[5] Hematopoiesis occurs in the extravascular part of the red marrow, with a single layer of epithelial cells separating the extravascular marrow compartment from the intravascular compartment (venous sinuses).[15] When new blood cells produced in the marrow are almost mature and ready to circulate in the peripheral blood, the migrating cells leave the marrow parenchyma by squeezing through cytoplasmic fenestrations in sinus endothelial lining cells and emerging into venous sinuses (see Chap. 2).

During infancy and early childhood, hematopoiesis takes place in the entire medullary space, with the volume of marrow in the newborn infant almost equaling the hematopoietic marrow space of adults.[5]

Hematopoiesis gradually decreases in the shaft of the long bones, and after the age of 4 years, fat cells begin to appear in the long bones.[5] Around age 18 to 20, hematopoietic marrow is found exclusively in the sternum, ribs, pelvis, vertebrae, and skull. Other bones contain primary fat (yellow marrow). After the age of 40, marrow in the sternum, ribs, pelvis, and vertebrae is composed of equal of amounts of hematopoietic tissue and fat.[3] Generally, hematopoiesis is sustained in a steady state as production of mature cells equals blood cell removal. When there is increased demand for blood cells, active hematopoiesis may again be found in the spleen, liver, and other tissues as a compensatory mechanism known as extramedullary hematopoiesis.[15]

Bone marrow hematopoietic activity can be divided into two separate pools—the stem cell pool and the bone marrow pool—with eventual release of mature cells into the peripheral blood (Fig. 1–17). It is assumed that in the bone marrow microenvironment there is a stem cell pool where morphologically unidentifiable multipotential stem cells (MSCs) and unipotential committed stem cells reside. In addition, there is a bone marrow pool, which can be divided into two distinct pools: cells that are proliferating and maturing, and cells that are stored for later release into the peripheral blood.

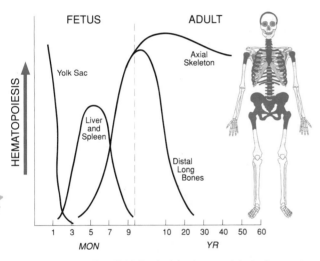

➤ **FIGURE 1–16** Location of active marrow growth in the fetus and adult. During fetal development, hematopoiesis is first established in the yolk sac mesenchyme, later moves to the liver and spleen, and finally is limited to the body skeleton. From infancy to adulthood, there is a progressive restriction of productive marrow to the axial skeleton and proximal ends of the long bones, shown as the shaded areas on the drawing of the skeleton. (From Hillman, RS, and Finch, CA: Red Cell Manual, ed 7. FA Davis, Philadelphia, 1996, p 2, with permission.)

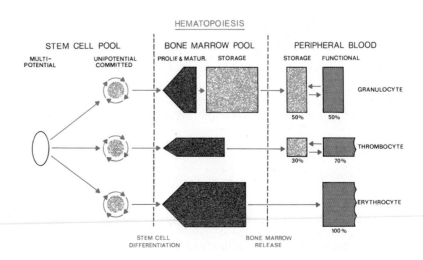

➤ **FIGURE 1–17** Hematopoiesis. (From Erslev, AJ, and Gabuzda, TG: Pathophysiology of Blood, ed 3. WB Saunders, Philadelphia, 1995, with permission.)

There are also two separate granulocytic pools in the peripheral blood: those that are functional within the circulation and those that exist in a storage form. In the granulocytic cell line in the bone marrow pool, there is a component for proliferation and maturation, as well as a storage component.[16] As seen in Figure 1–17,[13] the granulocytic cells in the peripheral blood also contain 50% of circulating cells and 50% of storage cells. The neutrophils that line the walls of the blood vessels are sometimes referred to as the marginating storage pool.[16]

For platelets (also known as thrombocytes), the peripheral blood contains 70% of platelets that circulate, with 30% being stored in the spleen. Figure 1–17 demonstrates that the bone marrow pool consists of only proliferating and maturating platelet precursor cells.[16]

One hundred percent of RBCs, known as erythrocytes, circulate in the peripheral blood in a functional state and in the bone marrow pool. Erythrocytes in various stages of development are a large component of proliferating and maturing red cell precursors found in the bone marrow.[16]

➤ ERYTHROPOIESIS

The term *erythropoiesis* identifies the entire process by which erythrocytes are produced in the bone marrow.[17,18] In response to erythropoietin, a growth factor that stimulates the erythroid precursors, erythropoiesis occurs in the central sinus beds of medullary marrow over a period of about 5 days through at least 3 successive reduction-divisions from rubriblast to prorubricyte to rubricyte, and finally to metarubricyte (orthochromatic normoblast). With successive developmental stages the following changes occur: reduction in cell volume, condensation of chromatin, decrease in N:C ratio, loss of nucleoli, decrease in ribonucleic acid (RNA) in the cytoplasm, decrease in mitochondria, and gradual increase in synthesis of hemoglobin (Fig. 1–18 and Color Plate 2).[17,18] Memorize the following developmental stages from "mother cell" to mature erythrocyte: rubriblast (pronormoblast) to prorubricyte (basophilic normoblast) to rubricyte (polychromatophilic normoblast) to metarubricyte (orthochromatic normoblast). The nucleus of the metarubricyte is eventually extruded, leaving a non-nucleated polychromatophilic (diffusely basophilic) erythrocyte, which is released into the circulating blood to mature in 1 to 2 days. Progressive cellular divisions of one rubriblast results in production of 14 to 16 erythrocytes.[17]

Rubriblast (Pronormoblast, Proerythroblast)

The rubriblast, the earliest recognizable cell of the erythrocytic series, has a round, primitive nucleus with visible nucleoli and chromatin strands that are distinct and dispersed. There is no evidence of clumped chromatin. The nucleus stains reddish-blue with Wright's stain. The cytoplasm stains a deep blue owing to the presence of RNA.[4] The nuclear-to-cytoplasmic (N:C) ratio in a rubriblast is 4:1 (Figs. 1–19A, 1–20A, 1–21, 1–22, and 1–23A, and Color Plates 19 through 23).

Rubriblasts range in size between 14 and 19 μm.[18] A rubriblast is usually slightly larger than a myeloblast and has more cytoplasm, which stains a deeper blue.[18] Rubriblasts constitute 1% or less of the cells observed in normal bone marrow (Table 1–5). Rubriblasts usually divide

within 12 hours to make daughter cells (prorubricytes).[17,18] The morphological characteristics of the erythrocytic series are summarized Table 1–6.

Prorubricyte (Basophilic Normoblast, Basophilic Erythroblast)

Prorubricytes, the daughter cells of rubriblasts, require about 20 hours to develop. In normal bone marrow there are about four times as many prorubricytes as rubriblasts.[17,18] The prorubricyte is differentiated from the rubriblast by the coarsening of the chromatin pattern and the nucleoli, which are ill-defined or not visible under light microscopy. As the prorubricyte matures, it accumulates more RNA and hemoglobin (Figs. 1–24, 1–25A, 1–26, and 1–27, and Color Plates 24 through 27). The predominant color of the cytoplasm is blue due to the staining of RNA, but there may be a pinkish tinge reflecting the presence of varying amounts of hemoglobin.[4] The N:C ratio in the prorubricyte is the same as that of its precursor (4:1). A prorubricyte is somewhat smaller than a rubriblast. Normal marrow contains from 1% to 4% prorubricytes (Table 1–5). The division of the prorubricytes forms rubricytes, which are smaller than prorubricytes but have twice the amount of hemoglobin.

Rubricyte (Polychromatophilic Normoblast, Polychromatophilic Erythroblast)

Rubricytes are smaller than prorubricytes (12 to 15 μm), having relatively more cytoplasm and a smaller nucleus than prorubricytes. The cytoplasm contains a varying mixture of pink due to hemoglobin and blue due to RNA; in the late rubricytes, the pinkish color is usually predominant.[4]

Nuclear chromatin is thickened and irregularly condensed in the rubricyte. Light-staining parachromatin areas are visible among the dark blue–staining, irregular pyknotic masses. Nucleoli are no longer visible.[4] The N:C ratio in a rubricyte is 4:1[18] (see Figs. 1–18, 1–19B, 1–20C, 1–25B, 1–28, and 1–29A, and Color Plates 2, 19, 20, 25, 28, and 29).

The maturation time for rubricytes in bone marrow is about 30 hours, and there are approximately 3 times as many rubricytes as prorubricytes in marrow. Marrow in a normal adult contains 10% to 20% rubricytes (Table 1–5). Rubricytes are *not* present in the normal peripheral blood of adults, but they may appear in small numbers in the peripheral blood of normal newborn infants.

Metarubricyte (Orthochromatic Normoblast, Orthochromatic Erythroblast)

Metarubricytes are formed from rubricytes and are recognized by the solid, blue-black, degenerated nucleus with a nonlinear clumped chromatin pattern (see Figs. 1–18, 1–20B, 1–25C, and 1–27, and Color Plates 2, 20, 25, and 27).[19] The metarubricyte nucleus is incapable of further DNA synthesis. The degenerated nucleus of the metarubricyte is destined to be extruded and will be phagocytized.[4,17,18] The N:C ratio in a metarubricyte is 1:1.

The cytoplasm is predominantly pink (or reddish) because of increasing hemoglobin synthesis, but there may remain minimal amounts of blue cytoplasm due to the presence of RNA.

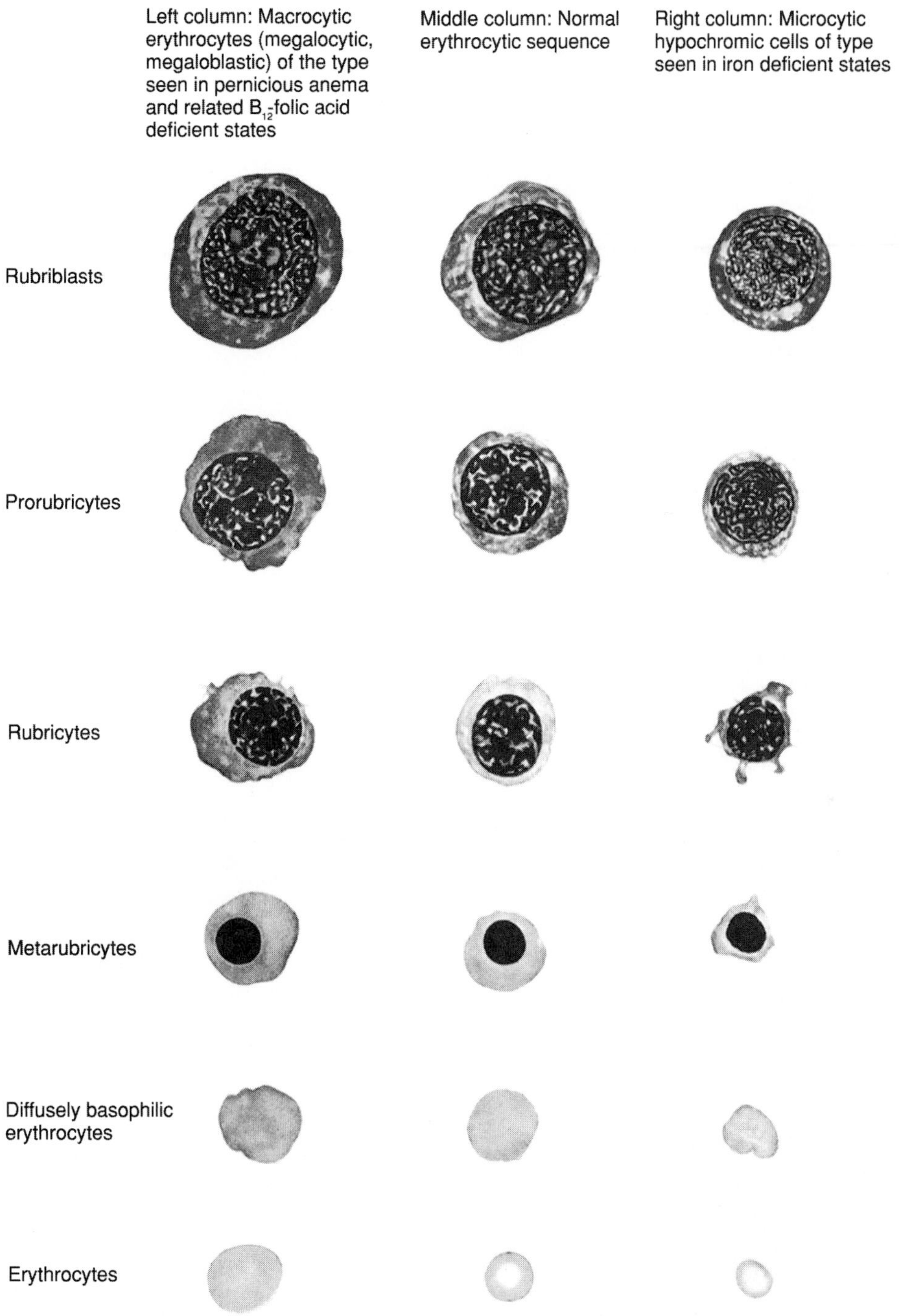

Left column: Macrocytic erythrocytes (megalocytic, megaloblastic) of the type seen in pernicious anema and related B$_{12}$-folic acid deficient states	Middle column: Normal erythrocytic sequence	Right column: Microcytic hypochromic cells of type seen in iron deficient states

Rubriblasts

Prorubricytes

Rubricytes

Metarubricytes

Diffusely basophilic erythrocytes

Erythrocytes

➤ FIGURE 1–18 Erythrocytic system. (From Diggs, LW, et al: The Morphology of Human Blood Cells, ed 5. Abbott Laboratories, Abbott Park, IL, 1985, pp 1–18, 25–27, with permission.)

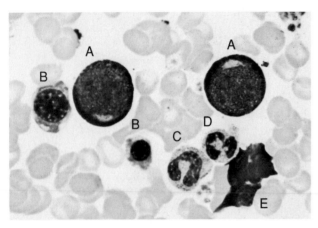

> **FIGURE 1–19**   *A*. Two rubriblasts (note the perinuclear halo). *B*. Two rubricytes. *C*. Neutrophilic band. *D*. Segmented neutrophil. *E*. Smudge cell.

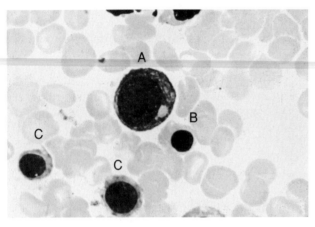

> **FIGURE 1–20**   *A*. Rubriblast. *B*. Metarubricyte. *C*. Two rubricytes.

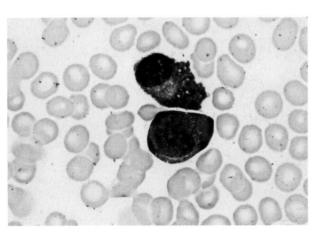

> **FIGURE 1–21**   Center: rubriblast; upper center: plasmacyte.

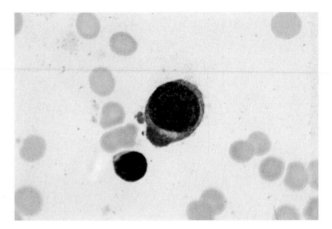

> **FIGURE 1–22**   Center: rubriblast; lower center: lymphocyte.

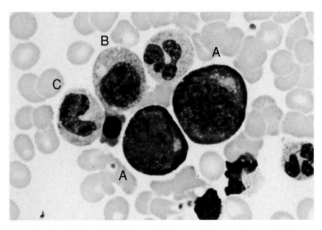

> **FIGURE 1–23**   *A*. Rubriblasts. *B*. Neutrophilic myelocyte. *C*. Neutrophilic metamyelocyte.

> **Table 1-5**
**BONE MARROW CELLS:
NORMAL ADULT VALUES**

Cell	Percent
Stem cell	0–0.01
Myeloblast	0–1
Promyelocyte	1–5
N. myelocyte	2–10
N. metamyelocyte	5–15
N. band	10–40
N. segmented	10–30
Eosinophil	0–3
Basophil	0–1
Lymphocyte	5–15
Plasmacyte	0–1
Monocyte	0–2
Other cells	0–1
Megakaryocyte	0.1–0.5
Rubriblast	0–1
Prorubricyte	1–4
Rubricyte	10–20
Metarubricyte	5–10
WBC: Nucleated RBC Ratio = 4:1	

Source: From Diggs, LW, et al: The Morphology of Human Blood Cells, ed 5. Abbott Laboratories, Abbott Park, IL, 1985, pp 1–18, 25–27, with permission.

The maturation time for metarubricytes is 48 hours.[17,18] The number of metarubricytes in normal marrow varies between 5% and 10% (Table 1–5). Metarubricytes are not observed in the normal peripheral blood of adults, but they can be found in the blood of normal newborn infants. The metarubricyte is the smallest of the nucleated erythrocyte precursors (8 to 12 μm). Morphological characteristics of metarubricytes are given in Table 1–6.

Diffusely Basophilic Erythrocyte (Polychromatophilic Erythrocyte)

The condensed, pyknotic nucleus of a metarubricyte is extruded, leaving a diffusely basophilic or polychromatophilic cell. The membrane of the erythrocyte seals itself. Some of the bluish-staining color remains because of the presence of RNA. The erythrocyte contains approximately two-thirds of its total hemoglobin content by the time the nucleus is lost. The RNA content soon begins to decrease.[4,17,18]

A diffusely basophilic erythrocyte is larger than a mature red cell (7 to 10 μm). It is released in 2 to 3 days from the marrow and circulates for 1 or 2 days before maturing into an erythrocyte. Only rarely are diffusely basophilic erythrocytes found in the blood of normal adults; however, polychromatophilic cells are frequently seen in the blood of normal newborn infants.[18]

When stained with new methylene blue, diffusely basophilic cells reveal ribosomes in a granulofilamentous arrangement (or network of strands and granules) and are classified as reticulocytes (Fig. 1–30 and Color Plate 30). As ribosomes disappear, the diffusely basophilic cell changes into a mature erythrocyte.[17,18]

> **Table 1-6**
MORPHOLOGICAL CHARACTERISTICS OF THE ERYTHROCYTIC SERIES

	Pronormoblast (Rubriblast)	Basophilic Normoblast (Prorubricyte)	Polychromatophilic Normoblast (Rubricyte)	Orthochromatic Normoblast (Metarubricyte)	Polychromatophilic Erythrocyte	Mature Erythrocyte
Cell size, μm	14–19	12–17	12–15	8–12	7–10	7–8
N:C ratio	4:1	4:1	4:1	1:1	n/a	n/a
Nuclear shape	Round	Round	Round	Round	n/a: nucleus has been extruded	n/a
Nuclear position	Central	Central	Central	Central	n/a	n/a
Nuclear color/chromatin	Reddish-blue finely stippled, granular chromatin	Increased, larger granularity of nuclear chromatin	Dark blue, smaller nucleus with parachromatin, increased clumped chromatin	Blue-purple, small nucleus with pyknotic degeneration/ condensed chromatin	n/a	n/a
Nucleoli	0–2	Usually none, occasional indistinct nucleolus	None	None	None	None
Color/amount of cytoplasm	Dark or royal blue/slight	Basophilic/slight	Bluish-pink/moderate	Pink/moderate	Clear gray-blue, polychromatophilic to pink	Pink
Cytoplasmic granules	None	None	None	None	None	None

Abbreviation: n/a = not applicable.

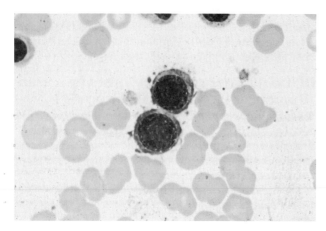

➤ **FIGURE 1-24**   Prorubricytes.

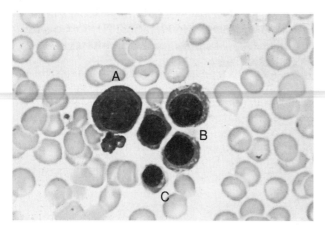

➤ **FIGURE 1-25**   *A.* Prorubricyte. *B.* Three rubricytes. *C.* Metarubricyte.

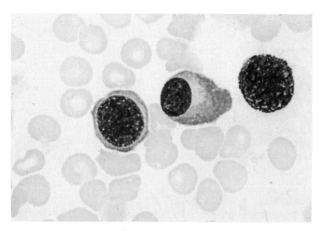

➤ **FIGURE 1-26**   Left: prorubricyte; center: plasmacyte; right: smudge.

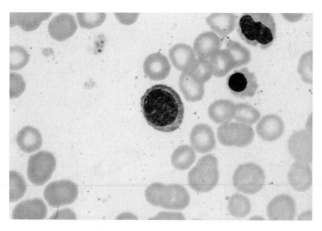

➤ **FIGURE 1-27**   Center: prorubricyte; right: metarubricyte.

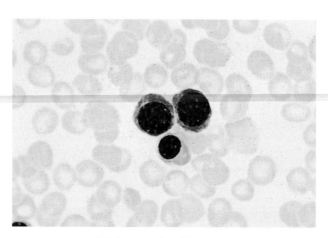

➤ **FIGURE 1-28**   Rubricytes: early and late stages.

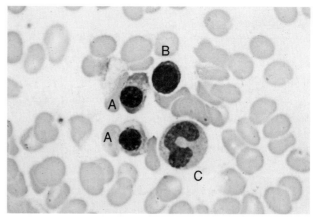

➤ **FIGURE 1-29**   *A.* Rubricytes. *B.* Lymphocyte. *C.* Segmented neutrophil.

➤ **FIGURE 1–30** Reticulocytes. New methylene blue stain of peripheral blood. Note reticulocytes with varying amounts of stained reticulum (RNA). Reticulocytosis is associated with increased erythropoietic activity reflected by polychromasia on the Wright's stain of the peripheral blood.

With anemia or hypoxia, erythropoietin stimulates marrow erythroid precursors to proliferate and to increase the number of early erythroid cells. An increased number of polychromatophilic cells are delivered early from the marrow and, therefore, the reticulocyte count is increased.[14]

Erythrocyte (Red Blood Cell, Discocyte)

The morphological characteristics of a normal erythrocyte are presented at the beginning of this chapter.

A mature erythrocyte is not able to synthesize hemoglobin, because it is without a nucleus, mitochondria, or ribosomes, but it has a unique, yet limited, metabolism to sustain itself while traversing the microvasculature. The erythrocyte carries oxygen from the lungs to the tissues where it is exchanged for carbon dioxide.[5] Erythrocytes are pliable or flexible and deformable, making them capable of unusual changes in shape that are necessary for the passage through the microcirculation to transport oxygen. Refer to Table 1–6 for a summary of the morphological characteristics of each stage of maturation of the red cell.

➤ MYELOPOIESIS (GRANULOCYTOPOIESIS)

Myelopoiesis or granulocytopoiesis refers to the production of neutrophils, eosinophils, and basophils (Fig. 1–31 and Color Plate 3). Mature neutrophils, eosinophils, and basophils have similar patterns of proliferation, differentiation, division, storage in marrow, and delivery to the blood. Maturation and division of the myeloid series in the marrow demonstrate a continuum of development from the blast to the most mature cell (segmented neutrophil), requiring from 7 to 11 days.[7,8,20,21]

Granulocyte production proceeds after cell lineage commitment has determined the identity of the maturing cell as a member of the myelocytic series. The system moves cells throughout passages and compartments where cellular stages occur in response to various stimuli. The proliferative or mitotic pool contains the committed stem cells, myeloblasts, promyelocytes, and myelocytes. These cells actively divide and mature, taking 1 to 2 days for each cellular cycle. The maturation pool is composed of metamye-

locytes and bands, and represents the end of DNA synthesis. The transformation of myelocyte to metamyelocyte to band takes about 8 to 9 hours after entry into the maturation pool. The storage pool retains mature cells for release into peripheral circulation.[5] These mature cells leave the marrow by moving through transiently formed pores in endothelial cells that separate marrow parenchyma from venous sinuses; when leaving blood for tissue, cells migrate between endothelial cells (diapedesis). After release, cells become part of the functional pool and reside as circulating cells or as marginated cells, which line blood vessel walls. Cells are released to enter the peripheral blood or vessel walls for a few hours, and then leave the blood to enter the tissues and body cavities. Under normal circumstances the rate at which these cells enter the blood and the rate at which they egress to tissue are in equilibrium.[5] As these cells exit the blood or the tissues, they are replaced by other cells from the marrow. Once in the blood, half of the released cells freely circulate while the other half are in a marginating pool on the walls of blood vessels, particularly those in lungs, liver, and spleen.[5,8] These latter cells leave the peripheral vessel to be directed by chemotactic factors to inflammatory or infectious tissue. After cells enter tissues, they do not reenter the circulation or the marrow.[7,8]

Morphological Changes

Many morphological changes occur during maturation of granulocytes. These include a reduction in nuclear volume, condensation of chromatin, change in nuclear shape, appearance and disappearance of primary granules, appearance of secondary granules, color changes in cytoplasm from blue to pinkish-red, and change in the size of cells[4,7,8] (Table 1–7).

Maturation of the granulocytic series of cells is characterized by the development of primary blue-staining granules, which are replaced by secondary granules that differ in their affinity for various dyes.[4,8] Cells with an affinity for basic dyes are basophils; the cells that stain reddish-orange with the acid dye eosin are eosinophils; the cells that do not stain intensely with either acid or basic dyes are called neutrophils. As these motile cells mature, the nucleus undergoes progressive changes from round to multilobular forms.[4,7,8]

Stages of Differentiation and Maturation

Neutrophils (Granulocytes)

Myeloblast

The earliest recognizable cell in the granulocytic series is a myeloblast. A myeloblast usually has a round nucleus that stains predominantly reddish-blue and has a smooth nuclear membrane. The interlaced chromatin strands are delicate, finely dispersed or stippled, and evenly stained, but are not clumped. One or more nucleoli of uniform size are usually demonstrable, but occasionally nucleoli may be barely visible.[4] A slight to moderate amount of bluish nongranular cytoplasm stains lighter next to the nucleus than at the periphery of the cell (see Figs. 1–31A and 1–32, and Color Plates 3 and 31). The N:C ratio in the myeloblast is 4:1. A myeloblast is smaller and has less blue cytoplasm than a rubriblast. After about three to five mitotic divisions, the myeloblast matures into a promyelocyte as primary granules become

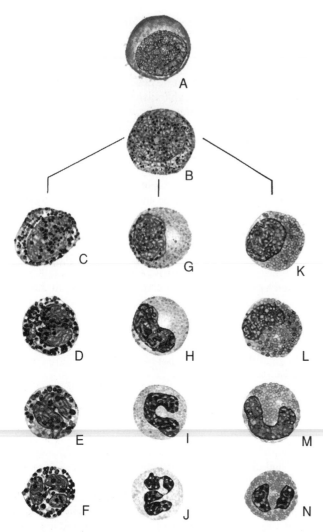

> **FIGURE 1–31** Granulocytopoiesis: myelocytic (granulocytic) system. *A.* Myeloblast. *B.* Promyelocyte (progranulocyte). *C.* Basophilic myelocyte. *D.* Basophilic metamyelocyte. *E.* Basophilic band. *F.* Segmented basophil. *G.* Neutrophilic myelocyte. *H.* Neutrophilic metamyelocyte. *I.* Neutrophilic band. *J.* Segmented neutrophil. *K.* Eosinophilic myelocyte. *L.* Eosinophilic metamyelocyte. *M.* Eosinophilic band. *N.* Segmented eosinophil. (From Diggs, LW, et al: The Morphology of Human Blood Cells, ed 5. Abbott Laboratories, Abbott Park, IL, 1985, pp 1–18, 25–27, with permission.)

visible. Ultrastructural studies of myeloblasts reveal numerous mitochondria, a Golgi area, and free ribosomes.[7,8,21]

Myeloblasts vary in size from 10 to 20 μm.[7] They are not present in normal peripheral blood. Normal marrow contains 1% or less myeloblasts (Table 1–5). The appearance of primary granules marks the maturation of the myeloblast into a promyelocyte.[4]

Promyelocyte (Progranulocyte)

The promyelocyte contains granules that stain dark blue or reddish-blue and may be round or irregular in shape. They appear scattered throughout the cytoplasm and may overlay the nucleus.[4,20] Primary granules are filled with lysosomal granules, which contain myeloperoxidase, acid phosphatase, hydrolytic enzymes, elastase, beta-glucuronidase, and other basic proteins (but not alkaline phosphatase).[7,21]

The nucleus of a promyelocyte is usually round and is large in relation to the cytoplasm. The chromatin of young promyelocytes is almost as finely granular as it is in a myeloblast. In older cells the chromatin structure is slightly coarser than that in a myeloblast. Nucleoli may be faintly visible but are not often distinct (see Figs. 1–31*B*, 1–33, and 1–34, and Color Plates 3, 32, and 33).[4] The N:C ratio in a promyelocyte is 3:1. The cytoplasm is blue, with a relatively light zone adjacent to the nucleus. The periphery of the cytoplasm is smooth and is not indented by neighboring cells.[4] The size of a promyelocyte may vary, depending on the stage of a given cell in the mitotic cycle, but it is often 20 μm and may be larger than a myeloblast.[4] Promyelocytes are not present in normal peripheral blood. From 1% to 5% promyelocytes are observed in normal bone marrow (Table 1–5). As the promyelocyte matures, nucleoli begin to fade, the chromatin becomes more condensed, and the granules are not as intensely stained. Specific secondary neutrophilic granules begin to appear, and the synthesis of primary granules ceases.[4,21] A few primary granules remain through division and maturation and may even appear in segmented neutrophils.[7,8]

Neutrophilic Myelocyte

When primary granules are no longer synthesized and smaller, less dense secondary neutrophilic granules can be identified, the cell has matured into a myelocyte. The first sign of neutrophilic differentiation has been called the "dawn of neutrophilia" or "beginning neutrophilia," which refers to a relatively light island of ill-defined or barely visible (reddish or pinkish) secondary lysosomal granules that develop adjacent to the nucleus and in proximity to the remaining primary granules. As myelocytes divide and age, the primary granules become fewer and the secondary (specific) neutrophilic granules predominate.[4] Secondary granules are considered to be specific granules for neutrophils, and they contain collagenase, lysozyme, lactoferrin, plasminogen activators, and aminopeptidase.[7,8]

The nuclei of myelocytes may be round, oval, or flattened on one side and usually are eccentrically located[4,20] (see Figs. 1–31*G* and 1–35*A*, and Color Plates 3 and 34). Chromatin strands become condensed, partly clumped, and thickened, and are unevenly stained. Nucleoli are absent or indistinct in myelocytes. The neutrophilic myelocyte is the last myeloid precursor capable of division.[4,8,21]

Neutrophilic myelocytes are often smaller than promyelocytes and have relatively large amounts of cytoplasm (N:C ratio is 2:1 or 1:1),[7,8] which gradually becomes less basophilic and more pinkish. The normal peripheral blood does not contain neutrophilic myelocytes. There are 2% to 10% myelocytes in normal bone marrow.

Neutrophilic Metamyelocyte

As maturation proceeds, the nucleus becomes slightly indented (bean- or kidney-shaped), and this shape serves to identify the cell as a metamyelocyte. The indentation is less than half the width of an arbitrary round nucleus (Fig. 1–36).[4] There is noticeable condensation with clumping of the chromatin, but the chromatin structure is not as dense as that of the segmented neutrophilic cell. Metamyelocytes do not divide, nor do they have nucleoli.[4] The N:C ratio is 1:1, and this ratio remains throughout the maturation sequence.[8,21]

Many small, pinkish secondary granules fill the cytoplasm, and there may be a few primary darker granules remaining (see Figs. 1–31*H*, 1–35*B*, and 1–37*A*, and Color Plates 3, 34,

> **Table 1-7**
MORPHOLOGICAL CHARACTERISTICS OF THE GRANULOCYTIC (NEUTROPHILIC) SERIES

	Myeloblast	Promyelocyte (Progranulocyte)	N. Myelocyte	N. Metamyelocyte	N. Band	N. Segmented
Cell size, μm	10–20	10–20	10–18	10–18	10–16	10–16
N:C ratio	4:1	3:1	2:1 or 1:1	1:1	1:1	1:1
Nuclear shape	Round	Round	Oval or round; slightly indented	Usually indented (kidney shaped)	Elongated, narrow band (horseshoe) shape of uniform thickness	2–5 distinct nuclear lobes
Nuclear position	Eccentric or central	Eccentric or central	Usually eccentric	Central or eccentric	Central or eccentric	Central or eccentric
Nuclear color/ chromatin	Light reddish-blue, fine meshwork with no aggregation of material	Light reddish-blue, fine meshwork, slight aggregation may be seen at nuclear membrane	Reddish-blue fine chromatin with slightly aggregated or granular pattern	Light blue-purple with basophilic chromatin easily distinguishable	Purplish-red, clumped granular chromatin	Purplish-red clumped granular chromatin
Nucleoli	1–3	1–2	May or may not have nucleolus	None	None	None
Color/amount of cytoplasm	Basophilic/slight	Basophilic/ increased	Bluish-pink/ moderate	Clear pink/ moderate	Pink/abundant	Pink/abundant
Cytoplasmic granules	Absent	Present, fine azurophilic, nonspecific granules	Present, azurophilic, *specific* granules	Present, (specific) granules, neutrophilic	Specific granules, fine violet-pink	Specific granules, fine violet-pink

and 35). These maturing cells remain in the bone marrow and represent a portion of the granulocytic reserve.[4,8,21]

Metamyelocytes are somewhat smaller than myelocytes (10 to 18 μm) and are larger than the band neutrophil or segmented cell. These cells are usually absent in normal peripheral blood.[4] There are approximately 5% to 15% metamyelocytes in normal bone marrow.

Band Neutrophil
When the stage is reached in which the nuclear indentation in the early granulocyte is greater than half the width of the nucleus (see Fig. 1–36), the cell is identified as a band neutrophil.[4]

The opposite edges of the nucleus become almost parallel, giving the appearance of a curved link of sausage. The shape of the nucleus of a band neutrophil is often folded or twisted, giving rise to difficulty in distinguishing a band from a segmented neutrophil. The nuclear chromatin is pyknotic, and there is usually a dark condensed mass at each end where the lobe is destined to be.[4] The small secondary neutrophilic granules are evenly distributed and stain various shades of pink (see Figs. 1–31*I* and 1–37*B*, and Color Plates 3 and 35). An occasional dark primary granule may be observed.

Neutrophilic band cells are often slightly smaller than metamyelocytes. Band forms constitute from 10% to 40% of the nucleated cells in the bone marrow.[4]

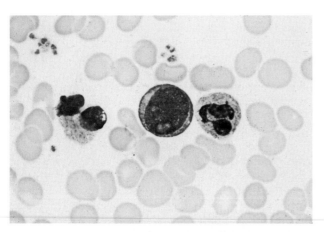

> FIGURE 1–32   Center: myeloblast; right: segmented neutrophil; left: disintegrated neutrophil.

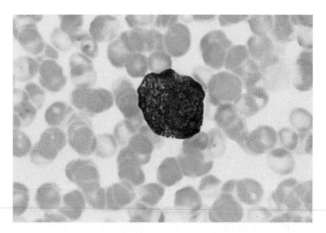

> FIGURE 1–33   Promyelocyte.

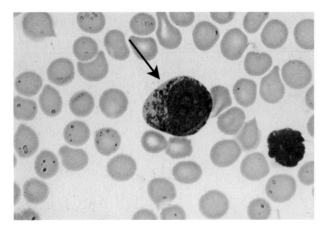

➤ FIGURE 1-34   Center: promyelocyte.

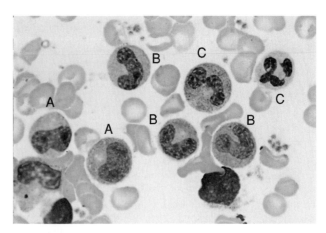

➤ FIGURE 1-37   *A.* Two neutrophilic metamyelocytes. *B.* Three neutrophilic bands. *C.* Two segmented neutrophils.

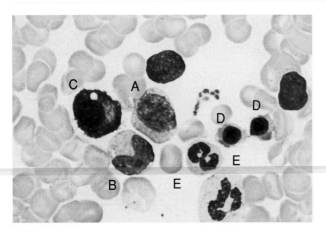

➤ FIGURE 1-35   *A.* Neutrophilic myelocyte. *B.* Neutrophilic metamyelocyte. *C.* Plasmacyte. *D.* Metarubricytes. *E.* Segmented neutrophils.

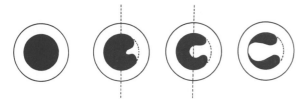

TERMINOLOGY   BASED   ON

INDENTATION   OF   NUCLEI

MYELOCYTE   METAMYELOCYTE   BAND   SEGMENTED

➤ FIGURE 1-36   Terminology based on indentation of nuclei: (left to right) myelocyte, metamyelocyte, band, segmented.

Segmented Neutrophil

As stated earlier in this chapter, the nucleus of the segmented neutrophil is divided into two to five (often three) lobes that are connected by a thin filament or strand (see Figs. 1–31*J*, 1–32, 1–35*E*, 1–36, 1–37*C*, and Color Plates 3, 31, 34, and 35). Approximately 10% to 30% segmented neutrophils are noted in normal bone marrow of older children and adults.

Because there is a gradual transition between the various stages of granulocytes, the division of neutrophils into developmental stages is somewhat arbitrary. This division is, however, necessary for morphological evaluation. Borderline cells that are difficult to distinguish from each other are often present. In this dilemma, the borderline cell should be classified as the more mature cell.[4] Differentiation of band neutrophil and segmented cells is described in the first part of this chapter on peripheral blood cells. Table 1–7 lists the morphological characteristics of the neutrophilic series.

Tissue Neutrophil

Tissue neutrophils are large marrow cells with ample cytoplasm having irregular, blunt pseudopods that are often multipointed and may have nebulous cytoplasmic streamers (Fig. 1–38 and Color Plate 36). These cells are readily indented by adjacent marrow cells or may be squeezed between adjacent cells. Often there are long and tenuous cytoplasmic extensions that seem to wrap around other cells. These cells are not phagocytic and seldom have cytoplasmic vacuoles. The cytoplasm stains light blue and has a fine latticelike structure. Granules vary in number and stain varying shades of red to blue, but the majority have a reddish-purple stain. Many of the granules tend to be arranged in chains. The beadlike granular aggregates extend into the cytoplasmic projections.[22,23]

The large, round, or oval nucleus has a coarse chromatin structure with a distinct linear pattern. Nucleoli are usually conspicuous and stain light blue.[22,23]

Tissue neutrophils are fixed or semifixed tissue cells. They are immobile end-stage cells that are probably derived from the same progenitor cells as neutrophils.[22,23]

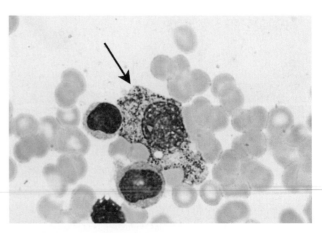

➤ FIGURE 1-38   Tissue neutrophil (large center cell).

Tissue neutrophils occur infrequently in normal bone marrow. However, they are found in increased numbers in bone marrow smears of patients who have conditions in which there is a proliferation of neutrophilic cells. These conditions include chronic myelocytic leukemia, myelocytic-monocytic leukemia, and myelofibrosis, as well as neutropenic states in which there is an arrest in the maturation and delivery of cells into the circulating blood.[22,23]

Eosinophil

Eosinophils pass through the same developmental stages as neutrophils: myelocyte, metamyelocyte, band, and segmented stages (see Figs. 1–31*K* through *N,* and Color Plate 3). The earliest eosinophil (eosinophilic myelocyte) has a few dark bluish primary granules intermingled with the few specific, reddish-orange granules (Fig. 1–39 and Color Plate 37). During development the bluish granules become less visible and disappear, and the round, specific, or secondary bright red eosinophilic granules fill the cytoplasm[4,9] (Figs. 1–40*A,* 1–41*A,* and 1–42*A,* and Color Plates 38, 39, and 40).

Eosinophils spend 3 to 6 days in production in the marrow before appearing in the peripheral blood. Bone marrow provides a storage area for eosinophils so that they can be rapidly mobilized when needed. The factors that regulate production and release of eosinophils into blood are probably different from those that regulate neutrophils. The mean transit time of these cells in the circulatory system of humans has been reported to be about 8 hours, but in some disease states with eosinophilia, the time may be longer. Much less is known about the stem cell kinetics of the eosinophil than of the neutrophil.

Eosinophils migrate from blood to tissue, such as bronchial mucosa, skin, gastrointestinal tract, and vagina in about 12 days. Eosinophils may migrate from tissue back into blood and marrow. Eosinophils, which are motile, can migrate between endothelial cells into the tissue or into an area of inflammation in the same manner as neutrophils.[7,9]

The granules of eosinophils contain various hydrolytic enzymes, including peroxidase, acid phosphatase, aryl sulfatase, β-glucuronidase, phospholipase, cathepsin, and ribonuclease, but they lack lysosome, cationic proteins, and alkaline phosphatase.[7,9]

Normal adult bone marrow contains 0 to 3% eosinophils. The morphological characteristics of the eosinophilic series are summarized in Table 1–8.

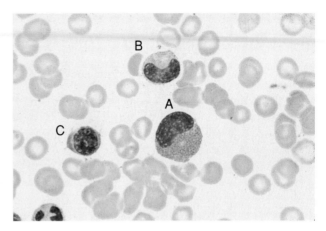

➤ **FIGURE 1–40**   *A.* Eosinophilic metamyelocyte. *B.* Neutrophilic band. *C.* Rubricyte.

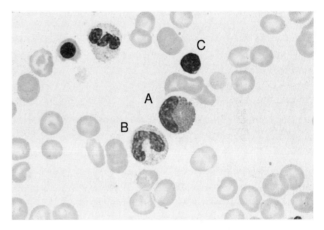

➤ **FIGURE 1–41**   *A.* Eosinophilic band. *B.* Neutrophilic band. *C.* Lymphocyte.

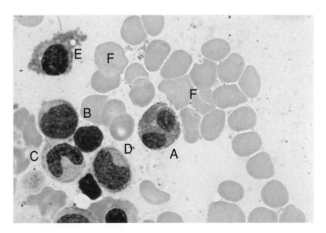

➤ **FIGURE 1–42**   *A.* Segmented eosinophil. *B.* Lymphocyte. *C.* Neutrophilic band. *D.* Neutrophilic metamyelocyte. *E.* Plasmacyte. *F.* Two diffusely basophilic red cells.

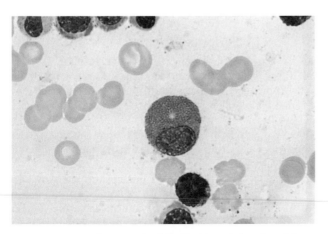

➤ **FIGURE 1–39**   Center: eosinophilic myelocyte; below: basophil.

TISSUE EOSINOPHIL

In smears of bone marrow, occasionally there may be a large cell with elongated and tapering cytoplasmic extensions, containing typical reddish-orange granules of the type seen in the eosinophils of the circulating blood[23] (Fig. 1–43 and Color Plate 41). The nucleus of such cells, instead of being indented or lobulated, is round or oval and has a well-

> **Table 1-8**
MORPHOLOGICAL CHARACTERIZATION OF THE GRANULOCYTIC (EOSINOPHILIC) SERIES

	Myeloblast	Promyelocyte (Proganulocyte)	E. Myelocyte	E. Metamyelocyte	E. Band	E. Segmented
Cell size, μm	10–20	10–20	10–18	10–16	10–16	10–16
N:C ratio	4:1	3:1	2:1 or 1:1	1:1	1:1	1:1
Nuclear shape	Round	Round	Oval or round; slightly indented	Usually indented (kidney shaped)	Elongated, narrow band shape of uniform thickness	2 distinct nuclear lobes
Nuclear position	Eccentric or central	Eccentric or central	Usually eccentric	Central or eccentric	Central or eccentric	Central or eccentric
Nuclear color/ chromatin	Light, reddish-blue, fine meshwork with no aggregation of material	Light reddish-blue, fine meshwork, slight aggregation may be seen at nuclear membrane	Reddish-blue find chromatin with slightly aggregated or granular pattern	Light blue-purple with basophilic chromatin easily distinguishable	Deep blue-purple, coarsely granular chromatin	Deep blue-purple, coarsely granular chromatin
Nucleoli	1–3	1–2	May or may not have nucleolus	None	None	None
Color/amount of cytoplasm	Basophilic/ scanty	Basophilic and increased	Bluish-pink/ moderate	Pink/moderate	Pink/moderate	Pink/moderate
Cytoplasmic granules	Absent	Present, fine azurophilic, nonspecific granules	Present, reddish-orange, uniform (specific) eosinophilic "granules	Present, reddish-orange, uniform (specific) eosinophilic granules	Present, red, uniform (specific) eosinophilic granules	Present, red, uniform, (specific) eosinophilic granules

defined reticular chromatin and, often, nucleoli. Such cells are identified as tissue eosinophils and are thought to be fixed tissue variants of the more motile eosinophils of the circulating blood.[23] Tissue eosinophils arise from the same progenitor cells as eosinophils in the marrow and blood.[23]

Basophil

Basophils may be identified as basophilic myelocytes, metamyelocytes, bands, and segmented cells based upon the shape of their nuclei. The shape of the nucleus is, however, often masked by large basophilic granules (see Figs. 1–31C through F, and Color Plate 3). The specific violet-blue granules of basophils are formed in the myelocytic state and continue to be produced throughout all later maturation stages (see Figs. 1–31C through F, and Color Plate 3). There are also some smaller granules that do not stain as darkly as the specific basophil granules but instead tend to be more reddish-blue.[4,10]

Maturation of basophils in the bone marrow takes place over 7 days.[10] Mature basophils rarely have more than two segments. Basophils circulate for a few hours in blood, then migrate into skin, mucosa, and other serosal areas.[10]

Basophils in all stages of maturation are smaller than promyelocytes and neutrophil myelocytes; their size approximates that of neutrophils. Table 1–9 summarizes the morphological characteristics of the basophilic series. Normal bone marrow has 0 to 1% basophils.

TISSUE BASOPHIL (MAST CELL)

Tissue basophils (mast cells) (Fig. 1–44 and Color Plate 42) and blood basophils are closely related in their functions and biochemical characteristics, but the relationship between them is still being studied.[10,23] Both cells participate in a similar manner in acute and delayed allergic reactions. The granules of both cells have similar morphological characteristics, and each cell contains histamine and heparin and is water soluble.[10,23]

Tissue basophils are derived from the pluripotential stem cell and are fixed tissue cells. The cytoplasm of the tissue basophils is filled with large, prominent, intensely stained violet-blue granules. The granules are usually round and about the same size (0.1 to 0.3 μm). They may overlay the

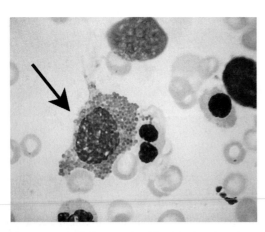

> **FIGURE 1–43**   Left: tissue eosinophils; right: binucleated metarubricyte.

> **Table 1-9**
MORPHOLOGICAL CHARACTERISTICS OF THE GRANULOCYTIC (BASOPHILIC) SERIES

	Myeloblast	Promyelocyte (Progranulocyte)	B. Myelocyte	B. Metamyelocyte	B. Band	B. Segmented
Cell size, μm	10–20	10–20	10–18	10–18	10–16	10–16
N:C ratio	4:1	3:1	2:1 or 1:1	1:1	1:1	1:1
Nuclear shape	Round	Round	Oval or round; slightly indented	Usually indented (kidney shaped), oval	Elongated, narrow band shape of uniform thickness	2 distinct nuclear lobes
Nuclear position	Eccentric or neutral	Eccentric or central	Commonly eccentric, may be central	Central or eccentric	Central or eccentric	Central or eccentric
Nuclear color/ chromatin	Light reddish-blue, fine meshwork with no aggregation of material	Light reddish-blue, fine meshwork, slight aggregation at nuclear rim	Reddish-blue, fine chromatin with slightly aggregated or granular pattern	Light blue-purple with basophilic chromatin easily distinguishable	Deep blue-purple, coarsely granular chromatin	Deep blue-purple, coarsely granular chromatin
Nucleoli	1–3	1–2	May/may not have nucleolus	None	None	None
Color/amount of cytoplasm	Basophilic/slight	Basophilic/ increased	Bluish pale, moderate	Pale blue, moderate	Pale blue, moderate	Pale blue, moderate
Cytoplasmic granules	Absent	Present, fine azurophilic, nonspecific granules	Present, coarse (*specific*) basophilic, nonuniform granules	Present, coarse violet-blue, nonuniform granules	Present, coarse violet-blue, nonuniform granules	Present, coarse violet-blue, nonuniform granules

margins of the palely stained nucleus or obscure the nucleus completely. The nucleus is small, round or oval, and not segmented.[10,23]

Tissue basophils are widely scattered in the connective tissue of various organs, bone marrow, and the mucosal area of serous membranes. In bone marrow tissue basophils are usually observed in the hypercellular area and can be located in the "squashed" smear made from a marrow particle. Some tissue basophils have spindle shapes and jagged margins resulting from trauma in the process of aspiration.[10,23]

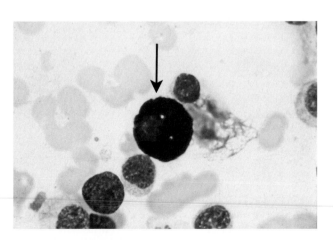

> **FIGURE 1–44** Tissue basophil (arrow).

► MONOPOIESIS

The mononuclear-phagocyte system (MPS) is composed of monocytes, macrophages, and their precursors—monoblasts and promonocytes.[12,24] The cells composing this system arise in the bone marrow from progenitor cells that are committed to monocyte-macrophage production.[24,25]

Monoblasts and Promonocytes

Monoblasts are large and have an eccentrically placed nucleus that may be minimally indented, one or two large prominent nucleoli, a fine, lacy nuclear chromatin, and a nongranular cytoplasm that stains a deep blue (Fig. 1–45B and Color Plate 6). The N:C ratio in these cells is 4:1. Monoblasts are nonmotile and nonphagocytic cells. Monoblasts divide and give rise to promonocytes and then to monocytes.[4,12,24,25]

Promonocytes also are large and have indented or folded nuclei and fine chromatin. They often have a visible nucleolus and sometimes contain a few peroxidase-positive granules. The N:C ratio in promonocytes is 3:1 or 2:1 (see Fig. 1–45E and Color Plate 6). Promonocytes are slightly motile and may infrequently take part in phagocytosis.[4,12,24,25]

Promonocytes and monoblasts are not easily identifiable in bone marrow or peripheral blood smears except in disorders in which there is marked proliferation of monocytic cells. The identification of early monocytic cells is based on slightly indented, or folded, large nuclei and on association with more mature cells that have pseudopods and brain-like convolutions in the nucleus.[4,24,25]

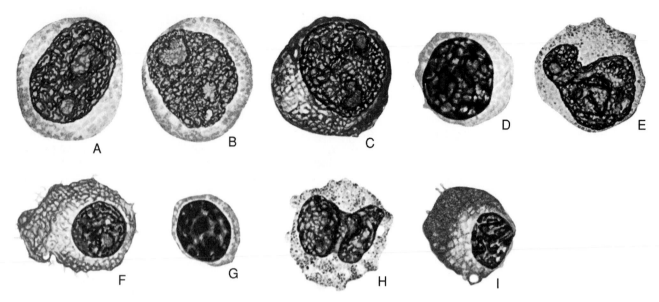

> **FIGURE 1-45**   Lymphocytic, monocytic, and plasmacytic systems. *A.* Lymphoblast. *B.* Monoblast. *C.* Plasmablast. *D.* Prolymphocyte. *E.* Promonocyte. *F.* Proplasmacyte. *G.* Lymphocyte with clumped chromatin. *H.* Monocyte. *I.* Plasmacyte. (From Diggs, LW, et al: The Morphology of Human Blood Cells, ed 5. Abbott Laboratories, Abbott Park, IL, 1985, pp 1–18, 25–27, with permission.)

Monocytes and Macrophages

Promonocytes develop into monocytes. Monocytes enter the circulation for a short time and then migrate into tissue to transform into tissue macrophages.[4]

The characteristic features of monocytes in normal peripheral blood are given in the earlier part of this chapter (see Fig. 1–10 and Color Plate 5). The scanning electron microscope shows the monocyte to have a ruffled plasma membrane with long, thin microvilli.[25]

As monocytes mature, they become too large to pass readily through capillaries, and so they move into tissue and convert into macrophages in many organs (e.g., pulmonary alveolar macrophages, peritoneal macrophages, splenic macrophages, Kupffer cells in the liver, and connective tissue macrophages).[12] This transformation involves rapid growth, enlargement, and intensified phagocytic activity. Macrophages do not normally reenter the bloodstream but may reenter the circulation during inflammation.[12,24,25]

Macrophages are large, irregularly shaped tissue cells (25 to 80 μm) with a round or reniform nucleus; and contain one or two nucleoli, clumped chromatin, abundant cytoplasm with vacuoles, and numerous azurophilic granules.[4,12,23–25] Macrophages are also called histiocytes (histio = tissue; cyte = cell). Table 1–10 summarizes the morphological characteristics of the monocytic-macrophage series.

> ## Table 1-10
> ## MORPHOLOGICAL CHARACTERISTICS OF THE MONOCYTIC SERIES

	Monoblast	Promonocyte	Mature Monocyte	Macrophage
Cell size, μm	12–20	12–20	15–18	25–80
N:C ratio	4:1	3:1 or 2:1	2:1 or 1:1	1:2 or 1:3
Nuclear shape	Round, oval, or slightly folded	Round with chromatin creases or cerebriform folding, more distinct	Increased folding or elongated	Round or reniform
Nuclear position	Eccentric	Central	Central	Eccentric
Nuclear color/ chromatin	Pale red-purple, fine, thready chromatin	Pale red-purple, reticular pattern	Blue-purple, finer reticular pattern than immature forms	Clumped chromatin
Nucleoli	1–2	0–2	None	1–2
Color/amount of cytoplasm	Basophilic/moderate	Paler gray basophilic/ abundant with "bleblike" pseudopodia at border	Pale gray-blue/ abundant "bleblike" pseudopodia	Abundant with vacuoles
Cytoplasmic granules	None	May or may not contain fine, red, dustlike particles	Numerous fine, pale red, dustlike particles throughout cytoplasm	Numerous azurophilic granules

➤ LYMPHOPOIESIS

The lymphoid progenitor cell is derived from the hematopoietic stem cell. The common lymphoid progenitor cell can differentiate into either T or B cells, depending on the microenvironment. T cells differentiate in the thymus, B cells in adult bone marrow. Null cells, or third-population cells, originate in the bone marrow, although the maturation sequence is unknown.[11] T, B, and null cells cannot be separately identified morphologically but can be distinguished functionally and by immunologic marker studies. (See the section on CD Nomenclature later in the chapter.)

In primary lymphoid organs such as the thymus and bone marrow, lymphocytes differentiate, proliferate, and mature into fully functional immune cells. In secondary lymphoid organs such as lymph nodes, spleen, and mucosal tissues (tonsils, Peyer's patches), lymphocytes communicate and interact with antigen-presenting cells (APCs), phagocytes, and macrophages in an active immune response.[11]

Lymphoblasts and Prolymphocytes

The earliest lymphocytes are identified as lymphoblasts and prolymphocytes. Lymphoblasts contain a large, round nucleus with a small or moderate amount of basophilic cytoplasm. The nuclear chromatin strands in lymphoblasts are thin, loose, evenly stained, and not clumped. One or several nucleoli are usually demonstrable.[4] These cells measure 10 to 20 μm in diameter (see Fig. 1–45A and Color Plate 6).

Prolymphocytes have an intermediate chromatin pattern that has clumps in some areas of the nucleus but does not appear as clumped as in mature lymphocytes.[4] Parachromatin, which appears reddish-purple, may be present in the nucleus. Nucleoli are less distinct than in lymphoblasts. Prolymphocytes are slightly smaller than lymphoblasts, approximately 9 to 18 μm (see Fig. 1–45D and Color Plate 6). Differences are subtle, and in case of doubt the cell should be called a lymphocyte.[4] The morphological characteristics of the lymphocytic series are summarized in Table 1–11.

Lymphocytes

The morphological description of lymphocytes may be found in the first part of this chapter.

Plasmablasts and Proplasmacytes

Cells designated as plasmablasts are similar to blast cells of other series. The nuclei are large in relation to the cytoplasm (N:C ratio is 4:1), appear round with fine, linear chromatin strands, and have a clearly visible nucleolus (see Fig. 1–45C and Color Plate 6). The cytoplasm is blue. Plasmablasts are identified primarily in the presence of proplasmacytes and plasmacytes but cannot be easily differentiated from other blasts. The plasmablast appears slightly larger than the more mature plasmacyte (16 to 25 μm).[11]

Proplasmacytes and plasmacytes differ from plasmablasts in that the color of the cytoplasm is deep blue, the juxtanuclear light areas are prominent, and the nuclei are eccentric. The chromatin structure of the nuclei in proplasmacytes is intermediate between that of plasmablasts and plasmacytes. In proplasmacytes the nucleolus may be ill defined or absent.[11,19] The N:C ratio in proplasmacytes is 3:1 (see Fig. 1–45F and Color Plate 6).

Plasmablasts and proplasmacytes, although not observed in normal bone marrow, are seen in diseases associated with abnormal immunoglobulin production, especially multiple myeloma.[11]

Plasmacytes (Plasma Cells)

Plasmacytes represent the end stage of B-lymphocyte lineage. They are not observed in the peripheral blood smears of normal individuals but constitute about 1% of the nucleated cells in normal marrow. Mature plasmacytes range in size from 10 to 18 μm.[10,19] They may be round or oval, with slightly irregular margins.

The cytoplasm is nongranular and usually stains a deep or vibrant blue that has been described as "corn flower" or "larkspur" blue. The cytoplasm adjacent to the nucleus is pale, with a perinuclear clear zone containing the Golgi apparatus, and at the cell periphery there are secretory vesi-

---

➤ Table 1-11
MORPHOLOGICAL CHARACTERISTICS OF THE LYMPHOCYTIC SERIES

	Lymphoblast	Prolymphocyte	Mature Lymphocyte
Cell size, μm	10–20	9–18	7–10
N:C ratio	4:1	4:1	4:1
Nuclear shape	Round	Round or indented	Round or indented
Nuclear position	Eccentric or central	Eccentric with scanty cytoplasm to one side or round	Eccentric with scanty cytoplasm to one side or round
Nuclear color/chromatin	Undifferentiated red-purple/ smooth chromatin	Condensed, clumped blue-purple chromatin with red-purple parachromatin	Homogenous, coarse blue-purple nuclear chromatin
Nucleoli	1–2	0–1	None
Color/amount of cytoplasm	Clear basophilic/scanty	clear basophilic/scanty	Light sky blue/scanty to moderate
Cytoplasmic granules	Absent	Absent	Usually absent, few azurophilic granules seen occasionally

cles. Fibrillar structures that stain blue may be demonstrable in the cytoplasm. One or several small vacuoles may be observed. There is no evidence of phagocytosis of visible particles.[19]

The nucleus of a plasmacyte is relatively small, round, or oval, and eccentrically placed in the cell. The nuclear chromatin is clumped or coarse and lumpy, similar to that of a lymphocyte[19] (see Figs. 1–45*I*, 1–46, and 1–47, and Color Plates 6, 43, and 44).

Plasmacytes in bone marrow are semifixed cells that may be torn in the process of aspiration and appear in marrow smears with irregular spiculate margins. Plasmacytes may cluster around large nongranular or finely granular tissue cells. This contact of plasmacytes with tissue cells is probably a manifestation of the immune response in which antigenic materials, processed by macrophages, are transferred to the plasmacytes, which in turn will manufacture immune globulins.[19]

Immune globulins manufactured by plasmacytes produce unusual morphological variants. The proteinaceous material appears in the form of round globules that are often red or pink, but may be blue or almost colorless, and are called Russell bodies (see Color Plate 245). The globules may fill the cytoplasm, giving the appearance of a bunch of grapes (berry, grape, or morula cells).[19]

In some cells, the globules are so numerous and so tightly packed that they assume a honeycomb configuration. In other cells, the redness has a diffuse distribution, producing cells called "flame cells," which are observed particularly in association with IgA (see Color Plate 247). The red-staining proteinaceous material may appear as granules or as pools at the margin; it also may crystallize and produce elongated crystalline structures that stain reddish.[19] Table 1–12 summarizes the morphological characteristics of the plasmacytic series.

➤ MEGAKARYOCYTOPOIESIS

The megakaryocyte is the largest hematopoietic cell in the bone marrow and descends from the same multipotential stem cell as do the other blood cells. The mission of megakaryocytes is to proliferate and then fragment their cytoplasm into platelets, when needed, in order to maintain a normal number of platelets (150,000 to 350,000/μL). The maturation of the megakaryocyte involves endoreduplica-

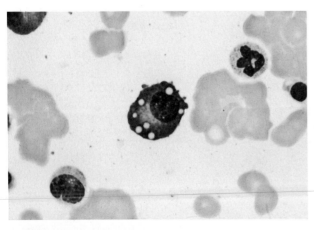

➤ FIGURE 1–46   Center: plasmacyte; upper right: segmented neutrophil, lower left: resting monocyte.

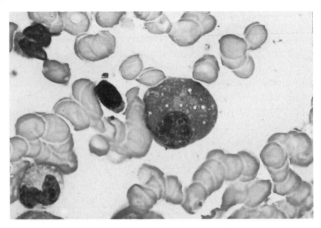

➤ FIGURE 1–47   Center: plasmacyte; left center: small lymphocyte.

tion (or endomitosis), which is a process whereby the nuclear material reduplicates but the nucleus does not divide. The result of endoreduplication is a polyploid nucleus. Each nuclear reduplication causes a doubling of the nuclear material. The cytoplasm increases in amount and in number of granules, but it does not divide. Megakaryoblasts are moderately sized cells in the range of 20 to 45 μm with a single, round (or slightly oval), primitive nucleus; one or two nucleoli; and blunt protrusions that stain blue and that may contain chromophobic globules. The scanty cytoplasm is nongranular and basophilic. The N:C ratio is 4:1.[26–28] The megakaryocytic series is shown in Figure 1–48 and Color Plate 7.

Pathologic alterations in megakaryoblasts are observed in myeloproliferative disease. The presence of micromegakaryoblasts is typical of acute megakaryocytic leukemia (classified as M7 in the French-American-British [FAB] classification of acute leukemia) (see Chap. 16). They may also be found in the blast crisis of chronic granulocytic leukemia, in myelofibrosis, and in other acute leukemias. Micromegakaryoblasts are small and difficult to distinguish from myeloblasts, but cytoplasmic blebs or budding (suggesting early platelet formation) helps to identify micromegakaryoblasts.[26]

As the megakaryoblast matures into a promegakaryocyte, it increases both the amount of nuclear material and the amount of cytoplasm itself[26] (N:C ratio is 4:1 to 1:1).

A promegakaryocyte not only increases the size of the nucleus but also becomes lobulated, with each lobe having a 2n complement of DNA. The size of the promegakaryoblast ranges from 20 to 80 μm. Reddish granules appear in the enlarging bluish cytoplasm. Electron micrographs reveal that demarcation membranes are beginning to develop as invaginations from the plasma membrane of the megakaryocyte. The demarcation membrane system establishes an outer limit of each platelet, which is released as a cytoplasmic fragment[27,28] (see Fig. 1–48 and Color Plate 7).

As endomitosis and DNA synthesis cease and maximum nuclear number (ploidy) is attained, the megakaryocyte has increased in volume with an abundant amount of pinkish cytoplasm and a multilobulated nucleus (Figs. 1–49 through 1–53, and Color Plates 45 through 49). The size of the megakaryocyte ranges from 30 to 100 μm. The majority of the cells are of the 8n, 16n, and 32n ploidy classes (16n average ploidy represents eight lobes).[27,28] The chromatin is linear and coarse. Numerous small, uniformly dis-

> **Table 1-12**
MORPHOLOGICAL CHARACTERISTICS OF THE PLASMACYTIC SERIES

	Plasmablast	Proplasmacyte	Mature Plasma Cell
Cell size, μm	16–25	15–20	10–18
N:C ratio	4:1	3:1	2:1 or 1:1
Nuclear shape	Round	Round or oval	Round or oval
Nuclear position	Central	Eccentric	Usually eccentric
Nuclear color/chromatin	Pale red-purple, fine stippled chromatin	Red-purple, increased granularity of chromatin	Blue-purple, dense chromatin with large clumps near nuclear margin
Nucleoli	1–3	0–1	None
Color/amount of cytoplasm	Pale blue/scanty to moderate, frequent perinuclear clear zone	Dark blue/moderate	Dark blue/moderate cytoplasm with perinuclear clear zone, may contain vacuoles
Cytoplasmic granules	None	None	None

tributed, dense granules that stain reddish-blue are present. The demarcation membrane system is uniform and its lumen open; the cytoplasm is divided into partitions that define platelet limits.[27,28] The N:C ratio at the megakaryocyte state of development ranges from 1:1 to 1:12. The morpho-

logical characteristics of the megakaryocytic series are given in Table 1–13.

After maturation is completed, the megakaryocyte membrane ruptures, the entire megakaryocyte cytoplasm fragments, and thrombopoiesis occurs. The polyploid naked

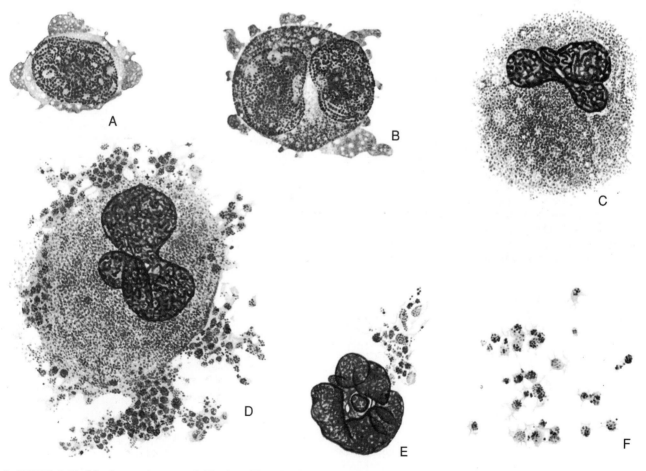

> FIGURE 1–48   Megakaryocytic system. *A.* Megakaryoblast with single oval nucleus, nucleoli, and bluish foamy marginal cytoplasmic structures. *B.* Promegakaryocyte with two nuclei, granular blue cytoplasm, and marginal bubbly cytoplasmic structures. *C.* Megakaryocyte with granular cytoplasm and without discrete thrombocytes (platelets). *D.* Megakaryocyte with multiple nuclei and with thrombocytes (platelets). *E.* Megakaryocyte nucleus with attached thrombocytes. *F.* Thrombocytes (platelets). (From Diggs, LW, et al: The Morphology of Human Blood Cells, ed 5. Abbott Laboratories, Abbott Park, IL, 1985, pp 33–34, 48–50, 85, with permission.)

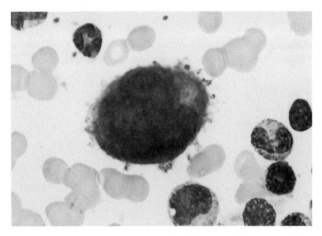

➤ FIGURE 1–49   Center: early megakaryocyte; top left: segmented neutrophil; bottom center: neutrophilic metamyelocyte.

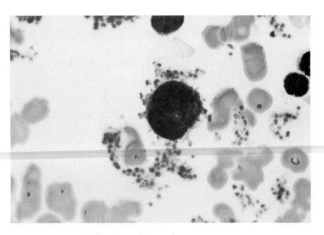

➤ FIGURE 1–50   Center: early megakaryocyte.

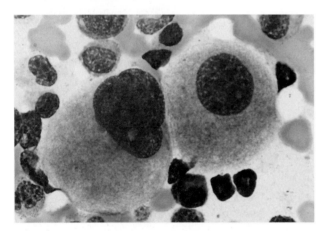

➤ FIGURE 1–51   Megakaryocytes without platelets.

nucleus (Fig. 1–54 and Color Plate 50) is soon to be engulfed by a macrophage.[27,28]

Some mature megakaryocytes are located adjacent to marrow sinuses and extend portions of their cytoplasm through the basement membrane and between endothelial cells of the marrow sinusoids in order to put platelets into the sinus. Membrane-bound platelets are released and swept into the bloodstream from these cytoplasmic projec-

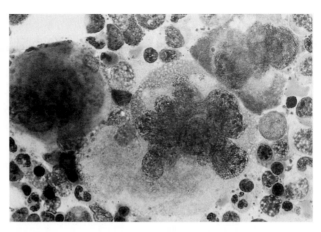

➤ FIGURE 1–52   Megakaryocytes tend to be in small groups with multilobulated single nuclei. Mature megakaryocytes have numerous fine cytoplasmic granules, and occasionally platelet units can be seen at their periphery (magnification ×640).

tions. Further fragmentation to form individual platelets occurs after release into the sinus. One megakaryocyte can release several thousand platelets.[27,28]

In the past, megakaryocytes were believed to shed platelets from their outer surface. However, transmission electron micrographs demonstrate that mature megakaryocytes have a well-defined marginal zone and that there are only a few channels of the demarcation membrane system in which platelets could be shed from the surface.[27,28] Therefore, during thrombocytopoiesis, the entire megakaryocyte cytoplasm fragments to form platelets.

Ultrastructural features and marker studies on megakaryocytes aid in identification of all stages. Ultrastructural features are the demarcation membrane, alpha (α) granules, and platelet peroxidase activity. Monoclonal antibodies for platelet glycoproteins Ib, IIb, and IIIa; factor VIII antigen; β-thromboglobulin, and factor V are markers for all stages of megakaryocytes.[27,28] In marrow smears of normal individuals, there are approximately 1 to 4 megakaryocytes per 100 nucleated cells, and these cells are in the late stage of maturation.[29] Table 1–13 summarizes the morphological characteristics of the megakaryocytic series.

➤ BONE-DERIVED CELLS

The formation of the bone marrow cavity results from a complex process in which hematopoietic cells migrate and

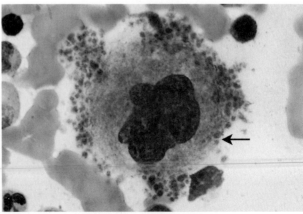

➤ FIGURE 1–53   Megakaryocyte with platelets.

> **Table 1-13**
> ## MORPHOLOGICAL CHARACTERISTICS OF THE MEGAKARYOCYTIC SERIES

	Megakaryoblast	Promegakaryocyte	Megakaryocyte	Thrombocyte
Cell size, μm	20–45	20–80	30–100	1–4
N:C ratio	4:1	4:1–1:1	1:1–1:12	n/a
Nuclear shape	Usually single round, oval, indented or kidney-shaped	Usually single round, oval indented or kidney-shaped	Lobulated (2 or more lobes)	n/a
Nuclear position	Central or eccentric	Central or eccentric	Central	n/a
Nuclear color/chromatin	Red-purple fine chromatin with distinct chromatin	Red-purple increased granularity of nuclear chromatin	Blue-purple, granular	n/a
Nucleoli	1–2	0–1, usually less than megakaryoblast	None	n/a
Color/amount of cytoplasm	Basophilic, pseudopodia frequent/scanty	Basophilic/abundant with pseudopodia	Pale blue with pink cast/abundant	Light blue, fragment of megakaryocyte cytoplasm
Cytoplasmic granules	Nongranular	Fine azurophilic granules	Numerous fine azurophilic granules	Reddish-blue, fine, evenly dispersed

Abbreviation: n/a = not applicable.

colonize spaces originally occupied by cartilage and bone. This process occurs both in the long bones of the limbs and in the membranous bones of the skull, which develop directly into bone. Studies have shown that bone formation and hematopoiesis are closely linked, in that the degree of hematopoiesis correlates with the rate of bone turnover. Two normal, nonhematopoietic cells that exhibit different functions, yet play essential roles in the formation of the bone cavity, are the osteoblast and the osteoclast. The hierarchy of cell maturation in bone-derived cells remains unclear.[26,30]

Osteoblasts

An osteoblast is a large cell that can measure up to 30 μm, with ample cytoplasm and a small, round, eccentrically placed nucleus. These cells may be traumatized in the process of marrow aspiration and smearing and often have irregular shapes and cytoplasmic streamers. The cells may have comet or tadpole shapes. The nucleus may be partially extruded, similar to a small, round head on a round body. The nuclear chromatin strands and nuclear margins are well defined and stain purple-red. Usually there is a distinct blue nucleolus[26] (Fig. 1–55 and Color Plate 51).

Throughout the blue cytoplasm there are small spherical bodies that are colorless and give a bubbly appearance to the cytoplasm. Within the cytoplasm there is a prominent round or oval chromophobic zone that stains lighter than the rest of the cytoplasm. This area is usually away from the nucleus but may be adjacent to it.[26]

Osteoblasts, more often seen in marrow from young children, are responsible for the formation, calcification, and maintenance of trabeculae and cancellous bone. Osteoblasts secrete large amounts of collagen and proteoglycans, contributing to structure of the bone and stromal matrix.[26,30]

Osteoblasts morphologically resemble plasmacytes, both having irregular shapes, eccentric nuclei, cytoplasmic protrusions, blue cytoplasmic fibrils, and vacuoles. The relatively unstained zone of the plasmacyte is adjacent to the nucleus and partially surrounds the nucleus like a collar, whereas the chromophobic zone of the osteoblast is often distinctly separate from the nuclear margin and, when adjacent to the nucleus, does not surround or enclose the nucleus.[26]

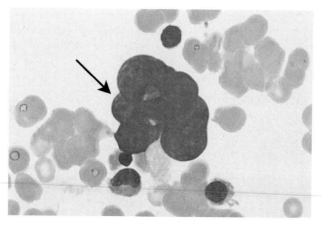

> **FIGURE 1–54** Naked nuclei, megakaryocyte.

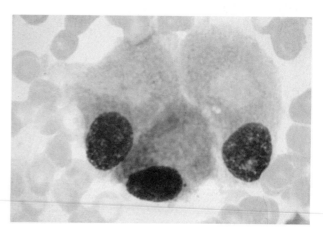

> **FIGURE 1–55** Three osteoblasts.

The protein secretions of the plasmacytes impart a reddish background color to the cells that is not demonstrable in osteoblasts. Osteoblasts that occur in clusters or aggregates may be misinterpreted as malignant cells (Fig. 1–56 and Color Plate 52). Malignant cells in a cluster are crowded and distorted, with indistinct margins, rendering it impossible to identify individual cells. Individual osteoblasts in a cluster can usually be identified. The size, shape, structure, and color of malignant cells are variable, whereas osteoblasts are more orderly and uniform. Chromophobic areas in the cytoplasm of osteoblasts are seldom demonstrable in malignant cells.[26]

It is thought that the mature osteoblast arises from the immature preosteoblast exhibiting mitotic activity. Other theories have placed osteoblast formation at the mesenchymal stem cells residing in the periosteum. It is probable, however, that there exist many intermediate stages in the development of the mature osteoblast as described by studies using monoclonal antibodies specific for bone phenotypes.[26,30]

Osteoclasts

Osteoclasts are giant (greater than 100 μm), multinucleated, irregularly shaped marrow phagocytes that are capable of absorption of bone.[26,30] Osteoclasts have from 2 to 50 nuclei, which are separate, usually round or oval, uniform in size, and haphazardly distributed within the cytoplasm. Osteoclasts have visible nucleoli[26] (Fig. 1–57 and Color Plate 53). Bone-absorbing osteoclasts are found by fusion of precursor cells derived from the monocyte-macrophage lineage.[26–30]

The abundant cytoplasm with ragged margins is bluish, with numerous reddish lysosomal granules containing acid phosphatase. In thin marrow smears it may be possible to demonstrate a ruffled cytoplasmic fringe consisting of diaphanous veils, fingerlike protrusions, and saccular invaginations.[26]

Osteoclasts and megakaryocytes are sometimes difficult to differentiate. Both cells are large with granular cytoplasm, irregular shapes, and multiple nuclei. The nuclei of megakaryocytes are connected by a nuclear strand, have irregular nuclear shapes, and may be superimposed, whereas the nuclei of osteoclasts are separated, uniform in size, and have no visible connections to each other (see Figs. 1–57 and 1–58, and Color Plate 53). The number of nuclei in normal megakaryocytes is even, whereas in osteoclasts it may be uneven. Table 1–14 compares the morphological characteristics of the multinucleated osteoclast and the multilobulated megakaryocyte.[26]

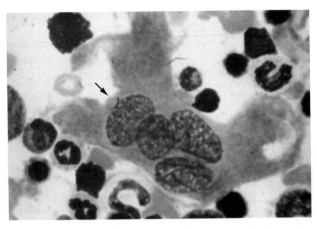

➤ FIGURE 1–57   The osteoclast is usually seen as a single giant cell with multiple and separated nuclei and basophilic granular cytoplasm (center) (magnification ×640).

Osteoclasts secrete enzymes that aid in dissolution of osteoid tissue and calcific bone. Osteoclast-activating factor (OAF), secreted by plasmacytes in myeloma, is a lymphokine that stimulates osteoclastic activity in the endosteum near groups of myeloma cells. The presence of OAF helps to explain the development of osteolytic bone lesions observed in myeloma.[30]

These cells are involved in the degradation (or reabsorption) of bone, which is essential for the formation of the bone marrow cavity and bone remodeling. Osteoclasts are thought to originate from hematopoietic stem cells based on in vivo studies; however, a general consensus to the immediate precursor has not been reached. Theories supporting osteoclasts as arising from the monocytic lineage have been well documented; both cells exhibit phagocytic activities and share common antigenic determinants.[30] In vivo and in vitro studies have demonstrated the fusion of monocytes and macrophages into multinucleated cells resembling osteoclasts, in addition to a growth factor acting in the generation of both cell types.[30] Table 1–15 compares the morphological characteristics of the osteoblast and osteoclast.

➤ MOLECULAR HEMATOLOGY AND ADVANCED CONCEPTS

Introduction to the Cell Cycle

The Generative (G) Cell Cycle Kinetics
When stimulated by hematopoietic growth factors (see the discussion of colony-stimulating factors and interleukins later in this section), hematopoietic cells undergo a continuous generative (G) cycle in which the cells divide, differ-

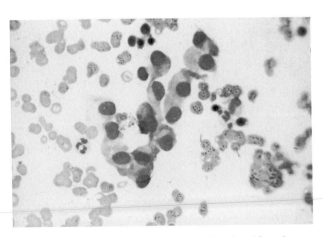

➤ FIGURE 1–56   Group of osteoblasts (center) aspirated from the marrow of a child (magnification ×400).

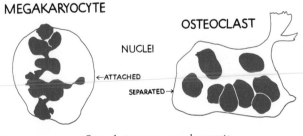

➤ FIGURE 1–58   Osteoclast versus a megakaryocyte.

> ## Table 1-14
> ## MORPHOLOGICAL CHARACTERISTICS OF OSTEOCLASTS AND MEGAKARYOCYTES

	Osteoclast	Megakaryocyte
Size, μm	> 100	30–100
Shape	Irregular	Irregular
Cytoplasm	Granular	Granular
Nuclei	Multiple, uniform in size, unconnected by nuclear strands	Multiple, connected by nuclear strands, not uniform in size
Number of nuclei	Odd number	Even number

entiate, or remain dormant (Fig. 1–59). The bone marrow contains cell populations in all phases of cell development. The generative cell cycle is divided into five phases: G_0, G_1, S, G_2, and M.[2,7] The cells able to proliferate enter a resting or dormant phase (G_0) after division. From the G_0 state the resting cell enters the G_1 phase, which is the postmitotic rest phase and which directly precedes the deoxyribonucleic acid (DNA) synthesis phase. The cell proceeds into the synthesis (S) phase of active DNA synthesis, where the DNA content is doubled. The next phase is the premitotic rest period (G_2) as the cell prepares to enter the mitotic period (M). During the final, or M, phase, there is cellular division of the chromosomes in the nucleus and the cytoplasm, resulting in two daughter cells.[2,7] T_g is the cycle of one complete mitotic division. After final differentiation, the cell leaves the cycle as a nondividing cell (G_{ND}) (see Fig. 1–59).

Specific Cell Line Ontogeny

Multipotential Stem Cells—Colony-Forming Units
The morphology of the recognizable stages of peripheral blood and marrow cells has been described. As stated earlier, these cells come from an unrecognizable pluripotential stem cell. The pluripotential stem cell has the capacity for continuous self-replication and also for differentiation into the multipotential stem cell and the lymphoid stem cell without capacity for self-renewal. The multipotential stem cell becomes committed to support progenitor cells for

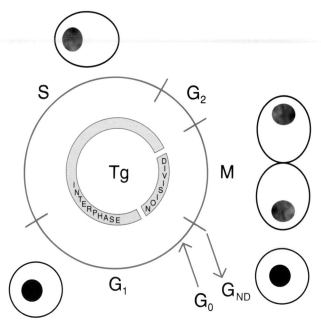

> FIGURE 1–59 Cell cycle kinetics. Tg = one complete mitotic cycle; G_0 = resting or dormant phase; G_1 = postmitotic rest period; S = active DNA synthesis phases; G_2 = premitotic rest period; M = mitotic period; G_{ND} = nondividing cell.

myelopoiesis, erythropoiesis, monopoiesis, and megakaryopoiesis. The lymphoid stem cell line supports lymphopoiesis.[7] The multipotential stem cell was shown to exist in a classic experiment in 1961 by Till and McCullock,[21] who irradiated mice to empty the hematopoietic organs and then injected a suspension of marrow cells intravenously. About a week later, nodules of injected marrow could be observed on the cut surface of the spleen colonies. All cell lines found in normal marrow were generated from the multipotential stem cells in the marrow suspension. The multipotential stem cell giving rise to several cell lines was called the colony-forming unit–granulocyte-erythrocyte-monocyte-macrophage-megakaryocyte (CFU-GEMM).[2,7]

The CFU-GEMM in a colony assay forms a series of progenitor cells (CFU-GM, CFU-Eo, CFU-Bas, CFU-Meg, BFU-E, CFU-E) under appropriate growth conditions (see Table 1–16 for acronyms). CFU-GM makes colonies of granulocytes and monocytes and/or macrophages. CFU-Eo forms colonies of eosinophils. CFU-Bas makes early ba-

> ## Table 1-15
> ## MORPHOLOGICAL CHARACTERISTICS OF OSTEOBLASTS AND OSTEOCLASTS

	Osteoblast	Osteoclast
Size, μm	Up to 30	> 100
Nuclei	Round, eccentric, uninuclear	Multinucleated, uniform size
Nucleolus	Present	Present
Cytoplasm	Chromophobic area, usually away from nucleus	Bluish, reddish lysosomal granules, cytoplasmic protrusions
Shape	Resemble plasmacytes	May be confused with megakaryocytes

> ## Table 1-16
> ## HEMATOPOIETIC PROGENITOR CELLS

Abbreviation	Full Name
CFU-GEMM	Colony-forming unit–granulocyte, erythrocyte, macrophage-monocyte, megakaryocyte
CFU-GM	Colony-forming unit–granulocyte, macrophage-monocyte
CFU-Eo	Colony-forming unit–eosinophil
CFU-Bas	Colony-forming unit–basophil
CFU-Meg	Colony-forming unit–megakaryocyte
BFU-E	Burst-forming unit–erythrocyte
CFU-E	Colony-forming unit–erythrocyte

sophils and mast cells. CFU-Meg forms megakaryocyte colonies. There are two colonies of erythroid progenitor cells: the early burst-forming unit–erythroid (BFU-E) and the more mature colony-forming unit–erythroid (CFU-E).

The lymphoid stem cell is also derived from the pluripotential stem cell. The lymphoid stem cell has the potential to differentiate into a T or B cell. T cells participate in immune functions of a cellular nature, either directly cytotoxic, or helping or suppressing immune activities through interaction with other immunocompetent cells. B cells differentiate into plasmacytes, which secrete specific immunoglobulins important in the host's defense against infection. Another population of lymphocytes, called null cells, has none of the characteristics of either the T or the B cells. The null cell category includes killer (K) cells, which interact with antibody to cause destruction of antibody-coated targets, and natural killer (NK) cells, which can lyse target cells through direct cytotoxic activity. Their differentiation is uncertain.[1] Table 1–17 lists the different types of lymphocytes and their functions.

Colony-Stimulating Factors and Interleukins

Each cell line is dependent on cytokines, which are soluble mediators secreted by cells for the purpose of cell-to-cell communication. Table 1–18 lists the different cell types and the cytokines they produce. Table 1–19 lists the characteristics of cytokines. Cytokines act on multipotential stem cells to stimulate their proliferation and differentiation to committed cell lines (Fig. 1–60 and Color Plate 8). For a cell to develop from a multipotential cell to a myeloblast, monoblast, erythroblast, or megakaryoblast, cytokines are necessary. Colony-stimulating factors (CSFs) or growth factors and interleukins (ILs) are two types of cytokines. Table 1–20 summarizes the cytokines involved in hematopoietic blood cell development, listing their sources and the target cells that they stimulate.

CSFs and interleukins regulate blood cell development by mediating proliferation, differentiation, and maturation of hematopoietic progenitor cells (see Fig. 1–60 and Color Plate 8).

➤ TRENDS IN THERAPEUTIC MANIPULATION OF HEMATOPOIESIS

Recombinant Cytokines

Many growth factors have been isolated, biochemically characterized, purified, genetically cloned, and produced through recombinant DNA technology.[22–28] During the past 10 years, growth factors G-CSF, GM-CSF, Epo, and

➤ Table 1-18
CELLULAR CYTOKINE PRODUCTION

Cell Type	Cytokine*
Endothelial cell	GM-CSF, G-CSF, M-CSF, IL-6
Monocyte-macrophage	GM-CSF, G-CSF, M-CSF, IL-3, IL-6, EPO, SCF
T cell	GM-CSF, IL-2, IL-3, IL-4, IL-5
Fibroblasts	GM-CSF, G-CSF, M-CSF, IL-6, SCF
NK cells	GM-CSF
Osteoblasts	IL-6, GM-CSF
PMN	G-CSF, GM-CSF
B cells	GM-CSF, M-CSF, IL-2, IL-5, IL-6
Marrow stroma	GM-CSF, G-CSF, M-CSF, IL-6, IL-3, SCF, IL-11
Renal parenchyma, liver, and marrow cells	EPO

*mRNA, protein, or specific biologic activity detected at baseline levels or immediately after induction.

the interleukins have been used for preclinical study and for clinical application.[26–28] In vivo, the regulation of hematopoiesis is under the control of cytokine production in the basal state, maintaining normal blood counts and the antigen stimulus state, eliciting cytokine stimuli above the basal state to combat infection. CSFs have been used to strengthen patients with cancer and acquired immunodeficiency syndrome (AIDS) and to guard against infection in bone marrow transplantation recipients. These factors have also been used to treat patients with anemia caused by either surgery or kidney failure. The blood counts of autologous donors can be raised for donation before surgical procedures. Interleukins are used clinically for wound healing, activating lymphocytes, and assisting in the growth of transplanted or damaged bone marrow.[29–31]

Clinical Trials of Recombinant Cytokines

Clinical trials of recombinant cytokines using biologic substances similar to those in the human body have provided new opportunities for evaluating their clinical usefulness in the treatment of hematologic and oncologic disorders.[29,30] Investigations have shown that recombinant human granu-

➤ Table 1-17
FUNCTIONS OF LYMPHOCYTES

Lymphocyte	Function
T cells	Cell-mediated immunity
B cell	Humoral immunity
Null cells (killer)	Antibody-dependent cell-mediated lysis
Natural killer (NK) cells	Direct cytotoxic activity

➤ Table 1-19
CYTOKINE CHARACTERISTICS

Glycoproteins

Produced by many cell types

Usually act on multiple cell lineages

Interact synergistically with one another

Activate receptors at very low concentrations

Usually act on the neoplastic counterpart of normal target cells

Usually act throughout the maturation hierarchy from stem cell to the terminally differentiated cell

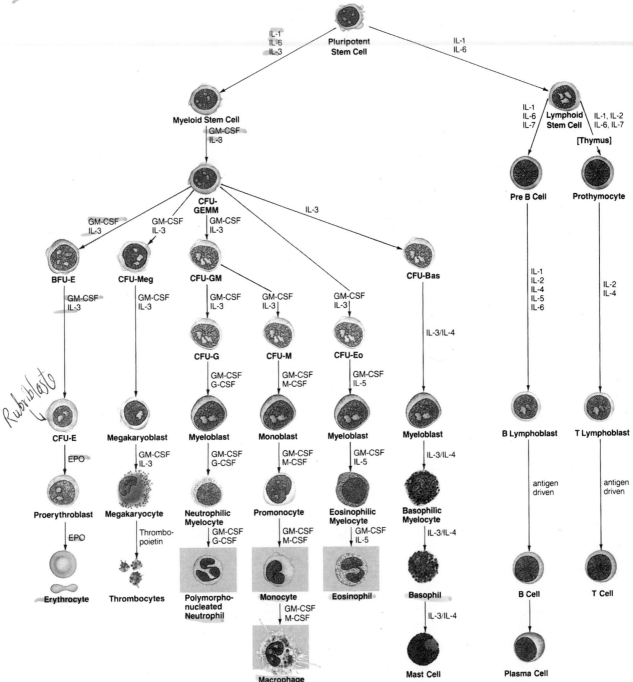

➤ **FIGURE 1–60**   Regulation of hematopoiesis by cytokines. BFU-E = burst-forming unit–erythroid; CFU-Bas = colony-forming unit–basophil; CFU-E = colony-forming unit–erythroid; CFU-Eo = colony-forming unit–eosinophil; CFU-G = colony-forming unit–granulocyte; CFU-GEMM = colony-forming unit–granulocyte, erythroid, monocyte macrophage, megakaryocyte; CFU-M = colony-forming unit–monocyte; CFU-Meg = colony-forming unit–megakaryocyte; EPO = erythropoietin; G-CSF = granulocyte colony-stimulating factor; GM-CSF = granulocyte-monocyte-macrophage–colony stimulating factor; M-CSF = monocyte–colony-stimulating factor; Meg-CSF = megakaryocyte–colony-stimulating factor. (Reprinted from Sandoz Pharmaceuticals Corporation and Schering-Plough, with permission.)

locyte CSF (rHuG-CSF) accelerates recovery from neutropenia induced by myelotoxic chemotherapy for different types of carcinoma.[32] RHuG-CSF has been given to patients receiving myelosuppressive chemotherapy and undergoing autologous bone marrow transplantation to accelerate the rate of neutrophil recovery.[7,33] Clinical trials are being conducted to determine whether rHuG-CSF is effective in correcting severe neutropenia in hematopoietic malignancies, such as hairy-cell leukemia, and also in non-

neoplastic hematopoietic diseases, such as aplastic anemia and cyclic neutropenia.[7,29,30]

Recombinant human GM-CSF appears to offer useful therapy with graft failure after bone marrow transplantation.[7,29] Hematopoietic growth factors can be combined with chemotherapy in treating both patients with advanced malignancies and bone marrow transplantation patients by increasing production of granulocytes and platelets.[23,24] Cytokines can augment mechanisms of host defense in pa-

> **Table 1-20**

CYTOKINES INVOLVED IN HEMATOPOIETIC BLOOD CELL DEVELOPMENT

	Synonym	Source	Target	Gene Location
GROWTH FACTORS				
Epo	Erythropoietin	Kidney, liver	Erythroid progenitors	7q
G-CSF	Granulocyte colony-stimulating factor	Macrophages, endothelial cells, fibroblasts	Stem cells, neutrophil precursors	17q
GM-CSF	Granulocyte-macrophage–colony-stimulating factor	T lymphocytes, macrophages, endothelial cells, fibroblasts	Progenitors for neutrophils, eosinophils, monocytes	5q
M-CSF	CSF-1, Monocyte-macrophage CSF	Endothelial cells, fibroblasts, B cells, monocytes-macrophages, stromal cells	Mononuclear phagocytes	5q
SCF	Stem cell factor, c-kit ligand	Fibroblasts	Stem cells	12q
INTERLEUKINS				
IL-1	Hematopoietic-1; response modulator	Macrophages, fibroblasts, endothelial cells	Mononuclear phagocytes progenitor cells	2q
IL-2	T-cell growth factor	T lymphocytes, macrophages	T cells, B cells	4q
IL-3	Multi-CSF	T lymphocytes	Precursors of neutrophils, platelets, monocytes, eosinophils, basophils, stem cells	5q
IL-4	B-cell stimulatory factor I	T lymphocytes	B cells, mast cells, T cells	5q
IL-5	B-cell growth factor II, eosinophil differentiation factor	T lymphocytes	B cells, eosinophils	5q
IL-6	Interferon β hybridoma growth factor	T lymphocytes, macrophages	Stem cells, B cells	7p
IL-7	Lymphopoietin-1	Stromal cells	Pre-B cells, T cells, early granulocytes	8q
IL-8	Granulocyte chemotactic factor	Monocytes, T cells, fibroblasts	Neutrophils, T cells, basophils	4q
IL-9	T-cell growth factor III	T cells	BFU-E, T cells, mast cells	5q
IL-10	Cytokine synthesis inhibitory factor	T cells, macrophages, B cells	B cells, macrophage, T cells, mast cells	1q
IL-11	Adipogenesis inhibitory factor	Stromal, fibroblasts	Megakaryocyte, B cells, mast cells	19q
IL-12	NK cell stimulatory factor	B cells, macrophages	T cells, NK cells	Not reported
IL-13	IL-13	T cells	B cells	5q
IL-14	High-molecular-weight B-cell growth factor	T cells	Activated B cells	Not reported

Abbreviations: BFU-E = burst-forming unit–erythroid; NK = natural killer cell.

tients with AIDS.[23,24] GM-CSF has been evaluated in HIV-infected (AIDS) patients and has been shown to increase the leukocyte count and to be effective when combined with antiretroviral agents such as AZT (azidothymidine or zidovudine, also Retrovir).[24,25]

IL-3, together with M-CSF, stimulates myelocytes, erythrocytes, and platelet production in aplastic anemia, myelodysplastic syndrome, and prolonged chemotherapy for malignancy.[34] Among patients with chronic anemia caused by renal failure, treatment with recombinant human erythropoietin (rHuEPO) has increased RBC production and alleviated anemia in more than 97% of patients.[23,24,31]

The rise in hematocrit is dose-dependent and is in proportion to the increase in RBC mass.[7,31] Clinical studies using stem cell factor (SCF) combined with other cytokines are now ongoing in patients with stage IV breast cancer and non–small cell lung cancer.[35] SCF produced from marrow fibroblasts acts on the hematopoietic stem cells, increasing the proliferation and differentiation to the committed cell lineages. In addition, SCF added to long-term cell culturing extends the growth period of a diverse population of cells.[35]

Clinical trials using other synthesized cytokines are currently in progress to determine activity in controlling hematopoiesis. Each factor needs to be purified and its function determined before the interactions between hematopoietic growth factors in the marrow microenvironment can be completely understood.

CD Nomenclature

The classification of cell surface antigens on hematopoietic cells has been aided by the development of monoclonal antibody technology. The rapid production of monoclonal antibodies and the development of multiple commercial sources under a variety of trade names and designations led to the development of a standardized nomenclature for human leukocyte differentiation antigens termed the *cluster designation (CD) nomenclature*. In 1989, at a series of international workshops on human leukocyte differentiation antigens sponsored by the World Health Organization, monoclonal antibodies having similar reactive patterns with tissue, cells, or molecules were assigned to a "cluster" and given a "cluster designation" (CD) number. CD numbers with a "w" indicate a provisional cluster that may or may not be promoted to full CD status at subsequent workshops. More than 160 CD antigens have been classified by the Seventh International Workshop on Leukocyte Typing held in Harrogate, England, in 2000.[36]

With the exception of lymphocytes, the current CD anti-gens for each cell lineage as determined by the Fifth International Workshop on Leukocyte Typing are given in Table 1–21. Table 1–22 lists the lymphocyte surface markers currently available.[36]

Clinical Applications of Cell Surface Markers

The use of monoclonal antibodies specific to cell surface markers (CDs) allows phenotypic characterization of cells in disease states. By using flow cytometry (see Chap. 30), cells labeled with monoclonal antibodies are sorted and enumerated to identify a specific population of cells.

Certain cell markers have been identified as being present on the cell surface in disease states such as the acute leukemias, autoimmune disease, and thromboembolytic disease. Cell markers have also been identified in the management of renal, cardiac, and bone marrow transplantation. Although diagnosis of disease states is dependent on clinical presentation, cytochemistry, and examination of morphology, flow-cytometry characterization of cells has added another dimension to disease classification. Monoclonal antibodies are used to characterize cells in the acute leukemias. Such markers allow for the differentiation of myeloblasts, lymphoblasts, monoblasts, megakaryoblasts, and erythroid ontogeny.

> **Table 1-21**
CD CELL MARKERS OF THE PROGENITOR, GRANULOCYTIC, MONOCYTIC, MEGAKARYOCYTIC, AND ERYTHROCYTIC CELL LINES

Progenitor	Myelocytes	Eosinophils	Basophils	Monocytes	Megakaryocytes	Erythrocytes
CD33	CD10	CD4*	CD9	CD4	CD9	CD35
CD34	CD11a,b,c	CD9	CD11a,b,c	CD9	CDw12	CD36†
CD38	CDw12	CD11a,b,c	CDw12	CD11,a,b,c	CD13	CD44
CD40	CD13	CDw12	CD13	CDw12	CD17	CD47
CD43	CD14	CD13	CDw17	CD13	CD23b	CD55
CD46	CD15	CD18	CD18	CD14	CD31	CD59
CD47	CD16	CD23b	CD24	CD15	CD36	CD71
CD54	CD17	CD24	CD29	CD16	CD41	CD75
CD59	CD18	CD29	CDw32	CD17	CD42	CD147
CD87	CD24	CD43	CD43	CD23b	CD43	
CD116	CD31	CD44	CD44	CD24	CD44	
CD117	CD32a,c	CD45	CD45	CD25	CD46	
CD119	CD33	CD46	CD46	CD28	CD47	
CD120a	CD35	CD47	CD47	CD31	CD51	
CD123	CD38	CD48	CD48	CD32	CD53	
CD124	CD43	CD49d	CD50	CD33	CD59	
CD126	CD44	CD50	CD52	CD35	CD60	
CD127	CD45	CD52	CD53	CD36	CD61	
CD135	CD45RO	CD53	CD55	CD37	CD62P	
CD155	CD45RA	CD58	CD58	CD38	CD63	
	CD45RB	CD59	CD59	CD39	CD69	
	CD46	CD69	CD69	CD40	CD84	
	CD47	CD89	CD89	CD43	CD87	
			CD92			

continued

CD CELL MARKERS OF THE PROGENITOR, GRANULOCYTIC, MONOCYTIC, MEGAKARYOCYTIC, AND ERYTHROCYTIC CELL LINES (Continued)

Progenitor	Myelocytes	Eosinophilis	Basophils	Monocytes	Megakaryocytes	Erythrocytes
	CD48	CD92	CD93	CD44	CD107	
	CD49d	CD93	CD97	CD45RO	CD109	
	CD50	CD98	CD98	CD45RA	CD120a	
	CD52	CD101*	CD99	CD45RB	CD141	
	CD53	CD116	CD101*	CD46	CD147	
	CD58	CD125	CD116	CD47	CD148	
	CD59	CD132	CD125	CD49a,d,e,f	CDw149	
	CD62L	CD147	CD128	CD50	CD151	
	CD65s	CD148	CD132	CD51	CD165	
	CD66f	CD156	CD147	CD53		
	CD68	CD157	CD148	CD54		
	CD69	CD162	CD156	CD55		
	CD88	CD164	CD157	CD58		
	CD89		CD162	CD59		
	CD92		CD164	CD60		
	CD93			CD62L,P		
	CD97			CD64		
	CD98			CD65s		
	CD101*			CD68		
	CD108			CD74		
	CD114			CD80		
	CD116			CD81		
	CD119			CD84		
	CD120a			CD87		
	CDw131			CD91		
	CD132			CD92		
	CDw136			CD97		
	CD139			CD98		
	CD141			CD93		
	CD147			CD101		
	CD148			CD102		
	CDw149			CD114		
	CD157			CD115		
	CD156			CD116		
	CD162			CD120a		
	CD164			CD122		
				CD123		
				CD127		
				CD132		
				CD136		
				CD139		
				CD142*		
				CD147		
				CD148		
				CDw149		
				CD155		
				CD156		
				CD157		
				CD161		

*Activated cells.
†Reticulocytes only.

> ➤ **Table 1-22**
> **CD CELL MARKERS OF THE LYMPHOCYTIC AND PLASMACYTIC CELL LINES**

B Cells		Plasma Cells	T Cells		Natural Killer Cells
CD1	CD71*	CD28	CD2	CD71*	CD2
CD5†	CD72	CD85	CD2R*	CD73	CD2R
CD10	CD73	CD138	CD3	CD81	CD5
CD11a,c	CD74		CD4	CD82	CD7
CD14	CD75*		CD5	CD87*	CD8
CD18	CD76		CD6	CD89	CD11b,c/18
CD19	CD77*		CD7	CD90	CD16
CD20	CD78*		CD8	CD95*	CD23b
CD21	CD79a,b		CD9*	CD96	CD25*
CD22	CD80*		CD11a/18	CD97*	CD27
CD23a	CD81		CD25*	CD98	CD28
CD24	CD82		CD26	CD99	CD29
CD25*	CD84		CD27	CD100*	CD38
CD26	CD85		CD28	CD101	CD39*
CD27	CD86		CD29	CD102	CD43
CD29	CD89		CD30*	CD109*	CD45RC
CD30*	CD95*		CD35	CD120a	CD46
CD32b	CD97*		CD38	CD122	CD47
CD35	CD98		CD39*	CD124	CD48
CD37	CD99		CD43	CD128	CD49d
CD38	CD100*		CD44	CD129	CD50
CD39*	CD102		CD45	CD132	CD56
CD40	CD120a		CD45RC	CD134*	CD57
CD44	CD122		CD46	CDw137*	CD58
CD45RC	CD123		CD47	CD146*	CD71
CD46	CD124		CD48	CD147	CD81
CD47	CDw125		CD49a,b,e,f	CD148	CD94
CD48	CD128		CD50	CDw149	CD96
CD49b,c,d	CDw131		CD52	CDw150	CD97
CD50	CD132		CD53	CD152*	CD98
CD51	CD135		CD56*	CD153*	CD99
CD52	CD139		CD58	CD154	CD102
CD53	CD147		CD60	CD158a	CD122
CD58	CDw149		CD63	CD161	CDw149
CD63	CDw150		CD68	CD162	CD158a,b
CD68			CD69*	CD164	CD161
CD69*			CD70*	CD165	CD165
CD70*				CD166*	

*Activated cells.
†B-CLL.

QUESTIONS

1. Which organ(s) is (are) the primary site(s) for hematopoiesis in the fetus?
   a. Liver
   b. Spleen
   c. Bone marrow
   d. All of the above

2. Which listing represents the proper cell sequence of erythropoiesis?
   a. Rubriblast, prorubricyte, rubricyte, metarubricyte, reticulocyte, erythrocyte
   b. Rubriblast, rubricyte, prorubricyte, metarubricyte, reticulocyte, erythrocyte
   c. Rubriblast, prorubricyte, metarubricyte, rubricyte, reticulocyte, erythrocyte
   d. Rubriblast, reticulocyte, prorubricyte, rubricyte, metarubricyte, erythrocyte

3. What is the best description of a metarubricyte?
   a. Solid, blue-black degenerated nucleus with nonlinear clumped chromatin pattern; no nucleoli; pink cytoplasm
   b. Round nucleus with visible nucleoli; indistinct and dispersed chromatin; blue cytoplasm
   c. Coarse chromatin; ill-defined or absent nucleoli; predominantly blue cytoplasm with pink tinge
   d. Small nucleus; thick and condensed nuclear chromatin; no nucleoli; mixture of pink and blue cytoplasm

4. What is the sequence for the maturation pools of granulocyte production?
   a. Maturation, proliferation, storage, functional (or marginated) pool
   b. Proliferation, maturation, storage, functional (or marginated) pool
   c. Storage, maturation, proliferation, functional (or marginated) pool
   d. Functional (or marginated) pool, storage, proliferation, maturation

5. Which listing represents the proper cell sequence of granulocytopoiesis?
   a. Myeloblast, myelocyte, promyelocyte, metamyelocyte, band, segmented cell
   b. Myeloblast, metamyelocyte, myelocyte, promyelocyte, segmented cell, band
   c. Myeloblast, promyelocyte, myelocyte, metamyelocyte, band, segmented cell
   d. Myeloblast, band, promyelocyte, myelocyte, metamyelocyte, segmented cell

6. Which granulocytic cell has a kidney-shaped nucleus with clumped chromatin and small, pink, secondary granules with a few primary dark granules?
   a. Band
   b. Myelocyte
   c. Promyelocyte
   d. Metamyelocyte

7. Which granulocytic cell has large, abundant violet-blue or purple-black granules?
   a. Eosinophil
   b. Basophil
   c. Neutrophil

8. What is the proper cell sequence for the monocyte-macrophage phagocytic system?
   a. Monoblast, macrophage, promonocyte, monocyte
   b. Monoblast, monocyte, promonocyte, macrophage
   c. Monoblast, promonocyte, monocyte, macrophage
   d. Monoblast, promonocyte, macrophage, monocyte

9. Which cell classification is described by the following statements: second most numerous cell in the blood; usually small and round; intensely blue cytoplasm; and nucleus with clumped dark purple chromatin?
   a. Monocyte
   b. Lymphocyte
   c. Null cell
   d. Plasmacyte

10. What is the average blood volume?
    a. 5 to 6 L
    b. 4 to 6 L
    c. 6 to 7 L
    d. 3 to 5 L

11. Which of the following is a plasma protein?
    a. Fibrinogen
    b. Globulin
    c. Albumin
    d. All of the above

12. What percent of the blood volume represents the formed elements?
    a. 55%
    b. 50%
    c. 60%
    d. 45%

SUMMARY CHART

➤ Blood is composed of 55% plasma, the liquid portion, and 45% cells, the formed elements (RBCs, WBCs, and platelets).

➤ The average blood volume in an adult is 4 to 6 L.

➤ Plasma contains mainly water (91.5%), proteins (7%), other solutes (1.5%).

➤ The plasma proteins are albumin, globulin, and fibrinogen.

➤ Erythrocyte morphology is evaluated in the thin area of every stained smear where red cells are evenly distributed, do not overlap, and are close together.

➤ Platelets should be evaluated in the same thin area of every stained blood smear where red cells are described by counting the number of platelets in 10 or more oil immersion fields. The normal finding is 7 to15 platelets per oil immersion field.

➤ Blood smears should be well made and well stained in order to properly differentiate leukocytes, platelets, and erythrocytes.

➤ Normal neutrophil segmented cells contain from two to five lobes (usually three) connected by a threadlike filament(s) and constitute 50% to 70% of mature neutrophils in an adult.

➤ Normal neutrophil band cells have a horseshoe-shaped nucleus without evidence of a filament and make up only 2% to 6% of the blood cells in an adult.

➤ Normal eosinophil granules are large, round, and stain orange to reddish-orange; eosinophils are found in 0 to 4% of the blood cells in an adult.

➤ The majority of lymphocytes on an adult blood smear are small, have a relatively round nucleus with clumped chromatin and a small amount of pale blue cytoplasm; lymphocytes comprise 20% to 44% of the blood cells in an adult.

➤ A monocyte is larger than the mature neutrophil; has abundant gray blue cytoplasm with fine, reddish or purplish, evenly distributed granules; and has a nucleus with folds or brain-like convolutions, and lacy, often delicate, chromatin. Monocytes comprise 2% to 9% of blood cells in an adult.

➤ Large lymphocytes may reveal a few well-defined purplish-red granules that can be easily counted, whereas numerous fine indistinct granules that cannot be enumerated are present in a monocyte.

➤ Hematopoiesis is defined as the dynamic processes of production and development of the various blood and marrow cells.

➤ Hematopoiesis begins in the mesoderm of the yolk sac and, after 2 months, migrates to the liver and spleen, where it remains until the seventh month, before finally shifting to the bone marrow, which becomes the major site of blood cell development in the fetus and after birth.

➤ Erythropoiesis identifies the entire process by which erythrocytes are produced in the marrow and develop from rubriblasts to diffusely basophilic cells and finally into a mature erythrocyte.

➤ Myelopoiesis refers to the production, proliferation, differentiation, division, storage, and delivery to the blood of neutrophils, eosinophils, basophils, and monocytes.

➤ A rubriblast differs little from a myeloblast: both have a round primitive nucleus, visible nucleoli, and chromatin strands that are distinct and dispersed; however, the rubriblast is slightly larger than a myeloblast and has more cytoplasm, which stains a deeper blue.

➤ A metarubricyte is recognized by the solid, blue-black, degenerated nucleus with nonlinear clumped chromatin and cytoplasm that is predominately pinkish because of increasing hemoglobin synthesis; however, there may remain a minimal amount of bluish cytoplasm owing to RNA.

➤ A promyelocyte has dark blue granules throughout the cytoplasm and sometimes lying over the nucleus, a large nucleus with slightly condensed chromatin, and often faintly visible nucleoli.

➤ A neutrophilic myelocyte is identified by a round or oval nucleus with condensed and unevenly stained chromatin strands and secondary pinkish-staining (neutrophilic) granules.

➤ A neutrophilic metamyelocyte has a bean-shaped nucleus with the indentation less than half the width of the arbitrary round nucleus, noticeable chromatin clumping, and cytoplasm filled with pinkish (neutrophilic) secondary granules.

➤ Lymphoblasts contain a large, round nucleus with thin, evenly stained, nonclumped chromatin strands; one or more nucleoli; and a small amount of blue cytoplasm.

➤ Monoblasts are large and demonstrate a large nucleus (sometimes minimally indented), one or two prominent nucleoli, fine lacy nuclear chromatin, and nongranular, often deep blue cytoplasm.

➤ Plasmacytes are characterized by an eccentrically placed, round, small nucleus with lumpy chromatin; nongranular deep or vibrant blue cytoplasm; perinuclear clear area; occasional vacuoles; and slightly irregular margins.

➤ The mature megakaryocyte, the largest of the hematopoietic cells (range is 30 to 100 μm) in the bone marrow, has a multilobulated nucleus with coarse linear chromatin and bluish cytoplasm, containing numerous small, dense, reddish-blue granules, which fragment to form platelets.

References

1. Perkins, SL: Examination of the blood and bone marrow. In Lee, GR, et al (eds): Wintrobe's Clinical Hematology, ed 10. Lea & Febiger, Philadelphia, 1998, pp 9–10, 19–22, 27.
2. Telen, MJ, and Kaufman, RE: The mature erythrocyte. In Lea, GR, et al (eds): Wintrobe's Clinical Hematology, ed 10. Lea & Febiger, Philadelphia, 1998, pp 193–198.
3. Williams, WJ, Morris, MW, and Nelson, DA: Examination of the blood. In Beutler, E, et al (eds): Williams' Hematology, ed 5. McGraw-Hill, New York, 1995, pp 10–14.
4. Diggs, LW, et al: The Morphology of Human Blood Cells, ed 5. Abbott Laboratories, Abbott Park, IL, 1985, pp 1–18, 25–27.
5. Bondurant, MC, and Koury, MJ: Origin and development of blood cells. In Lee, GR, et al (eds): Wintrobe's Clinical Hematology, ed 10. Lea & Febiger, Philadelphia, 1998, pp 145–148, 152–153.
6. Jandl, JH: Blood: Textbook of Hematology, ed 2. Little Brown, Boston, 1996, p 55.
7. Jandl, JH: Blood: Textbook of Hematology, ed 2. Little Brown, Boston, 1996, pp 615–620, 622–623.
8. Skulbitz, KM: Neutrophilic leukocytes. In Lee GR, et al (eds): Wintrobe's Clinical Hematology, ed 10. Lea & Febiger, Philadelphia, 1998, pp 301–318.
9. Moqbel, R, and Becker, AG: The human eosinophil. In Lee GR, et al (eds): Wintrobe's Clinical Hematology, ed 10. Lea & Febiger, Philadelphia, 1998, pp 351–352.

10. Befus, AD, and Denburg, JA: Basophilic leukocytes, mast cells and basophils. In Lee GR, et al (eds): Wintrobe's Clinical Hematology, ed 10. Lea & Febiger, Philadelphia, 1998, pp 362–365.

11. Paraskevas, F, and Foerster, J: The lymphatic system. In Lee GR, et al (eds): Wintrobe's Clinical Hematology, ed 10. Lea & Febiger, Philadelphia, 1998, pp 430–432, 436–438.

12. Jandl JH: Monocytes and macrophages. In Blood: Textbook of Hematology, ed 2. Little Brown, Boston, 1996, pp 651–656.

13. Koury, M, and Bondurant, M: News Physiol Sci 8:1993, pp. 170–174.

14. Hillman, RS, and Finch, CA: Red Cell Manual, ed 7. FA Davis, Philadelphia, 1996, p. 2.

15. Erslev, AJ, and Gabuzda, TG: Pathophysiology of Blood, ed 3. WB Saunders, Philadelphia, 1995.

16. Jandl, JH: Blood: Textbook of Hematology, ed 2. Little Brown, Boston, 1996, pp 30–32, 55.

17. Dessypris, EN: Erythropoiesis. In Lee, GR, et al (eds): Wintrobe's Clinical Hematology, ed 10. Lea & Febiger, Philadelphia, 1998, pp 169–177.

18. Bull, BS, and Breton-Gorius, J: The morphology of the erythron. In Beutler, E, et al (eds): Williams' Hematology, ed 5. McGraw-Hill, New York, 1995, pp 349–355.

19. Diggs, LW, et al: The morphology of Human Blood Cells, ed 5. Abbott Laboratories, Abbott Park, IL, 1985, pp 23–24, 33–35.

20. Williams, WJ, and Nelson, DA: Examination of the marrow. In Beutler E, et al (eds): Williams' Hematology, ed 5. McGraw-Hill, New York, 1995, pp 19–20.

21. Lisiewicz, J, and Bick, RL: Morphology and biochemistry of the myeloid series. In Bick RL, et al (eds): Hematology: Clinical and Laboratory Practice. Mosby, St. Louis, 1993, pp 1053–1057.

22. Diggs, LW, and Shibata, S: Ferrata cells. Tissue neutrophils, not artifacts. Lab Med 14:50, 1970.

23. Diggs, LW, et al: The Morphology of Human Blood Cells. Abbott Laboratories, Abbott Park, IL, 1985, pp 40–46.

24. Weinberg JB: Mononuclear phagocytes. In Lee, GR, et al (eds): Wintrobe's Clinical Hematology, ed 10. Lea & Febiger, Philadelphia, 1998, pp 377–383, 392.

25. Douglas, SD, and Wen-Zhe, HO: Morphology and monocytes and macrophages. In Beutler, E, et al (eds): Williams' Hematology, ed 5. McGraw-Hill, New York, 1985, pp 861–862, 864–865.

26. Diggs, LW, et al: The Morphology of Human Blood Cell, ed 5. Abbott Laboratories, Abbott Park, IL, 1985, pp 33–34, 48–50, 85.

27. Stenberg, PE, and Hill, RJ: Platelets and megakaryocytes. In Lee GR, et al (eds): Wintrobe's Clinical Hematology, ed 10. Lea & Febiger, Philadelphia, 1998, pp 616–617, 628–633.

28. Burstein, AS, and Breton-Gorius: Megakaryopoiesis and platelet formation. In Beutler, E, et al (eds): Williams' Hematology, ed 5. McGraw-Hill, New York, 1995, pp 349–355.

29. Jandl, JH: Blood: Textbook of Hematology, ed 2. Little Brown, Boston, 1996, pp 1301–1304.

30. Jandl, JH: Blood: Textbook of Hematology, ed 2. Little Brown & Co, Boston, 1996, pp 47–48.

31. Lappin, TRJ, and Rich, IN: Erythropoietin—the first 90 years. Clin Lab Hematol 18:137, 1996.

32. Takeyama, H, et al: In vitro growth and clinical response of leukemia cells to macrophage colony-stimulating factor (M-CSF) and granulocyte colony-stimulating factor (G-CSF) in acute leukemia. Gan To Kagaku Ryoho 27:873, 2000.

33. Gorin, NC: Acute myeloid leukemia: Autologous stem cell transplantation in acute myelocytic leukemia. American Society of Hematology Education Program, 1999, pp 119–137.

34. Rowe, JM: Concurrent use of growth factors and chemotherapy in acute leukemia. Curr Opin Hematol 7:197–202, 2000.

35. Ashman, LK: The biology of stem cell factor and its receptor C-kit. Int J Biochem Cell Biol 31:1037, 1999.

36. Seventh International Workshop on Leukocyte Typing, Harrogate, England, 6/20–6/24, 2000.

2 Bone Marrow

AAMIR EHSAN, MD

OBJECTIVES

At the end of this chapter, the learner should be able to:

1. Understand the process of hematopoiesis.
2. List indications for bone marrow studies.
3. Name the most common skeletal sites for hematologic studies.
4. Explain the role of the medical technologist during a bone marrow procedure.
5. Describe the preparation of bone marrow aspirate for laboratory examination.
6. Explain the effective use of different bone marrow preparations and specimen distribution.
7. List complications and contraindications of the bone marrow procedure.
8. Explain how to calculate the myeloid-to-erythroid (M:E) cell ratio.
9. Understand the difference between bone marrow aspirate and biopsy.
10. Explain how to estimate the bone marrow cellularity.
11. List the essential components of a bone marrow report.

The hematopoietic system consists of the bone marrow, liver, spleen, lymph nodes, and thymus. Hematopoiesis (blood cell production and maturation) can be seen at different anatomic locations (yolk sac, liver, spleen, axial and radial bones), depending on the gestational and postnatal period. In normal adults, hematopoiesis is seen mainly in the bone marrow. The bone marrow–derived pluripotential hematopoietic stem cells, under the influence of various cytokines or growth factors, or both, differentiate into myeloid (granulocytes, monocytes and megakaryocytes) erythroid and lymphoid cell lineages. Benign and malignant diseases related to these cells are called *hematolymphoid disorders*. Nonhematolymphoid diseases may also involve the bone marrow; therefore, examination of the bone marrow has a wide application in clinical medicine.

Because hematologic diseases involving the bone marrow can result in morphological abnormalities of the peripheral blood cells, the bone marrow examination should be interpreted in conjunction with a peripheral smear examination. Severe thrombocytopenia is generally not a contraindication to the procedure. In experienced hands and with the needles currently available, the bone marrow aspiration and biopsy carries minimal risk.

▶ BONE MARROW STRUCTURE

The bone marrow is one of the body's largest organs, representing 3.4 to 6 percent of total body weight and averaging about 1500 grams in adults.[1] The hematopoietic marrow is organized around the bone vasculature.[2,3] An artery entering the bone branches out toward the periphery to specialized vascular spaces called *sinuses* (Fig. 2–1). Several sinuses combine in a collecting sinus, forming a central vein that returns into the systemic circulation. Hematopoietic cords, in which hematopoiesis takes place, lie just outside of the sinuses. Following maturation in the cords, the hematopoietic cells cross the walls of the sinuses and enter the blood.[4–6] Hematopoietic cell colonies are compartmentalized in the cords. The structure of bone marrow consists of hematopoietic cells (erythroid, myeloid, lymphoid, and megakaryocyte), adipose tissue, bone and its cells (osteoblasts and osteoclasts), and stroma.

Erythropoiesis

Erythropoiesis takes place in distinct anatomic units called erythropoietic islands[7] (Fig. 2–2; see Color Plate 54). Each island consists of a macrophage surrounded by a cluster of maturing erythroblasts. Hemoglobin synthesis occurs as early as the pronormoblastic stage, but most hemoglobin synthesis occurs in the polychromatophilic stage. The average life span of circulating red cells is 120 days.

Granulopoiesis

Granulopoiesis is less conspicuously oriented toward a distinct reticulum cell, yet may be recognized as a unit[8] (Fig. 2–3 and Color Plate 55). Early granulocytic precursors are located deep in the cords and around the bone trabeculae. Neutrophils in the marrow can be divided into the proliferating pool and the maturation storage pool. The proliferating pool includes myeloblasts, promyelocytes, and myelocytes. The cells, which spend 3 to 6 days in this pool, are capable of DNA synthesis and undergo cell division. The maturation storage pool consists of nondividing metamye-

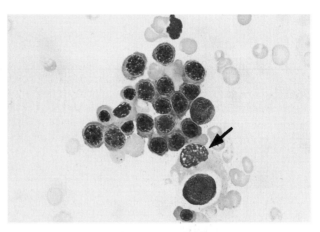

➤ FIGURE 2–2   Erythropoietic island composed mainly of polychromatophilic normoblasts. The nutrient-histiocyte (*arrow*) is slightly displaced off its central position by smearing of the particle. Its cytoplasmic slender processes envelop a basophilic normoblast, establishing intimate contact with the maturing red cell precursor (magnification ×640).

locytes, bands, and segmented neutrophils. The cells typically spend 5 to 7 days in this pool before entering into the circulation. Depending on the demand, the cells from the storage pool (representing 15 to 20 times as many cells as in the blood) can be released into the peripheral blood, thus increasing the total white blood cell (WBC) count in minutes or hours. The average life span of circulating neutrophils is 6 to 10 hours.

Megakaryopoiesis

Megakaryopoiesis occurs adjacent to the sinus endothelium. The megakaryocytes protrude as small cytoplasmic processes through the vascular wall, delivering platelets directly into the sinusoidal blood.[9] Megakaryocytes are situated close to marrow sinuses and, through a mechanism that is not entirely understood, shed platelets into the circulation. Approximately 5 days are required for the megakaryocytes to develop into platelets. Two-thirds of shed platelets are present in the circulation, whereas one-third is sequestered in the spleen. The average life span of platelets in the circulation is approximately 10 days.

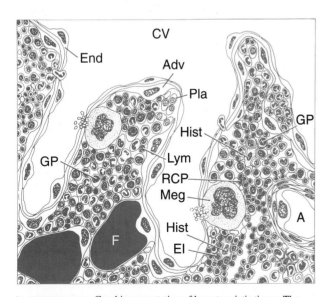

➤ FIGURE 2–1   Graphic presentation of hematopoietic tissue. The vascular compartment consists of arteriole (A) and central sinus (CV). The venous sinusoids are lined by endothelial cells (End), and their wall outside is supported by adventitial-reticulum cells (Adv). Fat tissue (F) is part of the marrow. The compartmentalization of the hematopoiesis is represented by areas of granulopoiesis (GP), areas of erythropoiesis (RCP), and erythropoietic islands (EI) with their nutrient histiocyte (Hist). The megakaryocytes protrude with small cytoplasmic projections through the vascular wall (Meg). Lymphocytes (Lym) are randomly scattered among the hemopoietic cells, whereas plasma cells (Pla) are usually situated along the vascular wall.

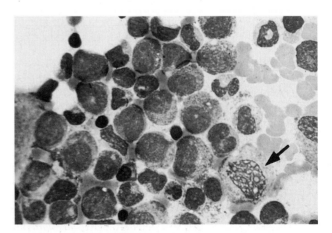

➤ FIGURE 2–3   Compartment of granulopoiesis. A reticulum cell (*arrow*) with open reticulated chromatin and light blue cytoplasm containing dustlike fine granules is situated among numerous granulocytic precursors, especially myelocytes (magnification ×640).

Lymphopoiesis

Marrow immunocytes consist of lymphocytes and plasma cells. Lymphocyte production is compartmentalized in lymphoid follicles, and lymphocytes are randomly dispersed throughout the cords. The lymphoid follicles (most often seen in elderly individuals) are unevenly distributed and tend to influence the variability of the lymphocyte count in aspirated bone marrow samples (Fig. 2–4 and Color Plate 56). Plasma cells are situated along the vascular wall.

Stem Cells

The marrow stem cells have two unique biologic characteristics: self-renewal and multilineage differentiation. These stem cells can be further subcategorized as pluripotential stem cells (which give rise to many different cell lines) and committed stem cells. Because committed stem cells are committed by lineage to one cell type and do not have the potential of self-renewal, they are also called progenitor cells. A progenitor is a cell committed to a single line of proliferation and differentiation. The stem cells on Wright's stain smears are morphologically indistinguishable from small lymphocytes. The stem cells in the presence of appropriate growth factors differentiate into myeloid and lymphoid cells that carry tissue and humoral immune functions, respectively. Some lymphoid progenitor cells produced in the marrow mature in the thymus as T lymphocytes;[10] others are produced and continue their maturation and differentiation in bone marrow as B lymphocytes from the 12th gestational week throughout life.[11] Therefore, the bone marrow and thymus are primary lymphoid organs of *antigen-independent* progenitor lymphoid cell proliferation and differentiation, which gives rise to new lymphocytes. These new lymphocytes may then populate the secondary lymphoid organs, lymph nodes, spleen, and lymphoid apparatus of the gastrointestinal tract. Under appropriate stimulation, the mature lymphocytes of the peripheral lymphoid organs undergo *antigen-dependent* effector cell proliferation, resulting in kinin and antibody production from T and B lymphocytes, respectively.

Hematogones

Hematogones are normal cellular constituents of bone marrow that resemble small- to intermediate-sized lympho-cytes. They range in size from 10 to 20 μm and have a high nuclear-to-cytoplasmic ratio and smooth, smudged homogeneous chromatin. Their cytoplasm is deeply basophilic and devoid of any granules or vacuoles (Fig. 2–5 and Color Plate 57). Hematogones are thought to be committed progenitor cells of lymphoid lineage. They are increased in normal infants, older children, and sometimes in adults (in regenerative marrow after chemotherapy and bone marrow transplantation). They are also increased in marrows of children with neuroblastoma with or without metastasis, iron-deficiency anemia, and idiopathic thrombocytopenic purpura.[12-15] These cells closely resemble blasts of lymphoblastic leukemia, and laboratory personnel should be aware of the conditions in which they can be increased.

Marrow Stromal Cells

The meshwork of stromal cells in which the hematopoietic cells are suspended is in a delicate semifluid state and is composed of reticulum cells, histiocytes, fat cells, and endothelial cells. The reticulum cells are associated with fibers that can be visualized after silver staining. They are adjacent to the sinus endothelial cells forming the outer part of the wall as an adventitial reticulum cell. Their fine cytoplasmic projections extend deep into the cords, making contact with similar projections of other cells. Occasionally, the nuclear region of these cells can be seen deep in the cords surrounded by granulopoiesis. Cytochemically, these cells are alkaline-phosphatase positive (Fig. 2–6 and Color Plate 58). The histiocytes or macrophage is seen as a perisinusoidal cell related to the bone marrow–blood barrier and as a central storage macrophage—part of the erythropoietic islands. Being a storage nutrient cell delivering iron to the growing immature erythroblasts, the storage macrophage sends out long, slender cytoplasmic processes that envelop the erythroid precursors. This extensive and intimate contact with the maturing erythropoietic cells is necessary in transferring iron from the macrophage to the red cell precursors. As phagocytic cells, the macrophages also undergo hyperplasia when there is increased destruction of hematopoietic cells. Histochemically, the macrophages are acid-phosphatase positive (Fig. 2–7 and Color Plate 59).

The stromal cells produce an extracellular matrix[16] composed of collagens, glycoproteins, proteoglycans, and other

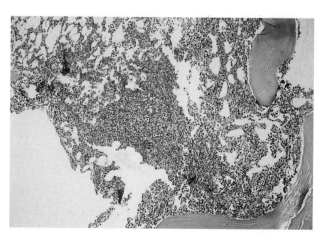

➤ **FIGURE 2–4** A lymphocytic nodule (follicle) in bone marrow as shown here may alter very significantly the marrow differential count when aspirated and give a false impression of lymphocytic malignancy (magnification ×250).

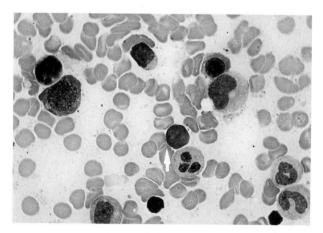

➤ **FIGURE 2–5** An arrow points toward a hematogone showing high nuclear-to-cytoplasmic ratio, homogenous chromatin, and scant cytoplasm. It can be confused with a blast of lymphoblastic leukemia (magnification ×1000).

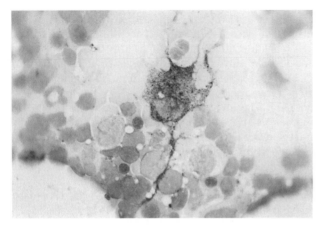

> **FIGURE 2–6**   An alkaline phosphatase–stained reticulum cell extends its slender cytoplasmic projections deep in the hemopoietic cord, maintaining an intimate contact with granulopoiesis. The background cells are stained with neutral red (magnification ×640).

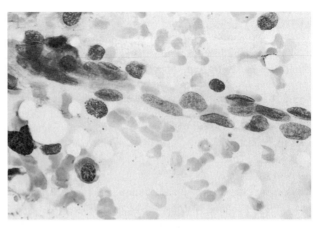

> **FIGURE 2–8**   A string of endothelial cells aspirated from hypocellular marrow. The nuclei are elongated and slightly tapered. The cytoplasm is transparent and barely visible (magnification ×640).

proteins. This extracellular matrix is essential in maintaining normal renewal and differentiation of marrow cells. The bone marrow consists of red marrow (hematopoietic active) and fatty yellow marrow (hematopoietic inactive). The marrow cellularity is estimated as a percentage of red marrow to total red and yellow marrow. The fatty yellow marrow (adipose cells) can vary in amount according to the age of the individual patient and the skeletal location from where the marrow is obtained. In young children, most of the marrow is composed of red, hematopoietic active marrow with only a few fat cells present. The adipose tissue gradually increases after 4 years of age. In adults, fat cells average about 50% of the total marrow volume in the vertebrae and flat bones of the pelvis. The marrow fat and the extracellular matrix are dynamic tissues similar to the hematopoietic tissue, and these may be altered rapidly in diseases.

The bone marrow is a highly vascularized tissue from which endothelial cells can occasionally be aspirated. Endothelial cells are more visible in hypoplastic marrows and should not be mistaken for metastatic tumors (Fig. 2–8 and Color Plate 60).

Mast Cells

Tissue mast cells (Fig. 2–9 and Color Plate 61), 6 to 12 μm in diameter, are connective tissue cells of mesenchymal origin, normally present in the bone marrow in varying numbers. They have a round or oval reticular nucleus and abundant blue-purple granules that obscure the nucleus. Their granules, in addition to all other substances that are present in the granules of basophils, contain serotonin and proteolytic enzymes. Mast cells can be increased in chronic infections, autoimmune diseases, chronic lymphoproliferative disorders, and especially in systemic mastocytosis.[17,18]

Bone-Forming Cells

In marrow aspirates, cells are occasionally seen originating from bone tissue. Osteoblasts are bone matrix–synthesizing cells usually found in groups. They are up to 30 μm in diameter and resemble plasma cells. The osteoblast nucleus has a fine chromatin pattern with a prominent nucleolus. A perinuclear halo, detached from the nuclear membrane with a cytoplasmic bridge, represents the Golgi apparatus area. Osteoblasts are alkaline-phosphatase positive. They are characteristically seen in bone marrow aspirates of children and patients with metabolic bone diseases.

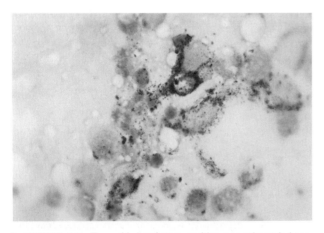

> **FIGURE 2–7**   Two acid phosphatase–positive macrophages in bone marrow of a patient treated with chemotherapeutic agents. Macrophages are also scavengers and cleaners of the hematopoietic tissue, so they increase in number during massive destruction of hematopoietic cells (magnification ×640).

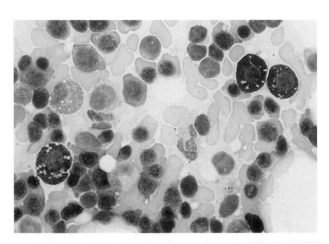

> **FIGURE 2–9**   Three mast cells, known also as tissue basophils, are shown in this marrow aspirate on a background of erythroid hyperplasia. Numerous regular round granules fill their cytoplasm and obscure the nuclear details (magnification ×640).

Osteoclasts, or bone remodeling cells, are multinucleated giant cells more than 100 μm in diameter, resembling megakaryocytes. The nuclei of the osteoclasts are separated from each other and may have nucleoli (compared with the megakaryocyte nucleus, which is multilobed). Their cytoplasm is well delineated and finely granular.

► BONE MARROW FUNCTION

The main function of the marrow is to supply mature hematopoietic cells into the peripheral blood in a steady-state condition as well as to respond to increased demands. A semidormant pool of pluripotential stem cells maintains a self-renewal property. Granulocytic, monocytic, eosinophilic, erythroid, and megakaryocyte progenitor cells are influenced in their differentiation by colony-stimulating factors (CSFs).[19–21] CSFs are produced by T lymphocytes— as well as stromal cells, fibroblasts, endothelial cells, and macrophages—when stimulated by monocyte interleukin-1 (IL-1) and tumor necrosis factor (TNF). Some CSFs, such as IL-3 and granulocyte-monocyte CSF, have a broad influence and are required throughout proliferation and differentiation of progenitor cells. Others, which include granulocyte, monocyte, and eosinophil CSFs, are lineage specific and regulate division and differentiation only of corresponding, committed progenitor cells. In addition, erythropoiesis is influenced by erythropoietin produced in the kidney.[22,23] In the process of cell egression from the cords to the circulation, a number of releasing factors are identified. The best characterized of these are granulocyte colony-stimulating factor (G-CSF) and granulocyte-macrophage colony-stimulating factor (GM-CSF), but other factors, such as components of a complement system, androgenic steroids, and endotoxins, may play a role.[24] The endothelial lining of the sinusoids forms a continuous, veil-like wall through which the mature cells migrate from extravascular sites into the circulation.[25] This is accomplished by close contact between mature hematopoietic cells and endothelial cells. A transient migration pore is formed during such contact through which the mature cells pass into the circulation without loss of plasma to the extravascular pool.[26] It is evident that the bone marrow is subjected to a complex regulation by many cellular and humoral systems of the body, and any disease that affects these systems is likely to affect hematopoiesis.

► INDICATIONS FOR BONE MARROW STUDIES

In 1929, Arinkin[27] introduced bone marrow studies in the diagnosis of hematopoietic disorders. Once a formidable task, obtaining bone marrow tissue has become, with current improved techniques, a standard procedure. Several techniques have been devised, each having its own merits and limitations. Bone marrow aspiration and bone marrow biopsy are usually performed concurrently.

Although obtaining the bone marrow for examination carries little procedural risk for the patient, the procedure is costly and can be quite painful. For this reason, bone marrow studies should be performed only when clearly indicated or whenever the physician expects a beneficial diagnostic result for his or her patient (Table 2–1). Hematologic diseases affecting primarily the bone marrow and causing a decrease or increase of any cellular blood elements are among the most

> ► **Table 2-1**
> **INDICATIONS FOR BONE MARROW STUDY**
>
> **Hematologic**
>
> - Anemias, erythrocytosis, polycythemia
> - Leukopenia and unexplained leukocytosis
> - Presence of blasts, immature, or abnormal cells in the circulation
> - Thrombocytopenia and thrombocytosis
>
> **Systemic Diseases**
>
> - Staging and management of solid malignant tumors arising elsewhere in the body, such as lymphomas, carcinoma, and sarcomas
> - Infections or fever of unknown origin, granulomas
> - Hereditary or acquired metabolic disorders
> - Systemic mast cell disease

common indications. It is not unusual for more than one blood element to be increased or decreased, as occurs in leukemias and some refractory anemias. In these situations, bone marrow study affords specific information, and it usually precedes any other diagnostic procedure.

Systemic diseases may affect the bone marrow secondarily and require bone marrow studies for diagnosis or monitoring patients' conditions. Patients having any of the solid malignant tumors may undergo bone marrow studies when the initial diagnosis is established for evaluation of the degree of tumor spread and clinical staging of disease. On occasion the bone marrow study may result in diagnosis of unsuspected disseminated malignant tumor. During the course of malignant disease, additional studies also are performed periodically to monitor the status of tumor spread and its therapeutic response.

Infections manifesting clinically as "fever of unknown origin" may exhibit granulomas, focal necrosis, or histiocytic proliferation. Intracytoplasmic organisms may be seen in the marrow. Material for morphological studies and bacterial cultures may be collected simultaneously during a single procedure. The suspected diagnoses of disseminated tuberculosis, fungal infections (particularly histoplasmosis, cryptococcosis), and some protozoan infections are frequently confirmed through such studies. Hereditary and acquired conditions occasionally involve the bone marrow histiocytes; for example Gaucher's disease, sea blue histiocytosis, hemophagocytic syndrome, and others. A simple procedure such as bone marrow aspiration or biopsy may establish the diagnosis.

► OBTAINING AND PREPARING BONE MARROW FOR HEMATOLOGIC STUDIES

The sites for bone marrow studies in adults are most commonly the posterior superior iliac crest, occasionally the sternum, and very rarely the anterior superior iliac crest and spinal processes or vertebral bodies (Fig. 2–10). Sternal aspiration should be avoided in children, as well as in patients with multiple myeloma and metastatic carcinoma, because these diseases can cause thinning and erosion of bone that

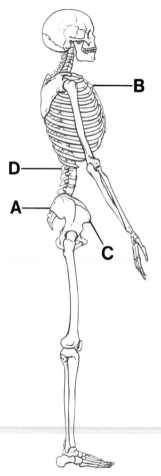

> **FIGURE 2–10**   Common sites from which bone marrow is obtained for studies. *A.* Posterior superior iliac crest. *B.* Sternum. *C.* Anterior superior iliac crest. *D.* Spinal processes.

plications include bleeding or infection at the biopsy site, transient neuropathy, and osteomyelitis. After the procedure, the patient is advised to lie on the biopsy site, which should be reevaluated in 15 to 30 minutes for any bleeding or oozing.

Bone marrow aspiration and biopsy can be performed on patients with severe thrombocytopenia, coagulation factor deficiencies (over 50% activity is required), and in those receiving anticoagulant therapy. The only valid contraindication is failure to meet the indication criteria (Table 2–1).

Equipment

The instrument tray used to perform a bone marrow procedure should contain enough equipment to complete the procedure and to prepare the tissues obtained for the appropriate studies (Table 2–2). Complete bone marrow trays are

> **Table 2-2**
> ## EXAMPLE OF A TRAY FOR BONE MARROW ASPIRATION AND BIOPSY

Required Materials

1. 30-mL syringes
2. 20-mL syringes
3. 10-mL syringes
4. 5-mL syringes
5. 2% lidocaine
6. Prepodyne prep
7. Alcohol (70%) or prep
8. 23-gauge needles
9. 21-gauge needles
10. Bone marrow biopsy/aspiration needle 11-gauge × 4 in.
11. Filter papers
12. Buffered formalin 10% with a pH of about 6.8 or other fixative for histologic processing of bone biopsy and marrow particles
13. Tube containing liquid EDTA anticoagulant
14. One box slides
15. One slide folder
16. One rubber bulb
17. Pasteur pipette
18. Petri dish
19. Sterile blades
20. Gloves (several pairs of different sizes)
21. Sterile gauze and cotton balls
22. Applicator sticks
23. Bandage
24. Culture bottles for bacterial culture (Note: Save some bone marrow specimen in syringe for tuberculosis and fungal cultures, when indicated)
25. Pencil to label slides
26. #11 Bard Parker blades

may increase the chance of perforation and can cause potential fatal cardiac complications. Occasionally, when a localized bone lesion is visualized on roentgenogram or computed tomographic (CT) scan, a directed or "open" bone marrow biopsy of the lesion may be done by a radiologist or surgeon in an operating room with the patient under anesthesia. In newborns and infants, bone marrow can be obtained from the upper end of the tibial bone.

Before performing the procedure, the physician should inform the adult patient or the parent or guardian of a child about the procedure, its risks, and its expected benefits for the diagnostic process. The bone marrow procedure cannot be performed until a consent form is signed and witnessed by a second person, usually the patient's nurse. The actual procedure is often performed with the assistance of a medical technologist. Although the physician performs the procedure, and the nurse attends to the patient, the medical technologist gives full attention to the processing of specimens. It is the medical technologist's responsibility to see that the samples are adequate. If they are not, the physician is informed immediately so that the procedure can be repeated before the patient is discharged. Samples are preserved appropriately for histologic, flow cytometric, cytogenetic, microbiologic, electron microscopic, molecular, and other studies as indicated in a particular case.

In experienced hands, complications of bone marrow biopsy and aspirate are very rare (0.1%). These rare com-

sold as disposable equipment, which may be convenient and also avoid risk of infectious disease transmission. Because of potential disease transmission, the sterile bone marrow trays are rarely used today.

Several different styles of aspiration and trephine bone biopsy needles or instruments are commonly used. Most instruments used today are patterned on the needle introduced by Jamshidi.[28] These instruments are produced in several sizes for both adult and pediatric patients. An example of the Jamshidi bone marrow biopsy/aspiration needle for adults is shown in Figure 2–11. Modifications of the original aspiration and trephine needles have been developed by different companies and are manufactured as disposable equipment.

Aspiration

A bone marrow aspiration may be performed as an independent procedure or in conjunction with a bone marrow biopsy. The procedure can be performed in the outpatient setting in clinics or in the physician's office. As a rule, children and very apprehensive patients receive a mild sedative prior to the procedure. The site selected is shaved, if hairy, and washed with soap. Then an antiseptic is applied, and the area is draped with sterile towels. A local anesthetic such as 1% to 2% lidocaine (Xylocaine) is infiltrated in the skin, in the intervening tissues between the skin and bone, and in the periosteum of the bone from which the marrow

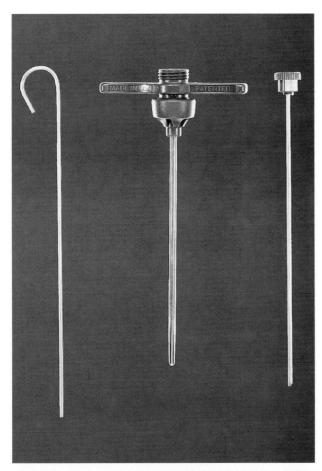

> **FIGURE 2–11** Adult-sized Jamshidi 11-gauge × 4-inch biopsy/aspiration needle showing stylet (left), biopsy needle (center), and probe (right).

is to be obtained. A cut of about 3 mm is made through the skin with a Bard-Parker blade to facilitate piercing skin and subcutaneous tissue.

The physician penetrates the bone cavity with an aspiration needle, assembled with guard and stylet locked in place. When the marrow cavity is penetrated, the stylet is removed, a syringe is attached to the free end of the needle, and the plunger is quickly pulled, drawing 1.0 to 1.5 mL of marrow particles and sinusoidal blood into the syringe. Because the vacuum created in the syringe is important for rapid and efficient suctioning of the cells and particles, the syringe should be 10 mL or larger with a well-fitting plunger. Despite the use of local anesthesia, the patient normally experiences discomfort during the aspiration process (aspiration pain). Accomplishing the aspiration with a quick and continuous pull on the plunger diminishes the patient's discomfort and decreases the chance of clotting the specimen. A clotted specimen is useless for smear preparation because the fibrin threads strip the cytoplasm off of the cells and hamper their spreading.

Keeping the volume of the initial aspirate small also prevents dilution of the sample with large amounts of sinusoidal blood, thus diminishing the quality of the aspirate. This first-aspirated material is used immediately for preparing smears. More aspirate may be obtained in additional syringes if needed for flow cytometry, chromosome studies, bacterial cultures, and other tests (Fig. 2–12). Once an adequate aspirate is obtained, the quality of the smear depends entirely on the technologist's skill and speed in preparing the smears and preserving the morphology of the marrow cells. Part of the first aspirate is used for the preparation of direct and marrow particle smears. The other part is placed in an ethylene diaminetetraacetic acid (EDTA) anticoagulant–containing tube for use later in the laboratory. If some aspirate still remains, it can be left to clot. The clot may be fixed in 10% buffered formalin or another chosen fixative and processed for histologic examination.

Preparation of Bone Marrow Aspirate

All necessary materials, preservatives, and slides should be meticulously clean and in readiness to avoid any delay. The aspirate in the first syringe contains mostly blood admixed with fat, marrow cells, and particles of marrow tissue, which should be used for smears. Several direct smears can be prepared immediately, using the technique for blood film preparation. A small drop is placed on a glass slide, and the blood and the particles are dragged behind a spreading slide with a technique similar to that for preparing blood film. Although this method of preparation preserves the cell morphology well, it is inadequate for the evaluation of the cells in relationship to each other and for the estimation of marrow cellularity.

Smears of marrow particles are prepared by pouring a small amount of the aspirate on a glass slide. The marrow tissue is seen as gray particles floating in blood and fat droplets. The particles are aspirated selectively with a plastic dropper or Oxford pipette and transferred to a clean glass slide. These are covered gently with another slide. The two slides are pulled in opposite and parallel directions to smear the particles without crushing the cells. Some people recommend an alternate technique using two cover glasses. In this process, the marrow particles are squashed between two coverslips, which are then gently pulled apart.

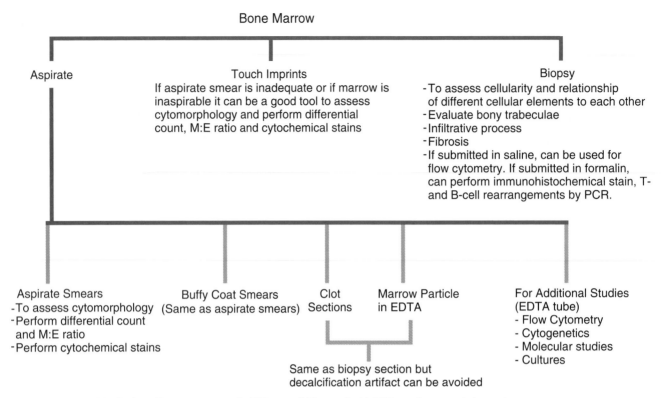

➤ FIGURE 2–12   Distribution of bone marrow sample. M:E = myeloid-to-erythroid; PCR = polymerase chain reaction.

Techniques for preparing particle smears vary from person to person and from laboratory to laboratory. The aspirate may be transferred into a watch glass and the particles collected with a capillary pipette or the broken end of a wooden stick applicator. With experience, technologists usually adapt a technique that facilitates production of high-quality slides. The technologist should prepare an adequate number of slides of smeared marrow particles. In cases of newly diagnosed acute leukemia, no fewer than 10 slides should be prepared. These are needed for histochemical stains such as myeloperoxidase, Sudan black B, naphthyl AS-D chloroacetate esterase, alpha-naphthyl butyrate esterase, and others.

Marrow particle smears are used in the evaluation of cellularity (usually marrow biopsy is ideal) and the relationship of the cells to each other. Well-prepared smears have the added advantage of excellent cell morphology, allowing subtle changes in cell maturation and cytoplasmic inclusions to be easily recognized.

All direct and particle smears should be labeled at the bedside with the patient's name, identification number, and the date and then quickly air-dried.

Measurement of Bone Marrow Aspirate

The EDTA-anticoagulated aspirate can be used for quantitative studies. About 1 mL of marrow aspirate is transferred to a Wintrobe tube and centrifuged at 2800 rpm (at 850 g) for 8 minutes. The fluid is separated into four layers, representing fat and perivascular cells, plasma, buffy coat of myeloid-erythroid cells, and erythrocytes (Fig. 2–13). Each layer is measured and read as a percentage directly from the Wintrobe tube, its volume correlating with a given basic element

of the marrow. Smears can be prepared from fat-perivascular and buffy coat layers[29] and used accordingly to study iron and hematopoietic cell and myeloid-to-erythroid (M:E) cell ratio. Such quantitative studies may be useful in estimating cellularity (fat versus buffy coat) when no histologic sections of bone biopsy and marrow particles are available.

Histologic Marrow Particle Preparation

The leftover marrow particles obtained during the aspiration procedure can be processed for histologic examination. The tissue particles, admixed with blood, may be left to clot, then fixed in 10% buffered formalin and processed for histologic sectioning. However, better results are obtained if the blood and particles are transferred to an EDTA anticoagulant–containing tube before clotting sets in. The blood and particles are then filtered through histo-wrap filter paper, and the concentrated particles enfolded in the paper are fixed in 10% buffered formalin. In the histology laboratory, these particles are collected by scraping the paper and then embedding the particles in paraffin for further processing.[30]

Bone Marrow Biopsy

A bone marrow biopsy is especially indicated when the marrow cannot be aspirated ("dry tap"), owing to pathologic alterations encountered in acute leukemias, myelofibrosis, hairy cell leukemia, and others. Trephine bone biopsy is also performed for the diagnosis of neoplastic and granulomatous diseases. For clinical staging of lymphomas and carcinomas and in multiple myeloma, bilateral posterior superior iliac crest biopsies are recommended as these increase the likelihood of diagnosing a

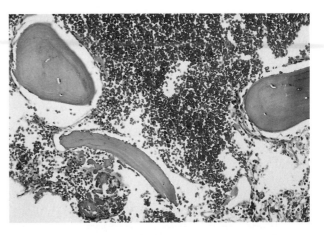

➤ **FIGURE 2–14** Bone marrow biopsy specimen showing an aspiration artifact that can affect the cellularity and alter the relationship of cells to each other (magnification ×200).

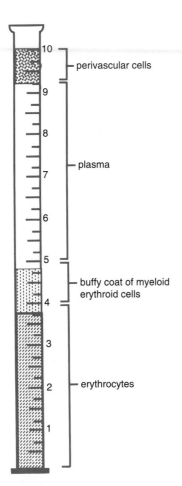

➤ **FIGURE 2–13** Quantitative measurement of bone marrow aspirate. A schematic presentation of the four marrow layers formed by centrifugation of aspirate in a Wintrobe tube.

The labels on the figure, top to bottom, read: perivascular cells, plasma, buffy coat of myeloid erythroid cells, erythrocytes.

focal process. An adequate biopsy sample is at least 15 mm in length.[31]

When a bone marrow biopsy is performed in conjunction with a marrow aspiration, customarily the biopsy sample is obtained after the aspirate. This sequence is usually achieved by changing the direction of the needle to avoid the aspiration artifact. However, this technique may result in an aspiration artifact with hemorrhage into the area of biopsy site, leading to difficulties in evaluating cellularity and morphology (Fig. 2–14 and Color Plate 62). Therefore, a core biopsy sample should be obtained before the aspiration or the marrow biopsy procedure is to be performed through a new puncture site in the anesthetized area. In some cases when flow cytometry is indicated, and the aspirate is difficult to obtain (e.g., in patients with hypercellular marrow, hairy cell leukemia, or marrow fibrosis) an additional core marrow biopsy may be obtained in normal saline or RPMI (Roswell Park Memorial Institute) solution. Adequate cell suspensions can then be made from this biopsy sample and processed for flow cytometric studies.

Preparation of Trephine Biopsy

Touch Preparation

The bone marrow core biopsy sample is supported lightly without pressure between the blades of forceps and touched several times on two or three clean slide surfaces. The biopsy

core sample should not be rubbed on the slide, because rubbing destroys the cells. The slides are air-dried. The touch preparations are fixed in absolute methanol and stained with Wright-Giemsa stain. In the absence of a good aspirate smear, the touch preparations may be the only source for studying cellular details and the maturation sequence of the bone marrow biopsy sample (Figs. 2–15 and 2–16, and Color Plates 63 and 64). Sometimes the touch preparations contain enough cells to obtain differential counts and blast evaluation, and to perform histochemical studies.[32]

Histologic Bone Marrow Biopsy Preparation

The biopsy specimen is immersed without delay in B-5 or 10% buffered formalin fixative. Histology laboratories may have a choice of other preferred fixatives such as Zenker's solution, Carnoy's solution, and others.[33,34] After fixation the biopsy specimen undergoes standard histologic processing of decalcification, dehydration, embedding in paraffin blocks, sectioning of 2- to 3-μm thick sections, and histologic staining. The advantage of the bone marrow biopsy is that it represents a large sample of marrow and bone structures in their natural relationship. A variety of different stains can be used to demonstrate marrow iron, reticulum, and collagen. However, because of decalcification, the core biopsy may not be a good method for studying marrow iron stores. Acid-fast organisms and fungi in granulomatous diseases may be detected quickly with specific stains, offering great advantages in diagnosing these infections (Figs. 2–17, 2–18, and 2–19, and Color Plates 65, 66, and 67). For instance, mycobacterial cultures may require weeks of incubation to show growth of organisms, whereas on tissue sections, the histologic and etiologic diagnosis may be made within 10 to 12 hours. When metastatic tumors and lymphomas are found in the bone marrow, immunohistochemical stains can be used on histologic sections to demonstrate specific tumor markers (Figs. 2–20, 2–21, and 2–22, and Color Plates 68, 69, and 70). Thus, a very precise diagnosis of the origin of a tumor can be made without elaborate, expensive, and invasive techniques.

A disadvantage of the bone marrow biopsy is that fine cellular details are lost in the processing; therefore, it is of little value in the diagnosis of leukemias and some refrac-

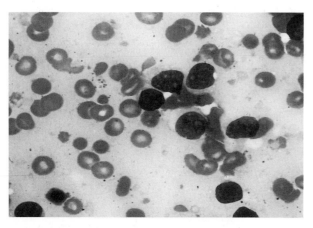

> ► FIGURE 2–15   Wright-stained bone marrow touch preparation from a patient with hairy cell leukemia. Aspirate was a "dry tap." A few diagnostic hairy cells are seen with abundant, fluffy, light blue cytoplasm and inconspicuous nucleoli (magnification ×1000).

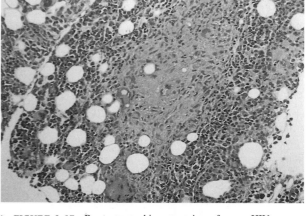

> ► FIGURE 2–17   Bone marrow biopsy specimen from an HIV-positive patient with tuberculosis shows a well-formed granuloma with epitheloid histiocytes (magnification ×200).

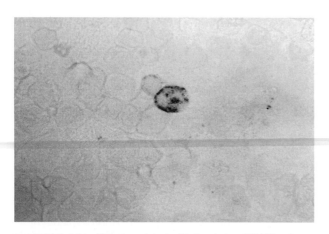

> ► FIGURE 2–16   Tartrate-resistant acid phosphatase (TRAP) stain showing a strong positive reaction in neoplastic cells of hairy cell leukemia (magnification ×1000).

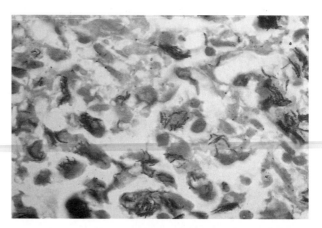

> ► FIGURE 2–18   Acid-fast stain on a bone marrow biopsy specimen from the same patient as in Figure 2–17 shows acid-fast organisms, confirming infection with *Mycobacterium* (magnification ×1000).

tory anemias. In these situations, the touch preparation from the biopsy may supply the missing morphological details. Multiple touch preparations also offer an opportunity for histochemical stains (myeloperoxidase, Sudan black B, naphthyl AS-D chloroacetate esterase, α-naphthyl butyrate esterase, etc.), which are essential in diagnosis and classification of leukemias. Polymerase chain reaction (PCR) can now be performed on paraffin-embedded, formalin, or B-5–fixed marrow biopsy specimens. PCR technology may be used to evaluate B-cell or T-cell gene rearrangements, various leukemias, and minimal residual disease, and to diagnose infectious diseases.

Trephine bone marrow biopsy specimens may be embedded in methyl methacrylate, a synthetic plastic medium, and sectioned into 1 to 2 μ thin sections without decalcification. The morphological quality of the cells is extremely well preserved, and a differential count can be done on hematoxylin-eosin (H & E) or Giemsa-stained slides.[35] However, this technique requires specially trained personnel, equipment, and separate handling in the histology laboratory, which increases the cost of the procedure. The processing time of the tissue also increases, which may not be acceptable for rapid diagnosis. In addition, tissue embedded in plastic media, instead of paraffin, may not be suitable for immunohistochemical studies of bone marrow.

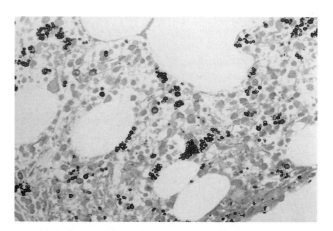

> ► FIGURE 2–19   GMS (Gomori's methenamine silver) stain on bone marrow biopsy specimen from an HIV-positive patient shows multiple budding yeasts consistent with histoplasmosis (magnification ×1000).

► BONE MARROW EXAMINATION

The examination of the bone marrow aspirate smears should start at low magnification with a dry objective of 10×. Scanning the slide permits selection of a suitable area for examination and differential count. "Bare nuclei" should be avoided; such nuclei result from destruction of the marrow

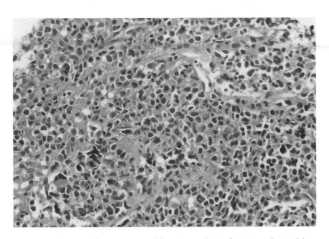

➤ **FIGURE 2–20** Bone marrow biopsy specimen from a patient with T-cell acute lymphoblastic leukemia shows an increased number of blasts. Note that the blasts are not cohesive and are individually scattered. This is a morphological feature of hematolymphoid malignancy (magnification ×640).

cells by squashing or stripping of their cytoplasm by fibrin threads. An area is selected in which the cells are well spread, intact, and not diluted by sinusoidal blood. When marrow particles are examined, such areas are found at the periphery of the particles. At this low magnification, marrow cellularity is also evaluated. The megakaryocytes are usually noted adjacent to a spicule, about five to ten per low-power field. Nonhematopoietic tumor cells infiltrating the bone marrow may also be seen at this magnification. These are usually larger than the granulocytic or erythropoietic precursors and are scattered in small groups and clusters (see Fig. 2–21 and Color Plate 69).

After the initial scan, immersion oil is applied to the slide and the examination continues on high magnification (oil immersion objective 50× or 100×). The high magnification provides details of the nuclear and cytoplasmic maturation process (Fig. 2–23 and Color Plate 71). The iron in histiocytes is visualized as brown-blue granules. Cytoplasmic inclusions of a diagnostic nature can be seen in histiocytes and granulocytes. Differential counts of bone marrow are performed with the oil immersion objective.

Estimation of Bone Marrow Cellularity

Cellularity is reflected in the ratio of nucleated hematopoietic cells to fat cells. Bone marrow cellularity normally varies with age, and the estimated cellularity must be compared to age-related normal ranges. At birth the normal marrow cellularity is 100%. Thereafter, the cellularity gradually decreases. Overall marrow cellularity in adults is about 50% (± 10%). The general rule to estimate age-related normal ranges is 100 minus age ± 10. For example, the estimated normal marrow cellularity of a 40-year-old person would be 100 − 40 ± 10 (i.e., a range from 50% to 70%).

Cellularity may vary from area to area, and, therefore, estimated cellularity should represent the average percentage. If hypercellular (90%) and hypocellular (10%) areas are seen, this finding should be mentioned descriptively in the report because in such cases an average cellularity may be difficult to estimate. The adjacent subcortical and paratrabecular area of bone marrow may normally be hypocellular compared with the deeper medullary area. Therefore, sections that contain predominantly subcortical bone may be suboptimal for assessing the marrow cellularity.

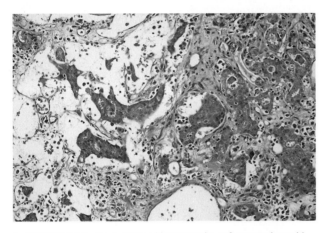

➤ **FIGURE 2–21** Bone marrow biopsy specimen from a patient with metastatic carcinoma shows glandular formation, a morphological feature of adenocarcinoma (magnification ×640).

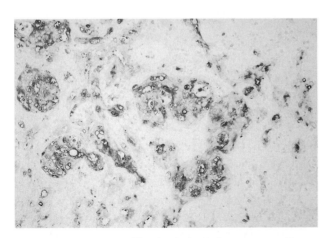

➤ **FIGURE 2–22** Immunohistochemical stain for prostate-specific antigen (PSA) performed on a marrow biopsy specimen from the same patient as in Figure 2–21. The specimen shows positive staining with PSA, thus confirming that the metastatic tumor is from prostate (magnification ×640).

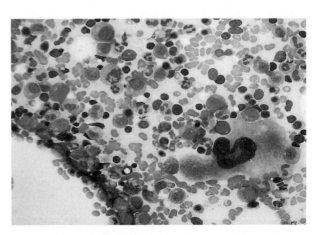

➤ **FIGURE 2–23** Smear of normal cellular marrow with normal maturation of erythropoietic, granulocytic, and megakaryocytic cells (magnification ×250).

The bone marrow biopsy specimen is most reliable for assessment of cellularity, because it offers a large amount of tissue for evaluation. However, the evaluation of cellularity can also be done on well-prepared aspirate smears or marrow particles. The best area for examination of cellularity in smears is the area between two uncrushed particles. The ratio of cells to fat is evaluated at low magnification (objective 10×), so that larger areas are included in the field of observation. The empty spaces that result from the spreading of the cells but are not occupied by fat cells are disregarded and treated as an artifact. The terms *decreased* or *increased* cellularity are used when fewer or more than the expected normal number of cells are found. Precise evaluation can be achieved with experience, and good reproducibility can be attained among several observers. The marrow cellularity can be expressed in percentages, but this is best done on histologic sections of biopsy specimens (Figs. 2–24, 2–25, and 2–26, and Color Plates 72, 73, and 74). Marrow cellularity has diagnostic value when it is related to the M:E ratio, which is calculated after a differential count is performed.

It is always important to look for any abnormal changes in the bony trabeculae. Various conditions can alter the morphological appearance of these trabeculae (Fig. 2–27 and Color Plate 75). Marked thickening of trabeculae (Fig. 2–28 and Color Plate 76) can be seen in myeloproliferative disorder (myelofibrosis with myeloid metaplasia), whereas thinning of trabeculae (Fig. 2–29 and Color Plate 77) can be seen in older adults, in patients with acquired immunodeficiency syndrome (AIDS) or other cachectic conditions, and after chronic steroid administration. Various metabolic disorders can also alter the morphology of bony trabeculae. Examples include mosaic pattern, seen in patients with Paget's disease, and resorption and cyst formation, in those with hyperparathyroidism and chronic renal failure.

When lymphoid aggregates are seen in the bone marrow biopsy specimen, the differential diagnosis include benign lymphoid aggregates and malignant lymphoma. Usually benign aggregates are small and well demarcated, nonparatrabecular, and composed predominantly of small, round lymphocytes with plasma cells at the periphery and blood vessels present within the aggregate. Conversely, malignant follicles are usually large with ill-defined borders, paratrabecular, composed of atypical lymphocytes, and

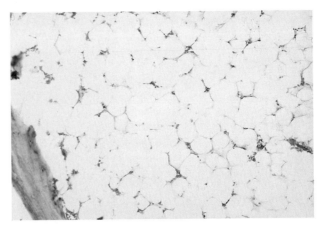

➤ **FIGURE 2–25**   Markedly hypocellular bone marrow biopsy specimen from a 20-year-old patient indicates severe aplastic anemia (low magnification).

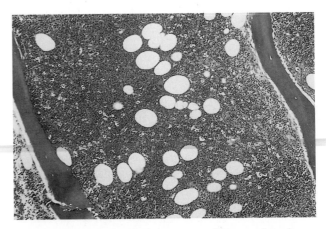

➤ **FIGURE 2–26**   Hypercellular bone marrow biopsy specimen from a 60-year-old patient with 80% cellular marrow. This patient was receiving growth factor therapy.

lack plasma cells at the periphery (Figs. 2–30 and 2–31, and Color Plates 78 and 79). However, the lymphoid infiltrate of lymphoma can also be interstitial, diffuse and patchy. In some cases, immunohistochemical stains can be done on the marrow biopsy to differentiate between benign lymphoid aggregates and malignant lymphoma.

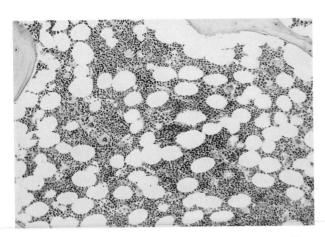

➤ **FIGURE 2–24**   Normal bone marrow biopsy specimen from a 50-year-old patient shows approximately 50% cellularity (low magnification).

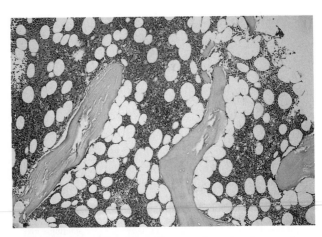

➤ **FIGURE 2–27**   Bone marrow biopsy specimen showing normal bony trabeculae (low magnification).

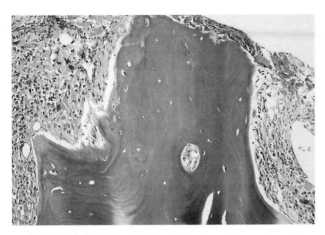

➤ **FIGURE 2–28** Bone marrow biopsy specimen from a patient with myelofibrosis and myeloid metaplasia shows marked thickening of bony trabeculae (osteosclerosis) (magnification ×200).

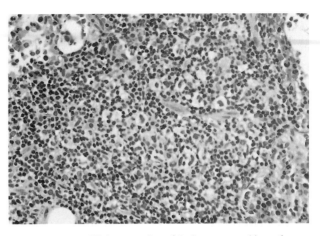

➤ **FIGURE 2–30** High-power view of the bone marrow biopsy from a 60-year-old patient shows lymphoid aggregate (low-power view is seen in Figure 2–4). Note the presence of blood vessel and plasma cells at the periphery of the lymphoid aggregate (magnification ×400).

Bone marrow fibrosis may be found in patients with hairy cell leukemia or myeloproliferative and myelodysplastic syndromes; sometimes in acute leukemia; after radiation; and following toxic injury to the marrow. If the marrow aspiration procedure results in a "dry tap" and flow cytometry is needed, it is a good practice to obtain two bone marrow biopsy samples. One biopsy sample can be put in formalin and processed for morphological examination. The other core biopsy sample can be put in saline or RPMI medium; a cell suspension is then made for flow cytometric studies. On routine H & E sections, streaming of marrow stroma and dilated sinusoids suggests marrow fibrosis; this finding can be confirmed and graded by performing reticulin and trichrome stains (Fig. 2–32 and Color Plate 80). Normally, occasional reticulin-positive fibers may be seen around the blood vessels. The fibrosis can be graded as mild, moderate, or severe. In addition, a description of the fibrosis as fine or coarse, and focal or diffuse, may be helpful, especially when following the improvement of a patient with myelofibrosis after treatment or bone marrow transplantation. Trichrome stain is usually performed to detect any collagenous fibrosis, which if present may indicate irreversible fibrosis.

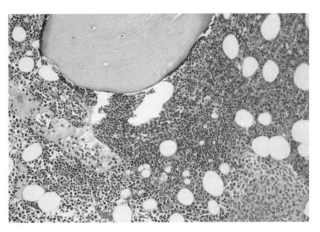

➤ **FIGURE 2–31** Bone marrow biopsy specimen shows paratrabecular lymphoid infiltrate. This pattern of infiltration is diagnostic of involvement of the marrow by malignant lymphoma (magnification ×200).

Bone Marrow Differential Count

A bone marrow differential count is an excellent tool for training a novice in bone marrow morphology and is widely used in diagnosing and following up patients with leukemias, refractory anemias, and myelodysplastic and myeloproliferative syndromes. Because of the compartmentalization of the hematopoietic cells and high cellularity of marrow, at least 500 to 1000 nucleated cells need to be classified for a representative differential count.

In infants during the first month after birth, dramatic alterations occur in the distribution of the different marrow compartments.[36] At birth there is a predominance of granulocyte precursors, which switches within a month to a predominance of lymphoid elements. In early infancy many lymphocytes have fine chromatin and a high nuclear-to-cytoplasmic ratio, and lack distinct nucleoli. They are called hematogones and represent normal lymphoid progenitor cells.[13] Hematogones may be misinterpreted as blasts if the observer is unfamiliar with these characteristics (see Fig. 2–5 and Color Plate 57). In children up to 3 years old, one-third or more of the marrow cellularity is made up of lymphocytes. The lymphocyte number gradually declines to the normal adult level thereafter.

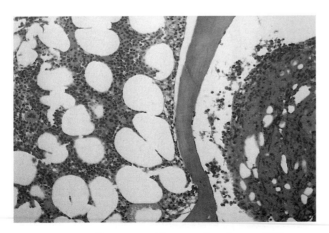

➤ **FIGURE 2–29** Bone marrow biopsy specimen from an HIV-positive patient shows thinning of bony trabeculae (osteopenia) (magnification ×200).

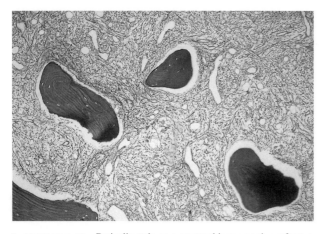

▶ **FIGURE 2–32**   Reticulin stain on a marrow biopsy specimen from a patient with hairy cell leukemia (same patient as in Figures 2–15 and 2–16), showing diffuse and severe fibrosis. Aspirate was "dry tap" (magnification ×200).

In adult marrow the lymphocytes are distributed both at random among the hematopoietic cells and in lymphoid follicles. This can introduce significant variation in the differential count from sample to sample in the same patient. The great mass of the adult marrow is composed of granulopoietic and erythropoietic precursors. For the purpose of the differential count, these are enumerated into different categories according to their stage of maturation. When adequate numbers of cells are tabulated, the percentage of each category is calculated. The ratio between all granulocytes and their precursors and all nucleated red cell precursors represents the M:E ratio.

Some hematologists prefer to exclude the segmented neutrophils from the differential count as being part of the neutrophil storage pool of the marrow. The normal M:E ratio in this case is between 1.5 and 3. However, pathologists and hematologists who interpret the bone marrow histologic sections of particle clot and biopsies in conjunction with marrow smears include the segmented neutrophils in the differential counts, because these cannot be excluded in the evaluation of histologic specimens and are part of the marrow cellularity. The normal M:E ratio then is slightly higher and ranges between 2 and 4. The granulopoietic tissue occupies two to four times greater marrow space than the erythropoietic precursors, owing to the shorter survival of the granulocytes in the circulation (i.e., neutrophils, 6 to 10 hours, versus erythrocytes, 120 days). Changes in the survival of granulocytes and erythrocytes are reflected in changes in the M:E ratio.

Megakaryocytes are unevenly distributed, and a differential count is a poor means for their evaluation. Megakaryocytes are not included in the differential count. Usually five to ten megakaryocytes are seen per microscopic field at low magnification (objective 10×). When clusters of megakaryocytes and promegakaryocytes are seen in every field, it is an indication of megakaryocytic hyperplasia. In normal cellular marrow, finding fewer than two megakaryocytes per field on screening may indicate megakaryocytic hypoplasia. A marked increase or decrease in the number of megakaryocytes is easy to evaluate, whereas slight to moderate changes are difficult to judge and are better estimated on histologic sections of biopsy and particle specimens.

Table 2–3 represents the data of normal marrow refer-

ence ranges used by the computer resources of the University Hospital and University of Texas Health Science Center at San Antonio, Texas.

Bone Marrow and Peripheral Blood Interpretation Based on Cellularity and M:E Ratio Changes

A bone marrow aspirate or biopsy sample represents a minute part of a very large and dynamic organ. Its activity and responses are reflected in blood changes; therefore, evaluation of the bone marrow should always be done in conjunction with evaluation of the peripheral blood. In adults with 50% marrow cellularity, about 30% to 40% represents granulopoiesis and 10% to 15% erythropoiesis, with an average M:E ratio of 4:1. An increase or a decrease in marrow cellularity with the normal M:E ratio usually indicates a balanced granulocytic and erythrocytic hyperplasia or hypoplasia, respectively. However, if cellularity changes occur simultaneously with the M:E ratio change, the interpretation requires a broader understanding of hematopoietic tissue physiology and its reactions during disease.

Cell morphology and the M:E ratio are well represented in random bone marrow specimens. The variations are not significant even when samples are compared from sternal and iliac crest aspirates.[37] However, marrow cellularity is poorly represented in random smears; thus, this interpretation should be considered with some degree of reservation. Even large biopsy specimens may have a great degree of variation in cellularity.[38] For this reason, in diseases where marrow cellularity is crucial for the diagnosis (aplastic anemia, marrow hypoplasia), more than one bone biopsy sample may need to be obtained.

Table 2–4 has been included to provide both a simple guide and some basic information to the reader. It cannot serve as a diagnostic tool without the addition of the patient's clinical history and a clinical evaluation of the disease. The reader is also cautioned that the variety of problems frequently presented by different patients with the same disease may not fit within such a simple schematic concept.

Bone Marrow Iron Stores

The storage iron of the bone marrow is in the form of hemosiderin. The iron content of hemosiderin is higher than that of ferritin. Other components of hemosiderin are protein, ferritin aggregates, some lipids, and membranes of cellular organelles. Hemosiderin can be seen on unstained smears as golden-yellow granules. On Wright-Giemsa–stained smears it appears as brownish-blue granules. However, for more precise evaluation Prussian blue reaction is used to demonstrate the intracytoplasmic iron of histiocytes and red cell precursors. The evaluation of marrow iron stores is essential in the diagnosis of anemias and especially in refractory and dyserythropoietic anemias. When the morphological characteristic of the iron particles in the storage nutrient histiocyte and erythroblastic precursors is an important diagnostic consideration (e.g., in sideroblastic anemias), an iron stain is performed on a particle smear. If the overall distribution of the amount of iron is of clinical importance (e.g., iron-deficiency anemia, anemia of chronic diseases, hemochromatosis, and others), then histologic sections of bone marrow biopsy sample, and/or marrow aspirate, and marrow clotted particles are stained

> ## Table 2-3
DIFFERENTIAL CELL COUNT OF BONE MARROW IN PERCENTAGE OF TOTAL NUCLEATED CELLS*

	At Birth	To 1 Month	Children	Adults
Undifferentiated cells	0–2	0–2	0–1	0–1
Myeloblasts	0–2	0–2	0–2	0–2
Promyelocytes	0–4	0–4	0–4	0–4
Myelocytes				
Neutrophilic	2–8	2–4	5–15	5–20
Eosinophilic	0–5	0–3	0–6	0–3
Basophilic	0–1	0–1	0–1	0–1
Metamyelocytes and bands				
Neutrophilic	15–25	5–10	5–15	5–35
Eosinophilic	0–5	1–5	1–8	0–5
Basophilic	0–1	0–1	0–1	0–1
Segmented neutrophils	5–15	3–10	5–15	5–15
Pronormoblasts	0–3	0–1	0–2	0–1.5
Basophilic normoblasts	0–5	0–3	0–5	0–5
Polychromatophilic normoblasts	6–20	5–50	5–11	5–30
Orthochromatic normoblasts	0–5	0–2	0–8	5–10
Lymphocytes	5–15	5–20	5–35	10–20
Plasma cells	0–2	0–2	0–2	0–2
Monocytes	0–2	0–2	0–2	0–5

*Normal reference ranges from the Laboratory Computing Resources of the University of Texas Health Science Center and University Hospital, San Antonio, TX.

for iron. The biopsy sample and the particles are a more reliable source of information, because they represent a large sample of hematopoietic tissue. Bone marrow biopsy samples for iron studies should be decalcified by the EDTA chelating method, which does not affect the storage iron.[39] Rapid-acid decalcifying solutions extract iron and must not be used in these cases.

After Prussian blue staining, hemosiderin and some ferritin aggregates are seen as bright blue specks and granules (Fig. 2–33 and Color Plate 81). Hemoglobin iron and dispersed ferritin do not stain. Normal marrow iron is seen as fine cytoplasmic granules within histiocytes, and 30% to 50% of marrow erythroblasts contain iron specks sideroblasts. Clumps of iron easily seen at scanning magnification (10×) indicate increased iron storage, whereas only a few specks of iron found after searching several microscopic fields (50× or 100× magnification) indicates decreased iron storage. When no stainable iron is detected on the bone marrow smear or tissue sections, this indicates iron storage depletion or absence.[39] The storage iron may be reported as

> ## Table 2-4
MARROW AND BLOOD INTERPRETATION BASED ON CELLULARITY AND M:E RATIO

Complete Blood Count	Bone Marrow Cellularity	M:E Ratio	Bone Marrow Interpretation
Normal	Increased or decreased*	Normal	Normal
Neutropenia	Decreased	Decreased	Granulocytic hypoplasia
Neutropenia	Normal or increased	Increased	Decreased neutrophilic survival or ineffective granulopoiesis
Neutrophilia	Normal or increased	Increased	Granulocytic hyperplasia
Anemia	Normal or decreased	Increased	Red cell hypoplasia
Anemia	Normal or increased	Decreased	Erythrocytic hyperplasia or ineffective erythropoiesis†
Erythrocytosis	Normal or increased	Decreased	Erythrocytic hyperplasia (polycythemia)
Pancytopenia	Decreased	Normal	Marrow hypoplasia
Pancytopenia	Increased	Normal, increased, or decreased	Ineffective myelopoiesis or hypersplenism

*Because of poor presentation of cellularity in random specimen.
†Reticulocyte count is necessary to differentiate between erythrocytic hyperplasia and ineffective erythropoiesis.

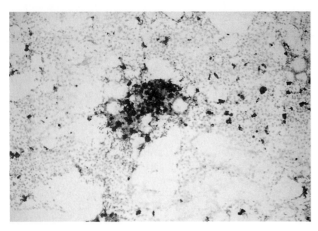

➤ **FIGURE 2–33** Iron stain of a bone marrow smear shows a marked increase in marrow storage iron, thus ruling out the possibility of iron-deficiency anemia (magnification ×200)

"absent," "decreased," "adequate," "moderately increased," and "markedly increased," or it can be given corresponding numerical values from 0 to 4, where 2 represents the normal or adequate iron stored in an adult.

➤ BONE MARROW REPORT

The bone marrow report usually encompasses the following (see the Case Study that follows):

1. The name of the laboratory or physician's office from which the report originates.
2. The patient's addressograph data, including age and relevant clinical summary or clinical diagnosis.
3. A description of material received for studies, such as smears of aspirate, marrow particles, and bone biopsy (or biopsies).
4. Data from the complete blood count (CBC) and WBC differential count, and a description of the blood smear preferably from the day on which the bone marrow specimen is obtained. A platelet count should be included, as well as a reticulocyte count, if available.
5. The bone marrow differential count.
6. A description of cellularity, M:E ratio, granulopoiesis, erythropoiesis, and megakaryopoiesis. Any change in the nonhematopoietic elements of marrow, such as hemophagocytosis, granulomas, microorganisms, metastatic tumor cells, histiocytic hyperplasia, or the appearance of bony trabeculae, is included in this section of the report. The status of iron stores and special staining procedures performed are reported.
7. A description of histologic sections of marrow particles or bone marrow biopsy.
8. The diagnostic conclusion. This should encompass separate diagnoses of blood and bone marrow even where the same diagnosis is applicable to both; for example: *Blood*—pancytopenia, *bone marrow left posterior iliac spine aspirate and biopsy*—myelodysplastic syndrome, refractory anemia with ringed sideroblasts; or *Blood*—acute myelogenous leukemia (FAB-M1), and *bone marrow left*

posterior iliac crest aspirate and biopsy—acute myelogenous leukemia (FAB-M1).

In summary, bone marrow can provide a representative picture of the disease process and has wide application in clinical medicine.[40,41] Marrow examination has a significant role in the evaluation of leukemias, lymphomas, plasma cell disorders, myeloproliferative disorders, myelodysplastic disorders, myelofibrosis, metastatic tumors, various anemias, granulomatous diseases, infectious diseases, and metabolic diseases; in evaluating the status of engraftment following bone marrow transplantation; and in assessing chemotherapy effects. The medical technologist's contribution in this phase consists of preparing the optimum blood and bone marrow slides and performing the differential count. Examination of the blood and the bone marrow, correlation with the clinical presentation, and diagnostic conclusions on each specimen are the responsibility of a physician who has adequate training and experience to integrate all of the available clinical and laboratory information in reaching the correct diagnosis.

➤ CASE STUDY

Patient Name: John Doe

Pathology Services, University Health System

Hospital Number: 123456

Surgical Pathology Accession Number: S01-1234

Physician: Dr. Z

Bone Marrow Examination
Gross Description
Specimen A: specimen label, patient's name and right posterior iliac crest biopsy. Received in formalin is a 1.2 cm × 0.2 cm × 0.2 cm bone marrow biopsy sample. Entirely submitted after decalcification: block A.

Specimen B: specimen label, patient's name and right posterior iliac crest aspirate. Received in EDTA are marrow particles with an aggregate of 0.8 cm × 0.5 cm × 0.2 cm. Entirely submitted: block B.

Aspirate smears: 14 unstained and 4 Wright-stained samples from the right posterior iliac crest, all labeled with the patient's name. Touch preparations: 3 unstained and 2 Wright-stained samples from the right posterior iliac crest, all labeled with patient's name.

Also received are 2 tubes of EDTA-anticoagulated bone marrow for flow cytometry and cytogenetic studies.

Microscopic Description
Peripheral Blood
CBC obtained from University Hospital on 2/22/01 reveals:

RBC: 3.0×10^{12}/L	WBC: 20×10^9/L
Hgb: 7.5 g/dL	**Manual differential**
Hct: 22%	Segmented neutrophils: 31%
MCV: 94.0 fL	Bands: 1%
MCH: 28 pg	Lymphocytes: 20%
MCHC: 32 g/dL	Monocytes: 2%

continued

RDW: 19.0

Platelet count
5.0 × 10⁹/L

Eosinophils: 1%
Basophils: 1%
Metamyelocytes: 4%
Myelocytes: 3%
Promyelocytes: 2%
Blasts: 35%

Anisocytosis: moderate with occasional microcytes and few macrocytes.

Poikilocytosis: mild with a few teardrop cells and rare schistocytes.

Polychromasia: mild. NRBCs are present 2/100 WBCs

The white blood cells display a left shift with increased number of circulating blasts. The blasts are of small size, show minimal variation, and have high nuclear-to-cytoplasmic ratio and fine and lacy chromatin with occasional small nucleoli. No Auer rods are seen.

The platelet count is 5.0 × 10⁹/L. Few giant platelets are seen. No platelet clumps are noted.

Bone Marrow

Examination of the bone marrow aspirate smears reveal hypercellular marrow with decreased megakaryocytes. Differential count performed on aspirate smears reveals:

Blasts: 65%	Pronormoblasts: 1%
Promyelocytes: 6%	Basophilic normoblasts: 4%
Myelocytes: 5%	Polychromatic normoblasts: 4%
Metamyelocytes and bands: 4%	Orthochromatic normoblasts: 7%
Segmented neutrophils: 2%	Monocytes: 1%
	Lymphocytes: 1%

Blasts are markedly increased. The morphology of blasts is the same as described in the peripheral smear. Residual myeloid and erythroid precursors showing progressive maturation are seen in the background. The M:E ratio is 5:1.

Cytochemical stains performed on the aspirate smears show that the blasts are negative for Sudan black B, myeloperoxidase, specific and nonspecific esterase, and acid phosphatase.

Sections from the right iliac crest biopsy and right particle preparation reveal hypercellular marrow (cellularity 90%) with complete involvement by leukemic blasts. Residual trilineage hematopoiesis is seen in the background. Bony trabeculae are unremarkable. Reticulin stain shows mild to moderate diffuse marrow fibrosis (2+).

Diagnosis

Blood

Acute lymphoblastic leukemia (ALL) (circulating blasts 35%); FAB: L1 subtype

Normochromic normocytic anemia—moderate

Thrombocytopenia—marked

Bone Marrow, Right Iliac Crest Aspirate Smears, Aspirate Particle Preparation, and Biopsy

Acute lymphoblastic leukemia (blasts 65%, cellularity 95%); FAB: L1 subtype (see Comment).

Comment

Flow cytometry performed on bone marrow reveals precursor B-cell phenotype. The blasts are positive for CD10, CD19, CD22, CD34, and HLA-DR and negative for CD20, kappa (κ) and lambda (λ) light chain and also negative for other T-cell and myelomonocytic markers. Refer to the separate Flow Report (not included here). Cytogenetic studies are pending and will be reported separately. Results called to Dr. Z at 6 PM on 2/22/01.

ACKNOWLEDGMENTS

The author would like to thank Beth D. Borders, BS, MT(ASCP). Her many hours of dedicated and meticulous review have ensured a more accurate and easily readable chapter.

QUESTIONS

1. Which of the following is most variable in normal marrow?
   a. Differential count of 500 cells
   b. M:E ratio
   c. Cellularity
   d. Iron storage

2. Bone marrow aspirate smears are preferred to bone biopsy in diagnosis and classification of:
   a. Granulomatous diseases
   b. Acute leukemias
   c. Metastatic carcinomas
   d. Gaucher's disease

3. When quantitative measurement of bone marrow is performed, the layer most suitable for iron study is:
   a. Fat and perivascular cells
   b. Plasma
   c. Buffy coat of nucleated myeloid and erythroid cells
   d. Erythrocytes

4. Occasionally, nonhematopoietic cells are seen in marrow aspirates. Which of the following is most likely to be misidentified as a megakaryocyte?
   a. Reticular cell
   b. Storage histiocyte
   c. Osteoclast
   d. Endothelial cell

5. Trephine marrow biopsy is most useful in initial diagnosis of all of the following except:
   a. Refractory anemia
   b. Disseminated tuberculosis
   c. Renal cell carcinoma staging
   d. Lymphoma staging

6. In early infancy the most numerous cells of the bone marrow are:
   a. Erythroblasts
   b. Granulocytic precursors

c. Lymphocytes

d. Histiocytes-monocytes

7. When is bone marrow biopsy not indicated?
   a. When circulating blasts are seen on the peripheral smear
   b. For pancytopenia
   c. In thrombocytopenia with no apparent cause
   d. Spurious thrombocytopenia

8. Which is true for hematogones?
   a. They are malignant cells
   b. They belong to granulocytic series
   c. Morphologically they mimic blasts of lymphoblastic leukemia
   d. Usually they are seen in elderly individuals

9. Which is/are true for lymphoid aggregates?
   a. Paratrabecular lymphoid aggregates are usually malignant
   b. Benign aggregates are usually nonparatrabecular
   c. Reactive lymphoid aggregates usually have plasma cells at the periphery.
   d. All of the above

10. The most appropriate site for bone marrow studies in adults is:
    a. Anterior superior iliac crest
    b. Posterior superior iliac crest
    c. Sternum
    d. Spinal processes

SUMMARY CHART

➤ The hematopoietic system consists of bone marrow, liver, spleen, lymph nodes, and thymus. In normal adults, hematopoiesis occurs mainly in the bone marrow.

➤ The bone marrow is one of the body's largest organs, representing 3.4% to 6% of total body weight and averaging about 1500 g in adults.

➤ The structure of the bone marrow consists of hematopoietic cells (erythroid, myeloid, lymphoid, and megakaryocytes), adipose tissue, bone and its cells (osteoblasts and osteoclasts), and stroma.

➤ Erythropoiesis takes place in distinct anatomic units called erythropoietic islands.

➤ Granulocytic precursors are located deep in the hematopoietic cords and around the bone trabeculae.

➤ Megakaryopoiesis occurs adjacent to the sinus endothelium; megakaryocytes protrude as small cytoplasmic processes through the vascular wall, delivering platelets directly to the sinusoidal blood.

➤ Lymphocyte production is compartmentalized in lymphoid follicles, and lymphocytes are randomly dispersed throughout the hematopoietic cords.

➤ Hematogones are normal cellular constituents of bone marrow that resemble small- to intermediate-

sized lymphocytes; they range in size from 10 to 20 μm, have a high N:C ratio and deeply basophilic cytoplasm, and are devoid of any granules or vacuoles.

➤ The meshwork of stromal cells in which the hematopoietic cells are suspended is in a delicate semifluid state and is composed of reticulum cells, histiocytes, fat cells, and endothelial cells.

➤ Among the most common indicators for bone marrow studies are diseases that affect the bone marrow, causing a decrease or increase in any of the cellular blood elements.

➤ In adults, the most common site for bone marrow aspiration or biopsy is the posterior superior iliac crest; in newborns and infants, bone marrow is obtained from the upper end of the tibial bone.

➤ In a bone marrow aspiration, 1.0 to 1.5 mL of marrow particles and sinusoidal blood is drawn into a syringe; all direct smears should be prepared from unclotted specimens and labeled at the bedside with the patient's name, identification number, and date.

➤ When marrow cannot be aspirated ("dry tap"), the common differential diagnosis includes leukemia, myelofibrosis, and hairy cell leukemia.

➤ In the estimation of marrow cellularity (ratio of nucleated hematopoietic cells to fat cells) low-power magnification is used. Overall marrow cellularity in adults is about 50% +/− 10%.

➤ When performing the marrow differential count, at least 500 to 1000 nucleated cells are classified; the oil immersion objective is used, and megakaryocytes are not included in the differential count.

➤ The normal M:E (myeloid-to-erythroid) ratio for adults is 4:1; granulopoietic tissue occupies a marrow space that is two to four times greater than that occupied by the erythropoietic precursors.

➤ The storage form of iron in the bone marrow is hemosiderin. On Wright-stained smears, iron appears as brownish-blue granules.

References

1. Bloom, W, and Fawcett, DW: A Textbook of Histology, ed 10. WB Saunders, Philadelphia, 1975, pp 204–232
2. Tavassoli, M, and Jossey, JM: Bone marrow, structure and function. Alan R. Liss, New York, 1978, p 43.
3. Lichtman, MA: The ultrastructure of the hemopoietic environment of the marrow: A review. Exp Hematol 9:391, 1981.
4. Tavassoli, M, and Shaklai, M: Absence of tight junctions in endothelium of marrow sinuses: Possible significance for marrow cell egress. Erythropoiesis in bone marrow. Br J Haematol 41:303, 1979.
5. Aoki, M, and Tavassoli, M: Dynamics of red cell egress from bone marrow after blood letting. Br J Haematol 49:337, 1981.
6. Aoki, M, and Tavassoli, M: Red cell egress from bone marrow in state of transfusion plethora. Exp Hematol 9:231, 1981.
7. Gulati, GL, et al: Structure and function of the bone marrow and hematopoiesis. Hematol Oncol Clin North Am 2:495, 1988.
8. Western, H, and Bainton, DF: Association of alkaline-phosphatase-positive reticulum cells in bone marrow with granulocytic precursors. J Exp Med 150:919, 1979.
9. Lichtman, MA, et al: Parasinusoidal location of megakaryocytes in marrow. A determinant of platelet release. Am J Hematol 4:303, 1978.
10. Claman, HN, et al: Immunocompetence of transferred thymus–marrow cell combinations. J Immunol 97:828, 1966.
11. Hassett, JM: Humoral immunodeficiency: A review. Pediatr Ann 16:404, 1987.
12. Caldwell, CW, et al: B-cell precursors in normal pediatric bone marrow. Am J Clin Pathol 95:816, 1991.
13. Longacre, TA, et al: Hematogones: A multiparameter analysis of bone marrow precursor cells. Blood 73:432, 1989.
14. Van den Doel, LJ, et al: Immunological phenotype of lymphoid cells in regen-

erating marrow of children after treatment for acute lymphoblastic leukemia. Eur J Haematol 41:170, 1988.

15. Kobayashi, SD, et al: The transient appearance of small blastoid cells in the marrow after bone marrow transplantation. Am J Clin Pathol 96:191, 1991.

16. Gordon, MY: Annotation. Extracellular matrix of the marrow microenvironment. Br J Haematol 70:1, 1988.

17. Hutchinson, RM: Mastocytosis and co-existent non-Hodgkin's lymphoma and myeloproliferative disorders. Leuk Lymphoma 7:29, 1992.

18. Travis, WD, et al: Systemic mast cell diseases. Analysis of 58 cases and literature review. Medicine 67:345, 1988.

19. Clark, SC, and Kamen, R: The human hematopoietic colony-stimulating factors. Science 236:1229, 1987.

20. Neinhuis, AW: Hematopoietic growth factors. Biologic complexity and clinical practice. N Eng J Med 318:916, 1988.

21. Ogawa, M: Differentiation and proliferation of hematopoietic stem cells. Blood 81:2844, 1993.

22. Erslev, AJ: Humoral regulation of red cell production. Blood 8:349, 1953.

23. Erslev, AJ: Erythropoietin coming of age. N Engl J Med 316:101, 1987.

24. Camille, AN, and Marshall, AL: Structure of marrow. In Beutler, E, et al (eds): Williams Hematology, ed 5. McGraw-Hill, New York, 1995, p 31.

25. Becker, RP, and de Bruyn, PPH: The transmural passage of blood cells into myeloid sinusoids and the entry of platelets into the sinusoidal circulation. A scanning electron microscopic investigation. Am J Anat 145:183, 1976.

26. de Bruyn, P, et al: The migration of blood cells of the bone marrow through the sinusoidal wall. J Morphol 133:417, 1971.

27. Arinkin, MJ: Intravitale Untersuchungsmethodik der Knochenmarks. Folia Haematol (Leipz) 38:233, 1929.

28. Jamshidi, K, and Swaim, WR: Bone marrow biopsy with unaltered architecture. A new biopsy device. J Lab Clin Med 77:335, 1971.

29. Izadi, P, et al: Comparison of buffy coat preparation to direct method for the evaluation and interpretation of bone marrow aspirates. Am J Hematol 43:107, 1993.

30. Rywlin, AM, et al: A simple technique for the preparation of bone marrow smears and sections. Am J Clin Pathol 53:389, 1970.

31. Brynes, RK, et al: Bone marrow aspiration and trephine biopsy, an approach to a thorough study. Am J Clin Pathol 70:753, 1978.

32. Humphries, JE: Dry tap bone marrow aspiration: Clinical significance. Am J Hematol 35:247, 1990.

33. Carson, FL: Histotechnology—A Self Instructional Text. ASCP Press, Chicago, IL, 1990, pp 10, 38.

34. Wilkins, BS, and O'Brien, CJ: Techniques for obtaining differential cell counts from bone marrow trephine biopsy specimens. J Clin Pathol 41:558, 1988.

35. Williams, WJ, and Douglas, NA: Examination of the marrow. In Beutler, E, et al (eds): Williams Hematology, ed 5. McGraw-Hill, New York, 1995, p 18.

36. Rosse, C, et al: Bone marrow cell population of normal infants: The predominance of lymphocytes. J Lab Clin Med 89:1225, 1977.

37. Rubinstein, MA: Aspiration of bone marrow from iliac crest comparison of iliac crest and sternal bone marrow studies. JAMA 137:1821, 1948.

38. Hartsock, RJ, et al: Normal variations with aging of the amount of hematopoietic tissue in bone marrow from anterior iliac crest. Am J Clin Pathol 43:326, 1965.

39. Lee, GR, et al (eds): Microcystosis and the anemias associated with impaired hemoglobin synthesis. In Wintrobe's Clinical Hematology, ed 9, vol I. Lea & Febiger, Philadelphia, 1993, pp 799–800.

40. Hyun, BH, et al: Bone marrow examination: Techniques and interpretation. Hematol Oncol Clin North Am 2:513, 1988.

41. De Wolf Peeters, C: Bone marrow trephine interpretation: Diagnostic utility and potential pitfalls. Histopathology 18:489, 1991.

See Bibliography at the back of this book.

3

The Red Blood Cell

Structure and Function

DENISE M. HARMENING, PhD, MT(ASCP), CLS(NCA)
VIRGINIA C. HUGHES, MS, MT(ASCP)
CARMEN DEL TORO, MS, MT

RED BLOOD CELL MEMBRANE
Red Blood Cell Membrane Proteins
Deformability
Permeability
Red Blood Cell Membrane Lipids
Phospholipids
Glycolipids and Cholesterol

HEMOGLOBIN STRUCTURE AND FUNCTION
Hemoglobin Synthesis
Abnormal Hemoglobins of Clinical Importance
Maintenance of Hemoglobin Function: Active Red
    Blood Cell Metabolic Pathways

ERYTHROCYTE SENESCENCE
Extravascular Hemolysis
Intravascular Hemolysis

OBJECTIVES

At the end of this chapter, the learner should be able to:

1. List the areas of red cell metabolism that are crucial to normal red cell survival and function.

2. Describe the chemical composition of the red cell membrane in terms of percentage of lipids, proteins, and carbohydrates.

3. List the two most important red blood cell (RBC) membrane proteins and describe their function and the characteristics of deformability and permeability.

4. List the abnormalities that may lead to a

change in RBC structure and name the associated RBC morphology.

5. List the major lipid components of the red cell membrane.

6. Define the primary function of hemoglobin.

7. List the criteria for normal hemoglobin synthesis.

8. List the structural components of normal hemoglobin.

9. Describe hemoglobin function.

10. Describe the assembly of the protoporphyrin ring.

11. List the globin chains found in HbA, HbA$_2$, and HbF, and their respective concentrations (%) found in vivo.

12. Describe hemoglobin function in terms of the oxygen dissociation curve.

13. Define "shift to the left" in relation to the hemoglobin-oxygen dissociation curve.

14. Define "shift to the right" in relation to the hemoglobin-oxygen dissociation curve.

15. Define P$_{50}$ and state normal in vivo levels.

16. Define the toxic levels for abnormal hemoglobins of clinical importance.

17. List the various metabolic pathways involved in red cell metabolism, stating the specific function of each one.

18. List the steps in the extravascular breakdown of senescent RBCs.

19. List the steps in the intravascular breakdown of senescent RBCs.

20. List the proteins that carry the following components in circulation: iron, hemoglobin, dimers, metheme, and bilirubin.

Three areas of red blood cell (RBC) metabolism are crucial for normal erythrocyte survival and function: the RBC membrane, hemoglobin structure and function, and cellular energetics (Table 3–1). Defects or problems associated with any of these areas will result in impaired RBC survival. A thorough working knowledge of these areas of RBC physiology will ensure basic understanding of the various complex erythrocyte functions.

➤ RED BLOOD CELL MEMBRANE

The best accepted paradigm of the lipid bilayer and protein interaction in plasma membranes is the *fluid-mosaic model* introduced by Singer and Nickelson in 1974.[1] This two-dimensional model conceptualizes interactions of the transmembrane and cytoplasmic proteins within the RBC membrane lipids. The model suggests that membranes are dynamic structures composed of proteins and phospho-

> **Table 3-1**
> **AREAS OF RED CELL METABOLISM IMPORTANT IN NORMAL RBC SURVIVAL AND FUNCTION**
>
> - RBC membrane
> - Hemoglobin structure and function
> - RBC metabolic pathways

lipids and that the lipid bilayer is a fluid matrix because the interactions between lipids and proteins are noncovalent, allowing individual lipid and protein molecules to move laterally in the plane of the membrane.

The RBC membrane viewed by transmission electron microscopy (TEM) appears as a trilaminar structure consisting of a dark-light-dark band arrangement of layers (Fig. 3–1). These layers represent (1) an outer hydrophilic portion chemically composed of glycolipid, glycoprotein, and protein; (2) a central hydrophobic layer containing protein, cholesterol, and phospholipid; and (3) an inner hydrophilic layer containing protein. The RBC membrane is highly elastic, responds rapidly to applied stresses of fluid forces, and is capable of undergoing large membrane extensions without fragmentation.[2]

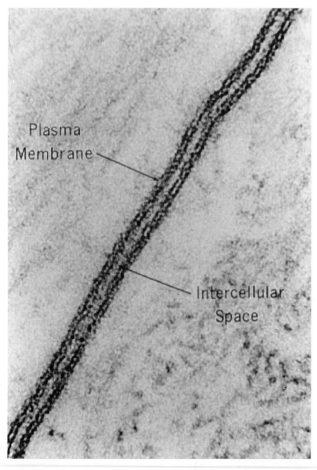

> **FIGURE 3–1**   Transmission electron microscopy (TEM) of plasma membrane.

The RBC membrane represents a semipermeable lipid bilayer supported by a meshlike cytoskeleton structure (Fig. 3–2). The RBC membrane cytoskeleton is a network of proteins on the inner surface of the plasma membrane that is responsible for maintaining the shape, stability, and deformability or flexibility of the RBC.[2] This fluid lipid matrix contains equal amounts of cholesterol and phospholipids with a mosaic of proteins interdispersed throughout at various intervals. Those proteins that extend from the outer surface and traverse the entire membrane to the inner cytoplasmic side of the RBC are termed *integral* membrane proteins. The other major class of RBC membrane proteins, called *peripheral* membrane proteins, is limited to the cytoplasmic surface of the membrane, which is beneath the lipid bilayer and forms the RBC cytoskeleton. Both the protein and the lipids are organized asymmetrically within the RBC membrane. The chemical composition of the membrane mass is approximately 40% lipids, 52% proteins, and 8% carbohydrates.[2]

Red Blood Cell Membrane Proteins

It is estimated that 10 major and 200 minor proteins are asymmetrically organized within the RBC membrane.[3] After solubilization of the RBC membrane with the detergent sodium dodecyl sulfate (SDS), membrane proteins can be separated by polyacrylamide gel electrophoresis and stained.[4] The separated RBC membrane proteins are numbered 1 through 8 when stained with Coomassie blue and 1 through 4 when stained with periodic acid–Schiff (PAS) stain, which forms the basis of their nomenclature (Fig. 3–3).[5] The proteins range in molecular weight from 16,000 to 244,000 daltons (d).

Two of the most important protein constituents include glycophorin, an integral membrane protein, and spectrin, a peripheral membrane protein. Table 3–2 lists the integral and peripheral membrane proteins.

Integral Membrane Proteins

Glycophorin is the principal RBC glycoprotein, representing approximately 20% of the total membrane protein.[6] The molecule contains approximately 60% carbohydrate and accounts for most of the membrane sialic acid, which gives the erythrocytes their negative charge, as a result of which they repel each other as they move through the circulation. Glycophorin, similar to other integral membrane proteins, spans the entire thickness of the lipid bilayer and appears on the external surface of the RBC membrane, accounting for the location of many RBC antigens. Four types of glycophorin have been described: A, B, and C (see PAS bands 1, 2, and 3), and D.[7] All glycoproteins are exposed on the outer RBC membrane surface and migrate primarily in band 3 of the SDS gel electrophoretic pattern stained with Coomassie blue (see Fig. 3–3). Most of these proteins, as mentioned previously, carry RBC antigens and are receptors (such as the glycophorins) or transport proteins (such as band 3, the anion exchange-channel glycoprotein). The plasma membrane envelope is anchored to the RBC cytoskeleton network of proteins through tethering sites of integral (transmembrane) proteins located in the lipid bilayer.[1] The condensed fluid lipid bilayer plus integral (transmembrane) proteins chemically isolates and regulates

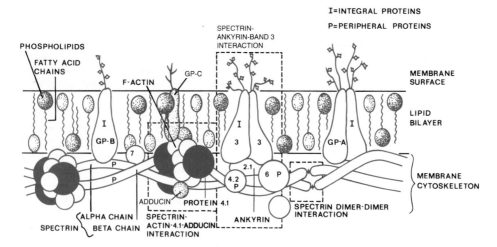

➤ **FIGURE 3–2** Schematic illustration of red blood cell membrane depicting the composition and arrangement of red cell membrane proteins. G = globin; GP-A = glycophorin A; GP-B = glycophorin B; GP-C = glycophorin C. Numbers refer to pattern of migration of sodium dodecyl sulfate (SDS) polyacrylamide gel pattern stained with Coomassie brilliant blue. Relations of proteins to each other and to lipids are purely hypothetical; however, the positions of the proteins relative to the inside or outside of the lipid bilayer are accurate. (Note: proteins are not drawn to scale, and many minor proteins are omitted.)

the cell interior. The RBC cytoskeleton network of proteins provides rigid support and stability to the lipid bilayer and is responsible for the deformability properties of the RBC membrane. It is speculated that band 3 and the glycophorins play a major role in anchoring the RBC membrane cytoskeleton to the lipid bilayer. As a result, lateral mobility of these integral proteins within the lipid bilayer is relatively restricted. Transmembrane (integral) proteins can also greatly influence mechanical stability and membrane rigidity.[3]

Peripheral Proteins

The major components of the red cell cytoskeleton include spectrin, ankyrin, protein 4.1, actin, and adducin.[8] Spectrin is clearly the most abundant peripheral protein of the RBC membrane cytoskeleton, comprising approximately 25% to 30% of the total membrane protein and 75% of the peripheral protein.[9]

Spectrin, a flexible rodlike molecule, is composed of a helix of two polypeptide chains, an alpha (α) chain (band 1, molecular weight 240,000 d) and a beta (β) chain (band 2, molecular weight 225,000 d).[9] These chains intertwined side to side form heterodimers, which link together with other αβ chains to form $(\alpha\beta)_2$ tetramers. Spectrin is an important factor in RBC membrane integrity, because it binds with other peripheral proteins such as actin (band 5), ankyrin (band 2.1), band 4.1, and adducin to form a skeletal network of microfilaments on the inner surface of the RBC membrane (see Fig. 3–2). These microfilaments strengthen the membrane, protecting the cell from being broken by circulatory shear forces, and also control the biconcave shape and deformability of the cell. In addition, the cytoskeletal network provides stability to the lipid bilayer interface.[1]

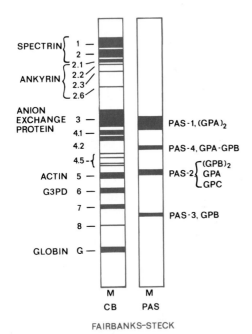

FAIRBANKS-STECK

➤ **FIGURE 3–3** Schematic illustration of SDS polyacrylamide gel electrophoresis patterns of red cell membrane proteins stained Coomassie brilliant blue (CB) and sialoglycoproteins stained with periodic acid-Schiff (PAS) stain. GPA, GPB, and GPC refer to glycophorins A, B, and C, respectively. $(GPA)_2$ and $(GPB)_2$ are the dimers, and GPA-GPB is the heterodimer of GPA and GPB.

➤ **Table 3-2**
RED CELL MEMBRANE INTEGRAL AND PERIPHERAL PROTEINS

Integral Proteins	Peripheral Proteins
Glycophorin A	Spectrin
Glycophorin B	Actin (band 5)
Glycophorin C	Ankyrin (band 2.1)
Glycophorin D	Band 4.1 and 4.2
Anion exchange-channel	Adducin
Protein (band 3)	p55

Two sets of spectrin complexes tie the RBC cytoskeleton network together and stabilize the spectrin-actin junction. A spectrin–actin–band 4.1–adducin complex and a spectrin-ankyrin complex bind to the integral protein, band 3, to anchor the skeleton to the overlaying lipid bilayer (see Fig. 3–2).[8] In addition, spectrin is also linked to the RBC lipid bilayer through the bonding of the complex 4.1, p55, and glycophorin C (GPC) in the erythrocyte membrane.[10] The phosphoprotein, p55, has recently been characterized as an obligate component of the protein 4.1–GPC complex, which regulates the stability and mechanical properties of the erythrocyte plasma membrane and is a member of a growing family of signaling and cytoskeletal proteins.[11] The preservation of the spectrin complexes, and thus the integrity of the RBC membrane, requires phosphorylation of spectrin by a protein kinase present in the membrane, which is energy-dependent, being catalyzed by adenosine triphosphate (ATP). Other peripheral membrane proteins that lack carbohydrates and are confined to the cytoplasmic membrane surface include certain enzymes such as glyceraldehyde-3-phosphate dehydrogenase (band 6) and structural proteins such as hemoglobin.

As mentioned earlier, the normal chemical composition, structural arrangement, and molecular interactions of the erythrocyte membrane are crucial to normal RBC survival. In addition, they play a critical role in two important RBC characteristics: deformability and permeability. Table 3–3 lists characteristics of the major components of the red cell membrane.

Deformability

RBC membrane deformability or flexibility is critical not only to RBC survival as the cell travels through the microvasculature, but also for its function of oxygen delivery.[12] Decreased cellular deformability and red cell shape changes have been recognized as distinguishing features of a number of congenital or hereditary hemolytic anemias leading to decreased RBC survival in these disorders (see Chaps. 9 and 10).

It has already been mentioned that a loss of ATP (energy) levels leads to a decrease in the phosphorylation of spectrin and, in turn, to a loss of membrane deformability. An accumulation or increase in deposition of membrane calcium also results, causing an increase in membrane rigidity and loss of pliability. These cells are at a marked disadvantage when they pass through the small (3- to 5-μm diameter) sinusoidal orifices of the spleen, one of the functions of which is extravascular sequestration and removal of aged, damaged, or less deformable RBC or fragments of their membrane (Fig. 3–4). The loss of RBC membrane is exemplified by the formation of spherocytes (Fig. 3–5), cells with a reduced surface-to-volume ratio, and the so-called bite cells (Fig. 3–6), in which the removal of a portion of membrane has left a permanent indentation in the remaining cell membrane. The survival time of these forms is also shortened.

Shape change from the normal symmetric and resilient discoid shape of the RBC can be stimulated by a variety of factors, which include both mechanically induced and chemically induced forces.[2] Spectrin molecules exist in a folded conformation in the membrane of the nondeformed red cell. During reversible membrane deformability, certain spectrin molecules become uncoiled and extended, whereas others become more compressed and folded, resulting in a rearrangement of the cytoskeletal network.[13] This reversible RBC membrane deformability results in a shape change while maintaining a constant surface area. The limit to reversible RBC membrane deformability oc-

> ## Table 3-3
CHARACTERISTICS OF THE MAJOR COMPONENTS OF THE RED CELL MEMBRANE

Protein	Size	Function
Spectrin*	0.1-μm heterodimeric filamentous protein consisting of a 240-kd α chain and a 225-kd β chain constitutes 25%–30% of the mass of membrane proteins	Principal structural element of RBC membrane, which plays a major role in the RBC cytoskeleton membrane organization
Ankyrin*	210-kd globular protein composed of 1879 amino acids	Primary determinant of mechanical coupling of the lipid bilayer to the membrane skeleton
Adducin*	Protein doublet of approximately 97 and 103 kd	Promotes the association of spectrin with F-actin in a manner similar to band 4.1
Band 4.1*	Composed of 622 amino acids, constitutes 5% of the mass of membrane proteins	Dual functions: promotes high-affinity association between spectrin and F-actin and may link the skeleton to the membrane by virtue of its associations with glycophorin and band 3
Band 3	Major RBC transmembrane protein and major integral protein that has two distinct domains: the transmembrane and cytoplasmic; 911-amino acid protein, comprising 15%–20% of the total membrane protein	Two separate functions: catalyzes chloride-bicarbonate exchange and contains binding sites for ankyrin, band 4.1, band 4.2, and several glycolytic enzymes
Band 4.2	Known to associate with the cytoplasmic domain of band 3	Actual function unknown; however, a deficiency of the protein is associated with several types of inherited hemolytic anemias

*Denotes major components of the red cell cytoskeleton.
Source: Data from Mohandes, N, and Chasis, JA: Red blood cell deformity, membrane material properties and shape: Regulation by transmembrane, skeletal and cytoplasmic proteins and lipids. Semin Hematol 30:171, 1993; and Cohen, CM, and Gascard, P: Regulation and post-translated modification of erythrocyte membrane and membrane-skeletal proteins. Semin Hematol 29:244, 1992.

curs when applied forces break the protein-to-protein associations, necessitating an increase in surface area.[9] RBC membrane deformability is characterized as irreversible when red cells are exposed to forces great enough to require an increase in surface area, leading to membrane fragmentation and instability of the cytoskeleton network.[13] Table 3–4 lists a wide variety of chemical changes that can induce shape changes in the red cell.

Permeability

The RBC membrane is freely permeable to water and anions; chloride (Cl^-) and bicarbonate (HCO_3^-) traverse the membrane in less than a second. It is speculated that this massive exchange of bicarbonate and chloride ions occurs through a large number of exchange channels formed by the integral membrane protein, band 3. In contrast, the RBC membrane is relatively impermeable to cations, with a half-time exchange of sodium (Na^+) and potassium (K^+) of more than 30 hours. It is primarily through the control of the sodium and potassium intracellular concentrations that the RBC maintains its volume and water homeostasis. The erythrocyte intracellular-to-extracellular ratios for sodium and potassium are 1:12 and 25:1, respectively. The passive influx of sodium

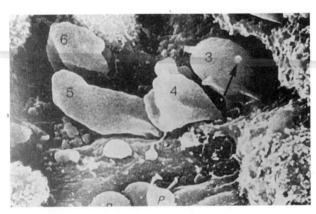

➤ **FIGURE 3–4** Scanning electron micrograph (SEM) of red cells (3 to 6) squeezing through fenestrated wall in transit from splenic cords to sinus. Epithelial linings of sinus wall to which platelets (P) adhere, along with "hairy" white cells, probably macrophages, are shown. (From Weiss, L: A scanning electron microscopic study of the spleen. Blood 43:665, 1974, with permission.)

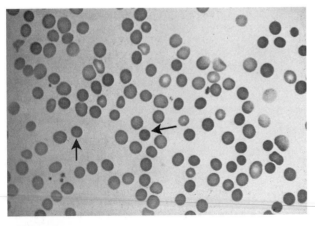

➤ **FIGURE 3–5** Spherocytes.

➤ **FIGURE 3–6** Bite cells.

and potassium is controlled by as many as 300 cationic pumps that actively transport sodium out of the cell and potassium into the cell. Like other cationic pumps, these sodium-potassium pumps are energy-dependent, requiring ATP. The functional active transport of these particular cations by these cationic pumps also requires the membrane enzyme sodium-potassium ATPase. It is interesting to note that full activation of the sodium-potassium-ATPase pumps requires the presence of the RBC membrane amino phospholipid phosphatidyl serine. Similarly, calcium (Ca^{2+}) is also actively pumped from the interior of the RBC and into the plasma through the energy-dependent calcium-ATPase cationic pump. Calmodulin, a cytoplasmic calcium-binding protein that contains four high-affinity calcium binding sites, is speculated to control these calcium-ATPase pumps. When calcium-calmodulin complexes form, the calcium-ATPase pump is activated, preventing excessive intracellular calcium buildup, which is deleterious to the RBC, resulting in shape changes and loss of deformability.[14] Moreover, studies have shown that calmodulin may have a more dynamic role in maintaining erythrocyte structure. When intracellular calcium is increased, calmodulin binds to its calcium-dependent site, causing a conformational change in protein 4.1 that decreases its affinity for both GPC and p55 and subsequently weakening the aforementioned spectrin-4.1 complexes, which leads to membrane instability.[10]

The permeability properties of the RBC membrane, as well as active cation transport, are crucial to the prevention of colloid osmotic hemolysis and controlling the volume of the RBC. In addition, ATP-depleted cells allow the accumulation of excess intracellular calcium and sodium fol-

➤ **Table 3-4**

BIOCHEMICAL CHANGES THAT CAN TRANSFORM RBC DISCS INTO CRENATED FORMS

- Low concentration of fatty acids and phospholipids
- A variety of amphoteric agents
- Elevated intracellular calcium concentration
- Decreased adenosine triphosphate (ATP) levels

lowed by potassium and water loss, resulting in a dehydrated, rigid cell subsequently sequestered by the spleen. The energy required for active transport and maintenance of membrane electrochemical gradients is provided by ATP. Any abnormality that increases membrane permeability or alters cationic transport may lead to a decrease in RBC survival.

Red Blood Cell Membrane Lipids

Phospholipids

The erythrocyte membrane lipid consists of a bilayer of phospholipids interspersed with molecules of unesterified cholesterol that are present in nearly equimolar quantities. Free fatty acids and glycolipids are present in small quantities.[2] Two groups of phospholipids, choline phospholipids and amino phospholipids, are known to possess a distinct asymmetry within the bilayer matrix of the RBC. The asymmetry allows selective movement of molecules into and out of the cell membrane.

Choline phospholipids, consisting of phosphatidyl choline and sphingomyelin, are primarily located on the outside half of the lipid bilayer, readily accessible to the external environment.[15] Because of their outward orientation in the lipid bilayer, the choline phospholipids may represent controlling points in the major pathways of lipid renewal, because there is an exchange between plasma fatty acids and the RBC membrane. Fatty acids are incorporated through an energy-dependent process into membrane phospholipids. Therefore, changes in body lipid transport and metabolism may cause abnormalities in the plasma phospholipid concentration that may alter the RBC membrane composition, resulting in a decreased RBC survival in circulation. In addition, cholesterol has a pronounced effect on membrane fluidity. Its interaction with phospholipids has been referred to as the "intermediate gel state," because membranes containing excess cholesterol are more viscous and less fluidic. This leads to a decrease in membrane deformability and RBC survival.[2]

In contrast, amino phospholipids, consisting of phosphatidylethanolamine and phosphatidylserine, are located almost exclusively on the inside half or cytoplasmic side of the RBC membrane along with phosphatidylinositol. The specific orientation of these phospholipids maintains a precise lipid pattern that is critical to normal RBC survival in circulation. Alteration of this arrangement, leading to the abnormal appearance of these amino phospholipids on the outer surface of the lipid bilayer, promotes activation of the clotting cascade and may result in extravascular hemolysis. Stabilization of this phospholipid asymmetry in the erythrocyte membrane is maintained through the interaction with specific peripheral membrane proteins (see the discussion under Red Blood Cell Membrane Proteins, earlier).

Glycolipids and Cholesterol

Most of the glycolipids are located in the outer half of the lipid bilayer and interact with glycoproteins to form many of the RBC antigens. Cholesterol is approximately equally distributed, being located on both sides of the lipid bilayer inserted between the choline and amino phospholipids. Cholesterol comprises 25% of the RBC membrane lipid and is present in a 1:1 molar ratio with phospholipids. RBC membrane cholesterol is in continual exchange with plasma cholesterol and is, therefore, affected by changes in body lipid transport.

As mentioned, accumulation of cholesterol results in a more viscous membrane with subsequent morphological changes in the RBCs such as target cells (Fig. 3–7), and may cause RBC membrane damage. Acanthocytes, RBCs with irregular, spiny projections called *spicules* (Fig. 3–8), have also been associated with an excess accumulation of membrane cholesterol in association with liver disease and inherited lipid disorders such as abetalipoproteinemia and lecithin-cholesterol acyltransferase deficiency (LCAT). The former disorder is caused by a decrease in apolipoprotein B (Apo B) in the blood with subsequent decreases in plasma and membrane lipids. The patient's red cells appear as acanthocytes with increased membrane rigidity.[16,17] LCAT deficiency results in a reduction of plasma cholesterol esters and increased free cholesterol in the plasma.[18,19] Target cell formation results from the subsequent increase in membrane cholesterol. All of these RBCs have a decreased survival rate because the excess lipid makes the cell membrane less deformable.

In general, all of these lipids are mobile within the plane of the erythrocyte membrane, and as a result of this phenomenon, the RBC membrane is characteristically a viscous, two-dimensional fluid. This lipid bilayer also acts as an impenetrable barrier. Consequently, most transport

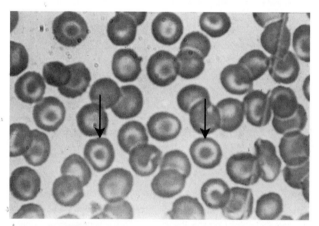

➤ **FIGURE 3–7** Target cells.

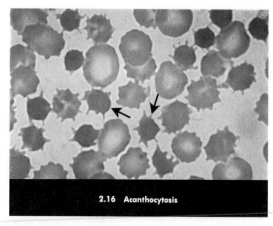

2.16 Acanthocytosis

➤ **FIGURE 3–8** Acanthocytes.

across the RBC membrane occurs through transport protein globules. Table 3–5 summarizes the abnormalities that can lead to a change in RBC morphology.

➤ HEMOGLOBIN STRUCTURE AND FUNCTION

Hemoglobin, a conjugated globular protein with a molecular weight of approximately 64.4 kilodaltons (kd), constitutes 95% of the RBC dry weight, or 33% of the RBC weight by volume.[20] Approximately 65% of the hemoglobin synthesis occurs during the nucleated stages of RBC maturation, and 35% occurs during the reticulocyte stage. Normal hemoglobin consists of globin (a tetramer of two pairs of unlike globin polypeptide chains) and four heme groups, each of which contains a protoporphyrin ring plus ferrous iron (Fe^{2+}).

Hemoglobin Synthesis

Normal hemoglobin production is dependent on three processes (Fig. 3–9):

1. Adequate iron delivery and supply
2. Adequate synthesis of protoporphyrins (the precursor of heme)
3. Adequate globin synthesis

Iron Delivery and Supply

Iron, in the ferric state (Fe^{3+}), is delivered to the membrane of the RBC precursor by the protein carrier transferrin. Most of the iron that crosses the membrane and enters the cytoplasm of the cell is committed to hemoglobin synthesis and thereby proceeds to the mitochondria (where ferric iron is reduced to ferrous [Fe^{2+}] for insertion into the protoporphyrin ring to form heme). Excess iron in the cytoplasm aggregates as ferritin, the amount of which depends on the ratio between the level of plasma iron and the amount of iron required by the erythrocyte for hemoglobin synthesis.[21] Two-thirds of the total body iron supply is bound to heme in the hemoglobin molecule (see Chap. 6 for a discussion of iron kinetics).

Synthesis of Protoporphyrins

Protoporphyrin synthesis begins in the mitochondria with the formation of delta-aminolevulinic acid (δALA) from the amino acid, glycine, and succinyl coenzyme A (CoA), which is the major rate-limiting step in heme biosynthesis (Fig. 3–10). The mitochondrial enzyme, δALA synthetase,

which mediates this reaction, is influenced by erythropoietin and requires the presence of the cofactor pyridoxal phosphate (vitamin B_6).[22]

Porphyrinogens, not porphyrins, are the intermediates of heme synthesis. Porphyrinogens are unstable tetrapyrroles that are readily and irreversibly oxidized to form porphyrins. In contrast, porphyrins are highly stable resonating molecules that are normally found in small quantities in the urine as a result of normal RBC catabolism.[23]

Excessive formation of porphyrins can occur if any one of the normal enzymatic steps in heme synthesis is blocked and can result in one of a number of metabolic disorders collectively called the *porphyrias*.[24]

Globin Synthesis

Globin chain synthesis occurs on RBC-specific cytoplasmic ribosomes, which are initiated from the inheritance of various structural genes. Each gene results in the formation of a specific polypeptide chain. Each somatic diploid cell, including the RBC, contains four alpha (α), two zeta (ζ), two beta (β), two delta (δ), two epsilon (ϵ), and four gamma (γ) genes.[2] The α and ζ genes are located on chromosome 16, and the β, δ, ϵ, and γ genes on chromosome 11 (Fig. 3–11). The resulting gene products formed have been called α, ζ, β, δ, ϵ, and γ globin chains. Throughout embryonic and fetal development, activation of the globin genes progresses from the ζ to the α gene and from the ϵ to the γ, δ, and β genes.[2]

The ϵ and ζ chains normally appear only during embryonic development (Table 3–6). These two chains, plus the α and γ chains, are constituents of embryonic hemoglobins: Hb Gower 1 ($\zeta_2\epsilon_2$), Hb Gower 2 ($\alpha_2\epsilon_2$), and Hb Portland ($\zeta_2\gamma_2$). The ϵ and ζ chains are produced up to approximately 3 months following conception. The α chain is always present. Production of γ chains is active from the third fetal month until 1 year postnatally. In the fetus, the major hemoglobin is $\alpha_2\gamma_2$ (hemoglobin F). The γ chains occur as a mixture of two types of chains, differing only by one amino acid at position 136. G-gamma ($^G\gamma$) contains glycine, whereas A-gamma ($^A\gamma$) has alanine at that position.[25] The ratio of $^G\gamma$ to $^A\gamma$ is approximately 3:1 at birth and 2:3 by 1 year of age.[17] By the age of 2 years, hemoglobin F comprises less than 2% of the total hemoglobin. Production of β chains rises gradually prenatally and reaches adult percentages between 3 and 6 months postnatally.[25] Figure 3–12 depicts the time sequence of globin chain synthesis during fetal development, birth, and infancy.

All normal adult hemoglobins are formed as tetramers consisting of two α chains plus two (non-α) globin chains. Normal adult RBCs contain the following types of hemoglobin:

- 95% to 97% of the hemoglobin is HbA, which consists of $\alpha_2\beta_2$ chains.
- 2% to 3% of the hemoglobin is HbA$_2$, which consists of $\alpha_2\delta_2$ chains.
- 1% to 2% of the hemoglobin is HbF (fetal hemoglobin), which consists of $\alpha_2\gamma_2$ chains.

In the cytoplasm, each synthesized globin chain links with heme (ferroprotoporphyrin IX) to form hemoglobin, which primarily consists of two α chains, two β chains, and four heme groups. Normal α chains consist of 141 amino acid residues linked together in a linear fashion, whereas normal β chains (as well as δ, γ, and ϵ) consist of 146 amino acid residues. Table 3–6 shows the composition of hemoglobin

➤ Table 3-5
ABNORMALITIES THAT CAN LEAD TO A CHANGE IN RBC MORPHOLOGY

Abnormality	RBC Morphology
Cholesterol accumulation in the RBC membrane (i.e., liver disease)	Target cells
Abetalipoproteinemia with cholesterol accumulation	Acanthocytes
LCAT deficiency with cholesterol accumulation	Hemolysis with red cell fragmentation
Decreased phosphorylated spectrin or altered spectrin	Bite cells and spherocytes

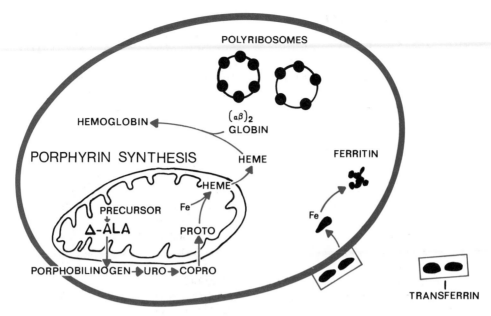

➤ **FIGURE 3–9** Hemoglobin synthesis in the reticulocyte. Δ-ALA = delta-aminolevulinic acid. URO = uroporphyrinogen, COPRO = coproporphyrinogen.

found during normal human development. The precise order of amino acids is critical to the structure and function of the hemoglobin molecule.

The rate of globin synthesis is directly related to the rate of porphyrin synthesis, and vice versa: protoporphyrin synthesis is reduced when globin synthesis is impaired. There is, however, no such relationship with iron uptake when either globin or protoporphyrin synthesis is impaired; iron accumulates in the RBC cytoplasm as ferritin aggregates. The iron-laden, nucleated RBC is termed a *sideroblast,* and the anucleated form, a *siderocyte,* when stained with Prussian blue for visualization of iron (see Fig. 6–11; see also Color Plate

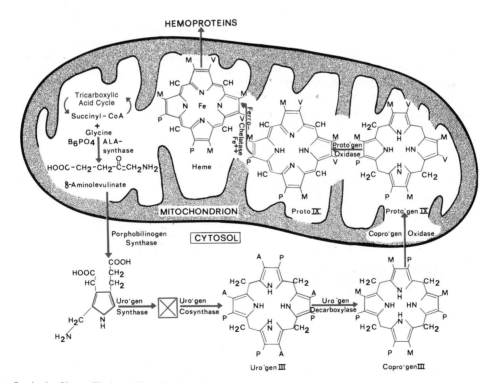

➤ **FIGURE 3–10** Synthesis of heme. The heme biosynthetic pathway, showing the distribution of enzymes between the mitochondria and the cytoplasm. Condensation of glycine and succinyl coenzyme A yields δALA, which is irreversible; two molecules of ALA undergo condensation by the enzyme *ALA dehydrase* to yield porphobilinogen (PBG). In the presence of *uroporphyrinogen III cosynthase* and *uroporphyrinogen I synthase,* PBG yields uroporphyrinogen III. Uroporphyrinogen III undergoes four decarboxylation steps, catalyzed by the enzyme *uroporphyrinogen decarboxylase,* to yield coproporphyrinogen III. Coproporphyrinogen III is transported from the cytosol into the mitochondria, where the enzyme *coproporphyrinogen oxidase* acts on the propionic acid side chains to yield protoporphyrinogen IX. Catalyzed by *protoporphyrinogen IX oxidase,* protoporphyrinogen IX is oxidized to protoporphyrin IX. Protoporphyrin IX combines with ferrous iron to yield heme (catalyzed by *heme synthase*). (Intermediates between uroporphyrinogen and coproporphyrinogen, designated by X, remain unidentified.) B_6PO_4 = pyridoxal phosphate. (From Tietz, MW: Textbook of Clinical Chemistry. WB Saunders, Philadelphia, 1986, with permission.)

GENE PRODUCTS (GLOBIN CHAINS)
HEMOGLOBINS (Hb)

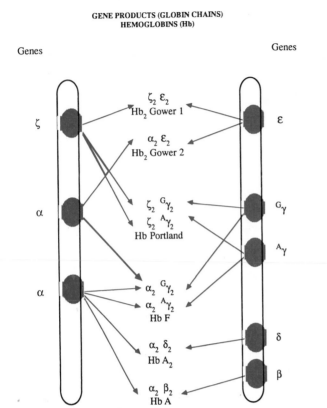

> FIGURE 3–11   Genetic control and formation of human hemoglobins.

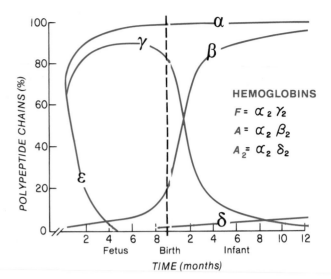

> FIGURE 3–12   Changes in globin chain synthesis during fetal development, birth, and infancy. (From Hillman, RF, and Finch, CA: Red Cell Manual, ed 7. FA Davis, Philadelphia, 1996, p 11, with permission.)

82). When protoporphyrin synthesis is impaired, the mitochondria become encrusted with iron, which is visible around the nucleus of the RBC precursor when stained with Prussian blue. Such an RBC is termed a *ringed sideroblast* and is diagnostic for a pathogenesis linked to deficient protoporphyrin synthesis (see Fig. 6–11; see also Color Plate 82).

Hemoglobin Function

Hemoglobin's primary function is delivery and release of oxygen to the tissues and facilitation of carbon dioxide excretion. Because of hemoglobin's multichain structure, the molecule is capable of a considerable amount of allosteric movement as it loads and unloads oxygen. One of the most

important controls of hemoglobin affinity for oxygen is the RBC organic phosphate 2,3-diphosphoglycerate (2,3-DPG). The unloading of oxygen by hemoglobin is accompanied by the widening of the space between β chains and the binding of 2,3-DPG on a mole-for-mole basis, with the formation of anionic salt bridges between the β chains.[26] The resulting conformation of the deoxyhemoglobin molecule is known as the tense (T) form, which has a lower affinity for oxygen. When hemoglobin loads oxygen and becomes oxyhemoglobin, the established salt bridges are broken and β chains are pulled together, expelling 2,3-DPG. This relaxed (R) form of the hemoglobin molecule has a higher affinity for oxygen.

These allosteric changes that occur as the hemoglobin loads and unloads oxygen are referred to as the *respiratory movement*.[27] The dissociation and binding of oxygen by hemoglobin are not directly proportional to the PO_2 of its environment, but instead exhibit a sigmoid-curve relationship—the hemoglobin-oxygen dissociation curve depicted in Figure 3–13. The shape of this curve is very important physiologically because it permits a considerable amount of oxygen to be delivered to the tissues with a small drop in oxygen tension. For example, in the environment of the lungs, where the PO_2 (oxygen tension), measured in millimeters of mercury (mm Hg), is nearly 100 mm Hg, the hemoglobin molecule is almost 100% saturated with oxygen (see Fig. 3–13, point A). As the RBCs travel to the tissues, where the PO_2 drops to an average 40 mm Hg (mean venous oxygen tension), the hemoglobin saturation drops to approximately 75%, releasing approximately 25% of the oxygen to the tissues (see Fig. 3–13, point B).

This is the normal situation of oxygen delivery at basal metabolic rate. In conditions such as hypoxia, a compensatory "shift to the right" of the hemoglobin-oxygen dissociation curve (Fig. 3–14) occurs to alleviate a tissue oxygen deficit. This rightward shift of the curve, mediated by increased levels of 2,3-DPG, results in a decrease in the affinity of hemoglobin for the oxygen molecule and an increase in oxygen delivery to the tissues. Note that the oxygen saturation of hemoglobin in the environment of the tissues (40 mm Hg PO_2; see Fig. 3–13, point B) is now only 50%; the other

> ## Table 3-6
> ## COMPOSITION OF HEMOGLOBIN FOUND IN NORMAL HUMAN DEVELOPMENT

Globin Chains	Hemoglobin	Stage of Development
$\alpha_2\epsilon_2$	Gower 2	Embryo
$\zeta_2\epsilon_2$	Gower 1	
$\zeta_2\gamma_2$	Portland	
$\alpha_2{}^A\gamma_2$	F	Fetus
$\alpha_2{}^G\gamma_2$	F	
$\alpha_2\beta_2$	A	Adult
$\alpha_2\delta_2$	A_2	

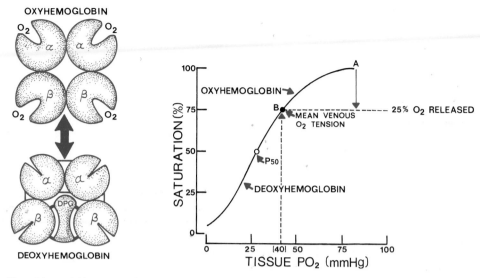

> ➤ **FIGURE 3–13**   Normal hemoglobin-oxygen dissociation curve. (From Hillman, RF, and Finch, CA: Red Cell Manual, ed 7. FA Davis, Philadelphia, 1996, p 18, with permission.)

50% of the oxygen is being released to the tissues. The RBCs thus have become more efficient in terms of oxygen delivery.

Therefore, a patient who is suffering from an anemia caused by a loss of RBCs may be able to compensate by shifting the oxygen dissociation curve to the right, making the RBCs, though fewer in number, more efficient. Some patients may be able to tolerate anemia better than others because of this compensatory mechanism. A shift to the right also may occur in response to acidosis or a rise in body temperature.[28] The shift to the right of the hemoglobin-oxygen dissociation curve is only one way in which patients may compensate for various types of hypoxia; other ways include increases in total cardiac output and in erythropoiesis.

A shift to the left of the hemoglobin-oxygen dissociation curve conversely results in an increase in hemoglobin-oxygen affinity and a decrease in oxygen delivery to the tissues (Fig. 3–15). With such a dissociation curve, RBCs are much less efficient because only 12% of the oxygen can be released to the tissues (point B). Among the conditions that can shift the oxygen dissociation curve to the left are alkalosis; increased quantities of abnormal hemoglobins, such as methemoglobin and carboxyhemoglobin; increased quantities of hemoglobin F; or multiple transfusions of 2,3-DPG–depleted stored blood (attesting to the importance of 2,3-DPG in oxygen release).[28]

Hemoglobin-oxygen affinity also can be expressed by P_{50} values, which designate the PO_2 at which hemoglobin is 50% saturated with oxygen under standard in vitro conditions of temperature and pH.[28] The P_{50} of normal blood is 26 to 30 mm Hg.[28] An increase in P_{50} represents a decrease in hemoglobin-oxygen affinity, or a shift to the right of the oxygen dissociation curve. A decrease in P_{50} represents an increase in the hemoglobin-oxygen affinity, or a shift to the left of the hemoglobin-oxygen dissociation curve. In addition to the reasons listed previously for shifts in the curve, inherited abnormalities of the hemoglobin molecule can result in either situation. These abnormalities are described by the P_{50} measurements. Abnormalities in hemoglobin structure or function can therefore have profound effects on the ability of RBCs to provide oxygen to the tissues.

Abnormal Hemoglobins of Clinical Importance

The hemoglobins previously described—oxyhemoglobin and reduced hemoglobin—are physiologic hemoglobins because they function in the transport and delivery of oxy-

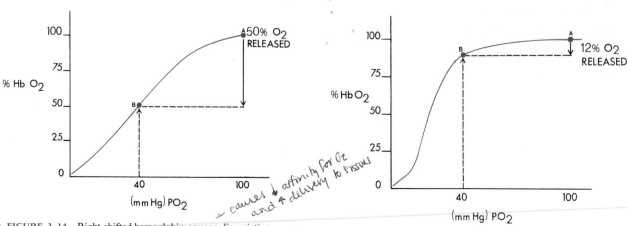

> ➤ **FIGURE 3–14**   Right-shifted hemoglobin-oxygen dissociation curve.

> ➤ **FIGURE 3–15**   Left-shifted hemoglobin-oxygen dissociation curve.

gen within the circulation. Abnormal hemoglobins of clinical significance that are unable to transport or deliver oxygen include the following:

1. Carboxyhemoglobin
2. Methemoglobin
3. Sulfhemoglobin

In carboxyhemoglobin, the oxygen molecules bound to heme have been replaced with carbon monoxide (CO). This replacement process is relatively slow and dependent on the concentration of carbon monoxide in the blood. Once attached, however, the binding of carbon monoxide to the heme of the hemoglobin molecule is 200 times tighter than the binding of oxygen to heme.[29] The concentration of carbon monoxide can be increased in a number of conditions, including that of chronic heavy smokers.

Methemoglobin is formed when the iron of the hemoglobin molecule is oxidized to the ferric (Fe^{3+}) state.[29] Normally, less than 1% of the total circulating hemoglobin is in the methemoglobin form. Increased formation of methemoglobin can occur as a result of an overload to oxidant stress, owing to the ingestion of strong oxidant drugs or to an enzyme deficiency (see the following section on RBC metabolic pathways).[30]

Sulfhemoglobin is formed when a certain situation or condition, such as ingestion of a sulfur-containing drug or chronic constipation, causes the sulfur content of the blood to build up.[31] Sulfhemoglobin is incapable of carrying oxygen and represents an irreversible change of the hemoglobin molecule that persists until the RBCs are removed from the circulation. Both carboxyhemoglobin and methemoglobin, however, can be reverted to oxyhemoglobin through the use of oxygen inhalation and the administration of strong reducing substances, respectively. Table 3–7 lists the toxic levels for each abnormal hemoglobin at which cyanosis, anemia, and death may result from a tissue oxygen deficit and increased concentration of circulating abnormal hemoglobin.

➤ MAINTENANCE OF HEMOGLOBIN FUNCTION: ACTIVE RED BLOOD CELL METABOLIC PATHWAYS

Active erythrocyte metabolic pathways are necessary for the production of adequate ATP levels. Such generated energy is crucial to RBC survival and function in that it is necessary for maintaining (1) hemoglobin function, (2) membrane integrity and deformability, (3) RBC volume, and (4) adequate amounts of reduced pyridine nucleotides.

RBCs generate energy almost exclusively through the anaerobic breakdown of glucose, because the metabolism of the anucleated erythrocyte is more limited than that of

other body cells. The adult RBC possesses little ability to metabolize fatty acids and amino acids. Additionally, mature RBCs contain no mitochondrial apparatus for oxidative metabolism (Table 3–8). The RBC metabolic pathways are mainly anaerobic, fortunately, because the function of the RBC is to deliver oxygen and not to consume it. Four pathways of RBC metabolism will be considered: the anaerobic glycolytic pathway, and three ancillary pathways that serve to maintain the function of hemoglobin (Fig. 3–16). All of these processes are essential if the RBC is to transport oxygen and maintain the physical characteristics required for its survival in circulation.

Of the ATP needed by RBCs, 90% is generated by the Embden-Meyerhof glycolytic pathway.[29] Here, the metabolism of glucose results in the net generation of two molecules of ATP. Although this ATP synthesis is inefficient when compared with cells that use the Krebs cycle (aerobic metabolism), it provides sufficient ATP for the requirements of the RBCs. Glycolysis also generates NADH from NAD^+, which is important in some of the other RBC metabolic pathways.

Another 5% to 10% of glucose is metabolized by the hexose monophosphate shunt (also called the *phosphogluconate pathway*).[29] This pathway produces the pyridine nucleotide NADPH from $NADP^+$. NADPH, together with reduced glutathione, provides the main line of defense for the RBC against oxidative injury.[32] Oxidant drugs, as well as infections, can cause the accumulation of hydrogen peroxide and other oxidants, which can be toxic to cell proteins. The sequence of biochemical reactions shown in Figure 3–17 occurs within the normal RBC with adequate levels of appropriate enzymes and substrate to prevent the accumulation of these agents.

When the hexose monophosphate pathway is functionally deficient, the amount of reduced glutathione becomes insufficient to neutralize intracellular oxidants. This results in globin denaturation and precipitation as aggregates (Heinz bodies) within the cell. If this process sufficiently damages the membrane, cell destruction occurs. Inherited defects in the pentose phosphate glutathione pathway, the most common of which is glucose-6-phosphate dehydrogenase (G6PD) deficiency, result in the formation of Heinz bodies with subsequent extravascular hemolysis.[33] (Glutathione is not only crucial to keeping hemoglobin in a functional state but it is also important in maintaining RBC integrity by reducing sulfhydryl groups of hemoglobin, membrane protein, and enzymes subsequent to oxidation.)

The methemoglobin reductase pathway is another important component of RBC metabolism. Two methemoglobin reductase systems are important in maintaining heme iron in the reduced (Fe^{2+}, ferrous) functional state.[8] Both pathways depend on the regeneration of reduced pyridine nucleotide and are referred to as the NADH and NADPH methemoglobin reductase pathways. In the absence of the enzyme methemoglobin reductase and the reducing action of the pyridine nucleotide NADH, there is an accumulation of methemoglobin, resulting from the conversion of the ferrous iron of heme to the ferric form (Fe^{3+}). Methemoglobin is a nonfunctional form of hemoglobin, having lost oxygen transport capabilities, as the metheme portion cannot combine with oxygen. Normal efficiency of the methemoglobin reductase pathway is exemplified by the fact that usually no more than 1% of RBC hemoglobin exists as methemoglobin in the RBCs of healthy individuals.[25]

➤ Table 3-7
TOXIC LEVELS FOR ABNORMAL HEMOGLOBINS OF CLINICAL IMPORTANCE

Abnormal Hemoglobin	Toxic Level (g%)
Carboxyhemoglobin	5.0
Methemoglobin	1.5
Sulfhemoglobin	0.5

> **Table 3-8**

COMPARISON OF RED BLOOD CELL METABOLIC ACTIVITIES DURING VARIOUS STAGES OF MATURATION

	Nucleated RBC	Reticulocyte	Adult RBC
Replication	+	0	0
DNA synthesis	+	0	0
RNA synthesis	+	0	0
Lipid synthesis	+	+	0
RNA present	+	+	0
Heme synthesis	+	+	0
Protein synthesis	+	+	0
Mitochondria	+	+	0
Krebs' tricarboxylic acid cycle	+	+	0
Embden-Meyerhof pathway	+	+	+
Pentose phosphate pathway	+	+	+
Maturation and/or senescence	+	+	+

Another important pathway that is crucial to RBC function is the Leubering-Rapoport shunt. This pathway causes an extraordinary accumulation of the RBC organic phosphate 2,3-DPG, which is important because of its profound effect on the affinity of hemoglobin for oxygen. Stores of this organic phosphate can serve as a reserve for additional ATP generation.

> ## ERYTHROCYTE SENESCENCE

The RBC, a 6- to 8-μm biconcave disc (Fig. 3–18), travels 200 to 300 miles during its 120-day life span. During this time, circulating RBCs undergo the *process* of senescence or aging. Various metabolic and physical changes associated with the aging of RBCs are listed in Table 3–9. Each day 1%

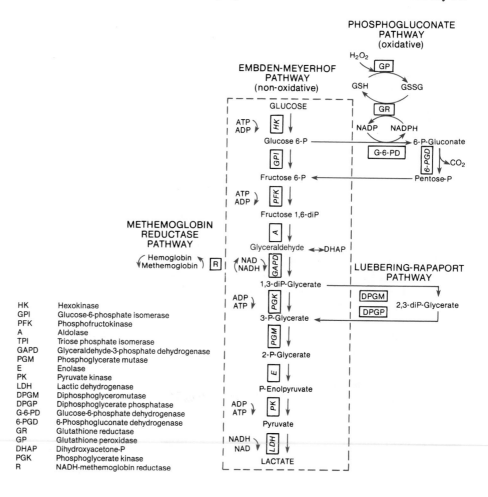

HK	Hexokinase
GPI	Glucose-6-phosphate isomerase
PFK	Phosphofructokinase
A	Aldolase
TPI	Triose phosphate isomerase
GAPD	Glyceraldehyde-3-phosphate dehydrogenase
PGM	Phosphoglycerate mutase
E	Enolase
PK	Pyruvate kinase
LDH	Lactic dehydrogenase
DPGM	Diphosphoglyceromutase
DPGP	Diphosphoglycerate phosphatase
G-6-PD	Glucose-6-phosphate dehydrogenase
6-PGD	6-Phosphogluconate dehydrogenase
GR	Glutathione reductase
GP	Glutathione peroxidase
DHAP	Dihydroxyacetone-P
PGK	Phosphoglycerate kinase
R	NADH-methemoglobin reductase

> FIGURE 3–16 Red cell metabolism. (From Hillman, RF, and Finch, CA: Red Cell Manual, ed 7. FA Davis, Philadelphia, 1996, p 15, with permission.)

Reaction A.   RBC + infection or oxidant $\longrightarrow$ H_2O_2

Reaction B. H_2O_2 + 2GSH (reduced glutathione) $\xrightarrow{\text{Glutathione peroxidase}}$ GSSG (oxidized glutathione)+$2H_2O$

Reaction C.   GSSG + NADPH (reduced form) + H^+ $\xrightarrow{\text{Glutathione reductase}}$ 2GSH+ $NADP^+$ (oxidized form)

Reaction D.   G-6-P (glucose-6-phosphate) + $NADP^+$ $\xrightarrow{\text{Glucose-6-Phosphate dehydrogenase}}$ 6-PG (6-phosphogluconate) + NADPH + H^+

➤ **FIGURE 3–17**   Reactions with erythrocytes to prevent accumulation of oxidants.

of the old RBCs in circulation are taken out by a system of fixed macrophages in the body known as the *reticuloendothelial system* (*RES*). These RBCs are replaced by the daily release of 1% of the younger RBCs reticulocytes, from the bone marrow storage pool. As erythrocytes become older, certain glycolytic enzymes decrease in activity, resulting in a decrease in the production of energy and loss of deformability. At a certain critical point, the RBCs are no longer able to traverse the microvasculature and are phagocytized by the RES cells. Although RES cells are located in various organs and throughout the body, those of the spleen, called *littoral cells*, are the most sensitive detectors of RBC abnormalities.[34]

Extravascular Hemolysis

Ninety percent of the destruction of senescent RBCs occurs by the process of extravascular hemolysis (Fig. 3–19). During this process, old or damaged RBCs are phagocytized by the RES cells and digested by their lysosomes. The hemoglobin molecules are disassembled and broken down into their various components. The iron recovered is salvaged and returned by the plasma protein carrier, transferrin, to the erythroid precursors in the marrow for synthesis of the new hemoglobin. Globin is broken down into amino acids and redirected to the amino acid pool of the body. Finally, the protoporphyrin ring of heme is disassembled, and its α carbon exhaled in the form of carbon monoxide. The opened tetrapyrrole, biliverdin, is converted to bilirubin and carried by the plasma protein albumin to the liver.[35] In the liver, bilirubin is conjugated to bilirubin glucuronide and excreted along with bile into the intestines. Here it is further converted through bacterial action into urobilinogen (stercobilinogen) and excreted in the stool. A small amount of urobilinogen is reabsorbed through enterohepatic circulation, filtered by the kidneys, and excreted in small amounts in the urine. Both unconjugated (prehepatic) and conjugated (posthepatic) bilirubin can be measured in the

➤ **Table 3-9**
CHANGES OCCURRING DURING AGING OF RBCS

Increases	Decreases
Membrane-bound IgG	Several enzyme activities
Density	Sialic acid
Spheroidal shape	Deformability
MCHC	MCV
Internal viscosity	Phospholipid
Agglutinability	Cholesterol
Na^+	K^+
Methemoglobin	Protoporphyrin
Oxygen affinity	

Abbreviations: MCHC = mean cell hemoglobin concentration; MCV = mean cell volume.

Source: Garratty, G: Basic mechanisms of in vivo cell destruction. In Bell, C (ed): A Seminar in Immune-Mediated Cell Destruction. American Association of Blood Banks, Bethesda, MD, 1981, with permission.

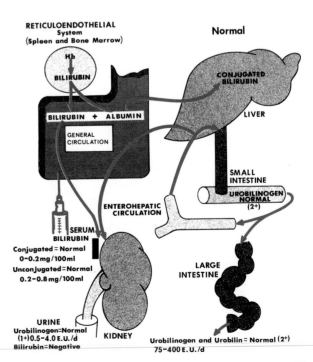

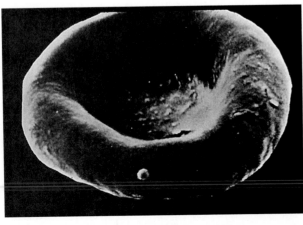

➤ **FIGURE 3–18**   SEM of a normal red cell.

➤ **FIGURE 3–19**   Normal extravascular hemolysis. (From Tietz, MW: Textbook of Clinical Chemistry. WB Saunders, Philadelphia, 1986, with permission.)

plasma as indirect and direct bilirubin, respectively, and used to monitor the amount of hemolysis.[35]

Intravascular Hemolysis

Only 5% to 10% of normal RBC destruction occurs through intravascular hemolysis (Fig. 3–20).[35] During this process, RBC breakdown occurs within the lumen of the blood vessels. The RBC ruptures, releasing hemoglobin directly into the bloodstream. The hemoglobin molecule dissociates into $\alpha\beta$ dimers and is picked up by the protein carrier, haptoglobin.[35] The haptoglobin-hemoglobin complex prevents renal excretion of the hemoglobin and carries the dimers to the liver cell for further catabolism. The hepatocyte uptake and processing are identical at this point to the process previously described for extravascular hemolysis (see Fig. 3–19). Haptoglobin levels, therefore, fall in plasma as haptoglobin is removed via the hemoglobin-haptoglobin complex. It is estimated that as little as 1 to 2 mL of the RBC intravascular hemolysis can totally deplete the amount of plasma haptoglobin.[36] Normally, 50 to 200 mg/dL of plasma haptoglobin is available and represents the hemoglobin-dimer binding capacity.[36] As haptoglobin is depleted, unbound hemoglobin dimers appear in the plasma (hemoglobinemia) and are filtered through the kidneys and reabsorbed by the renal tubular cells. The renal tubular uptake capacity is approximately 5 g per day of filtered hemoglobin.[36] Beyond this level, free hemoglobin appears in the urine (hemoglobinuria).

Hemoglobinuria is always associated wit hemoglobinemia. A normal plasma hemoglobin level is approximately 2 to 5 mg/dL, which is released as a result of excessive intravascular hemolysis.[36] Depending on the amount of hemolysis and type of hemoglobin, the plasma may be pink, red, or brown. Likewise, in hemoglobinuria the urine also may be pink, red, brown, or black. Two hemoglobin pigments, oxyhemoglobin and methemoglobin, are produced by auto-oxidation of the hemoglobin in the urinary tract when the urine is acidic.[36] Oxyhemoglobin is bright red, and methemoglobin is dark brown. The color of the urine, therefore, depends on the amount of hemolysis and the concentration and relative proportions of these two pigments.

> **Table 3-10**
> **PROTEIN CARRIERS**

Protein	Substance Carried
Transferrin	Iron
Haptoglobin	Hemoglobin dimers
Hemopexin	Metheme
Albumin	Bilirubin

Oxyhemoglobin predominates in alkaline urine, and methemoglobin predominates in acidic urine.

Hemoglobin that is neither processed by the kidneys nor bound to haptoglobin is oxidized to methemoglobin, which is further disassembled as metheme groups are released and globin degradated. Free metheme is quickly bound by another transport protein, hemopexin, and is carried to the liver cell to be catabolized, as previously described. The heme-binding capacity of hemopexin is approximately 50 to 100 mg/dL; when this is exceeded, the metheme groups combine with albumin to form methemalbumin.[36] Albumin cannot transfer the metheme across the membrane of the hepatocyte for subsequent degradation. As a result, the methemalbumin circulates until additional hemopexin is produced by the liver to serve as the protein carrier. It is this circulating methemalbumin that imparts a brown tinge to the plasma or blood (Table 3–10). Intravascular hemolysis that occurs as a result of RBC senescence is so minimal that it is limited to the involvement of only haptoglobin, which is rarely depleted. Hemoglobinemia and hemoglobinuria, as well as the other processes discussed, come into play only with excessive intravascular hemolysis, which can occur in patients having various hemolytic anemias (see Chaps. 9 through 14).

This chapter has outlined and described three important areas of RBC structure and metabolism: the red cell membrane, hemoglobin structure and function, and red cell metabolic pathways. An understanding of these aspects of the RBC is important to appreciating the development and pathogenesis of the many forms of inherited and acquired RBC defects that result in hemolytic anemias.

QUESTIONS

1. Which of the following is not a crucial area of RBC survival and function?
   a. Integrity of RBC cellular membrane
   b. Cell metabolism
   c. Intravascular hemolysis
   d. Hemoglobin structure

2. Which abnormal RBC is not caused by a structural membrane defect?
   a. Spherocyte
   b. Target cell
   c. Siderocyte
   d. Acanthocyte

3. Which list represents the complete set of processes necessary for normal hemoglobin production?

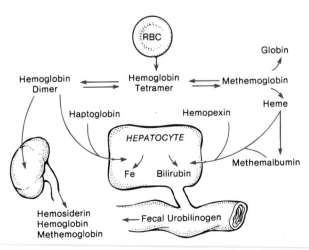

> **FIGURE 3–20** Intravascular hemolysis. (From Hillman, RF, and Finch, CA: Red Cell Manual, ed 7. FA Davis, Philadelphia, 1996, p 23, with permission.)

a. Iron delivery and supply, synthesis of protoporphyrins, and globin synthesis
b. Iron salvage, synthesis of conjugated bilirubin, and haptoglobin synthesis
c. Iron accumulation, synthesis of hemopexin, and globin catabolism
d. Iron catabolism, synthesis of uroporphyrinogen, and ferritin synthesis

4. What is the correct list for the number and type of globin chains in normal adult hemoglobin?
   a. Four α, two β, and two δ chains
   b. Two α and two non-α chains
   c. Two α, four β, one δ, and one ϵ chain
   d. Two α, two β, two δ, and one ϵ chain

5. What is the composition of normal adult hemoglobin?
   a. 92% to 95% HbA; 5% to 8% HbA$_2$; 1% to 2% HbF
   b. 90% to 92% HbA; 2% to 3% HbA$_2$; 2% to 5% HbF
   c. 80% to 85% HbA; 2% to 3% HbA$_2$; 1% to 2% HbF
   d. 95% to 97% HbA; 2% to 3% HbA$_2$; 1% to 2% HbF

6. Which of the following cells is caused by iron accumulation?
   a. Acanthocyte
   b. Ringed sideroblast
   c. Burr cell
   d. Bite cell

7. Which of the following is a complete list of abnormal hemoglobins that are unable to transport or deliver oxygen?
   a. Carboxyhemoglobin and methemoglobin
   b. Methemoglobin and fetal hemoglobin
   c. Carboxyhemoglobin, sulfhemoglobin, and fetal hemoglobin
   d. Carboxyhemoglobin, methemoglobin, and sulfhemoglobin

8. Which metabolic pathway generates 90% of the ATP needed by RBCs?
   a. Methemoglobin reductase pathway
   b. Hexose monophosphate shunt
   c. Embden-Meyerhof pathway
   d. Leubering-Rapoport shunt

9. What steps occur in the extravascular breakdown of senescent RBCs?
   a. RES cells phagocytize red cells; iron is coupled to transferrin and returned to marrow; globin is returned to amino acid pool; biliverdin is converted to bilirubin; bilirubin is coupled to albumin and transported to liver; bilirubin glucuronide is converted to urobilinogen and excreted
   b. RBCs break down in lumen of vessel; haptoglobin-hemoglobin complex goes to the liver; unbound hemoglobin dimers are excreted through the kidney as hemosiderin, hemoglobin, or methemoglobin; haptoglobin is broken down to be excreted as urobilinogen
   c. RES cells phagocytize red cells; iron is coupled to transferrin and returned to marrow; globin is

returned to amino acid pool; haptoglobin-hemoglobin complex goes to liver; unbound hemoglobin dimers are excreted through kidney as hemosiderin, hemoglobin, or methemoglobin; haptoglobin is broken down to be excreted as urobilinogen
   d. RBCs break down in lumen of vessel; haptoglobin picks up dissociated hemoglobin; haptoglobin-hemoglobin complex goes to the liver; biliverdin is converted to bilirubin; bilirubin is coupled to albumin and transported to liver; bilirubin glucuronide is converted to urobilinogen and excreted

10. What steps occur in the intravascular breakdown of senescent RBCs? (Use answer choices for question 9.)

SUMMARY CHART

➤ Glycophorin is the major integral membrane protein, representing 20% of the total RBC membrane protein.
➤ Spectrin is the most abundant peripheral protein of the RBC membrane cytoskeleton, comprising 25% to 30% of the total membrane protein and 75% of the peripheral protein.
➤ The loss of ATP and subsequent decrease in the phosphorylation of spectrin leads to a decrease in deformability and RBC survival.
➤ The RBC membrane is freely permeable to water and anions while relatively impermeable to cations (Na$^+$, K$^+$).
➤ The erythrocyte intracellular-to-extracellular ratios for sodium and potassium are 1:12 and 25:1, respectively.
➤ RBC membrane lipids consist of a bilayer of phospholipids interspersed with molecules of unesterified cholesterol and glycolipids present in equimolar quantities.
➤ Cholesterol comprises 25% of the RBC membrane lipid and is present in a 1:1 molar ratio with phospholipids.
➤ Hemoglobin is a conjugated globular protein consisting of globin (two pairs of polypeptide chains) and four heme groups, each of which contains a protoporphyrin ring plus ferrous iron.
➤ Normal hemoglobin synthesis is dependent on adequate iron delivery and supply, adequate synthesis of protoporphyrins, and adequate globin synthesis.
➤ Iron is delivered to the membrane of the RBC precursor by the protein carrier transferrin; two-thirds of total body iron is bound to heme in the hemoglobin molecule.
➤ Globin chain synthesis occurs on RBC-specific cytoplasmic ribosomes, which are initiated from the gene inheritance.
➤ Normal adult hemoglobin consists of 95% to 97% HbA, 2% to 3% HbA$_2$, and 1% to 2% HbF.

➤ The primary function of hemoglobin is delivery and release of oxygen to the tissues and facilitation of carbon dioxide excretion.

➤ A shift to the left of the hemoglobin-oxygen dissociation curve results in a decrease in oxygen delivery to the tissues.

➤ A shift to the right of the hemoglobin-oxygen dissociation curve results in a decrease of oxygen affinity for hemoglobin and increased oxygen delivery to the tissues.

➤ Abnormal hemoglobins, which are unable to carry oxygen, include carboxyhemoglobin, methemoglobin, and sulfhemoglobin.

➤ Ninety percent of RBC senescence occurs by extravascular hemolysis, whereas 5% to 10% occurs through intravascular hemolysis.

➤ Ninety percent of ATP needed for RBC survival is generated via the Embden-Meyerhof glycolytic pathway.

➤ The abnormal hemoglobins of clinical importance are carboxyhemoglobin, methemoglobin, and sulfhemoglobin.

References

1. Singer, SJ, and Nicholson, GL: The fluid mosaic model of the structure of cell membranes. Annu Rev Biochem 43:805, 1974.
2. Telen, MJ, and Kaufman, RE: The mature erythrocyte. In Lee, et al (eds): Wintrobe's Clinical Hematology, ed 10. Williams & Wilkins, Baltimore, 1999, pp 194–200.
3. Cabantchik, ZI: Erythrocyte membrane transport. Novartis Found Symp 226:6, 1999.
4. Pincus, MR: Physiological structure and function of proteins. In Sperelakis, N (ed): Cell Physiology Source Book, ed 2. Academic Press, New York, 1998, p 30.
5. Steck, TL: The organization of proteins in the human red blood cell membrane. J Cell Biol 62:1, 1974.
6. Mohandas, N, and Evans, E: Mechanical properties of the red cell membrane in relation to molecular structure and genetic defects. Annu Rev Biophys Biomol Struct 23:787, 1994.
7. Hemming, et al: Localization of the protein 4.1-binding site on human erythrocyte glycophorins C and D. Biochem J 299:191, 1994.
8. Murray, RK, et al: Harper's Biochemistry, ed 25. Appleton & Lange, Stamford, 2000, pp 768–769.
9. Cherry, L, et al: Spin label EPR structural studies of the N-terminus of alpha-spectrin. FEBS Lett 466:341, 2000.
10. Nunomura, W, et al: Regulation of protein 4.1R, p55, and glycophorin C ternary complex in human erythrocyte membrane. J Biol Chem Aug 11; 275(32):24540-6 2000.
11. Chishti, AH: Function of p55 and its nonerythroid homologues. Curr Opin Hematol 5:116, 1998.
12. Bossi, D, and Russo, M: Hemolytic anemias due to disorders of red cell membrane skeleton. Mol Aspects Med 17:171, 1996.
13. Marikovsky, Y: The cytoskeleton in ATP-depleted erythrocytes: The effect of shape transformation. Mech Ageing Dev 86:137, 1996.
14. Sleight, RG, and Lieberman, MA: Signal transduction. In Sperelakis, N (ed): Cell Physiology Source Book, ed 2. Academic Press, New York, 1998, p 125.
15. Murray, RK, and Granner, DK: Membranes: Structure, assembly, and function. In Murray, RK et al (eds): Harper's Biochemistry, ed 25. Appleton & Lange, Stamford, 2000, p 509.
16. Yang, XP, et al: Abetalipoproteinemia caused by maternal isodisomy of chromosome 4q containing an intron 9 splice acceptor mutation in the microsomal triglyceride transfer protein gene. Arterioscler Thromb Vasc Biol 19:1950, 1999.
17. Raabe, M, et al: Using genetically engineered mice to understand apolipoprotein-B deficiency syndromes in humans. Proc Assoc Am Physicians 110:521, 1998.
18. Teh, EM, et al: Classical LCAT deficiency resulting from a novel homozygous dinucleotide deletion in exon 4 of the human lecithin: Cholesterol acyltransferase gene causing a frameshift and stop codon at residue 144. Atherosclerosis 146:141, 1999.
19. Li M, Kuivenhoven JA, Ayyobi AF, Pritchard PH: T→G or T→A mutation introduced in the branchpoint consensus sequence of intron 4 of lecithin:cholesterol acyltransferase (LCAT) gene: Intron retention causing LCAT deficiency. Biochim Biophys Acta 1391:256, 1998.
20. Bunn, HF: Hemoglobin structure, function, and assembly. In Embury, SH, et al (eds): Sickle Cell Disease: Basic Principles and Clinical Practice. Raven Press, New York, 1994.
21. Rand, ML, and Murray, RK: Plasma proteins, immunoglobulins, and blood coagulation. In Murray, RK, et al (eds): Harper's Biochemistry, ed 25. Appleton & Lange, Stamford, 2000, p 742.
22. Dessypris, EN: Erythropoiesis. In Lee, GR (ed): Wintrobe's Clinical Hematology, ed 10. Williams & Wilkins, Baltimore, 1999, p 181.
23. McBride, LJ: Textbook of Urinalysis and Body Fluids. Lippincott, Philadelphia, 1998, pp 151–152.
24. Sassa, S, and Kappas, A: Molecular aspects of the inherited porphyrias. J Intern Med 247:169, 2000.
25. Williams, WJ, et al: Hematology, ed 5. McGraw-Hill, New York, 1995.
26. Rodwell, VW: Proteins: Myoglobin and hemoglobin. In Murray, RK, et al (eds): Harper's Biochemistry, ed 25. Appleton & Lange, Stamford, 2000, pp 69–70.
27. Green, R, and Deloach, JR: Resealed erythrocytes as carriers and bioreactors. In: Proceedings of the Third International Meeting held at the Gwinn Estate, Cleveland, OH. Pergamon Press, New York, 1991.
28. Bell, SG: An introduction to hemoglobin physiology. Neonatal Netw 18:9, 1999.
29. Stevens, ML: Fundamentals of Clinical Hematology. WB Saunders, Philadelphia, 1997, pp 154–155.
30. Akintonwa, DA: Theoretical mechanistic basis of oxidants of methaemoglobin formation. Med Hypotheses 54:312, 2000.
31. Noor, M, and Beutler, E: Acquired sulfhemoglobinemia. An underreported diagnosis? West J Med 169:386, 1998.
32. Bossi, D, and Giardina, B: Red cell physiology. Mol Aspects Med 17: 117, 1996.
33. Verle, P, et al: Glucose-6-phosphate dehydrogenase deficiency in northern Vietnam. Trop Med Int Health 5:203, 2000.
34. Cotran, RS, et al: Robbins Pathologic Basis of Disease, ed 5. WB Saunders, Philadelphia, 1994.
35. Deiss, A: Destruction of erythrocytes. In Lee, GR, et al (eds): Wintrobe's Clinical Hematology, ed 10. Williams & Wilkins, Baltimore, 1999, pp 276–277.
36. Burtis, CA, and Ashwood, ER: Tietz Fundamentals of Clinical Chemistry, ed 4. Saunders, Philadelphia, 1996.

4 Anemia

Diagnosis and Clinical Considerations

ARMAND B. GLASSMAN, MD

OBJECTIVES

At the end of this chapter, the learner should be able to:

1. Describe clinical signs of anemia.

2. List causes of anemia.

3. Use laboratory criteria for the diagnosis of anemia.

4. Explain the most common method for the measurement of hemoglobin on automated instruments.

5. Explain how the hematocrit is calculated on automated hematology instruments.

6. Calculate the significance of red blood cell indices as related to the diagnosis of anemia.

7. Describe the appearance of the peripheral blood smear in various anemias.

8. Explain the diagnostic value of the reticulocyte count.

9. List factors to be evaluated in the interpretation of a bone marrow aspirate smear.

➤ DEFINITION OF ANEMIA

Anemia in its broadest sense is the inability of the blood to supply the tissue with adequate oxygen for proper metabolic function.[1] Clinically, the diagnosis of anemia is made by patient history, physical examination, signs and symptoms, and hematologic laboratory findings. Determining the specific cause of an anemia in a patient is important to the physician so that he or she can base the appropriate therapy and prognosis on the natural history of the disease in that patient. Anemia is usually associated with decreased levels of hemoglobin or a decreased packed red blood cell (RBC) volume, also known as the hematocrit. Under rare circumstances, certain abnormal hemoglobins have very strong oxygen-binding capacities or oxygen is not released normally to tissue, resulting in all the clinical signs and symptoms of anemia even though the hemoglobin or hematocrit value is normal or even raised. From a practical laboratory standpoint, however, the usual diagnostic criterion for anemia is a decreased hemoglobin (Hgb), hematocrit (Hct), or RBC count.[2]

Because most patients with anemia have lowered hemoglobin levels, the anemia may be classified arbitrarily as either moderate (7 to 10 g Hgb/dL) or severe (less than 7 g Hgb/dL).[2] Moderate anemias do not usually produce clinically evident signs or symptoms, especially if the onset is slow. However, depending on the patient's age or cardiovascular condition, even moderate amounts of anemia may be associated with exertional dyspnea (difficulty breathing), light-headedness, vertigo, muscle weakness, headache, or general lethargy. Anemia of rapid onset, such as that resulting from gastrointestinal hemorrhage, may be associated with significant clinical symptoms, such as hypotension, tachycardia, and dyspnea. These symptoms are usually associated with the precipitous loss of intravascular volume as well as the oxygen-carrying capacity of the RBCs.

➤ CONSIDERATIONS BY AGE, SEX, AND OTHER FACTORS

Newborn infants (younger than 1 week old) have a hemoglobin value of 18 ± 4 g/dL as a reference range. At approximately 6 months of age, the reference range is 12.5 ± 1.5 g/dL. Childhood levels from the ages of 1 to 15 years have a reference range of approximately 13.0 ± 2 g/dL. Adult hemoglobin reference ranges are approximately 16.0 ± 2 g/dL for men and 14.0 ± 2 g/dL for women (Table 4–1). In the geriatric age group, the difference between hemoglobin levels of men and women narrows. Hemoglobin levels of geriatric men usually decrease slightly, and those of postmenopausal woman approach those of men. The reference ranges used by each laboratory should be obtained, because they best reflect the patient population served.

Other factors, including geographic elevation, influence individual "normal" hemoglobin levels. Persons living at elevations above 8000 feet may have persistently increased hemoglobin values secondary to decreased oxygen saturation in the ambient atmosphere. Lung diseases may alter oxygen diffusion at the lung alveolar membranes. A compensatory sequence to chronic lung disease may result in increased hemoglobin levels (secondary polycythemia).

Various diseases and disorders are associated with lower than usual hemoglobin levels; these include nutritional deficiencies, external or internal blood loss, accelerated destruction of RBCs, ineffective or decreased production of RBCs, abnormal hemoglobin synthesis, bone marrow replacement by infection or tumor, and bone marrow suppression by toxins, chemicals, or radiation.[3]

➤ CAUSES OF ANEMIA

Anemia has many causes (Table 42). These can be broadly classified as nutritional deficiency (e.g., folate or vitamin B_{12} deficiencies), blood loss (hemorrhage), accelerated destruction of RBCs (immune and nonimmune hemolysis), bone marrow replacement (e.g., by cancer), infection, toxicity, hematopoietic stem cell arrest or damage, and hereditary or acquired defect. Categories may be simplified to embrace conditions of increased RBC destruction, abnormal or decreased RBC production, or some combination thereof.

➤ Table 4-1
REFERENCE RANGE VALUES FOR HEMOGLOBIN

Age Group	Hemoglobin (g/dL)
Infants	
Newborns (< 1 wk old)	14.0–22.0
6 mo old	11.0–14.0
Children (1–15 yr old)	11.0–15.0
Adults	
Men	14.0–18.0
Women	12.0–16.0

➤ Table 4-2
CATEGORIES OF ANEMIA BY CAUSE

- Blood loss (hemorrhage)
- Accelerated destruction of RBCs (immune and nonimmune hemolytic)
- Nutritional deficiency (folate or vitamin B_{12})
- Bone marrow replacement (e.g., by cancer)
- Infection
- Toxicity
- Hematopoietic stem cell arrest or damage
- Hereditary or acquired defect
- Unknown

➤ SIGNIFICANCE OF ANEMIA AND COMPENSATORY MECHANISMS

Red Blood Cell and Hemoglobin Production

In a healthy ambulatory person, approximately 1% of the senescent circulating RBCs are lost daily. Normally, the bone marrow continues to produce RBCs. A laboratory measure of this replacement is the reticulocyte count. In healthy people, reticulocytes, early circulating RBCs containing residual ribonucleic acid (RNA), account for 0.5% to 2.0% of the circulating RBCs. Replacement of RBCs requires a bone marrow with adequate functioning stem cells, normal RBC maturation processes, and the ability to release mature RBCs from the bone marrow. Proper hemoglobin and RBC production require a variety of nutritional factors, including iron, vitamin B_{12}, and folic acid, and normal pathways of hemoglobin synthesis.[4] The role of hemoglobin synthesis in anemias is covered in greater detail in Chapter 11.

In severe anemias (less than 7 g Hgb/dL), symptoms of functional impairment of a number of organ systems may be evident. With minimal exercise, the patient's cardiac and respiratory rates may increase dramatically. If the anemia is secondary to blood loss and decreased intravascular volume, the patient's blood pressure may drop significantly when he or she is raised from the reclining to a sitting or standing position. The heart rate will increase in order to elevate the cardiac output to keep pace with peripheral tissue oxygen demands in the face of a decreased oxygen-carrying capacity of the lowered hemoglobin level. Respiratory symptoms, including dyspnea on exertion, may also occur with anemia.

An interesting compensatory mechanism in response to anemia is an increase in the 2,3-diphosphoglycerate (2,3-DPG) levels. This compound is a remarkable physiologic regulator of normal hemoglobin oxygen-carrying capacity and tissue oxygen delivery. In the presence of 2,3-DPG, hemoglobin can more readily release the oxygen it is carrying to peripheral tissues. This enhanced release occurs regardless of pH or blood arterial oxygen level.

A normal individual responds to anemia with elevated levels of erythropoietin (Epo) (see Chap. 1). The Epo level is sometimes used as an ancillary diagnostic aid in the differential diagnosis of anemia. Epo is a hormone of approximately 31,000 daltons (d). It has a plasma half-life of between 6 and 9 hours and is produced by the peritubular complex of the kidney. In patients with anemia, Epo levels vary as a result of altered oxygen tension in the tissues of the kidney. Increased Epo production occurs when there is a decreased hemoglobin level, a hemoglobin structural problem in which oxygen is not released, or low ambient oxygen tension at high altitude. On the other hand, high oxygen levels in the kidney result in a decrease in Epo production. Recombinant Epo is now available for treatment of certain types of anemias, particularly end-stage renal disease, anemia associated with human immunodeficiency virus, and certain other chronic disorders.[5] Bone marrow production of new RBCs in response to proper nutrients, vitamins, and other factors may be evaluated by the reticulocyte count.

▶ CLINICAL DIAGNOSIS OF ANEMIA

The clinical diagnosis of anemia is made by a combination of factors, including patient history, physical signs, and changes in the hematologic profile. The signs and symptoms of anemia are generally nonspecific, such as fatigue and weakness, and may include gastrointestinal symptoms such as nausea, constipation, or diarrhea. The patient may complain of dyspnea after a level of exertion that previously had not caused any problems.[6–9]

A patient example may be useful here. A man who had been able to climb three flights of stairs without difficulty or significant shortness of breath might report that now he must stop after climbing one flight of stairs and is then very short of breath. Subsequent information indicates that the patient has passed very dark stools (melena) over the past week. Measurement of his hemoglobin reveals a level of 8 g/dL. The diagnostic impression from the clinical information is that the patient's anemia is secondary to gastrointestinal bleeding.

Physical signs of anemia are usually not specific for the underlying disease. Occasionally, however, the underlying diagnosis may be suspected from certain physical findings. One example would be signs of malnutrition and neurologic changes with loss of proprioception (position sense) and vibration awareness in a patient with vitamin B_{12} deficiency. Another example would be severe pallor, smooth tongue, and an esophageal web in a patient with severe iron-deficiency anemia.[9] Light-skinned patients who are anemic may appear to have pale coloration of mucosal membranes, nail beds, and skin. Occasionally, the temperature may be slightly elevated, particularly in patients having certain types of hemolytic anemia. In the presence of anemia, heart murmurs may be heard; these are sometimes secondary to the cause of the anemia and sometimes related to the increased cardiac workload required to bring oxygen to the tissues. Patients with bacterial endocarditis have fever, heart murmurs, and anemia. Bacterial endocarditis is a clinical example in which the damaged myocardial valve and heart murmur are related etiologically to the anemia. Prosthetic heart valves, arterial grafts, or disseminated intravascular coagulation (DIC) can cause a form of mechanical hemolytic anemia known as *microangiopathic hemolytic anemia*.

A broad category of anemias includes those termed *aplastic*. Aplastic anemia is defined as pancytopenia resulting from bone marrow production failure. Additional information concerning aplastic anemia is found in Chapter 8.

In general, there are two types of aplastic anemia. The first type includes congenital and so-called idiopathic acquired forms. The second type is secondary or acquired. Causes of secondary aplastic anemia include exposure to chemicals (benzene and some other fluorocarbons), therapeutic agents (especially cancer chemotherapy agents), infection (some types of hepatitis and parvovirus infections), and ionizing radiation. This chapter deals primarily with the decrease in the RBC and oxyhemoglobin carrying capacity. It should be noted that aplastic anemia is a pancytopenia involving the red cell, white cells, and platelets.

▶ CLASSIFICATION OF ANEMIA

The individual types of anemias can be classified according to several different criteria. A functional classification would be hypoproliferative or accelerated destruction (hemolytic), or a combination of the two (sometimes called *ineffective hematopoiesis*). Anemias are often classified clinically according to their associated causes, such as blood loss, iron deficiency, hemolysis, infection, metastatic bone marrow replacement, or nutritional deficiency. Anemias can also be categorized quantitatively by their hematocrit, hemoglobin level, blood cell indices, or reticulocyte count.[7–9] The clinical laboratory scientist is frequently involved in these quantitative measurements and in subsequent evaluations.

Hemoglobin and Hematocrit

Measurement of the hemoglobin level and packed cell volume is the usual method of determining whether a patient has anemia. As discussed earlier, reference ranges may vary by age and sex (Table 4–1) as well as state of hydration, patient positioning, and local laboratory patient population determinations. Hemoglobin assays are based on the spectrophotometric absorbance readings of cyanmethemoglobin compared with known amounts (a standard curve). Several companies manufacture automated instruments that include these determinations as part of a hematologic profile. The hematocrit, or packed red blood cell volume (PCV), is determined by centrifugation of blood of either capillary or venous origin or can be calculated on some automated instruments. The reference PCV for adult men varies by institution (i.e., 47% ± 5%). For adult women during the reproductive years, the PCV reference range is 42% ± 5%. On the basis of hemoglobin or PCV values and the duration of onset, anemias may be classified as mild, moderate, or severe, and as either acute or chronic. The approximate relationship of the hemoglobin level to hematocrit is 1:3, a ratio that may vary with the cause of the anemia and the effect of that cause on the RBC indices, particularly the mean corpuscular volume (MCV).

Microscopic examination of a properly prepared peripheral blood smear is a requirement for the clinical and laboratory evaluation of anemia. This technique is discussed later under the tests in the diagnosis of anemia. Histologic examinations of the bone marrow smear and aspirate are adjuncts to further elucidate the cause of the anemia.

Red Blood Cell Indices

The RBC indices are the mean corpuscular volume (MCV), mean cell hemoglobin (MCH), and mean cell hemoglobin concentration (MCHC).[10] The MCV is used as an estimation of the average size of the RBC. It may be calculated by dividing the hematocrit by the number of RBCs or measured directly using automated cell counters. If the MCV is within the reference range, the RBCs are considered normocytic; if less than normal, microcytic; and if greater than normal, macrocytic. Both MCH and MCHC values are used to determine the content of hemoglobin in RBCs. Most automated hematology instruments also provide an RBC distribution width (RDW) value. The RDW is an index of size variation and has been used to quantitate the amount of anisocytosis seen on a peripheral blood smear. The reference range for RDW is 11.5% to 14.5% for both men and women. The MCV is not dependable when RBCs vary markedly in size. If MCHC is normal, the RBCs are referred to as normochromic; hypochromic RBCs have a less than normal MCHC; and there are no truly hyperchromic RBCs.

Red Blood Cell Indices and Other Tests

The RBC indices are accurately calculated by the automated blood profiling machines. These instruments provide precise numeric values for hemoglobin levels, the numbers of RBCs, and the MCV. Although less precise, careful microscopic examination of a peripheral blood smear can tell the examiner whether the RBCs are normocytic, microcytic, macrocytic, normochromic, or hypochromic. A proper specimen is required to obtain accurate answers.[11] RBC index calculations and reference ranges are:

MCV equals Hct (in %) multiplied by 10, divided by RBC count (in millions/μL); reference range: 90 $\pm$ 10 fL.

$$MCV = \frac{Hct\,(\%) \times 10}{RBC\ count\ (millions/\mu L)}$$

MCH equals Hgb (in g/dL) multiplied by 10, divided by RBC count (in millions/μL); reference range: 29 $\pm$ 2 pg.

$$MCH = \frac{Hgb\,(g/dL) \times 10}{RBC\ count\ (millions/\mu L)}$$

MCHC equals Hgb (in g/dL) multiplied by 100, divided by Hct (as a percentage); reference range: 34 $\pm$ 2%.

$$MCHC = \frac{Hgb\,(g/dL) \times 100}{Hct\,(\%)}$$

Use of the RBC indices in the differential diagnosis of anemia can provide a general idea as to what is occurring

clinically (Table 4–3). A normocytic normochromic anemia may be the result of bone marrow failure, hemolytic anemia, or some subset of either of these conditions.

Making the differential diagnosis of bone marrow failure requires information about RBC production. This information can be obtained from the reticulocyte count, which indicates whether there is bone marrow capacity for increased RBC production. Because RBC destruction may exceed production, the reticulocyte count, in fact, measures effective RBC production. Hemolytic anemia occurs when there is decreased RBC survival, which in turn may be the result of extravascular elimination, intravascular destruction, or a combination of the two.

Macrocytic normochromic anemias usually occur in association with folate or vitamin B_{12} deficiency. The most commonly encountered anemias are the microcytic hypochromic anemias, usually related to iron-deficiency anemia. Beta-thalassemia, an inherited defect of hemoglobin synthesis, is another cause of microcytosis. Less frequently seen are the sideroblastic anemias, which are also associated with decreased MCV.

The differential diagnosis of anemia is based on a combination of laboratory findings (Table 4–3) and clinical symptoms (Table 4–4). An abbreviated flowchart for the diagnosis of anemia using the RBC indices is provided in Figure 4–1.

➤ OVERVIEW OF THE TREATMENT OF ANEMIAS

Anemia is treated according to its causes. The cause should be considered before beginning either supportive therapy (such as a transfusion) or replacement therapy. Table 4–3 and Figure 4–1 represent only some of the possible causes of anemia. Indeed, more than one cause of anemia can exist in a patient. Obtaining the proper diagnostic studies in the shortest and most cost-effective manner is the responsibility of the attending physician and the laboratory professionals. More details concerning the appropriate treatment of anemias are provided in Chapters 6 through 14.

The natural history of anemia depends on its cause. For example, a patient with an iron-deficiency anemia associated with carcinoma of the colon may present with signs of an iron-deficiency anemia associated with blood loss from the tumor. Later, with more extensive tumor involvement, the anemia may have a bone marrow failure component because of bone marrow replacement by the tumor (a myelophthisic anemia). Patients with pernicious anemia require a lifetime of parenteral vitamin B_{12} supplementation.

➤ Table 4-3 CLASSIFICATION OF ANEMIA BY RBC INDICES		
Size (MCV) (fL)	**Hgb Content (MCHC) (%)**	**Possible Causes**
Normocytic (80–100)	Normochromic (32–36)	Bone marrow failure, hemolytic anemia chronic renal disease, leukemia, metastatic malignancy
Macrocytic (> 100)	Normochromic (32–36)	Megaloblastic and nonmegaloblastic macrocytic anemias (e.g., liver disease, myelodysplasias)
Microcytic (< 80)	Hypochromic (< 32)	Iron deficiency, sideroblastic anemia, thalassemia, lead poisoning, chronic diseases, chronic infection or inflammation, unstable hemoglobins

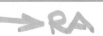

> ## Table 4-4
> ## CLINICAL SYMPTOMS OF ANEMIA
>
> - Pallor
> - Weakness
> - Fatigue
> - Lethargy or malaise
> - Exercise dyspnea
> - Palpitation
> - Pica (consumption of substance such as ice, starch, or clay, frequently found in iron deficiency anemia)
> - Syncope (particularly following exercise)
> - Dizziness
> - Headache
> - Tinnitus or vertigo
> - Irritability
> - Difficulty sleeping or concentrating
> - Gastrointestinal symptoms

Patients with other forms of megaloblastic anemia may need only a balanced diet and replacement of folic acid.[9]

Transfusions can obscure and confuse the findings of diagnostic tests in patients with anemia. Transfusions can suppress erythropoiesis; alter vitamin B_{12}, folate, and iron levels; and thwart the interpretation of diagnostic tests seeking the specific cause of the anemia. It is important that a diagnosis be made, if at all possible, before transfusions are given.

Other Factors in Red Blood Cell Production

Bone marrow stem cells require various other factors to continue to synthesize hemoglobin and permit proper maturation of erythrocytes and other cells. These include cytokines, for example, stem cell factor, erythropoietin, interleukin-3 (IL-3), and other interleukins. The hormones of the androgen group and thyroxin are also necessary. Many vitamins, such as vitamin B_{12}, folate, vitamin C, vitamin E, pyridoxine (B_6), thiamin, riboflavin, and pantothenic acid, play roles in bone marrow productivity. Certain metals, such as iron, manganese, and cobalt, are part of the production process for RBCs and other bone marrow cellular components.

Some factors act as growth-inhibiting agents. Among these are transforming growth factor-beta (TGF-β), which

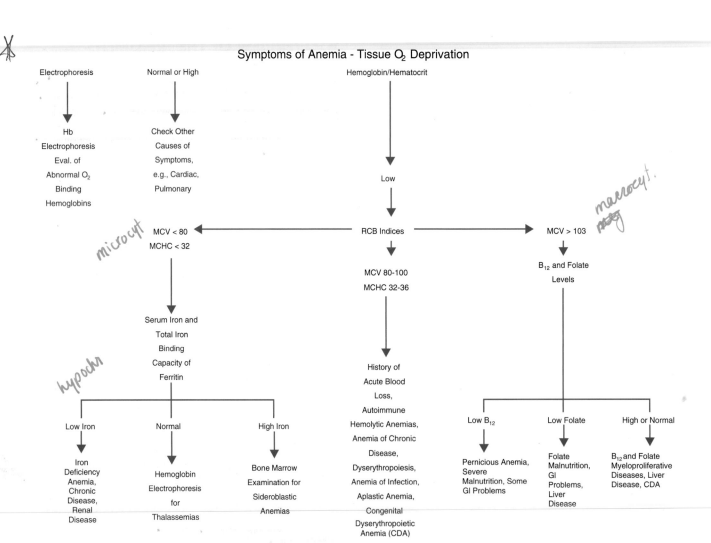

> ➤ **FIGURE 4–1**   Decision-making flowchart (algorithm) for symptoms of anemia

causes inhibition of growth of hematopoietic stem cells. Myeloid progenitors are known to be inhibited by tumor necrosis factor (TNF) and interleukin-4 (IL-4).

➤ TESTS IN THE DIAGNOSIS OF ANEMIA

Hemoglobin

Hemoglobin is the main component of the RBC. It is the physiologic carrier of oxygen to tissues and acts as a buffer to handle carbon dioxide formed in metabolic activities.[12] The three methods for measuring hemoglobin are the cyanmethemoglobin method, the oxyhemoglobin method, and the method in which iron content is measured. The cyanmethemoglobin method as modified in 1978 is recommended by the International Committee for Standardization in Hematology and will be the only one discussed. In this technique, blood is diluted in a solution of potassium ferricyanide and potassium cyanide, which oxidizes the hemoglobin to form methemoglobin. Subsequently, methemoglobin forms cyanmethemoglobin in the presence of the potassium cyanide. Because the absorption maximum occurs at a wavelength of 540 nm, the absorbance of the solution is read in a spectrophotometer at 540 nm and compared with a standard cyanmethemoglobin solution. The advantages of this method are that most forms of hemoglobin are measured, the sample can be directly compared with a standard, the solutions are stable, and the coefficient of variation for the method is less than 2% at physiologic ranges.

Errors in the measurement of hemoglobin can be produced by improperly drawing or handling the specimen, by poorly prepared or stored reagents, faulty equipment, and operator error.

Hematocrit

The hematocrit, or packed RBC volume, is the ratio of the volume of RBCs to the volume of whole blood. Hematocrit is usually expressed as a percentage (e.g., 42%) but is expressed in Standard International (SI) units as a decimal fraction (e.g., 0.42 L/L). The venous hematocrit agrees closely with the central blood hematocrit but is greater than the total body hematocrit. Anticoagulants—usually ethylene diaminetetraacetic acid (EDTA), oxalate, or heparin—are used to prevent the blood from clotting so that the hematocrit may be measured.

Measurement of the hematocrit may be done by centrifugation or through calculations performed on many automated hematology instruments. The calculated hematocrit is the product of the MCV and the RBC count.

The adult reference range for hematocrit is 42% to 52% in men and 37% to 47% in women. Different reference ranges are required for neonates, very young children, and male and female patients, and may vary among institutions.

Problems in the measurement of hematocrit include incorrect centrifuge calibration, choice of sample site, incorrect ratio of anticoagulant to blood owing to improper amount of blood drawn, and reading error—particularly for hematocrit values determined after centrifugation. In our laboratory, the coefficient of variation for hematocrit, within the reference range, is approximately 2%. With centrifuge hematocrit techniques, the lower hematocrit values are associated with the higher coefficients of variation.

Red Blood Cell Indices

RBC indices were introduced earlier. The MCV is the average volume, expressed in femtoliters (fL), of RBCs, and is measured directly or calculated from the hematocrit and RBC count. The MCH is the content of hemoglobin in the average RBC. MCH is calculated from the hemoglobin concentration and the RBC count. MCHC, the average concentration of hemoglobin in a volume of packed RBCs, is calculated from the hemoglobin concentration and the hematocrit.[10]

RBC indices are readily available from the automated hematology counting devices. In those devices in which the MCV is derived from the voltage changes formed during the RBC count and the hemoglobin is measured by spectrophotometric determination of the cyanmethemoglobin, the values are calculated as follows: the hematocrit equals the MCV times the RBC count, the MCH equals the hemoglobin divided by the RBC count, and the MCHC equals the hemoglobin divided by the hematocrit. The reference range for MCV is 80 to 100 fL; for MCH it is 27 to 31 pg; and for MCHC it is 32% to 36%.

In various anemic states, the indices may be altered as follows: in microcytic anemia, from an MCV of less than 80 fL down to a low of approximately 50 fL; from an MCH of less than 25 pg to approximately 15 pg; and from an MCHC of less than 30% to 22%. In the macrocytic anemias, MCV values are usually greater than 100 fL and may be as high as, and sometimes even higher, than 120 fL; the MCHC may be normal or decreased. The MCHC may be increased only in the presence of spherocytosis, if at all.

Peripheral Blood Smear

Much information concerning the cause of an anemia can be determined from a peripheral blood smear. Coexistent neutropenia, thrombocytopenia, and anemia may indicate bone marrow failure or a lack of a nutritional substance to provide adequate bone marrow production. The size and shape of the RBCs can be noted. Alteration in size of the RBCs results in anisocytosis; alterations in their shape result in poikilocytosis. The hemoglobin (chromatic) content of the RBCs can be inspected visually on the peripheral smear. In addition, cytologic details on the peripheral smear may provide clues to the etiology of the anemia, the bone marrow response, or both. The white cells may be evaluated. For example, excess lobulations of the polymorphonuclear leukocytes are seen in the hypersegmented granulocytes of macrocytic anemias (see Chap. 7).

Basophilic stippling in the RBCs may suggest the presence of increased bone marrow production and reticulocytosis (see Fig. 1–30 and Color Plate 30). It may also indicate that there are remnants of RNA, which may be associated with lead poisoning and some malignancies. Howell-Jolly bodies (see Chap. 12), which are small, round, blue inclusions seen in RBCs, are the result of leftover fragments of deoxyribonucleic acid (DNA). Howell-Jolly bodies are often seen in hyposplenism or asplenism, pernicious anemia, and some hemoglobinopathies—particularly thalassemia.[13–16] Pappenheimer bodies, which are iron-containing or siderotic granules, appear as purplish-blue granules with Wright's stain and as coarse blue granules with Prussian blue iron stain. The clinical disorders associated with Pappenheimer bodies include sideroblastic anemia, alcoholism, thalassemia, and some myelodysplastic syndromes. Nucleated RBCs with iron granules are known as sideroblasts, and RBCs containing iron granules but without a nucleus are referred to as siderocytes. Ringed sideroblasts are those in which more than five granules are arranged in a ring around the nucleus of an orthochromatic normoblast (Fig. 4–2 and Color Plate 82). Ringed sideroblasts are indicative of ineffective erythropoiesis.

A threadlike blue ring contained entirely within an abnormal RBC, which may or may not have a "figure-of-8" and a round or oval configuration, is known as a Cabot ring (see Fig. 7–6). This is a remnant of the nuclear membrane. This infrequent finding may be seen in several clinical disorders, including pernicious anemia, lead poisoning, and other severe anemias. Heinz bodies (Fig. 4–3 and Color Plate 83) are small, rounded, angular inclusions about 1 μm in diameter that are aggregates of denatured hemoglobin and are negative when stained with Prussian blue or other iron stains. Heinz bodies can be demonstrated only by using supravital stains (e.g., methylene blue) and are not visible with the usual Wright's stain. The clinical disorders that have been associated with Heinz bodies include glucose-6-phosphate dehydrogenase (G6PD) deficiency after exposure to oxidizing drugs, a variety of unstable hemoglobinopathies, and alpha-thalassemia; they can also be seen after splenectomy.

Reticulocyte Count

The reticulocyte count is useful in determining the response and potential of the bone marrow. Reticulocytes are non-nucleated RBCs that still contain RNA. Reticulocytes may be visualized after incubation with a variety of so-called supravital dyes, including new methylene blue or brilliant cresyl blue (see Chap. 28). RNA is precipitated as a dye-protein complex. Reticulocytes under normal circumstances lose their RNA a day or so after reaching the bloodstream from the marrow. Reticulocyte activity can be expressed as an absolute count, a production index, or a percentage. The reference values for reticulocytes range from 0.5% to 2.0% as a percentage of all RBCs. Because anemia should be accompanied by increased bone marrow activity, the reticulocytes should be expected to increase. One may correct the reticulocyte count for the following formula:

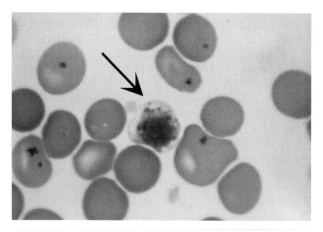

➤ **FIGURE 4–2**   Ringed sideroblast (center) and siderocytes (surrounding cells). (From Bell, A: Hematology. Listen, Look and Learn. Health and Education Resources, Inc., Bethesda, MD, with permission.)

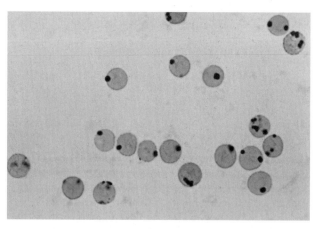

➤ **FIGURE 4–3**   Heinz bodies. (From Bell, A: Hematology. Listen, Look and Learn, Health and Education Resources, Inc., Bethesda, MD, with permission.)

Corrected reticulocyte %

$$= \frac{\text{Patient PCV} \times \text{Reticulocyte \%}}{\text{Reference PCV mean}}$$

Manual reticulocyte counting is associated with poor reproducibility. In the reference range, the coefficient of variation is said to be as great as 50%. Automated reticulocyte counting using fluorescent compounds and automated instruments results in better reproducibility.[2,10]

Interpretation of the reticulocyte count must take into account the age and nutritional status of the patient. Normal adults have a reticulocyte count between 0.5% and 2.0%, or from 24 to 100 $\times$ 10^9 reticulocytes per liter. The newborn infant has a higher reticulocyte count, which falls to the adult range usually by the second or third week of life. Sources of error in the reticulocyte count include sampling error resulting from counting relatively few reticulocytes in a large number of erythrocytes. The 95% confidence level when counting 100 RBCs, where the true reticulocyte count is 1%, ranges from 0.4% to 1.6%; obviously, there is a very high coefficient of variation unless large numbers of RBCs are counted. Usually 1000 cells are counted for a reticulocyte count.

Bone Marrow Smear and Biopsy

Bone marrow aspiration and biopsy are important diagnostic tools in the determination of anemia. Bone marrow interpretation and evaluation are covered in Chapter 2. Factors to be evaluated in interpretation of a bone marrow aspirate smear and biopsy include maturation of the red and white cell series, presence of megakaryocytes, ratio of myeloid to erythroid series, abundance of iron stores, presence or absence of granulomas, tumor cells, and overall estimate of bone marrow activity.

Interpretation requires a differential count of the myeloid, lymphoid, and erythroid series; an iron stain; and other appropriate techniques, such as immunohistochemical stains if a differential diagnosis of lymphoproliferative or myeloproliferative disorders is being considered. Other appropriate specific stains may be indicated if metastatic tumor or infection is suspected or being evaluated.[17–19] Table 4–5 lists the other tests that may be performed in the diagnosis of anemias and the chapters in which these tests are discussed.

> **Table 4-5**
OTHER TESTS THAT MAY BE PERFORMED IN THE DIAGNOSIS OF ANEMIAS

Test	Diagnostic Use	Chapter
Hemoglobin electrophoresis	Hemoglobinopathies Thalassemia syndromes	11, 28
Antiglobulin testing	Hemolytic anemias	13
Osmotic fragility test	Hereditary spherocytosis* Severe iron deficiency Sickle cell disease β Thalassemia	9, 28
Sucrose hemolysis test (sugar-water test)	Paroxysmal nocturnal hemoglobinuria* Hypoplastic anemias Myelodysplastic syndromes	13, 28
Acidified serum test (Ham's test)	Paroxysmal nocturnal hemoglobinuria Dyserythropoietic anemia, type II	13, 28
Tests for red blood cell enzymes	Hemolytic anemias G6PD deficiency PK deficiency	10
Serum iron and iron-binding capacity	Iron-deficiency anemia	6
Folate and vitamin B_{12} measurements	Megaloblastic anemias	7

*Primary use.
Abbreviations: G6PD = glucose-6-phosphate dehydrogenase; PK = pyruvate kinase.

Anemia has physiologic, functional, and quantitative parameters that may be related to hemoglobin or hematocrit levels. The differential diagnosis of anemia requires careful consideration of a wide variety of marrow, extramedullary, and interrelating disease states. A large armamentarium of tests is available to aid in the differential diagnosis of the multiple types of anemia. Successful studies of causes of anemia require broad knowledge of clinical laboratory techniques and medicine.

Patient Studies of Anemia
Individual patient studies of anemia are addressed in Chapters 6 to 14.

QUESTIONS

1. Which of the following laboratory results would not be a usual criterion for making a diagnosis of anemia?
   a. Decreased hemoglobin level
   b. Decreased hematocrit level
   c. Decreased platelet count
   d. Decreased RBC count

2. What condition is not a cause of anemia?
   a. Dietary deficiency
   b. Moderate exercise
   c. Decreased RBC production
   d. Increased RBC destruction or loss

3. Which response represents the most complete and correct listing of the most common clinical signs of anemia?
   a. Fatigue, weakness, dyspnea, pallor
   b. Urticaria, hypertension, inflammation, nausea

   c. Nausea, hypertension, temperature elevation, melena
   d. Rapid pulse, inflammation, temperature elevation, dehydration

4. What is the most commonly accepted method for measuring hemoglobin?
   a. Conversion of hemoglobin to oxyhemoglobin, followed by spectrophotometric measurement
   b. Iron content measured by radioimmunoassay technique
   c. Copper sulfate measured by specific gravity
   d. Conversion of hemoglobin to cyanmethemoglobin, followed by spectrophotometric measurement

5. How is hematocrit measured on automated hematology instruments?
   a. Centrifugation
   b. Photometrically
   c. Calculation (MCV × RBC count)
   d. Calculation (MCH × Hgb)

6. A patient has the following results: Hct 26%; Hgb 8 g/dL; and RBC count $3.5 \times 10^6/\mu L$. Calculate the RBC indices—MCV, MCH, and MCHC—and determine the classification of the anemia.
   a. MCV 88 fL; MCH 30 pg; MCHC 33 g/dL; normocytic, normochromic
   b. MCV 101 fL; MCH 33 pg; MCHC 35 g/dL; macrocytic, normochromic
   c. MCV 74 fL; MCH 22 pg; MCHC 31 g/dL; microcytic, hypochromic

7. Which of the following would not be characteristically found on a peripheral blood smear in a case of anemia?
   a. Anisocytosis and/or poikilocytosis
   b. Basophilic stippling, Howell-Jolly bodies, and Pappenheimer bodies
   c. Cabot rings and Heinz bodies
   d. Döhle bodies and toxic granules

8. What is the diagnostic value of the reticulocyte count in the evaluation of anemia?
   a. Determines response and potential of the bone marrow
   b. Determines compensation mechanisms for anemia
   c. Determines the corrected RBC count after calculation
   d. Determines the potential sampling error for RBC count

9. Which of the following is a lesser factor to be considered in the interpretation of a bone marrow aspirate smear?
   a. Maturation of red and white blood cell series
   b. M:E ratio
   c. Type and amount of hemoglobin
   d. Estimate of bone marrow activity

➤ SUMMARY CHART

➤ Anemia is usually characterized by decreased RBC count, hemoglobin, and/or hematocrit levels.

➤ Moderate anemias (7 to 10 g Hgb/dL) that develop slowly may have few clinical symptoms.

➤ Severe anemias or those that develop rapidly (e.g., following acute blood loss) may be associated with dyspnea, general lethargy, and orthostatic hypotension.

➤ Hemoglobin levels vary with age and sex. Reference ranges should be determined and reported for infants, children, and adult men and women.

➤ There are many causes of anemia. They include nutritional deficiencies, blood loss, increased destruction or decreased production of RBCs, infections, toxicity, heredity, and acquired defects.

➤ Chronic anemia is usually compensated for by increased levels of 2,3-DPG, which enables enhanced release of oxygen from hemoglobin.

➤ Reference range values for red cell indices can be used to aid in the classification and diagnosis of anemias.

➤ Treatment of anemia varies with the cause. Generally, the causes should be determined before a treatment is instituted.

➤ The cyanmethemoglobin method is the reference method for measuring hemoglobin.

➤ Morphological examinations of the peripheral blood smear and bone marrow preparations are valuable aids in the diagnosis of anemias.

➤ Clinical symptoms associated with anemia may include vertigo, light-headedness, muscle weakness, headache, or dyspnea.

➤ Adult hemoglobin reference ranges are approximately 14 to 18 g/dL for men and 12 to 16 g/dL for women.

➤ Persons living at elevations above 8000 feet may have persistently increased hemoglobin values secondary to decreased oxygen saturation in ambient atmosphere.

➤ Erythropoietin, a hormone produced in the kidney, is increased in states of anemia.

➤ The hematocrit (Hct), or packed red cell volume, is determined by centrifugation of blood of either capillary or venous origin; it can be calculated by the mean corpuscular volume (MCV) multiplied by the RBC count.

➤ The ratio between the hemoglobin and hematocrit values is 1:3.

➤ The hematocrit reference range of adult males is $47\% \pm 5\%$; for women, it is $42\% \pm 5\%$

➤ The MCV is used as an estimation of the average size of the RBC, and is calculated by the hematocrit multiplied by 10, divided by the RBC count (reference range: 80 to 100 fL).

➤ The mean corpuscular hemoglobin (MCH) is a measure of hemoglobin content and is calculated by the hemoglobin multiplied by 10, divided by the RBC count (reference range: 27 to 31 pg).

➤ The mean corpuscular hemoglobin concentration (MCHC) is derived by hemoglobin multiplied by 100, divided by the hematocrit (reference range: 32% to 36%).

➤ The red cell distribution width (RDW) is an index of size variation and has been used to quantitate the amount of anisocytosis seen on the peripheral blood smear (reference range: 11.5% to 14.5%).

➤ Anemias may be classified as normocytic and normochromic, microcytic and hypochromic, or macrocytic and normochromic.

➤ The reticulocyte count is useful in determining the response and potential of the bone marrow. Staining techniques include new methylene blue or brilliant cresyl blue. Normal adult values are 0.5% to 2.0%. The count can be determined by automated or manual methods.

➤ The corrected reticulocyte count is determined by patient packed corpuscular volume (PCV) multiplied by the reticulocyte count (%), divided by the reference PCV.

References

1. Beck, WS: Hematology, ed 3. MIT Press, Cambridge, MA, 1981, p 16.
2. Reiss, RF: Laboratory diagnosis of erythroid disorders. In Tilton, RC, et al (eds): Clinical Laboratory Medicine. Mosby-Year Book, St. Louis, 1992, pp 898–937.
3. Hoffbrand, AV, et al: Erythropoiesis and general aspects of anaemia. In Hoffbrand, AV, and Pettit, JE (eds): Essential Haematology, ed 3. Blackwell Scientific, Oxford, 1993, pp 12–35.
4. Woodson, RD, et al: Introduction to hemopoiesis. In MacKinney, AA, Jr (ed): Pathophysiology of Blood. John Wiley & Sons, New York, 1984, pp 12–15.
5. Nathan, DG: Hematologic diseases. In Wyngaarden, JB, et al (eds): Cecil Textbook of Medicine, ed 19, vol 1. WB Saunders, Philadelphia, 1992, pp 817–822.

6. Lindenbaum, J: An approach to the anemias. In Wyngaarden, JB, et al (eds): Cecil Textbook of Medicine, ed 19, vol 1. WB Saunders, Philadelphia, 1992, pp 822–831.

7. Kushner, JP: Normochromic, normocytic anemias. In Wyngaarden, JB, et al (eds): Cecil Textbook of Medicine, ed 19, vol 1. WB Saunders, Philadelphia, 1992, pp 837–839.

8. Kushner, JP: Hypochromic anemias. In Wyngaarden, JB, et al (eds): Cecil Textbook of Medicine, ed 19, vol 1. WB Saunders, Philadelphia, 1992, pp 839–846.

9. Allen, RH: Megaloblastic anemias. In Wyngaarden, JB, et al (eds): Cecil Textbook of Medicine, ed 10, vol 1. WB Saunders, Philadelphia, 1992, pp 846–856.

10. Savage, RA, et al: The red cell indices: Yesterday, today, and tomorrow. Routine Hematologic Testing. Clin Lab Med 13:773, 1993.

11. Jones, BA, et al: Complete blood count specimen acceptability. A college of American pathologists Q-probes study of 703 laboratories. Arch Pathol Lab Med 119:203, 1995.

12. Benz, EJ: Structure, function, and synthesis of the human hemoglobins. In Wyngaarden, JB, et al (eds): Cecil Textbook of Medicine, ed 10, vol 1. WB Saunders, Philadelphia, 1992, pp 872–877.

13. Benz, EJ: Classification and basic pathophysiology of the hemoglobinopathies. In Wyngaarden, JB, et al (eds): Cecil Textbook of Medicine, ed 19, vol 1. WB Saunders, Philadelphia, 1992, pp 877–879.

14. Benz, EJ: Hemoglobinopathies with altered solubility or oxygen affinity. In Wyngaarden, JB, et al (eds): Cecil Textbook of Medicine, ed 10, vol 1. WB Saunders, Philadelphia, 1992, pp 879–883.

15. Nienhuis, AW: The thalassemias. In Wyngaarden, JB, et al (eds): Cecil Textbook of Medicine, ed 19, vol 1. WB Saunders, Philadelphia, 1992, pp 883–888.

16. Forget, BG: Sickle cell anemia and associated hemoglobinopathies. In Wyngaarden, JB, et al (eds): Cecil Textbook of Medicine, ed 19, vol 1. WB Saunders, Philadelphia, 1992, pp 888–893.

17. Brunning, RD, and McKenna, RW: Atlas of Tumor Pathology. Tumors of the Bone Marrow. Armed Forces Institute of Pathology, Washington, DC, 1994, p 496.

18. Young, NS: Aplastic anemia and related bone marrow failure syndromes. In Wyngaarden, JB, et al (eds): Cecil Textbook of Medicine, ed 19, vol 1. WB Saunders, Philadelphia, 1992, pp 831–837.

19. Ross, DW: Laboratory evaluation of the patient with hematologic disease. In Bick, RL, et al (eds): Hematology. Clinical and Laboratory Practice, vol I. Mosby-Year Book, St. Louis, 1993, pp 7–16.

5 Evaluation of Cell Morphology and Introduction to Platelet and White Cell Morphology

Betty E. Ciesla, MS, MT(ASCP)SH
Peggy Simpson, MS, MT(ASCP)

THE NORMAL RED BLOOD CELL

ASSESSMENT OF RED CELL ABNORMALITY

SIZE VARIATIONS

Macrocytes

Microcytes

COLOR VARIATIONS

Hypochromia

Polychromasia

SHAPE VARIATIONS

Target Cells (Codocytes)

Spherocytes

Ovalocytes and Elliptocytes

Stomatocytes

Sickle Cells (Drepanocytes)

Acanthocytes

Fragmented Cells (Schistocytes, Burr Cells, Helmet Cells)

Teardrop Cells

VARIATIONS IN RED CELL DISTRIBUTION

Agglutination

Rouleaux

RED CELL INCLUSIONS

Howell-Jolly Bodies

Basophilic Stippling

Siderotic Granules and Pappenheimer Bodies

Heinz Bodies

Cabot Rings

EXAMINATION OF PLATELET MORPHOLOGY

WHITE BLOOD CELL MORPHOLOGY

CASE STUDY

OBJECTIVES

At the end of the chapter, the learner should be able to:

1. Define anisocytosis and poikilocytosis.

2. List the clinical conditions in which a variable red cell size is observed.

3. Define the terms *normochromic* and *hypochromic* according to red cell indices.

4. Name and describe the clinical disorders that result in hypochromia.

5. Describe the clinical conditions that may produce polychromatophilic cells.

6. Indicate which clinical conditions may show target cells, spherocytes, ovalocytes, elliptocytes, and stomatocytes.

7. List diseases that may show fragmented red cells and describe their pathophysiology.

8. Discuss agglutination and rouleaux and specify the particular clinical conditions associated with these abnormalities.

9. Describe the most common red blood cell inclusions and relate each inclusion to a clinical condition.

10. Describe normal platelet morphology and specify some platelet abnormalities seen in pathologic conditions.

11. Specify conditions showing leukocyte cytoplasmic changes, such as toxic granulation, toxic vacuolization, or Dohle bodies.

Automation in hematology has dramatically shifted work patterns. Staff technologists in hematology laboratories or core laboratories are expected to maintain quality, efficiency, and morphological acuity as they respond to continuing changes in laboratory services. Less and less time is spent reviewing normal blood smears, because according to the flagging codes of most automated instruments, only those samples with quantitative abnormalities and some qualitative abnormalities are "flagged."[1] Once a sample is flagged, it must be resolved either through reflex testing or prior history. As part of reflex testing, nonroutine samples are those that are given a slide review or slide screen (usually fewer than 100 white cells) and if, necessary, a complete differential count. If a sufficiently strict set of critical values is in place, combined with the internal instrument flagging criteria, technologists usually feel comfortable with alternatives to the full differential, such as slide reviews.[2] Although red cell morphology is still being assessed by most institutions, its significance in terms of discovery has diminished. Red cell morphology linked to red blood cell indices and the red cell distribution width (RDW) is fairly reliable; therefore, the only smears that are reviewed are those that fall out of autoverification.[3]

From the educational perspective, it is essential that students be trained to recognize cellular abnormalities, because most of the blood smears they review will be abnormal. From the practitioner perspective, however, students graduating from some programs will become familiar with automated differential instruments only through their clinical rotations. Because of the high cost of purchasing automated differential instruments, few programs have the luxury of owning and subsequently training their students on automated cell counting equipment. The easy and natural progression from student laboratory to training or clinical affiliate laboratory will be lost. Training at the laboratory site will need to include comprehensive and detailed training on automated instruments.

This chapter guides the student in interpretation of red cell, platelet, and white cell morphology. Basic mechanics in assessing red blood cell morphology are reviewed (Table 5–1); however, the emphasis is on recognizing a distinct morphology and relating it to the clinical condition. *Physiologic mechanisms* are explained for each morphology to give the reader a better understanding about a particular abnormality. This description of blood cell morphology maximizes the ability of each slide reviewer to recognize and correlate the blood morphology to the clinical pathology and abnormal results.

➤ THE NORMAL RED BLOOD CELL

The mature erythrocyte (red blood cell, normocyte, erythron) has a remarkable structure. Its simplistic appearance is deceiving. It is one of the few cells that pass from a nucleated to a nonnucleated status on maturity, with decreasing size, and a dramatic change in cytoplasmic color. On a Wright-stained blood smear, this mature red cell has a reddish-orange appearance. The red cell has an average diameter of 7 to 8 μm and an average volume of 90 fL. The area of central pallor is approximately 2 to 3 μm in diameter (Fig. 5–1), and the size variation of red cells from a normal patient is approximately 5%. Fundamental to the red cell is the formation of hemoglobin, which functions primarily in an oxygen-carrying capacity for the cell. Additionally, a minimum amount of hemoglobin is required for maintenance of structural integrity. The red cell membrane is a lipid bilayer, the skeleton of which is composed of glycophorin and spectrin. Glycophorin, an integral red cell membrane, spans the entire diameter of the red cell membrane and contains most of the membrane sialic acid on which many red cell antigens are located. Spectrin, the dominant peripheral membrane protein, consists of two high-molecular-weight polypeptides and functions prominently in the maintenance of cell shape and deformability.

➤ ASSESSMENT OF RED CELL ABNORMALITY

A well-stained and well-distributed blood smear is essential for any peripheral blood smear review. When a blood smear is inspected for abnormal morphology, two criteria must be met. Firstly, is the abnormal morphology seen in every field to be examined? Secondly, is the morphology pathologic and not artificially induced? If these criteria are met, then the reviewer must make a general assessment of whether the morphology is due to shape change (poikilocytosis) or size change (anisocytosis). Most assessments of anisocytosis are performed in concert with the red cell indices and the RDW rating. A reviewer takes into account the percentage of cells that vary in size in at least 10 oil immersion fields. For example, if the mean corpuscular volume (MCV) was 65 fL, the reviewer would expect to see a majority of small cells. If, however, the MCV was 80 fL with a high RDW rating (normal RDW is 11.5% to 14.5%), the reviewer would expect to see a mixture of large and small cells.[4]

The majority of institutions use either qualitative remarks (few or marked) or a numerical grading (1+ to 4+) based on percentage of variation to describe the type of cell or cells that have caused the variation from the normal. Using this

➤ Table 5-1
GRADING SCALE FOR RED CELL MORPHOLOGY (ANISOCYTOSIS/POIKILOCYTOSIS)

Percentage of Cells That Differ in Size or Shape from Normal Red Blood Cells

Normal	5%
Slight	5%–10%
1+	10%–25%
2+	25%–50%
3+	50%–75%
4+	>75%

At the level of 4+, the suffix "-cytosis" is acceptable, rather than a numerical grading.

Sample Situations

2+ microcytes	Few schistocytes
1+ macrocytes	Few burr cells
	1+ target cells
3+ anisocytosis	
	2+ poikilocytosis

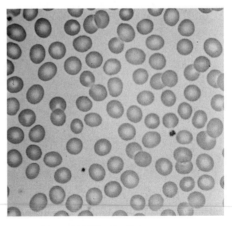

➤ FIGURE 5–1 Normal red blood cells.

method, a reviewer can present to the clinician a series of objective ratings that can translate to a visual impression of a patient's peripheral smear. Refer to Table 5–1 for guidelines in grading red cell morphology. Figure 5–2 is a composite chart of normal and abnormal red cell morphology.

Included in this chapter are flowcharts that correlate the abnormal morphology with a possible pathology. This scheme should enable the learner to more easily associate an abnormal morphology with the clinical condition.

➤ SIZE VARIATIONS

Macrocytes

Macrocytes may be defined as cells that are approximately 9 μm or larger in diameter, having an MCV of greater than 100 fL.[5] They may arrive in the peripheral circulation by several mechanisms. Three of the most distinct are (1) impaired deoxyribonucleic acid (DNA) synthesis leading to a decreased number of cellular divisions, consequently a larger cell (megaloblastic erythropoiesis); (2) accelerated erythropoiesis yielding a premature release of reticulocytes, in the Wright-stained smear manifested as polychromatophilic macrocytes; and (3) conditions in which membrane cholesterol and lecithin are increased. However, this last mechanism may not be reflective of a "true" macrocytosis (obstructive liver disease). Macrocytes should be evaluated for shape (oval versus round) as shown in Figure 5–3, color (red versus blue), pallor (if present), and the presence or absence of inclusions.

Figure 5–4 lists the more common conditions in which macrocytes may be seen: the megaloblastic processes, liver disease, and regenerative bone marrow. Additionally, macrocytic cells may be seen in metastatic marrow infiltration in neonatal blood, hypothyroidism, and postsplenectomy.

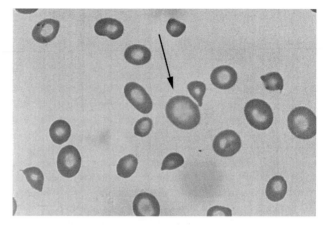

➤ **FIGURE 5–3**   Note the different size (anisocytosis) and shape (poikilocytosis) of the red cells. Compare the largest (macrocytic) cell below the arrow in the center of the field with the smaller (microcytic) cells.

Microcytes

A microcyte is defined as a small cell having a diameter of less than 7 μm and an MCV of less than 80 fL.[6] Any defect that results in impaired hemoglobin synthesis will result in a microcytic, hypochromic blood picture. When developing, erythroid cells are deprived of any of the essential elements in hemoglobin synthesis (see Chap. 6); the result is increased cellular divisions and consequently a smaller cell in the peripheral blood. Hemoglobin synthesis involves multiple steps, and microcytosis develops from (1) ineffective iron utilization, absorption, or release, and (2) decreased or defective globin synthesis. Effective porphyrin synthesis is, of course, vital for hemoglobinization; however, the porphyrias generally do not cause a microcytic erythrocyte.

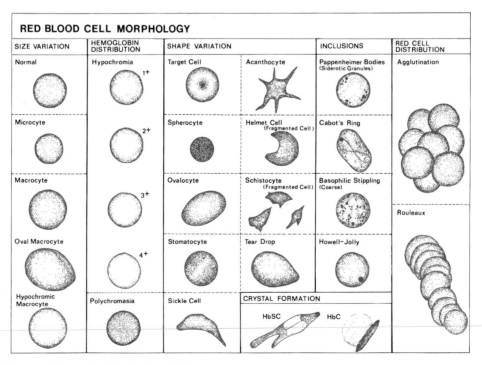

➤ FIGURE 5–2   Normal and abnormal red blood cell morphology.

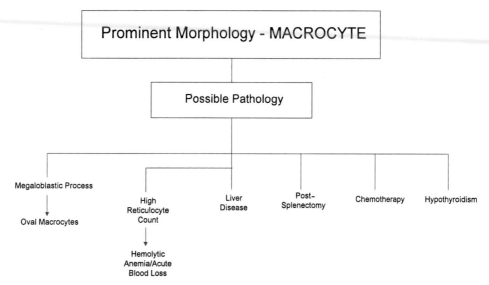

➤ FIGURE 5–4   Correlation of macrocytes to pathologic processes.

Figure 5–5 illustrates clinical conditions in which microcytes may be seen as the predominant cell morphology.

➤ COLOR VARIATIONS

Hypochromia

Any red blood cell having a central area of pallor of greater than 3 μm is said to be hypochromic. There is a direct relationship between the amount of hemoglobin deposited in the red cell and the appearance of the red cell when properly stained. For this reason, any irregularity in hemoglobin synthesis will lead to some degree of hypochromia. Most clinicians choose to assess hypochromia based on the mean corpuscular hemoglobin concentration (MCHC), which by definition measures hemoglobin content in a given volume of red cells (100 mL). In general, this is very reliable; however, it does not take into account the situation in which a true hypochromia is observed in the presence of a normal MCHC. Suffice it to say that not all hypochromic cells are microcytic. Target cells possess some degree of hypochromia, and there are macrocytes and normocytes that can be distinctly hypochromic.

Peripheral Blood Observations

The most common condition manifesting hypochromia is iron-deficiency anemia. In severe cases of iron-deficiency anemia, red cells exhibit an inordinately thin band of hemoglobin. Patients with iron deficiency have many hypochromic cells, depending on the magnitude of the deficiency. Hypochromia in the alpha (α) and beta (β) trait thalassemia syndromes is much less pronounced. However red cells in the α thalassemias and β thalassemia homozygous states show significant amounts of pallor.[7] The sideroblastic anemias show a prominent dimorphic blood picture—macrocytic, normocytic, and microcytic cells together, only some of which show true hypochromia. Some hypochromic cells may be seen in patients with lead poisoning; however, the association of microcytosis with lead poisoning irrespective of any other underlying process is being questioned. The morphologist should not be unduly influenced by the red blood cell indices in the evaluation of hypochromia. In many cases, the MCHC will not be concordant with what is observed on the peripheral smear. True hypochromia will appear as a delicate shaded area of pallor as opposed to pseudohypochromia (the water artifact), in which the area of pallor is distinctly outlined. Refer to Table 5–2 for a guideline to grading hypochromia.

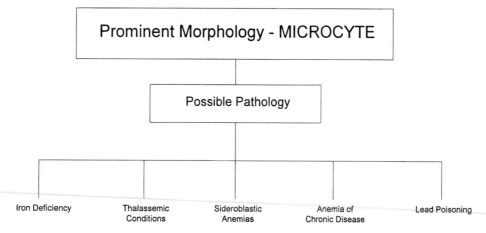

➤ FIGURE 5–5   Correlation of microcytes to pathologic processes.

> **Table 5-2**
> **HYPOCHROMIA GRADING**

1+	Area of central pallor is one-half of cell diameter
2+	Area of pallor is two-thirds of cell diameter
3+	Area of pallor is three-quarters
4+	Thin rim of hemoglobin

> **Table 5-3**
> **POLYCHROMASIA GRADING**

Percentage of Red Cells That Are Polychromatophilic

Slight	1%
1+	3%
2+	5%
3+	10%
4+	>11%

Polychromasia

When red blood cells are delivered to the peripheral circulation prematurely, their appearance in the Wright-stained smear is distinctive. Red cells showing polychromatophilia are gray-blue in color and are usually larger than normal red cells (Fig. 5–6; see also Color Plate 84). The basophilia of the red cell is the result of the residual ribonucleic acid (RNA) involved in hemoglobin synthesis.[8] Polychromatophilic macrocytes are actually reticulocytes; however, the reticulum cannot be visualized without supravital staining.

Peripheral Blood Observations

It is not uncommon to find a few polychromatophilic cells in a normal peripheral blood smear, because regeneration of red cells is a dynamic process. The reticulocyte count should reflect the degree of polychromasia. In the blood smear, polychromatophilic red cells come in varying shades of blue. Any clinical condition in which the marrow is stimulated, particularly red blood cell regeneration, will produce a polychromatophilic blood picture. This represents effective erythropoiesis. Examples of several conditions in which polychromasia is noted include acute and chronic hemorrhage, hemolysis, and any regenerative red cell process. The degree of polychromasia is an excellent indicator of therapeutic effectiveness when a patient is given iron or vitamin therapy as a treatment for anemia. Refer to Table 5–3 for a guideline to polychromasia grading.

➤ SHAPE VARIATIONS

Target Cells (Codocytes)

Target cells appear on the peripheral blood as a result of an increase in red blood cell surface membrane. Their true circulating form is a bell-shaped cell. In air-dried smears, however, they appear as "targets," with a large portion of hemoglobin displayed at the rim of the cell and a portion of hemoglobin that is central, eccentric, or banded (Fig. 5–7). Target cells are always hypochromic.

The mechanism of targeting is related to excess membrane cholesterol and phospholipid and decreased cellular hemoglobin. This is well documented in patients with liver disease, in whom the cholesterol-phospholipid ratio is altered. Mature red cells are unable to synthesize cholesterol and phospholipid independently. As cholesterol accumulates in the plasma, as occurs in liver dysfunction, the red cell is expanded by increased membrane lipid, resulting in increased surface area. Consequently, the osmotic fragility is also decreased. Figure 5–8 shows the more common conditions in which target cells are observed.

Spherocytes

Spherocytes have several distinctive properties and, in contrast to target cells, the lowest surface area-to-volume ratio. They are smaller than the normal red cell, their hemoglobin content seems to be relatively concentrated, and they have no visible central pallor. Because of their density (intense color) and smaller size, they are easily distinguished in a peripheral smear. Their shape change is irreversible. There are several mechanisms for the production of spherocytes, each sharing the mutual defect of loss of membrane. In the normal aging process of red cells, spherocytes are produced as a final stage before senescent red cells are detained in the spleen and trapped by the reticuloendothelial system. Coating of the red cells with antibodies and the detrimental effect of complement activation will produce spherocytes as the red cell membrane loses cholesterol, and secondarily surface area, as a result of splenic sequestration.

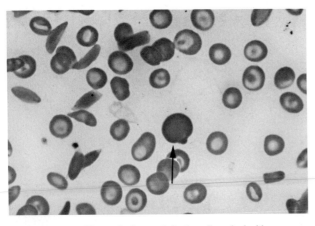

➤ FIGURE 5–6   Note polychromasia in the cell marked with an arrow.

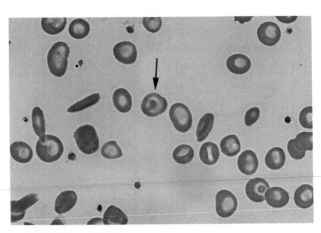

➤ FIGURE 5–7   Note the target cell at the arrow.

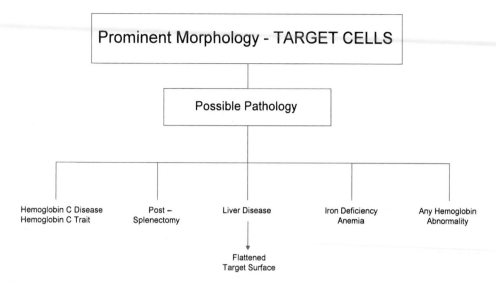

➤ **FIGURE 5-8**   Correlation of target cells to pathologic processes.

Perhaps the most detailed mechanism for sphering is the congenital condition known as hereditary spherocytosis. This is an inherited, autosomal dominant condition, and it is an intrinsic defect in the red cell membrane protein, spectrin, which is decreased in quantity and functionally abnormal.[9] This defect causes the spheroidal red cell to be prematurely trapped and destroyed in the spleen. Erythrocytes from patients with hereditary spherocytosis have a mean influx of sodium twice that of normal cells, but their potassium and water content is decreased. Consequently, when these cells reach the microenvironment of the spleen, the active-passive transport system is unbalanced and the cells swell and hemolyze (see Chap. 9). In over one-half of these patients, the MCHC is greater than 36%. Yet for those individuals not exhibiting an increased MCHC, a careful observation of their peripheral smear is the key to diagnosis.[9] Figure 5–9 lists the more common pathologic conditions in which spherocytes are seen, and Figure 5–10 shows a blood smear from a patient with hereditary spherocytosis.

Ovalocytes and Elliptocytes

The ovalocyte is a cell of many capabilities. It can appear normochromic or hypochromic, normocytic or macrocytic. The exact physiologic mechanism is not well defined. When these erythrocytes are incubated in vitro, they reduce adenosine triphosphate (ATP) and 2,3-diphosphoglycerate (2,3-DPG) more rapidly than do normal cells. Hemoglobin seems to have a bipolar arrangement in these cells, and there seems to be a reduction in membrane cholesterol.

Many investigators consider the terms *ovalocyte* and *elliptocyte* to be interchangeable; however, for the purposes of this discussion, they are viewed as distinct and separate. Ovalocytes are more egg-shaped and have a greater tendency to vary in their hemoglobin content. Elliptocytes, on the other hand, are pencil-shaped and invariably not hypochromic. Hereditary elliptocytosis is an inherited condition with many subsets and degrees of clinical severity. In the most common form, there is a membrane defect in spectrin and protein 4.1, which may cause hemolysis.[10] Refer to Figure 5–11 for a description of pathologic processes associated with ovalocytes and elliptocytes.

Stomatocytes

The stomatocyte is defined as a red cell of normal size that, in wet preparation, appears bowl-shaped (Fig. 5–12). This peculiar shape is manifested in air-dried smears as a slitlike area of central pallor. The exact physiologic mechanism of stomatocytosis has yet to be clarified. Many chemical agents can induce stomatocytosis in vitro (phenothiazine and chlorpromazine); however, these changes are reversible. Stoma-

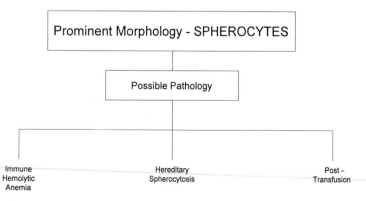

➤ **FIGURE 5-9**   Correlation of spherocytes to pathologic processes.

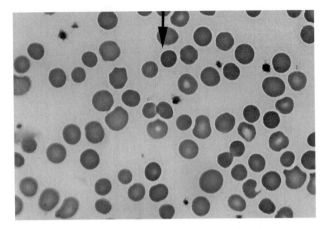

➤ FIGURE 5–10 Note the spherocyte at arrow in a blood smear from a patient with hereditary spherocytosis.

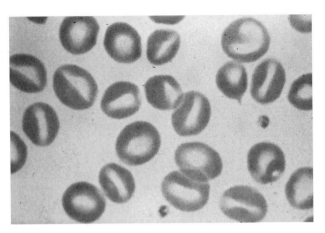

➤ FIGURE 5–12 Stomatocytes in peripheral blood.

tocytes are known to have an increased permeability to sodium; consequently, their osmotic fragility is increased.

Stomatocytes are more often artifactual than a true manifestation of a particular pathophysiologic process. The artifactual stomatocyte has a distinct slitlike area of central pallor, whereas the area of pallor in the genuine stomatocyte appears shaded. Several of the associated disease states in which stomatocytes may be found are hereditary spherocytosis (the stomatospherocyte is best viewed in wet preparations); hereditary stomatocytosis, which is usually a benign condition; occasionally hemolytic, acute alcoholism; and in patients with the Rh null phenotype.

Sickle Cells (Drepanocytes)

Sickle cells, or drepanocytes, are red cells that have been transformed by hemoglobin polymerization into rigid, inflexible cells with at least one pointed projection (Fig. 5–13). Patients may be homozygous or heterozygous for the presence of the abnormal hemoglobin, hemoglobin S. In the homozygous patient, physiologic conditions of low oxygen tension (in vivo or in vitro) cause the abnormal hemoglobin to polymerize, forming tubules that line up in bundles to deform the cell. The surface area of the transformed cell is much greater, and the normal elasticity of the cell is severely restricted.

Most sickled cells possess the ability to revert to the discocyte shape when oxygenated; however, approximately 10% are incapable of reverting to their normal shape. These irreversibly sickled cells (ISCs) are the result of repeated sickling episodes. In the peripheral smear, they appear as crescent-shaped cells with long projections. When reoxygenated, the ISCs may undergo fragmentation. During a symptomatic period, the percentage of ISCs varies tremendously, and, consequently, it does not correlate with symptomatology. Sickle cells are not usually seen in the peripheral smears of individuals who are heterozygous (carriers).

Classically sickled cells are best seen in wet prepara-

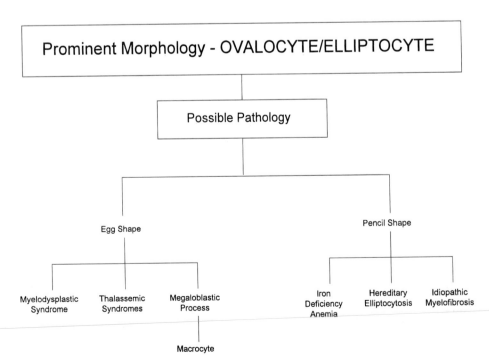

➤ FIGURE 5–11 Correlation of ovalocytes and elliptocytes to pathologic processes.

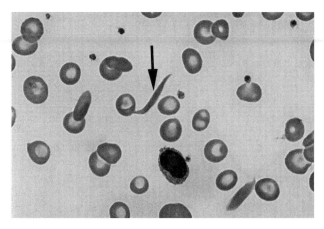

➤ FIGURE 5–13   Irreversibly sickled cells.

tions. Many of the cells observed in the Wright-Giemsa stain are the oat cell–shaped form of the sickled cell (Fig. 5–14). In this form, the projections are much less pronounced and the central area of the cell is fairly broad. This shape is reversible.[11] The more prominent pathologic conditions in which sickle cells may be observed are listed in Figure 5–15. In this figure, a morphological distinction is made between ISCs and reversibly sickled cells.

Acanthocytes

An acanthocyte is defined as a cell of normal or slightly reduced size, possessing 3 to 12 spicules of uneven length distributed along the periphery of the cell membrane. The uneven projections of the acanthocyte are blunt rather than pointed, and the acanthocyte can easily be distinguished from the peripheral smear background because it appears to be saturated with hemoglobin. The MCHC is, however, always in the normal range.

A specific mechanism related to the formation of acanthocytes is unknown. There are, however, some details about these peculiar cells that are of interest. Acanthocytes contain an excess of cholesterol and have an increased cholesterol-to-phospholipid ratio. Their surface area is increased. The lecithin content of acanthocytes is decreased. The only inherited condition in which acanthocytes are seen in high numbers is congenital abetalipoproteinemia; however, acanthocytes may be observed in patients with anorexia nervosa.[12] Most cases of acanthocytosis are acquired, such as the deficiency of lecithin-cholesterol acyltransferase, which

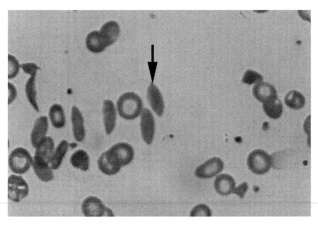

➤ FIGURE 5–14   Reversible, oat-shaped sickle cell.

has been well documented in patients with severe hepatic disease. This enzyme is synthesized by the liver and is directly responsible for esterifying free cholesterol; when this enzyme is deficient, cholesterol is increased in the plasma.

The red cell responds to this excess cholesterol in one of two ways, depending on the balance of other lipids in the membrane. It will become a target cell or an acanthocyte. Once an acanthocyte is formed, it is very liable to splenic sequestration and fragmentation, and the fluidity of the membrane is directly affected. Figure 5–16 lists the most prominent pathologies in which acanthocytes may be observed.

Fragmented Cells (Schistocytes, Burr Cells, Helmet Cells)

It may seem unusual to include these three red cell forms under the same heading; however the choice for such a grouping becomes reasonable with an expanded definition of fragmentation. Fragmentation may be defined as loss from the cell of a piece of membrane that may or may not contain hemoglobin. These events may occur repeatedly without the loss of hemoglobin; however, each successive loss of membrane (each fragmentation that occurs) leaves the red cell more rigid and more likely to become entrapped in the splenic sinuses.

It is recognized that not all membrane alterations occur pathologically. Indeed, the echinocytic transformation of normal red cells in stored plasma is known to be reversible. Likewise, discocyte-to-echinocyte transformation is part of normal red cell senescence. However, there are certain triggering events in disease that invariably lead to fragmentation. Two pathways are recognized. Firstly, alteration of normal fluid circulation occurs, which may predispose to fragmentation. Examples of this include vasculitis, malignant hypertension, thrombotic thrombocytopenic purpura, and heart valve replacement. Secondly, intrinsic defects of the red cell make it less deformable and, therefore, more likely to be fragmented as it traverses the microvasculature of the spleen. Spherocytes, antibody-altered red cells, and red cells containing inclusions have significant alterations that decrease their red cell survival, and these serve as examples of the second pathway.

Burr cells (echinocytes) are red cells with approximately 10 to 30 rounded spicules evenly placed over the surface of the red cells (Fig. 5–17). They are normochromic and normocytic, for the most part. They may be observed as an artifact, usually as a result of specimen contamination, in which case they will appear in large numbers and will present with spiky projections. "True" burr cells occur in small numbers in uremia, heart disease, cancer of the stomach, bleeding peptic ulcer, immediately following an injection of heparin, and in a number of patients with untreated hypothyroidism. In general, they may occur in situations that cause a change in tonicity of the intravascular fluid (e.g., dehydration and azotemia).

Helmet cells (bite cells) are recognized by their distinctive projections, usually two, surrounding an empty area of the red cell membrane that looks as if it has been bitten off (see Fig. 5–17). In hematologic conditions in which large inclusion bodies are formed (Heinz bodies), helmet cells are visible in the peripheral smear. Fragmentation occurs by the pitting mechanism of the spleen. Helmet cells may also be seen in patients with pulmonary emboli, myeloid metaplasia, and disseminated intravascular coagulation (DIC).

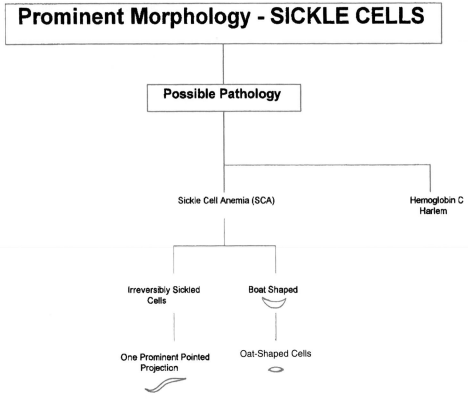

> FIGURE 5-15   Correlation of sickle cells to pathologic processes.

Schistocytes are the extreme form of red cell fragmentation (see Fig. 5–17). Whole pieces of red cell membrane appear to be missing, and bizarre red cells are apparent. Schistocytes may be occur in patients with microangiopathic hemolytic anemia, DIC, heart valve surgery, hemolytic uremic syndrome, thrombotic thrombocytopenic purpura,[13] as well as in severe burn cases.

Refer to Figure 5–18 for a flowchart correlation of the fragmented cells matched to the pathologic processes in which they may be observed.

Teardrop Cells

Teardrop cells appear in the peripheral circulation as pear-shaped red cells (Fig. 5–19). The extent to which a portion of

the red cells form tails is variable, and these cells may be normal, reduced, or increased in size. The exact physiologic mechanism is unknown, yet teardrop formation from inclusion-containing red cells is well documented. As cells containing large inclusions attempt to pass through the microcirculation, the portion of the cells containing the inclusion gets pinched, leaving a tailed end. For some reason, the red cell is unable to maintain the discocyte shape once this has occurred.

Teardrop cells are seen most prominently in idiopathic myelofibrosis with myeloid metaplasia. This type of morphological finding can also be seen in patients with the thalassemia syndromes, in iron deficiency, and in conditions in which inclusion bodies are formed. Refer to Figure 5–2 for a composite of abnormal red cell morphology.

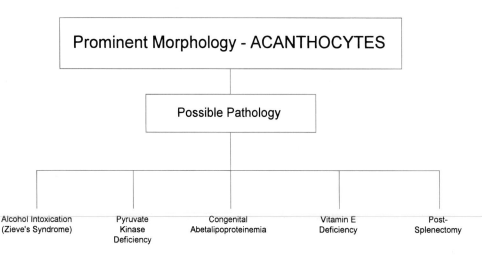

> FIGURE 5-16   Correlation of acanthocytes to pathologic processes.

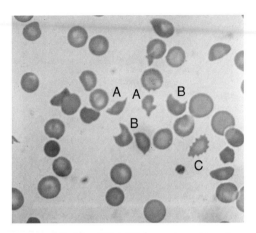

➤ FIGURE 5–17 Peripheral blood from a patient with malignant hypertension. Note the presence of fragmented cells: (*A*) schistocytes, (*B*) helmet cells, and (*C*) a burr cell. (From Bell, A: Hematology. In: Listen, Look, and Learn. Health and Education Resources, Inc., Bethesda, MD, with permission.)

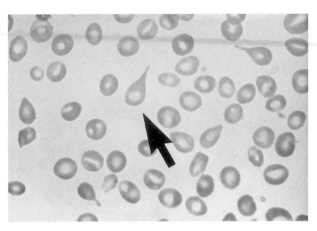

➤ FIGURE 5–19 Teardrop cells (peripheral blood).

➤ VARIATIONS IN RED CELL DISTRIBUTION

Agglutination

If an erythrocyte antibody is present in a patient's plasma and a corresponding erythrocyte antigen is represented, agglutination will take place. Such is the case with cold antibody syndromes such as cold hemagglutination disease and paroxysmal cold hemoglobinuria. The agglutination occurs at room temperature in sample preparation and appears as interspersed areas of clumping throughout the peripheral smear (see Color Plate 116). The use of saline will not disperse these agglutinated areas; however, warming the sample helps to break up the agglutinins. The MCHC is usually falsely elevated in response to the agglutinin formation.

Rouleaux

Rouleaux formation is the result of elevated globulins or fibrinogen in the plasma. Red cells that are constantly bathed in this abnormal plasma appear as stacks of coins in the peripheral smear (see Color Plate 244). These stacks are rather evenly dispersed throughout the smear. The use of a saline dilution of the serum disperses rouleaux. Rouleaux formation correlates well with a high erythrocyte sedimentation rate and occurs as a direct result of protein deposition or adsorption on the erythrocyte membrane. This lowers the zeta (ζ) potential, thus facilitating the stacking effect.

Rouleaux is seen in patients with multiple myeloma, Waldenstrom's macroglobulinemia, chronic inflammatory disorders, and some lymphomas.

➤ RED CELL INCLUSIONS

Howell-Jolly Bodies

Howell-Jolly bodies (Fig. 5–20 and Color Plate 85) are nuclear remnants containing DNA. They are 1 to 2 μm in size and may appear singly or doubly in an eccentric position on the periphery of the cell membrane. They are thought to develop in periods of accelerated or abnormal erythropoiesis.

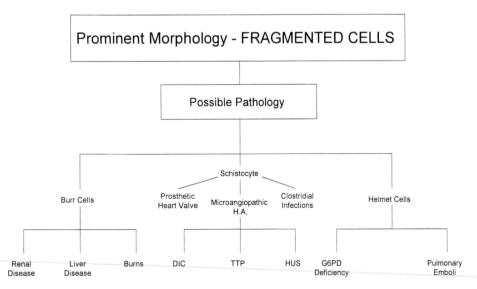

➤ FIGURE 5–18 Correlation of fragmented cells to pathologic processes. HA = hemolytic anemia; DIC = disseminated intravascular coagulation; HUS = hemolytic uremic syndrome; TTP = thrombotic thrombocytopenic purpura.

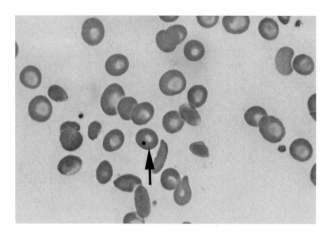

► FIGURE 5–20   Howell-Jolly body.

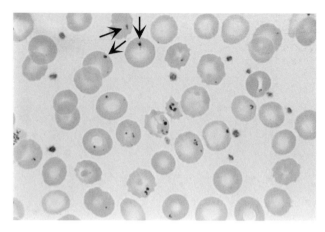

► FIGURE 5–21   Pappenheimer bodies (Wright stain).

A fragment of the chromosome becomes detached and is left floating in the cytoplasm after the nucleus has been extruded. Under ordinary circumstances, the spleen effectively pits these nondeformable bodies from the cell. However, during periods of erythroid stress, the pitting mechanism cannot keep pace with inclusion formation.

Howell-Jolly bodies may be seen following splenectomy, in patients with thalassemic syndromes, hemolytic anemias, and megaloblastic anemias, and in functional hyposplenia.

Basophilic Stippling

Red cells that contain ribosomes can potentially form stippled cells; however, it is thought that the actual stippling is the result of the drying of cells in preparation for microscopic examination. Coarse, diffuse, or punctate basophilic stippling may occur and consist of ribonucleoprotein and mitochondrial remnants (see Color Plate 122).

Diffuse basophilic stippling appears as a fine blue dusting, whereas coarse stippling is much more clearly outlined and easily distinguished. Punctate basophilic stippling is a coalescing of smaller forms and is very prominent and easily identifiable.

Stippling may be found in any condition showing defective or accelerated heme synthesis, lead intoxication, and thalassemia syndromes.

Siderotic Granules and Pappenheimer Bodies

Siderotic granules are small, irregular magenta inclusions seen along the periphery of red cells. They usually appear in clusters, as if they have been gently placed on the red cell membrane. Their presence is presumptive evidence for the presence of iron. However, the Prussian blue stain is the confirmatory test for determining the presence of these inclusions. These granules in red blood cells are nonheme iron, resulting from an excess of available iron throughout the body. They are designated *Pappenheimer bodies* when seen in a Wright-stained smear (Fig. 5–21 and Color Plate 86) and *siderotic granules* when seen in Prussian blue stain.

Siderotic granules are found in sideroblastic anemias and in any condition leading to hemochromatosis or hemosiderosis. They may also be seen in the hemoglobinopathies (e.g., sickle cell anemia and thalassemia) and in patients following splenectomy.

Heinz Bodies

Heinz bodies are formed as a result of denatured or precipitated hemoglobin. They can be formed experimentally by incubation with phenylhydrazine. They are large (0.3 to 2 μm) inclusions that are rigid and severely distort the cell membrane. Upon initial exposure to phenylhydrazine, small crystalline bodies appear, coalesce, and migrate to an area beneath the cell membrane. They may not be visualized in Wright's stain but may be seen with crystal violet and brilliant cresyl blue.

Heinz bodies may be seen in the α-thalassemic syndromes, glucose-6-phosphate dehydrogenase (G6PD) deficiency under oxidant stress, and in any of the unstable hemoglobin syndromes (hemoglobin Köln, hemoglobin Zurich). They may also be seen in red cell injury resulting from chemical insult.

Cabot Rings

The exact physiologic mechanism in Cabot ring formation has yet to be elucidated. Cabot rings are found in heavily stippled cells and appear in a figure-of-eight conformation similar to the beads of a necklace (see Chap. 7, Color Plate 94). They are not composed of DNA, but they do contain arginine-rich histone and nonhemoglobin iron. Cabot rings may be found in megaloblastic anemias and homozygous thalassemia syndromes, and postsplenectomy. Table 5–4 summarizes abnormal red cell morphologies and associated disease states and red blood cell inclusions.

► EXAMINATION OF PLATELET MORPHOLOGY

The normal platelet has several distinctive morphological characteristics. This structure measures approximately 2 to 4 μm, with a discoid shape and even blue granules dispersed throughout a light-blue cytoplasm. In pathologic states, platelets may appear as blue or gray agranular discs; they may be extremely large and may show tailing or streaming of the cytoplasm. In rare instances, one may see megakaryocytic fragments in the peripheral circulation.

A close and thorough examination of platelet morphology provides important information about the patient's hemostatic capability. Gross variation in platelet morphology may be seen in infiltrative disease of the bone marrow (e.g., idiopathic myelofibrosis or metastatic infiltrates). Large platelets may be seen in any disorder associated with in-

> **Table 5-4**
> **SUMMARY OF ABNORMAL RED CELL MORPHOLOGIES AND DISEASE STATES THAT MAY BE ASSOCIATED WITH THESE ABNORMAL MORPHOLOGIES**

Microcytes

- Iron-deficiency anemia
- Thalassemias
- Lead poisoning
- Sideroblastic anemia

Macrocytes

- Megaloblastic anemias
- High reticulocyte count
- Liver disease
- Myelodysplatic syndromes

Target Cells

- Liver disease
- Hemoglobinopathies
- Thalassemias
- Sideroblastic anemia

Spherocytes

- Hemolytic anemias
- Posttransfusion
- Hereditary spherocytosis

Elliptocytes

- Hereditary elliptocytosis
- Iron-deficiency anemia
- Thalassemias

Stomatocyte

- Acute alcoholism
- Malignancies

Sickle Cells

- Sickle cell anemia
- Sickle thalassemia

Acanthocytes

- Congenital abetalipoproteinemia
- Vitamin E deficiency
- Alcohol intoxication
- Postsplenectomy

Burr Cells

- Liver disease
- Renal disease
- Severe burns
- Bleeding gastric ulcers

Helmet Cells

- G6PD deficiency
- Pulmonary embol

Schistocytes

- Disseminated intravascular coagulopathy (DIC)
- Thrombotic thrombocytopenic purpura (TTP)
- Hemolytic uremic syndrome

Teardrop Cells

- Severe anemias
- Myeloproliferative disorders
- Pernicious anemia

creased platelet turnover, such as may occur with idiopathic thrombocytopenic purpura or bleeding disorders. In addition to the elevated platelet count, morphological changes may also occur postsplenectomy.

> ## WHITE BLOOD CELL MORPHOLOGY

White blood cells (WBCs, leukocytes) may exhibit several morphological changes, and neutrophils are the cell type primarily affected. Most of these neutrophilic changes originate in the cytoplasm in response to various pathologic processes. Severe infections, inflammatory conditions, or other leukemoid reactions may be accompanied by toxic granulation, toxic vacuolization, or the presence of Dohle bodies (see Chap. 15). Toxic granulation and Dohle bodies are generally considered nonspecific reactive changes, whereas vacuolization strongly indicates a serious bacterial infection.

Toxic granulation describes medium to large granules that are evenly scattered throughout the cytoplasm of segmented polymorphonuclear neutrophil leukocytes. These granules are seen in metabolically active neutrophilia and are composed of peroxidases and acid hydrolases. Although nonspecific, they may occur in patients with severe bacterial infections, toxemia of pregnancy, or vasculitis, or in patients receiving chemotherapy. Toxic vacuolization refers to the round, clear unstained areas that are dispersed randomly throughout the cytoplasm of neutrophils in patients with overwhelming infections. Additional cytoplasmic inclusions—Dohle bodies—are oval, blue, single or multiple inclusions originating in RNA, and are 1 to 3 μm

in diameter. Dohle bodies may be seen in peripheral blood smears of patients with severe infections, in patients with severe burns, in pregnant women, and in patients receiving chemotoxic drugs. In these conditions, they represent toxic changes; however, Dohle bodies are also characteristically observed in certain congenital qualitative WBC disorders such as the May-Hegglin anomaly and the Chédiak-Higashi disorder (see Chap. 15).

In addition to these morphological changes, severe bacterial infections are also commonly associated with a moderate leukocytosis and a shift to the left in granulocytes. Mild infections are characterized by a slight leukocytosis, with or without the shift to the left. "Shift to the left" implies a release of younger granulocytes—specifically bands and metamyelocytes—from the bone marrow storage pool. These particular cell populations may often be observed during an infection or inflammatory process. The presence of more immature forms such as promyelocytes or myeloblasts, in the absences of severe infection, strongly suggests direct marrow architectural involvement. This may indicate an infiltrative, neoplastic, or myeloproliferative process.

The degree of leukocytosis or neutrophilia is useful in discriminating among bacterial, viral, or fungal conditions. Leukocytosis commonly refers to an increase in peripheral blood leukocyte (WBC) concentration of greater than 10,000 cells/μL. Because acute infection can rapidly mobilize the neutrophilic nondividing marrow storage pool, the patient usually has a WBC count below 50,000 cells/μL (average is 25,000 cells/μL). A shift to the left is seen in the peripheral blood smear; however, it is unusual to see cells as immature as myelocytes in the peripheral blood. Fungal infections may also be associated with neutrophilia and an increased WBC count, but a monocytosis is more commonly observed. Viral infections usually are not associated with neutrophilia but rather with lymphocytosis (see Chap. 15).

Leukemoid reactions are characterized by a peripheral neutrophilia that may resemble an emerging leukemia. The WBC count is between 50,000 and 100,000 cells/μL, with immaturity observed in one or more cell types. However, a high blast count is not part of the WBC differential picture, which can be helpful in eliminating leukemia as part of the differential diagnosis. Acute infections, chronic infections such as tuberculosis and chronic osteomyelitis, as well as severe metabolic inflammatory and neoplastic processes have all been associated with leukemoid reactions. Extremely elevated WBC counts (greater than 100,000 cells/μL) are more suggestive of a myeloproliferative process (see Chap. 18), although exceptions have been reported.

Physiologic leukocytosis is defined as an increased WBC count without a shift to the left or any associated morphological changes previously described for granulocytes. This transient condition may be associated with such stimuli as exercise, intense emotional stress, or the administration of epinephrine or glucocorticoids.

➤ CASE STUDY

A 57-year-old woman admitted to the hospital for a hysterectomy had a recent Pap smear and biopsy that revealed the persistence of dysplasia. The patient had not experienced any blood loss and appeared to be healthy. The preadmission workup included an electrocardiogram (ECG), chest x-ray, complete blood count (CBC), and type and screen. The CBC results were as follows:

	Patient Results	Reference Range
WBC	11.7×10^9/L	$4.5–11.0 \times 10^9$/L
RBC	5.77×10^{12}/L	$4.50–5.90 \times 10^{12}$/L
Hgb	11.1 g/dL	12.0–15.0 g/dL
Hct	33.7%	36.0–45.0%
MCV	62.9 fL	80.0–96.0 fL
MCH	20.8 pg	27.0–32.0 pg
MCHC	33.1%	32.0–36.0%
RDW	13.0%	11.5–14.5%
PLT	274×10^9/L	$140–440 \times 10^9$/L
Additional tests ordered:		
Serum ferritin	175 μg/dL	30–300 μg/dL
Hemoglobin A_2	5.8%	1.5–4.0%

Questions
1. Describe the red blood cell (RBC) morphology expected on the peripheral blood smear?
2. Do the CBC results comply with the "rule of three" for evaluation prior to verification and reporting to the physician?
3. What condition is consistent with this CBC?
4. Why are the RBCs microcytic in this condition?

The MCV of 62.9 fL is consistent with a red cell population that is predominantly microcytes. The RDW is normal, which indicates a uniform microcytic population. The MCV and MCH are decreased, but the normal MCHC indicates that the RBCs contain a normal amount of hemoglobin for their size. The expected RBC morphology is microcytic, normochromic.

The CBC results do not correlate with the "rule of three," which states that the RBC count multiplied by three should approximate the hemoglobin value, and the hemoglobin value multiplied by three should equal the hematocrit. Applying the "rule of three" to check the results indicates a problem. The RBC count multiplied by three ($5.77 \times 3 = 17.3$) does not equal the reported hemoglobin value of 11.1. Additionally, the results of $11.1 \times 3 = 33.3$ do not correlate with the actual hematocrit value of 33.7%. The RBC count is out of proportion to the hemoglobin and the hematocrit.

An iron-deficiency anemia is a common microcytic anemia. In the earlier stages of iron-deficiency anemia, a microcytosis without hypochromia may be seen. To differentiate this condition from an iron-deficient condition, iron stores are evaluated. The normal ferritin level indicates normal storage iron in this patient. Because the impaired hemoglobin synthesis is not caused by an iron deficiency, globin chain synthesis is evaluated and hemoglobin A_2 is analyzed. The elevated hemoglobin A_2 is an indication of an increase in delta (δ) globin chain synthesis. This is characteristic of β thalassemia minor. The increase in hemoglobin A_2 and the normal RBC count out of proportion to the slightly decreased hemoglobin and hematocrit are also consistent with β thalassemia minor. Refer to Figure 5–5 for a correlation of microcytosis to the pathologic process.

The RBCs are microcytic in β thalassemia minor owing to the impairment of hemoglobin synthesis. Because there is a decrease in the synthesis of β chains, there is a net decreased synthesis of hemoglobin A. With less hemoglobin A available to the red cells, the result is a microcytic anemia. Whereas in iron deficiency microcytosis occurs because there is not enough heme, in thalassemia minor, the microcytic condition occurs because there is not enough globin.[14]

QUESTIONS

1. The elliptocyte is a morphological feature in:
   a. Myeloid metaplasia
   b. Hemolytic anemia
   c. Iron-deficiency anemia
   d. Sickle cell anemia

2. Which of the following conditions would show oval macrocytes?
   a. Thalassemia syndromes
   b. Megaloblastic processes
   c. Anemia of chronic disorders
   d. Myelodysplastic syndromes

3. All but one of the following are possible mechanisms for the production of macrocytes:

a. Liver disease

b. Postsplenectomy status

c. Pernicious anemia

d. Thalassemia minor

4. The blood smear of a patient with a prosthetic heart valve may show:

a. Target cells

b. Burr cells

c. Schistocytes

d. Elliptocytes

5. Oat-shaped cells may be associated with:

a. Myelofibrosis

b. Hereditary spherocytosis

c. Burns

d. Sickle cell anemia

6. How would a cell be classified that has a diameter of 9 μm and an MCV of 104 fL?

a. Macrocytic

b. Microcytic

c. Normal

d. Either normal or slightly microcytic

7. Abnormal platelet morphology may be observed most prominently in:

a. Idiopathic myelofibrosis

b. Anemia of chronic disorders

c. Hereditary spherocytosis

d. Septic shock

8. Which type of red cell inclusion is a DNA remnant?

a. Heinz body

b. Howell-Jolly body

c. Pappenheimer body

d. Cabot ring

9. Which type of cell is most prominently seen in idiopathic myelofibrosis?

a. Acanthocyte

b. Burr cell

c. Schistocyte

d. Teardrop cell

10. In a patient with an MCHC of 36%, one would expect to observe:

a. Target cells

b. Spherocytes

c. Helmet cells

d. Elliptocytes

11. Precipitates of denatured hemoglobin found primarily in patients with hemolytic anemia resulting from oxidant stress describes:

a. Howell-Jolly bodies

b. Heinz bodies

c. Basophilic stippling

d. Pappenheimer bodies

12. Pappenheimer inclusions form from:

a. Excess α chains

b. Excess β chains

c. Excess iron

d. Oxidant stress

13. Helmet cells suggest the presence of which RBC inclusion?

a. Howell-Jolly bodies

b. Heinz bodies

c. Basophilic stippling

d. Pappenheimer bodies

14. When an RBC containing an inclusion becomes entrapped in microvasculature, it may work free and transform from a discocyte into a:

a. Teardrop cell

b. Stomatocyte

c. Schistocyte

d. Target cell

SUMMARY CHART

➤ A variation in cell size is termed *anisocytosis*.

➤ A variation in cell shape is termed *poikilocytosis*.

➤ On an automated cell counter, a flag is a signal that a significant abnormality may be present in the sample.

➤ In a peripheral smear, only red cell abnormalities that are present in each observed field are significant.

➤ Microcytes are associated with an MCV of less than 80 fL and are seen in iron-deficiency anemia, thalassemias, sideroblastic anemias, and anemia of chronic disease.

➤ Macrocytes are associated with an MCV of more than 100 fL and are seen in megaloblastic and nonmegaloblastic processes.

➤ Macrocytes are associated with high reticulocyte counts and liver disease; oval macrocytes are associated with megaloblastic processes.

➤ Spherocytes are associated with hereditary spherocytosis and an MCHC that is greater than 36% in many cases.

➤ Spherocytes may also be seen in autoimmune hemolytic anemia (AIHA) and posttransfusion.

➤ There are two types of sickle cells, irreversible sickle cells (ISCs) and oat-shaped, reversible sickle cells.

➤ Any regenerative red cell process will result in inclusions such as Howell-Jolly bodies, basophilic stippling, and Pappenheimer bodies.

➤ Howell-Jolly bodies are seen in patients postsplenectomy.

➤ Helmet cells are seen in patients with G6PD syndrome and occur as a result of Heinz body formation.

➤ Heinz bodies cannot be seen on a Wright-stained peripheral smear.

➤ Abnormal platelet morphology includes lack of granulation, giant platelets, and megakaryocytic fragments.

References

1. Koepke, J: Let's improve the flagging of abnormal hematology specimens. MLO 26:11, 1994.
2. Cornbleet, J, et al: Streamline your automated hematology laboratory. MLO 29:68, 1997.
3. Davis, GM: Autoverification of the peripheral blood count. Lab Med 25:528, 1994.
4. Shojana, AM: Protein synthesis in megaloblastic disorders. In Gross, S, and Roath, S (eds): Hematology: A Problem Oriented Approach. Williams & Wilkins, Baltimore, 1996, p 27.
5. Glassey, E (ed): Color Atlas of Hematology. College of American Pathologists, Hematology and Clinical Microscopy Resource Committee, Northfield, IL, 1998, p 86.
6. McKenzie, S: Textbook of Hematology. Williams & Wilkins, Baltimore, 1996, p 108.
7. Orkin, SH, Nathan, DG: The thalassemias. In Nathan and Oski's Hematology of Infancy and Childhood, ed 5. WB Saunders, Philadelphia, 1998, p 818.
8. Turgeon, ML: Clinical Hematology: Theory and Procedures, ed 3. Lippincott, Williams & Wilkins, Baltimore, 1998, p 89.
9. Jandl, JH: Blood—Textbook of Hematology, ed 2. Little, Brown, Boston, 1996, p 364.
10. Cochran, DL, and Burnside, LK: Detecting and identifying hereditary pyropoikilocytosis. Lab Med 30:26, 1999.
11. Camilo, N, and Ravindranath, Y: Hemoglobinopathies: Abnormal structure in hematology. In Gross, S, and Roath, S (eds): Hematology: A Problem Oriented Approach. Williams & Wilkins, Baltimore, 1996, p 77.
12. Gallagher, PG, et al: Disorders of the erythrocyte membrane. In Nathan and Oski's Hematology of Infancy and Childhood, ed 5. WB Saunders, Philadelphia, 1998, p 626.
13. Womack, EP: Treating thrombotic thrombocytopenic purpura with plasma exchange. Lab Med 30:276, 1999.
14. Uthman, MD (ed): Hemoglobinopathies and thalassemias. April 30, 2000, p 13. Available from: http://www.neosoft.com/~Euthman/hemoglobinopathy/hemoglobinopathy.html.

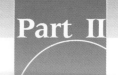

Part II

Anemias

6 Iron Metabolism and Hypochromic Anemias

JERRY W. HUSSONG, DDS, MD

NORMAL IRON METABOLISM
  Requirements and Distribution
  Absorption, Storage, and Reutilization
HYPOCHROMIC ANEMIAS
  Disorders of Iron Metabolism and Utilization
  Disorders of Heme Synthesis
  Disorders of Globin Protein Chain Synthesis

CASE STUDY 1

CASE STUDY 2

CASE STUDY 3

OBJECTIVES

At the end of this chapter, the learner should be able to:

1. List the three components of the hemoglobin molecule.
2. State the function of iron in relationship to hemoglobin.
3. Describe the distribution of body iron.
4. List several increased iron consumptive states.
5. Trace absorption and utilization of body iron.
6. List numerous causes of hypochromic anemia.
7. Describe the peripheral blood findings in iron-deficiency anemia.
8. List the complete blood count (CBC) indices that are used to distinguish among the hypochromic anemias.
9. Describe the bone marrow iron-staining pattern in anemia of chronic disease.
10. List several causes of sideroblastic anemia.

The production of red blood cells (erythropoiesis) is a highly regulated process that begins early in fetal development and continues throughout adult life. Hemoglobin synthesis is an integral part of erythropoiesis and requires the production and assembly of three key components. They include iron, globin protein chains, and protoporphyrin. It is the protoporphyrin-iron complex or heme portion of the hemoglobin molecule that is responsible for the binding of oxygen and carbon dioxide and their transport to and from the tissues of the body. This chapter begins with a review of normal iron metabolism. This is followed by a discussion of iron-deficiency and iron-utilization disorders and their associated hypochromic anemias.

➤ NORMAL IRON METABOLISM

Requirements and Distribution

The average adult has a total body iron content of approximately 3500 mg. Two-thirds of this iron is present as he-

moglobin iron, and about one-third is present as tissue iron (Table 6–1). Nearly 90% of the total tissue iron is storage iron and available for utilization in the form of ferritin or hemosiderin. Ten percent of tissue iron is nonavailable or elemental iron and includes the iron in myoglobin and the cytochrome enzymes. A very small amount of iron is also present as plasma or transport iron and other body iron.

Iron metabolism and maintenance of body stores is a tightly regulated process. Daily iron intake, absorption, and losses are usually very small. Body iron is repeatedly recycled, and the small amount of iron that is lost each day is replaced by the diet (Fig. 6–1). The normal life span of the red blood cell (RBC) is 120 days. Therefore, healthy adults with a blood volume of 4500 to 5000 mL will lose the RBCs in 37 to 42 mL of whole blood per day. Because 2 mL of blood contains 1 mg of iron, 18.5 to 21 mg of iron is needed each day to replace the iron lost by senescent RBCs. The majority of this iron comes from recycling, because nearly 100% of the iron from RBC turnover is taken up by the mononuclear phagocytic system and reutilized. The small

➤ Table 6-1
TOTAL BODY IRON

	% Total	mg*
Hemoglobin iron	66	2310
Tissue iron, total	33	1155
Storage or available	(30)*	(1050)
Essential or nonavailable	(3)	(105)
Plasma and transport iron, other body iron	1	35
	100%	3500 mg

*mg = approximate milligrams; ( ) = portion of total tissue iron.

amount of iron that is lost through cellular shedding and sweating (approximately 1 mg/day) is typically replaced through the diet.[1,2] In a nonmenstruating adult, this 1 mg of iron represents the minimum daily requirement (MDR) (Table 6–2). In pregnant and lactating women, the MDR is even greater. The average western diet contains about 6 mg of elemental iron per 1000 calories. Therefore, if a typical adult consumes a 2500-calorie diet, approximately 15 mg of iron is ingested per day. Of this 15 mg of ingested iron, only about 5% to 10%, or 1 mg, is absorbed each day (Fig. 6–2). Despite the excess of iron in the western diet, iron deficiency continues to be a significant cause of morbidity in North America and throughout the world.[3–6] Many food products, including flour and baby formulas, are now supplemented with iron to help alleviate the problem.

Daily iron requirements are affected by a number of physiologic and pathologic states, including menstruation, pregnancy, growth, and iron deficiency (Table 6–3). During menstruation, the average woman loses about 40 to 50 mL of blood per menstrual cycle. Within each milliliter of blood, there is about 0.5 mg of iron; therefore, 20 to 25 mg of iron is lost by the average woman each month. This represents a loss of about 0.8 mg of iron per day, in addition to the 1 to 2 mg typically lost daily through cellular shedding and sweating. The extent of menstrual bleeding is extremely variable, and some women may lose up to 1.5 to 2.5 mg of iron per day as a result of menstruation.

Iron requirements are substantially increased during pregnancy and lactation.[7,8] In the second and third trimesters, the daily requirement of iron can increase to as high as 5 to 6 mg. Although the cessation of menstruation during pregnancy spares approximately 200 mg of iron from being lost (20 to 25 mg per month for 9 months), the increased demands from pregnancy far outshadow this saving. During pregnancy, expansion of the mother's blood volume and hemoglobin mass is accompanied by an increased requirement for the fetus, pla-

Daily Iron (Fe) Turnover and Distribution

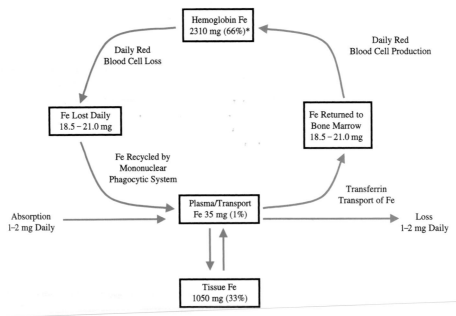

*( ) = percentage of total body iron

➤ FIGURE 6–1   Bodily iron distribution and turnover. Sixty-six percent of the total body iron is present as hemoglobin iron, 33% as tissue iron, and 1% as plasma or transport iron. Approximately 1 mg of iron is absorbed each day to replace daily losses.

> **Table 6-2**
MINIMUM DAILY REQUIREMENT (MDR) FOR IRON

Population	MDR
Infant	1.0
Child	0.5
Menstruating woman	2.0
Pregnant or lactating woman	3.0
Adult man or nonmenstruating woman	1.0

> **Table 6-3**
FACTORS AFFECTING DAILY IRON REQUIREMENTS

- Growth spurts
- Menstruation
- Pregnancy
- Lactation and breast-feeding
- Iron deficiency

centa, and umbilical cord. In addition, at delivery there is a loss of about 600 to 700 mL of blood. In total, during pregnancy approximately 1000 mg of iron is utilized. This equals and at times exceeds the amount of storage iron in an average woman of childbearing age. Lactation and breast feeding also contribute to the loss of iron associated with pregnancy.

During infancy as well as adolescence, iron requirements are substantially increased.[9,10] A newborn infant weighing 7.5 lbs has approximately 250 mg of total body iron. The vast majority of this iron is contained in hemoglobin. During the first year of life, absorption of 150 to 175 mg of iron is required to maintain an appropriate hemoglobin concentration. Because milk is a poor source of iron, many baby formulas are supplemented with iron. Infants who are fed only mothers' breast milk are at a significant risk of developing iron-deficiency anemia. In addition, if the fetus loses substantial amounts of blood at delivery, is a twin, or is born to an iron-deficient mother, it is at increased risk for development of iron-deficiency anemia.

Absorption, Storage, and Reutilization

Of the iron ingested in the diet, 5% to 10% is absorbed. The vast majority is absorbed in the duodenum and first portion of the jejunum. Regulation of iron absorption occurs within the intestinal mucosa of the small bowel. Iron molecules within the diet and iron complexes within the body can be present in various iron states (Table 6–4). Ferric iron (Fe^{3+}) is the most common dietary form of iron. It is typically converted into the ferrous state (Fe^{2+}) by the acid of the stomach. Ferrous iron within the intestinal lumen readily enters the mucosal cells (Fig. 6–3). Within the mucosal cells

ferrous iron is reoxidized to ferric iron, some of which creates complexes with the protein apoferritin to form ferritin.

Ferritin is the primary storage compound for iron and is commonly found within the liver, spleen, and bone marrow. Ferritin iron is easily mobilized by the body for utilization. Serum ferritin levels can be measured and used as an indirect measure of iron stores. Hemosiderin, another form of storage iron, is made up of precipitated aggregates of ferritin. The iron in hemosiderin is released more slowly than that from ferritin and is less readily available for utilization. Hemosiderin can be easily identified as golden granules in tissue samples through hematoxylin-eosin (H & E) staining (Fig. 6–4; see also Color Plate 87). Prussian blue staining also accentuates the aggregates of hemosiderin.

The remainder of the ferric iron from within the mucosal cells combines with apotransferrin to form transferrin. Transferrin is a beta$_1$ (β_1) globulin protein that is responsible for transporting iron through the bloodstream to the various organs of the body.

The rate at which iron is transferred from the intestinal mucosal cell to the bloodstream is regulated by the body's iron levels and requirements. It has been postulated that, as ferritin levels decrease (e.g., in iron deficiency), iron absorption increases.

In addition to the ferrous and ferric iron molecules in the diet, heme iron is also present. It is derived from myoglobin and hemoglobin in dietary meat and is absorbed by the mucosal cells as intact heme molecules. Only after absorption of the heme molecule is the iron freed from the porphyrin ring and available for utilization. Absorption of heme iron is not under the same influences from the diet as the inorganic and nonheme irons and is not inhibited by compounds such as tannins and polyphenols.

Daily Iron (Fe) Intake and Absorption in Western Diet

$$\frac{6 \text{ mg Fe}}{1000 \text{ cal}} \quad \times \quad \frac{2500 \text{ cal diet}}{\text{day}} \quad = \quad \frac{15 \text{ mg Fe ingested}}{\text{day}}$$

> FIGURE 6–2 Calculation of daily absorption of iron based on an average western diet and assuming a 5% to 10% absorption rate.

$$\frac{15 \text{ mg ingested Fe}}{\text{day}} \quad \times \quad 5\text{-}10\% \text{ absorption rate} \quad = \quad \frac{\text{Approx. 1 mg Fe absorbed}}{\text{day}}$$

> **Table 6-4**
IRON (FE) MOLECULES AND COMPOUNDS

Fe Molecule/Compound	Fe State	Location	Function
Dietary Fe	Fe^{2+} or Fe^{3+}	Upper GI tract	Hemoglobin, myoglobin, enzyme synthesis
Hemoglobin	Fe^{2+}	RBCs	Bind oxygen
Transferrin	Fe^{3+}	Serum	Transport Fe
Ferritin	Fe^{3+}	Serum and tissue sites	Fe storage
Hemosiderin	Fe^{3+}	Bone marrow and other tissue sites	Fe storage

Iron, because of its electron state, is ideally suited to form chelates or complexes with heterocyclic rings and proteins. It is the ability of iron to chelate or form complexes with various molecules that enables its absorption, transport, storage, and function. The interaction of iron with protoporphyrin allows the formation of heme (Fig. 6–5). Ferrous iron combines with protoporphyrin in the mitochondria of the RBC to form heme. Protoporphyrin is produced through a sequence of steps that starts with aminolevulinic acid (ALA) formation from glycine and succinyl coenzyme A (CoA). This is the rate-limiting step in heme synthesis. Two ALA molecules combine to form porphobilinogen, and four porphobilinogen molecules join together to form uroporphyrinogen III. Decarboxylation of uroporhyrinogen III forms coproporphyrinogen III, which is oxidized to protoporphyrin (Fig. 6–6). Also within the cytoplasm of the RBC, alpha (α) and beta (β)

globin protein chains are synthesized. The two α and two β globin protein chains combine with four heme groups and four oxygen molecules to form an intact functional hemoglobin molecule (Fig. 6–7).

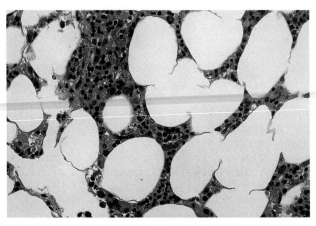

> **FIGURE 6–4**   Bone marrow core biopsy specimen with abundant golden-brown hemosiderin granules (H & E stain, ×400).

Iron (Fe) Absorption and Transport

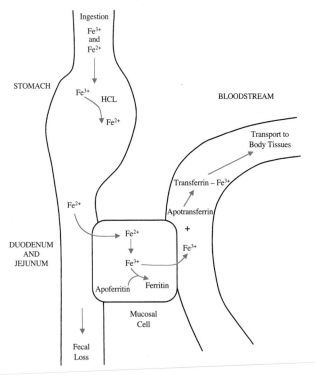

> **FIGURE 6–3**   Schematic of iron intake and absorption through the mucosal cells in the small intestine. Absorbed iron is converted to ferritin for storage or transported bound to transferrin for distribution to body tissues.

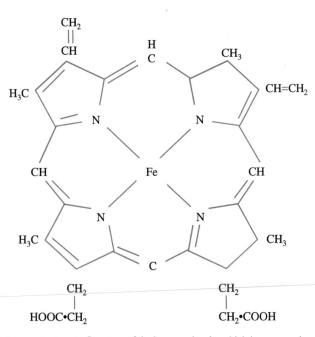

> **FIGURE 6–5**   Structure of the heme molecule, which is composed of iron and protoporphyrin rings.

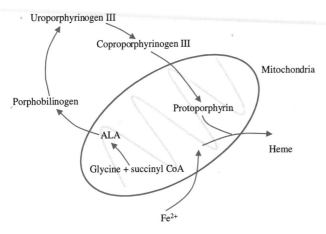

> **FIGURE 6–6**   Synthesis of heme within the mitochondria and cytoplasm of the erythroid precursors. Protoporhyrin combines with iron to form heme.

> **Table 6-5**
> **CAUSES OF HYPOCHRONIC ANEMIAS**

Disorders of iron metabolism and utilization

Iron deficiency

Chronic disease states

Disorders of heme synthesis

Hereditary sideroblastic anemias

Acquired sideroblastic anemias

  Primary

    Myelodysplasia

  Secondary

    Toxins including lead, alcohol and drugs

Disorders of globin protein chain synthesis

α Thalassemia

β Thalassemia

➤ HYPOCHROMIC ANEMIAS

The hypochromic anemias represent a related group of disorders in which there is a quantitative defect in hemoglobin synthesis.[11] DNA synthesis occurs normally, and as the erythroid precursors divide, the lack of hemoglobin results in hypochromic red blood cells that are usually smaller than normal. The etiology of the hypochromic anemias includes disorders that affect iron metabolism and utilization, heme synthesis, and globin protein chain synthesis (Table 6–5).

Processes that impair normal iron metabolism and utilization include iron deficiency and chronic disease states such as neoplasia, infection, and autoimmune disorders. Iron deficiency and chronic disease states are the most common causes of hypochromic anemias. Disorders of heme synthesis result in sideroblastic anemias, which can be acquired or inherited. Acquired sideroblastic anemias include refractory anemia with ringed sideroblasts (RARS), a myelodysplastic syndrome, and disorders of toxic insult. Toxins such as lead, alcohol, and various other drugs are well-known causes of

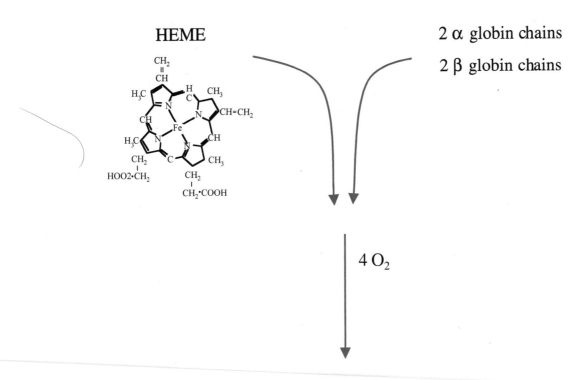

> **FIGURE 6–7**   Formation of hemoglobin from heme, α and β globin protein chains, and oxygen.

sideroblastic anemias. Disorders that affect globin protein chain synthesis include the thalassemic syndromes, such as α and β thalassemia.

Evaluation of anemias requires the measurement of several key indices in addition to morphological assessment. The most commonly measured indices and features used to evaluate the hypochromic anemias are summarized in Table 6–6.

Disorders of Iron Metabolism and Utilization

Iron-Deficiency Anemia

Iron-deficiency anemia is the most commonly recognized cause of hypochromic anemia. It is characterized by a decrease in hemoglobin concentration, hematocrit, and mean corpuscular volume (MCV).[12] Iron-deficiency anemia is frequently associated with hypochromasia and microcytosis of the RBCs. The latter finding is reflected by the decreased MCV. The hypochromasia can occasionally be evidenced by a decreased mean corpuscular hemoglobin concentration (MCHC), but it is usually more apparent by morphological examination.

Iron-deficiency anemia results after there is total or near total depletion of the body iron stores. The depletion of iron stores and the development of iron-deficiency anemia occurs through a sequential series of steps (Table 6–7). Firstly, there is depletion of body iron stores as is recognized by lack of stainable iron in the reticuloendothelial cells of the bone marrow (Fig. 6–8A and Color Plate 88). This is accompanied by a decreased serum ferritin level, decreased serum iron level, and increased total iron-binding capacity (TIBC). As erythropoiesis continues, there is inadequate iron for hemoglobin

---

➤ Table 6-6
COMMONLY USED INDICES AND FEATURES TO EVALUATE THE HYPOCHROMIC ANEMIAS

Indices	Comments
RBC count	Enumeration of RBC number; decreased with anemias; increased with polycythemia
Hemoglobin (Hgb) concentration	Concentration of Hgb measured by spectrophotometry
Hematocrit (Hct)	Represents % of blood volume occupied by RBCs
MCV	Average measurement of RBC volume or size; useful in classifying anemias
MCH	Average weight of Hgb in the RBC; calculated by dividing the Hgb concentration by the RBC count
MCHC	Calculated by dividing the Hgb concentration by the hematocrit ×100; represents an average value
Red cell distribution width (RDW)	Measurement of RBC anisocytosis
Serum Fe	Fe circulates bound to transferrin; it has a diurnal variation and is typically measured in a morning blood draw
Serum ferritin	Correlates with Fe stores; may be elevated out of proportion to Fe stores with tissue damage, malignancy, infection
TIBC	Indirect measure of transferrin; equals sum of the serum iron plus additional Fe that serum transferrin can bind
% saturation	Calculated by dividing serum Fe by the TIBC × 100; transferrin is normally 33% saturated
Free erythrocyte protoporphyrin (FEP)	Free protoporphyrin combines with Fe to form heme; FEP is increased with Fe deficiency and lead poisoning; lead blocks the formation of heme from Fe and protoporphyrin
Serum soluble transferrin receptor	Levels of serum soluble transferrin receptor are proportional to cellular receptor levels; levels are increased with iron deficiency; levels do not appear to be altered by inflammatory states
Peripheral Blood and Bone Marrow Features	
Anisocytosis	Variability in RBC size
Poikilocytosis, including target cells	Variability in cell shape; target cells are seen with excess cell membrane as with liver disease, postsplenectomy, and in hemoglobinopathies
Basophilic stippling	Results from increased precipitation of RNA; course basophilic stippling may be seen in lead poisoning and thalassemia; fine stippling may be seen in various anemias
Stainable bone marrow iron	Represent body Fe stores; usually present in the reticuloendothelial cells
Marrow sideroblasts/ringed sideroblasts	Normally 20%–40% of red blood cell precursors are sideroblasts (contain identifiable iron granules); ringed sideroblasts (iron granules extending around 3/4 of the nuclear circumference) can be seen in sideroblastic anemias

➤ Table 6-7
SEQUENTIAL STEPS IN THE DEVELOPMENT OF IRON-DEFICIENCY ANEMIA

1. Depletion of iron stores
   - Decrease or absence of stainable bone marrow iron
   - Decreased serum ferritin level
   - Increased TIBC
2. Iron-deficient erythropoiesis
   - Decreased hemoglobin in developing RBCs without frank anemia
   - Early microcytosis
   - Decreased transferrin saturation
3. Iron-deficiency anemia
   - Decreased hemoglobin synthesis with anemia and significant microcytosis (decreased MCV)
   - Anisocytosis of the RBCs
   - Increased serum soluble transferrin receptor levels

synthesis, resulting in hypochromasia. In addition, there is decreased transferrin saturation with iron and beginning microcytosis. Frank anemia, however, is not yet present. The final stage is the development of iron-deficiency anemia. It is characterized by hypochromasia and microcytosis of the red blood cells (decreased MCV) with mild to moderate anisopoikilocytosis (Fig. 6–9 and Color Plate 90). At this stage, serum soluble transferrin receptor levels are increased. The features and indices associated with iron-deficiency anemia are summarized in Table 6–8.

Anemia of Chronic Disease

The anemias that occur in patients with a chronic disease state often are multifactorial in origin.[13,14] They commonly are associated with infections, malignant neoplasms, and autoimmune disorders[15,16] (Table 6–9). Anemia of chronic disease (ACD) is defined by an aggregate of clinical, morphological, and laboratory findings (Table 6–10). The ane-

mia is usually present for 1 to 3 months following the onset of a chronic disease state. Examination of the peripheral blood smear reveals normocytic red blood cells (normal MCV) that are hypochromic or normochromic (Fig. 6–10). The MCHC is usually within the normal range. Anisopoikilocytosis and polychromasia are mild or absent. Within the bone marrow there are adequate numbers of erythrocytic precursors. Storage iron is increased and sideroblasts are decreased (see Fig. 6–8B and Color Plate 89). It has been suggested that chronic disease states block the transfer of storage iron to maturing erythoid precursors within the bone marrow. Ringed sideroblasts are typically absent. Laboratory studies reveal decreased serum iron, decreased TIBC, and decreased saturation of transferrin. Serum ferritin levels, however, are normal to increased.

Disorders of Heme Synthesis

Sideroblastic Anemias

The sideroblastic anemias are a heterogenous group of disorders that are characterized by ineffective erythropoiesis, increased levels of serum and tissue iron, and increased numbers of ringed sideroblasts within the marrow. The pathogenesis of the sideroblastic anemias is incompletely understood. Several investigators have identified enzyme deficiencies, including deficiencies of ALA synthase and uroporphyrinogen decarboxylase, in patients with sideroblastic anemia. No one defect, however, can account for all inherited and acquired disorders. Irrespective of the etiology, the result is an abnormal deposition of iron or siderotic granules within the mitochondria. Because the mitochondria of erythroid precursors are located around the nucleus, the deposition of iron within these organelles results in identifiable ringed sideroblasts with Prussian blue staining (Fig. 6–11 and Color Plate 82).

The sideroblastic anemias can be inherited or acquired.[17–21] The inherited sideroblastic anemias include sex-linked congenital sideroblastic anemia and autosomal recessive sideroblastic anemia. The acquired sideroblastic anemias can be primary (also referred to as idiopathic) or secondary (Table 6–11). The secondary sideroblastic anemias typically are the result of toxins or drugs.

The hereditary sideroblastic anemias are rare. The X-linked type is more common than the autosomal recessive

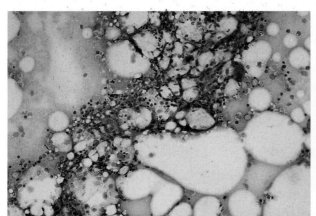
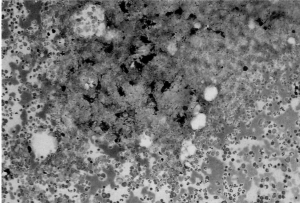

➤ **FIGURE 6–8** *A.* Markedly decreased reticuloendothelial iron in a patient with iron-deficiency anemia (Prussian blue stain, ×200). *B.* Increased reticuloendothelial iron in a patient with anemia of chronic disease (Prussian blue stain, ×200).

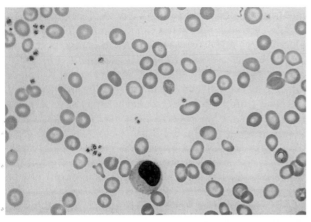

> ➤ FIGURE 6–9 Iron-deficiency anemia characterized by hypochromic, microcytic red blood cells (Wright's stain, ×400).

> ## ➤ Table 6-9
> ## DISORDERS ASSOCIATED WITH ANEMIA OF CHRONIC DISEASE (ACD)
>
> **Infections**
>
> Tuberculosis
>
> Chronic osteomyelitis
>
> Fungal infections
>
> **Neoplasms**
>
> Carcinomas
>
> Malignant lymphoma
>
> Multiple myeloma
>
> **Autoimmune Disorders**
>
> Systemic lupus erythematosus (SLE)
>
> Rheumatoid arthritis
>
> Sarcoidosis

variant. The anemias typically appear early, usually within the first few months or years of life. Pallor and splenomegaly are often seen associated with the anemia. Examination of the peripheral blood smear commonly reveals microcytic, hypochromic RBCs. Dimorphic populations of RBCs are commonly seen with prominent anisopoikilocytosis (Fig. 6–12 and Color Plate 91). Serum iron and ferritin are usually increased as is transferrin saturation and free erythrocyte protoporphyrin. TIBC may be normal or decreased. Serum soluble transferrin receptor levels are usually normal or decreased. Increased storage iron and ringed sideroblasts are seen within the bone marrow after staining with Prussian blue. Treatment for these patients

has included pyridoxine therapy and, rarely, bone marrow transplantation.

The acquired sideroblastic anemias can be primary or secondary. The primary or "idiopathic" sideroblastic anemias are exemplified by refractory anemia with ringed sideroblasts (RARS), one of the myelodysplastic syndromes. Clinically, patients are typically older than 50 years of age and present with weakness, pallor, and fatigue in addition to anemia. The peripheral blood often exhibits a dimorphic RBC population with a prominent hypochromic component.

> ## ➤ Table 6-8
> ## INDICES AND FEATURES OF IRON-DEFICIENCY ANEMIA
>
> **Clinical**
>
> Clinical findings depend on severity of the anemia
>
> Severe anemias may be associated with pallor, weakness, and dyspnea
>
> **Morphological**
>
> Usually hypochromic, microcytic RBC
>
> Mild to moderate anisopoikilocytosis
>
> Decreased storage iron
>
> Decreased sideroblasts
>
> Absent ringed sideroblasts
>
> **Laboratory**
>
> Decreased serum iron
>
> Decreased serum ferritin
>
> Decreased % transferrin saturation
>
> Increased TIBC
>
> Increased FEP
>
> Increased serum soluble transferrin receptor levels

> ## ➤ Table 6-10
> ## INDICES AND FEATURES OF ANEMIA OF CHRONIC DISEASE
>
> **Clinical**
>
> Anemia present for several months following development of a chronic disease state
>
> **Morphological**
>
> Usually normocytic RBCs (normal MCV)
>
> May be hypochromic or normochromic
>
> Normal number of bone marrow erythrocytic precursors
>
> Increased storage iron
>
> Decreased sideroblasts
>
> Rare to absent ringed sideroblasts
>
> **Laboratory**
>
> Decreased serum iron
>
> Decreased TIBC
>
> Decreased % transferrin saturation
>
> Normal to increased serum ferritin levels
>
> Normal serum soluble transferrin receptor levels

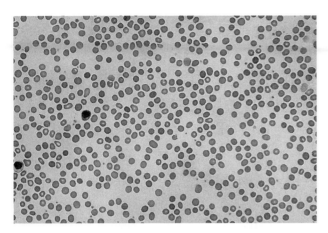

➤ **FIGURE 6–10** Normochromic, normocytic red blood cells in a patient with anemia of chronic disease (Wright's stain, ×200).

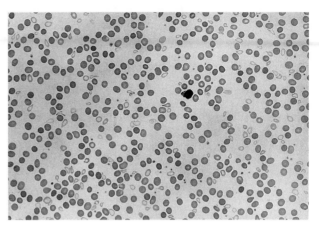

➤ **FIGURE 6–12** Dimorphic population of red blood cells with a striking hypochromic component in a patient with sideroblastic anemia. Moderate anisopoikilocytosis is also present (Wright's stain, ×200).

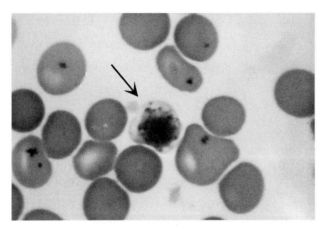

➤ **FIGURE 6–11** Ringed sideroblast as detected by Prussian blue staining of a bone marrow aspirate (Prussian blue stain, ×1000).

➤ **Table 6-12**
CLINICAL AND MORPHOLOGICAL FEATURES OF REFRACTORY ANEMIA WITH RINGED SIDEROBLASTS (RARS)

Clinical

Usually older than 50 years of age

Weakness, pallor, fatigue with associated with anemia

Morphological

Dimorphic RBC population with prominent hypochromic component

Anisopoikilocytosis of RBCs, which may be associated with basophilic stippling

Hypercellular bone marrow with erythroid hyperplasia

More than 15% ringed sideroblasts

➤ **Table 6-11**
COMMON CAUSES OF SIDEROBLASTIC ANEMIA

Inherited

Congenital sideroblastic anemia, sex-linked

Autosomal recessive sideroblastic anemia

Acquired

Primary or idiopathic

    Myelodysplasia (RARS)

Secondary

    Lead

    Alcohol

    Drugs, including isoniazid and chloramphenicol

The secondary sideroblastic anemias are the result of ingestion of alcohol, lead, and various medications. The medications that commonly cause sideroblastic anemia include isoniazid, chloramphenicol, pyrazinamide, and cycloserine. Many of these and other medications antagonize or decrease the level of pyridoxine to exert their effect. The secondary sideroblastic anemias are often severe but improve rapidly with the discontinuation of the offending medication or with pyridoxine administration. Examination of the peripheral blood smear often reveals a hypochromic anemia and a dimorphic appearance of the RBCs.

Lead poisoning impairs heme synthesis at several steps, including incorporation of iron into protoporphyrin. This results in the formation of ringed sideroblasts. Coarse basophilic stippling of the RBCs is also a common feature of lead poisoning. Severe alcoholism often results in the formation of ringed sideroblasts, which usually disappear after the withdrawl of alcohol. A comparison of the features and indices of iron deficiency anemia, anemia of chronic disease, and sideroblastic anemia is presented in Table 6–13.

Anisopoikilocytosis and basophilic stippling may be seen. The bone marrow is typically hypercellular with erythroid hyperplasia and dyserythropoiesis. Iron stains reveal more than 15% ringed sideroblasts. The clinical and morphological features seen with RARS are summarized in Table 6–12.

> Table 6-13
SUMMARY AND COMPARISON OF INDICES AND FEATURES IN IRON-DEFICIENCY ANEMIA, ANEMIA OF CHRONIC DISEASE, AND SIDEROBLASTIC ANEMIA

Indices	Iron-Deficiency Anemia	Anemia of Chronic Disease	Sideroblastic Anemia
RBC count	Decreased	Decreased	Decreased
Hemoglobin (Hgb) concentration	Decreased	Decreased	Decreased
Hematocrit (Hct)	Decreased	Decreased or normal	Variable
MCV	Decreased	Normal or decreased	Variable
MCH	Decreased	Usually normal	Variable
MCHC	Decreased	Usually normal	Variable
Red cell distribution width (RDW)	Increased	Usually normal	Normal or increased
Serum Fe	Decreased	Decreased	Increased
Serum ferritin	Decreased	Normal to increased	Increased
TIBC	Increased	Decreased	Decreased or normal
% saturation	Decreased	Decreased	Increased
Free erythrocyte protoporphyrin (FEP)	Increased	Increased	Increased
Serum soluble transferrin receptor levels	Increased	Usually normal	Decreased or normal
Peripheral Blood and Bone Marrow Features			
Anisocytosis	Yes	No	Yes*
Poikilocytosis, including target cells	Yes	No	Yes*
Basophilic stippling	No	No	Yes
Stainable bone marrow iron	Decreased or absent	Increased	Increased
Marrow sideroblasts/ringed sideroblasts	Decreased	Decreased	Increased

*In hereditary forms.

Disorders of Globin Protein Chain Synthesis

The thalassemic syndromes are a group of disorders that result in variable impairment of the synthesis of globin protein chains. Typically, they are characterized by decreased overall hemoglobin synthesis, unbalanced synthesis of globin protein chains, and increased levels of hemoglobin A₂ or hemoglobin F, or both. The α thalassemias result from α gene deletion with a subsequent decrease in α globin protein chain synthesis. The β thalassemias result from β gene deletion and a decrease in the production of β globin protein chains. The severity of the thalassemic syndrome is directly related to the number of globin protein chain genes that are deleted. The overall impairment in hemoglobin synthesis frequently results in microcytic, hypochromic RBCs with associated anisopoikilocytosis, including target cells, ovalocytes, and basophilic stippling. The reader is referred to Chapter 12 for a more complete discussion of the thalassemias.

> **CASE STUDY 1**

The patient is a 33-year-old woman who presented to her physician with complaints of fatigue and increased shortness of breath with exercise. Medical history revealed heavy menstrual bleeding of several years' duration. On physical examination, the patient appeared pale and was tachycardic with a resting heart rate of 96 beats per minute. Results of laboratory tests included WBC, 6.9×10^9/L; Hgb, 10.8 g/dL; Hct, 31.3%; MCV, 78 fL; PLT, 250×10^9/L. Examination of the peripheral blood smear revealed microcytic, hypochromic red blood cells with only minimal anisopoikilocytosis.

Questions
1. What is the most likely explanation of this patient's anemia?
   a. α Thalassemia
   b. Lead poisoning
   c. Iron-deficiency anemia
   d. Refractory anemia with ringed sideroblasts
2. What additional test may useful in confirming the diagnosis?
   a. Hemoglobin electrophoresis
   b. Vitamin B₁₂ and folate levels
   c. Measurement of serum iron, ferritin, and TIBC
   d. Chromosome analysis
3. Iron-deficiency anemia is associated with:
   a. Decreased hemoglobin, increased MCV, increased serum ferritin, and decreased serum iron
   b. Decreased hemoglobin, decreased hematocrit, decreased serum ferritin, and increased stainable bone marrow iron
   c. Decreased hemoglobin, decreased hematocrit,

increased serum iron, increased serum ferritin, and marked anisopoikilocytosis

   d. Decreased hemoglobin, decreased serum iron, decreased ferritin, increased TIBC, and decreased transferrin saturation

4. Assuming the patient has normal dietary iron absorption, the minimum dietary requirement of iron for this patient would be:
   a. 12 mg/day
   b. 0.5 mg/day
   c. 2 mg/day
   d. 1 mg/day

5. Prussian blue staining of the bone marrow in this patient would reveal:
   a. Increased storage and increased sideroblastic iron
   b. Increased storage and decreased sideroblastic iron
   c. Decreased storage and decreased sideroblastic iron
   d. Increased ringed sideroblasts

Answers
   1. c
   2. c
   3. d
   4. c
   5. c

➤ CASE STUDY 2

A 78-year-old man who was diagnosed 3 months earlier with non-Hodgkin's lymphoma has undergone an extensive staging workup. The patient has not yet received chemotherapy, and staging studies suggest localized disease. The results of laboratory tests included WBC, 10.3 $\times 10^9$/L; Hgb, 12.0 g/dL; Hct, 33.1%; MCV, 81 fL; PLT, 221 $\times 10^9$/L. Examination of the peripheral blood revealed normocytic, hypochromic red blood cells without significant anisopoikilocytosis. A bone marrow biopsy was performed to rule out involvement by malignant lymphoma. Examination of the bone marrow specimen revealed no evidence of malignant lymphoma, and iron stains were performed.

Questions
1. What is the best explanation for this patient's anemia?
   a. Iron-deficiency anemia
   b. Sideroblastic anemia
   c. Anemia of chronic disease
   d. Lead poisoning

2. If serum iron studies were performed on this patient, they would reveal:
   a. Decreased serum iron, decreased serum ferritin, and increased TIBC
   b. Decreased serum iron, normal to increased serum ferritin, and decreased TIBC
   c. Increased serum iron, increased serum ferritin, and decreased or normal TIBC
   d. Increased serum iron, increased serum ferritin, and increased TIBC

3. Prussian blue staining of a bone marrow aspirate specimen from this patient would reveal:

   a. Decreased stainable bone marrow iron and decreased ringed sideroblasts
   b. Decreased stainable bone marrow iron and increased ringed sideroblasts
   c. Increased stainable bone marrow iron and decreased marrow sideroblasts
   d. Increased stainable bone marrow iron and increased ringed sideroblasts

Answers
   1. c
   2. b
   3. c

➤ CASE STUDY 3

The patient is a 57-year-old woman with a 1-year history of anemia. The patient had no other associated medical conditions, and a previous workup for iron-deficiency anemia was negative. The patient had previously been followed without therapy but required red blood cell transfusion recently for a worsening anemia. A bone marrow biopsy was performed. The bone marrow was hypercellular with an erythroid hyperplasia. There was moderate dyserythropoiesis. Iron staining of the bone marrow aspirate revealed increased bone marrow iron as well as increased ringed sideroblasts.

Questions
1. What is the most likely cause of this patient's anemia?
   a. Iron-deficiency anemia
   b. Anemia of chronic disease
   c. Acquired sideroblastic anemia, primary (refractory anemia with ringed sideroblasts)
   d. Metastatic carcinoma

2. The serum iron studies in this patient would reveal:
   a. Increased serum iron, increased serum ferritin, and decreased to normal TIBC
   b. Decreased serum iron, normal to increased serum ferritin, and decreased TIBC
   c. Decreased serum iron, decreased serum ferritin, and increased TIBC
   d. Increased serum iron, decreased serum ferritin, and increased TIBC

3. Iron stains performed on the bone marrow aspirate specimen would reveal:
   a. Decreased stainable bone marrow iron and increased sideroblasts
   b. Decreased stainable bone marrow iron and decreased sideroblasts
   c. Increased stainable bone marrow iron and decreased sideroblasts
   d. Increased stainable bone marrow and increased ringed sideroblasts

Answers
   1. c
   2. a
   3. d

QUESTIONS

1. The average adult has a total body iron content of:
   a. 2500 mg
   b. 1000 mg
   c. 350 mg
   d. 3500 mg

2. Two-thirds of the total body iron is present as:
   a. Hemosiderin
   b. Ferritin
   c. Transferrin
   d. Hemoglobin iron

3. The normal life span of the red blood cell is:
   a. 120 days
   b. 80 days
   c. 140 days
   d. 180 days

4. One milligram of blood contains:
   a. 2 mg of iron
   b. 1 mg of iron
   c. 0.5 mg of iron
   d. 10 mg of iron

5. On average, what percentage of the ingested iron is absorbed each day?
   a. 25% to 35%
   b. 5% to 10%
   c. 80% to 90%
   d. 100%

6. Dietary iron is predominantly absorbed in the:
   a. Stomach
   b. Duodenum and first part of the jejunum
   c. Transverse colon
   d. Sigmoid colon

7. The globulin protein responsible for transporting iron in the bloodstream is:
   a. Hemoglobin
   b. Hemosiderin
   c. Transferrin
   d. Ferritin

8. The hypochromic anemias represent a related group of disorders with:
   a. A quantitative defect in hemoglobin synthesis
   b. A qualitative defect in globin protein chains
   c. Excess hemoglobin synthesis
   d. Vitamin B_{12} and folate deficiency

9. The most common cause of hypochromic anemia is:
   a. Sideroblastic anemia
   b. Megaloblastic anemia
   c. Iron deficiency anemia
   d. Lead poisoning

10. Microcytosis of red blood cells is reflected by:
    a. Increased MCV
    b. Decreased MCV
    c. Increased hemoglobin concentration
    d. Decreased hemoglobin concentration

11. Anemia of chronic disease is commonly associated with each of the following except:
    a. Infections
    b. Malignant neoplasms
    c. Autoimmune disorders
    d. A congenital defect

12. Each of the following are causes of secondary sideroblastic anemias except:
    a. Alcohol
    b. Lead
    c. Medications
    d. Radiation therapy

13. β Thalassemia is associated with:
    a. An increase in the production of β globin protein chains
    b. An increased production of α globin protein chains
    c. A deletion of the α gene
    d. A decrease in the production of β globin protein chains

SUMMARY CHART

➤ The three key components of the hemoglobin molecule are iron, globin protein chains, and protoporphyrin.
➤ The average adult total body iron content is approximately 3500 mg.
➤ The majority of the total body iron is present as hemoglobin iron.
➤ Ninety percent of tissue iron is present as storage iron in the form of ferritin or hemosiderin.
➤ The normal life span of the red blood cell is 120 days.
➤ Approximately 5% to 10% of the ingested iron is absorbed per day.
➤ The minimum daily requirement for iron for an adult man and nonmenstruating woman is 1 mg.
➤ Increased iron consumptive states include growth spurts, menstruation, pregnancy, lactation, and iron deficiency.
➤ Ferrous iron (Fe^{2+}) is easily absorbed into intestinal mucosa cells.
➤ Ferritin is the primary storage compound for iron.
➤ Transferrrin is a globulin protein responsible for transporting iron within the bloodstream.
➤ Because of its electron state, iron readily combines with heterocyclic rings and proteins to form chelates or complexes.
➤ Ferrous iron combines with protoporphyrin in the mitochondria of the red blood cell to form heme.
➤ The rate-limiting step in heme synthesis is the formation of aminolevulinic (ALA) from glycine and succinyl CoA.
➤ Hemoglobin is formed from two α and two β

globin protein chains, four heme groups, and four oxygen molecules.

➤ Hypochromic anemias represent a group of disorders in which there is a quantitative defect in hemoglobin synthesis.

➤ Iron-deficiency anemia is the most common cause of hypochromic anemia.

➤ Serum ferritin levels are an indirect measure of body iron stores.

➤ The MCV represents the average measurement of red blood cell volume or size and is useful in classifying anemias.

➤ Iron-deficiency anemia is characterized by hypochromic and microcytic red blood cells.

➤ Bone marrow evaluation of anemia of chronic disease reveals increased storage iron and decreased sideroblastic iron.

➤ Sideroblastic anemias are disorders of heme synthesis and may be inherited or acquired.

References

1. Dallman, PR: Iron deficiency: Does it matter. J Intern Med 226:367, 1989.
2. Bothwell, TH, et al: Nutritional iron requirements and food iron absorption. J Int Med Res (Engl) 226:357, 1989.
3. Nimeh, N, and Bishop, RC: Disorders of iron metabolism. Med Clin North Am 64:631, 1981.
4. Finch, CA, and Huebers, H: Perspectives in iron metabolism. N Engl J Med 306:1520, 1981.
5. Moore, DF, Jr, and Sears, DA: Pica, iron deficiency, and the medical history. Am J Med 97:390, 1994.
6. Baynes, RD, and Cook, JD: Current issues in iron deficiency. Curr Opin Hematol 3(2):145, 1996.
7. Provan, D: Mechanisms and management of iron deficiency anaemia. Br J Haematol Suppl 1:19, 1999.
8. Singh, K, et al: The role of prophylactic iron supplementation in pregnancy. Int J Food Sci Nutr 49(5):383, 1998.
9. Cohen, AR: Choosing the best strategy to prevent childhood iron deficiency. JAMA 281(23):2247, 1999.
10. Blot, I, et al: Iron deficiency in pregnancy: Effects on the newborn. Curr Opin Hematol 6(2):65, 1999.
11. Eldinbany, MM, et al: Usefulness of certain red blood cell indices in diagnosing and differentiating thalassemia trait from iron-deficiency. Am J Clin Pathol 111(5):676, 1999.
12. Means, RT, Jr: Pathogenesis of the anemia of chronic disease: A cytokine mediated anemia. Stem Cells (Dayt) 13(1):32, 1995.
13. Bain, BJ: Pathogenesis and pathophysiology of anemia in HIV infection. Curr Opin Hematol 6(2):89, 1999.
14. Jurado, RL: Iron, infections, and anemia of inflammation. Clin Infect Dis 25(4):888, 1997.
15. Mijovic, A, and Mufti, GJ: The myelodyspastic syndromes: Towards a functional classification. Blood Rev 12(2):73, 1998.
16. Olivieri, NF: The beta-thalassemias. N Engl J Med 341(2):99, 1999.
17. Fitzsimons, EJ, and May, A: The molecular basis of sideroblastic anemias. Curr Opin Hematol 3(2):167, 1996.
18. Koc, S, and Harris, JW: Sideroblastic anemias: Variations on imprecision in diagnostic criteria, proposal for an extended classification of sideroblastic anemias. Am J Hematol 57(1):1, 1998.
19. Bridges, KR: Sideroblastic anemia: A mitochondrial disorder. J Pediatr Hematol Oncol 19(4):273, 1997.
20. Atlay, C, and Gumruk, F: Pyridoxine-responsive sideroblastic anemia in four children. Pedriatr Hematol Oncol 12(2):205, 1995.
21. May, A, and Bishop, DF: The molecular biology and pyridoxine responsiveness of X-linked sideroblastic anaemia. Haematologica 83(1):56, 1998.

7

Megaloblastic Anemias

Mitra Taghizadeh, MS, MT(ASCP)

OBJECTIVES

At the end of this chapter, the learner should be able to:

1. Define megaloblastic anemia.

2. Compare and contrast the morphological characteristics of megaloblasts and normoblasts.

3. Characterize the peripheral blood morphology of megaloblastic anemia.

4. Identify the bone marrow morphology of megaloblastic anemia.

5. Describe pernicious anemia, including the pathophysiology and clinical and laboratory findings.

6. Describe the Schilling test as a diagnostic tool for pernicious anemia.

7. List the causes of vitamin B$_{12}$ and folate deficiencies.

8. Evaluate laboratory tests used for differential diagnosis of megaloblastic anemia.

9. Compare and contrast the treatment for vitamin B$_{12}$ and folate deficiencies.

10. Using the peripheral blood findings, differentiate the anemia of liver disease from a megaloblastic anemia caused by vitamin B$_{12}$ or folate deficiency.

Megaloblastic anemia is a subgroup of macrocytic anemia characterized by defective nuclear maturation caused by impaired deoxyribonucleic acid (DNA) synthesis. This defect is manifested by the presence of megaloblasts (large and abnormal red cell precursors) in the bone marrow and macroovalocytes in the peripheral blood. The granulocyte precursors tend to be larger than normal, with giant metamyelocytes as a striking feature. An abnormal nuclear pattern in megakaryocytes may be seen in severe anemia. The megaloblastic changes are not limited to the hematopoietic cells; changes are also present in other nucleated actively prolifer-ating cells, such as skin, vaginal, uterine, cervical, and buccal cells.

➤ BIOCHEMICAL ASPECT

The defective nuclear maturation and the megaloblastic morphology are caused by a decrease in thymidine triphosphate (TTP) synthesis from uridine monophosphate (UMP). This deficiency interferes with nuclear maturation, DNA replication, and cell division. When TTP is not present in adequate amounts, deoxyuridine triphosphate incorporates into the

112

DNA instead[1-5] (Fig. 7–1). This misincorporation causes fragmentation of the nucleus and, ultimately, destruction of immature cells.

The primary causes for lack of thymidine and consequently defective DNA synthesis are vitamin B_{12} and folic acid deficiencies. These vitamins, in the form of cofactors, play important roles in some key reactions involved in DNA synthesis. In addition, drugs that interfere with the metabolism of these vitamins also cause DNA impairment.

➤ CLINICAL MANIFESTATIONS OF MEGALOBLASTIC ANEMIA

Certain clinical manifestations are common to all patients with megaloblastic anemias regardless of the cause. The degree of anemia may be mild to severe, with the symptoms of weakness, fatigue, shortness of breath, and lightheadedness. Congestive heart failure may or may not be present, depending on the degree of anemia. In severe anemia, the patient may have a lemon-yellow skin tint because of mild jaundice and pallor. Increased bilirubin is reported in about 30% of patients as a result of intramedullary hemolysis caused by ineffective erythropoiesis.[3]

➤ HEMATOLOGIC FEATURES

Ineffective Hematopoiesis

Megaloblastic anemia is associated with ineffective erythropoiesis and hemolysis. The mean corpuscular volume (MCV) is greater than 100 femtoliters (fL). Patients with megaloblastic anemia may have MCV values as high as 160 fL. This elevated MCV reflects the megaloblastic picture of the bone marrow. Increased erythrocyte precursors in the bone marrow and their decreased release into the peripheral blood indicate ineffective erythropoiesis, which is supported by decreased reticulocytes.

The megaloblastic erythrocyte progenitors have a much shorter life span than the normal erythrocyte progenitors. They are more fragile and, therefore, die prematurely in the marrow. Evidence of intramedullary hemolysis includes increased values for serum bilirubin, serum lactate dehydrogenase (LDH—in particular, LDH-1 and LDH-2 isomers), and serum iron.[1,6] The cell death occurs primarily at the later stages of the megaloblast maturation (i.e., basophilic and polychromatophilic stages), causing a decrease in production and release of mature erythrocytes. A decreased level of erythrocytes in the circulation stimulates erythropoietin release, which in turn stimulates production of red cell progenitors.[4]

Ineffective granulopoiesis is defined by increased bone marrow white cell precursors and failure to release mature forms into the peripheral blood. The giant metamyelocytes do not mature to circulating neutrophils but, rather, die prematurely in the bone marrow. The elevated serum muramidase is a result of this increased turnover of white cells.

Ineffective thrombopoiesis is manifested by the presence of increased abnormal megakaryocytes in the bone marrow and thrombocytopenia in the peripheral blood.

Bone Marrow Morphology

Patients with megaloblastic anemia have a hypercellular bone marrow. The myeloid-to-erythroid (M:E) ratio is decreased (Fig. 7–2; see also Color Plate 92) and may be as low as 1:1 to 1:3. The degree of increased cellularity (megaloblastic picture) depends on the severity of the anemia. Megaloblasts are large cells with increased ribonucleic acid (RNA) per DNA unit. Their nuclear chromatin appears loose and less mature than the nuclear chromatin of the normal red cells at the same stage of maturation (Fig. 7–3 and Color Plate 93). The cytoplasm maturation is, however, normal. This phenomenon is referred to as nuclear to cytoplasm asynchrony. The mature megaloblastic red cells entering the circulation usually have a shorter life span than normal, mature red cells.

Megaloblastic changes are manifested in white cell precursors by the presence of large bands (see Fig. 7–2B) and giant metamyelocytes in the bone marrow. The nucleus of the giant bands may show abnormal staining characteristics. These white cell abnormalities are not seen in the megaloblastic bone marrow present in patients with myelodysplastic syndrome or erythroleukemia.[7] Megakaryocytes are also affected in severe megaloblastic anemia. They may have abnormal nuclear or cytoplasm morphology, such as increased nuclear lobulation and hypogranulation.[8]

Peripheral Blood Morphology

Megaloblastic anemia is a macrocytic, normochromic anemia. Depending on the degree of anemia, the MCV may range from 100 to 160 fL. The mean corpuscular hemoglobin (MCH) is elevated but the mean corpuscular hemoglobin concentration (MCHC) is normal. Not all patients with macrocytosis have megaloblastic anemia (i.e., alcoholism and liver disease), and not all megaloblastic anemias are macrocytic. A normal MCV may be present in patients with megaloblastic anemia and coexisting iron deficiency or thalassemia.

The hemoglobin value may be normal to low. In a severe anemia the hemoglobin may drop to below 7 to 8 g/dL. The

➤ FIGURE 7–1   Thymidine synthesis pathway from uridine nucleotide. Uracil is incorporated into DNA in the absence of thymine. UDP = uridine diphosphate; dUDP = deoxyuridine diphosphate; dUTP = deoxyuridine triphosphate; dUMP = deoxyuridine monophosphate; dTMP = deoxythymidine monophosphate; dTDP = deoxythymidine diphosphate; dTTP = deoxythymidine triphosphate; CH_2THF = methylene tetrahydrofolate.

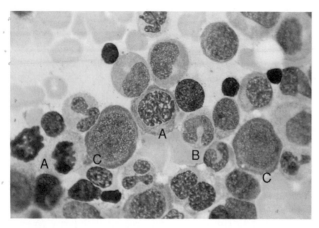

➤ **FIGURE 7–2** *A.* Mitotic figures in megaloblastic marrow. *B.* Large megaloblastic band neutrophil. *C.* Megaloblastic pronormoblast with open, sievelike chromatin. The myeloid-to-erythroid (M:E) ratio is decreased because of the increase in megaloblastic erythroid precursors labeled A and C.

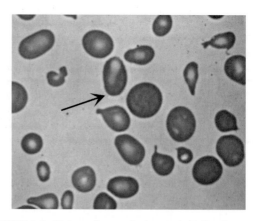

➤ **FIGURE 7–4** Extreme degree of anisocytosis (+4) and poikilocytosis (+4) with oval macrocytosis (*arrow*) in a patient with severe pernicious anemia. (From Bell, A: Hematology. In: Listen, Look and Learn. Health and Education Resources, Inc., Bethesda, MD, with permission.)

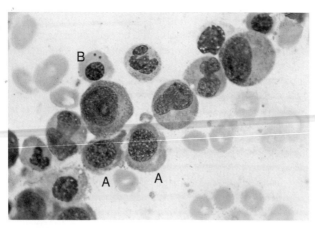

➤ **FIGURE 7–3** Bone marrow. *A.* Polychromatophilic megaloblasts. *B.* Orthochromic megaloblast with multiple Howell-Jolly bodies.

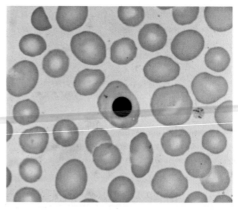

➤ **FIGURE 7–5** Howell-Jolly body in an orthochromic megaloblast in pernicious anemia (*center*). (From Bell, A: Hematology. In: Listen, Look and Learn. Health and Education Resources, Inc., Bethesda, MD, with permission.)

erythrocyte count is generally decreased. The leukocyte count may be normal at the early stage of anemia but may decrease to as low as 1 to 3×10^9/L. Although platelets are the least affected cell line, platelet counts below 100×10^9/L have been reported in patients with severe anemia.[6]

The peripheral smear is pancytopenic with the presence of macrocytes and macro-ovalocytes (Fig. 7–4) The degree of anisocytosis and poikilocytosis varies with the severity of anemia. Other poikilocytes, such as schistocytes, teardrop-shaped cells, spherocytes, and target cells, may also be seen on the peripheral blood smear. Increased anisocytosis causes an elevated red cell distribution width (RDW) as determined by an automated cell counter. Dimorphic red cell morphology may be present in patients who have iron-deficiency anemia, thalassemia, anemia of chronic disease, or hyperthyroidism in addition to the megaloblastic anemia. A trimorphic blood smear may be seen in transfused patients. Red cell inclusions such as Howell-Jolly bodies and basophilic stippling are frequently present (Fig. 7–5; see also Color Plate 85). Cabot rings and megaloblastic nucleated red cells may be seen on the peripheral blood smear (Fig. 7–6 and Color Plate 94). The absolute reticulocyte count is decreased with a reticulocyte production index (RPI) of less than 2, indicating ineffective erythropoiesis. With treatment, the number of

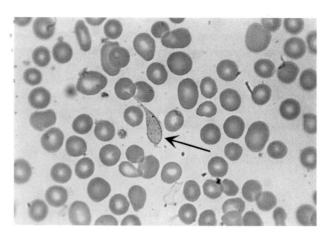

➤ **FIGURE 7–6** Cabot ring in pernicious anemia (*center*).

reticulocytes increases along with increased numbers of nucleated red cells.

In patients with untreated megaloblastic anemia, the macrocytes have a shortened survival time (27 to 75 days) compared with the survival time of normal red cells (110 to 120 days). The survival of normal red cells is shortened when transfused to a patient with severe and untreated megaloblastic anemia, which is indicative of extracorpuscular hemolysis.[6]

Multilobed neutrophils, termed hypersegmented neutrophils, are seen in the peripheral smear in 98% of cases.[9] (Fig. 7–7 and Color Plate 95). Hypersegmented neutrophils refer to one or more neutrophils with six lobes, or five or more neutrophils with five or more lobes.[7] They are larger than normal mature neutrophils. The number of the hypersegmented neutrophils counted per 100 white cells as determined by the differential should be reported. Although hypersegmented neutrophils appear early in the peripheral blood, they are the last morphological feature to disappear. Their absence does not rule out the diagnosis of megaloblastic anemia.

Other notable abnormal laboratory tests are elevated LDH, indirect bilirubin and urobilinogen, decreased haptoglobin, increased serum iron and ferritin, and increased erythropoietin.[4,6,10]

The diagnosis of megaloblastic anemia is usually based on the morphological characteristics of the peripheral blood, and the results of other biochemical tests. The bone marrow examination is generally not required. Bone marrow aspirates are performed for diagnosis of other disorders with a megaloblastic picture, such as myelodysplastic syndrome or erythroleukemia. The clinical features of megaloblastic anemia are summarized in Table 7–1.

➤ ETIOLOGY

The major causes of the megaloblastic anemias are vitamin B_{12} deficiency, folic acid deficiency, or a combination of both. Megaloblastic anemia can also be present in non–vitamin-deficient diseases, such as myelodysplastic syndromes and acute leukemias. Drug-induced megaloblastic anemia is caused by drugs that interfere with the metabolism of either vitamin B_{12} or folic acid. Examples of these drugs include chemotherapeutic agents and anticonvulsants.

➤ VITAMIN B_{12} DEFICIENCY

Sources and Requirements

Vitamin B_{12} is the only vitamin produced by microorganisms and fungi. It is present in foods of animal origin such

> **Table 7-1**
> ## CLINICAL FEATURES OF MEGALOBLASTIC ANEMIA

Bone Marrow

Hypercellular

Low M:E ratio

Megaloblasts

Giant bands and metamyelocytes

Peripheral Blood

Pancytopenia

Macro-ovalocytes

Hypersegmented neutrophils

Biochemical Changes

Elevated LDH

Elevated indirect bilirubin

Increased serum iron and ferritin

Increased erythropoietin

as liver, fish, poultry, meat, eggs, and dairy products. Liver is a major source of vitamin B_{12}. Vegetables do not contribute B_{12} to the diet. Vitamin B_{12} is commercially available for treatment of deficiencies.

In the United States, the daily diet contains an average of 5 to 30 µg of vitamin B_{12}, of which 1 to 5 µg is absorbed. The recommended dietary intake of vitamin B_{12} for adults is 5 µg/day.[1] This requirement increases in pregnancy, infancy, during growth and increased metabolic stages, and in the elderly. Vitamin B_{12} is lost through the urine and feces. The rate of loss is about 0.1% per day. Body storage of vitamin B_{12} is about 1 to 5 mg, of which approximately 1 to 2 mg is stored in the liver.[1] Because the daily requirement of vitamin B_{12} is low and the storage rate is high, it takes several years for a person to develop vitamin B_{12} deficiency as a result of malabsorption.

Structure

Vitamin B_{12} (cobalamin) is a large, water-soluble molecule. It consists of a corrin nucleus composed of four pyrrol rings (A to D) with a cobalt atom at the center (Fig. 7–8), similar to porphyrin nucleus (see Chap. 6). The corrin ring is attached to the nucleotide 5,6-dimethylbenzimidazole. The cobalt atom can be attached to several different molecules, such as adenosyl (5-deoxyadenoside), methyl, cyanide, and hydroxy, to form the biologically active forms of cobalamins (see Fig. 7–8).

Transport and Metabolism

Two important proteins are involved in the transport of vitamin B_{12} from duodenum to ileum and from ileum to tissues: the intrinsic factor (IF) and transcobalamin II.[7,9] The dietary cobalamin is released from the food by gastric acids and intestinal enzymes. On release, it binds to a carrier protein called R protein (fast-moving protein electrophoretically). Upon entering the duodenum, B_{12} releases from the R protein by the action of pancreatic enzymes. The released

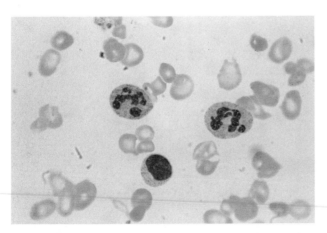

➤ **FIGURE 7–7** Neutrophil hypersegmentation in pernicious anemia.

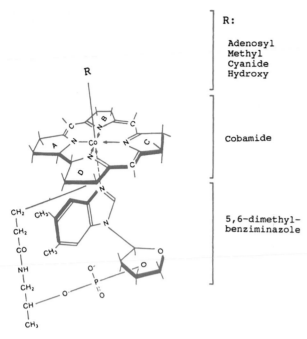

R:

Adenosyl
Methyl
Cyanide
Hydroxy

Cobamide

5,6-dimethyl-
benziminazole

➤ **FIGURE 7–8** Structure of vitamin B_{12} (cobalamin). When R is adenosyl, the compound is adenosylcobalamin (AdoCb); when R is methyl, it is methylcobalamin (MeCb); when R is cyanide, it is cyanocobalamin (CNCb); and when R is hydroxy, it is hydroxocobalamin (OHCb).

vitamin B_{12} then binds to IF, a glycoprotein with molecular weight of approximately 44,000 d.[1] The gene for IF is located on chromosome 11.[7] IF is secreted by parietal cells of the stomach. The parietal cells also secrete hydrochloric acid and other gastric juices. IF binds to vitamin B_{12} and forms B_{12}-IF complex. This complex allows vitamin B_{12} to be absorbed through the receptors present on the brush borders of the ileum (the distal half of the small intestine) (Fig. 7–9). IF is not absorbed by the ileum and, therefore, cannot be reutilized. It is degraded on release from vitamin B_{12}.[1,11] The released vitamin B_{12} then enters the portal vein.

When vitamin B_{12} leaves the ileum and enters the portal vein, it attaches to three proteins, transcobalamin I (TC I), transcobalamin II (TC II), and transcobalamin III (TC III). About 70% to 90% of vitamin B_{12} is bound to TC I, TC III,

and other R proteins, whereas only about 10% to 25 % of vitamin B_{12} is bound to TC II.[1,7] TC II is the main transport protein of cobalamin to the tissues. It is a polypeptide with a molecular weight of 43,000 d.[7] TC II is synthesized by ileal cells, endothelial cells, liver, spleen, heart, and macrophages, and is secreted into the plasma.[1,7,9] TC II transports vitamin B_{12} to the liver for storage and to the bone marrow and other tissues for DNA synthesis (see Fig. 7–9). The deficiency of TC II causes megaloblastic anemia. It is suggested that the functions of TC I and TC III are to bind to vitamin B_{12} preventing its losses in the urine.[1,12,13]

Vitamin B_{12} plays an important role in two key reactions in the body. Firstly, it is necessary in the synthesis of methionine from homocysteine. In this biochemical reaction, both vitamin B_{12} and folic acid are involved. Vitamin B_{12} acts as a coenzyme, methylcobalamin (MeCb), for the enzyme methyltransferase (Fig. 7–10). Secondly, vitamin B_{12} is important in conversion of methylmalonyl CoA, a Krebs cycle intermediate, to succinyl CoA. In this reaction vitamin B_{12} also acts as a coenzyme, adenosylcobalamin (AdoCb), for the enzyme methylmalonyl CoA mutase. Adenosylcobalamin acts as a hydrogen (H) carrier, taking the H from methylmalonyl CoA to make succinyl CoA (Fig. 7–11).

Causes of Vitamin B_{12} Deficiency

Vitamin B_{12} deficiency progresses through four stages: stage I, negative vitamin B_{12} balance; stage II, vitamin B_{12} depletion; stage III, vitamin B_{12}-deficient erythropoiesis; and stage IV, vitamin B_{12}-deficient anemia. Stages I and II are referred to as the depletion stages. Stages III and IV are referred to as the deficient stages.[14]

Dietary Vitamin B_{12} Deficiency

Nutritional vitamin B_{12} deficiency is uncommon in western countries and is limited to strict vegetarians. In this group, the decrease in vitamin B_{12} is accompanied by an increased plasma folate level.

It is worth noting that the children born to a vegan mother (one who consumes no animal food) or to a mother who has an untreated vitamin B_{12} deficiency are vitamin B_{12} deficient, especially if they are breast-fed.[7] Untreated infants are severely megaloblastic, with retarded growth and psychomotor development. Neurologic complications, such as

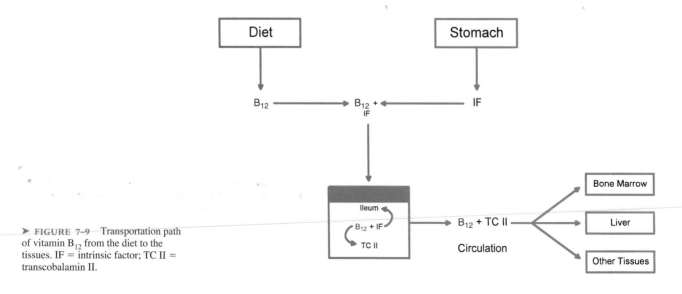

➤ **FIGURE 7–9** Transportation path of vitamin B_{12} from the diet to the tissues. IF = intrinsic factor; TC II = transcobalamin II.

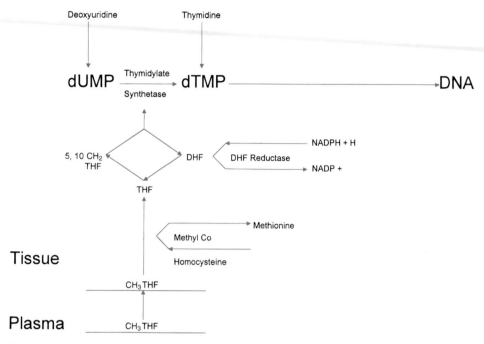

➤ FIGURE 7–10 The role of vitamin B_{12} and folate in DNA synthesis. CH_2THF = methylene tetrahydrofolate; THF = tetrahydrofolate; DHF = dihydrofolate; CH_3THF = methyl tetrahydrofolate; dUMP = deoxyuridine monophosphate; dTMP = deoxythymidine monophosphate.

irritability, anorexia, and failure to thrive, have been reported in severely vitamin B_{12}-deficient infants.[7,15]

The major cause of vitamin B_{12} deficiency is malabsorption. The most common form of intestinal malabsorption is pernicious anemia. Other causes of vitamin B_{12} deficiency are summarized in Table 7–2 and discussed later.

Pernicious Anemia

Definition

Pernicious anemia is the common cause of vitamin B_{12} deficiency. It is a chronic disease caused by the deficiency of IF. The cause for a decrease in IF is gastric parietal cell atrophy, which is associated with a concomitant decrease in other gastric juices. Lack of IF leads to defective vitamin B_{12} absorption and, consequently, megaloblastic anemia.

Pernicious anemia is more common in people of Scandinavian, English, and Irish descent, with a prevalence in women (female-to-male ratio of 4:1).[6] Pernicious anemia is more common after age 50. In blacks, the disease may start earlier.[6,16] Pernicious anemia occurs rarely in children, and, if it occurs, it may be in the congenital form. Congenital pernicious anemia is characterized by the total absence of IF and normal secretion of other gastric juices. There are no antibodies present against IF or the parietal cells. Juvenile pernicious anemia is similar to adult pernicious anemia, with the age of onset in the second decade.[6]

Pathophysiology

The main cause of pernicious anemia is atrophic gastritis characterized by atrophy of the gastric mucosa with decrease of gastric secretions and IF. The cause of gastric atrophy is probably autoimmune, with poorly defined genetic predisposition.[6] IF is essential for absorption of vitamin B_{12}. In the absence of IF, only a small amount of vitamin B_{12} is absorbed, causing a gradual deficiency in vitamin B_{12}.

➤ FIGURE 7–11 Conversion of methylmalonyl CoA to succinyl CoA. AdoCo = adenosylcobalamin.

> **Table 7-2**
CAUSES OF VITAMIN B$_{12}$ DEFICIENCY

Dietary Deficiency

Strict vegans

Malabsorption

Pernicious anemia

Gastrectomy (total or partial)

Blind loop syndrome

Fish tapeworm (*Diphyllobothrium latum*)

Diseases of ileum

Chronic pancreatic disease

Other Disorders

Hemodialysis

Human immunodeficiency virus (HIV) infection

Acquired immunodeficiency syndrome (AIDS)

Drugs

Alcohol

Nitrous oxide (N$_2$O)

Para-aminosalicylic acid (PAS)

GENETIC FACTORS

The congenital form of pernicious anemia is inherited as an autosomal-recessive trait and is primarily seen in children before age two.[6,17] The genetic contribution to the adult form of pernicious anemia is supported by (1) the concordant presence of pernicious anemia in identical twins, (2) the increased risk in relatives of patients with pernicious anemia, (3) the presence of achlorhydria with or without malabsorption in relatives of patients with pernicious anemia, and (4) the findings that relatives of patients with pernicious anemia may produce antibody to gastric parietal cells (24%, as compared with 3.8% in patients with a negative family history).[1,6,12]

The exact cause for the genetic predisposition of pernicious anemia is not yet clear. A weak association has been made between pernicious anemia and the human leukocyte antigen (HLA) is not conclusive. An association between HLA-B7 and pernicious anemia has been reported in whites. The association of HLA-D antigens Dw2, Dw5, and DR2 with pernicious anemia is more significant than that of other HLA antigens.[6,12] IF antibodies are associated with HLA-Dw2.[6]

IMMUNOLOGIC FACTORS

The serum of patients with pernicious anemia contains autoantibodies to parietal cells, to IF, and to thyroid tissue. The parietal cell antibodies are found in the serum of approximately 84% of all patients with pernicious anemia and in 50% of patients with atrophic gastritis. The antibodies are also present in the gastric juices of 75% of patients with pernicious anemia. This antibody is specific for the parietal cells only, and does not show any cross-reactivity.[6]

Antibodies to IF are demonstrated in the serum of approximately 56% of patients with pernicious anemia. These antibodies are more specific for diagnosis of anemia than

antiparietal antibodies. Two types of IF antibodies have been reported. Type I, or blocking antibodies, prevent IF-B$_{12}$ complex formation. Type II, or binding antibodies, are usually present with blocking antibodies. Binding antibodies are of two varieties. One type binds to free IF and IF-B$_{12}$ complex, and the other binds to the complex, only.[6,12]

Thyroid antibodies have often been found in the serum of patients with pernicious anemia or their relatives.[6]

Lymphocytotoxic antibodies have also been detected in one-third of patients with pernicious anemia. A decrease in suppressor T cells and an increase in the CD4:CD8 ratio support the presence of cell-mediated immunity in patients with pernicious anemia.[6]

An association between pernicious anemia and other autoimmune diseases, such as thyroid disease, diabetes mellitus, and rheumatoid arthritis, has also been noted.[6] The positive response to steroids in some patients with pernicious anemia supports the autoimmune mechanism.[6]

The *Helicobacter pylori* microorganism has been identified as a major cause of gastritis and peptic ulcers. However, its role in pernicious anemia is not yet clear.[1]

Clinical Manifestations of Vitamin B$_{12}$ Deficiency

The onset of pernicious anemia is generally insidious. Patients with pernicious anemia and other vitamin B$_{12}$ deficiencies have all the signs and symptoms of megaloblastic anemia mentioned earlier. Fever is usually present in severe anemia. Loss of appetite is a common complaint. Glossitis (sore tongue) is reported in 50% of patients.[6] Although the initial presentations may vary among patients with vitamin B$_{12}$ deficiency, the classic symptoms include weakness, glossitis, and paresthesias.[6]

The bone marrow morphology of patients with vitamin B$_{12}$ deficiency is megaloblastic, and the peripheral smear has macro-ovalocytes.

In addition to hematologic abnormalities, vitamin B$_{12}$ deficiency is associated with gastrointestinal, thrombotic, psychiatric, and neurologic complications.

Neurologic Manifestations

Neurologic problems are more common in pernicious anemia than in other types of vitamin B$_{12}$ deficiencies. The degree of neurologic involvement is not directly related to the degree of anemia. Neurologic manifestations in the absence of hematologic abnormalities have been reported in many cases.[18]

The neurologic abnormalities may be mild, moderate, or severe and may involve degeneration of peripheral nerves, posterior columns of the spinal cord, and posterior and lateral columns of the spinal cord (Table 7–3). Because multiple neuropathies are involved, the terms *subacute combined degeneration* (SCD) and *combined system disease* may be used.[6,19]

> **Table 7-3**
NEUROLOGIC MANIFESTATIONS IN PERNICIOUS ANEMIA

- Degeneration of peripheral nerves
- Degeneration of posterior columns
- Degeneration of posterior and lateral columns

In the earlier stage of pernicious anemia, the peripheral nerves are affected, causing paresthesia and areflexia.[19,20] The patient often experiences symmetric tingling or "pins-and-needle" sensations in the toes and later in all four limbs. Less often, the patient may complain of numbness. At the later stage, the posterior spinal columns may be involved. At this stage, the patient may complain of clumsiness and have an incoordinate gait. The lateral spinal columns become involved in the most severe stage of illness, with manifestations of severe weakness and stiffness of limbs, impairment of memory, and depression. Severe psychiatric symptoms are less common and include stupor, hallucinations, paranoia, and severe depression, referred to as "megaloblastic madness." Less frequent neurologic problems include ophthalmoplegia. Bilateral retinal bleeding in severe anemia with thrombocytopenia has been reported in some patients.[6,21] Patients with SCD respond well with proper and adequate treatment. Neurologic manifestations of less than 3 months' duration are reversible; complete improvement in 47% of patients and partial improvement in 53% have been reported.[6,22] However, some degree of dysfunction may remain. In untreated patients, the neurologic symptoms are progressive, and the degree of severity is directly proportional to the duration of symptoms.[6,22]

The basic underlying cause for the neuropathy associated with vitamin B_{12} deficiency is not exactly known. However, the impairment of methionine synthetase reaction has been indicated as the possible cause for the neuropathy. The rationale for this hypothesis is that the deficiency of methionine leads to decreased production of S-adenosyl methionine (SAM), a key intermediate in methylation reactions of myelin. The impairment of methylation in myelin could result in demyelination and, consequently, in clinical neuropathy.[6,23–26]

Other Causes of Vitamin B_{12} Deficiency

Gastrectomy

Many other causes of malabsorption can lead to vitamin B_{12} deficiency (see Table 7–2). In a gastrectomy procedure, the IF-producing cells are removed. Vitamin B_{12} deficiency develops in these patients within several years in the absence of vitamin B_{12} therapy. Vitamin B_{12} deficiency has been reported in 30% to 40% of patients with partial gastrectomy.[6]

Blind Loop Syndrome

In blind loop syndrome, an anatomic abnormality of the small intestine, there is an overgrowth of bacteria in the small bowel. These microorganisms take up the vitamin B_{12} and make it unavailable for absorption by the ileum. Tetracycline therapy for 10 days normalizes the vitamin B_{12} level.[6,12]

Fish Tapeworm

Fish tapeworm (*Diphyllobothrium latum*) is a parasite that competes for vitamin B_{12} by splitting B_{12} from IF. This type of vitamin B_{12} deficiency is common in Scandinavian countries and is reported in 1.9% to 3.0% of carriers of the fish tapeworm.[6,12] The malabsorption type of vitamin B_{12} deficiency is normally corrected when vitamin B_{12} or B_{12} and IF are given to the patients.

Diseases of Ileum

Vitamin B_{12} deficiency can also be seen in diseases of the ileum, such as ileal resection or bypass, and in regional enteritis.[6]

Chronic Pancreatic Disease

In pancreatic disease, vitamin B_{12} deficiency develops as a result of a decrease in the proteases necessary for release of vitamin B_{12} from salivary and gastric R proteins for absorption. A low level of free calcium, which is necessary for calcium-dependent ileal absorption, can cause vitamin B_{12} deficiency in patients with chronic pancreatic disease.[6,14]

Other Disorders

Vitamin B_{12} deficiency has also been reported in patients who are on hemodialysis and in patients with human immunodeficiency virus (HIV) infection and with acquired immunodeficiency syndrome (AIDS), especially in those receiving zidovudine therapy.[6,7]

Drug-Induced Vitamin Deficiency

Other causes of vitamin B_{12} deficiency are drugs such as alcohol, anesthetics, nitrous oxide (N_2O), and the antituberculosis drug para-aminosalicylic acid (PAS).[7,14,24]

► FOLIC ACID DEFICIENCY

Sources and Requirements

Folic acid, also known as folate or pteroylglutamic acid, is a water-soluble vitamin present in a variety of foods. The highest concentration is present in green leafy vegetables, fruits, dairy products, cereals, and also in animal foods such as liver and kidney. The average daily diet contains about 400 to 600 μg of folate; however, folate is a heat-labile vitamin and, therefore, is easily destroyed in overcooked vegetables.[1] The recommended dietary intake of folic acid for adults is approximately 50 to 100 μg/day.[1,6] This requirement increases significantly during infancy, pregnancy, and lactation. Folate deficiency during early pregnancy (first trimester) can cause renal tube defects in the fetus and is associated with paralysis and brain damage.[1,27–30] The body storage is about 5 to 10 mg,[6] of which almost 80% is stored in the liver. The amount of folic acid absorbed is about 80% of intake. It is absorbed through the duodenum and jejunum. Folate is lost via body secretions such as bile, urine, and sweat. Folic acid has a higher turnover time and a higher rate of loss compared to vitamin B_{12} and, therefore, it takes only a few months to develop dietary folate deficiency.

Structure

Folic acid consists of three components: pteridine, para-aminobenzoic acid, and glutamic acid (Fig. 7–12). Folic acid derived from the diet is not biologically active. Once absorbed through the intestinal lumen, it is hydrolyzed, reduced, and methylated to form methyl tetrahydrofolate (CH_3THF). Other biologically active forms of folic acid are tetrahydrofolate (THF) and its coenzyme, N^5N^{10}-methylene tetrahydrofolate ($N^5N^{10}CH_2THF$).

Serum folate is in the form of CH_3THF and enters all tissue cells in this form.

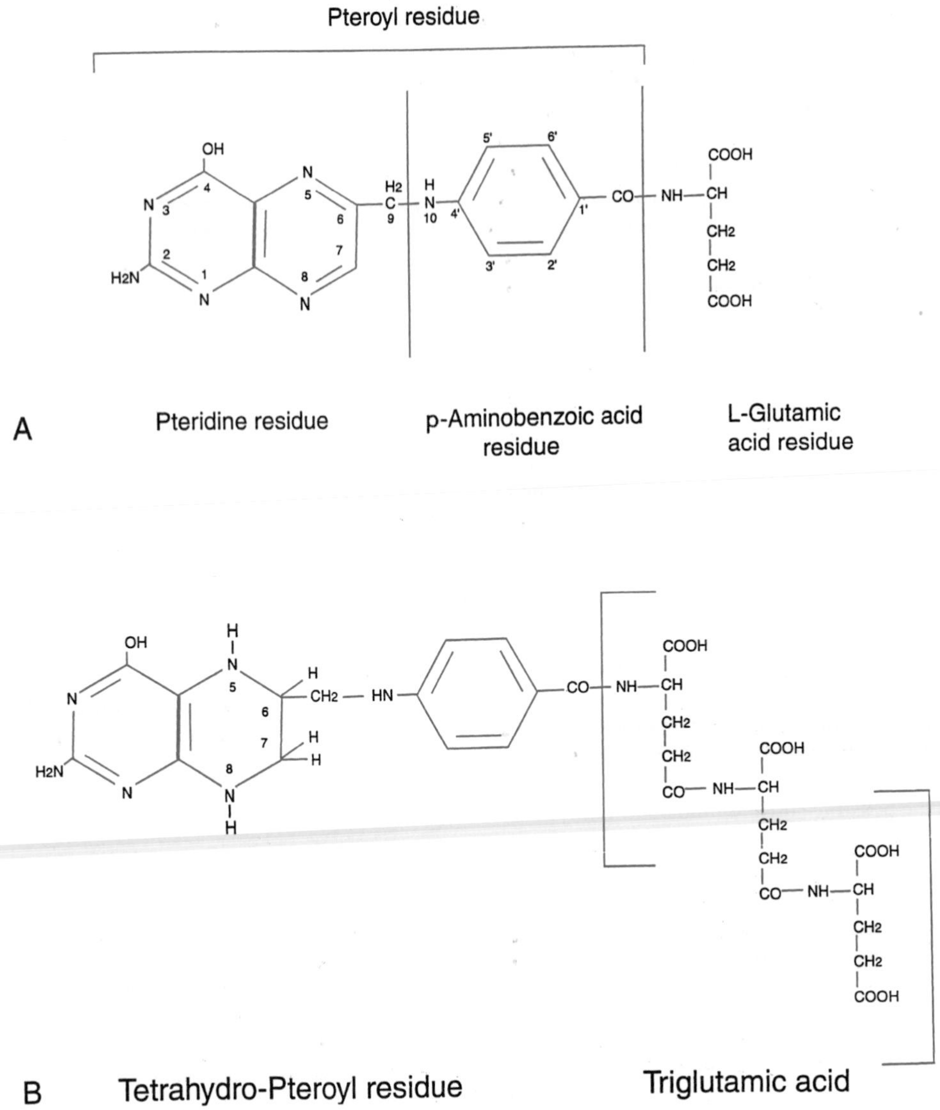

> **FIGURE 7–12**   Structure of folic acid and its derivative. *A.* Folic acid (pteroylglutamic acid). The three components are defined by vertical lines. *B.* Tetrapteroyltriglutamic acid (tetrahydrofolate triglutamate), the active form of folate present in the tissues.

Absorption and Metabolism

Dietary folic acid is in the form of polyglutamic acid (many glutamic acid residues). Once in the intestinal lumen, it is acted on by the enzyme folate deconjugase, which is present in the epithelial cells of intestine, to form monoglutamic acid (single glutamic acid residue) (Figs. 7–13 and 7–14). Monoglutamic acid is then reduced and methylated to CH$_3$THF. This compound is then released into the circulation (see Fig. 7–13) Most of the circulatory folic acid is in the form of CH$_3$THF.[11] When CH$_3$THF is absorbed from the circulation into the tissue cells, it transfers its methyl group to homocysteine to form methionine and THF. The THF formed reconjugates with additional glutamic acid residues to form the cellular THF (see Figs. 7–12 and 7–13). The THF is then methylated to form coenzyme methylene THF (N^{5}N^{10}CH$_2$THF) necessary for the formation of thymidine monophosphate from uridine monophosphate. This is the key reaction for DNA synthesis (see Fig. 7–10).

Causes of Folic Acid Deficiency

Dietary Deficiency

The main cause of folic acid deficiency is decreased dietary intake. Other causes are malabsorption, increased requirement, and drug-induced folate deficiencies (Table 7–4). Nutritional folate deficiency is usually a consequence of poverty, old age, alcoholism, pregnancy, and chronic diseases. In the United States, folic acid has been added to cereal grains, rice, and milled flour to increase the average adult's intake by 100 μg.[20] The government urges women planning to become pregnant and in early pregnancy to eat a diet rich in folic acid or take vitamin supplements to prevent the adverse effects of folic acid deficiency on their fetus.

Malabsorption

The most common causes of folate malabsorption are tropical sprue and gluten-sensitive enteropathy. Tropical sprue is

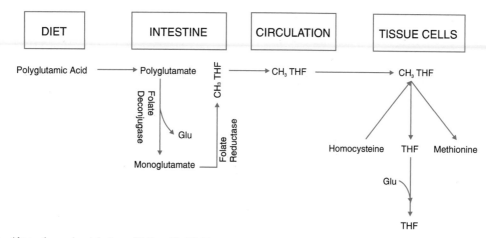

➤ FIGURE 7-13   Absorption and metabolism of folic acid. CH_3THF = methyl tetrahydrofolate; Glu = glutamic acid; THF = tetrahydrofolate.

an infection that causes intestinal atrophy with clinical manifestations of weakness, weight loss, and steatorrhea. Tropical sprue affects the entire intestine and, therefore, causes a wide variety of nutritional deficiencies, including vitamin B_{12} deficiency.[6] Affected individuals respond well to antibiotics.

Gluten-sensitive enteropathy has the same clinical manifestations as those mentioned for tropical sprue. It includes both nontropical sprue and childhood celiac disease. Affected individuals cannot digest gluten, a protein found in wheat and other grains. Lesions are most severe in the proximal intestine. Childhood celiac disease is a malabsorption syndrome resulting in anemia caused by iron deficiency and, to a lesser degree, by vitamin B_{12} and folate deficiencies.

The requirement for folic acid also increases during rapid cellular proliferation in hematologic diseases such as sickle cell anemia, thalassemia, hereditary spherocytosis, and autoimmune hemolytic anemia.

Drug-Induced Folate Defiiency

Drug-induced folate-deficient megaloblastic anemia has been reported with a variety of drugs such as methotrexate, pyrimethamine, phenytoin, alcohol, isoniazid, and oral contraceptives[6,12] (see Table 7-4).

Clinical Manifestations of Folic Acid Deficiency

Clinical manifestations of folate deficiency are the same as those for vitamin B_{12} deficiency, mentioned earlier. The on-set of anemia is insidious, with the distinct morphology characteristic of megaloblastic anemia in the bone marrow and in the peripheral blood. Although neuropathy is mainly characteristic of vitamin B_{12} deficiency, several cases of neurologic abnormalities, such as depression, dementia, and peripheral neuropathy associated with folic acid deficiency, have been reported.[25] Some of these neuropathies, in particular depression, have responded favorably to treatment with folate.[25,31-33]

Folic acid and vitamin B_{12} are both necessary cofactors to the enzyme methionine synthase, which converts homocysteine to methionine. The deficiency of these vitamins causes an increased level of plasma homocysteine. Hyperhomocysteinemia is a risk factor for thrombosis.[30,34] An association between folate deficiency and development of leukemia in high-risk patients has been reported.[35]

➤ LABORATORY DIAGNOSIS OF MEGALOBLASTIC ANEMIA

Several important factors in differential diagnosis of megaloblastic anemias are the patient's physical examination, medical history, drug history, family history, and laboratory tests.

The most common laboratory screening tests and results that are used in the diagnosis of megaloblastic anemias are low hemoglobin level, elevated MCV, and peripheral smear morphology, such as macro-ovalocytes and hypersegmented

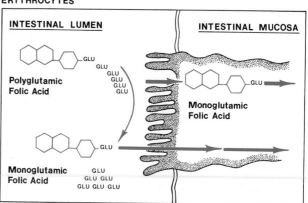

➤ FIGURE 7-14   Intestinal absorption of the folate derivatives of food. (From Streiff, RR: Intestinal absorption of the folate derivatives of food. JAMA 214:105, 1970, with permission.)

> **Table 7-4**
> **CAUSES OF FOLIC ACID DEFICIENCY**

Dietary Deficiency

Poverty

Old age

Alcoholism

Chronic diseases

Malabsorption

Tropical sprue

Gluten-sensitive enteropathy

Childhood celiac disease

Increased Requirement

Pregnancy

Infancy

Malignancy

Drugs

Methotrexate

Pyrimethamine

Phenytoin

Alcohol

Isoniazid

Oral contraceptives

Others

neutrophils. Once the diagnosis of megaloblastic anemia is established, the exact cause of the anemia should be determined for appropriate and effective treatment. Figure 7–15 demonstrates the proper selection and interpretation of laboratory tests in the differential diagnosis of megaloblastic anemia.

Differential Diagnosis of Vitamin B_{12} and Folic Acid Deficiencies

Diagnostic tests used for vitamin B_{12} and folate deficiencies are serum B_{12} and serum and red cell folate levels. Red cell folate is a better indicator of tissue folate levels (Table 7–5). The methods available for quantitation of these vitamins are microbiologic assay and immunoassays (radioimmunoassay and chemiluminescence). However, the microbiologic assay is time-consuming and is now replaced by immunoassay methods. Vitamin B_{12} and folic acid can be measured simultaneously by both immunoassay methods.

Low levels of serum B_{12} in the absence of vitamin B_{12} deficiency have been reported in patients with folate deficiency, pregnancy, oral contraceptive use, and decreased TC I level. Normal or elevated serum B_{12} is associated with myeloproliferative disorders, chronic myelocytic leukemia, and liver disease.[9,12,14]

In patients with folate deficiency, both serum folate and red cell folate are decreased. However, in patients with both folate and B_{12} deficiencies, the serum folate is increased while the red cell folate is decreased. In this case, the increased serum folate level is caused by increased CH_3THF

in the serum (the methyl trap hypothesis), resulting from the lack of vitamin B_{12} necessary for conversion of homocysteine to methionine and methyl THF to THF (see Fig. 7–10). Serum folate may also increase following ingestion of foods high in folate. False low serum folate levels have been reported in patients taking antibiotics or certain cytotoxic drugs.[21]

Other Laboratory Tests

Other laboratory tests that may support a diagnosis of vitamin B_{12} or folate deficiency are gastric achlorhydria, antibodies to IF, vitamin B_{12} absorption (Schilling) test, methylmalonic acid (MMA) assay, homocysteine assay, and the deoxyuridine (dU) suppression test. These tests are useful when the other laboratory tests are inconclusive.

Gastric Achlorhydria

Gastric achlorhydria (low gastric acidity) is present in almost all patients with pernicious anemia. Achlorhydria following histamine stimulation supports the diagnosis of pernicious anemia. However, this test is not specific, because achlorhydria has also been reported in patients without pernicious anemia.

Antibodies to Intrinsic Factor

Antibodies to IF are present in the serum of about 56% of patients with pernicious anemia. Although testing for the presence of antibodies is not sensitive, it is specific for the diagnosis of pernicious anemia. Decreased serum B_{12} and the presence of the antibody to IF are indicative of pernicious anemia.

Schilling test

The Schilling test evaluates absorption of vitamin B_{12} from the intestinal tract. The test is specific for vitamin B_{12} and is performed to pinpoint the cause of vitamin B_{12} malabsorption. The Schilling test is done in two parts (Fig. 7–16).

In part I, the patient is given 0.5 to 2.0 μg of labeled (^{57}Co or ^{58}Co) vitamin B_{12} orally. Two hours later, a flushing dose (1000 μg) of unlabeled vitamin B_{12} is injected intramuscularly to saturate all of the circulating cobalamin binders. The amount of the labeled vitamin B_{12} is then measured in a 24-hour urine collection. If IF is present and the normal absorption takes place, the labeled vitamin B_{12} absorbed through the intestine is rapidly excreted into the urine. The urinary excretion varies, depending on the dosage given. In normal absorption, about 5% to 35% of labeled B_{12} is excreted in the urine.[7] An abnormal result in part I indicates that B_{12} was not absorbed through the intestine. In this case, testing proceeds to part II to find the cause of malabsorption (see Fig. 7–16).

In part II, the test is repeated with the addition of IF to the oral dose to determine if malabsorption is caused by the lack of IF. If the Schilling test is corrected in part II, a deficiency of IF is confirmed. If the Schilling test is still abnormal, other causes of malabsorption should be investigated (see Fig. 7–16). Parts I and II can be done simultaneously if B_{12} and B_{12} + IF are labeled with different isotopes. Reliability of the Schilling test depends on normal renal function and proper urine collection.

Serum and Urine Methylmalonic Acid

Serum and urine MMA levels are both elevated in patients with vitamin B_{12} deficiency. As discussed earlier, vitamin

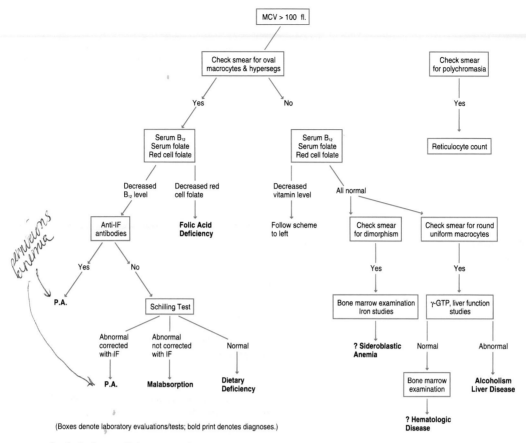

> **FIGURE 7–15** Logical scheme of laboratory testing in cases of macrocytosis. Boxes denote laboratory evaluations or tests; bold type denotes diagnoses. IF = intrinsic factor; PA = pernicious anemia.

B_{12} in the form of adenosylcobalamin is necessary for conversion of methylmalonyl CoA to succinyl CoA (see Fig. 7–11). In the absence of vitamin B_{12}, the level of methylmalonyl CoA will be increased in the serum and consequently in the urine. Falsely elevated results have been reported in non–vitamin-deficient patients with renal disease and with inborn errors of metabolism.

Measurement of urinary MMA by a gas chromatograph–mass spectrophotometer (GC-MS) is a highly specific and sensitive test. This test can be used for evaluation of tissue vitamin B_{12} deficiency in the absence of decreased serum B_{12} and lack of clinical manifestations of megaloblastic anemia.[36]

Normal individuals excrete approximately 9 mg MMA in the urine in 24 hours. Patients with B_{12} deficiency may excrete as much as 300 mg/day.[6]

Serum and Urine Homocysteine
Serum and urine homocysteine levels are elevated in patients with both vitamin B_{12} and folate deficiencies, because both vitamins are necessary in the conversion of homocysteine to methionine. Serum homocysteine is also increased in the short-term folate-restricted diet and in patients with congenital homocysteinuria.[2,37–39]

Deoxyuridine Suppression Test
The dU suppression test measures the level of 5,10-CH_2THF. It is an indirect measurement of thymidylate synthesis in vitro and is abnormal in both vitamin B_{12} and folate deficiencies (see Fig. 7–10). The principle of this test is based on the fact that B_{12}- or folate-deficient cells cannot convert deoxyuridine to deoxythymidine and, therefore, the radioactive-labeled thymidine will be incorporated into DNA. In patients with normal levels of B_{12}- or folate, deoxyuridine is converted to thymidine. This conversion suppresses the labeled thymidine incorporation into the DNA.[9,24] Specificity of the deficient vitamin can be determined by addition of vitamin B_{12} or folate to the test system and a correction of the original abnormal result. This test is relatively time-consuming and, therefore, despite its sensitivity, is not used as a diagnostic test.

> **Table 7-5**
DIAGNOSIS OF VITAMIN DEFICIENCIES

	Serum B_{12}	Serum Folate	Red Cell Folate
Vitamin B_{12} deficiency	Decreased	Increased–normal	Decreased–normal
Folate deficiency	Normal	Decreased	Decreased
Vitamin B_{12} and folate deficiencies	Decreased	Decreased	Decreased

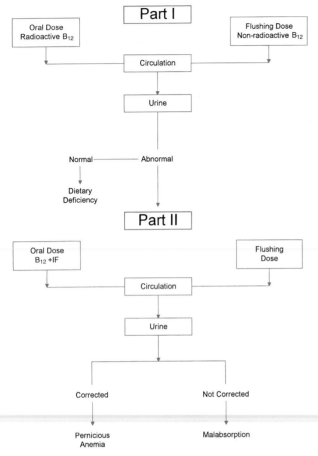

> ➤ FIGURE 7–16   The two-part Schilling test. IF = intrinsic factor.

Many studies have shown that some patients with vitamin B_{12} deficiency may seek medical help because of complications other than the classical features of megaloblastic anemia. Examples of these complications are retinopathy, neuropathy, vascular disorders, infertility, and physical and mental growth retardations in infancy.[15,25,30,37,40,41] However, these conditions have been reversed upon early treatment with vitamin B_{12}. To prevent these complications, numerous attempts have been made at early diagnosis of vitamin B_{12} and folate deficiencies.

The laboratory tests that are helpful for early detection of vitamin B_{12} and folate deficiencies are urinary methylmalonyl assay and serum homocysteine assay, respectively.[39]

The diagnosis of vitamin B_{12} may be inconclusive in the absence of hematologic and neurologic abnormalities.[42] However, vitamin B_{12} deficiency should be included in the differential diagnosis in patients with neurologic and neuropsychiatric problems.[22]

➤ TREATMENT

Transfusion is rarely required in patients with megaloblastic anemia unless the anemia is severe (hematocrit of less than 15%) or is associated with congestive heart failure.

Vitamin B_{12} Deficiency

Most people with a vitamin B_{12} deficiency require lifelong vitamin therapy. Cyanocobalamin and hydroxocobalamin are the two therapeutic forms of vitamin B_{12}. Hydroxocobalamin is preferred by some physicians because it has a longer half-life. Cyanocobalamin is less expensive and converts to the physiologic form.

Vitamin B_{12} can be administered orally to patients with dietary vitamin deficiency or to those who cannot tolerate parenteral treatment. Several studies have shown that oral vitamin therapy can be as effective and efficient as parenteral therapy in conducting hematologic and neurologic remissions and in maintaining normal serum B_{12}.[6,20,43] In patients with pernicious anemia, about 1% of the oral dose is absorbed.[1,43] Therefore, high doses of oral vitamin (1000 to 2000 µg/day) is sufficient to replace the parenteral therapy. The efficiency of the treatment should be checked by occasional measurement of serum B_{12} in patients undergoing the oral therapy.[1,43]

Vitamin B_{12} is injected intramuscularly or subcutaneously. Although the treatment protocol varies, the initial dose administered is higher in order to saturate the body storage. Vitamin B_{12} may be given as 100 to 1000 µg/day over a 1- to 2-week period monitored by daily reticulocyte counts. If a positive response is achieved, the intervals can be extended to every other day and later by once every 3 to 4 days until hematologic values are normalized. The maintenance therapy is administered in lower doses with longer intervals (every 1 to 2 months) for life.[1]

Folic Acid Deficiency

The recommended therapeutic dose for folate deficiency is 1 to 5 mg/day for 2 to 3 weeks.[1,6] Folic acid vitamin is water soluble and is given orally. Lifelong therapy is not required because it is usually possible to treat folate deficiency in a short period of time.[1,24] Folic acid may be given along with vitamin B_{12} when both vitamins are deficient or in therapeutic trial when the exact cause of megaloblastic anemia is not known. In this case, folate therapy will correct the hematologic abnormalities in vitamin B_{12} patients, but the neurologic manifestations will progress.

Folic acid given as prophylaxis (0.25 to 0.5 mg/day) is recommended during pregnancy and dialysis and may be required in patients with hemolytic anemia and in patients who are on antifolate drugs.[1,12,30,31] Folic acid can be injected to hospitalized patients and those who cannot take the medication by mouth.

➤ RESPONSE TO THERAPY

The initial sign of a positive response to therapy is an increase in the reticulocyte count. The number of circulatory reticulocytes increases 2 to 3 days after therapy, with a peak at about 5 to 8 days.[1,6] The reticulocyte count may increase to 50% to 70% initially.[9] The megaloblastic morphology of the bone marrow disappears within the first 24 to 48 hours after therapy. The hematocrit rises in about 5 to 7 days after therapy, reaching normal levels in 4 to 8 weeks. Giant metamyelocytes and hypersegmented neutrophils disappear within 2 weeks. The entire therapeutic response process may take only 3 to 6 weeks, depending on the severity of the disease.[9,11]

➤ VITAMIN-INDEPENDENT MEGALOBLASTIC CHANGES

This group of disorders is characterized by the presence of megaloblastic changes in the bone marrow and in the peripheral blood that are refractory to vitamin B$_{12}$ and folic acid treatments. The megaloblastic changes in this group of patients may occur because of an inherited or acquired predisposition, or they may be drug induced (Table 7–6).

Inherited

Orotic aciduria is a rare inherited disorder of pyrimidine metabolism characterized by increased excretion of orotic acid in the urine. Lesch-Nyhan syndrome is an X-linked disorder of purine metabolism. Megaloblastic changes are also noted in inherited dihydrofolate reductase deficiency, a disorder of folate metabolism and methyl tetrahydrofolate transferase. Inherited disorders of transcobalamin II deficiency or abnormal transcobalamin II molecule, and congenital IF deficiency are associated with megaloblastic anemia. In congenital dyserythropoiesis, the megaloblastic changes are limited only to erythrocyte precursors of the bone marrow and red cells in the peripheral smear. White blood cells and platelets are normal.[9] About 11 different inherited disorders are associated with methylmalonic aciduria, homocysteinuria, or both. In these disorders, pancytopenia is present with or without megaloblastic pictures.[6]

> **Table 7-6**
VITAMIN-INDEPENDENT MEGALOBLASTIC ANEMIAS

Inherited

Orotic aciduria

Lesch-Nyhan syndrome

Dihydrofolate reductase deficiency

Methyl tetrahydrofolate transferase deficiency

Transcobalamin deficiency

Abnormal cobalamin molecule

Congenital IF deficiency

Methylmalonic aciduria

Homocysteinuria

Congenital dyserythropoiesis

Acquired

Myelodysplastic syndrome

Erythroleukemia

Drugs

Folate antagonist (methotrexate)

Purine or pyrimidine antagonists (6-mercaptopurine, cytosine arabinoside, and hydroxyurea)

Nitrous oxide

Azidothymidine (AZT)

Others

Toxic Materials

Arsenic

Chlordane

Others

Acquired

Megaloblastic changes may be secondary to hematologic disorders such as myelodysplastic syndromes and erythroleukemia. The exact mechanism responsible for the defects in the hematologic disorders is not known.[24]

Drug and Toxin Induced

A wide variety of drugs with differing modes of action are associated with megaloblastic anemia. Methotrexate is an example of a folate antagonist drug. Drugs such as 6-mercaptopurine, cytosine arabinose, and hydroxyurea interfere with purine or pyrimidine metabolism. Nitrous oxide (N$_2$O), an anesthetic gas, inactivates vitamin B$_{12}$.[1,6,9,24] Azidothymidine (AZT) is associated with megaloblastic changes. Exposure to toxic materials such as arsenic and chlordane can also cause megaloblastic anemia.[9]

> ## MACROCYTIC NONMEGALOBLASTIC ANEMIAS

Macrocytic anemias may be megaloblastic or nonmegaloblastic. Differentiation between the two is important. In macrocytic, normoblastic anemias, the MCV is more than 100 fL, but not as high as in megaloblastic anemias (where the MCV is more than 110 fL). The red cells on the peripheral blood smear appear large and round, but not oval. The neutrophils are not hypersegmented. The bone marrow is normocellular or hypercellular with erythroid hyperplasia. The red cell precursors in the marrow are normoblastic and not megaloblastic. The mechanism responsible for the macrocytic morphology may be associated with an increase in both red cell membrane cholesterol and phospholipid. Increased lipid deposition onto the red cell membrane and altered maturation time of the red cell precursors are among the possible causes.[10,24]

Causes of Macrocytic Nonmegaloblastic Anemias

The most common causes of macrocytic anemia are chronic liver disease and alcoholism. In 40% to 96% of alcoholics, macrocytosis is present in the absence of anemia, and in this case, alcohol has a direct toxic effect on the red cells rather than causing folate deficiency. The finding of macrocytosis is a valuable screening test for early detection of alcoholism.[6,12] Megaloblastic changes have been reported in 20% to 40% of alcoholics.[6,10] Liver function tests such as serum LDH and bilirubin are helpful in the diagnosis. Although 50% of patients with liver disease have macrocytic anemia, normocytic and microcytic anemias have also been reported.[10]

Macrocytic anemia with an elevated reticulocyte count is associated with hemolytic anemia or acute blood loss. Macrocytic anemia may also be associated with aplastic anemia, chronic myeloproliferative disorders, and sideroblastic anemia. In sideroblastic anemia, a dimorphic red cell population may be observed (see Fig. 6–12). Bone marrow examination is often required for differential diagnosis.

Macrocytosis has also been reported in patients taking immunosuppressive drugs as well as arsenic and chlordane intoxication. Causes of macrocytic nonmegaloblastic anemia are summarized in Table 7–7.

> **Table 7-7**
CAUSES OF MACROCYTIC NONMEGALOBLASTIC ANEMIAS

Chronic liver disease

Alcoholism

Acute hemorrhage

Hypothyroidism

Hematologic disorders

  Hemolytic anemia

  Aplastic anemia

  Chronic myeloproliferative disorders

Immunosuppressive drugs

Arsenic and chlordane intoxication

> ## CASE STUDY

A 50-year-old woman visited her physician because she had experienced weakness, fatigue, and shortness of breath for the past few months. Physical examination revealed a tall, slender woman with "lemon-yellow skin" and a smooth, red tongue. No hepatosplenomegaly was noted. She had experienced a loss of vibratory sense and had some problem with gait coordination. Her family history and her past medical history were unremarkable. The patient was not taking any medications.

A complete blood count with WBC differential was ordered and the results were as follows: WBC = 7.4 × 10^9/L (4.4 to 11); RBC = 2.2 × 10^{12}/L (4.1 to 5.1); Hgb = 8.5 g/dL (12.3 to 15.3); Hct = 25% (36 to 45); MCV = 114 fL (87 to 98); MCHC = 34% (32 to 36); RDW = 15.2% (11.5 to 14.5); Platelet = 170 × 10^9/L (150 to 400). Differential: 67% segmented neutrophils (5% hypersegmented); 25% lymphocytes; 5% monocytes; 3% eosinophils. RBC morphology: macrocytic with few macro-ovalocytes and few schistocytes. RBC inclusions: few Howell-Jolly bodies. Reticulocytes = 0.2% (0.5 to 1.5).

Chemistry test results were as follows: total bilirubin = 4.0 mg/dL (0.2 to 1.0); indirect bilirubin = 2.9 mg/dL (0.2 to 0.8); serum LDH = 720 U/L (100 to 190); serum iron = 220 μg/dL (50 to 170); TIBC = 215 μg/dL (250 to 450); serum B_{12} = 50 pg/dL (100 to 700); red cell folate = 200 ng/mL (130 to 628).

Questions
1. These laboratory findings are representative of what type of anemia?
2. How would you classify this anemia based on the RBC indices?
3. What does the decreased reticulocyte count represent?
4. What is the cause of this anemia?
5. What test is used to evaluate vitamin B_{12} malabsorption?

Comments

The diagnosis of megaloblastic anemia was made based on the patient's physical examination and the highlights of the laboratory results. Physical findings reveal that the patient had the signs and symptoms of anemia, with the "lemon-yellow skin" caused by anemia and jaundice. The low hemoglobin and hematocrit levels in combination with an elevated MCV and normal MCHC are suggestive of macrocytic, normochromic anemia, a characteristic of megaloblastic anemia. The macro-ovalocytes and hypersegmented neutrophils present on the peripheral smear are striking features of megaloblastic anemia. Howell-Jolly bodies are the red cell inclusions commonly seen in this type of anemia. The low reticulocyte value is indicative of ineffective erythropoiesis. The white blood cell (WBC) and platelet counts are normal in this patient, as is expected in early stages of megaloblastic anemia.

The elevated bilirubin, serum LDH, and serum iron levels can all be attributed to red cell hemolysis. In megaloblastic anemia, the red cells are fragile and have a shortened life span, and are thus prematurely destroyed in the bone marrow and in the peripheral blood.

The most common causes of megaloblastic anemia are vitamin B_{12} and folate deficiencies. In this patient, the serum B_{12} level was decreased, whereas the red cell folate level was normal. These findings indicate that B_{12} deficiency was the probable cause for the megaloblastic anemia. The patient was eating a balanced diet and had no past medical history. Vitamin B_{12} deficiency because of malabsorption was suspected, and a two-part Schilling test was ordered to evaluate the cause of B_{12} malabsorption. In part I, the patient excreted 2% labeled B_{12} in her 24-hour urine, and in part II, she excreted 8%. This result supported the diagnosis of pernicious anemia.

The initial doses of hydroxocobalamin were administered intramuscularly for several weeks, followed by maintenance doses. After 2 months of therapy, the patient had completely recovered. Her hemoglobin and hematocrit had returned to normal and her abnormal blood cell morphologies had disappeared. The patient was advised to continue the vitamin B_{12} therapy to prevent relapse of the symptoms, because lack of IF in patients with pernicious anemia prevents absorption of dietary B_{12}.

QUESTIONS

1. The pathophysiology of megaloblastic anemia is:
    a. Defective RNA synthesis and abnormal cytoplasm maturation
    b. Defective DNA synthesis and abnormal nuclear maturation
    c. Defective RNA synthesis and abnormal nuclear maturation
    d. Defective DNA synthesis and abnormal cytoplasm maturation

2. All of the following laboratory findings coincide with megaloblastic anemia except:
   a. Increased serum bilirubin
   b. Increased serum iron
   c. Decreased muramidase
   d. Increased LDH-1

3. Megaloblastic anemia is associated with:
   a. Ineffective erythropoiesis and increased reticulocytes
   b. Ineffective erythropoiesis and decreased reticulocytes
   c. Ineffective erythropoiesis and decreased LDH
   d. Ineffective erythropoiesis and decreased erythropoietin

4. According to the morphological classification of anemias, megaloblastic anemia is a:
   a. Macrocytic, hypochromic anemia
   b. Macrocytic, hyperchromic anemia
   c. Macrocytic, normochromic anemia
   d. Normocytic, normochromic anemia

5. Which of the following are not seen on the peripheral smear of a patient with megaloblastic anemia?
   a. Macro-ovalocytes
   b. Hypersegmented neutrophils
   c. Hyposegmented neutrophils
   d. Howell-Jolly bodies

6. Which of the following are the characteristic findings of the bone marrow in a patient with megaloblastic anemia?
   a. Hypocellular with low M:E ratio
   b. Hypercellular with high M:E ratio
   c. Hypocellular with high M:E ratio
   d. Hypercellular with low M:E ratio

7. The glycoprotein necessary for absorption of vitamin B_{12} is:
   a. Albumin
   b. Transcobalamin II
   c. Haptoglobin
   d. Intrinsic factor

8. All of the following are clinical manifestations of both B_{12} deficiency and folate deficiency except:
   a. Anemia and jaundice
   b. Weakness and shortness of breath
   c. Thrombocytopenia and bleeding
   d. Hemoglobinuria

9. Which of the following Schilling test results corresponds to a diagnosis of pernicious anemia?
   a. Part I abnormal, part II not corrected
   b. Part I abnormal, part II corrected
   c. Part I and part II abnormal
   d. Part I normal, part II corrected

10. Which of the following is not a cause of vitamin B_{12} deficiency?
   a. Atrophic gastritis
   b. Total gastrectomy
   c. Blind loop syndrome
   d. Chronic glossitis

SUMMARY CHART

➤ Megaloblastic anemia is a macrocytic anemia characterized by defective nuclear maturation caused by impairment of DNA synthesis.
➤ Megaloblastic anemia is associated with ineffective erythropoiesis, ineffective granulopoiesis, and ineffective thrombopoiesis.
➤ The bone marrow of patients with megaloblastic anemia is hypercellular with a low M:E ratio (1:1 to 1:3), high number of megaloblasts, and giant bands and metamyelocytes.
➤ The peripheral blood is characterized by pancytopenia, macrocytes, macro-ovalocytes, and hypersegmented neutrophils.
➤ Other biochemical changes are increased levels of lactate dehydrogenase (LDH), indirect bilirubin, serum iron and ferritin, and erythropoietin.
➤ The major causes for megaloblastic anemias are vitamin B_{12} deficiency, folic acid deficiency, or both.
➤ Vitamin B_{12} and folic acid in the form of cofactors are essential for two key reactions in the body.
➤ Intrinsic factor enhances vitamin B_{12} absorption through the receptors present on the brush borders of the ileum.
➤ Transcobalamin II transfers vitamin B_{12} to the tissues.
➤ The main cause of vitamin B_{12} deficiency is pernicious anemia.
➤ Pernicious anemia is the lack of intrinsic factor.
➤ Clinical manifestations that are often associated with vitamin B_{12} deficiency are anemia, fever, glossitis, and neurologic symptoms.
➤ Other causes of vitamin B_{12} deficiency are dietary malabsorption secondary to diseases and drugs.
➤ The main cause of folic acid deficiency is a poor diet.
➤ Other causes of folic acid deficiency are malabsorption, increased requirement, and drugs.
➤ Clinical manifestations associated with folic acid deficiency are similar to those in vitamin B_{12} deficiency, with neuropathies not being the prominent features.
➤ Laboratory tests used for the differential diagnosis of vitamin B_{12} and folate deficiencies are serum B_{12}, and serum and red cell folate.
➤ Other laboratory tests that may be useful are gastric achlorhydria, antibodies to intrinsic factor, Schilling test, serum and urine methylmalonic acid serum and urine homocysteine, and deoxyuridine suppression test.

➤ Vitamin B$_{12}$ deficiency can be treated with cyanocobalamin or hydroxocobalamin, and folate deficiency can be treated with folic acid supplementation.
➤ The initial response to therapy is increased reticulocyte counts.
➤ Vitamin-independent megaloblastic anemias can be inherited or acquired.
➤ Macrocytic nonmegaloblastic anemias are characterized by a high MCV, macrocytes in the peripheral blood, and normocellular or hypercellular bone marrow with erythroid hyperplasia.
➤ The most common causes of macrocytic anemia are liver disease and alcoholism.

References

1. Williams, WJ, et al: Hematology, ed 5. McGraw-Hill, New York, 1995, pp 381–390, 471–484.
2. Wickramasinghe, SN, and Fida, S: Bone marrow cells from vitamin B$_{12}$ and folate deficient patients misincorporate uracil into DNA. Blood 83:1656, 1994.
3. Jandl, JH: Blood, Text Book of Hematology, ed 2. Little, Brown, Boston, 1996, p 254.
4. Koury, MJ, et al: Apoptosis of late-erythroblasts in megaloblastic anemia: Association with DNA damage and macrocyte production. Blood 89:4617, 1997.
5. Ingram, CF, et al: Evaluation of DNA analysis for evidence of apoptosis in megaloblastic anemia. Br J Haematol 96:576, 1997.
6. Lee, GR, et al: Wintrobe's Clinical Hematology, ed 10, vol 1. Lea & Febiger, Philadelphia, 1999, pp 942–959, 965–977.
7. Nathan, DG, and Oski, AF: Hematology of Infancy and Childhood, ed 5, vol 1. WB Saunders, Philadelphia, 1998, pp 388–396.
8. Heckner, F, et al: Practical Microscopic Hematology, ed 4. Lea & Febiger, Philadelphia, 1994, pp 47, 50–53.
9. Bick, RL: Hematology, Clinical and Laboratory Practice, vol 1. CV Mosby, St. Louis, 1993, p 460.
10. McKenzie, SB: Text Book of Hematology, ed 2, Williams & Wilkins, Baltimore, 1998, pp 184–196.
11. Babior, BM, and Stossel, TP: Hematology, A Pathophysiological Approach, ed 3. Churchill Livingstone, New York, 1994, p 87.
12. Spivak, JL, and Eichner, ER: The Fundamentals of Clinical Hematology, ed 3. Johns Hopkins University Press, Baltimore, 1993, p 31.
13. Simmons, A: Hematology, A Combined Theoretical and Technical Approach, ed 2, Butterworth-Heinemann, Boston, 1997, p 48.
14. Herbert, V: Staging vitamin B$_{12}$ (cobalamin) status in vegetarians. Am J Nutr 59:1214S, 1994.
15. Graham, SM, et al: Long-term neurologic consequences of nutritional vitamin B$_{12}$ deficiency in infants. J Pediatr 1:710, 1992.
16. Pippard, MJ: Megaloblastic anemia: Geography and diagnosis. Lancet 344:7, 1994.
17. Kozyraki, R, et al: The human intrinsic factor-vitamin B$_{12}$ receptor, cubilin: Molecular characterization and chromosomal mapping of the gene 10p within the autosomal recessive megaloblastic anemia (MGA1) region. Blood 91:3593, 1998.
18. Van Den Berg, H: Vitamin B$_{12}$. Int J Vitam Nutr Res 63:283, 1993.
19. Yamada, K, et al: A case of subacute combined degeneration: MRI finding. Neuroradiology 40:398, 1998.
20. Stabler, SR: Vitamin B$_{12}$ deficiency in older people: Improving diagnosis and preventing disability. JAGS 46:1317, 1998.
21. Hoggarth, K: Macrocytic anemia. Practitioner 237:331, 1993.
22. Hemmer, B, et al: Subacute combined degeneration: Clinical, electrophysiological, and magnetic resonance imaging findings. J Neurol Neurosurg Psychiatry 65:822, 1998.
23. Metz, J: Pathogenesis of cobalamin neuropathy: Deficiency of nervous system s-adenosylmethionin. Nutr Rev 51:12, 1993.
24. Hoffbrand, AV, and Pettit, JE: Essential Haematology, ed 3. Blackwell Scientific, Oxford, 1993, p 64.
25. Alpert, JE, Fava, M: Nutrition and depression: The role of folate. Nutr Rev 55:145, 1997.
26. Ramaekers, VTh, et al: Central pontine myelolysis associated with acquired folate depletion. Neuropediatrics 28:126, 1997.
27. Hibbard, BM: Folate and fetal development. Br J Obstet Gynaecol 100:307, 1993.
28. Wald, NJ, and Bower, C: Folic acid, pernicious anemia, and prevention of neural tube defects. Lancet 343:307, 1994.
29. Lockith, G: Handbook of Diagnostic Biochemistry and Hematology in Normal Pregnancy. CRC Press, Ann Arbor, 1993, p 125.
30. Morgan, SL: Folic acid supplementation prevents deficient blood folate levels and hyperhomocysteinemia during longterm, low dose methotrexate therapy for rheumatoid arthritis: Implications for cardiovascular disease prevention. J Rheumatol 25:441, 1998.
31. Wevers, RA, et al: Folate deficiency in cerebrospinal fluid associated with a defect in folate binding protein in the central nervous system. J Neurol Neurosurg Psychiatry 57:223, 1994.
32. Crellin, R, et al: Folate and psychiatric disorders, clinical potential. Drugs 45:624, 1993.
33. Skerritt, UM: A prevalence study of folate deficiency in a psychiatric inpatient population. Acta Psychiatr Scan 97:228, 1998.
34. Ballas, SK, and Saidi, P: Thrombosis, megaloblastic anemia, and sickle cell disease: A unified hypothesis. Br J Haematol 96:872, 1997.
35. Koury, MJ: Folate deficiency delays the onset but increases the incidence of leukemia in friend virus-infected mice. Blood 90:4054, 1997.
36. Joosten, E, et al: Is metabolic evidence for vitamin B-12 and folate deficiency more frequent in elderly patients with Alzheimer's disease? J Gerontol Med Sci 52A:M76, 1997.
37. Ubbnik, JB, et al: Vitamin B12, vitamin B6, and folate nutritional status in men with hyperhomocysteinemia. Am J Clin Nutr 57:47, 1993.
38. Savage, DG, et al: Sensitivity of serum methylmalonic acid and total homocysteine determinations for diagnosing cobalamin and folate deficiencies. Am J Med 96:239, 1994.
39. Joostan, E, et al: Metabolic evidence that deficiencies of vitamin B12 (cobalamin), folate, and vitamin B6 occur commonly in elderly people. Am J Clin Nutr 58:468, 1993.
40. Rees, MM, and Rodgers, GM: Homocysteinemia: Association of a metabolic disorder with vascular disease and thrombosis. Throm Res 71:337, 1993.
41. Menachem, Y, et al: Cobalamin deficiency and infertility. Am J Hematol 469:152, 1994.
42. Miller, A: Food-bound B$_{12}$ absorption and serum total homocysteine in patients with low serum B$_{12}$ levels. Am J Hematol 59:42, 1998.
43. Kuzminski, AM: Effective treatment of cobalamin deficiency with oral cobalamin. Blood 92:1191, 1998.

See the Bibliography for this chapter at the back of the book.

8 Aplastic Anemia (Including Pure Red Cell Aplasia and Congenital Dyserythropoietic Anemia)

SHERRIE L. PERKINS, MD, PHD

OBJECTIVES

At the end of this chapter the learner should be able to:

1. Define aplastic anemia.

2. Understand the etiologic subclassification of aplastic anemia.

3. List four causes of acquired aplastic anemia and identify the most common cause.

4. Name the most common congenital disorder associated with the development of aplastic anemia.

5. Describe the clinical and laboratory features associated with aplastic anemia.

6. Describe the bone marrow findings in aplastic anemia.

7. List the treatment modalities used in aplastic anemia and identify the best therapy for younger patients.

8. List clinical and laboratory features associated with this pure red cell aplasia.

9. Describe the common characteristics seen in congenital dyserythropoietic anemias (CDAs).

➤ DEFINITION

Aplastic anemia is a disorder (or group of disorders) characterized by cellular depletion and fatty replacement of the bone marrow. The concomitant decreases in hematopoietic progenitors lead to diminished production of erythrocytes, leukocytes, and platelets and development of peripheral blood cytopenias or pancytopenia. The loss of functional bone marrow occurs following a variety of bone marrow insults that include drugs, chemicals, irradiation, infections, and immune dysfunction. Though the inciting mechanisms vary, all lead to the loss of bone marrow precursor cells or damage of the bone marrow microenvironment required to sustain bone marrow cell growth and differentiation. Thus, the hematopoietic progenitor cells that give rise to the various peripheral blood elements lose their ability to self-renew and produce progeny, leading to a loss of bone marrow cellular mass and bone marrow failure. Clinical criteria that have been used to define aplastic anemia include (1) marrow of less than 25% normal cellularity; and (2) at least two blood cytopenias defined as neutrophil count less than 500/μL or platelets less than 20,000/μL or anemia with corrected reticulocyte count of less than 1%.[1]

➤ PATHOGENESIS

The basic defect in aplastic anemia is a failure of blood cell production by the bone marrow, involving erythrocytes, leukocytes, and platelets. Blood cell production within the bone marrow is dependent on the growth, differentiation, and self-renewal of a common, pluripotential stem cell

(CFU-S).[2] To proliferate and differentiate into mature blood elements, the CFU-S responds to cytokines and other growth factors produced in the bone marrow microenvironment.[3] Thus, bone marrow failure may develop as a consequence of decreased hematopoietic stem cells resulting from decreased self-renewal or cellular destruction. Alternatively, a disruption of the bone microenvironment, leading to decreased signal for cellular proliferation and differentiation, could lead to bone marrow aplasia (Fig. 8–1).

Most studies to date show decreases in bone marrow stem cells rather than a defective microenvironment to be the underlying defect in development in most cases of aplastic anemia.[1-4] Because the bone marrow is unable to respond to the developing peripheral blood cytopenias by increased hematopoietic activity, it has been classified as a refractory or aregenerative process. No clear-cut cause for the loss of blood cell production is applicable to all causes of aplastic anemia. Postulated mechanisms for the development of aplastic anemia include direct toxic effects on the bone marrow, immune-mediated destruction of the marrow, and congenital disorders. However, in most cases a clear-cut mechanism for the development of bone marrow failure is not known (Table 8–1).[1,4-6]

➤ ETIOLOGY

Clinically, it is useful to divide aplastic anemia into acquired or congenital (hereditary) types (Table 8–2).[1] The vast majority (more than 95%) of the cases are acquired. Of these cases, most (40% to 70%) are primary or idiopathic in nature, because no clear-cut etiologic agent can be identified. The remaining acquired cases of aplastic anemia are considered to be secondary, resulting from documentable exposure to chemicals, drugs, irradiation, or infection. In addition, some cases of aplastic anemia have been attributed to immune dysfunction, leading to immunologic attack on and ultimate "rejection" of the marrow. The antibodies against bone marrow cells may be induced by drugs, some infections or states of altered immunity, such as pregnancy or collagen vascular disorders. Hereditary cases of

aplastic anemia are extremely rare, with the most common group designated as Fanconi's anemia.[4-6]

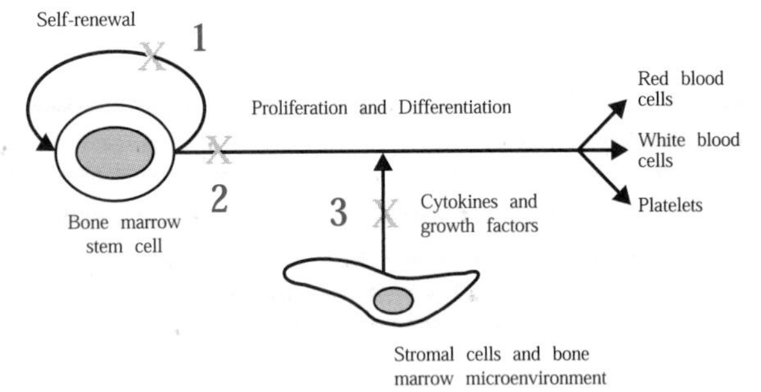

➤ ACQUIRED APLASTIC ANEMIA

Idiopathic or Primary

Aplastic anemia is most often thought to be idiopathic in nature, because no clear-cut cause of the bone marrow failure can be identified despite a careful search. Idiopathic aplastic anemia makes up about 40% to 70% of the cases of nonhereditary aplastic anemia seen in western populations.[1,4-6]

> **Table 8-1**
POSTULATED PATHOGENIC MECHANISMS IN DEVELOPMENT OF APLASTIC ANEMIA

Idiopathic or unknown
Direct bone marrow toxic effects
  Radiation
  Drugs (i.e., chemotherapy drugs, other drugs)
  Benzene
  Toxins or chemicals
  Starvation
  Some bone marrow infections
Immune-mediated bone marrow damage
  Drug-induced autoantibodies
  Autoimmune disorders
  Pregnancy
  Some bone marrow infections
Congenital bone marrow defects
  Fanconi's anemia
  Dyskeratosis congenita

> **Table 8-2**
ETIOLOGIES ASSOCIATED WITH DEVELOPMENT OF APLASTIC ANEMIA

Acquired (> 95%)
Idiopathic or primary (40%–70%)
Secondary
  Chemical agents
  Drugs
  Ionizing radiation
  Infections
  Miscellaneous causes
Congenital (Hereditary) (< 5%)
Fanconi's anemia
Dyskeratosis congenita

> **FIGURE 8–1** Schematic representation of possible defects in hematopoiesis that may give rise to aplastic anemia. It is postulated that decreased numbers of bone marrow stem cells and/or changes in the bone marrow microenvironment that alter cytokine levels, or both, may cause aplasia to develop. Most evidence points to decreased stem cells caused by the lack of self-replication (1) or direct destruction of stem cells (2), rather than changes in the bone marrow microenvironment (3), as pathogenetic mechanisms for development of aplastic anemia.

Secondary Causes

A wide variety of chemical, physical, and infectious agents have been associated with the development of aplastic anemia (Table 8–3). Usually these agents are divided into those that regularly produce bone marrow aplasia upon sufficient exposure (e.g., benzene, irradiation, and chemotherapeutic agents) and those for which development of aplasia is considered a rare or idiosyncratic event (e.g., chloramphenicol, phenylbutazone) (Table 8–4).[4–6]

Chemical Agents

Some of the chemical agents linked with bone marrow failure or aplastic anemia include benzene, trinitrotoluene, arsenic, insecticides, and weed killers. Many of these compounds have a benzene ring as part of their chemical structure. Modification of the benzene ring moiety with the nitroso or nitro group is highly associated with development of aplastic anemia.[7,8]

Benzene has been known to cause varying degrees of bone marrow failure for nearly 100 years, since the original description by Santesson of four cases of fatal aplastic anemia occurring in workers in a bicycle tire factory. Benzene has a variety of industrial applications, including use as a solvent for rubber, fats, and alkaloids, and in the manufacture of drugs, dyes, and explosives. Because most benzene compounds are volatile, they are easily absorbed by inhalation.[8]

Benzene may induce a wide spectrum of bone marrow suppression, ranging from mild anemia or thrombocytopenia to fatal pancytopenia. There is wide diversity in individual

> **➤ Table 8-3**
> ## CAUSES OF SECONDARY ACQUIRED APLASTIC ANEMIA

Chemical agents

   Benzene

   Insecticides

   Weed killers

Drugs

   Chloramphenicol

   Phenylbutazone

   Anticonvulsants

   Sulfonamides

   Gold

   Chemotherapeutic agents

Ionizing radiation

Infections

   Hepatitis

   Epstein-Barr virus

   Cytomegalovirus

Miscellaneous causes

   Pregnancy

   Malnutrition

   Immunologic dysfunction

susceptibility to benzene compounds, with bone marrow suppression occurring shortly after initial exposure in some people, or as long as 10 years after exposure in others. Often bone marrow suppression is reversible after discontinuation of benzene exposure.[9] It is thought that benzene acts to inhibit synthesis of deoxyribonucleic acid (DNA) and ribonucleic acid (RNA), inhibiting cellular proliferation and differentiation of bone marrow cells.[10,11] Benzene has also been associated with accumulation of chromosomal abnormalities and development of acute leukemia in some patients.[12]

Drugs

A wide variety of drugs have been associated with development of aplastic anemia, often the result of a nonpredictable or idiosyncratic reaction to a drug.[1,4–6,13] As discussed previously, this may be a result of direct toxicity or development of an abnormal immune reaction whereby antibodies against a drug cross-react with bone marrow cells. The antibiotic chloramphenicol and the anti-inflammatory drug phenylbutazone are probably the best-documented examples of drugs causing aplastic anemia. The toxicity associated with these drugs is usually *not* related to the total dosage of the drug received, and drug-induced antibodies have only been identified in a few patients. Thus, the association between the drug and development of aplastic anemia is dependent on epidemiologic data and a temporal relationship to drug ingestion and development of bone marrow failure.[13] The mechanism of drug-induced bone marrow failure suppression is usually unknown, and it is impossible to identify which patients will react adversely to a drug. Luckily, such idiosyncratic reactions to drugs are relatively rare. It is estimated that 1 person in 20,000 to 30,000 may have an idiosyncratic reaction to chloramphenicol, which is about 10 times the incidence of developing aplastic anemia for the general population not taking chloramphenicol.[14]

Chloramphenicol has been shown to cause two types of bone marrow effects.[15] The most common reaction is a reversible bone marrow suppression that occurs while the patient is receiving the drug and is associated with vacuolization of bone marrow precursor cells (Fig. 8–2; see also Color Plate 96) and increased serum iron levels. The second reaction seen is development of an irreversible aplastic anemia that occurs weeks to months after drug exposure. This more severe reaction is not predictable by the dose, duration, or route of administration of the drug. Because of the strong association with development of aplastic anemia, chloramphenicol use has decreased, and the drug is administered only for specific indications when no other reasonable alternative exists.[14,15]

A wide variety of other drugs have been implicated as direct suppressors of hematopoiesis and are occasionally associated with development of bone marrow aplasia. The incidence and predictability of bone marrow suppression vary with the type of drug (Table 8–4). For example, chemotherapeutic agents are well known to regularly cause bone marrow hypoplasia in a dose-related manner, whereas other drugs (antibiotics, anticonvulsants, analgesics) are much less predictable. Knowledge of potential bone marrow side effects must be kept in mind when using these drugs and appropriate monitoring of peripheral blood indices performed. Often, drug-induced bone marrow hypoplasia is fully reversible on removal of the drug, although some patients may develop irreversible damage.[4,5,13]

➤ **Table 8-4**
AGENTS ASSOCIATED WITH APLASTIC ANEMIA

Agents That Regularly Produce Bone Marrow Hypoplasia with Sufficient Doses

Ionizing radiation

Benzene and benzene derivatives

Chemotherapeutic agents (e.g., busulfan, vincristine)

Agents That Produce Bone Marrow Hypoplasia in an Idiosyncratic Manner

TYPE OF DRUG	RELATIVELY FREQUENT	RARE
Antimicrobials	Chloramphenicol	Streptomycin
	Penicillin, Tetracyline	Amphotericin B
		Sulfonamides
Anticonvulsants	Methylphenylethylhydantoin	Methylphenylhydantoin
	Trimethadione	Diphenylhydantoin
		Primidone
Analgesics	Phenylbutazone	Aspirin
		Tapazole
Hypoglycemic agents		Tolbutamide
		Chlorpropamide
Insecticides		Chlorophenothane
		Parathion
Miscellaneous		Colchine
		Acetazolamide
		Hair dyes

Ionizing Radiation

It is well known that ionizing radiation has an acute destructive effect on the rapidly dividing cells of the bone marrow, which is predictable based on the radiation dosage.[16] High doses of radiation, in the range of 300 to 500 rads, lead to complete loss of hematopoietic cells that is irreversible and lethal. Lesser doses lead to reversible anemia, leukopenia, and thrombocytopenia with full recovery of counts in 4 to 6 weeks. Hematopoietic cells are most susceptible to penetrating forms of radiation, such as those found in gamma rays and x-rays. However, chronic ingestion of lower-energy radiation sources (such as was seen in watch dial painters who ingested radium by wetting their brushes in their mouths and inhaling radium dust) may also cause bone marrow effects.[17]

Ionizing radiation affects bone marrow and other rapidly proliferating cells by disrupting chemical bonds, leading to the formation of free radicals and other biologically active compounds. These interact with DNA to cause breaks or cross-linking of the DNA strands, leading to cellular death or genetic abnormalities.[18]

In addition to the immediate dose-dependent effects of irradiation on hematopoietic cells, there may also be delayed or long-term effects that are less predictable. Aplastic anemia may occur months to years after radiation exposure, although development of bone marrow dysplasia and acute leukemias is more common.[19]

Infections

Many infections have suppressive effects on the bone marrow. Acute, self-limited infections may suppress bone marrow activity for 10 to 14 days with minor effects on the peripheral blood counts. Chronic infections may have more severe effects on hematopoiesis. Several viral infections, including hepatitis,[20] Epstein-Barr virus,[21,22] and cytomegalovirus,[22,23] have been associated with the development of aplastic anemia. Of these, hepatitis from an uncharacterized hepatitis virus (i.e., non–A, non–B, non–C type) has the strongest association with the development of a refractory aplastic anemia.[20] Although the mechanism whereby viruses

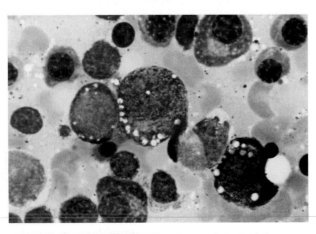

➤ **FIGURE 8–2** Vacuolization of bone marrow hematopoietic precursor cells indicating toxicity in a patient being treated with chloramphenicol (Wright-Giemsa stain, ×1000 magnification).

cause aplastic anemia is unknown, it has been suggested that the virus may directly infect the hematopoietic stem cell, or induce an autoimmune reaction against bone marrow.[1,4,5] Other systemic infections, such as miliary tuberculosis,[24] have also been associated with the development of aplastic anemia or bone marrow dysfunction.

Miscellaneous Causes

Aplastic anemia has been associated with a number of conditions of altered immunity, including eosinophilic fasciitis,[25] pregnancy,[26] and graft-versus-host disease.[27] This suggests that autoimmune targeting of the hematopoietic stem cell may provide a mechanism for the development of the disease. Other cases of aplastic anemia have been associated with malnutrition, such as in cases of anorexia nervosa[28] or pancreatic insufficiency (Schwachman-Diamond syndrome).[29] These are associated with stem cell necrosis and degenerative changes within the bone marrow stromal cells, termed gelatinous transformation.

➤ CONGENITAL APLASTIC ANEMIA

Fanconi's Anemia

Congenital aplastic anemia is characterized by hematologic abnormalities that have been present since birth, a familial occurrence, and the frequent presence of associated congenital defects. Several identifiable clinical entities are known, of which the best described is Fanconi's anemia.[30] Over 400 cases have been reported in the literature and show variable clinical features and an autosomal recessive inheritance pattern. Often these patients have a variety of associated physical abnormalities, including one or more of the following: skeletal defects (usually aplasia or hypoplasia of the thumb), cutaneous hyperpigmentation, renal abnormalities, microcephaly, mental retardation, and poor growth. Patients develop pancytopenia that progresses with age and is usually symptomatic within 5 to 10 years after birth. Anemia (usually macrocytic or normochromic and normocytic) and thrombocytopenia usually precede development of leukopenia. There may be increased expression of i antigen on red cells, increased fetal hemoglobin levels, and elevated erythropoietin levels, suggesting a stress erythropoiesis pattern. The bone marrow may be originally normocellular or hypercellular, but over time hypoplasia develops.[30,31]

Fanconi's anemia is characterized by a number of chromosomal abnormalities, as noted on cytogenetic analysis, and special studies show a high number of chromosomal breakages and defective DNA repair. It is therefore not surprising that these patients may also have an increased incidence of acute myelogenous leukemia and other malignancies, leading to characterization as a genetic cancer syndrome.[30,31] Molecular analysis of patients with Fanconi's anemia has shown a diverse range of mutations. Several Fanconi's anemia–associated genes have been cloned, but none have homology to known hematopoietic genes. Some reports have suggested mutational defects in apoptosis or control of mitosis, but further characterization is needed.[31,32]

Untreated, patients with Fanconi's anemia usually die from infections or hemorrhage secondary to blood cytopenias. Some patients respond to cytokine or corticosteroid therapy. Currently, most patients are treated with allogeneic or cord blood bone marrow transplantation, although chemotherapy or irradiation conditioning regimens are associated with high levels of toxicity as a result of the DNA repair defects.[33] The development of other possible treatment approaches, such as gene therapy, may offer hope to these patients in the future.[31,32]

Other congenital causes of aplastic anemia are much more rarely seen than Fanconi's anemia. Dykeratosis congenita is an X-linked disorder in which approximately half of the affected patients develop aplastic anemia. It is not associated with chromosomal instability or development of acute leukemia.[34]

➤ CLINICAL MANIFESTATIONS OF APLASTIC ANEMIA

Aplastic anemia often presents as an insidious process, owing to the gradual decrease in bone marrow production of erythrocytes, leukocytes, and platelets. It may occur in all age groups. Most patients present with symptoms of progressive fatigue, dyspnea, and palpitations. However, bleeding or infection may also be seen. Physical examination may reveal pallor secondary to the anemia or evidence of thrombocytopenia, including petechiae, purpura, ecchymoses, and mucosal bleeding. Signs of infection, resulting from the decrease in leukocytes, are usually late manifestations of the disease. Other physical findings are minimal. Mild lymphadenopathy may be seen, but splenomegaly is unusual.[1] A detailed history of drug ingestion, toxic exposure, or infection is essential, as well as a family history of similar hematologic problems.

➤ LABORATORY EVALUATION

The laboratory studies to evaluate a patient with aplastic anemia are aimed at defining the degree of bone marrow dysfunction and at excluding other possible causes of cytopenias for which other therapies are available.[1,4,5] Laboratory evaluation usually involves a complete blood count (CBC) and reticulocyte count, peripheral smear, and bone marrow examination, as well as ancillary biochemical tests to evaluate renal and hepatic function, in addition to cultures or serologic tests looking for infectious agents (Table 8–5). The CBC shows pancytopenia of varying degrees, often with anemia being the most notable (Table 8–6). The hemoglobin concentration is usually 70 g/L or lower, and the anemia is usually normochromic and normocytic, although the cells may occasionally be macrocytic with moderate anisocytosis and poikilocytosis. The corrected reticulocyte count is characteristically low (less than 1%, or less than 25×10^9/L absolute reticulocyte count), reflecting the lack of bone marrow regenerative activity. The white cells, in particular the myeloid and monocytic cells, as well as platelets are decreased. Lymphocytes may be normal or decreased in number.

There is no specific morphological abnormality of the blood smear that is diagnostic of aplastic anemia. Examination of the blood smear confirms a normochromic, normocytic anemia with little or no evidence of regeneration such as polychromatophilic cells, basophilic stippling, or nucleated red cells seen. White cells usually show a relative lymphocytosis of up to 70% to 90%, because of decreased numbers of myeloid and monocytic cells. If the white cell count falls below 1.5×10^9/L, an absolute lymphopenia may also be present. Rarely, immature myeloid cells such as myelocytes and metameyelocytes are seen, but large numbers of

> ## Table 8-5
> ### LABORATORY EVALUATION FOR APLASTIC ANEMIA

Test	Purpose
CBC and differential	Establish severity of cytopenias
Peripheral blood examination	Exclude malignancy and other causes of cytopenias
Reticulocyte count	Establish decreased marrow regeneration
Bone marrow examination	Rule out leukemia, other causes of cytopenias (i.e., myelodysplasia, storage disorder, metastatic diseases, granulomas, fibrosis); establish hypoplasia of bone marrow
Biochemical testing	Liver function, renal function
Cultures	Document possible infection
Serologic testing	Document infection

these cells would call into doubt the diagnosis of aplastic anemia. Platelets are usually decreased, and it is unusual to find large or abnormal forms. When thrombocytopenia is present, bleeding time is prolonged and clot retraction poor.

Because of the lack of specific features in the CBC data and peripheral smear, a wide differential diagnosis for causes of pancytopenia must usually be considered (Table 8–7), and a bone marrow examination must be performed to arrive at a diagnosis. The bone marrow aspiration is often markedly hypocellular or is a dry tap (Fig. 8–3 and Color Plate 97). Small numbers of lymphocytes, plasma cells, and rare hematopoietic precursor cells are seen. The bone marrow biopsy specimen most commonly shows a very hypocellular bone marrow with marked reductions in the myeloid, erythroid, and megakaryocytic lineages. Compared to a normocellular bone marrow biopsy specimen (Fig. 8–4A and Color Plate 98), a markedly hypocellular bone marrow biopsy sample shows only residual stroma and fat (Fig. 8–4B). Scattered lymphocytes and plasma cells (Fig. 8–5 and Color Plate 99) or occasional lymphoid aggregates (Fig. 8–6 and Color Plate 100) may be seen. It should be noted that patients with aplastic anemia often have residual islands of normal marrow or focal areas of bone marrow hyperplasia adjacent to hypoplastic areas that may mimic the findings of myelodyspla-

> ## Table 8-7
> ### DIFFERENTIAL DIAGNOSIS FOR PANCYTOPENIA

Infiltration of the bone marrow

    Tumors—leukemias, lymphomas, metastatic disease

    Fibrosis—myelofibrosis

    Granulomatous infections—mycobacteria, fungi

    Other processes—sarcoid, storage disorders such as Gaucher's disease

Inhibition of hematopoiesis or ineffective hematopoiesis

    Myelodysplasia or paroxysmal nocturnal hemoglobinuria

    Vitamin B_{12} or folate deficiency

    Myelosuppressive drugs

Increased splenic activity (hypersplenism)

    Congestion

    Splenic infiltrative disorders—Gaucher's disease, Niemann-Pick disease

    Infections

    Primary hypersplenism

Aplastic anemia

sia or other processes (Fig. 8–7 and Color Plate 101). It is crucial to remember that there may be variations within each bone marrow biopsy specimen and between different biopsy sites in aplastic anemia, perhaps necessitating multiple sequential biopsies to establish the diagnosis.

> ## Table 8-6
> ### CHARACTERISTIC ABNORMAL CBC VALUES SEEN IN SEVERE APLASTIC ANEMIA

Red Blood Cells

Hematocrit ≤ 0.20–0.25 (L/L) or 20%–25%

Hemoglobin concentration ≤ 70 g/L

Absolute reticulocyte count ≤ 25 × 10⁹/L

Corrected reticulocyte count < 1%

White Blood Cells

Total leukocyte count ≤ 1.5 × 10⁹/L

Absolute neutrophil count ≤ 0.5 × 10⁹/L

Platelets

Platelet count ≤ 20–60 × 10⁹/L

> ## TREATMENT, CLINICAL COURSE, AND PROGNOSIS

Untreated aplastic anemia has an extremely poor prognosis, as the patients undergo progressive decreases in blood counts and subsequent lethal infection or bleeding.[1,35] However, some patients recover spontaneously. Until the early 1970s, patients with severe aplastic anemia were treated by supportive transfusions, possible treatment with androgens or

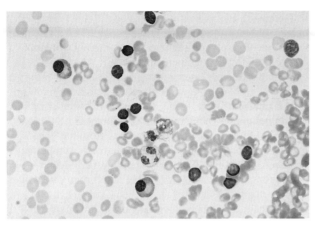

➤ **FIGURE 8–3** Hypocellular bone marrow aspirate containing primarily lymphocytes and plasma cells, reflecting bone marrow aplasia (Wright-Giemsa stain, ×500 magnification).

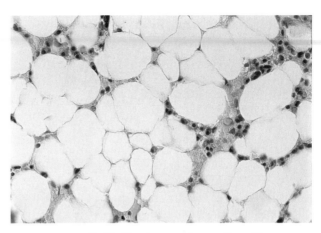

➤ **FIGURE 8–5** Residual lymphocytes, plasma cells, and bone marrow stroma with marked decrease in hematopoietic cells in a bone marrow biopsy specimen from a patient with aplastic anemia (H & E stain, ×200 magnification).

anabolic steroids to stimulate hematopoiesis, and an extensive search for the possible etiologic agent to prevent further exposure. Even so, the course was usually progressive, with a 5-year mortality rate of about 70% and only 10% of patients fully recovering.[36]

Currently, the treatment of choice for aplastic anemia in patients younger than 50 years of age is allogeneic bone marrow transplantation, usually with peripheral stem cells. This therapy is optimal if bone marrow from an HLA-matched sibling is used, although unrelated donors are becoming more readily available. Long-term survival rates of 65% to 85% have been reported following bone marrow transplantation, usually with full functional bone marrow recovery.[35,37,38] It should be noted that the chances of successful transplantation diminish in patients who have received multiple transfusions (more than 20), probably as a result of autoimmunization, which increases the chance of graft rejection. Thus, to minimize the numbers of supportive transfusions, many patients receive bone marrow transplantation early in the course of the disease.[37]

For patients who are unable to receive bone marrow transplantation because of age or lack of a suitable donor, immunomodulatory therapy has been utilized. This type of therapy makes use of antithymocyte or antilymphocyte globulin, cyclosporine, or cyclophosphamide in an attempt

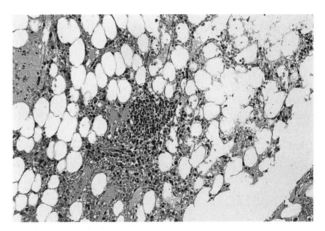

➤ **FIGURE 8–6** Lymphoid aggregate seen in a bone marrow biopsy specimen from a patient with aplastic anemia (H & E stain, ×100 magnification).

to inhibit a presumed immune attack on the bone marrow stem cell. Up to 75% survival after 5 years has been seen with this therapy, although relapses may occur.[35,39] Other alternative approaches include long-term stimulation with hematopoietic growth factors, usually in association with

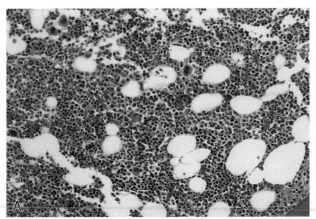
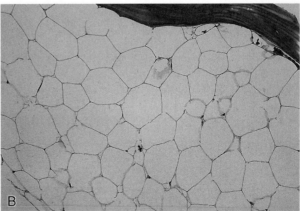

➤ **FIGURE 8–4** Panel *A:* Normocellular bone marrow. Panel *B:* Markedly hypocellular bone marrow biopsy specimen from a patient with aplastic anemia (hematoxylin-eosin [H & E] stain, ×500 magnification).

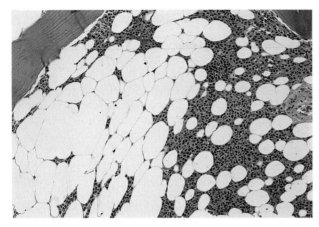

➤ **FIGURE 8–7**   Focal area of bone marrow hyperplasia adjacent to a hypoplastic area in early aplastic anemia (H & E stain, ×100 magnification).

immunosuppressive therapy. There is a variable increase in neutrophil count, often dependent on the severity of the bone marrow aplasia, with much less effective stimulation of erythrocyte or platelet production.[40]

The prognosis for patients with aplastic anemia has markedly improved with the advent of such therapeutic options as bone marrow transplantation. The outcome is still variable and depends primarily on the severity of the anemia at the time of presentation, supportive care such as blood product transfusions, and the treatment modality employed.[1,35,37–40]

➤ RELATED DISORDERS

Pure Red Cell Aplasia

Pure red cell aplasia is an uncommon disorder in which the erythroid cells in the bone marrow are selectively destroyed, giving rise to an anemia without other associated cytopenias. Over 600 cases have been reported in the world's literature. This may be an acquired or congenital process (Table 8–8). The disease is characterized by severe, chronic, normocytic to slightly macrocytic anemia. Reticulocytes are decreased and may be absent. There is no evidence of hemolysis or hemorrhage. White cells and platelets are normal. A bone marrow biopsy usually demonstrates normal cellularity with a notable absence of erythroid precursor cells. Erythropoietin levels are often markedly increased as the body attempts to compensate for the profound anemia.[41,42]

Acquired causes of pure red cell aplasia are most common, and may be short-lived acute illnesses or have a more prolonged chronic course. Viral illnesses have been associated with development of a transient cessation of red cell production and disappearance of erythroblasts from the bone marrow. In most patients this would be relatively asymptomatic; however, in patients with long-standing hemolytic disease and rapid cell turnover (e.g., sickle cell disease, hereditary spherocytosis), this loss of red cell production causes a precipitous decrease in hematocrit or an aplastic crisis. In some cases, aplastic crisis has been associated with parvovirus B19 infection (the causative agent of erythema infectiosum, or fifth disease, observed in children). Parvovirus B19 selectively infects red blood cell precursors, leading to an absence of late erythroblasts and subsequent stages of erythroid differentiation. Some erythroblasts may contain viral inclusions (Fig. 8–8 and Color Plate 102). Parvovirus B19 infection may also cause a transient anemia in immunocompromised patients or patients with severe malnutrition. Usually the patient recovers erythropoietic capacity, as evidenced by the appearance of reticulocytes, within 7 to 10 days although chronic anemia may persist in some patients. Most immunocompetent patients, without conditions of rapid cell turnover, only experience a brief, transient fall in hematocrit.[43]

Another frequent cause of pure red cell aplasia is an idiosyncratic reaction to a drug. Several drugs have been implicated, and these are usually the same drugs that give rise to aplastic anemia, including phenytoin, isoniazid, and azathioprine. Both direct inhibition of erythroid cells by the drug and development of drug-induced antibodies have been implicated as pathogenetic mechanisms.[44] Other etiologies associated with development of pure red cell aplasia include malnutrition, chronic infections, vitamin deficiency in children, and the presence of a thymoma in adults. In adults with persistent red cell aplasia, more than 50% have a thymoma, although it may not be detected until several years after the development of anemia. Removal of the thymic tumor causes a resolution of the anemia in about one-third of the patients.[45] Pure cell aplasia has also been associated with B- or T-cell lymphoproliferative disorders, such as chronic lymphocytic leukemia or T-cell large gran-

> **Table 8-8**
> **CAUSES OF PURE RED CELL APLASIA**

Acquired

Infections—parvovirus B19

    Aplastic crisis in patients with hemolytic disorders

    Immunocompromised patients

    Malnutrition

Drugs

Thymoma or lymphoid neoplasms

Idiopathic

Congenital

Diamond-Blackfan anemia

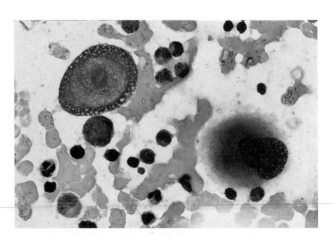

➤ **FIGURE 8–8**   Erythroid precursors containing parvovirus B19 viral inclusions (Wright-Giemsa stain, ×500 magnification).

ular lymphocytosis. This association of pure red cell aplasia with these neoplasms is usually a result of production of antibodies that cross-react with erythroid precursors immune etiology, and some response to immunosuppressive therapies has been noted in these patients.[46]

A congenital form of pure red cell aplasia was described in 1938 and bears the name Diamond-Blackfan anemia. It is characterized by a chronic, moderate to severe anemia that usually manifests early in infancy and is associated with normal numbers of white cells and platelets. The anemia is usually macrocytic but may occasionally be normocytic. The reticulocyte count is decreased. Bone marrow examination shows a normocellular bone marrow with erythroid hypoplasia. Usually normal or increased numbers of proerythroblasts are present in the marrow; however, later differentiational stages of erythroid cells stages are markedly decreased. Minor congenital abnormalities of the head and upper limbs may be present, similar to Fanconi's anemia. The mode of inheritance is uncertain, with sporadic cases making up 75%. Both recessive and dominant inheritance patterns have been described. There is a wide variation in the age of onset, severity, and natural course of the disease. Spontaneous remissions have been noted in up to 25% of patients, often following many years of anemia.[47] Most patients respond to steroids and are able to maintain adequate hemoglobin levels, but some patients may become transfusion dependent and develop possible iron overload from long-term transfusion therapy. Bone marrow transplantation is curative.[48] There is a marked increase in the incidence of acute myelogenous leukemia late in the course of the disease. Although the pathogenetic mechanism underlying Diamond-Blackfan anemia is not clear, most studies point to a molecular defect in signal transduction in the erythroid bone marrow progenitors that leads to decreased responsiveness to erythropoietin or other cytokines.[46,48]

Congenital Dyserythropoietic Anemias

Congenital dyserythropoietic anemias (CDAs) are a rare group of familial disorders in which anemia and ineffective erythropoiesis are associated with bizarre binuclear and multinuclear erythroblasts (Fig. 8–9 and Color Plate 103). Three types of CDA have been well described (Table 8–9), and other rare cases of types of congenital anemia have been described. All of the CDAs present clinically with anemia, erythroid hyperplasia with variable degrees of dyserythropoiesis, and indirect hyperbilirubinemia or mild jaundice.[49]

Type 1 CDA is characterized by a mild to moderate macrocytic anemia with prominent anisocytosis and poikilocytosis. Bone marrow erythroblasts show megaloblastic maturation and the presence of a small number (1% to 3%) of marrow erythroblasts that are binucleated or contain chromatin bridges (thin, fiberlike connections between the nuclei). It is inherited as an autosomal recessive trait.

Type 2 CDA gives rise to a mild to severe normocytic anemia in which 10% to 50% of the erythroblasts in the marrow are binucleated or multinucleated. This form is also characterized by an autosomal recessive mode of inheritance and is the most commonly seen form of CDA. Type 2 CDA red cells will lyse in acidified serum (Ham's test), giving rise to the alternative name for this disorder of *HEMPAS* (*hereditary erythroblast multinuclearity with a positive acid serum test*). Because of red cell lysis in an acidified serum test, a diagnosis of paroxysmal nocturnal hemoglobinuria (PNH) may be entertained. However, unlike PNH, the cells of CDA type 2 do not lyse in a sugar water test, nor do they have the characteristic flow cytometric finding of decreased levels of CD55 and CD59.[50] In addition, type 2 CDA cells have been found to be strongly agglutinated by anti-i, and the i antigen is persistently expressed on all of the erythrocytes in HEMPAS.

Type 3 CDA presents as a mild to moderate macrocytic anemia. It differs from type 1 CDA by having as many as 30% multinucleated bone marrow erythroid cells, some containing as many as 12 nuclei (gigantoblasts). This disorder appears to be inherited in an autosomal dominant fashion. The anemias associated with the well-described types of CDA are mild to moderate, and most patients may be treated with transfusions and supportive therapy. Some patients may develop splenomegaly requiring a splenectomy.[49]

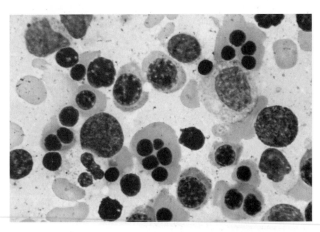

➤ FIGURE 8–9   Multinucleated erythroid precursors in type 2 congenital dyserythropoietic anemia (HEMPAS) (Wright-Giemsa stain, ×500 magnification).

> ### ➤ CASE STUDY

A 20-year-old woman was seen by her physician for fatigue, pallor, and easy bruising. Physical examination was unremarkable except for pallor, widespread petechiae, ecchymosis, and bleeding gums. The spleen was not enlarged. There was no history of recent exposure to drugs, toxins, or radiation. There was no history of any other illness, and she had been in good health until the past 2 weeks.

Laboratory data revealed a normochromic, normocytic anemia with a hematocrit of 20%, WBC of $20 \times 10^9/L$, and platelets of $20 \times 10^9/L$. The peripheral blood showed 9% neutrophils, 90% lymphocytes, and 1% monocytes. The corrected reticulocyte count was 0.5%. A bone marrow aspirate and biopsy specimen was markedly hypocellular, with less than 5% cellularity composed of lymphocytes and plasma cells admixed with a rare myeloid or erythroid precursor. No megakaryocytes were noted. No dysplastic changes were noted in the few hematopoietic cells seen, and there was no increase in the number of blasts. Further studies failed to identify an underlying

continued

> **Table 8-9**
CONGENITAL DYSERYTHROPOIETIC ANEMIAS

	Type 1	Type 2 (HEMPAS)	Type 3
Degree of anemia	Mild to moderate	Mild to severe	Mild
Red blood cell size	Macrocytic	Normocytic	Macrocytic
Bone marrow features	Megaloblastic maturation with 1%–3% binucleated or chromatin bridges in erythroid precursors	10%–50% binucleated or multinucleated erythroid precursors	Extreme multinucleation of erythroid precursors (gigantoblasts)
Genetic inheritance pattern	Autosomal recessive	Autosomal recessive	Autosomal dominant
Acid serum test	Negative	Positive	Negative
Sugar water test	Negative	Negative	Negative

Abbreviation: HEMPAS = hereditary erythroblast multinuclearity with positive acid serum test.

etiology for the patient's pancytopenia. The patient was followed for the next 3 months with no resolution of her symptoms and no improvement in her blood count. She received two transfusions of red blood cells as a result of worsening anemia.

The patient's family was tested, and she was found to have a sister who was HLA compatible. The sister had collection of peripheral stem cells for an allogeneic transplantation. The stem cells were infused into the patient following conditioning with cyclophosphamide to deplete the patient's immune system. The patient had one bout of acute graft-versus-host disease approximately 35 days after transplantation that was successfully treated with cyclosporine therapy. Her counts 1 year after the transplantation showed a hematocrit of 42%, WBC of 6.0 $\times$ 10^9/L, and platelets of 210 $\times$ 10^9/L. The WBC differential showed 71% neutrophils, 21% lymphocytes, 6% monocytes, and 2% eosinophils. A bone marrow biopsy specimen showed a bone marrow cellularity of 50%, with all cell lineages present and maturing normally. The patient has had no further episodes of graft-versus-host disease, bleeding, or infection.

This is a fairly typical history for development of an idiopathic aplastic anemia in a young patient. Currently, if an HLA-related bone marrow donor can be found, most of these patients proceed to bone marrow transplantation. This procedure usually occurs relatively early in the course of the disease to minimize the numbers of transfusions, as the latter have been found to negatively impact the graft survival. If the transplantation is successful, these patients often lead normal lives without a need for chronic immunosuppression or the development of other hematologic problems.

QUESTIONS

1. How is aplastic anemia best defined?
   a. A condition in which bone marrow production of red cells, white blood cells, and platelets has failed
   b. A condition in which severe anemia is seen
   c. A condition in which platelets are decreased
   d. A condition in which there is pancytopenia with a hypercellular bone marrow

2. Which is the most common cause of aplastic anemia?
   a. Drug ingestion
   b. Toxin exposure
   c. Idiopathic or unknown
   d. Ionizing radiation

3. Which of the following represents the most complete list of etiologies causing aplastic anemia?
   a. Secondary and congenital
   b. Idiopathic and congenital
   c. Secondary and idiopathic
   d. Secondary, idiopathic, and congenital

4. Which of the following has not been associated with an acquired type of aplastic anemia?
   a. Ionizing radiation
   b. Increased chromosomal breakage
   c. Chemical agents
   d. Drugs

5. The aplastic anemia associated with benzene exposure is characterized by which of the following statements?
   a. Always occurs while the exposure to benzene is occurring
   b. Is always irreversible
   c. Always causes fatal, severe aplastic anemia
   d. May cause a spectrum of disease that may not manifest until several years following the benzene exposure

6. Which of the following statements about chloramphenicol-induced aplastic anemia is true?
   a. The onset of the bone marrow aplasia is not predictable by the dose or the duration of drug exposure
   b. Low doses of chloramphenicol never lead to aplastic anemias
   c. People who receive chloramphenicol are 500 times more likely to develop aplastic anemia than the general population
   d. The longer a patient receives chloramphenicol, the more likely it is that he or she will develop aplastic anemia

7. Which of the following drugs is not associated with the development of aplastic anemia?
   a. Chloramphenicol
   b. Phenylbutazone
   c. Aspirin
   d. Chemotherapeutic agents

8. Ionizing radiation causes aplastic anemia by which of the following mechanisms?
   a. A dose-dependent destruction of bone marrow stem cells
   b. An idiosyncratic delayed development of bone marrow aplasia
   c. Disruption of chemical bonds to form free radicals that damage bone marrow cells
   d. All of the above

9. What is the most common congenital disorder associated with aplastic anemia?
   a. Fanconi's anemia
   b. Thrombocytopenia-absent radius (TAR) syndrome
   c. Congenital dyserythropoietic anemia, type 1
   d. Diamond-Blackfan anemia

10. Which of the following is not seen in the peripheral blood of patients with aplastic anemia?
    a. Normochromic, normocytic anemia
    b. Increased reticulocyte count
    c. Relative lymphocytosis
    d. Decreased neutrophils

11. What is the appearance of the bone marrow in aplastic anemia?
    a. Hypercellular
    b. Normocellular
    c. Hypocellular
    d. Fibrotic

12. The differential diagnostic considerations for bone marrow hypoplasia do not include which of the following disorders?
    a. Severe malnutrition
    b. Myeloproliferative disorder
    c. Aplastic anemia
    d. Recent chemotherapy

13. What is the treatment of choice for severe aplastic anemia in patients who are younger than age 50?
    a. Multiple transfusions
    b. Androgens
    c. Bone marrow transplantation
    d. Erythropoietin therapy

14. What is the definition of pure red cell aplasia?
    a. Lack of hematopoietic precursors in the bone marrow
    b. Abnormal, giant normoblasts in the bone marrow
    c. Lack of erythroid precursors with normal white blood cell and megakaryocytic precursors
    d. Dysplastic red cell precursors with normal white cell and megakaryocytic precursors

15. What features do the congenital dyserythropoietic anemias (CDAs) have in common?
    a. Anemia, microcytosis, erythroid hyperplasia, and abnormal erythroblasts
    b. Anemia, erythroid hyperplasia with abnormal erythroblasts, and indirect hyperbilirubinemia.
    c. Anemia, lysis in acidified serum, and indirect hyperbilirubinemia
    d. Anemia, macrocytosis, erythroid hyperplasia with abnormal erythroblasts, and indirect hyperbilirubinemia

SUMMARY CHART

➤ Aplastic anemia is defined as a failure of bone marrow and loss of bone marrow cellularity leading to decreased production of erythrocytes, leukocytes, and platelets, and development of peripheral blood cytopenias.

➤ Clinical criteria defining aplastic anemia include a bone marrow cellularity of less than 25% and at least two peripheral blood cytopenias.

➤ Aplastic anemia usually arises as a result of acquired damage, although rare cases are hereditary. The underlying cause of aplastic anemia is idiopathic, or unknown, in the majority of cases.

➤ Of those cases of aplastic anemia in which an etiologic agent can be identified, drugs, chemicals (especially benzene-type compounds), irradiation, and some infections have been implicated as causes of aplastic anemia.

➤ Drug-induced aplastic anemia is usually an idiosyncratic (not dose-related) reaction; the most commonly implicated drugs are chloramphenicol and phenylbutazone.

➤ Ionizing radiation usually causes bone marrow aplasia in an immediate dose-dependent manner, although late effects may also be seen.

➤ Infections and altered or autoimmune states may also cause bone marrow aplasia, probably as a result of immune destruction of the bone marrow hematopoietic precursor or stem cell.

➤ The congenital form of aplastic anemia, Fanconi's anemia, is characterized by an autosomal recessive inheritance pattern and progressive development of pancytopenia and bone marrow hypoplasia as well as an increased incidence of acute leukemia and other malignancies.

➤ Fanconi's anemia is characterized at a molecular and cytogenetic level by increased chromosomal breakage and defective DNA repair.

➤ Blood findings in aplastic anemia include normochromic, normocytic anemia with low numbers of reticulocytes (hypoproliferative anemia), leukopenia (especially of myeloid and monocytic cells) and thrombocytopenia. Lymphocyte counts may be normal or decreased.

➤ Bone marrow examination is required for diagnosis of aplastic anemia to document bone marrow

➤ hypocellularity and exclude other causes (i.e., metastatic tumor) for pancytopenia.

➤ Aplastic anemia in patients younger than 50 years of age is usually treated by bone marrow transplantation. Patients unsuitable for transplantation therapy may be treated with supportive transfusion therapy, immunomodulatory therapy, or androgens.

➤ Pure red cell aplasia is defined as a selective loss of bone marrow red cell precursors and presents clinically as an isolated hypoproliferative anemia. Causes of pure red cell aplasia include infections (parvovirus B19), reactions to drugs, and immune abnormalities. A congenital form is recognized, called Diamond-Blackfan anemia.

➤ Congenital dyserythropoietic anemias (CDAs) are familial or inherited anemias that are characterized by ineffective erythropoiesis, bone marrow erythroid hyperplasia, and bizarre erythroid precursors with multiple nuclei and intranuclear chromatin bridges.

➤ Type 2 CDA is associated with an abnormal lysis in acidified serum (Ham's test). It is also known as HEMPAS (hereditary erythroblast multinuclearity with positive acid serum test) and is inherited in an autosomal recessive fashion.

➤ Type 3 CDA often has large numbers of erythroid cells with multiple nuclei (gigantoblasts) and is inherited in an autosomal dominant fashion.

References

1. Guinan, EC: Clinical aspects of aplastic anemia. Hematol Oncol Clin N Amer 6:1025, 1997.
2. Maciejewski, JP, et al: Phenotypic and functional analysis of bone marrow progenitor cell compartment in bone marrow failure. Br J Haematol 87:227, 1994.
3. Kojima, S: Hematopoietic growth factors and marrow stroma in aplastic anemia. Int J Hematol 68:19, 1998.
4. Young, NS, and Maciejewski, JP: The pathophysiology of acquired aplastic anemia. N Engl J Med 19:1365, 1997.
5. Dessypris, EN: Aplastic anemia and pure red cell aplasia. Curr Opin Hematol 1:157, 1994.
6. Nissen, C: The pathophysiology of aplastic anemia. Semin Hematol 28:313, 1991.
7. Kalf, GF: Recent advances in the metabolism and toxicity of benzene. CRC Crit Rev Toxicol 18:141, 1987.
8. Rangan, U, and Snyder, R: Scientific update on benzene. Ann NY Acad Sci 837:105, 1997.
9. Goldstein, BD: Benzene toxicity. Occup Med 3:541, 1988.
10. Farris, GM, et al: Benzene-induced hematoxicity and bone marrow compensation in B6C3F1 mice. Fundam Appl Toxicol 36:119, 1997.
11. Wanatabe, KH, et al: Benzene toxicokinetics in humans: Exposure of bone marrow to metabolites. Occup Environ Med 51:414, 1994.
12. Smith, MT, et al: Increased translocations and aneusomy in chromosomes 8 and 12 among workers exposed to benzene. Canc Res 58: 2176, 1998.
13. Malkin, D, and Koren, EF: Drug-induced aplastic anemia: Pathogenesis and clinical aspects. Am J Pediatr Hematol Oncol 12:402, 1990.
14. Flegg, P, et al: Chloramphenicol. Are concerns about aplastic anemia justified? Drug Saf 7:167, 1992.
15. Yunis, AA: Chloramphenicol toxicity: 25 years of research. Am J Med 87:44N, 1989.
16. Vorobiev, AI: Acute radiation disease and biological dosimetry in 1993. Stem Cells 15:269, 1997.
17. Amrtland, HS: Occupational poisoning in manufacture of luminous watch dials. JAMA 92:466, 1929.
18. Lavin, MF: Radiation-induced cell death and its implications in human disease. Results Probl Cell Differ 24:213, 1998.
19. Cronkite, EP: Radiation-induced aplastic anemia. Semin Hematol 4:273, 1967.
20. Brown, KE, et al: Hepatitis-associated aplastic anemia. N Engl J Med 336:1059, 1997.
21. Baranski, B, et al: Epstein-Barr virus in the bone marrow of patients with aplastic anemia. Ann Int Med 109:695, 1988.
22. Young, N, and Mortimer, P. Viruses and bone marrow failure. Blood 63:729, 1984.
23. Knobel, B, et al: Infection of hematopoietic progenitor cells by human cytomegalovirus. Blood 80:170, 1992.
24. Maciejewski, JP, et al: Pancytopenia: A rare complication of miliary tuberculosis. Isr J Med Sci 19:555, 1983.
25. Helfman, T, and Falanga, V: Eosinophilic fasciitis. Clin Dermatol 12:449, 1994.
26. Asarelli, MH, et al: Aplastic anemia and immune-mediated thrombocytopenia: Concurrent complications encountered in the third trimester of pregnancy. Obstet Gynecol 91:803, 1998.
27. Ferrera, JLM, and Deeg, HJ: Graft versus host disease. N Engl J Med 324, 1991.
28. Commerci, GD: Medical complications of anorexia nervosa and bulimia nervosa. Med Clin N Amer 74:1293, 1990.
29. Smith, OP, et al: Haematologic abnormalities in Schwachman-Diamond syndrome. Br J Haematol 94:279, 1996.
30. Lui, J, et al: Fanconi's anemia and novel strategies for therapy. Blood 73:391, 1994.
31. Kupfer, GM, et al: Molecular biology of Fanconi anemia. Hematol Oncol Clin N Amer 11:1045, 1997.
32. D'Andrea, AD, and Grompe, M: Molecular biology of Fanconi anemia: Implications for diagnosis and therapy. Blood 90:1725, 1997.
33. Gluckman E, et al: Bone marrow transplantation for Fanconi anemia. Blood 86:2856, 1995.
34. Dokal, I: Severe aplastic anemia including Fanconi's anemia and dyskeratosis congenita. Curr Opin Hematol 3:453, 1996.
35. Brodsky, RA: Biology and management of acquired severe aplastic anemia. Curr Opin Oncol 10:95, 1998.
36. Najean, Y, and Pecking, A: Prognostic factors in aplastic anemia. Am Med J 67:564, 1979.
37. Passweg, JR, et al: Bone marrow management of acquired severe aplastic anemia. Curr Opin Oncol 10:95, 1998.
38. Deeg, HJ, et al: Long-term outcome after marrow transplantation for severe aplastic anemia. Blood 91:3637, 1998.
39. Gillio, AP, et al: Comparison of long-term outcome of children with severe aplastic anemia treated with immunosuppression versus bone marrow transplantation. Biol Blood Marrow Transplant 3:18, 1997.
40. Kumar, M, and Alter, BP: Hematopoietic growth factors for the treatment of aplastic anemia. Curr Opin Hematol 5:226, 1998.
41. Mamiya, S, et al: Acquired pure red cell aplasia in Japan. Eur J Haematol 59:199, 1997.
42. Desspyris, EN: The biology of pure red cell aplasia. Semin Hematol 28: 275, 1991.
43. Brown, KE, and Young, NS: Parvovirus B19 in human disease. Annu Rev Med 48:59, 1997.
44. Thompson, DF, and Gales, MA: Drug-induced pure red cell aplasia. Pharmacotherapy 16:1002, 1996.
45. Matsudas, M, et al: Pure red cell aplasia with thymoma: Evidence of T-cell clonal disorder. Am J Hematol 54:324, 1997.
46. Pritsch, et al: Basic biology of autoimmune phenomena in chronic lymphocytic leukemia. Semin Oncol 25:34, 1998.
47. Krijanovski, OI, and Sieff, CA: Diamond-Blackfan anemia. Hematol Oncol Clin N Amer 11:1061, 1997.
48. Dianzani, I, et al: Diamond-Blackfan anemia: A congenital defect in erythropoiesis. Hematologica 81:560, 1996.
49. Wickramasinghe, SN: Dyserythropoiesis and congenital dyserythropoietic anemias. Br J Haematol 98:785, 1997.
50. Nishimura, JI, et al: Paroxysmal nocturnal hemoglobinuria: Molecular pathogenesis and molecular therapeutic approaches. Hematopathol Mol Hematol 11:119, 1998.

See Bibliography for this chapter at the back of the book.

9 Introduction to Hemolytic Anemias

Intracorpuscular Defects

I Hereditary Defects of the Red Cell Membrane

THERESA L. COETZER, PHD
STAN ZAIL, MBBCH, MD, FRCPATH

OBJECTIVES

At the end of this chapter, the learner should be able to:

1. Define intracorpuscular and extracorpuscular red cell defects as related to hemolytic processes.
2. List laboratory tests that reflect increased red cell destruction.
3. Calculate a reticulocyte production index.
4. Name laboratory tests that help to classify the cause of red cell hemolysis.
5. Identify the red cell membrane abnormalities associated with hereditary spherocytosis.
6. Recognize abnormal laboratory results associated with hereditary spherocytosis.
7. Name the functional abnormalities affecting membrane skeleton proteins in hereditary elliptocytosis.
8. Recall laboratory findings associated with hereditary elliptocytosis.
9. Identify the abnormalities that cause the severe fragmentation and microspherocytosis characteristic of hereditary pyropoikilocytosis.
10. List rare disorders of membrane cation permeability.

➤ CLASSIFICATION OF HEMOLYTIC ANEMIAS

A hemolytic state exists when the in vivo survival of the red cell is shortened. The presence of anemia in an individual patient is, however, dependent on the degree of hemolysis and the compensatory response of the erythroid elements of the bone marrow. Normal bone marrow is able to increase its output about six- to eightfold, so that anemia is not manifest until this capacity is exceeded, corresponding to a red cell life span of about 15 to 20 days or less. Anemia may, however, occur with more moderate shortening of the red cell life span if there is an associated depression of bone marrow function, which may occur with certain systemic diseases or exposure to chemicals or drugs.

A useful classification of the hemolytic anemias entails their subdivision into those disorders associated with an intrinsic (intracorpuscular) defect of the red cell and those associated with an extrinsic (extracorpuscular) abnormality. Red cells from a patient with an intracorpuscular defect have a shortened survival in both the patient and a normal recipient, whereas normal donor red cells survive normally in the patient. In contrast, normal red cells are destroyed more rapidly when transfused into a patient with an extracorpuscular abnormality. The patient's red cells, when transfused into a healthy recipient, have normal survival, provided that they have not been irreversibly damaged. Hemolytic states have also traditionally been regarded as intravascular or extravascular; that is, sequestration occurs in reticuloendothelial tissue. However, vigorous extravascular hemolysis may often be associated with signs of hemoglobin release into the plasma such as hemoglobinemia and decreased haptoglobin levels. The distinction still is useful from a clinical standpoint because certain hemolytic states are associated with predominantly intravascular hemolysis (e.g., paroxysmal nocturnal hemoglobinuria and infections caused by *Clostridia* or *Plasmodium falciparum*).

Hemolytic anemias may be classified as follows:

1. Intracorpuscular defects
   a. Hereditary defects
      (1) Defects in the red cell membrane
      (2) Enzyme defects
      (3) Hemoglobinopathies
      (4) Thalassemia syndromes
   b. Acquired defects
      (1) Paroxysmal nocturnal hemoglobinuria
2. Extracorpuscular defects
   a. Immune hemolytic anemias
   b. Infections
   c. Chemicals and toxins
   d. Physical agents
   e. Microangiopathic and macroangiopathic hemolytic anemias
   f. Splenic sequestration (hypersplenism)
   g. General systemic disorders (in which hemolysis is not the dominant feature of the anemia)

► APPROACH TO DIAGNOSIS OF A HEMOLYTIC STATE

The approach to diagnosis of a hemolytic state initially involves establishing the fact that the rate of red cell destruction is increased and then focuses on determining the cause of hemolysis.

Establishing the Presence of Hemolysis

Diagnostic tests used to establish the presence of hemolysis rely on the fact that hemolysis is characterized by both increased cell destruction and increased production.

Tests Reflecting Increased Red Cell Destruction

The most frequently used tests in this category are the serum unconjugated (indirect) bilirubin and serum haptoglobin determinations. The serum unconjugated bilirubin level seldom exceeds 3 to 4 mg/dL in uncomplicated hemolytic states and reflects the catabolism of heme derived from red cells phagocytosed by the reticuloendothelial system (Fig. 9–1). The test is, however, relatively insensitive, as is the measurement of fecal sterobilinogen and urine urobilinogen that represents further stages in the disposition of unconjugated bilirubin by the liver (see Fig. 9–1). Because the unconjugated bilirubin is bound to albumin it cannot pass the glomerular filter, and the jaundice is said to be "acholuric." On the other hand, a decreased serum haptoglobin level is a very sensitive test of both intravascular and extravascular hemolysis, and reflects the rapid clearance by the reticuloendothelial system of a complex formed between liberated hemoglobin and circulatory haptoglobin. Drawbacks to the use of serum haptoglobin levels are that low levels may occur in hepatocellular disease, reflecting decreased synthesis by the liver, and that some individuals, particularly in black populations, may have a genetically determined deficiency of haptoglobin. Increased synthesis of haptoglobin in acute inflammatory states or malignancy may also mask depletion of serum haptoglobin owing to hemolysis.

Other tests that reflect increased red cell destruction, particularly if it is primarily intravascular, are those that test for

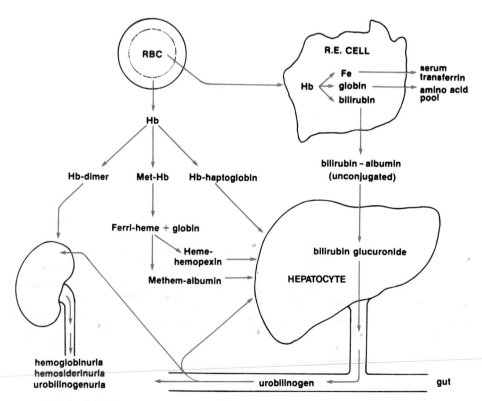

► **FIGURE 9–1** Diagrammatic representation of the degradation of hemoglobin after intravascular or extravascular destruction of red cells. Fe = iron; Hb = hemoglobin; RBC = red blood cell; R.E. = reticuloendothelial cell.

the presence of hemoglobinemia, hemoglobinuria, and hemosiderinuria. The assessment of hemoglobinemia requires stringent precautions in the prevention of hemolysis during blood collection. Once the hemoglobin-binding capacity of serum haptoglobin is exceeded, hemoglobin passes through the glomerulus as alpha-beta ($\alpha\beta$) chain dimers, reassociates to $\alpha_2\beta_2$ tetramers in the tubule, where the hemoglobin is reabsorbed and degraded. The liberated iron is conserved as ferritin and hemosiderin. When the tubular reabsorptive capacity for hemoglobin is exceeded, hemoglobinuria ensues and is detectable by either spectroscopic examination or commercially available dipsticks that detect heme. Staining of the urine sediment for iron (e.g., with Prussian blue) will detect the hemosiderin- and ferritin-containing renal tubular cells that are sloughed several days after a hemolytic episode. Some of the free plasma hemoglobin may be oxidized to methemoglobin with subsequent dissociation of ferri-heme, which combines with albumin to form methemalbumin. Methemalbumin can be detected spectroscopically by the Schumm's test. This test is relatively insensitive and is seldom positive in mild hemolytic states. In routine practice, determination of red cell survival using ^{51}Cr-labeled red cells is seldom required to document an increased rate of red cell destruction. The fate of hemoglobin when processed intravascularly or extravascularly is shown diagrammatically in Figure 9–1.

Tests Reflecting Increased Red Cell Production

The compensatory bone marrow response to hemolysis results in the delivery of young red cells in the form of reticulocytes into the circulation. These young cells contain RNA, which stains supravitally with dyes such as new methylene blue or brilliant cresyl blue. The normal reticulocyte count has a range of 0.5% to 2.0%. This reflects the fact that each day approximately 1% of the red cell mass is destroyed and replaced by young red cells from the bone marrow, because red cell survival is approximately 120 days. The reticulocyte count is always elevated in a hemolytic state in which there is a normal compensatory bone marrow response. However, a more accurate assessment of red cell production is required, because the percentage of reticulocytes may be "spuriously" elevated as the reticulocytes may be diluted into a lesser number of total circulating red cells. In addition, in response to the anemia, reticulocytes may leave the bone marrow prematurely and mature in the circulation for longer than the normal maturation time of 1 day, again leading to a falsely elevated reticulocyte count. These cells (so-called shift reticulocytes) are recognizable as large bluish-gray erythrocytes on Romanowsky stains.

The reticulocyte production index (RPI) corrects the hematocrit to a normal value of 45% and takes into account the maturation time of the reticulocyte at a particular hematocrit (approximately 1.0 day at a hematocrit of 45%, 1.5 days at 35%, 2.0 days at 25%, and 2.5 days at 15%).[1]

$$\text{RPI} = \frac{\%\ \text{Reticulocytes}}{\text{Reticulocyte maturation time}} \times \frac{\text{Hematocrit}}{45}$$

For example, an RPI of 5.3 is calculated for a patient suspected of having a hemolytic state with the following indices: hemoglobin, 12.0 g/dL; hematocrit, 36%; reticulocyte count, 10%; shift cells present.

An RPI of greater than 2.5 to 3.0 is generally regarded as indicative of a hemolytic state, but it is very important to exclude the presence of hemorrhage in a particular patient, as this too may lead to an elevated RPI. Although the RPI is probably the single most useful test to detect a hemolytic state, a cautionary note is in order, as the test may not be sensitive enough to detect mild hemolytic states (see Chap. 28).

Establishing the Cause of Hemolysis

Once having documented the presence of hemolysis, it is our experience that the approach followed by Lux and Glader[2] in establishing the cause of hemolysis is pragmatic and logical, and this is the technique that is followed in this chapter. The initial step consists of separating patients into Coombs test–positive (i.e., immunohemolytic anemias) and Coombs test–negative groups. The latter group is then further divided into "smear-positive" and "smear-negative" subgroups. It is fundamentally important to assess morphology in peripheral smears that are free of artifact. On the basis of the classification according to the predominant morphology criteria associated with a particular disease state (Table 9–1), it is possible to considerably narrow the differential diagnosis and then institute further appropriate tests to make a definitive diagnosis.

It is also worth emphasizing that many hemolytic states are associated with an underlying disease, as will become apparent in the ensuing chapters, and this should not be lost sight of in the assessment of the individual patient.

➤ HEREDITARY DEFECTS OF THE RED CELL MEMBRANE

Red Cell Membrane Structure

An understanding of the etiology and pathophysiology of hemolytic states caused by defects of the red cell membrane requires some knowledge of its structural organization. The membrane consists of a relatively fluid lipid bilayer stabilized by interactions with integral membrane proteins within the bilayer and with the underlying membrane protein skeleton. The membrane provides the red cell with the necessary strength and flexibility to survive the circulatory shear stress and numerous passages through the spleen during its 4-month life span. The ability of the red cell to deform and to subsequently regain its original biconcave disc shape is determined by three factors: (1) cell surface area-to-volume ratio; (2) the viscoelastic properties of the membrane, which depend on the structural and functional integrity of the membrane skeleton; and (3) the cytoplasmic viscosity, which is determined primarily by hemoglobin.

The structural organization of the protein and lipid components of the red cell membrane has been reviewed in Chapter 3, and only some aspects of the membrane proteins implicated in the pathogenesis of hemolytic anemia are emphasized here.

The red cell membrane *skeleton* underlies the lipid bilayer and is a loosely knit two-dimensional protein network consisting mainly of the structural proteins, α and β spectrin, actin, and protein 4.1.[3] Negatively stained stretched skeletons viewed by high-resolution electron microscopy[4] reveal a hexagonal lattice of predominantly spectrin tetramers with some hexamers joined together by junctional protein complexes (Fig. 9–2). These junctional complexes are com-

➤ **Table 9-1**

PREDOMINANT RED CELL MORPHOLOGY COMMONLY ASSOCIATED WITH NONIMMUNE HEMOLYTIC DISORDERS

Spherocytes

Hereditary spherocytosis

Acute oxidant injury (HMP shunt defects during hemolytic crisis, oxidant drugs and chemicals)

Clostridium welchii septicemia

Severe burns, other red cell thermal injuries

Spider, bee, and snake venoms

Severe hypophosphatemia

Bizarre Poikilocytes

Red cell fragmentation symdrome (microangiopathic and macroangiopathic hemolytic anemias)

Hereditary elliptocytosis in neonates

Hereditary pyropoikilocytosis

Elliptocytes

Hereditary elliptocytosis

Thalassemias

Iron deficiency

Megaloblastic anemia

Stomatocytes

Hereditary stomatocytosis and related disorders

Stomatocytic elliptocytosis

Irreversibly Sickled Cells

Sickle cell anemia

Symptomatic sickle syndromes

Intraerythrocytic Parasites

Malaria

Babesiosis

Bartonellosis

Prominent Basophilic Stippling

Thalassemias

Unstable hemoglobins

Lead poisoning

Pyrimidine-5'-nucleotidase deficiency

Spiculated or Crenated Red Cells

Acute hepatic necrosis (spur cell anemia)

Uremia

Infantile pyknocytosis

Abetalipoproteinemia

McLeod blood group

Target Cells

Hemoglobins S, C, D, and E

Thalassemias

Hereditary xerocytosis

Nonspecific or Normal Morphology

Embden-Meyerhof pathway defects

HMP shunt defects

Adenosine deaminase hyperactivity with low red cell ATP

Unstable hemoglobins

Paroxysmal nocturnal hemoglobinuria

Dyserythropoietic anemias

Copper toxicity (Wilson's disease)

Cation permeability defects

Erythropoietic porphyria

Vitamin E deficiency

Hypersplenism

Abbreviations: ATP = adenosine triphosphate; HMP = hexose monophosphate.

---

posed of protein 4.1, short F-actin filaments, as well as the minor actin-binding proteins adducin, dematin (protein 4.9), tropomyosin, and tropomodulin.[5] The skeleton is linked to the lipid bilayer by interactions with the integral membrane proteins, band 3 and glycophorin C. The primary attachment occurs via a high-affinity interaction with ankyrin, which binds to both band 3 and β spectrin.[6] Protein 4.2 (pallidin) also participates in this complex.[7] Secondary attachment sites of lower affinity are provided by interactions between band 3 and protein 4.1,[8] as well as among glycophorin C, protein 4.1, and protein p55.[9] Spectrin and protein 4.1 also interact directly with the lipid bilayer.

Red cell *spectrin,* the major skeletal protein, is an elongated flexible heterodimer composed of stoichiometric amounts of two structurally related, but functionally distinct, α and β polypeptides that are encoded by separate genes.[10–12] Both α and β spectrin can be subdivided into structural domains (αI to αV and βI to βIV, respectively) that are resistant to mild proteolysis by trypsin[13] (Fig. 9–3A). α Spectrin contains 22 tandem 106–amino acid repeats, known as a spectrin motif, each composed of a coiled triple helix.[14,15] Repeat 10 is atypical and is an SH3 domain, whereas the C terminal has an EF hand motif.[11] β Spectrin is composed of an N-terminal protein 4.1–actin-binding domain and 17 repeats of which repeats 15 and 16 bind ankyrin[10,12] (see Fig. 9–3A). The α and β monomers interact along their length in an antiparallel fashion starting at nucleation sites at the tail end of the molecules.[16] The head regions of the αβ heterodimers self-associate into tetramers via an interaction between two helices from the phosphorylated C-terminal repeat of the βI domain and a third helix from the N-terminal repeat of the αI domain to form a complete triple helix.[17] An important aspect in the biogenesis of the membrane skeleton is that α spectrin is synthesized in approximately threefold excess over β spectrin[18] and undergoes slower degradation,[19] indicating that β spectrin is the rate-limiting component in spectrin assembly.

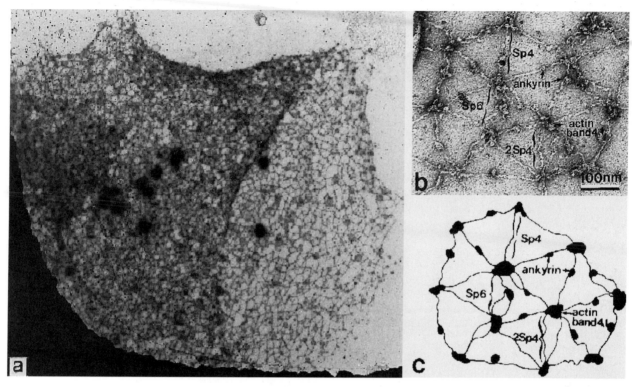

> ➤ FIGURE 9–2   Transmission electron micrographs of negatively stained membrane skeletons. *A*. An area of spread skeleton network. *B* and *C*. The hexagonal lattice made up of spectrin tetramers (Sp4), hexamers (Sp6), or double tetramers (2Sp4). Cross-linking junctional complexes are thought to contain short F-actin filaments and protein 4.1. Globular ankyrin structures are bound to spectrin filaments about 80 nm from their distal ends. (From Liu, SC, et al: Visualization of the hexagonal lattice in the erythrocyte membrane skeleton. J Cell Biol 104:527, 1987, with permission.)

Red cell *band 3*, the major integral membrane protein, is the anion exchanger.[20] It performs an important transport function by regulating HCO_3^-/Cl^- exchange and facilitating the transfer of carbon dioxide from tissues to lungs. It is divided into two structurally and functionally distinct domains. The 43-kd N-terminal cytoplasmic domain contains binding sites for ankyrin and proteins 4.1 and 4.2, and also binds glycolytic enzymes and hemoglobin. The 52-kd C-terminal region has 12 to 14 transmembrane segments intercalated in the lipid bilayer that form the anion exchange channel.[20]

Ankyrin is the major connecting protein that links the membrane skeleton to the bilayer.[21] It is a pyramid-shaped protein with an N-terminal 89-kd band 3–binding domain, formed by a series of 24 repeats containing 33 amino acids each. Spectrin binds to the central 62-kd domain of ankyrin, whereas the 55-kd C-terminal portion is a regulatory domain that is alternatively spliced, yielding ankyrin isoforms.

Protein 4.1 has four structural domains.[22] A 10-kd domain enhances the spectrin-actin interaction by binding to both proteins, and the N-terminal 30-kd domain interacts with glycophorin C and protein p55.

The genes coding for the major membrane proteins have been cloned and sequenced and their chromosomal localization identified (Table 9–2). Mutations in any of these genes that alter the amount or function of the expressed proteins, compromise the integrity of the membrane and manifest in altered red cell morphology. These cells are unable to survive passage through the spleen, resulting in hemolytic anemia.

Classification

The hereditary hemolytic anemias may be classified according to the morphological abnormality of the red cells. Four main groups are delineated:

1. Hereditary spherocytosis (HS)
2. Hereditary elliptocytosis (HE) and morphologically related disorders, including hereditary pyropoikilocytosis (HPP) and Southeast Asian ovalocytosis (SAO)
3. Hereditary stomatocytosis
4. Hereditary xerocytosis

By far the most common and well-characterized groups of disorders are HS and HE, and this chapter focuses on these

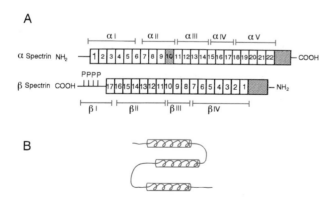

> ➤ FIGURE 9–3   Schematic representation of spectrin structure. *A*. The subunit structure of α and β spectrin, showing the antiparallel arrangement of the N and C terminals, the homologous repeat units (open squares), and the trypsin-resistant domain structure are indicated above the α chain and below the β chain. α Spectrin has 5 domains (αI to αV) and 22 repeats. β Spectrin has 4 domains (βI to βIV) and 17 repeats. The hatched squares indicate nonhomologous regions. *B*. Diagrammatic triple α helical structure of one of the spectrin repeats.

> ➤ Table 9-2
PROPERTIES OF SELECTED RED CELL MEMBRANE PROTEIN IMPLICATED IN HEMOLYTIC ANEMIA

Protein	SDS PAGE Band*	Molecular Weight† (kD)	Gene Symbol	Chromosomal Localization	Diseases
Skeletal proteins					
α Spectrin	1	281	SPTA 1	1q22→q23	HS, HE, HPP
β Spectrin	2	246	SPTB	14q23→q24.2	HS, HE, HPP
Protein 4.1	4.1	66	EL 1	1p33→p34.2	HE
Integral proteins					
Band 3	3	102	EPB 3	17q12→q21	HS, SAO
Stomatin	7	32	EPB7.2	9q34.1	HSt
Glycophorin C	PAS-2	14	GYPC	2q14→q21	HE
Connecting proteins					
Ankyrin	2.1	206	ANK 1	8p11.2	HS
Protein 4.2	4.2	77	EPB 4.2	15q15→q21	HS

*Proteins are separated by sodium dodecyl sulfate polyacrylamide gel electrophoresis (SDS PAGE) and stained with Coomassie blue or periodic acid–Schiff's reagent (PAS).
†Molecular weight is calculated from the amino acid sequence.
Abbreviations: HS = hereditary spherocytosis; HE = hereditary elliptocytosis; HPP = hereditary pyropoikilocytosis; HSt = hereditary stomatocytosis; SAO = Southeast Asian ovalocytosis.

entities. In recent years there have been major advances in our understanding of the molecular basis of these disorders. To gain insight into their pathogenesis and to enable a correlation of the genotype with the observed morphological phenotype, it is useful to divide the interactions between the red cell membrane components into two categories, as follows:

1. Vertical interactions occur between the membrane skeleton and the bilayer and mainly involve spectrin-ankyrin–band 3 associations, as well as weak contacts between spectrin and the negatively charged lipids of the inner half of the membrane bilayer.
2. Horizontal interactions occur between components of the membrane skeleton and include spectrin dimer self-association and spectrin-actin–protein 4.1 complex formation.

As first predicted by Palek in 1984[23] and subsequently verified by mutation analyses, defects in vertical interactions manifest as spherocytosis, whereas defects in horizontal interactions lead to elliptocytosis.

Hereditary Spherocytosis

Mode of Inheritance

Hereditary spherocytosis (HS), characterized by osmotically fragile, spherical red cells, is the most common hereditary hemolytic anemia in people of northern European origin (Fig. 9–4). It has been documented in other race groups, such as the Japanese and southern African blacks, but with a lower prevalence. In at least 75% of cases it follows a classic autosomal-dominant pattern of inheritance, but in the remaining families both parents are clinically normal, suggesting autosomal-recessive inheritance or variable penetrance of a dominant gene or a de novo mutation.

Molecular Defects

The underlying molecular defects in HS are heterogeneous and several genetic loci have been implicated.[24,25] In the vast majority of cases the abnormalities are quantitative with decreased amounts of the membrane proteins involved in vertical interactions between the bilayer and the skeleton (Table 9–3).

Spectrin deficiency is a common underlying cause of HS in population groups originating from northern Europe and is also found in the vast majority of southern African blacks. It was first documented by Agre and coworkers,[26] who noted that the number of spherocytes, severity of the disease, and response to splenectomy correlated closely with the reduced spectrin content. Spectrin deficiency is often secondary to a decreased amount of ankyrin (see later discussion) because

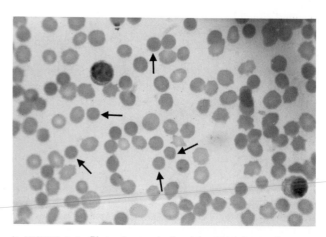

➤ FIGURE 9–4 Photomicrograph of peripheral blood smear from a patient with hereditary spherocytosis (HS). Note the microspherocytes (small condensed spherocytes with no central pallor) and the pincered (mushroom-shaped) cell.

> **Table 9-3**

DEFECTS OF RED CELL MEMBRANE PROTEINS IN HEREDITARY SPHEROCYTOSIS

Protein Deficiencies

Spectrin

Ankyrin

Spectrin and ankyrin

Band 3

Protein 4.2

Protein Dysfunction

β Spectrin-4.1 interaction

Band 3–pallidin interaction

the loss of ankyrin attachment sites prevents binding of spectrin to band 3. Mutations in the α-spectrin gene have no effect in the heterozygous state, because α-spectrin is synthesized in excess. However, frameshift errors caused by splice-site mutations in both α-spectrin alleles have been implicated in severe recessive HS.[27] β-Spectrin defects are associated with dominant HS because β-spectrin synthesis is rate limiting in the assembly of spectrin in the membrane. Several different mutations have been described in individual families. These include splice-site mutations, as well as deletions and insertions, that ultimately result in a shift in the reading frame of the gene, creating abnormal stop codons that terminate translation prematurely. These, together with nonsense mutations, as well as a point mutation in the translation initiation codon that prevents translation of the peptide, silence the expression of the mutant allele and manifest as null mutations. Truncated β spectrins also cause spectrin deficiency in HS. Several missense β-spectrin point mutations have also been documented and one of these, Sp$_{Kissimmee}$, impairs the binding of β spectrin to protein 4.1.[28]

Ankyrin deficiency, resulting in a concomitant decrease in spectrin, was first described by Coetzer and coworkers,[29] and subsequently shown to be caused by decreased ankyrin mRNA production and synthesis of an unstable molecule.[30] A combined ankyrin and spectrin deficiency is the most common abnormality underlying HS in Europe and North America.[24,25] Interstitial deletions of chromosome 8 involving the ankyrin gene (8p11.2), as well as balanced translocations involving chromosome 8p11, have been reported.[31,32] Nonsense and frameshift mutations are prevalent in dominant HS, resulting in either unstable mRNA transcripts or truncated proteins with functional abnormalities or decreased stability. In recessive HS, the defects are usually missense or promoter mutations.

Band 3 deficiency is found in approximately 20% of American and European HS patients but is more common among Japanese and South African whites, in whom it comprises nearly half of the cases. The decreased band 3 content often results in a secondary deficiency of protein 4.2. Null mutations are common and may be caused by single nucleotide insertions or deletions that alter the reading frame of the mutant band 3 allele or by nonsense mutations or splicing defects. Small in-frame deletions or insertions have been documented in a few cases. Band 3 missense mu-

tations are very common, and these often result in substitution of highly conserved amino acids that play a crucial role in the stabilization of the protein and its insertion into the membrane. The abnormal amino acids may also influence the anion transport function of band 3 if they are located in the transmembrane domain, or alter the binding of protein 4.2 if they occur in the cytoplasmic domain. Arginine substitutions are common[33] and arginine 760 (encoded by CGG) appears to be a mutation "hotspot," because it is frequently mutated to either CAG (glutamine) or TGG (tryptophan).[34]

Protein 4.2 deficiency is rare in Europeans but relatively common in the Japanese population, mainly because of protein 4.2$_{Nippon}$, which is caused by a point mutation that alters mRNA processing.[35]

Pathophysiology

The fundamental expression of the membrane defect in HS is a loss of surface area of the red cell, resulting in a decreased surface-to-volume ratio. This is manifested morphologically as spherocytosis, although it should be noted that the majority of HS cells are spherostomatocytic rather than truly spherocytic. Such cells tolerate less swelling than normal red cells and are osmotically fragile. The decrease in surface-to-volume ratio also makes the cells less deformable than normal. This has a particularly deleterious effect on their survival in the spleen and explains one of the hallmarks of HS, which is the excellent clinical response to splenectomy in most, but not all cases (see later discussion). The exact mechanism of spherocyte formation and subsequent hemolysis is not yet fully elucidated, but a postulated pathway of the pathophysiology of HS is summarized in Figure 9–5. The primary red cell membrane protein defects in HS are thought to weaken the vertical interactions between the skeleton and the bilayer. Spectrin- or band 3–deficient areas destabilize the membrane and allow the skeleton to be uncoupled from the bilayer. This results in loss of membrane in the form of microvesicles, which reduces the membrane surface area and decreases the surface-to-volume ratio of the cell. These cells are selectively trapped and "conditioned" in the spleen, where they progressively lose more surface area and are ultimately destroyed.

Clinical Manifestations

The classic presenting features of patients with HS are the triad of jaundice, anemia, and enlarged spleen, but many patients do not show all these signs. The age of presentation can vary from within a day or two after birth to old age, and sometimes the condition is only diagnosed during family studies or investigation for other reasons. Approximately two-thirds of HS patients present with the classic signs and a mild, uncompensated hemolytic anemia. Characteristically the jaundice is said to be "acholuric," because unconjugated bilirubin cannot pass the glomerular filter. Many of these patients have pigment gallstones, presumably caused by increased concentrations of bilirubin in the bile. About one-quarter of HS patients have a mild hemolytic state that is compensated for, and such patients are not anemic and are usually asymptomatic. A minority of patients (about 10%) have a severe hemolytic anemia that may require blood transfusion. Aplastic crises, in which erythropoiesis is suppressed leading to more pronounced anemia, occurs particularly in this group but may supervene in patients with milder forms of the disease. The usual cause of such crises

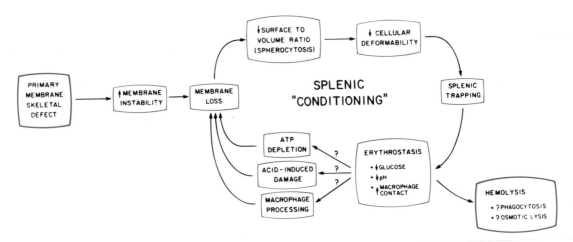

> ► FIGURE 9–5   Postulated mechanisms of "conditioning" and destruction of HS red cells in the spleen. (ATP = adenosine triphosphate.) (From Lux, SE, and Glader, BE: Disorders of the red cell membrane. In Nathan, DG, and Oski, FA (eds): Hematology of Infancy and Childhood, ed 2. WB Saunders, Philadelphia, 1981, with permission.)

is infection of erythropoietic precursors by parvovirus B19. An uncommon complication of prolonged hemolysis, which is not limited to HS, is chronic leg ulceration.

An interesting observation is that the clinical severity may vary in patients with the same gene mutation, implying that other factors influence the clinical presentation. These factors may include a second mutation or polymorphism inherited either in *cis* or in *trans* to the affected allele, which influences either its level of expression[27] or its stability or function.[25]

Clinical Laboratory Findings
Evidence of Hemolytic Process

The laboratory features of extravascular hemolysis, outlined earlier, are usually apparent. Hyperbilirubinemia is found in about half the patients, and haptoglobins are variably reduced. Classic features of intravascular hemolysis such as hemoglobinemia, hemoglobinuria, or hemosiderinuria do not occur. The reticulocyte production index is elevated above 2.5 in most cases (presplenectomy).

Red Cell Indices

Anemia is usually mild. The mean level of hemoglobin in several series is about 12 to 13 g/dL, but individual cases may vary widely depending on the severity of hemolysis and the degree of compensation. The mean corpuscular volume (MCV) is usually within normal range both before and after splenectomy but can be low, normal, or high. The mean corpuscular hemoglobin (MCH) tends to parallel the MCV. Although the MCV is usually normal, because of the red cell's spheroidal shape, the diameter of some cells is substantially decreased and these appear as dark, rounded microspherocytes on the peripheral smear (see Fig. 9–4). The mean corpuscular hemoglobin concentration (MCHC) is elevated (higher than 36%) in about 50% of cases and probably reflects mild cellular dehydration, particularly of cells that have undergone splenic conditioning and that have low levels of cell water and potassium (see the earlier section on Pathophysiology).

Morphology of Peripheral Smear

The morphological hallmark of HS is the spherocyte (see Fig. 9–4). Although in many instances the detection of these cells may present no difficulty, in some patients their detection may provoke argument even among experienced hematologists. It is particularly important to examine well-prepared smears free of any artifact. In typical cases prior to splenectomy there may be varying degrees of polychromasia, poikilocytosis, and anisocytosis with many normal discoid cells, but the overriding impression is one of increased numbers of uniformly round cells (see Fig. 9–4). Some of the cells appear as microspherocytes and are dark, round, and lack central pallor. Pincered or mushroom-shaped cells are often, but not exclusively, found in band 3–deficient patients. An interesting observation is the presence of acanthocytes on the peripheral blood smears of HS patients with β-spectrin defects.

Special Laboratory Tests
OSMOTIC FRAGILITY TEST

This test is essentially a measure of the surface-to-volume ratio of the red cell. If the test is performed on fresh red cells, it is then also a measure of the proportion of cells that have undergone splenic conditioning. When red cells are placed in a series of graded hypotonic salt solutions, water rapidly enters the cells and osmotic equilibrium is achieved. The cells swell and become spherical, and eventually a critical volume is reached at which point the cellular contents (hemoglobin) leak out and ultimately the cell may burst. Red cells of patients with HS, because of their decreased surface area-to-volume ratio, can tolerate less swelling than normal cells and lyse at higher concentrations of salt than do normal cells. About 25% of HS patients have normal osmotic fragility of fresh red cells, particularly in the very group that is mildly affected and is difficult to diagnose on morphological grounds. Generally, patients in the latter group, as well as patients with more typical cases, have abnormal osmotic fragility of red cells that have been stressed by prior sterile incubation for 24 hours. During the 24-hour incubation, HS cells have greater loss of membrane surface because of the relative membrane instability. A corollary of the use of the incubated osmotic fragility test is that if the test result is normal, it is highly unlikely that one is dealing with a patient with HS. Representative osmotic fragility curves for fresh and incubated normal and HS red cells are shown in Figure 9–6. Increased osmotic fragility is independent of the cause of spheroidal cells; for

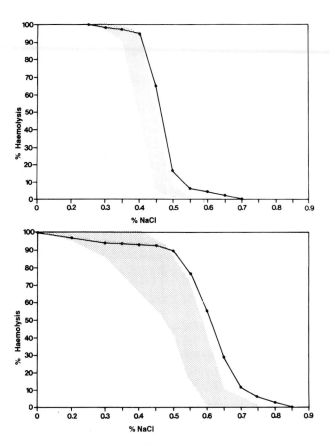

> **FIGURE 9–6** Osmotic fragility curves of fresh blood (*top*) and incubated blood (*bottom*) obtained from a patient with HS. The normal range is shown by dotted areas. Note the increased fragility of the HS red cells to osmotic lysis.

example, it may be found in autoimmune hemolytic anemia, burns, and so on (see Chap. 28).

AUTOHEMOLYSIS TEST

This relatively sensitive test in the diagnosis of HS measures the structural and metabolic integrity of the HS red cell membrane under conditions of erythrostasis and relative glucose depletion, that is, sterile incubation of red cells in their own plasma for 48 hours at 37°C. The HS red cell is leaky to sodium. To "keep its head above water," the cell utilizes adenosine triphosphate (ATP) and glucose to drive the cation pump to a greater extent than normal. Associated with the increased activity of the pump, there is a greater turnover of membrane phospholipids and associated membrane fragmentation with a decrease in surface-to-volume ratio until the critical hemolytic volume is reached and autohemolysis occurs. The usual range of autohemolysis in HS cells is variable and is about 10% to 50%, compared with control values of 0.2% to 2.0%. However, a minority of patients show only minimally elevated autohemolysis or may even be within the normal range. In most HS patients, addition of glucose markedly diminishes autohemolysis but not usually to within the normal range of samples incubated with glucose (0% to 1.0%). A minority of patients show no correction of autohemolysis with glucose, a finding also obtained with many patients with spherocytosis associated with autoimmune hemolytic anemia. It should be noted that many laboratories do not use this test routinely (see Chap. 28 for a description of the procedure).

RED CELL MEMBRANE STUDIES

Densitometric quantitation of red cell membrane proteins separated by sodium dodecyl sulfate polyacrylamide gel electrophoresis (SDS PAGE) reveals the underlying quantitative defect in the majority of HS patients. The abnormality in the remaining cases may either be a subtle deficiency in one of the proteins, which is not detected by SDS PAGE, or an altered functional interaction between membrane proteins. Once the defective protein has been identified, deoxyribonucleic acid (DNA) and ribonucleic acid (RNA) analyses are required to elucidate the causative mutations.

Treatment

From the foregoing discussion of the pathophysiology of the HS red cell and the central role of the spleen in "conditioning" such cells and ultimately leading to their destruction, it should not be surprising that splenectomy is functionally curative in the majority of patients with this disease. In the relatively rare patient with severe spectrin deficiency (less than 40% spectrin), clinical improvement occurs after splenectomy but ongoing hemolysis and anemia may continue. In the usual case, although spherocytosis persists, "conditioned" microspherocytes are no longer seen and red cell life span is normal or very near normal. At one time, many authorities recommended splenectomy uniformly in all patients with HS because of the risks of biliary tract disease and the development of aplastic crises, but this view has been considerably tempered in recent years. Patients with mild, compensated cases of HS are usually not offered splenectomy unless the previously mentioned complications intervene. An important consideration in infants and young children is the risk of postsplenectomy sepsis, particularly with *Streptococcus pneumoniae,* so that most authorities recommend deferment of splenectomy until about 6 years of age. In severe cases, however, splenectomy may have to be performed earlier; but in either event, treatment with pneumococcal vaccine is recommended, preferably starting before splenectomy. Younger children may also require prophylactic penicillin or other antibiotics postsplenectomy, but the latter course is controversial. Failure of splenectomy is almost always associated with an accessory spleen not removed at surgery, or more rarely is caused by autotransplantation of splenic tissue in the peritoneal cavity, leading to splenosis.

> ## CASE STUDY 1

A 40-year-old woman presented to her physician with an attack of acute cholecystitis. Physical examination revealed a palpable spleen in addition to the signs of acute cholecystitis. On investigation she was found to have numerous gallstones, and a routine blood count showed a mild, compensated hemolytic state: Hgb, 13.8 g/dL; Hct, 38%; MCV, 80 fL; MCHC, 36%; reticulocyte count, 7%; shift cells present; RPI, 3.9. The peripheral smear showed moderate numbers of spherocytes and a few microspherocytes. The Coombs test was negative. Unconjugated bilirubin was 2.5 mg/dL, and the conjugated bilirubin was 0.5 mg/dL. Haptoglobin concentration was less than 10

continued

mg/dL (normal range is 25 to 180 mg/dL). Further investigation revealed that osmotic fragility of both fresh and incubated venous blood was increased. Autohemolysis was 25% after 48 hours' incubation, corrected to 3% in the presence of glucose. After the acute episode had settled, an elective cholecystectomy was performed. A diagnosis of hereditary spherocytosis was made and confirmed in a subsequent study of the patient's family when two of her three children were found to have mild, compensated hemolytic states associated with spherocytosis. In view of the risk of recurrence of common bile duct calculi, an elective splenectomy was performed 6 months later, curing the hemolytic state.

Questions

1. Why was a Coombs test performed on this patient?
2. What type of hemolysis is occurring in this patient?
3. What is the surface-to-volume ratio of these red cells as indicated by the osmotic fragility test?
4. In what type of hemolytic anemia is the osmotic fragility uncorrected by glucose?
5. Which of the red blood cell (RBC) indices is typically increased in HS?

Hereditary Elliptocytosis

Mode of Inheritance

Hereditary elliptocytosis (HE) is a group of disorders found in all race groups and characterized by the presence of elliptical red cells in the peripheral blood (Fig. 9–7). The HE syndrome is heterogeneous in terms of inheritance, clinical manifestations, and underlying molecular defects. It is usually inherited in an autosomal dominant fashion, except for hereditary pyropoikilocytosis (HPP), which is a recessive and very severe HE variant.

Clinical Phenotypes

Three major clinical and morphological phenotypes have been delineated by Palek and Lux: common HE, including HPP; spherocytic HE; and Southeast Asian ovalocytosis (SAO).[23,24] *Common HE* is the most prevalent, especially in African populations. There is marked clinical and morphological heterogeneity, ranging from an asymptomatic carrier state with normal morphology to homozygous HE and HPP with severe hemolysis and bizarre poikilocytic and microspherocytic morphology (Fig. 9–8; see also Color Plate 104). The most frequently occurring clinical form is mild HE with no or minimal hemolysis. *Spherocytic HE* is a rare phenotypic hybrid of HE and HS, in which the clinical course resembles HS and responds well to splenectomy. *Southeast Asian ovalocytosis* is very common in Melanesian and other Southeast Asian population groups because of the protective effect toward malaria; it also occurs in the Cape Coloured population of South Africa.[36]

Common Hereditary Elliptocytosis

Molecular Defects

The underlying abnormality in HE resides in the red cell membrane skeleton and usually involves spectrin or protein 4.1 (Table 9–4).

Spectrin mutations that impair the self-association of spectrin dimers into tetramers are the most common. This functional defect is caused by an alteration in the structure of the spectrin self-association site, usually involving the N-terminal domain of α spectrin, or less frequently, the C-terminal domain of β spectrin. This disrupts the 106–amino acid spectrin repeats and alters the partial tryptic cleavage pattern of spectrin. The affected domain, as well as the size of the abnormal tryptic peptide, is used in the nomenclature of these defects, and SpαI/74, SpαI/65, and SpαI/46 are the most common. The extent of impairment of spectrin dimer self-association and the amount and type of abnormal tryptic peptide correlate with the clinical severity.[37] Several mutations have been described in both α- and β-spectrin genes.

Point mutations in the α-*spectrin* gene, resulting in single amino acid substitutions close to the tryptic cleavage site, are most common. Codon 28 of the α-spectrin gene, CGT, is a "hotspot" for mutations, and the normal arginine is replaced by one of four different amino acids, causing SpαI/74.[38] Interestingly, a histidine (CAT) substitution predominates in American blacks who originated from West Africa, whereas southern African blacks have a cysteine (TGT) mutation. SpαI/65 is invariably caused by a duplication of codon 154, which inserts an additional leucine into the protein, and is

➤ FIGURE 9–7   Photomicrograph of peripheral blood smear from a patient with mild hereditary elliptocytosis (HE). Note the high percentage of elliptocytes.

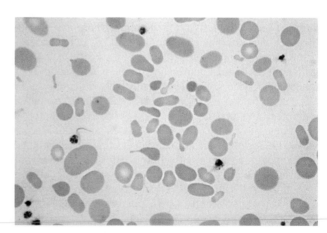

➤ FIGURE 9–8   Photomicrograph of peripheral blood smear from a patient with hereditary pyropoikilocytosis (HPP). Note the bizarre micropoikilocytosis, red cell budding, and lack of elliptocytes.

> ➤ **Table 9-4**
> ## DEFECTS OF RED CELL MEMBRANE PROTEINS IN HEREDITARY ELLIPTOCYTOSIS
>
> **Protein Deficiencies**
>
> Protein 4.1
>
> Glycophorin C
>
> Spectrin (HPP)
>
> **Protein Dysfunction**
>
> Spectrin dimer self-association
>
>   α Spectrin mutations
>
>   β Spectrin mutations
>
> Truncated α or β spectrin
>
> Spectrin-ankyrin interaction
>
> Protein 4.1–spectrin interaction
>
> Band 3 (SAO)

Abbreviations: HPP = hereditary pyropoikilocytosis; SAO = Southeast Asian ovalocytosis.

common in Central and North Africa.[39,40] In-frame deletions have been documented in α spectrin; for example, in Sp_{Dayton} the insertion of a novel mobile element into the α-spectrin gene causes skipping of exon 5.[41] $Sp_{St. Claude}$ has a single point mutation in intron 19 of α spectrin, which creates two different RNA splice forms. At the protein level this ultimately has long-range negative effects on tetramer formation and on the binding of β spectrin to ankyrin.[42,43]

Mutations in β *spectrin* include missense point mutations, as well as frameshift errors caused by small deletions,

insertions, or splice-site mutations that result in mutant β-spectrin molecules with truncated C-terminal domains.[25]

A decreased amount of *protein 4.1* has also been implicated in HE. This is usually the result of mutations influencing the translation initiation site, or more rarely, of deletions that shorten the protein or abolish spectrin binding.[22,25]

Hereditary Pyropoikilocytosis
HPP is an interesting, relatively rare, severe hemolytic disease that is part of the HE group of disorders. The peripheral blood smear is characterized by microspherocytosis, micropoikilocytosis, fragments, and relatively few, if any, elliptocytes (see Fig. 9–8 and Color Plate 104). Persons with HPP are compound heterozygotes, and all cases thus far investigated exhibit two genetic defects:

1. A mutant α or β spectrin that shows severe impairment of spectrin dimer self-association.[37]
2. A partial spectrin deficiency resulting from decreased synthesis of α spectrin, which causes the characteristic microspherocytosis.[44,45]

Pathophysiology of Common HE and HPP
The molecular defects in common HE involve horizontal interactions between proteins of the membrane skeleton (Fig. 9–9). Defective spectrin dimer self-association or protein 4.1 deficiency weakens the skeleton and, under the influence of shear stress in the circulation, the cells become distorted and progressively lose their ability to regain their original disc shape, resulting in elliptocytes and poikilocytes. The clinical expression of HE is variable and can differ between individuals of the same family with the identical mutation, implying that other mutations or polymorphisms influence

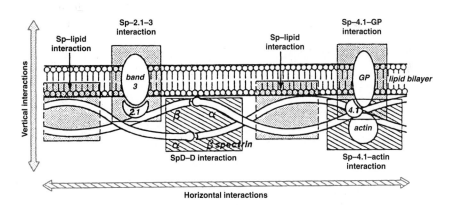

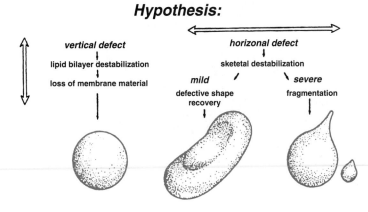

➤ **FIGURE 9–9** Pathophysiology of the red cell lesion in hereditary spherocytosis (HS), hereditary elliptocytosis (HE), and hereditary pyropoikilocytosis (HPP). The top section is a diagrammatic illustration of the vertical and horizontal interactions between the red cell membrane components. The bottom left-hand section illustrates a defect in a vertical interaction resulting in spherocytes and HS. The bottom right-hand section illustrates a defect in a horizontal interaction resulting in elliptocytes and poikilocytes (HE and HPP). (From Palek, J: Disorders of red cell membrane skeleton: An overview. In Kruckeberg, WL, et al (eds): Erythrocyte Membranes 3: Recent Clinical and Experimental Advances. Liss, New York, 1984, p 177, with permission.)

the expression of the mutant allele. A low expression α spectrin allele, Sp_{Lely}, is an example of a modifying polymorphism that exacerbates the clinical phenotype when inherited in *trans* to a mutant α-spectrin allele.[46]

In the case of HPP, the clinical severity and morphology are thought to result from a combination of horizontal and vertical defects. Spectrin self-association (horizontal defect) is severely impaired in HPP, which markedly decreases the strength and stability of the skeleton, resulting in poikilocytes and fragmentation. Spectrin deficiency impairs the vertical interaction of the skeleton with the lipid bilayer and gives rise to microspherocytes as described for HS (see Fig. 9–9).

Southeast Asian Ovalocytosis

SAO is a very common, asymptomatic condition in ethnic Southeast Asian populations. It also occurs in the Cape Coloured population of South Africa, where it can be associated with mild hemolysis.[36] SAO is characterized by rigid, spoon-shaped ovalocytes (Fig. 9–10) that are resistant to invasion by malaria parasites and provide an example of the selective pressure of malaria.[47] The underlying molecular defect is a deletion of 27 base pairs in exon 11 of the band 3 gene, resulting in the absence of nine amino acids at the junction of the cytoplasmic and transmembrane domains of the band 3 protein.[48,49] This alters the structure and function of the mutant band 3, causing increased binding to ankyrin,[50] an inability to transport anions,[51] and markedly restricted lateral and rotational mobility in the membrane.[52]

Clinical Laboratory Findings

Evidence of Hemolytic Process

The usual picture in the most common variant (mild HE) is that of a very mild, compensated hemolytic anemia in which the only features may be a slight reticulocytosis and decreased haptoglobin levels. Many patients show no biochemical evidence of a hemolytic process. In the more severe cases, such as in spherocytic HE, HE with infantile poikilocytosis, homozygous HE, and HPP, the usual features of extravascular hemolysis outlined earlier are found.

Morphology of Peripheral Smear

The morphology of the peripheral smear varies with the clinical phenotypes of HE. In the usual variant of *mild HE*

with no hemolysis or a compensated hemolytic state, the red cells show prominent uniform elliptocytosis, the cells being elliptical rather than oval or egg shaped (see Fig. 9–7). Usually, more than 30% of the red cells are elliptocytic, but many patients have a higher proportion of elliptocytes, for example, more than 75%. Very elongated or rod-shaped cells are characteristic and often constitute more than 10% of the red cells. In patients with uncompensated hemolysis (mild HE with sporadic hemolysis), the red cells show more prominent poikilocytosis, and a small proportion of elliptocytes may have budlike projections.

Infants with *mild HE and poikilocytosis* of infancy exhibit prominent poikilocytosis, microspherocytosis, fragmentation, budding of red cells, and a variable degree of elliptocytosis (Fig. 9–11). By the time the infant reaches the age of 1 to 2 years, the morphology has changed to that characteristic of mild HE. In the neonatal period, the red cells show increased thermal sensitivity (which is also a characteristic of HPP), but the diagnosis is suggested by finding evidence of mild HE in one parent.

The rare patients with *homozygous HE* or *HPP* (see Fig. 9–8 and Color Plate 104) present with marked microspherocytosis, micropoikilocytosis, fragments, and very few, if any, elliptocytes.

Red cell morphology in *spherocytic HE* is very variable, but the hallmarks are less prominent elliptocytosis with spherocytes and microspherocytes. The proportion of spherocytes and elliptocytes varies in different kindred and even within the same kindred. Patients with stomatocytic HE or *SAO* have very distinctive red cell morphology. The elliptocytes are more rounded and oval and are often quite large with a transverse bar that divides the central pale space (see Fig. 9–10).

Red Cell Indices

In the common variants of mild HE with compensated and uncompensated hemolysis, the MCV is usually normal or slightly elevated, the latter finding probably reflecting an associated reticulocytosis. MCH and MCHC are also usually within the normal range. In infants with HE and poikilocytosis, the MCV may be decreased and the MCHC is either normal or slightly elevated. In HPP, the MCV is always decreased and the MCHC is usually elevated.

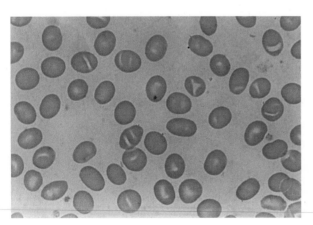

➤ FIGURE 9–10 Photomicrograph of peripheral blood smear from a patient with Southeast Asian ovalocytosis (SAO). Note the characteristic spoon-shaped oval cells with a band across the central area.

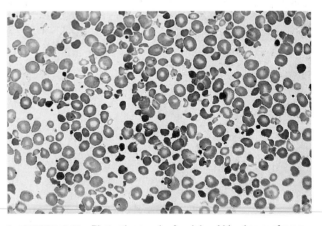

➤ FIGURE 9–11 Photomicrograph of peripheral blood smear from a patient with mild HE and poikilocytosis of infancy. Note the poikilocytosis and fragmentation.

Special Laboratory Tests

OSMOTIC FRAGILITY AND AUTOHEMOLYSIS

The osmotic fragility and autohemolysis tests are useful additional tests in delineating some of the HE phenotypes. In patients with mild HE (compensated and uncompensated) both the preincubation and the postincubation osmotic fragility and autohemolysis results are normal. Rarely, patients with mild HE and uncompensated hemolysis, may have increased autohemolysis corrected by glucose. However, in HPP, pre- and postincubation osmotic fragility is markedly increased, and autohemolysis is increased and unaffected by glucose. Pre- and postincubation osmotic fragility are uniformly increased in spherocytic HE, and autohemolysis is characteristically increased but corrected by glucose. Children with HE and infantile poikilocytosis have increased osmotic fragility and autohemolysis in the early neonatal period that revert to normal with the development of more prominent elliptocytosis.

RED CELL MEMBRANE STUDIES

Red cell membrane protein deficiencies or size abnormalities may be detected by SDS PAGE and quantitation, as described earlier for HS. Spectrin dimer self-association is analyzed by extracting spectrin from the membrane at 4°C followed by nondenaturing PAGE and quantitation of spectrin dimers and tetramers.

Treatment

Patients with compensated mild HE and no splenomegaly have a benign disorder and require no therapeutic intervention. Those with HE and uncompensated hemolysis usually benefit from splenectomy, which is also uniformly beneficial to patients with HPP and spherocytic HE. Patients with HE and infantile poikilocytosis should be recognized and treated symptomatically, because they will improve spontaneously with the development of a clinical picture indistinguishable from mild HE.

➤ CASE STUDY 2

A 45-year-old woman presented to her physician complaining of malaise and tiredness on mild exertion. On physical examination, she was found to have slight scleral icterus and a two-finger splenomegaly. A blood count revealed the following: Hgb, 11.0 g/dL; Hct, 32%; MCHC, 34.3%; MCV, 100 fL; reticulocyte count, 12.0%; shift cells on peripheral smear; and RPI, 5.7. The peripheral smear showed about 80% elliptocytes with some poikilocytosis consisting of a few fragmented cells and budding elliptocytes. Unconjugated bilirubin was 3.5 mg/dL, conjugated bilirubin, 0.6 mg/dL, and haptoglobin, 15 mg/dL (normal range is 25 to 180 mg/dL). Preincubation and postincubation osmotic fragility and autohemolysis were within the normal range. Examination of the patient's family showed striking elliptocytes with normal hemoglobin and reticulocyte count in her father and in one of her three children. A diagnosis of mild HE with sporadic hemolysis was made, and a good response to splenectomy was obtained.

Questions

1. How can the anemia presented here be classified?
2. What parameter(s) is (are) suggestive of effective erythropoiesis?
3. Do the laboratory values presented here indicate hemolysis in this patient?
4. What is the significance of the RPI value?

➤ DISORDERS OF MEMBRANE CATION PERMEABILITY

Hereditary Stomatocytosis (Hydrocytosis) and Hereditary Xerocytosis

This is a heterogeneous group of rare disorders characterized by alterations in the permeability of the red cell membrane to cations.[24] Two main clinical and morphological syndromes have been described: hereditary stomatocytosis (hydrocytosis), in which the red cells are swollen (Fig. 9–12); and hereditary xerocytosis, in which the cells are markedly dehydrated (Fig. 9–13). Several intermediate syndromes have been described, but these syndromes are not considered here.

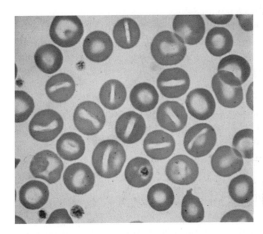

➤ FIGURE 9–12 Photomicrograph of peripheral blood smear from a patient with hereditary stomatocytosis. Note the high percentage of red cells with a central slit of pallor. (From Bell, A: Hematology. In: Listen, Look and Learn. Health and Education Resources, Inc., Bethesda, MD, with permission.)

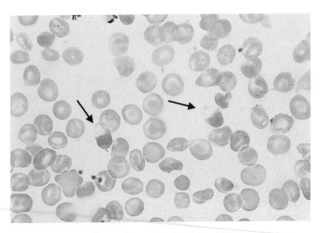

➤ FIGURE 9–13 Photomicrograph of peripheral blood smear from a patient with hereditary xerocytosis. Note the characteristic target cells and cells with hemoglobin concentrated on one side of the cell.

Mode of Inheritance

Hereditary stomatocytosis is inherited in an autosomal dominant fashion, but some patients with severe hemolysis show autosomal recessive inheritance. Hereditary xerocytosis is inherited by autosomal dominant transmission.

Etiology and Pathophysiology

An important determinant of the water content of red cells is the total intracellular concentration of the monovalent cations, sodium and potassium. To maintain osmotic equilibrium, water enters cells in which the total cation content is increased, leading to swelling and hydrocyte formation. In contrast, a net loss of cations results in a movement of water out of the cell with formation of dehydrated cells (xerocytes).

The basic abnormality of *stomatocytic* red cells is a marked increase in the passive permeability of sodium into the cell and of potassium out of the cell. The defect in sodium permeability is greater than that for potassium. Although the sodium-potassium pump is stimulated by the influx of sodium, it cannot cope with the influx, and the total cation content of the cell increases, with resultant water influx and formation of hydrocytes. A deficiency of one component of band 7, designated stomatin (see Table 9–2), has been reported in these patients,[53] although the DNA sequence of the gene is normal. How this relates to the permeability lesion is unknown, but one possibility is that stomatin associates with another protein, which is required for insertion or stabilization of stomatin in the membrane. This protein may be the true defective protein. Because of the influx of water, stomatocytes have an increased volume with a decreased surface-to-volume ratio and the attendant consequences of decreased red cell deformability and susceptibility to splenic sequestration. Although splenectomy is predictably beneficial in most patients with hereditary stomatocytosis, paradoxically some patients with severe permeability defects do not have significant hemolysis, suggesting that other, still unknown factors may be important in the destruction of these cells.

Stomatocytes are also found in Rh null disease, a hemolytic anemia characterized by an absence of the Rh antigens. This disorder is clinically and biochemically heterogeneous, and the molecular pathophysiology is not completely understood.

Red cells from patients with hereditary *xerocytosis* have an increased efflux of potassium that approximates sodium influx. Although the sodium-potassium pump is stimulated by the influx of sodium, it is insufficient to correct the loss of potassium. Irreversible potassium and total cation loss occurs with resultant dehydration and formation of xerocytes. The underlying molecular pathology is not understood. Xerocytes have an increased surface-to-volume ratio, an increased MCHC, and presumably increased cell viscosity, which make them less deformable and liable to sequestration in the reticuloendothelial system. The red cells are not specifically sequestered in the spleen, so that splenectomy does not have a beneficial effect.

Clinical Laboratory Findings

Morphology of Peripheral Smear

The characteristic morphological features of hereditary *stomatocytosis* are a tendency toward macrocytosis and the presence of stomatocytes on the peripheral smear. These are red cells with a central slit or stoma (see Fig. 9–12). On phase contrast or scanning electron microscopy, the cells have a bowl-like appearance. In hereditary *xerocytosis*, target cells are present, reflecting the greater surface-to-volume ratio of these cells. Small spiculated echinocytes and cells with hemoglobin concentrated in one part of the cell are also features of hereditary xerocytosis (see Fig. 9–13).

Red Cell Indices

The MCV in both hereditary stomatocytosis and hereditary xerocytosis is elevated, despite the cellular dehydration in the latter condition. The MCHC is decreased in hereditary stomatocytosis and increased in hereditary xerocytosis.

Special Laboratory Tests

Osmotic fragility is increased in hereditary *stomatocytosis* and reflects the decreased surface-to-volume ratio. Red cell sodium concentration is markedly elevated, and potassium concentration is decreased. Total monovalent cation content is increased. In contrast, red cells in hereditary *xerocytosis* have strikingly decreased osmotic fragility, reflecting the increased surface-to-volume ratio. Red cell potassium concentration is markedly decreased, sodium concentration may be normal or increased, and total cation concentration is decreased.

Treatment

Most patients with hemolysis caused by hereditary stomatocytosis respond well to splenectomy. However, patients with hereditary xerocytosis do not benefit from splenectomy, presumably because of more generalized sequestration of these cells.

> ## ➤ CASE STUDY 3

A 6-year-old boy was noted by his mother to have slight scleral icterus and was referred for further investigation. He complained of some tiredness on exertion but was otherwise symptom-free. Physical examination showed only a one-finger splenomegaly. A blood count showed the following: Hgb, 10.8 g/dL; Hct, 29%; MCHC, 37%; MCV, 100 fL; reticulocyte count, 10%. Numerous target cells, some spiculated cells, and a few cells showing eccentric concentration of hemoglobin at one pole of the red cell were seen on the peripheral smear. The unconjugated bilirubin level was mildly elevated, and serum haptoglobin levels were decreased. There was no hemoglobinemia or hemosiderinuria. The osmotic fragility curve was strikingly decreased. Determination of red cell cation concentrations revealed a markedly decreased red cell potassium level of 65 mEq/L of RBCs (normal is 90 to 104 mEq/L) and a slightly elevated red cell sodium level of 15 mEq/L of RBCs (normal is 5 to 12 mEq/L). Similar findings were obtained in the child's father, who had previously been diagnosed at another center as having an "unusual" form of anemia. A diagnosis of hereditary xerocytosis was made. Splenectomy was not advised, and the child has maintained a hemoglobin level varying between 9.5 and 11.0 g/dL over the past 2 years.

continued

Questions
1. How can this anemia be classified, as indicated by the RBC indices?
2. What does the decreased osmotic fragility represent?
3. Why would a splenectomy not be beneficial in this case?
4. Why are these red cells (xerocytes) said to be dehydrated with regard to osmotic equilibrium?

QUESTIONS

1. What happens when normal donor red cells are transfused into a patient with an intracorpuscular red cell defect?
   a. Donor cells are destroyed
   b. Donor cells have normal survival
   c. Depends on the severity of the defect
   d. Depends on the severity of the anemia

2. Which of the following tests is not used to determine increased red cell destruction?
   a. Unconjugated (indirect) bilirubin
   b. Serum haptoglobin
   c. Schumm's test
   d. Reticulocyte count

3. An anemic patient investigated for a hemolytic state has the following laboratory findings: hemoglobin, 8 g/dL; hematocrit, 23%; reticulocyte count, 8%; shift cells on peripheral smear. What is the RPI?
   a. 8
   b. 4
   c. 2
   d. 1

4. What tests are useful in the classification of the cause of red cell hemolysis?
   a. Direct Coombs test
   b. Indirect Coombs test and hemoglobin level
   c. Reticulocyte count and hemoglobin electrophoresis
   d. Red cell enzyme studies and iron-binding capacity

5. Which of the following red cell membrane protein deficiencies does not cause hereditary spherocytosis?
   a. Ankyrin
   b. Protein 4.1
   c. Spectrin
   d. Protein 4.2
   e. Band 3

6. Which of the following laboratory tests would not be typical of hereditary spherocytosis?
   a. Increased osmotic fragility
   b. Spherocytes on peripheral smear
   c. Decreased MCHC
   d. Increased RPI

7. Which is the most frequent functional abnormality affecting membrane skeleton proteins in common hereditary elliptocytosis?
   a. Defective binding of spectrin to ankyrin
   b. Defective spectrin tetramer assembly
   c. Defective binding of ankyrin to protein 3
   d. Deficiency of protein 4.1

8. Which of the following abnormalities is (are) thought to cause the severe fragmentation and microspherocytes characteristic of hereditary pyropoikilocytosis?
   a. Susceptibility of spectrin to thermal denaturation
   b. Defective membrane spectrin tetramer assembly and spectrin deficiency
   c. Unstable membrane lipids
   d. Membrane ankyrin deficiency

9. Which disorders are classified as disorders of membrane cation permeability?
   a. Hereditary stomatocytosis and hereditary xerocytosis
   b. Sideroblastic anemia and myelofibrosis
   c. Autoimmune hemolytic anemia and microangiopathic hemolytic anemia
   d. Ehlers-Danlos syndrome and Bernard-Soulier syndrome

SUMMARY CHART

➤ Anemia may occur with a moderate shortening of the red cell life span if there is an associated depression of bone marrow function, which may occur with certain systemic diseases or exposure to chemicals.
➤ Hemolytic anemias may be classified as follows:
  ➤ **Intracorpuscular**
    • *Hereditary defects*
      • Defects in the red cell membrane
      • Enzyme defects
      • Hemoglobinopathies
      • Thalassemia syndromes
    • *Acquired defects*
      • Paroxysmal nocturnal hemoglobinuria
  ➤ **Extracorpuscular**
    • *Immune hemolytic anemias*
    • *Infections*
    • *Chemicals or toxins*
    • *Physical agents*
    • *Microangiopathic or macroangiopathic*
    • *Splenic sequestration (hypersplenism)*
    • *General systemic disorders*
➤ The most frequently used test reflecting increased red cell destruction is the serum unconjugated (indirect) bilirubin and serum haptoglobin determinations. Other tests, if primarily intravascular, are those that test for the presence of hemoglobinemia, hemoglobinuria, and hemosiderinuria.

> The reticulocyte production index (RPI) is calculated by the following equation:

$$RPI = \frac{\% \text{ Reticulocytes}}{\text{Reticulocyte maturation time}} \times \frac{\text{Hematocrit}}{45}$$

> The red cell membrane skeleton consists of structural proteins, α and β spectrin, actin, and protein 4.1.

> Hereditary hemolytic anemias are broken into four main groups:
> > **Hereditary spherocytosis (HS)**
> > **Hereditary elliptocytosis (HE) and hereditary pyropoikilocytosis (HPP)**
> > **Hereditary stomatocytosis**
> > **Hereditary xerocytosis**

> Hemolytic anemias characteristically have a mean corpuscular volume (MCV) that is normal (but can be low or high); a mean corpuscular hemoglobin that parallels the MCV; and a mean corpuscular hemoglobin concentration (MCHC) that is elevated (above 36%).

> Osmotic fragility measures the surface-to-volume ratio of the red blood cell. RBCs of patients with HS tolerate less swelling than normal cells and lyse at a higher concentration of salt.

References

1. Hillman, RS, and Finch, CA: Red Cell Manual, ed 7. FA Davis, Philadelphia, 1996.
2. Lux, SE, and Glader, BE: Disorders of the red cell membrane. In Nathan, DG, and Oski, FA (eds): Hematology of Infancy and Childhood, ed 2. WB Saunders, Philadelphia, 1981.
3. Liu, SC, and Derick, LH: Molecular anatomy of the red blood cell membrane skeleton: Structure-function relationships. Semin Hematol 29:231, 1992.
4. Liu, SC, et al: Visualization of the hexagonal lattice in the erythrocyte membrane skeleton. J Cell Biol 104:527, 1987.
5. Gilligan, DM, and Bennett, V: The junctional complex of the membrane skeleton. Semin Hematol 30:74, 1993.
6. Bennett, V, and Stenbuck, PJ: The membrane attachment protein for spectrin is associated with band 3 in human erythrocyte membranes. Nature 280:468, 1979.
7. Cohen, CM, et al: Human erythrocyte membrane protein 4.2 (Pallidin). Semin Hematol 30:119, 1993.
8. Pasternack, GR, et al: Interactions between protein 4.1 and band 3: An alternative binding site for an element of the membrane skeleton. J Biol Chem 260:3676, 1985.
9. Marfatia, SM, et al: In vitro binding studies suggest a membrane-associated complex between erythroid p55, protein 4.1, and glycophorin C. J Biol Chem 269:8631, 1994.
10. Gallagher, PG, and Forget, BG: Spectrin genes in health and disease. Semin Hematol 30:4, 1993.
11. Sahr, KE, et al: The complete cDNA and polypeptide sequences of human erythroid α spectrin. J Biol Chem 265:4434, 1990.
12. Winkelmann, JC, et al: Full length sequence of the cDNA for human erythroid β spectrin. J Biol Chem 265:11827, 1990.
13. Speicher, DW, et al: A structural model of human spectrin: Alignment of chemical and functional domains. J Biol Chem 257:9093, 1982.
14. Speicher, DW, and Marchesi, VT: Erythrocyte spectrin is comprised of many homologous triple helical segments. Nature 311:177, 1984.
15. Yan, Y, et al: Crystal structure of the repetitive segments of spectrin. Science 262:2027, 1993.
16. Speicher, DW, et al: Properties of human red cell spectrin heterodimer (side-to-side) assembly and identification of an essential nucleation site. J Biol Chem 267:14775, 1992.
17. Speicher, DW, et al: Location of the human red cell spectrin tetramer binding site and detection of a related "closed" hairpin loop dimer using proteolytic footprinting. J Biol Chem 268:4227, 1993.
18. Hanspal, M, and Palek, J: Biogenesis of normal and abnormal red blood cell membrane skeleton. Semin Hematol 29:305, 1992.
19. Woods, CM, and Lazarides, E: Degradation of unassembled alpha and beta spectrin by distinct intracellular pathways: Regulation of spectrin topogenesis by beta spectrin degradation. Cell 40:959, 1985.
20. Tanner, MJA: The structure and function of band 3 (AE1): Recent developments. Mol Membr Biol 14:155, 1997.
21. Peters, LL, and Lux, SE: Ankyrins: Structure and function in normal cells and hereditary spherocytes. Semin Hematol 30:85, 1993.
22. Conboy, JG: Structure, function, and molecular genetics of erythroid membrane skeletal protein 4.1 in normal and abnormal red blood cells. Semin Hematol 30:58, 1993.
23. Palek, J: Disorders of red cell membrane skeleton: An overview. In Kruckeberg, WL, et al (eds): Erythrocyte Membranes 3: Recent Clinical and Experimental Advances. Liss, New York, 1984, p 177.
24. Lux, SE, and Palek, J: Disorders of the red cell membrane. In Handin, RI, et al (eds): Blood: Principles and Practice of Hematology. Philadelphia, Lippincott, 1995, p 1701.
25. Tse, WT, and Lux, SE: Red blood cell membrane disorders. Br J Haematol 104:2, 1999.
26. Agre, P, et al: Inheritance pattern and clinical response to splenectomy as a reflection of erythrocyte spectrin deficiency in hereditary spherocytosis. N Engl J Med 315:1579, 1986.
27. Wichterle, H, et al: Combination of two mutant α spectrin alleles underlies a severe spherocytic hemolytic anemia. J Clin Invest 98:2300, 1996.
28. Becker, PS, et al: βSpectrin Kissimmee: A spectrin variant associated with autosomal dominant hereditary spherocytosis and defective binding to protein 4.1. J Clin Invest 92:612, 1993.
29. Coetzer, TL, et al: Partial ankyrin and spectrin deficiency in severe atypical hereditary spherocytosis. N Engl J Med 318:230, 1988.
30. Hanspal, M, et al: Molecular basis of spectrin and ankyrin deficiencies in severe hereditary spherocytosis: Evidence implicating a primary defect of ankyrin. Blood 77:165, 1991.
31. Lux, SE, et al: Hereditary spherocytosis associated with deletion of the human ankyrin gene on chromosome 8. Nature 345:736, 1990.
32. Bass, EB, et al: Further evidence for localization of the spherocytosis gene on chromosome 8. Ann Intern Med 99:192, 1983.
33. Jarolim, P, et al: Mutations of conserved arginines in the membrane domain of erythroid band 3 lead to a decrease in membrane-associated band 3 and to the phenotype of hereditary spherocytosis. Blood 85:634, 1995.
34. Van Zyl, C, et al: Codon 760 of the erythrocyte anion exchanger is a "hotspot" for mutations in hereditary spherocytosis. In press.
35. Bouhassira, EE, et al: An alanine to threonine substitution in protein 4.2 cDNA associated with a Japanese form of hereditary hemolytic anemia (protein 4.2 Nippon). Blood 79:1846, 1992.
36. Coetzer, TL, et al: Southeast Asian Ovalocytosis (SAO) in a South African kindred with hemolytic anemia. Blood 87:1656, 1996.
37. Coetzer, TL, et al: Molecular determinants of clinical expression of hereditary elliptocytosis and pyropoikilocytosis. Blood 70:766, 1987.
38. Coetzer, TL, et al: Four different mutations in codon 28 of α spectrin are associated with structurally and functionally abnormal spectrin α I/74 in hereditary elliptocytosis. J Clin Invest 88:743, 1991.
39. Sahr, KE, et al: Sequence and exon-intron organization of the DNA encoding the αI domain of human spectrin. Application to the study of mutations causing hereditary elliptocytosis. J Clin Invest 84:1243, 1989.
40. Roux, AF, et al: Molecular basis of SpαI/65 hereditary elliptocytosis in North Africa: Insertion of a TTG triplet between codons 147 and 149 in the α spectrin gene from five unrelated families. Blood 73:2196, 1989.
41. Hassoun, H, et al: A novel mobile element inserted in the α spectrin gene: Spectrin Dayton. A truncated α spectrin associated with hereditary elliptocytosis. J Clin Invest 94:643, 1994.
42. Zail, SS, and Coetzer, TL. Defective binding of spectrin to ankyrin in a kindred with recessively inherited hereditary elliptocytosis. J Clin Invest 74:753, 1984.
43. Burke, JPWG, et al: Reduced spectrin-ankyrin binding in a South African hereditary elliptocytosis kindred homozygous for Spectrin St Claude. Blood 92:2591, 1998.
44. Coetzer, TL, and Palek, J: Partial spectrin deficiency in hereditary pyropoikilocytosis. Blood 67:919, 1986.
45. Hanspal, M, et al: Molecular basis of spectrin deficiency in hereditary pyropoikilocytosis. Blood 82:1652, 1993.
46. Wilmotte, R, et al: Low expression allele α LELY of red cell spectrin is associated with mutations in exon 40 (αV/41 polymorphism) and intron 45 and with partial skipping of exon 46. J Clin Invest 91:2091, 1993.
47. Mohandas, N, et al: Rigid membranes of Malayan ovalocytes: A likely genetic barrier against malaria. Blood 63:1385, 1984.
48. Tanner, MJA, et al: Melanesian hereditary ovalocytes have a deletion in red cell band 3. Blood 78:2785, 1991.
49. Jarolim, P, et al: Deletion in erythrocyte band 3 gene in malaria-resistant Southeast Asian ovalocytosis. Proc Natl Acad Sci USA 88:11022, 1991.
50. Liu, S-C, et al: Molecular defect of the band 3 protein in Southeast Asian ovalocytosis. N Engl J Med 323:1530, 1990.
51. Schofield, AE, et al: Defective anion transport activity of the abnormal band 3 in hereditary ovalocytic red blood cells. Nature 355:836, 1992.
52. Mohandas, N, et al: Molecular basis for membrane rigidity of hereditary ovalocytosis. A novel mechanism involving the cytoplasmic domain of band 3. J Clin Invest 89:686, 1992.
53. Lande, WM, et al: Missing band 7 membrane protein in two patients with high Na, low K erythrocytes. J Clin Invest 70:1273, 1982.

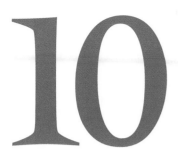

Hemolytic Anemias
Intracorpuscular Defects

II Hereditary Enzyme Deficiencies

ARMAND B. GLASSMAN, MD

OBJECTIVES

At the end of this chapter, the learner should be able to:

1. Name the most common glycolytic enzyme deficiency associated with the hexose monophosphate shunt or pentose phosphate pathway.

2. Name the most common glycolytic enzyme deficiency associated with the Embden-Meyerhof pathway.

3. Identify the red blood cell cytoplasmic inclusions associated with oxidative denaturation of hemoglobin.

4. List laboratory test results that would suggest a deficiency of glucose-6-phosphate dehydrogenase (G6PD).

5. Identify a laboratory test result that would indicate a pyruvate kinase (PK) deficiency.

6. Name the deficiency that causes hemoglobin to be oxidized from the ferrous to the ferric state.

➤ HISTORY

In 1926, 72 plantation workers in Panama suffered acute hemolysis after receiving the antimalarial drug 8-aminoquinoline. Subsequent reports from widely scattered geographic locations added credence to the relationship of hemolysis, cyanosis, and methemoglobinemia with the ingestion of certain antimalarial drugs. In 1953 Dacie and associates[1] evaluated apparently heterogeneous cases of congenital hemolytic anemias that had several common characteristics. There was no detectable abnormal hemoglobin, the antiglobulin test result was negative, and the osmotic fragility was normal. The term *hereditary nonspherocytic hemolytic anemia* (*HNSHA*) was used to describe the group, which was later found to be associated with red cell enzyme abnormalities. Biochemical and molecular studies rapidly advanced the further characterization of these anemias.

The most common anemia in this group is caused by deficiency of glucose-6-phosphate dehydrogenase (G6PD), an enzyme in the hexose monophosphate pentose phosphate or shunt pathway. The second most frequent enzyme deficiency is that of pyruvate kinase (PK), an essential enzyme in the Embden-Meyerhof pathway. Many other enzyme deficiencies of these pathways have also been identified. They are variably associated with HNSHA. Laboratory testing is directed toward identification of the specific enzyme deficiency. Treatment is generally supportive, although experimental gene therapy may have a future role.

➤ SPECIFIC ENZYMOPATHIES

Glucose-6-Phosphate Dehydrogenase Deficiency

G6PD deficiency, one of the most common genetic abnormalities known, is thought to affect over 400 million people worldwide. Carson and associates[2] identified the enzyme G6PD deficiency in 1956 in an individual who developed hemolytic anemia following the administration of the antimalarial drug primaquine (8-aminoquinoline). Yoshida[3] first purified the enzyme from human red cells in 1966. Further progress characterized the diverse variants of G6PD by sequencing of amino acids, cloning of cDNA, and sequencing of nucleotides.

More than 400 variants of G6PD enzyme have been described on the basis of biochemical and genetic analyses.[4–6] Recent advances in molecular biology have enabled classification of the variants into approximately 50 gene mutation groups.[6,7] Nearly all of these variants are the result of point mutations[8] that produce structurally abnormal or functionally defective enzymes, or both.

Mode of Inheritance

G6PD deficiency is transmitted by a mutant gene located on the X chromosome.[9] The gene encoding G6PD has been mapped to the Xq28 region in humans.[10] The disorder is fully expressed in men who are hemizygous when they inherit the mutant gene from their mothers, who are usually silent carriers. In women, full expression of the disorder occurs when two mutant genes (homozygous) are inherited. The heterozygous woman has a mosaic of one red blood cell population with normal enzyme activity and another with deficient enzyme activity.[11] The expression of G6PD deficiency varies markedly among heterozygotes, which is explained in part by the X-inactivation hypothesis.[12] In females, one of the two X chromosomes (maternally or paternally derived) becomes randomly inactivated in each cell of the early embryo. Thus, each somatic cell in a heterozygote expresses either one or the other Gd allele. The ratio of the two cells types may vary widely, not only in different individuals but also among different tissues, even within the same individual.[13]

Distribution of the mutant gene for G6PD deficiency is worldwide; however, the highest incidence occurs in the darkly pigmented racial and ethnic groups. In fact, most of the studies of G6PD variants have been performed on samples from African Americans, people of Mediterranean ancestry, and Asians. Normally active G6PD, type Gd B, is the most common form of the enzyme in all populations and exists in 99% of whites in the United States. Another variety of the G6PD enzyme, Gd A+, is commonly found in Africans, has normal activity, but differs from Gd B by a single amino acid substitution that alters its electrophoretic mobility.[14] The Gd A+ variant is found in about 20% of African men.[15,16] Among African Americans who possess the Gd A+ gene, there is a reduced activity variety designated Gd A−, which can be demonstrated in 10% to 15% of the men. Approximately 20% of African-American women are heterozygous for the Gd A− gene. Gd A− is the prototype of the mild form of G6PD deficiency.

Among whites, G6PD Mediterranean (G6PD Med) is the most common variant, although the overall prevalence is low. Among Kurdish Jews, however, the incidence of G6PD Med may be as high as 50% to 60%. G6PD Med (also known as G6PD B−) is the prototype of a more severe enzyme deficiency associated with acute hemolytic anemia, including favism. The variant Gd Canton is more commonly found in native people of Southeast Asia and China. There is a high frequency of G6PD deficiency in Taiwan and southern China. Approximately 20% to 40% of neonatal jaundice in these areas is related to G6PD deficiency, whereas neonatal jaundice is rarely attributed to G6PD deficiency in the United States.[17] Table 10–1 lists the type of G6PD variant found in selected populations.

The variants have been generally designated by geographic names. With the use of modern techniques of molecular biology, these variants have been reclassified in terms of the exact sites of nucleotide substitutions. Using this nomenclature, Gd A+ would be designated as G6PD A^{376G} to indicate the presence of guanine at nucleotide 376.[18]

Pathogenesis

G6PD catalyzes the first step in the hexose monophosphate shunt (or pentose phosphate) aerobic glycolytic pathway. Oxidative catabolism of glucose is accompanied by reduction of nicotinamide adenine dinucleotide phosphate (NADP) to NADPH (Fig. 10–1), which is subsequently required to reduce glutathione. Reduced glutathione (GSH) is an important source of reducing potential that protects hemoglobin from oxidative denaturation.

The activity of G6PD is highest in young erythrocytes and decreases with cell aging. Under normal conditions, the individual with G6PD deficiency compensates for the shortened life span of the erythrocytes by producing more early red cells (reticulocytosis). Oxidative stress, however, can lead to a mild to severe hemolytic episode. A deficiency of GSH results in oxidative destruction of certain erythrocyte

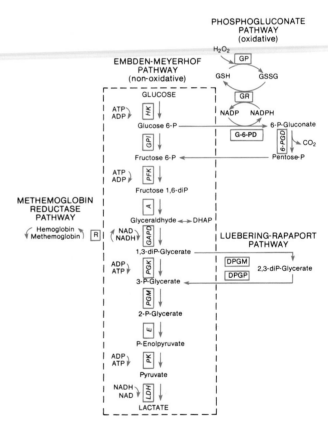

> FIGURE 10–1   Red cell metabolic pathways. The nucleated red cell depends almost exclusively on the breakdown of glucose for energy requirements. The Embden-Meyerhof (nonoxidative or anaerobic) pathway is responsible for most of the glucose utilization and generation of adenosine triphosphate (ATP). In addition, this pathway plays an essential role in maintaining pyridine nucleotides in a reduced state to support methemoglobin reduction (the methemoglobin reductase pathway) and 2,3-diphosphoglycerate synthesis (the Luebering-Rapaport pathway). The phosphogluconate pathway couples oxidative metabolism with pyridine nucleotide and glutathione reduction. It serves to protect red cells from environmental oxidants. (From Hillman, RS, and Finch, C: Red Cell Manual, ed 7. FA Davis, Philadelphia, 1996, p 15, with permission.)

> Table 10-1

DISTRIBUTION OF SOME COMMON G6PD VARIANTS

Enzyme Type	Population Usually Associated
Gd B (normal)	All
Gd Med (also known as Gd B−)	Whites (Mediterranean area)
Gd A+	Africans (~16% of African Americans)
Gd A−	Africans
Gd Canton	Asians

components, including sulfhydryl groups of globin chains and the cell membrane.[19-21] In addition, more than 50 chemical agents may induce hemolysis in G6PD-deficient erythrocytes. Table 10–2 lists the drugs that have more commonly been reported to induce hemolysis in individuals with G6PD deficiency. The hemolytic episode results when G6PD-deficient erythrocytes fail to maintain adequate levels of GSH.[21,22] The resulting oxidation of hemoglobin leads to progressive precipitation of irreversibly denatured hemoglobin (Heinz bodies) (see Color Plate 83). The cells lack normal deformability when sulfhydryl groups are oxidized and consequently encounter difficulties passing through the microcirculation. Premature destruction of the cells results when they undergo intravascular lysis or are sequestered and destroyed in the liver and spleen. This early destruction may sometimes be detected in the peripheral blood smear with the formation of small, condensed bite- or helmet-shaped red cells (Fig. 10–2).

Certain G6PD-deficient individuals also exhibit sensitivity to the fava bean (favism) (Fig. 10–3; see also Color Plate 105). These individuals develop severe hemolysis after ingesting the fava bean or even after inhaling the plant's pollen. Favism is found in some individuals with G6PD deficiency of the Mediterranean and Canton types. Some chemicals isolated from fava beans destroy red cell glutathione, leading to symptomatic hemolysis in susceptible G6PD-deficient individuals.

Clinical Manifestations

The majority of G6PD-deficient persons are asymptomatic most of the time and go through life without ever being aware of their genetic trait. G6PD enzymatic activity that is 20% of normal or even slightly less is sufficient for normal red cell function and survival under ordinary circumstances. However, newborns with this intrinsic defect and adults who take certain therapeutic drugs or develop infections may suffer various degrees of hemolysis from these challenges to the G6PD-deficient erythrocytes.

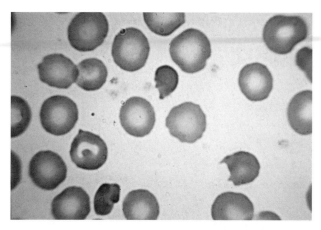

➤ **FIGURE 10–2** Peripheral blood smear from a patient with a G6PD deficiency. Note the small, condensed "bite" or "helmet" cells.

Symptoms of the disorder are related to the severity of the hemolytic episode. Two to three days after the administration of the offending drug, the erythrocyte count decreases, along with the hemoglobin content. The anemia appears normochromic and normocytic, and there is an increase in reticulocytes. The patient may experience back pain. Hemoglobinuria and jaundice may also be evidence of the hemolytic process. Table 10–3 compares the clinical features of the two most common variants.

The hemolytic episode in Gd A– is usually self-limiting. Young cells that are produced in response to the anemia have levels of G6PD that are nearly normal[23] and have better survival characteristics. Hemolysis associated with G6PD Med is more easily induced, usually more severe, and has been reported to result in death on occasion. Red blood cell transfusions may be indicated for hemolytic episodes in patients with G6PD Med.

Laboratory Testing

G6PD deficiency should be suspected after a clinical episode of acute hemolysis after administration of chemical or therapeutic agents known to cause the reaction in patients with the disorder. Laboratory changes of nonspecific type include a fall in hemoglobin (and hematocrit), hemoglobinuria (urine can turn brown to almost black secondary to presence of hemoglobin), Heinz bodies in the erythrocytes, evidence of he-

➤ Table 10-2 **DRUGS AND CHEMICALS ASSOCIATED WITH HEMOLYTIC ANEMIA IN G6PD DEFICIENCY**	
Acetanilide	Pamaquine
Chloramphenicol	Pentaquine
Dapsone	Phenylhydrazine
Daunorubicin	Primaquine
Doxorubicin	Sulfacetamide
Methylene blue	Sulfamethoxazole (Gantanol)
Nalidixic acid (Neg Gram)	Sulfanilamide
Naphthalene	Sulfapyridine
Niridazole (Ambilhar)	Thiazolesulfone
Nitrofurantoin (Furadantoin)	Toluidine blue
	Trinitrotoluene (TNT)

Source: Modified from Beutler, E, and Yoshida, A: Genetic variation of glucose-6-phosphate dehydrogenase: A catalog and future prospects. Medicine 67: 311, 1988.

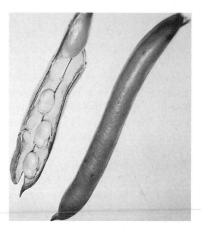

➤ **FIGURE 10–3** Fava beans.

> ### Table 10-3
> ## COMPARISON OF CLINICAL FEATURES OF Gd A− AND Gd MED (Gd B−)

Clinical Feature	Gd A−	Gd Med
Cells affected by defect	Aging erythrocytes	All erythrocytes
Hemolysis with drugs	Unusual	Common
Hemolysis with infection	Common	Common
Favism	No	Occasionally
Degree of hemolysis	Moderate	Severe
Transfusions required	No	Occasionally
Chronic hemolysis	No	No
Hemolytic disease of newborn	Rare	Occasionally

molysis in the serum, elevated serum bilirubin levels, and markedly decreased or absent haptoglobin levels. Generally there are no significant alterations in leukocyte or platelet counts or function.

Laboratory investigation of hemolytic anemia when there is evidence (family history or drug sensitivity, or both) of G6PD deficiency may include several screening procedures. Oxidative denaturation of hemoglobin results in formation of Heinz bodies. These small particles of precipitated hemoglobin can be visualized by supravital staining using certain basic dyes such as crystal violet (see Color Plate 83). Heinz bodies will appear as small (1- to 4-μm) purple inclusions, usually on the cell periphery. They are not seen with Romanowsky stains such as Wright's stain. Although Heinz bodies may be seen in some other enzyme deficiencies, they are not seen in PK deficiency, which is the second most common RBC enzyme deficiency. Some unstable hemoglobins also form Heinz bodies after incubation of erythrocytes at 37°C for 48 hours.

Other test procedures that may be used to screen for G6PD deficiency include the methemoglobin reduction test[24] and the ascorbate-cyanide test.[25] In the methemoglobin reduction test which is a simple and sensitive screening procedure, G6PD-deficient erythrocytes fail to reduce methemoglobin in the presence of methylene blue. The ascorbate-cyanide test, which measures perioxidative denaturation of hemoglobin, is not specific for G6PD deficiency, because it will yield moderately positive results if the patient has PK deficiency or certain unstable hemoglobins.

The fluorescent spot test and the specific G6PD assay are positive only with G6PD deficiency.[26] When a mixture of glucose-6-phosphate, NADP, saponin, and buffer is mixed with blood and is placed on filter paper, G6PD converts the NADP to its reduced form, NADPH. When the filter paper is observed under fluorescent light, those erythrocytes that fail to convert NADP to NADPH (i.e., are deficient in G6PD) will lack fluorescence. The quantitative assay of G6PD is based on the measurement of the rate of reduction of NADP to NADPH measured at 340 nm.[27] G6PD variants can also be identified by electrophoretic methods.

The diagnosis of G6PD deficiency during an acute hemolytic episode may be difficult. The deficiency may be obscured by the younger erythrocyte population (which has more G6PD) as the older G6PD-deficient erythrocytes are destroyed.

➤ PYRUVATE KINASE DEFICIENCY

In 1960 DeGruchy and associates[28,29] reported that some patients with hereditary nonspherocytic hemolytic anemia (HNSHA) had elevated red blood concentrations of 2,3-diphosphoglycerate (2,3-DPG). This elevation suggested a block in anaerobic glycolysis further down the pathway (see Fig. 10–1). The enzyme was identified in 1961, when a severe deficiency of red blood cell PK was found in three patients with HNSHA.[30] PK catalyzes one of the reaction steps in the Embden-Meyerhof pathway of anaerobic glycolysis. Because mature red blood cells lack mitochondria, they are dependent on anaerobic glycolysis for the generation of adenosine 5'-triphosphate (ATP). The diminished capacity to generate ATP in PK-deficient red blood cells results in cell membrane fragility and a hemolytic anemia.

Since its discovery in 1961, more than 300 cases of PK deficiency have been reported, and many of these were cases of variant enzymes with different biochemical characteristics.[31,32] The nucleotide sequence of cDNA for the human PK gene and sequences of several of the mutations that cause HNSHA have been described.[33,34] PK deficiency is the most common enzymatic disease involving anaerobic glycolysis of the red blood cell. Together, G6PD deficiency and PK deficiency constitute most cases of HNSHA arising from red blood cell enzyme deficiencies.

Mode of Inheritance

PK deficiency is inherited as an autosomal recessive trait, but true homozygotes are rare and are restricted to children of consanguineous parents. The most common mode of inheritance is that of double heterozygosity; that is, when two mutant variants of the PK enzyme are simultaneously inherited from each parent.[32,35,36] To date, approximately 20 different mutations of the PK gene are known to produce hemolytic anemia.[37] Thus, the clinical symptoms of PK deficiency are observed both in true homozygotes and in double heterozygotes for the PK gene. Both sexes appear to be affected equally. There is increasing evidence that PK deficiency is worldwide in distribution, with most of the cases reported to date in northern Europe, the United States, and Japan. Other cases have been reported in Australia, Canada, China, Costa Rica, Hong Kong, Italy, Mexico, the Near East, New Zealand, the Philippines, Saudi Arabia, Spain, and Venezuela.[35,38–41]

The Pennsylvania Amish have a high frequency of PK deficiency, which has been traced back to a single immigrant couple. In affected families, consanguinity is common. Thus the PK deficiency in the Amish population is the result of a true homozygote condition.[42]

Pathogenesis

PK deficiency results in a decreased capacity to generate ATP (see Fig. 10–1). The ATP-requiring membrane pumps that maintain the proper electrochemical gradients begin to fail with decreasing concentrations of ATP. This results in cell water loss with cell shrinkage, distortion of cell shape, and increased membrane rigidity.[43,44] These membrane abnormalities lead to premature destruction of the red blood cells in the spleen and liver with consequent anemia. It has been shown that PK-deficient reticulocytes consume six to seven times more oxygen than normal reticulocytes.[44] In most cells, the drop in ATP regeneration because of a block in the glycolytic pathway would be compensated for by oxidative phosphorylation, but that capacity is lost in red blood cells as they mature and they lose mitochondria.

Clinical Manifestations

The severity of the hemolytic disease associated with PK deficiency varies from mild to severe, depending on the properties of the mutant enzymes.[35,45,46] True homozygotes are anemic and jaundiced at birth and may require repeated transfusions during life. Less severely affected patients may come to clinical attention later in childhood or early adulthood because of anemia, jaundice, or an enlarged spleen. The hemolytic anemia is often more pronounced during periods of infection or other stresses. There is an increased incidence of pigmented gallstone formation in these patients, as is true with all chronic hemolytic disorders.

Interestingly, these patients may tolerate exercise to a greater degree than might be expected from the extent of their anemia. Red blood cell concentrations of 2,3-DPG are increased up to three times the normal levels in patients with PK deficiency because of the enzyme block[35] (see Fig. 10–1). The increase of 2,3-DPG decreases the affinity for O_2, which is more readily released to the tissues where it is needed. For this reason, transfusion therapy should be based on the patient's tolerance of the anemia. Removal of the spleen benefits some patients because it increases the life span of the altered red blood cells.

Laboratory Testing

The peripheral blood smears of patients with PK deficiency typically show a normochromic, normocytic anemia with varying degrees of reticulocytosis. Accelerated erythropoiesis may result in polychromasia, poikilocytosis, anisocytosis, and nucleated red blood cells. Both the hemoglobin and the hematocrit levels are decreased from normal. The serum usually has a moderate increase in unconjugated bilirubin, and the haptoglobin level is decreased or absent.[46,47]

Several screening tests may be used to distinguish the nonspherocytic anemia of PK deficiency from the anemias of hereditary spherocytosis and the unstable hemoglobinopathies. These tests are nonspecific and serve only as a mechanism for classifying the type of anemia. Diagnosis is made on the basis of specific testing for the PK enzyme.

Screening tests may include the osmotic fragility test and the autohemolysis test (see Chap. 28), as well as the antiglobulin test and red blood cell survival tests. Erythrocytes that are PK-deficient show osmotic fragility near normal when the test is performed on freshly drawn blood. If the blood is incubated, some patients exhibit an increase in osmotic fragility.[19] Sterile defibrinated blood is used to perform the test for autohemolysis. When normal erythrocytes are incubated in their own serum at 37°C, they gradually lyse, showing up to 3.5% lysis after 48 hours. Erythrocytes from patients with nonspherocytic anemias, as well as those with hereditary spherocytosis, demonstrate an increased amount of autohemolysis. When glucose is added before incubation, erythrocytes from the patient with hereditary spherocytosis demonstrate a decreased amount of autohemolysis. The addition of glucose does not correct the increased autohemolysis of PK-deficient erythrocytes (Fig. 10–4). The antiglobulin test in PK deficiency is negative, and the red blood cell survival is decreased.

A fluorescence screening test, which is relatively simple and sensitive, is used for the diagnosis of PK deficiency. It is based on the following coupled enzyme assay:

$$PEP + ADP + Mg^{2+} \xrightarrow{PK\ enzyme} Pyruvate + ATP$$

$$Pyruvate + NADH + H^+ \xrightarrow{LDH\ enzyme} Lactate + NAD^+$$
$$(UV\ fluorescence) \qquad\qquad (No\ fluorescence)$$

This assay takes advantage of the fact that NADH fluoresces when it is illuminated with long-wave ultraviolet (UV) light, whereas NAD does not fluoresce. Phosphoenolpyruvate (PEP), NADH, adenosine diphosphate (ADP), Mg^{2+}, and lactate dehydrogenase (LDH) are added to a patient sample of blood, which is spotted on filter paper and examined with a UV light. If the blood lacks PK enzyme, NADH will not be oxidized and the fluorescence will persist for 45 minutes to an hour. If the blood is normal and has the PK enzyme, the fluorescence will disappear in 15 minutes, because NAD^+ does not fluoresce.[35,47] It should be noted that leuko-

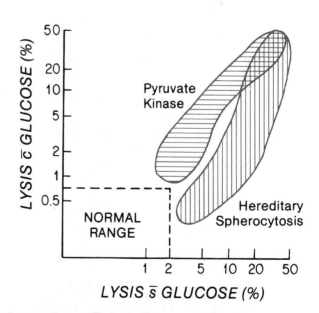

➤ **FIGURE 10–4** The incubation hemolysis test provides a further measure of cell resistance to hemolysis. Pyruvate kinase–deficient blood demonstrates an abnormal rate of hemolysis that is independent of the presence or absence of glucose in the incubation medium. In contrast, the blood from a patient with hereditary spherocytosis shows more marked hemolysis when glucose is absent. (From Hillman, RS, and Finch, C: Red Cell Manual, ed 7. FA Davis, Philadelphia, 1996, p 124, with permission.)

cytes contain a PK isoenzyme that will also catalyze the same reaction. Therefore, blood must be centrifuged and plasma and buffy coat removed prior to testing the erythrocytes. In addition, patients who have recently been transfused may have enough donor cells remaining in circulation to give erroneous test results.

Any abnormal fluorescence spot test should be followed with a confirmatory quantitative PK enzyme assay. This involves the same coupled reaction mechanisms as previously described, but the conversion of NADH to NAD$^+$ is measured spectrophotometrically at 340 nm under standard conditions. Most PK-deficient individuals have 5% to 25% of normal activity.[35,47]

Methemoglobin Reductase Deficiency

Hemoglobin that is oxidized from the ferrous to the ferric state is called *methemoglobin*. Normally, about 1% of the circulating hemoglobin is in the form of methemoglobin. The balance between methemoglobin formation and reduction is maintained by the NADH-methemoglobin reductase (also called diaphorase) pathway. Methemoglobinemia may occur either when there is decreased enzyme activity or when production of methemoglobin exceeds the reducing capacity of the enzyme system. Hereditary deficiency of NADH-methemoglobin reductase results in increased levels of methemoglobin. This congenital deficiency is inherited as an autosomal recessive trait.[48] The heterozygote does not usually show signs of methemoglobinemia unless challenged with certain drugs.

The major clinical feature of methemoglobinemia is cyanosis. Because methemoglobin cannot carry oxygen, some patients exhibit symptoms similar to those of anemia, and some patients develop a compensatory mild polycythemia (see Chap. 18). The course of this disorder is generally benign, and patients are treated only for cosmetic reasons. In cases of severe cyanosis, methylene blue is administered intravenously to activate the NADH-methemoglobin reductase system.

In addition to the hereditary deficiency of NADH-methemoglobin reductase, methemoglobinemia may be caused by the hemoglobin M diseases (see Chap. 11).

The laboratory differentiation of the types of methemoglobinemia is shown in Table 10–4. Methemoglobin has a maximum absorbance band at 630 nm. The addition of cyanide causes the band to disappear, and the change in absorbance is directly proportional to the concentration of methemoglobin.[49] Methemoglobin is increased to varying degrees in all three disorders; enzyme activity is decreased only in hereditary NADH-methemoglobin reductase deficiency. Hemoglobin electrophoresis produces normal-appearing results in patients with methemoglobinemia except in the hemoglobin M diseases.

Other Enzyme Deficiencies

Except for the deficiencies of G6PD and PK, reports of hereditary enzyme deficiencies have been limited to a few rare cases. In a study of 350 cases of suspected enzyme-deficient hemolytic anemia, Beutler[50] reported 13.9% G6PD deficiencies and 9.9% PK deficiencies. Glucose phosphate isomerase (GPI) was the third most commonly identified enzyme deficiency (1.7%). Although there have been reports of other enzyme deficiencies (glycolytic and nonglycolytic), not all such deficiencies have been associated with hemolytic anemia.

Laboratory tests are available to assay many of the specific enzymes. Some of these tests may be available only through reference laboratories. Most laboratories, however, will be able to screen patients with a suspected hemolytic anemia caused by enzyme deficiency. The antiglobulin, erythrocyte survival, autohemolysis, osmotic fragility, and Heinz body tests can all be useful in distinguishing the enzyme deficiencies from hereditary spherocytosis and the unstable hemoglobinopathies.

> ## CASE STUDY

A 26-year-old African-American man was referred to the clinical laboratory for investigation of reported hemoglobinuria. The patient had recently been diagnosed as having infectious mononucleosis. The following laboratory data were obtained:

RBC	3.7×10^{12}/L
Hgb	11.0 g/dL
Hct	32%
MCV	86.0 fL
MCHC	34.0 g/dL
WBC	9.5×10^9/L

Differential

Segmented neutrophils	40%
Bands	3%
Lymphocytes	48% (many atypical)
Monocytes	7%
Eosinophils	2%
Platelets	Adequate
Reticulocytes	14.5% (uncorrected)

The red blood cell (RBC) morphology was normochromic and normocytic. Polychromasia was noted. A

> ## Table 10-4
LABORATORY DIFFERENTIATION OF METHEMOGLOBINEMIA

Methemoglobinemia Resulting From	Methemoglobin Level	Enzyme Activity	Hemoglobin Electrophoresis
Hereditary enzyme deficiency	Increased	Decreased	Normal
Toxic substance exposure	Increased	Normal	Normal
Hemoglobin M disease	Increased	Normal	Abnormal

slight poikilocytosis was also noted, with some red cells showing irregular protrusions. On further investigation, the antiglobulin test result was found to be negative. On the basis of the antiglobulin test, the hemolytic process was considered not to be the result of an immune reaction. A normal hemoglobin electrophoresis was reported.

The hematologist suggested that the patient return in 30 days for testing for erythrocyte enzyme deficiency. At that time the patient was found to have an adequate erythrocyte G6PD content. Spuriously elevated G6PD levels may be found during or immediately after the hemolytic episode because of the presence of younger red blood cells.

Questions

1. What does the reticulocyte count in this patient represent?
2. What is the corrected reticulocyte count?
3. What type of G6PD correlates to this patient's familial background?
4. What RBC inclusion might also be found on the peripheral blood smear with supravital stains?
5. What further testing can be performed in diagnosing G6PD deficiency?
6. What type of hemolysis is present here?

ACKNOWLEDGMENT

This work was supported in part by the Olla Stribling Fund.

QUESTIONS

1. What is the most common glycolytic enzyme deficiency associated with the pentose phosphate pathway (aerobic pathway)?
   a. PK deficiency
   b. G6PD deficiency
   c. Hexokinase deficiency
   d. Glutathione reductase deficiency

2. What is the most common glycolytic enzyme deficiency associated with the Embden-Meyerhof pathway (anaerobic pathway)? (Use answer choices for question 1.)

3. Oxidative denaturation of hemoglobin results in formation of small particles that are visualized with supravital staining. What is the term for these particles?
   a. Basophilic stippling
   b. Howell-Jolly bodies
   c. Pappenheimer bodies
   d. Heinz bodies

4. In the evaluation of a patient for G6PD deficiency, which of the following test results would indicate a deficiency of the enzyme?
   a. Increased formation of Heinz bodies
   b. Lack of fluorescence in the fluorescent spot test
   c. Failure to reduce methemoglobin in the presence of methylene blue
   d. All of the above

5. Which laboratory test result would indicate a patient who is PK-deficient?
   a. Abnormal rate of hemolysis that is independent of the presence or absence of glucose in the incubation medium of the autohemolysis test
   b. Lack of fluorescence in the fluorescent spot test
   c. A change in the indicator from red to yellow in the orthocresol red test
   d. Increase in osmotic fragility

6. What deficiency causes hemoglobin to be oxidized from the ferrous to the ferric state?
   a. G6PD deficiency
   b. PK deficiency
   c. NADH-methemoglobin reductase deficiency
   d. Lactate dehydrogenase deficiency

SUMMARY CHART

➤ Hereditary nonspherocytic hemolytic anemia (HNSHA) encompasses a group of disorders associated with red blood cell (RBC) abnormalities.
➤ Glucose-6-phosphate dehydrogenase (G6PD) enzyme abnormalities are the most common cause of HNSHA.
➤ G6PD is an enzyme in the hexose monophosphate (or pentose phosphate) shunt pathway.
➤ G6PD enzyme variants are noted for their association with particular racial and ethnic backgrounds.
➤ Pyruvate kinase, an essential enzyme of the Embden-Meyerhof pathway, is the second most common enzyme abnormality associated with HNSHA.
➤ There are over 400 G6PD variants. The gene for G6PD is mapped to chromosome Xq28.
➤ Clinical expression of G6PD deficiency is more often evident in men because it is a sex-linked (X chromosome) abnormality.
➤ Deficient G6PD activity results in reduced glutathione levels, which cause increased oxidative denaturation of hemoglobin and subsequent hemolysis.
➤ Patients with G6PD abnormalities are usually asymptomatic until exposed to conditions of lowered oxygen tension, certain chemicals or substances (including fava beans), and some medications.
➤ G6PD is diagnosed by clinical symptoms and laboratory determinations. Laboratory testing includes finding the presence of Heinz bodies in

erythrocytes (not specific), electrophoresis of G6PD, and, where indicated, molecular genetic studies.
➤ PK deficiency, which was first identified in 1961, is associated with a diminished capacity to generate ATP, resulting in fragile red blood cells and a hemolytic anemia.
➤ Laboratory diagnosis of PK deficiency requires specific testing of PK activity. A fluorescent screening test is used.
➤ Other red cell enzyme deficiencies include methemoglobin reductase and glucose phosphate isomerase deficiencies. Almost any enzyme of the aerobic and anaerobic metabolic pathways has been implicated in HNSHA, although presence or levels of hemolysis are quite variable and may be entirely absent.

References

1. Dacie, JR, et al: Atypical congenital haemolytic anemia. Q J Med 22:79, 1953.
2. Carson, PE, et al: Enzymatic deficiency in primaquine sensitive erythrocytes. Science 124:484, 1956.
3. Yoshida, A: Glucose-6-phosphate dehydrogenase of human erythrocytes. I. Purification and characterization of normal (B+) enzyme. J Biol Chem 241:4966, 1966.
4. Beutler, E, and Yoshida, A: Genetic variation of glucose-6-phosphate dehydrogenase: A catalog and future prospects. Medicine 67:311, 1988.
5. Beutler, E: The genetics of glucose-6-phosphate dehydrogenase deficiency. Semin Hematol 27:137, 1990.
6. Hirono, A, and Miwa, S: Human glucose-6-phosphate dehydrogenase: Structure and function of normal and variant enzymes. Haematologia 25:85, 1993.
7. Vulliamy, TJ, et al: Diverse point mutations in the human glucose-6-phosphate dehydrogenase gene cause enzyme deficiency and mild or severe hemolytic anemia. Proc Natl Acad Sci USA 85:5171, 1988.
8. Kletzien, RF, et al: Glucose-6-phosphate dehydrogenase: A "housekeeping" enzyme subject to tissue-specific regulation by hormones, nutrients, and oxidant stress. FASEB J 8:174, 1994.
9. Desorges, JF: Genetic implications of G-6-PD deficiency. N Engl J Med 294:1438, 1976.
10. Pai, GS, et al: Localization of loci for hypoxanthine phosphoriboxyltransferase and glucose-6-phosphate dehydrogenase and biochemical evidence of non-random X-chromosome expression from studies of a human X-autosome translocation. Proc Nat Acad Sci USA 77:2810, 1980.
11. Beutler, E, et al: The normal human female as a mosaic of X-chromosome activity: Studies using the gene for G-6-PD deficiency as a marker. Proc Nat Acad Sci, USA 48:9, 1962.
12. Beutler, E: Biochemical abnormalities associated with hemolytic states. In Weinstein, IM, and Beutler, E (eds): Mechanisms of Anemia in Man. McGraw-Hill, New York, 1962, p 195.
13. Luzzatto, L: Glucose-6-phosphate dehydrogenase: Genetic and haematological aspects. Cell Biochem Funct: 5:101, 1987.
14. Takizawa, T, et al: A single nucleotide base transition is the basis of the common human glucose-6-phosphate dehydrogenase variant A(+). Genomics 1:228,1987.
15. Beutler, E: Glucose-6-phosphate dehydrogenase deficiency. N Engl J Med 324:169, 1991.
16. Beutler, E: The molecular biology of G6PD variant and other red cell enzyme defects. Annu Rev Med 43:47, 1992.
17. Chiu, DTY, et al: Molecular characterization of glucose-6-phosphate dehydrogenase (G6PD) deficiency in patients of Chinese descent and identification of new base substitution in the human G6PD gene. Blood 81:2150, 1993.
18. Beutler, E: Glucose-6-phosphosphate dehydrogenase: New prospectives. Blood 73:1397, 1989.
19. Beutler, E: Glucose-6-phosphate dehydrogenase deficiency. In Williams, WJ, et al (eds): Hematology, ed 2. McGraw-Hill, New York, 1977, p 466.
20. Arese, P, and De Flora, A: Pathophysiology of hemolysis in glucose-6-phosphate dehydrogenase deficiency. Semin Hematol 27:1, 1990.
21. Johnson, RM, et al: Oxidant damage to erythrocyte membrane in glucose-6-phosphate dehydrogenase deficiency: Correlation with in vivo reduced glutathione concentration and membrane protein oxidation. Blood 83:1117, 1994.
22. Beutler, E: Glucose-6-phosphate dehydrogenase deficiency. In Stanbury, JB, et al (eds): The Metabolic Basis of Inherited Disease. McGraw-Hill, New York, 1978, p 1430.
23. Beutler, E, et al: The hemolytic effect of primaquine. IV. The relationship of cell age to hemolysis. J Lab Clin Med 44:439, 1954.
24. Grewer, GJ, et al: The methemoglobin reduction test for primaquine-type sensitivity of erythrocytes: A simplified procedure for detecting a specific hypersusceptibility to drug hemolysis. JAMA 180:386, 1962.
25. Jacob, HS, and Jandl, JH: A simple visual screening test for glucose-6-phosphate dehydrogenase deficiency employing ascorbate and cyanide. N Engl J Med 274:1162, 1966.
26. Beutler, E, et al: International committee for standardization in hematology: Recommended screening test for glucose-6-phosphate dehydrogenase (G-6-PD) deficiency. Br J Haematol 43:465, 1979.
27. Beutler, E: Red Cell Metabolism. A Manual of Biochemical Methods, ed 2. Grune & Stratton, New York, 1975.
28. De Gruchy, GC, et al: Non-spherocytic congenital hemolytic anemia. Blood:1371, 1960.
29. Robinson, MA, et al: Red cell metabolism in non-spherocytic congenital haemolytic anaemia. Br J Haematol 7:327, 1961.
30. Valentine, WN, et al: A specific glycolytic enzyme defect (pyruvate kinase) in three subjects with congenital nonspherocytic hemolytic anemia. Trans Assoc Am Physicians 74:100, 1961.
31. Miwa, S, and Fujii, H: Pyruvate kinase deficiency. Clin Biochem 23:155, 1990.
32. Miwa, S, et al: Concise review: Pyruvate kinase deficiency: Historical perspective and recent progress of molecular genetics. Am J Hematol 42:31, 1993.
33. Tani, K, et al: Human liver type pyruvate kinase: Complete amino acid sequence and the expression in mammalian cells. Proc Natl Acad Sci 85:1792, 1988.
34. Baronciani, L, and Beutler, E: Analysis of pyruvate kinase-deficiency mutations that produce nonspherocytic hemolytic anemia. Proc Natl Acad Sci 90:4324, 1993.
35. Lukens, J: Hereditary hemolytic anemias associated with abnormalities of erythrocyte anaerobic glycolysis and nucleotide metabolism. In Lee, GR, et al (eds): Wintrobe's Clinical Hematology, ed 9. Lea & Febiger, Philadelphia, 1993, chap 34.
36. Lakomek, M, et al: Erythrocyte pyruvate kinase deficiency: A kinetic method for differentiation between heterozygosity and compound-heterozygosity. Am J Hematol 31:225, 1989.
37. Baronciani, L, and Beutler, E: Prenatal diagnosis of pyruvate kinase deficiency. Blood 84:2354, 1994.
38. Feng, CS, et al: Prevalence of pyruvate kinase deficiency among the Chinese: Determination by the quantitative assay. Am J Hematol 43:271, 1993.
39. de Medicis, E, et al: Hereditary nonspherocytic hemolytic anemia due to pyruvate kinase deficiency: A prevalence study in Quebec, Canada. Hum Hered 42:179, 1992.
40. Fonella, A, et al: Iron status in red-cell pyruvate kinase deficiency: Study of Italian cases. Br J Haematol 83:485, 1993.
41. Wei, DC, et al: Homozygous pyruvate kinase deficiency in Hong Kong ethnic minorities. J Paediatr Child Health, 28:334, 1992.
42. Kanno, G, et al: Molecular abnormality of erythrocyte pyruvate kinase deficiency in the Amish. Blood 83:2311, 1994.
43. Keith, AS: Pyruvate kinase deficiency and related disorders of red cell glycolysis. Am J Med 41:762, 1966.
44. Mentzer, WC, Jr, et al: Selective reticulocyte destruction in erythrocyte pyruvate kinase deficiency. J Clin Invest 50:688, 1971.
45. Lakomek, M, et al: Erythrocyte pyruvate kinase deficiency: Relations of residual enzyme activity, altered regulation of defective enzymes and concentrations of high-energy phosphates with the severity of clinical manifestations. Eur J Haematol 49:82, 1992.
46. Rapaport, SI: Introduction to Hematology, ed 2. JB Lippincott, Philadelphia, 1987, chaps 6 and 7.
47. Kjeldsberg, C (ed): Practical Diagnosis of Hematologic Disorders, rev ed. ASCP Press, Chicago, 1991, chap 9.
48. Jaffe, ER: Hereditary methemoglobinemias associated with abnormalities in the metabolism of erythrocytes. Am J Med 41:786, 1966.
49. Evelyn, KA, and Maloy, HT: Micro determination of oxyhemoglobin, methemoglobin and sulfhemoglobin in a single sample of blood. J. Biol Chem 126:655, 1938.
50. Beutler, E: Red cell enzyme defects as nondiseases and as diseases. Blood 54:1, 1979.

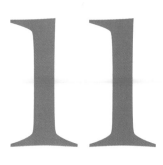

Hemolytic Anemias
Intracorpuscular Defects
III The Hemoglobinopathies

DENISE M. HARMENING, PhD, MT(ASCP), CLS(NCA)
HALLYE ZERINGER, MT(ASCP), SH
CARLO BRUGNARA, MD

OBJECTIVES

At the end of this chapter, the learner should be able to:

1. Characterize hemoglobinopathies.
2. Define qualitative and quantitative hemoglobin defects.
3. Explain the nomenclature for abnormal hemoglobins.
4. Name the amino acid substitution found in sickle cell anemia.
5. List factors contributing to the sickling process.
6. Name and describe the three types of sickle cell anemia.
7. List tests useful in the laboratory diagnosis of sickle cell disease.
8. Describe the effects on hemoglobin S cells when parasitized by *Plasmodium falciparum*.
9. List characteristics for sickle cell trait.
10. Describe the goals of treatment for sickle cell anemia.
11. Name the amino acid substitution found in hemoglobin C disease.
12. List findings for hemoglobin C disease.
13. Identify the laboratory findings that provide a diagnosis of hemoglobin SC disease.
14. List characteristics for hemoglobin D, hemoglobin E, and other variants and combinations such as hemoglobin O$_{Arab}$ and hemoglobin SD.
15. Identify causes of methemoglobinemia.
16. Recognize useful techniques for studying hemoglobin variants with altered oxygen affinity.

Hemoglobinopathies are defined in the broadest sense as conditions in which there are either qualitative or quantitative abnormalities in the synthesis of hemoglobin. More than 625 hemoglobin variants have been described.[1] Most of these hemoglobin variants were discovered coincidentally and are of no clinical significance. However, approximately one-third (200) of these variants represent hemoglobinopathies with clinically significant hemolytic anemia, because the abnormality results in a defect in the structural integrity or function of the hemoglobin molecule. The hemoglobinopathies are either inherited according to classic mendelian genetics or arise from new genetic mutations.

More than 90% of the hemoglobin variants are single amino acid substitutions in the alpha (α), beta (β), delta (δ), or gamma (γ) globin chains as a result of a single-point mutation in one of the globin genes. When both parents carry one gene that codes for an abnormal hemoglobin (such as HbS), there is a 25% chance with each pregnancy that the infant will be homozygous (inheriting two genes for HbS), resulting in sickle cell anemia[2] (Fig. 11–1, block C). A total of eight genes are inherited on two homologous chromosomes that code for polypeptide globin chains. The α and zeta (ζ) globin genes are located on chromosome 16, with two α and one ζ globin gene per chromosome. The β, δ, γ, and epsilon (ϵ) globin genes are located on chromosome 11, with one β, δ, ϵ, and two γ globin genes per chromosome (Fig. 11–2).

➤ REVIEW OF NORMAL HEMOGLOBIN STRUCTURE

A brief review of normal hemoglobin structure is provided here to aid in understanding the hemoglobinopathies; however, the reader is referred to Chapter 3 for a more detailed discussion.

Hemoglobin is a conjugated protein composed of iron, pro-

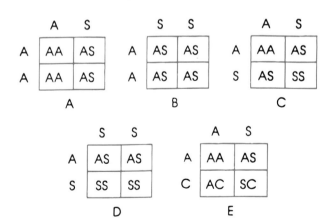

➤ **FIGURE 11–1**   Inheritance of abnormal hemoglobins. *A.* With one parent heterozygous for an abnormal hemoglobin, the offspring have a one-in-two chance of carrying the trait. *B.* With one parent homozygous for an abnormal hemoglobin, all offspring will carry the trait because that parent can contribute only an abnormal gene. *C.* With both parents heterozygous for the abnormality, the chances are one in four for normal, two in four for heterozygous, and one in four for homozygous. *D.* With both parents carrying the same abnormal hemoglobin—one homozygous and one heterozygous—the offspring have a 50–50 chance of being either homozygous or heterozygous. *E.* With parents carrying two different abnormal hemoglobins, offspring have a one-in-four chance of not inheriting an abnormality, a one-in-two chance of carrying the trait for one or the other abnormality, and a one-in-four chance of carrying both abnormalities in codominance.

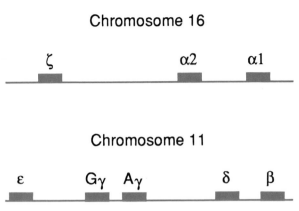

➤ **FIGURE 11–2**   Location of the globin genes on chromosomes 16 and 11.

toporphyrin IX type III, and globin. The combination of iron and protoporphyrin is referred to as the *heme* moiety. The globin portion of the molecule consists of four polypeptide chains, each with an attached heme group. These heme moieties are positioned so that they are suspended in the center of the polypeptide chains. This configuration provides an environment where iron can exist in the reduced (ferrous) state, a feature that is critical for oxygen transport and delivery.

There are six known polypeptide chains that make up the different globin portions of the hemoglobin molecule. These chains are α, β, γ, δ, ϵ, and ζ. The latter two represent embryonic globin chains. The structure of the chains and the resulting hemoglobin molecule is described in the following four steps:

1. The primary structure relates to the number and sequence of amino acids constituting each globin chain. α chains have 141 amino acids; the non–α chains have 146 amino acids. The sequence of amino acids is different in each chain.
2. The secondary structure occurs with the twisting of the amino acid chain around an axis in a helical conformation.
3. The tertiary structure consists of bending the twisted amino acid chain into a three-dimensional shape resembling an "irregular pretzel." The polar groups are oriented outward, and the nonpolar groups are interior. The heme molecule is nestled in a nonpolar pocket and attached to a proximal histidine residue.
4. The quaternary structure is the assembling of the four three-dimensional chains with their respected heme groups. The result is a completed, functional hemoglobin molecule.

Table 11–1 reviews the composition of normal physiologic hemoglobins.

➤ CLASSIFICATION

Classification of hemoglobinopathies is somewhat arbitrary. Hemoglobin disorders may be divided into two very broad categories: qualitative and quantitative hemoglobinopathies. In the qualitative category, hemoglobins differ in the sequence of the amino acids composing the globin chain. This category is the one usually referred to in the general discussion of hemoglobinopathies. Quantitative defects are those characterized by decreased production of

➤ **Table 11-1**
COMPOSITION OF NORMAL PHYSIOLOGIC HEMOGLOBINS

Globin Chains	Hemoglobin	Normal (%)	Stage of Development
$\alpha_2\epsilon_2$	Gower 2		
$\zeta_2\epsilon_2$	Gower 1		Embryo
$\zeta_2\gamma_2$	Portland		
$\alpha_2{}^A\gamma_2$	F	60–90	
$\alpha_2{}^G\gamma_2$	F		Fetus
$\alpha_2\beta_2$	A	95–97	
$\alpha_2\delta_2$	A_2	2–3	Adult

hemoglobin resulting from a decreased synthesis of one particular globin chain, which is commonly known as thalassemia (see Chap. 12).

A more inclusive method of classification allows division of the hemoglobinopathies into five major categories:

1. Abnormal hemoglobins without clinical significance
2. Aggregating hemoglobins (i.e., sickle cell anemia)
3. Unbalanced synthesis of hemoglobin (thalassemia)
4. Unstable hemoglobins
5. Hemoglobins with abnormal heme function

Table 11–2 summarizes this classification of hemoglobinopathies.

➤ HEMOGLOBINOPATHIES

The majority of hemoglobinopathies (hemoglobin variants) result from β-chain abnormalities. Many of these variants have no associated physiologic consequences. There also can be α-, γ-, and δ-chain abnormalities, but these conditions are usually clinically benign. Some individuals with β-chain abnormalities present with abnormal physical properties resulting in clinical disease. From the first description of a sickle cell by Herrick in 1910,[3] research efforts continue to define, understand, and treat these abnormalities associated with inherited abnormal hemoglobins.

Most hemoglobinopathies arise from a single amino acid substitution. For example, when valine substitutes for glutamic acid in the sixth position of the β chain, hemoglobin S

➤ **Table 11-2**
CLASSIFICATION OF HEMOGLOBINOPATHIES

- Abnormal hemoglobins without clinical significance
- Aggregating hemoglobins (structural abnormalities with amino acid substitution *away* from the crevice of the heme, i.e., HbS, HbC)
- Unbalanced synthesis of hemoglobin (thalassemia)
- Unstable hemoglobins
- Hemoglobins with abnormal heme function (structural abnormalities with amino acid substitutions *near* the crevice of the heme)

(HbS) is produced rather than hemoglobin A (HbA). When lysine replaces glutamic acid at position six of the β chain, hemoglobin C (HbC) is produced. These changes truly represent a molecular alteration; a feature that was initially appreciated by Linus Pauling in the late 1940s when he won the Nobel prize for defining sickle cell anemia as a molecular disease.[4] The abnormality was demonstrated by electrophoresis to be located in the protein portion of the hemoglobin molecule. Other substitutions can cause instability of hemoglobin, such as deformation of the three-dimensional structure, oxidation of the ferrous iron, or alteration in residues that interact with heme, with 2,3-diphosphoglycerate (2,3-DPG), or at subunit contact points.[1]

At the molecular level, a single-base deoxyribonucleic acid (DNA) substitution in the corresponding triplet codon produces one amino acid change, which is the most common cause of a hemoglobinopathy. Other molecular changes that are more rare include (1) multiple-base substitutions, (2) the production of long or short subunits, and (3) the occurrence of fusion subunits.[1]

➤ NOMENCLATURE

Investigators began naming the abnormal hemoglobins with capital letters; but with the end of the alphabet rapidly approaching, they changed to the use of names of places. A letter plus a place name indicates identical mobility on electrophoresis, but there are different substitutions. It should be noted, in general, that there is more than one abnormal hemoglobin with the same letter designation (i.e., $HbC_{Georgetown}$, HbC_{Harlem}, $HbG_{Philadelphia}$, $HbG_{San\ Jose}$, HbO_{Arab}, $HbO_{Indonesia}$).[1] The description of the variant can also involve identifying the chains and the substitution. For example, homozygous HbS is $\alpha_2\beta_2{}^S$ or $\alpha_2\beta_2{}^{6Val}$ or $\alpha_2\beta_2{}^{6Glu\text{-}Val}$. Hemoglobin $G_{Philadelphia}$, the most common α-chain variant in the black population, is written $\alpha_2{}^{GPhil}\beta_2$ or $\alpha_2{}^{68Lys}\beta_2$ or $\alpha_2{}^{68Asn\text{-}Lys}\beta_2$. Additionally, the exact helix of the secondary structure and the position in that helix can be indicated. For example, the designations would be $\alpha_2\beta_2{}^{6(A3)}$ for HbS and $\alpha_2{}^{68(E17)}\beta_2$ for $HbG_{Philadelphia}$.

➤ SICKLE CELL ANEMIA

Historic Overview

In 1910, a 20-year-old black student from the West Indies was described by Herrick[3] to be suffering from a severe hemolytic anemia in which peculiarly elongated, "sickled" red cells were found on his peripheral blood smear. The classic hematologic features included not only the presence of sickle cells on the peripheral blood smear but also nucleated red cells indicative of a severe anemia, cardiac enlargement, icterus, and leukocytosis. The presence of target cells as well as a normocytic, normochromic anemia is also generally associated with hemoglobinopathies. Sickle cell anemia represents the most common type of severe hemoglobinopathy, with an estimated prevalence in the United States of 1 in 375 African-American live births.[5] It is estimated to affect more than 50,000 Americans.[2,5]

Definition

The term *sickle cell disease* is used generically to describe a group of genetic disorders characterized by the production of the abnormal HbS.[2,5] Sickle cell anemia (HbSS disease) is the most common type of sickle cell disease and represents the homozygous form, in which the individual inherits a double dose of the abnormal gene that codes for HbS. This type of hemoglobin differs from normal hemoglobin by the single amino acid substitution of valine for glutamic acid in the sixth position from the NH_2-terminal end of the β chain (Fig. 11–3). The structural formula for sickle cell anemia (HbSS) is $\alpha_2\beta_2^{6Glu-Val}$. The formula alternatively may be written as $\alpha_2\beta_2^S$ or $\alpha_2\beta_2^{6Val}$. The gene for HbS occurs with greatest frequency in tropical Africa, particularly Central Africa. Many social and historic factors, such as slavery and conquest, are responsible for the appearance of this hemoglobin in North American and Middle Eastern populations.[2] In the United States, the birth incidence of the homozygous state (HbSS), is approximately 0.26% (1 in 375 African-American babies).[2,6] It is estimated that 8% to 10% of American blacks carry the trait (one gene) for HbS.

Although in the United States sickle cell disease is most commonly found in persons of African ancestry, it has also been found in individuals from the Caribbean, South and Central America, Mediterranean (Turkey, Greece), the Middle East, and India. Table 11–3 lists the other common variants of sickle cell disease with their estimated incidence.

Pathophysiology

HbS is soluble and usually causes no problem when properly oxygenated. However, when the oxygen tension decreases, this single amino acid substitution in the β-globin chain of HbS polymerizes, forming tactoids or fluid polymers (Fig. 11–4).[7] As these polymers realign, they cause the red cell to deform into the characteristic sickle shape (Fig. 11–5). The sickling process is dependent on the degree of oxygenation, pH, and dehydration of the patient.[7] Decreases in oxygenation and pH, as well as dehydration, promote sickling. Sickled cells in circulation increase the viscosity of the blood, which slows circulation, thereby increasing the time of exposure to a hypoxic environment, particularly in the small vasculature of the spleen. This effect then promotes further sickling. There are two types of sickled cells: reversible and irreversible.[7] Sickling of the

> **Table 11-3**
> ## SICKLE CELL DISEASE (A GROUP OF GENETIC DISORDERS CHARACTERIZED BY THE PRODUCTION OF HbS)

Disorder	Incidence in African-American Live Births
Sickle cell anemia (HbSS)	1 in 375 (0.26%)
Sickle cell disease (HbSC)	1 in 835 (0.12%)
Sickle β thalassemia	1 in 1,667 (0.06%)

Source: Sickle Cell Disease Guideline Panel. Sickle cell disease: Screening, diagnosis, management, and counseling in newborns and infants. Clinical Practice Guideline No 6. AHCPR Pub No 93-0562. US Department of Health and Human Services, Rockville, MD, April 1993.

cell is reversible up to a point. However, repeated sickling eventually damages the red blood cell (RBC) membrane permanently. The formation of rigid sickled cells is likely to plug small blood vessels, further lowering the pH and oxygen tension and increasing the number of sickled cells, resulting in both acute and chronic tissue damage. The tissue injury is secondary to the obstruction of blood flow and

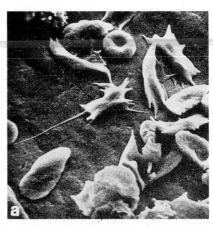

> FIGURE 11–4   Scanning electron micrograph (SEM) of sickle cells. (From Bell, A: Hematology. In: Listen, Look and Learn. Health Education Resources, Inc., Bethesda, MD, with permission.)

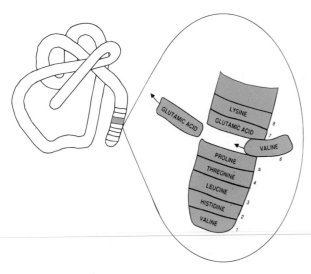

> FIGURE 11–3   Amino acid substitution in hemoglobin S.

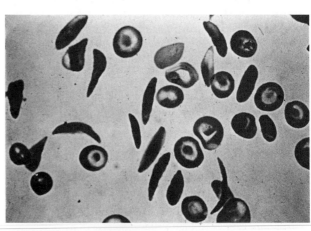

> FIGURE 11–5   Sickle cell disease (peripheral blood). Note the sickle-shaped red cells and target cells. (From Bell, A: Hematology. In: Listen, Look and Learn. Health Education Resources, Inc., Bethesda, MD, with permission.)

hypoxia produced by the abnormally shaped, sickled red cells. This injury leads to painful crises and infarction of organs. It should be noted that the presence of hemoglobin F (HbF) and HbA in red cells with HbS modifies the degree or severity of the sickling.[2,6–8] Table 11–4 lists other factors affecting the severity of HbS.

Clinical Features

The hallmark features of sickle cell disease are chronic hemolytic anemia and vaso-occlusion, resulting in ischemic tissue injury.[5–7] All tissues and organs within the body are at risk for damage as a result of the vascular obstruction produced by the sickled red cells. Organs at greatest risk include the spleen, kidney, and bone marrow because, in these organs, blood flow is slow in the venous sinuses and there is a reduced oxygen tension and low pH.[9] The eye and head of the femur are also target sites for ischemic injury because of the limited terminal arterial blood supply to these areas.

Sickle cell anemia is usually diagnosed early in life, when the level of HbF declines. HbSS disease typically presents as a severe chronic hemolytic anemia, with hemoglobin levels in the range of 6 to 8 g/dL. Characteristically the patient demonstrates an asthenic physique and is mildly jaundiced (Fig. 11–6; see also Color Plate 106). Many complications are associated with the disease, with the major manifestations being "sickle crises." There are three types of crises: aplastic, hemolytic, and painful (vaso-occlusive).[5,6,10]

An aplastic crisis is usually associated with infections, particularly to parvoviruses, which cause a temporary suppression of erythropoiesis. The marrow is simply overworked as a result of the stress related to the continuous stimulus for production of new red cells. With an already shortened red cell life span, even a temporary decrease or arrest in red cell production causes a drastic anemia. During the evaluation of the febrile patient, a fall in the reticulocyte count can also indicate the onset of aplastic crisis, which requires future monitoring of the hemoglobin level in the HbSS disease patient. Aplastic crises usually spontaneously resolve within 5 to 10 days.[5,6]

A hemolytic crisis reflects an acute exacerbation of the anemia with a resulting fall in hemoglobin and hematocrit, an increased reticulocyte count, and jaundice.[5,6,10] Acute splenic sequestration is the cause, resulting in a decrease in hemoglobin and hematocrit, which usually occurs in infants and young children between 5 months and 2 years of age.[5,6] Intrasplenic pooling of vast amounts of blood results in enlarged spleens of some children with HbSS disease. The usual clinical features of a hemolytic crisis include sudden

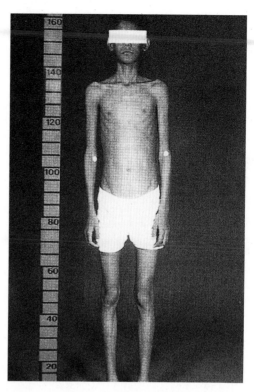

➤ **FIGURE 11–6** Asthenic physique with mild jaundice. (Reproduced with permission from Sandoz Pharmaceuticals Corporation.)

weakness, rapid pulse, faintness, pallor of the lips and mucous membranes, and abdominal fullness caused by the enlarged spleen.[5,6,10] In contrast to this process, multiple infarctions and subsequent fibrosis lead to a process termed *autosplenectomy* in adult patients with HbSS disease, which results in a small, fibrotic and nonfunctional spleen.

Vaso-occlusive or painful crisis is the hallmark of sickle cell anemia.[5,6,10] The crisis is usually associated with severe pain, caused by occlusion of small blood vessels mediated by the adhesion of sickled cells to endothelium, resulting in tissue damage and necrosis.[9] The decreased blood flow causes regional hypoxia and acidosis, further exacerbating the ischemic injury. A painful crisis usually lasts 4 to 6 days but sometimes persists for weeks.[5,6] Painful crisis can be precipitated by infection, fever, acidosis, dehydration, and exposure to extreme cold. Some patients have reported that even emotional states such as anxiety, stress, and depression may cause their painful crises.

Generally, three principles of therapy are applied in the management of painful crisis: adequate rehydration, pain relief using sufficient analgesics, and antibiotic therapy to treat any precipitating or underlying illness such as infection.[5,6,10,11] In severe cases, exchange transfusion may be necessary to reduce the hemoglobin S content in the blood of the patients with HbSS disease. However, the mainstay of therapy for painful crises is hydration (administration of fluid volumes) to correct fluid and electrolyte deficits in an attempt to maintain normal serum electrolyte concentrations.

Symptoms and clinical manifestations of HbSS disease are many and varied. Table 11–5 lists the most prominent types of clinical manifestations associated with sickle cell anemia. As mentioned previously, these clinical presentations represent the sequelae of repeated infarction. Table 11–6 provides a more comprehensive list, dividing the clin-

➤ **Table 11-4**
FACTORS AFFECTING THE SEVERITY OF HbS

Amount of HbS	Vascular stasis
Other hemoglobins	Temperature
Thalassemia	pH
G6PD deficiency	Viscosity
Deoxygenation	MCHC
Amount of HbF	Dehydration

Abbreviations: G6PD = glucose-6-phosphate dehydrogenase; MCHC = mean corpuscular hemoglobin concentration.

> ## Table 11-5
> ## CLINICAL MANIFESTATIONS OF SICKLE CELL ANEMIA

Cutaneous manifestations (leg ulcers)

Cardiac enlargement

Joint and skeletal problems

Arthritis

Renal complications (renal papillary necrosis)

Bone marrow infarctions

Conjunctival vascular abnormalities

Gastrointestinal symptoms

Hepatomegaly

Autosplenectomy

Cholelithiasis

Priapism (persistent, painful penile erection)

> ## Table 11-6
> ## CLINICAL FEATURES OF SICKLE CELL ANEMIA BY CATEGORY

Hematologic

- Aplastic crisis
- Hemolytic crisis
- Vaso-occlusive crisis

Nonhematologic

- Abnormal growth
- Bone and joint abnormalities
  - Pain
  - *Salmonella* infection
  - Hand-foot dactylitis
- Genitourinary
  - Renal papillary necrosis
  - Priapism
- Spleen and liver
  - Autosplenectomy
  - Hepatomegaly
  - Jaundice
- Cardiopulmonary
  - Enlarged heart
  - Heart murmurs
  - Pulmonary infarction
- Eye
  - Retinal hemorrhage
- Central nervous system
- Leg ulcers
- Risky pregnancy

ical features of HbSS disease into hematologic and non-hematologic categories.

Vasculopathy

Occlusion of blood vessels and tissue ischemia can occur virtually anywhere in the body: in bones, joints, lungs, liver, kidneys, eye, central nervous system, and spleen.[5,6] In the lungs, sickling in the pulmonary microvasculature produces the acute chest syndrome in HbSS disease patients. It is a common cause of hospital admission and in some cases represents a medical emergency. The acute chest syndrome represents an acute illness characterized by fever, chest pain, prostration, and the presence of pulmonary infiltrates on the chest x-ray.[6,12] The syndrome in adults is characteristically a result of pulmonary infarction, although other causes such as bacterial or viral infection have been reported. This contrasts with the acute chest syndrome in children with HbSS disease, which is usually caused by an infectious agent. Pleuritic chest pain is the dominant symptom of acute chest syndrome in adults, whereas fever, cough, and tachypnea are often the only complaints in infants and young children who are affected.[5,6]

The most common cutaneous manifestation in HbSS disease is the development of ulcers or sores on the lower leg (Fig. 11–7 and Color Plate 107). Approximately 8% to 10% of patients develop leg ulcers, which are usually manifested between 10 and 50 years of age and are very difficult to resolve.[5,6,10] There are important differences in the tendency of patients to develop leg ulcers; Jamaican patients have a much greater incidence of leg ulcers than patients in North America.[10]

Bones and joints in HbSS disease are frequent sites of pathology, with musculoskeletal pain being the most com-

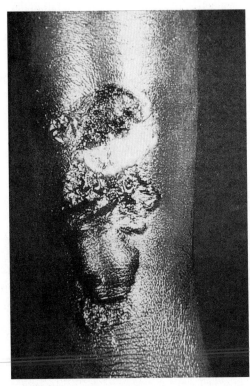

> FIGURE 11–7 Leg ulcers in a patient with sickle cell anemia. (Reproduced with permission from Sandoz Pharmaceuticals Corporation.)

mon symptom. There can be bone marrow hyperplasia, infection, or infarction. Infarction is also commonly responsible for the symptoms of the hand-foot syndrome observed in sickle cell anemia. Dactylitis (the painful swelling of the hands and feet) occurs commonly in infants and young children with HbSS disease and is observed exclusively in patients in that age group.[5,6,10] In many infants it is the first manifestation of the disease. The characteristic "hand-foot" syndrome develops later in life as a result of microinfarction of small bones of the hands and feet, which leads to unequal growth and bone deformities of the fingers and toes (Fig. 11–8). In addition, episodes of painful swollen joints and aseptic necrosis of the femoral head and other articulating bones are caused by the process of infarction.

Infections

Serious bacterial infections remain a major cause of morbidity and mortality in patients with HbSS disease. Table 11–7 lists the organisms implicated in causing infections in these patients.

The most significant cause of death during early childhood is the severe overwhelming septicemia and meningitis caused by *Streptococcus pneumoniae*.[5,6,10, 13] In HbSS disease, splenic dysfunction develops during infancy and predisposes the infant to overwhelming infections from encapsulated bacteria, such as *S. pneumoniae* and *Haemophilas influenzae*.[5,6,10] After the first decade of life, anaerobic and enteric organisms become important pathogens, causing infections in adult patients with HbSS disease. Repeated splenic infarcts result in autosplenectomy by the adult years. These patients then become more prone to serious infections with encapsulated organisms such as *S. pneumoniae* and *H. influenzae*. Infections in patients with HbSS disease cause greater morbidity, disseminate more rapidly, and are more difficult to resolve than infections in healthy individuals. In particular, pyelonephritis recurs regularly in these patients, is difficult to treat, and is often associated with septicemia.[5,6,10] This infection results in a predisposition to sickling in the renal papilla, ultimately causing renal papillary necrosis, which frequently develops along with the pyelonephritis (see the following discussion of Sickle Cell Nephropathies).

Table 11–8 outlines the multiple factors responsible for the increased susceptibility to infection in patients with HbSS disease.

The relationship between the incidence of the malarial parasite and the frequency of the abnormal HbS gene requires further explanation. Malaria, caused by a parasite of the *Plasmodium* species, is still a serious disease in tropical areas, with *Plasmodium falciparum* being responsible for the most life-threatening situations. The original geographic distribution of sickle cell disease overlaps with that of malaria. As in thalassemias, these hemoglobinopathies are believed to provide some kind of selective advantage for malaria. This is applicable only to subjects carrying one abnormal HbS gene (sickle cell trait). The precise mechanism of this protective effect from malaria is not known.[10] Cells carrying HbS, when parasitized by *P. falciparum*, may sickle more quickly than will nonparasitized cells. The sickling could affect the cycle of the parasite in one of two ways: directly, by killing the parasite; or indirectly, by causing the parasitized sickle cells to be sequestered in the spleen. The fact that persons homozygous for the HbS gene often lack splenic function by the time they reach adulthood (autosplenectomy or functional asplenia) may be one reason why malaria is exceptionally severe, and often fatal, in these cases. Thus, HbS confers a relative degree of protection from malaria only in the heterozygous (trait) state.

Sickle Cell Nephropathies

In the kidney, intravascular sickling occurs more rapidly than in any other organ owing to deoxygenation of HbS in the acidic and hyperosmolar environment of this organ.[7] The combination of hypoxia, hypertonicity, and acidosis in the kidney causes sickling, stasis, and ischemia of the renal medulla and papillary tip, leading to progressive renal events. Eventually, over time, a number of sickle cell nephropathies develop. Hyposthenuria, the inability of the kidney to concentrate the urine, is the earliest and most common nephropathy in sickle cell disease, occurring usually in the first decade.[10,14] Progressive renal pathology occurs in patients with HbSS disease as renal tubular dysfunction and atrophy presents itself in the second decade of life. The third decade in HbSS disease is characterized by interstitial nephritis, papillary necrosis, pyelonephritis, and the nephrotic syndrome, to name a few of the renal disorders that may develop. In the fourth decade and beyond, end-stage renal disease develops as one or more of the sickle cell nephropathies results in chronic renal failure.[5,6,10]

It should be noted that hyperuricemia and gross hema-

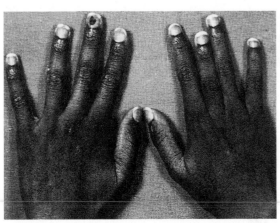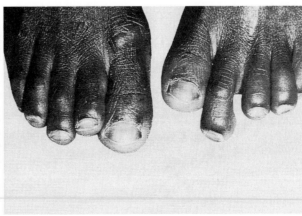

➤ **FIGURE 11–8** Hand-foot syndrome in a patient with sickle cell anemia. (Reproduced with permission from Sandoz Pharmaceuticals Corporation.)

> **Table 11-7**
ORGANISMS IMPLICATED IN CAUSING INFECTIONS IN PATIENTS WITH SICKLE CELL ANEMIA

Bacterial	Viral	Fungal	Parasitic
Streptococcus pneumoniae	Rubeola	*Coccidioides immitis*	*Plasmodium* species
Haemophilus influenzae	Cytomegalovirus	*Histoplasma capsulatum*	
Neisseria meningitidis			
Mycoplasma pneumoniae			
Staphylococcus aureus			
Streptococcus pyogenes			
Mycobacterium tuberculosis			
Escherichia coli			
Salmonella species			

turia occur commonly in patients with HbSS disease. Hyperuricemia occurs in approximately 15% of children and 40% of adults with HbSS disease because of the increased urate production associated with the accelerated erythropoietic rate and decreased renal clearance of urate.[10] Gross hematuria occurs commonly not only in sickle cell anemia but also in sickle cell trait because of the sickling, stasis, ischemia, and extravasation of blood in the kidney.[10,14]

Stroke

Stroke occurs in 6% to 12% of patients with HbSS disease.[6,11,13,15] Stroke represents an array of neurologic complications caused by an ischemic or hemorrhagic lesion in a specific cerebral vessel.[15] The neurologic manifestations may be focal, such as hemiparesis, or more generalized, such as coma or seizure.[10] Recurrent episodes of stroke cause progressively greater impairment and increased mortality. The most common cause of stroke in children is cerebral infarction.[10] With age, subarachnoid and intracerebral hemorrhage become increasingly common. A distinguishing pathologic feature of arterial vessels involved in stroke is the presence of intimal and medial proliferation, which results in severe restriction of blood flow. Most likely this is owing to the interaction of sickled cells with endothelium, which results in endothelial damage, inflammation, and the local release of growth factors that stimulate proliferation of subintimal and medial cells.

Patients with a characteristic abnormality of cerebral blood flow (higher than normal velocity of flow on transcranial Doppler ultrasonography) have been shown to be at much greater risk to develop stroke.[15] These patients have also been shown to benefit from a prophylactic treatment with chronic red cell transfusions.[15]

Infarction strokes recur in at least two-thirds of HbSS disease patients who are *not* chronically transfused. HbSS diseased patients with hemorrhagic stroke (intracerebral or subarachnoid hemorrhage) have a high mortality rate during the acute stage (may be as high as 50%).[5,6,10]

► SICKLE CELL TRAIT

In sickle cell trait (Fig. 11–9), the heterozygous form of the disease, individuals inherit both a normal β-globin gene and a sickle globin gene (β^S). As a result, individuals with sickle cell trait produce both normal HbA and HbS, with a predominance of HbA in an approximate ratio of 60:40.[2,7] The structural formula is $\alpha_2\beta_1\beta_1^{6Glu-Val}$. The frequency of this heterozygous condition in American blacks is approximately 8%.[2,5] Individuals with HbS trait are usually asymptomatic, but occasionally episodes of hematuria and hyposthenuria occur as a complication of sickle cell trait because of sickling in the kidney. The potential for sickling exists, therefore, and drastic lowering of pH or reduction in oxygen tension can precipitate a crisis. Causes for these include severe respiratory infections, air travel in unpressurized aircraft, anesthesia, and congestive heart failure. Even excessive exercise can lead to a significant buildup of lactic acid,

> **Table 11-8**
FACTORS RESPONSIBLE FOR THE INCREASED SUSCEPTIBILITY OF PATIENTS WITH SICKLE CELL ANEMIA TO INFECTIONS

- Reticuloendothelial blockage caused by increased hemolysis
- Stasis of sickled RBCs in the sinusoids of the liver and spleen
- Secondary splenic dysfunction
- Deficiency of nonantibody serum opsonic activity

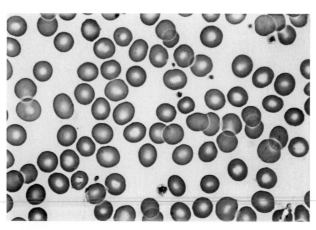

> **FIGURE 11–9**   Sickle trait (peripheral blood). Note the normal-appearing smear.

resulting in sickling and subsequent infarction. Several deaths of American black soldiers with sickle cell trait have been reported as a result of rigorous basic training at altitudes greater than 4000 feet, which led to a buildup of lactic acid, followed by acidosis and subsequent organic infarction.[16]

➤ LABORATORY DIAGNOSIS

The following laboratory tests should be performed to diagnose sickle cell disease: the complete blood count, a reticulocyte count, evaluation of the peripheral smear, hemoglobin electrophoresis, and measurement of hemoglobins A_2 and F.[5,17]

The chronic anemia of HbSS typically is quite severe, with hemoglobins ranging between 6 and 8 g/dL. The RBC indices are normochromic and normocytic. The peripheral red blood picture can be striking, with numerous target cells, fragmented red cells, polychromasia, nucleated red cells, and usually sickled cells (see Fig. 11–5). Siderotic granules and Howell-Jolly bodies may be seen in the red cells as a result of rapid RBC turnover and "stressed" erythropoiesis. The average reticulocyte count is between 5% and 20%. This count decreases, however, during an aplastic crisis; indeed, a falling reticulocyte count may herald the onset of such a crisis. There may be a neutrophilic leukocytosis with a shift to the left and thrombocytosis. The bone marrow reflects marked erythroid hyperplasia, except during an aplastic crisis.

In individuals with the trait, sickled cells are not present on the peripheral blood smear. On rare occasions, however, sickled cells may be observed in the peripheral blood smear during a crisis episode.

Laboratory Screening for Sickle Cell Disease

According to the Clinical Practice Guideline on Sickle Cell Disease published by the U.S. Department of Health and Human Services in April 1993, all newborns, regardless of race or ethnic background should be screened for the presence of HbS (Table 11–9).[5]

Newborn screening for sickle cell disease began in the United States in the early 1970s. The initial screening programs grew out of the recognition that sickle cell anemia was associated with significant morbidity and mortality.

Today newborn hemoglobinopathy screening is performed in more than 40 states, the District of Columbia, Puerto Rico, and the Virgin Islands.[5]

The first step most commonly used to characterize hemoglobin is electrophoresis. Cellulose acetate and isoelectric focusing (IEF) are the most commonly used electrophoretic methods.[5] Electrophoresis separates different hemoglobins by electrical charge.

The definitive test for HbS is hemoglobin electrophoresis on cellulose acetate at alkaline pH, followed if necessary by electrophoresis on citrate agar at acid pH (Fig. 11–10). Hemoglobin separation by citrate agar electrophoresis depends on both the charge of the hemoglobin and the ability of the hemoglobin to combine with components in the agar gel mixture. The patient with sickle cell anemia produces no normal β chains; therefore, there will be no HbA on electrophoresis (unless the patient has been recently transfused). HbS constitutes 80% or more of hemoglobin, with HbF ranging from 1% to 20%.[2,7,8,10] When HbF levels are higher than 20%, there is a decrease in the severity of the disease.[8] High levels of HbF are seen transiently in newborns and in hereditary persistence of fetal hemoglobin (HPFH). In sickle cell anemia, the HbA_2 level may be slightly increased, with a mean of 3.4%.[2,17] Hemoglobins with similar charges have similar migration patterns during electrophoresis, especially on cellulose acetate. Hemoglobins D and G both migrate to the same position as HbS at alkaline pH. Hemoglobin E (HbE) and hemoglobin O_{Arab} (HbO_{Arab}) migrate in the same position as HbC. Citrate agar electrophoresis is very useful, because it clearly separates HbS from HbG and HbD, and HbC from HbE and HbO_{Arab}, at acid pH.[17]

Citrate agar electrophoresis is rarely used as the primary electrophoretic method for screening, but it is used by many laboratories to confirm the presence of abnormal hemoglobins detected by other methods.[17] This practice of employing two laboratory methods is called a two-tier screening technique.[5] In sickle cell trait, hemoglobin electrophoresis at alkaline pH shows 60% HbA, 40% HbS, and usually elevated HbA_2 (mean is 3.6%).[5,17] At acid pH, one band is present in the A position ($HbA + HbA_2$), whereas the other band migrates to the S position (see Fig. 11–10).[5,17]

It should be noted that most hemoglobin variant traits, without coexistent conditions such as iron deficiency, or thalassemia, have alkaline electrophoretic patterns with an

---

➤ **Table 11-9**
SCREENING METHODS

Criteria	Cellulose Acetate Electrophoresis	Isoelectric Focusing	High-Performance Liquid Chromatography
Equipment cost	$2500	$4000	$30,000
Cost per test (consumables)	$0.15–0.25	$0.35–0.50	$0.10–1.75
Samples run per hour	200	72	5–20
Advantages	Semiquantitative	Sharper bands	Automated
	Simple to operate		Quantitative
Disadvantages	Densitometer for quantitation	Densitometer for quantitation	Complex to use

Note: Labor costs vary with number of samples per run.
  Source: Sickle Cell Disease Guideline Panel: Sickle cell disease: Screening, diagnosis, management, and counseling in newborns and infants. Clinical Practice Guideline No 6. AHCPR Pub No 93-0562. US Department of Health and Human Services, Rockville, MD, April 1993.

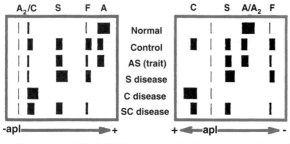

A. Cellulose Acetate (pH 8.4)   B. Citrate Agar (pH 6.0-6.5)

▶ FIGURE 11–10   Electrophoretic patterns of hemoglobin on (A) cellulose acetate, run at pH 8.4, and (B) citrate agar, run at pH 6.0 to 6.5. apl = point of application.

approximate 60:40 ratio of normal to abnormal hemoglobin. This is because of the effect of charge on assembly of globin chains: relatively positively charged globins, such as S (+1) and C (+2) have a slight disadvantage in assembling with the α chains to form αβ dimers compared with normal β globin. For this reason, HbS comprises less than 50% of the hemoglobin in heterozygotes, and a further reduction is seen in HbC trait.

Two previously used screening tests should *not* be used for newborn screening. These are (1) the sickle cell preparation using sodium metabisulfite, and (2) solubility tests using a concentrated phosphate buffer, a hemolyzing agent, and sodium dithionate. These tube solubility tests either isolate HbS at an interface or cause the abnormal hemoglobin to precipitate (Fig. 11–11). Both tests depend on the concentration of HbS in the red cell or hemolysate.[5,17]

The low level of HbS in cells of the neonate is believed to explain the unreliability of these tests during the newborn period. Although sickle cell disease should not be diagnosed from either a sickle cell preparation or solubility test, because neither of these tests will reliably distinguish sickle cell trait from sickle cell anemia, many hospitals still perform these tests on adult patients.[17] It is important to note that some rare hemoglobins also sickle, giving positive solubility tests. Table 11–10 lists some of the rare hemoglobins that sickle. Because HbS, HbG, and HbD all migrate in the same position on cellulose acetate electrophoresis, it is helpful to know that HbG and HbD do not give a positive tube solubility test.

Some authors have advocated DNA analysis as an additional testing method for detection of the sickle cell gene.[17] However, at present, this method is both costly and limited in the number of genotypes that can be identified.

▶ TREATMENT

With advances in the diagnosis, treatment, and prevention of complications, the life expectancy of individuals with sickle cell disease has improved. There is an 85% chance that infants born in the United States with HbSS disease will survive to age 20.[5,6,11] Delay in diagnosis and treatment resulting from lack of appropriate health services plays an important role in overall morbidity and mortality in developing countries. It is believed that in Africa, 50% of infants with sickle cell disease die in the first year of life. A large number of young African children also die in the first decade of life from pneumococcal sepsis, malaria, meningitis, acute splenic sequestration, or aplastic crisis.[17]

The principal causes of death in infants with HbSS disease in the United States include overwhelming infections with *S. pneumoniae*, cerebrovascular accidents, and acute splenic sequestration crises.[6,13] One of the greatest advances in therapy of sickle cell disease has been the introduction of prophylactic penicillin therapy, which has virtually eliminated pneumococcal sepsis, one of the major causes of death in children with sickle cell disease.[18] Twice-daily administration of oral penicillin reduces both morbidity and mortality from pneumococcal infection in HbSS disease in infants.[5,6,18] In addition, administration of age-appropriate immunizations should be given, including pneumococcal, conjugated *H. influenzae*, and hepatitis B vaccines.[5,6]

A variety of drugs are being tested for their potential in ameliorating the effects of sickle cell anemia. Development of drug therapies is based on the pathophysiology of sickle cell disease.[7,11] Studies in vitro have shown that increasing

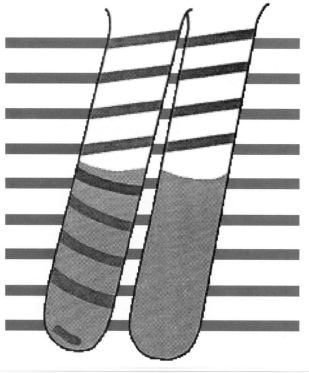

Negative   Positive

▶ FIGURE 11–11   Tube solubility screening test for sickle cell anemia.

▶ Table 11-10
EXAMPLES OF RARE HEMOGLOBINS THAT SICKLE AND GIVE A POSITIVE TUBE SOLUBILITY TEST

HbC$_{Harlem}$ (HbC$_{Georgetown}$)

HbC$_{Ziguinchor}$

HbS$_{Memphis}$

HbS$_{Travis}$

Hb$_{Alexandra}$

Hb$_{Porto-Alegre}$

HbF decreases HbS polymerization; this effect is based on the reduction in concentration of HbS and on a direct inhibition of polymerization by HbF. Several candidate agents for increasing HbF have been evaluated in the past 15 to 20 years. Several studies in small groups of patients with HbSS disease showed an increase in HbF levels and an increase in the fraction of cells containing HbF (F cells) with hydroxyurea therapy. These findings were dramatically confirmed in the randomized, double-blind multicenter study of hydroxyurea in patients with sickle cell disease (MSH).[19] This study demonstrated a 50% reduction in the frequency of painful crises, and of the incidence of acute chest syndromes, transfusion of blood, and hospitalization.[19] Hydroxyurea had much less dramatic effects on the chronic anemia of sickle cell disease, inducing a significant but modest (on average, 0.7 g/dL) increase in hemoglobin levels. Half of the patients had no increase or only trivial increments in HbF levels.[20] The benefit induced by the hydroxyurea therapy on the polymerization tendency of HbS (estimated with measurements of the delay time for HbS polymerization) is of a magnitude to transform HbSS disease into the milder but still clinically relevant HbSC disease.[21] Thus, the erythrocytes of hydroxyurea-treated patients maintain a very significant polymerization capability. In addition, the percentage of dense, dehydrated cells, which is most likely associated with organ damage and vaso-occlusion, is reduced but not totally abolished by hydroxyurea therapy. Therefore, a significant proportion of cells that can readily polymerize is still present in hydroxyurea-treated patients. There are also concerns regarding the short-term marrow toxicity and long-term possible carcinogenic potential of hydroxyurea. These concerns are heightened by the use of hydroxyurea in children, in whom it has been shown to provide significant clinical benefits.[22,23] It is thus still necessary to improve on the positive response induced by hydroxyurea with similar or different drugs.

Other therapeutic approaches have attempted to increase HbF by using intravenous argine butyrate, Na⁴-phenylbutyrate, or oral butyramide. Increases in HbF have been noted in patients treated with valproic acid.[24–28] Yet other studies have attempted to use compounds that improve the fluidity of the membrane, or alter the cellular metabolism of sickle erythrocytes. There have been some preliminary reports on the use of artificial hemoglobin in patients with sickle cell disease. Table 11–11 lists the goals of these therapeutic approaches to the treatment of sickle cell anemia. Table 11–12 lists various approaches to specific therapy with a specific drug.

Blood transfusions may be required for acute situations and for prevention of certain complications of HbSS disease, such as stroke.[15] Simple transfusion has little or no benefit for treatment of acute sickle vasculopathies, unless it is associated with removal of sickle erythrocytes. In fact, transfusion only increases blood viscosity and further compromises peripheral blood flow. Exchange transfusions are indicated in the acute setting.[5,6] For HbSS patients with higher hematocrits (20% or greater in children, 25% or higher in adults) an exchange transfusion technique may be safer than a simple blood transfusion.[5,6] Table 11–13 lists the general considerations and indications for blood transfusions in HbSS disease. Chronic blood transfusions have been shown to reduce the risk of stroke.[15] When discontinuing chronic transfusions becomes necessary (for iron overload concerns, presence of multiple alloantibodies, or other reasons) patients should be carefully followed, because they have an increased risk for intracranial hemorrhage.[29]

Bone marrow transplantation is currently being investigated in the United States and in Europe for the treatment of sickle cell anemia and may represent a potential cure.[30–33] A national trial of bone marrow transplantation has been conducted on selected patients with HbSS disease having severe symptoms of sickle-induced vasculopathy.[30,32,33] Although marrow transplantation has been recognized since the 1980s as a potential cure,[31] the risks (high mortality) associated with this procedure created considerable caution for use as a treatment.[30,32,33] However, the risks appear sufficiently reduced today, and marrow transplantation should be considered in selected cases as an alternative to conventional supportive care and pharmacologic treatment, such as hydroxyurea and transfusion therapy. Initial studies have indicated that bone marrow transplantation is effective in reducing pain and morbidity from vaso-occlusive crises, ameliorating osteonecrosis, and reversing reticuloendothelial dysfunction after transplantation in patients with HbSS disease.[32,33] On a worldwide level, experience with bone marrow transplantation for HbSS disease has been more limited.[33] The first report on the use of cord blood transplantation involving a girl with sickle cell disease transplanted with cord blood obtained from her HLA-matched sister born with sickle cell trait was published in 1996.[33] The experience on the use of cord blood transplantation for sickle cell disease is limited to only a few cases.

It is now possible to efficiently diagnose the presence or absence of sickle cell disease in embryos obtained with in vitro fertilization, prior to implantation.[34] This powerful technique may help carrier couples by allowing them to select a healthy child without facing the decision of aborting an affected fetus.

The future treatment of gene therapy for HbSS disease as well as other hemoglobinopathies is also currently under investigation.[35–38] The success of gene therapy for hemoglobinopathies depends on the ability of researchers to isolate, enrich, and insert genes into hematopoietic pluripotential stem cells.[35,37,38] Gene therapies based on repairing the genetic defect and inserting the normal hemoglobin gene into the patient's own hematopoietic stem cells may one day become feasible.[38]

> ## Table 11-11
> ### TREATMENT OF SICKLE CELL ANEMIA: GOALS OF THERAPEUTIC APPROACHES

Increase the production of fetal hemoglobin in the adult

Decrease microvascular entrapment of sickle cells

Modify the oxygen affinity or solubility of sickle hemoglobin

Change the volume of the sickle erythrocyte

Alter expression of the abnormal sickle gene

➤ HEMOGLOBIN C (HbC) DISEASE AND TRAIT

HbC disease is found almost exclusively in the black population. HbC differs from normal HbA by the single amino acid

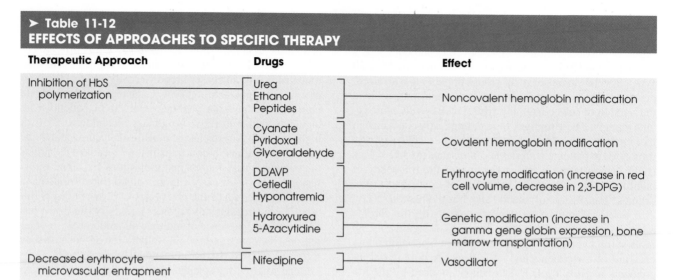

> **Table 11-12**
EFFECTS OF APPROACHES TO SPECIFIC THERAPY

Therapeutic Approach	Drugs	Effect
Inhibition of HbS polymerization	Urea Ethanol Peptides	Noncovalent hemoglobin modification
	Cyanate Pyridoxal Glyceraldehyde	Covalent hemoglobin modification
	DDAVP Cetiedil Hyponatremia	Erythrocyte modification (increase in red cell volume, decrease in 2,3-DPG)
	Hydroxyurea 5-Azacytidine	Genetic modification (increase in gamma gene globin expression, bone marrow transplantation)
Decreased erythrocyte microvascular entrapment	Nifedipine	Vasodilator

Abbreviation: DDAVP = 1-Deamino-8-d-arginine vasopressin.

substitution of lysine for glutamic acid in the sixth position from the NH_2 terminal end of the β chain (Fig. 11–12). This represents the same substitution point as in HbS but with a positively charged amino acid. The structural formula for HbC, the presence of which is often referred to as HbC disease, is $\alpha_2\beta_2^{6Glu-Lys}$. HbC is seen with great frequency in West Africa, particularly northern Ghana, where the incidence is 17% to 28%.[1,39] In the United States, only 0.02% of blacks have HbC disease.[1,39] The clinical manifestations are mild chronic hemolytic anemia with associated splenomegaly and abdominal discomfort. The red cell morphology is typically normocytic, and normo- or hyperchromic, with numerous target cells (50% to 90%) and occasionally microspherocytes, fragmented cells, and folded cells (Fig. 11–13). HbC crystals (Fig. 11–14 and Color Plate 108) or "bar of gold" crystals occur more often in the red cells of individuals who have undergone splenectomy than in those whose spleen is intact. Figure 11–15 is a scanning electron micrograph (SEM) of hemoglobin C crystals. These crystals can be demonstrated in wet preparations by washing the red cells and then suspending them in a sodium citrate solution.[14] The reticulocyte count is slightly increased. Hemoglobin bands, at alkaline pH, reveal approximately 95% HbC plus A_2, less than 7% HbF, and no HbA. Hemoglobins E, O_{Arab}, C, and A_2 all migrate to the same position at alkaline pH. HbC can be separated from these other hemoglobins at acid pH (see Fig. 11–10).

HbC trait, $\alpha_2\beta_1\beta_1^{6Glu-Lys}$, is present in 2% to 3% of American blacks, and these individuals are clinically

> **Table 11-13**
GENERAL CONSIDERATIONS AND INDICATIONS FOR BLOOD TRANSFUSION IN PATIENTS WITH SICKLE CELL ANEMIA

Consideration	Indications
To improve the oxygen-carrying transport in red cells by simple transfusions	Severely anemic as reflected by dyspnea, postural hypotension, high-output cardiac failure, angina, or cerebral dysfunction
	Sudden fall in hemoglobin or hematocrit levels during acute splenic or hepatic sequestration crisis
	Hemoglobin level < 5.0 g/dL or hematocrit of 15% in patients who exhibit fatigue and dyspnea along with erythroid hypoplasia or aplasia
To improve microvascular perfusion by decreasing the number of red cells containing HbS by partial exchange transfusion	Life-threatening events, such as cerebrovascular accidents including stroke and transient ischemic attacks (TIAs)
	Arterial hypoxia syndrome (fat embolization)
	Acute progressive lung disease
	Unresponsive acute priapism
	Eye surgery when performed under local anesthesia and in the nonanemic patient

Source: Charache, S, et al (eds): Management and Therapy of Sickle Cell Disease. US Department of Health and Human Services, Public Health Service, National Institutes of Health. NIH Pub 91:2117, August 1991.

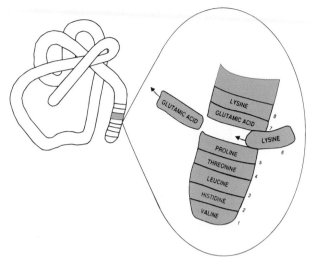

> **FIGURE 11-12** Amino acid substitution in hemoglobin C.

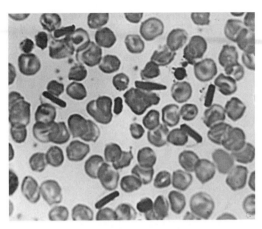

> **FIGURE 11-14** Hemoglobin C disease (peripheral blood). Note the particular crystals: "bar of gold" and numerous target cells (postsplenectomy). (From Bell, A: Hematology. In: Listen, Look and Learn. Health and Education Resources, Inc., Bethesda, MD, with permission.)

asymptomatic.[39] The only significant finding on the peripheral blood smear is targeting. At alkaline pH, there is approximately 60% HbA and 40% HbC plus A_2.

➤ HEMOGLOBIN D (HbD) DISEASE AND TRAIT

HbD has several variants. The most common variant in American blacks is HbD$_{Punjab}$, which is synonymous with HbD$_{Los Angeles}$. Its frequency is less than 0.02%.[39] Both the homozygous ($\alpha_2\beta_2{}^{121Glu-Gln}$) and the heterozygous ($\alpha_2\beta_1\beta_1{}^{121Glu-Gln}$) states are asymptomatic. The peripheral blood smear is unremarkable, except for a few target cells. HbD migrates electrophoretically to the same position as HbS and HbG at alkaline pH but migrates with HbA at acid pH. HbD is a nonsickling soluble hemoglobin.

➤ HEMOGLOBIN E (HbE) DISEASE AND TRAIT

HbE occurs with greatest frequency in Burma, Thailand, Cambodia, Laos, Malaysia, and Indonesia.[1,39] This variant is now prevalent in the United States because of the influx of refugees from Southeast Asia. The homozygous state ($\alpha_2\beta_2{}^{26Glu-Lys}$) presents with little or no anemia, target cells, and microcytic, hypochromic red cell indices. Alkaline electrophoresis reveals approximately 95% to 97% HbE plus A_2, and the remainder of the hemoglobin is HbF. HbE migrates with HbC and HbO$_{Arab}$ at alkaline pH, but migrates with HbA at acid pH. HbE trait ($\alpha_2\beta_1\beta_1{}^{26Glu-Lys}$) is asymptomatic clinically. Microcytosis, target cells, and approximately 70% HbA and 30% HbE plus A_2 are noted on routine electrophoresis.[1,39] HbE is slightly *unstable,* and there is an associated thalassemic component with this hemoglobin variant. This is responsible for the microcytosis, and the lower than expected quantified value of HbE in HbAE.[40]

It has been postulated that HbE may protect against malaria, because areas such as Thailand that are highly endemic for malaria also have a high incidence of the HbE gene. Some authors attribute this effect to the fact that the parasite *P. falciparum* multiplies more slowly in HbE red cells than in the HbAE or HbAA red cells.[39]

➤ HEMOGLOBIN O$_{ARAB}$ (HbO$_{ARAB}$) DISEASE AND TRAIT

HbO$_{Arab}$ is a rare hemoglobin variant that occurs infrequently in black, Arab, and Sudanese populations. Homozygous O$_{Arab}$ ($\alpha_2\beta_2{}^{121Glu-Lys}$) disease exhibits a mild he-

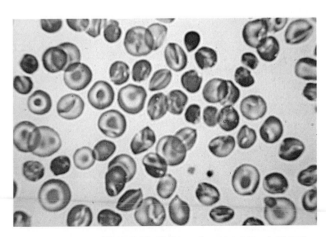

> **FIGURE 11-13** Hemoglobin C disease (presplenectomy). Note the numerous target and envelope forms.

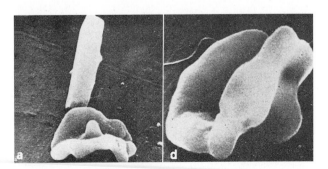

> **FIGURE 11-15** SEM of hemoglobin C crystals. (From Bell, A: Hematology. In: Listen, Look and Learn. Health and Education Resources, Inc., Bethesda, MD, with permission.)

molytic anemia with slight splenomegaly and target cells on the peripheral blood smear. This hemoglobin migrates electrophoretically with HbC, HbE, and HbA_2 at alkaline pH but separates at acid pH, migrating in the HbA position (see Fig. 11–10). In the heterozygous state of HbO_{Arab} ($\alpha_2\beta_1\beta_1^{121Glu-Lys}$), the patient is asymptomatic.[39]

➤ HEMOGLOBIN S WITH OTHER ABNORMAL HEMOGLOBINS

As mentioned previously, *sickle cell disease* is a generic term for a group of genetic disorders that includes sickle cell anemia and hemoglobinopathies in which HbS is found in association with another abnormal hemoglobins, and the sickle β thalassemia syndromes.[1,2,10,40–42] This section focuses on defining the disorders that have HbS and another abnormal hemoglobin. Sickle β thalassemia is briefly mentioned at the end of this section. Table 11–14 lists the common and uncommon forms of sickle cell disease.

Hemoglobin SC (HbSC) Disease

Hemoglobin SC disease ($\alpha_2\beta_1^{6Val}\beta_1^{6Glu-Lys}$) occurs when the gene for HbS is inherited from one parent and that for HbC from the other. About 0.12% of black Americans have SC disease.[1,10,39] Patients with HbSC disease are generally less anemic and experience a milder course than those with HbSS disease. However, because of increased blood viscosity, this condition has a greater incidence of retinal hemorrhage, renal papillary necrosis, and necrosis of the femoral head.[10] Peripheral blood smear findings include target cells, folded red cells, and occasionally glove-shaped intracellular crystals (Fig. 11–16 and Color Plate 109).[41] The solubility test results are positive owing to the presence of HbS. Hemoglobin electrophoresis at alkaline pH separates HbS and HbC in approximately equal amounts (Fig. 11–17 and Color Plate 110). HbF is usually less than 2% compared with average HbF levels of about 6% in sickle cell anemia. Electrophoresis at acid pH confirms the S and C hemoglobins (see Fig. 11–10). Table 11–15 compares the incidence of the most common hemoglobinopathies found in American blacks.

Hemoglobin SD (HbSD) Disease

The combination of HbS and HbD, although rare, presents an interesting diagnostic problem. Because these hemoglobins migrate together at alkaline pH, the electrophoretic pattern is similar to that of HbSS disease. Solubility tests are positive.

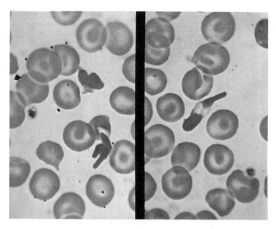

➤ **FIGURE 11–16**   Hemoglobin SC disease (peripheral blood). Note the type of "Washington monument" crystals and target cells. (From Bell, A: Hematology. In: Listen, Look and Learn. Health and Education Resources, Inc., Bethesda, MD, with permission.)

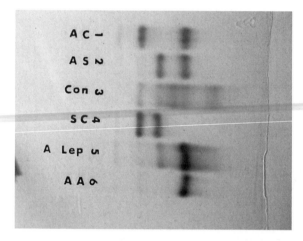

➤ **FIGURE 11–17**   Hemoglobin electrophoretic patterns: (1) HbAC, (2) HbAS, (3) commercial control, (4) HbSC, (5) HbA-Lepore, and (6) HbAA normal control.

The clinical severity of HbSD disease, however, falls between that of sickle cell anemia and that of sickle cell trait.[1,10,39,40] Acid electrophoresis separates these two hemoglobins. HbS has its own migration point, whereas HbD migrates with HbA in the same position (see Fig. 11–10).

➤ **Table 11-14**
COMMON AND UNCOMMON FORMS OF SICKLE CELL DISEASE

Common	Uncommon
(HbSS) sickle cell anemia	(HbSD) hemoglobin SD disease
(HbSC) sickle-HbC disease	($HbSO_{Arab}$) hemoglobin SO_{Arab}
(HbSβ¹) sickle β⁺ thalassemia	(HbSE) hemoglobin SE disease
(HbSβ⁰) sickle β⁰ thalassemia	(HbS-Lepore) hemoglobin S Lepore

➤ **Table 11-15**
INCIDENCE OF COMMON HEMOGLOBINOPATHIES IN AMERICAN BLACKS

Condition	Genotype	Incidence (All Ages)
Hemoglobin C disease	$\alpha_2\beta^C\beta^C$	0.02% (1 in 4500)
Hemoglobin C trait	$\alpha_2\beta^A\beta^C$	3.0% (1 in 33)
Sickle cell anemia	$\alpha_2\beta^S\beta^S$	0.26% (1 in 375)
Sickle cell trait	$\alpha_2\beta^A\beta^S$	8.0% (1 in 13)
Sickle C disease	$\alpha_2\beta^S\beta^C$	0.12% (1 in 835)
Sickle β thalassemia	$\alpha_2\beta^S\beta^0$	0.06% (1 in 1667)

Hemoglobin SO$_{Arab}$ (HbSO$_{Arab}$) and S-Oman (HbS-Oman) Disease

The combination of HbS and HbO$_{Arab}$ can have a clinical presentation that is similar in severity to that of HbSS disease. The anemia is severe, with typical sickled cells seen on the peripheral blood smear. This condition might initially be confused with HbSC on routine electrophoresis; however, differentiation can be made with acid electrophoresis (see Fig. 11–10).

HbS-Oman is a unique hemoglobin variant that carries both the classic sickle mutation in β^6 and one additional mutation in $\beta^{121Glu-Lys}$, which is the same substitution observed in HbO$_{Arab}$. Heterozygotes for this variant express between 14% and 20% of the abnormal hemoglobin. The higher levels of expression are associated with a sickle cell anemia clinical syndrome of moderate intensity.[43]

Hemoglobin S/β Thalassemia Combination

The severity of HbS combined with β thalassemia depends on the degree of suppression of β-globin chain synthesis. Hemoglobin S/β^0 thalassemia is a severe condition that clinically resembles sickle cell anemia; on the other hand, HbS/β^+ thalassemia generally has a milder clinical presentation. The reader is referred to Chapter 12 for a detailed discussion of HbS/β thalassemia and other hemoglobin variants that occur in combination with thalassemia.[42]

Laboratory Diagnosis of HbS with Other Abnormal Hemoglobins

When HbS is found in association with another abnormal hemoglobin, the diagnosis in many instances can be made from hemoglobin electrophoresis alone. However, it may be difficult to distinguish between HbSS disease and some of the sickle β thalassemia syndromes such as HbSβ^0 thalassemia, HbSβ^+ thalassemia, HbSδβ thalassemia, and HbS in association with hereditary persistence of fetal hemoglobin syndrome (HbS HPFH).[1,2,40,42] In these cases, the electrophoresis demonstrates only HbS, HbF, and HbA$_2$. It is important to properly diagnose these disorders because the clinical manifestations and subsequent treatment are different. For example, HbSβ^0 thalassemia is similar in severity to HbSS disease. Patients with HbSδβ thalassemia have few symptoms; HbS/β^+ thalassemia is a milder form, and HbS HPFH is usually asymptomatic with no anemia. Measurement of HbF and HbA$_2$ may be helpful in distinguishing these conditions, because patients with HbSS, HbSβ^0 thalassemia, HbSδβ thalassemia, and HbS HPFH all have similar electrophoretic patterns.[40,42] In HbSβ^0 thalassemia, HbA$_2$ levels are greater than 3.5% whereas they are low in patients with HbSδβ thalassemia and HbS HPFH.[17,40,42] Generally, HbF levels are higher in all the HbSβ thalassemias in comparison with HbSS. Assessment of HbF in the parents may be indicated when HbS HPFH is suspected.[17,40,42] Table 11–16 summarizes the clinical and hematologic findings in the common variants of sickle cell disease.

➤ HEMOGLOBIN VARIANTS WITH ALTERED OXYGEN AFFINITY

High-affinity hemoglobins, which are inherited as an autosomal dominant disorder, are seen in the heterozygous state. These hemoglobins bind oxygen more readily and release it less easily to the tissues. The result is tissue hypoxia, which stimulates increased erythropoietin production. This, in turn, causes a compensatory increase in red cell mass, with increases in red count, hemoglobin, and hematocrit, producing erythrocytosis and congenital polycythemia. Other hematologic parameters are normal. There is a shift to the left in the oxygen dissociation curve, and a diagnosis is established by measuring P$_{50}$ levels (Fig. 11–18). Individuals with these hemoglobin variants are asymptomatic.[39] For a review of P$_{50}$ refer to Chapter 3.

Hemoglobins with decreased oxygen affinity release oxygen quite readily to the tissues. There is a shift to the right in the oxygen-dissociation curve (see Fig. 11–18). As more oxygen is released per gram of hemoglobin, erythropoietin concentrations fall. This can result in decreased hemoglobin concentration with the development of a mild anemia. There may also be mild cyanosis associated with a decreased oxygen saturation level. Hemoglobins with increased or decreased oxygen affinities are listed in Table 11–17. In cases of unexplained erythrocytosis or cyanosis, oxygen affinity studies may be helpful.[39]

➤ UNSTABLE HEMOGLOBINS

More than 180 unstable hemoglobins (Fig. 11–19 and Color Plate 111) have been described and less than 50% are associated with a hemolytic disorder.[39] Unstable hemoglobins are hemoglobin variants in which amino acid substitutions or deletions have weakened the binding forces that maintain the structure of the molecule. The instability may cause hemoglobin to denature and precipitate in the red cells as Heinz bodies. Most unstable hemoglobin variants are inherited as autosomal dominant disorders.[39] However, absence of a positive family history is not always helpful, as new mutations are common. Many mutations producing unstable hemoglobinopathies are single amino acid substitutions in either the α-, β-, γ-, or δ-globin chains that affect a few key areas of the hemoglobin structure. By far the majority of these substitutions are in the β-globin chain, followed by an α-chain substitution and only a few in γ or δ chains. Many of the unstable hemoglobins have high oxygen affinity and, therefore, may not cause anemia, making diagnosis in this group of patients particularly difficult. When anemia is present, the degree of hemolysis associated with an unstable hemoglobin varies considerably.[39] Some patients experience severe chronic hemolysis with jaundice and splenomegaly. However, most patients have a mild compensated condition and seek medical attention only after exacerbation of the hemolysis caused by infection and increased temperature or exposure to oxidative drugs.[41] Reticulocytosis is variable. Hypochromia may be apparent on the peripheral blood smear, and the mean red cell hemoglobin (MCH) content can be low in some cases because the unstable hemoglobin may be denatured and "pitted" out of the cell by the mononuclear phagocytic cells of the spleen.

Hemoglobin electrophoresis is usually not a very helpful laboratory method to detect unstable hemoglobins; however, subtle indications of an abnormality may be observed.[39,40] These include an increased level of HbA$_2$, a common finding in unstable β-chain hemoglobins, and the presence of minor electrophoretic components such as free

> **Table 11-16**

CLINICAL AND HEMATOLOGIC FINDINGS IN THE COMMON VARIANTS OF SICKLE CELL DISEASE AFTER THE AGE OF 5 YEARS

| Disease Group | Clinical Severity | Hemoglobin Electrophoresis | | | | Hematologic Values* | | | |
		S (%)	F (%)	A₂ (%)	A (%)	Hb (g/dL)	Retic (%)	MCV (fL)	RBC Morphology
SS	Usually marked	> 90	< 10	< 3.5	0	6–10	5–20	> 80	Sickle cells
									nRBCs
									Normochromic, normocytic
									Anisocytosis
									Poikilocytosis
									Target cells
									Howell-Jolly bodies
Sβ⁰ Thal	Marked to moderate	> 80	< 20	> 3.5	0	6–10	5–20	< 80	Sickle cells nRBCs
									Hypochromic
									Microcytosis
									Anisocytosis
									Poikilocytosis
									Target cells
Sβ⁺ Thal	Mild to moderate	> 60	< 20	> 3.5	20 (A)	9–12	5–10	< 75	No sickle cells
									Hypochromic
									Microcytosis
									Anisocytosis
									Poikilocytosis
									Target cells
SC	Mild to moderate	50	< 5	—	50 (C)	10–15	5–10	75–95	Occasional SC crystals
									Anisocytosis
									Poikilocytosis
									Target cells
S HPFH	Asymptomatic	> 70	> 30	< 2.5	—	12–14	1–2	< 75	No sickle cells
									Anisocytosis
									Poikilocytosis
									Rare target cells

*Hematologic values are approximate. There is a tremendous variability between disease groups and between individual patients of the same group, particularly with regard to clinical severity.

Abbreviations: SS = sickle cell anemia; Sβ⁰Thal = sickle beta no thalassemia; Sβ⁺Thal = sickle beta plus thalassemia; S HPFH = HbS in association with the hereditary persistence of fetal hemoglobin syndrome; SC = hemoglobin SC disease; nRBCs = nucleated red blood cells.

Source: Charache, S, et al (eds): Management and Therapy of Sickle Cell Disease. US Department of Health and Human Services, Public Health Service, National Institutes of Health. NIH Pub 91:2117, August 1991.

α-globin chains, indicative of an unstable β globin (Table 11–18).[39,40]

Most hospitals still perform the isopropanol precipitation or heat denaturation test for detection of unstable hemoglobins. Newer techniques such as IEF can resolve many hemoglobin mutations with only a very slight alteration in their isoelectric point, and globin chain analysis can be performed by reversed phase high-performance liquid chromatography (HPLC).[39,40]

> ## METHEMOGLOBINEMIA

Methemoglobinemia is a clinical condition with methemoglobin levels greater than 1% of the total hemoglobin.[39] Methemoglobin contains the oxidized ferric form of iron (Fe^{3+}) rather than ferrous form (Fe^{2+}). In this state, the molecule is unable to bind oxygen and results in cyanosis. The blood is chocolate-brown. In general, there are three causes of methemoglobinemia:

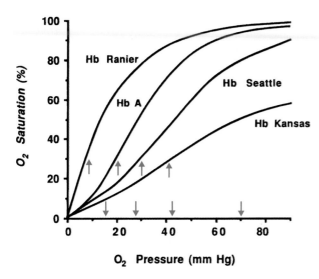

> **FIGURE 11–18** Oxygen equilibrium curve of whole blood from subjects with hemoglobin$_{Rainer, Seattle,}$ and $_{Kansas}$ and from normal controls.

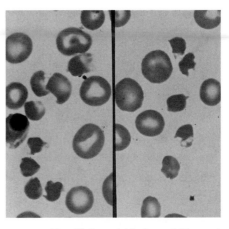

> **FIGURE 11–19** Unstable hemoglobin: hemoglobin$_{Zurich}$ (peripheral blood). (From Bell, A: Hematology. In: Listen, Look and Learn. Health and Education Resources, Inc., Bethesda, MD, with permission.)

1. Hemoglobin M variants (dominant inheritance)
2. NADH-diaphorase deficiency (recessive inheritance)
3. Toxic substance (acquired)

There are five variants of hemoglobin M (Table 11–19), which result from a single amino acid substitution in the globin chain that stabilizes iron in the ferric form. If the substitution occurs in the α chain, cyanosis is present at birth. Cyanosis does not occur with a β-chain substitution until approximately 6 months of age.[39] This correlates with the switch from γ to β chains. The presumptive diagnosis of HbM is made from the absorption spectra of hemolysates, and hemoglobin electrophoresis on agar gel at pH 7.1.[39] Patients have obvious cyanosis but otherwise are generally asymptomatic. No specific treatment is indicated or possible.

The enzyme NADH-diaphorase reduces cytochrome b5, which converts the naturally occurring ferric iron back to the ferrous state. To confirm NADH-diaphorase deficiency, a quantitative enzyme assay is necessary. Although nearly all enzyme-deficient individuals are asymptomatic, some find their lifelong cyanosis to be a cosmetic hardship. The level of methemoglobin can be reduced with the administration of ascorbic acid or methylene blue.[39]

Acquired methemoglobinemia can occur in healthy individuals when drugs or other toxic substances oxidize hemoglobin in circulation. Patients who appear to be symptomatic from methemoglobinemia should be treated promptly with intravenous methylene blue.

➤ GENERAL SUMMARY OF LABORATORY DIAGNOSIS

Hemoglobinopathies usually cannot be correctly diagnosed with a single laboratory procedure. It is usually necessary to correlate the results of a complete blood count and indices with additional laboratory tests such as a reticulocyte count, peripheral smear evaluation, hemoglobin electrophoresis, and, if necessary, measurement of hemoglobins A_2 and F. Selected patient information such as age, gender, ethnic background, family history, and physical symptoms is helpful.

Most abnormal hemoglobins are associated with RBC indices that are normocytic and normochromic. Microcytosis and hypochromia are seen in some variants (e.g., HbE). Abnormal red cell morphology may or may not be noted on the peripheral blood smear, and reticulocyte counts are often elevated. Screening tests include hemoglobin electrophoresis, IEF, and HPLC.[17,40]

Cellulose acetate electrophoresis at alkaline pH (see Fig. 11–17) is commonly performed first. Electrophoresis on citrate agar at acid pH can further differentiate abnormal hemoglobins. HbF quantitation should be done, following the newborn period, when this hemoglobin is seen on cellulose acetate.

IEF, a type of sensitive electrophoresis, separates hemoglobins according to their isoelectric points. Superior IEF resolution differentiates some hemoglobins that migrate to the same electrophoretic point at alkaline and acid pH. On the initial patient visit other laboratory tests should also be performed; these include urinalysis, liver function tests, urea, creatinine, and electrolytes. In addition, a chest x-ray should be obtained.

➤ Table 11-17
HEMOGLOBINS ASSOCIATED WITH ALTERED OXYGEN AFFINITY

Increased O$_2$ Affinity and Polycythemia		Decreased O$_2$ Affinity— May Have Mild Anemia or Cyanosis	
Hb$_{Chesapeake}$	$\alpha_2^{92Leu}\beta_2$	Hb$_{Kansas}$	$\alpha_2^{102Thr}\beta_2$
HbJ$_{Cape Town}$	$\alpha_2^{92Gln}\beta_2$	Hb$_{Titusville}$	$\alpha_2^{94Asn}\beta_2$
Hb$_{Malmö}$	$\alpha_2\beta_2^{97Gln}$	Hb$_{Providence}$	$\alpha_2\beta_2^{82Asn,Asp}$
Hb$_{Yakima}$	$\alpha_2\beta_2^{99His}$	Hb$_{Agenogi}$	$\alpha_2\beta_2^{90Lys}$
Hb$_{Kempsey}$	$\alpha_2\beta_s^{99Asn}$	Hb$_{Beth Israel}$	$\alpha_2\beta_2^{102Ser}$
Hb$_{Ypsi (Ypsilanti)}$	$\alpha_2\beta_2^{99Tyr}$	Hb$_{Yoshizuka}$	$\alpha_2\beta_2^{108Asp}$
Hb$_{Hiroshima}$	$\alpha_2\beta_2^{146Asp}$	Hb$_{Seattle}$	$\alpha_2\beta_2^{70Asp}$
Hb$_{Rainier}$	$\alpha_2\beta_2^{145Cys}$		
Hb$_{Bethesda}$	$\alpha_2\beta_2^{145His}$		

➤ Table 11-18
UNSTABLE HEMOGLOBINS*

α-Chain Abnormalities			β-Chain Abnormalities		
Hb$_{Torina}$	$\alpha_2{}^{43Val}\beta_2$		Hb$_{Leiden}$	$\alpha_2\beta_2{}^{6or7}$	(Glu deleted)
Hb$_{L-Ferrara}$	$\alpha_2{}^{47Gly}\beta_2$		Hb$_{Sogn}$	$\alpha_2\beta_2{}^{14Arg}$	
Hb$_{Hasharon}$	$\alpha_2{}^{47His}\beta_2$		Hb$_{Freiburg}$	$\alpha_2\beta_2{}^{23}$	(Val deleted)
Hb$_{Ann\ Arbor}$	$\alpha_2{}^{80Arg}\beta_2$		Hb$_{Riverdale\ Bronx}$	$\alpha_2\beta_2{}^{24Arg}$	
Hb$_{Etobicoke}$	$\alpha_2{}^{84Arg}\beta_2$		Hb$_{Genova}$	$\alpha_2\beta_2{}^{28Pro}$	
Hb$_{Dakar}$	$\alpha_2{}^{112Gln}\beta_2$		Hb$_{Tacoma}$	$\alpha_2\beta_2{}^{30Ser}$	
Hb$_{Bibba}$	$\alpha_2{}^{136Pro}\beta_2$		Hb$_{Philly}$	$\alpha_2\beta_2{}^{35Phe}$	
			Hb$_{Louisville}$	$\alpha_2\beta_2{}^{42Leu}$	
			Hb$_{Hammersmith}$	$\alpha_2\beta_2{}^{42Ser}$	
			Hb$_{Zurich}$	$\alpha_2\beta_2{}^{63Arg}$	
			Hb$_{Toulouse}$	$\alpha_2\beta_2{}^{66Glu}$	
			Hb$_{Bristol}$	$\alpha_2\beta_2{}^{67Asp}$	
			Hb$_{Sydney}$	$\alpha_2\beta_2{}^{67Ala}$	
			Hb$_{Shepherd's\ Bush}$	$\alpha_2\beta_2{}^{74Asp}$	
			Hb$_{Seattle}$	$\alpha_2\beta_2{}^{70Asp}$	
			Hb$_{Boras}$	$\alpha_2\beta_2{}^{88Arg}$	
			Hb$_{Santa\ Ana}$	$\alpha_2\beta_2{}^{88Pro}$	
			Hb$_{Gun\ Hill}$	$\alpha_2\beta_2{}^{91-95}$	(5 a.a. deleted)
			Hb$_{Sabine}$	$\alpha_2\beta_2{}^{91Pro}$	
			Hb$_{Köln}$	$\alpha_2\beta_2{}^{98Met}$	
			Hb$_{Kansas}$	$\alpha_2\beta_2{}^{102Thr}$	
			Hb$_{Wein}$	$\alpha_2\beta_2{}^{130Asp}$	
			Hb$_{Olmsted}$	$\alpha_2\beta_2{}^{141Arg}$	

*Hemoglobins that may precipitate as Heinz bodies after splenectomy: congenital Heinz body hemolytic anemia.
Abbreviation: a.a. = amino acids.

➤ Table 11-19
HEMOGLOBINS ASSOCIATED WITH METHEMOGLOBINEMIA AND CYANOSIS

HbM$_{Boston}$	$\alpha_2{}^{58Tyr}\beta_2$
HbM$_{Iwate}$	$\alpha_2{}^{87Tyr}\beta_2$
HbM$_{Saskatoon}$	$\alpha_2\beta_2{}^{63Tyr}$
HbM$_{Milwaukee}$	$\alpha_2\beta_2{}^{67Glu}$
HbM$_{Hyde\ Park}$	$\alpha_2\beta_2{}^{92Tyr}$

➤ CASE STUDY

A 13-year-old black girl was admitted to the hospital appearing acutely ill with fever and abdominal pain. On physical examination, an enlarged spleen was evident. Laboratory test results were as follows:

Hgb	5.0 g/dL
Hct	15%
RBC	1.4×10^{12}/L

WBC	2.2×10^9/L
Reticulocyte count	1%

Differential

Segmented neutrophils	62%
Bands	12%
Lymphocytes	19%
Monocytes	4%
Eosinophils	2%
Basophils	1%
RBC indices	Normal
Platelet count	400×10^9/L
Peripheral blood smear	(see Fig. 11-16)

Hemoglobin electrophoresis, alkaline pH, showed one band in the HbS position and one band in the HbC position. The hemoglobins were quantified as 55% HbS and 45% HbC plus A$_2$. Hemoglobins S and C were confirmed by electrophoresis at acid pH.

continued

Questions

1. Describe the morphological features of this peripheral blood smear.
2. In reviewing the electrophoretic data, what diagnosis is suggested?
3. Comment on crystal formation in this condition.
4. Discuss the clinical presentation of the patient. Is it consistent with HbSC disease?
5. This girl's parents have no hematologic problems; therefore, for her to have HbSC disease, what would be their most likely genotypes?
6. The inheritance of structurally abnormal hemoglobins follows simple mendelian laws. With parents having the trait form of HbS and HbC, what would be the expected genotypes in each of four children?

Answers

1. Numerous target cells are present on the peripheral blood smear along with some cells that appear to have shadows of precipitating intraerythrocytic crystals.
2. The data suggest a diagnosis of HbSC disease.
3. The crystals in HbSC disease appear to be only partially formed, or there may be more than one formation. The crystals in the red cells often are described as having a glove-shaped appearance with several "fingers" protruding.
4. Generally HbSC disease has a milder presentation than HbSS disease; however, this patient appears to be experiencing a severe episode of SC crisis. This is indicated by her acute illness, abdominal pain, and decrease in hemoglobin and hematocrit without an increase in the reticulocyte count.
5. With no hematologic problems, one parent would be expected to have HbS trait (HbAS), whereas the other would most likely have HbC trait (HbAC).
6. The probability for offspring would be one child with HbAA, one with HbAS, one with HbAC, and one with HbSC.

QUESTIONS

1. Which of the following is not a characteristic of hemoglobinopathies?
   a. Conditions in which abnormal hemoglobins are synthesized
   b. Result from inherited abnormalities or genetic mutations
   c. All are manifested in clinically significant conditions
   d. Result in a defect in structural integrity or function of the hemoglobin molecule

2. Which of the following are used in the nomenclature system for abnormal hemoglobins?
   a. Capital letters
   b. Names of places
   c. Names of chains and substitutions
   d. All of the above

3. What is the amino acid substitution found in sickle cell anemia?
   a. Substitution of valine for glutamic acid in the sixth position from the NH_2-terminal β chain
   b. Substitution of lysine for glutamic acid in the sixth position from the NH_2-terminal β chain
   c. Substitution of lysine for glutamic acid in the 26th position from the NH_2-terminal β chain
   d. Substitution of valine for glutamic acid in the 121st position from the NH_2-terminal β chain

4. What factors contribute to the sickling of RBCs?
   a. Increase in pH and oxygenation
   b. Decrease in pH and oxygenation, and dehydration
   c. Increase in pH and decrease in oxygenation
   d. Decrease in dehydration, and increase in pH and oxygenation

5. Which of the following are crises associated with sickle cell anemia?
   a. Aplastic crisis with low reticulocyte count, and infections
   b. Hemolytic crisis with splenic sequestration, decreased hemoglobin and hematocrit, increased reticulocyte count, and jaundice
   c. Vaso-occlusive or painful crises with severe pain, tissue damage, and necrosis
   d. All of the above

6. What are the therapeutic goals in the treatment of sickle cell anemia?
   a. Decrease microvascular entrapment of sickled cells or change the volume of RBCs
   b. Modify oxygen affinity or solubility of sickle hemoglobin
   c. Increase production of fetal hemoglobin
   d. All of the above

7. What is the amino acid substitution found in HbC disease?
   a. Substitution of valine for glutamic acid in the sixth position from the NH_2-terminal β chain
   b. Substitution of lysine for glutamic acid in the sixth position from the NH_2-terminal β chain
   c. Substitution of lysine for glutamic acid in the 26th position from the NH_2-terminal β chain
   d. Substitution of valine for glutamic acid in the 121st position from the NH_2-terminal β chain

8. Which of the following is not true for HbC disease?
   a. Mild anemia
   b. Numerous target cells
   c. Crystals in red cells
   d. HbC can be separated from other hemoglobins at an alkaline pH

9. Which finding would be most useful in establishing a diagnosis of HbSC disease?
   a. Target cells and sickled cells on peripheral blood smear
   b. Severe anemia; increased reticulocyte count
   c. Hemoglobin electrophoresis at alkaline pH
   d. RBC indices

10. Which of the following is a cause of methemoglobinemia?
    a. HbM variants
    b. NADH-diaphorase deficiency
    c. Toxic substances
    d. All of the above

SUMMARY CHART

➤ More than 90% of the hemoglobin variants are single amino acid substitutions in the alpha- (α), beta- (β), delta- (δ), or gamma- (γ) globin chains as a result of a single-point mutation.

➤ Hemoglobin S (HbS) is produced when valine substitutes for glutamic acid in the sixth position of the β chain.

➤ Hemoglobin C (HbC) is produced when lysine replaces glutamic acid at position six of the β chain.

➤ Sickle cell anemia (HbSS disease) is the most common type of sickle cell disease and represents the homozygous form in which the individual inherits a double dose of the abnormal gene that codes for HbS.

➤ The characteristic morphology in HbSS disease is the sickled cell, which increases the viscosity of the blood, leading to hypoxia, painful crises, and infarction of the spleen, kidney, and bone marrow.

➤ The three types of crises associated with sickle cell disease are aplastic, hemolytic, and vaso-occlusive (painful).

➤ HbS constitutes 80% or more of the hemoglobin content in addition to HbF plus A_2.

➤ Sickle cell trait represents the heterozygous form of sickle cell disease in which individuals inherit both a normal β-globin gene and a sickle globin gene.

➤ Individuals with sickle cell trait produce both HbA and HbS in a ratio of 60:40.

➤ In sickle cell disease (HbSS) the red blood cell (RBC) indices are normochromic and normocytic, with hemoglobins ranging from 6 to 8 g/dL, target cells, sickled cells, nucleated red cells, and polychromasia.

➤ The definitive test for HbS is hemoglobin electrophoresis on cellulose acetate or citrate agar.

➤ HbC disease presents with a normocytic and normo- or hyperchromic anemia, and numerous target cells, microspherocytes, schistocytes, folded cells, and "bar of gold" crystals.

➤ Electrophoresis in HbC disease shows 95% HbC plus A_2, and less than 7% HbF.

➤ Hemoglobin SC (HbSC) disease occurs when an HbS gene is inherited from one parent and an HbC gene is inherited from the other; morphology includes target cells, folded red cells, and glove-shaped intracellular crystals.

➤ Methemoglobinemia occurs when levels exceed 1% of total hemoglobin and may be the result of hemoglobin M (HbM) variants, NADH-diaphorase deficiency, or toxic substances.

➤ Unstable hemoglobins are hemoglobin variants in which amino acid substitutions or deletions have weakened the binding forces that maintain the structure of the molecule.

➤ High-affinity hemoglobins, associated with a shift to the left, bind oxygen more readily and release it less easily to the tissues.

➤ Low-affinity hemoglobins, associated with a shift to the right, release oxygen quite readily to the tissues.

References

1. Huisman, TH, et al: A syllabus of human hemoglobin variants, ed 2. The Sickle Cell Anemia Foundation, Augusta, GA, 1998.
2. Steinberg, MH: Genetic modulation of sickle cell anemia. Proc Soc Exper Biol Med 209:1, 1995.
3. Herrick, JB: Peculiar elongated and sickle-shaped red corpuscles in a case of severe anemia. Arch Intern Med 6:517, 1910.
4. Pauling, L, et al: Sickle cell anemia, a molecular disease. Science 110:543, 1949.
5. Sickle Cell Disease Guideline Panel: Sickle cell disease: Screening, diagnosis, management, and counseling in newborns and infants. Clinical Practice Guideline No 6. AHCPR Pub No 93-0562. Agency for Health Care Policy and Research, Public Health Service, US Department of Health and Human Services, Rockville, MD, April 1993.
6. Steinberg, MH: Management of sickle cell disease. N Engl J Med 340:1021, 1999.
7. Eaton, WA, and Hofrichter, J: Sickle cell hemoglobin polymerization. Adv Protein Chem 40:63, 1990.
8. Steinberg, MH: Sickle cell anemia and fetal hemoglobin. Am J Med Sci 308(5):259, 1994.
9. Hebbel, RP: Beyond hemoglobin polymerization: The red blood cell membrane and sickle disease pathophysiology. Blood 77:214, 1991.
10. Embury, SH, et al: Sickle Cell Disease: Basic Principles and Clinical Practice. Raven Press, New York, 1994.
11. Bunn, HF: Pathogenesis and treatment of sickle cell disease. N Engl J Med 337:762, 1997.
12. Castro, O, et al: The acute chest syndrome in sickle cell disease: Incidence and risk factors. The Cooperative Study of Sickle Cell Disease. Blood 84:643, 1994.
13. Platt, OS, et al: Mortality in sickle cell disease. Life expectancy and risk factors for early death. N Engl J Med 13:331(15):1022, 1994.
14. Falk RJ, et al: Prevalence and pathologic features of sickle cell nephropathy and response to inhibition of angiotensin-converting enzyme. N Engl J Med 326:910, 1992.
15. Adams RJ, et al: Prevention of a first stroke by transfusion in children with sickle cell anemia and abnormal results on transcranial Doppler ultrasonography. N Engl J Med 339:5, 1998.
16. Kark, JA, et al: Sickle-cell trait as a risk factor for sudden death in physical training. N Engl J Med 317:781, 1987.
17. Sandhaus, LM, and Harvey, FG: Laboratory methods for the detection of hemoglobinopathies in the community hospital. Clin Lab Med 13(4):801, December 1993.
18. Gaston, MH, et al: Prophylaxis with oral penicillin in children with sickle cell anemia: A randomized trial. N Engl J Med 314:1593, 1986.
19. Charache, S, et al: Effect of hydroxyurea on the frequency of painful crises in sickle cell anemia. N Engl J Med 18:322(20):1372, 1995.
20. Steinberg, MH, et al: Fetal hemoglobin in sickle cell anemia: Determinants of response to hydroxyurea. Multicenter Study of Hydroxyurea. Blood 89(3):1078, 1997.
21. Bridges, KR, et al: A multiparameter analysis of sickle erythrocytes in patients undergoing hydroxyurea therapy. Blood 88:4701, 1996.
22. Ferster, A, et al: Hydroxyurea for treatment of severe sickle cell anemia: A pediatric clinical trial. Blood 88(6):1960, 1996.
23. Maier-Redelsperger, M, et al: Fetal hemoglobin and F-cell responses to long-term hydroxyurea treatment in young sickle cell patients. The French Study Group on Sickle Cell Disease. Blood 91(12):4472, 1998.
24. Perrine, SP, et al: A short-term trial of butyrate to stimulate fetal-globin-gene expression in the beta-globin disorders. N Engl J Med 328:81, 1993.
25. Sher, GD, et al: Extended therapy with intravenous arginine butyrate in patients with β-hemoglobinopathies. N Engl J Med 332:1606, 1995.
26. Dover, GJ, et al: Induction of fetal hemoglobin production in subjects with sickle cell anemia by oral sodium phenybutyrate. Blood 84:339, 1994.
27. Bunn, HF: Induction of fetal hemoglobin in sickle cell disease. Blood 93:1787, 1999.
28. Ataweh, G, et al: Sustained induction of fetal hemoglobin by pulse butyrate therapy in sickle cell disease. Blood 93:1790, 1999.
29. Wang, WC, et al: High risk of recurrent strokes after discontinuance of five to twelve years of transfusion therapy in patients with sickle cell disease. J Pediatr 118:377, 1991.
30. Johnson, FL, et al: Bone marrow transplantation for sickle cell disease: The United States experience. Am J Pediatr Hematol Oncol 16:22, 1994.

31. Thomas, ED: Marrow transplantation for non-malignant disorders. N Engl J Med 312:46, 1985.
32. Vermylen, C, and Cornu, G: Bone marrow transplantation for sickle cell anemia. Curr Opin Hematol 3(2):163, 1996.
33. Walters, MC, et al: Collaborative multicenter investigation of marrow transplantation for sickle cell disease: Current results and future directions. Biol Blood Marrow Transplant 3(6):310, 1997.
34. Xu, K, et al: First unaffected pregnancy using preimplantation genetic diagnosis for sickle cell anemia. JAMA 281:1701, December 1999.
35. Walsh, CE, et al: Gene therapy for human hemoglobinopathies. Proc Soc Exper Biol Med 204(3):289, December, 1993.
36. Walsh, CE, et al: Regulated high level expression of a human gamma-globin gene introduced into erythroid cells by an adeno-associated virus vector. Proc Natl Acad Sci 89:7257, 1992.
37. Mulligan, RC: The basic science of gene therapy. Science 260:926, 1993.
38. Kiem, HP, et al: Retrovirus-mediated gene transduction into canine peripheral blood repopulating cells. Blood 83:1467, 1994.
39. Nagel, RL: Disorders of hemoglobin function and stability. In Handin, RJ, et al (eds): Blood: Principles and Practice of Hematology. Lippincott-Raven, Philadelphia, pp 1591–1644, 1995.
40. Lubin, BH, et al: Laboratory diagnosis of hemoglobinopathies. Clin Biochem 24(4):363, August, 1991.
41. Lawrence, C, et al: The unique red cell heterogeneity of SC disease: Crystal formation, dense reticulocytes, and unusual morphology. Blood 78:2104, 1991.
42. Huisman, THJ: Combinations of β chain abnormal hemoglobins with each other or with β-thalassemia determinants with known mutations. Influence on phenotype. Clin Chem 43:1850,1997.
43. Nagel, RL, et al: HbS-Oman heterozygote: A new dominant sickle syndrome. Blood 92:4375, 1998.

12 Hemolytic Anemias:
Intracorpuscular Defects

IV Thalassemia

Chantal Ricaud Harrison, MD

GENETICS OF HEMOGLOBIN SYNTHESIS

PATHOPHYSIOLOGY OF THALASSEMIA

Beta Thalassemia

Alpha Thalassemia

Delta-Beta Thalassemias and Hemoglobin Lepore
Syndrome

Hereditary Persistence of Fetal Hemoglobin

Thalassemia Associated with Hemoglobin Variants

CLINICAL COURSE AND THERAPY

Hemoglobin Bart's Hydrops Fetalis

Thalassemia Major

Thalassemia Intermedia

Thalassemia Minor

BLOOD TRANSFUSION IN THALASSEMIA

LABORATORY DIAGNOSIS OF THALASSEMIA

Routine Hematology Procedures

Hemoglobin Electrophoresis

Hemoglobin Quantitation

Routine Chemistry

**DIFFERENTIAL DIAGNOSIS OF MICROCYTIC,
HYPOCHROMIC ANEMIA**

CASE STUDY

OBJECTIVES

At the end of this chapter, the learner should be able to:

1. Name the hemoglobin defect of thalassemia.

2. Describe the different types of mutation involved in alpha (α) and beta (β) thalassemia.

3. Describe the clinical expression of different gene combinations of α and β thalassemia.

4. Describe the condition known as hereditary persistence of fetal hemoglobin (HPFH).

5. List the complications of a regular blood transfusion program for patients with thalassemia major.

6. Name the most characteristic laboratory findings for the diagnosis of thalassemia.

7. List red cell indices that help to distinguish thalassemia from iron deficiency.

8. Describe the appearance of the peripheral smear in thalassemia.

9. Name the test used as a population screening test for thalassemia carriers.

10. List conditions in which quantitation of hemoglobin F is important.

11. Describe the use of routine chemistries for differentiation of thalassemia from iron-deficiency anemia.

The thalassemia syndromes consist of a diverse group of inherited disorders, which clinically manifest themselves as anemia of varying degrees. These disorders are the result of a defective production of the globin portion of the hemoglobin.

In 1925 Thomas B. Cooley and Pearl Lee described the first cases of severe thalassemia in several North American children of Mediterranean origin.[1] "Cooley's anemia" is still a commonly used term for this form of severe thalassemia, which is also termed *thalassemia major*. The name *thalassemia* was actually applied to these clinical syndromes a few years later. The term is derived from the Greek word *thalassa,* which means sea, because at that time, all of the cases described were from the Mediterranean coastal region. It is now well known that the distribution of thalassemia is world-

wide and not restricted to the Mediterranean Sea area. It was later realized that the original severe clinical disease described by Cooley was the result of a homozygous defect in hemoglobin production, whereas many milder cases described as "thalassemia minima" or "thalassemia minor" were manifestations of a heterozygous defect.

In contrast with hemoglobinopathies such as sickle cell disease, hemoglobin C, or hemoglobin E, in which the genetic defect results in a structurally abnormal globin chain, the thalassemia syndromes result from an abnormality in the rate of synthesis of one of the globin chains. With a few minor exceptions, the globin chains produced are structurally normal, but there is an imbalance in production of the two different types of chain, resulting in an absolute decrease in the amount of normal hemoglobin formed, as well as an excess production of one type of chain that may precipitate and induce hemolysis.

There are two major types of thalassemia: alpha (α) thalassemia, which is caused by a defect in the rate of synthesis of α chains; and beta (β) thalassemia, caused by a defect in the rate of synthesis of β chains. The original cases described by Cooley were cases of homozygous β thalassemia. The world distribution of thalassemia is summarized in Figure 12–1. In North and South America and northern Europe, thalassemia has been imported and is present in immigrant populations originating mostly from Italy, Greece, West Africa, and Southeast Asia. For all practical purposes, thalassemia is absent from American Indian populations. The marked similarity in worldwide distribution of thalassemia with malignant malaria caused by *Plasmodium falciparum* has been attributed to the process of gene selection secondary to a protective effect against *P. falciparum* malaria brought about by the heterozygous state of thalassemia.[2]

Because the hemoglobin structural variants (such as hemoglobin S and hemoglobin C in West Africans and African Americans or hemoglobin E in Southeast Asians) occur in the same population in which α or β thalassemia is frequent, the two types of genetic defects may be found in the same person, resulting in variability of clinical expression of the two defects.

➤ GENETICS OF HEMOGLOBIN SYNTHESIS

All normal human hemoglobins have a general tetrameric structure consisting of two alpha-like (alpha or zeta, respectively abbreviated as α or ζ) and two beta-like (beta, delta, A-gamma, G-gamma, or epsilon, respectively abbreviated as β, δ, $^A\gamma$, $^G\gamma$, and ϵ) chains (see Chap. 3). In the normal adult, the majority (95% to 97%) of the hemoglobin is $\alpha_2\beta_2$ (hemoglobin A) and a minor fraction (about 2.5%) is $\alpha_2\delta_2$ (hemoglobin A_2). A small amount of hemoglobin F, $\alpha_2\gamma_2$, (always less than 2%) may also be found (see Fig. 3–12). Table 12–1 lists the different normal hemoglobins found throughout human development, as well as the abnormal hemoglobins found in patients with thalassemia.

The ζ- and α-globin genes are found on chromosome 16 and the genes for ϵ, $^G\gamma$, $^A\gamma$, δ, and β globins on chromosome 11 (see Fig. 3–11). All globin genes consist of three exons separated by two introns, with 5' promoter sequences and untranslated regions in 5' and 3' directions. Each globin gene spans approximately 1.5 kilobases (kb).

There are two closely linked genes, both active and coding for identical α-globin chains, although at different levels of activity in the normal adult. The α_2-globin gene is expressed at two to three times the rate of the α_1-globin gene.[3] Detailed mapping of the deoxyribonucleic acid (DNA) shows great similarity between the two α genes and between the two regions immediately upstream (5') of each α gene.[4] There are three areas of homology in DNA blocks called x, y, and z (Fig. 12–2), including or juxtaposed to the α genes. These homologous blocks render this area more susceptible to mispairing. Crossing over in this area of chromosome 16 may result in deletions of all or part of one α gene. Occasionally a chromosome with three α genes can be produced. This explains why the majority of α thalassemias are the result of a gene deletion.

On the other hand, the majority of β thalassemias are the result of point mutation affecting the regulation of the rate of production of the β-globin chain. A diagram of the β-globin gene fine structure, including the areas involved in the regulation of expression, is depicted in Figure 12–3. Between 5 to 20 kb upstream of the ϵ gene is a β-locus control region (β-LCR), which is mainly involved in the regulation of the switching on and off of the different β-like genes. Between 30 and 105 bases upstream of the β gene lie the three classic promoter sequences TATA, CAT, and CAC boxes. The point mutations resulting in β thalassemia can be classified

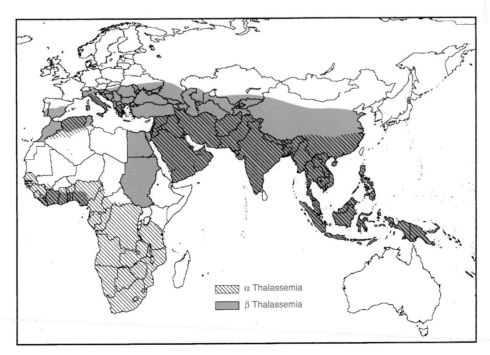

➤ FIGURE 12–1 World distribution of alpha (α) and beta (β) thalassemia.

> **Table 12-1**
COMPOSITION OF HEMOGLOBINS FOUND IN NORMAL HUMAN DEVELOPMENT AND ABNORMAL HEMOGLOBINS FOUND IN THALASSEMIA

Globin Chains	Hemoglobin	State
$\alpha_2\beta_2$	A	Adult
$\alpha_2\delta_2$	A_2	
$\alpha_2{}^A\gamma_2$	F	Fetus
$\alpha_2{}^G\gamma_2$	F	
$\alpha_2\epsilon_2$	Gower 2	Embryo
$\zeta_2\epsilon_2$	Gower 1	
$\zeta_2\gamma_2$	Portland	
β_4	H	α Thalassemia
γ_4	Bart's	
α_2 Precipitate	—	β Thalassemia

into the following categories: (1) transcriptional mutants affecting one of the promoter sequences; (2) RNA processing mutants, usually affecting introns at the splice junction sites or in the consensus sites; (3) RNA translational mutants due to nonsense or frameshift mutations, which produce premature termination and consistently result in complete lack of production of β chains; and (4) miscellaneous mutations affecting initiation codon, Cap site, or cleaving or polyadenylation sites at the 3' end.[5,6] In all cases the final result is a decreased or absent production of the β-globin chain.

➤ PATHOPHYSIOLOGY OF THALASSEMIA

In thalassemia, a defect in the rate of production of one of the globin chains causes a decrease in the amount of normal physiologic hemoglobin produced, resulting in a microcytic, hypochromic anemia. There is also an excess of globin chains produced by the unaffected genes. In the case of α thalassemia, the excess γ chains and β chains can form stable tetramers: hemoglobin Bart's (γ_4) and hemoglobin H (β_4), respectively. However, these hemoglobins are physiologically useless and will precipitate in older red cells, causing a shortened red cell life span. In the case of β thalassemia, the excess α chains form α_2 precipitates, which cause hemolysis of the red cell precursors in the bone marrow, resulting in ineffective erythropoiesis.

Beta Thalassemia

In β thalassemia the disease does not manifest itself until the switch from γ-chain to β-chain synthesis has been completed. This usually occurs several months after birth. Thus,

the clinical presentation of a patient with this disease usually occurs during the first year of life. There often is a compensatory absolute or relative increase in production of γ chains and δ chains, resulting in an increased level of hemoglobin F and hemoglobin A_2. The genetic background for β thalassemia is very heterogeneous. Almost 200 different mutations have been described; however, only some 20 alleles account for over 80% of all β-thalassemia genes worldwide. A specific group of mutations (four to six) is characteristically found in each geographic area.[6] Clinically, these alleles may be broadly subdivided into β^0 and β^+ thalassemia.

β^0 Thalassemia
This gene results in complete absence of production of β chains. This particular gene expression is commonly found in the Mediterranean area, particularly in northern Italy, Greece, Algeria, and Saudi Arabia. It is also common in Southeast Asia.

β^+ Thalassemia
The β^+-thalassemia genes produce a reduced amount of β chains. There is heterogeneity in β^+ thalassemia, and at least three different groups of genes have been described. The type 1 β^+-thalassemia gene produces the least amount of β chains (about 10% of normal production) and is found throughout the Mediterranean region, the Middle East, the Indian subcontinent, and Southeast Asia. The type 2 β^+-thalassemia gene produces a greater amount of β chains (about 50% of normal production) and is characteristically found in blacks of North America and West Africa. The type 3 β^+-thalassemia gene produces an even greater amount of β chains and causes a much milder form of β thalassemia. It is found sporadically in Italy, Greece, and the Middle East.

Clinical Expression of the Different Gene Combinations
Homozygosity for a β^0- or β^+-thalassemia gene, or compound heterozygosity for these genes, causes a severe form of thalassemia called *thalassemia major*. The only exception is perhaps the homozygous type 2 or type 3 β^+ thalassemia, which causes a milder form of thalassemia that is called *thalassemia intermedia*. In thalassemia major a severe hypochromic, microcytic anemia develops during the first year of life (Fig. 12–4; see also Color Plate 112). The hemoglobin level is usually less than 7 g/dL and consists mostly of hemoglobin F and hemoglobin A_2.

Heterozygosity for the β^0- or β^+-thalassemia gene causes a mild form of chronic hypochromic, microcytic anemia that has been called *thalassemia minor* (Fig. 12–5 and Color Plate 113). Although the degree of anemia is variable, with hemoglobin levels from 10.5 to 13.9 g/dL, it is impossible to determine whether the patient has the β^0 or β^+ gene on clinical grounds alone. In general, the levels of hemoglobin F and hemoglobin A_2 are mildly elevated. The patient with

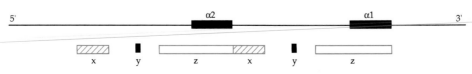

➤ FIGURE 12–2   The areas of homology (x, y, and z) can lead to mispairing.

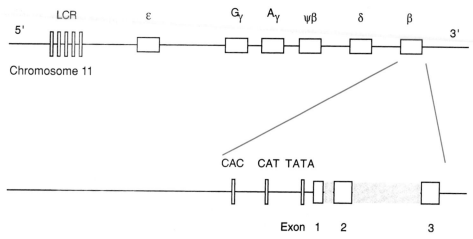

➤ **FIGURE 12–3** Diagram of the β-globin gene expression: (*top*) schematic of the location of the β-like genes on chromosome 11 with the locus control region (LCR) on the 5' end; (*bottom*) exploded β gene depicting the 3 exons and 2 introns with the three promoter areas upstream.

heterozygous type 3 β⁺ thalassemia usually shows no clinical or laboratory evidence of anemia and, for this reason, has been called the silent carrier.

Alpha Thalassemia

In contrast to β thalassemia, α thalassemia is usually manifested immediately at birth and even in utero, as the α genes are activated early in fetal life. Another characteristic of α thalassemia is its wide range of clinical expression. Because each chromosome 16 carries two α genes, the total normal complement of α genes is 4. Thus, there will be a greater variety in severity of disease, as there may be one, two, three, or four α genes affected in one patient.

Owing to the wide variety of genetic backgrounds and the difficulty in defining the heterozygous carrier state, there has been much confusion in the classification and nomenclature of α thalassemias. Much of this confusion is the result of the indiscriminate use of a phenotypic or genotypic classification without clear definition. In this chapter, a genotypic classification that parallels the classification used for β thalassemia is used.

Another characteristic of α thalassemia is the fact that the decreased or absent α-chain production will result in excess γ chains during fetal life and at birth and in excess β chains later on. This causes formation of stable tetramers, such as γ₄ (hemoglobin Bart's) and β₄ (hemoglobin H), which can be detected by hemoglobin electrophoresis. These stable, nonfunctional tetramers precipitate in older red cells, forming inclusion bodies and interfering with membrane function, which results in decreased red cell survival and may induce a hemolytic crisis during infectious episodes.

α⁰ Thalassemia (α Thalassemia 1)

α⁰ Thalassemia and *α thalassemia 1* have been used interchangeably in the past to describe a genetic determinant. However, because α thalassemia 1 has been also used to describe the phenotypic or clinical expression of a disease, α⁰ *thalassemia* is the preferred term for the description of the genetic determinant. This gene complex (or haplotype) results in complete absence of production of α chains. This means that both α genes on chromosome 16 are nonfunctional. Studies have shown that the α⁰ determinant is the result of α-gene deletions. In addition, they also demonstrated that there are at least 21 major haplotypes, resulting in α⁰ thalassemia, depending on the amount of DNA that has been deleted from the chromosome.[6] Each haplotype appears to

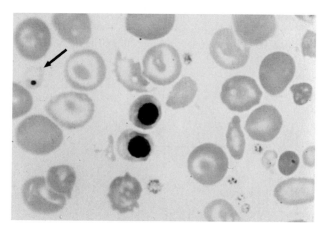

➤ **FIGURE 12–4** Peripheral smear from a patient with β-thalassemia major. Note the nucleated red cells, Howell-Jolly body in the hypochromic microcyte (*arrow*), numerous target cells, and moderate anisocytosis and poikilocytosis (Wright's stain). (Bell, A: Hematology. In: Listen, Look and Learn. Health and Education Resources, Inc., Bethesda, MD, with permission.)

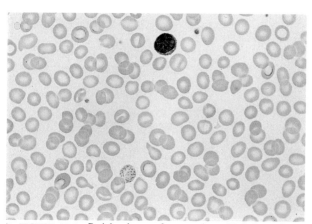

➤ **FIGURE 12–5** Peripheral smear from a patient with thalassemia minor. Note the microcytosis and hypochromia with mild anisocytosis and poikilocytosis. A few target cells and basophilic stippling are present (Wright's stain, magnification ×400).

be characteristic of a certain population in the world. α^0-Thalassemia genes are found frequently in Southeast Asia and less frequently in the Mediterranean area. They also occur sporadically in other parts of the world. This gene may be recognized in adults through the detection of small amounts of ζ-globin chain.[7]

α^+ Thalassemia (α Thalassemia 2)

Again, α^+ *thalassemia* is the better term to describe the genetic determinant, because α *thalassemia 2* has been used to describe both the genetic determinant and a phenotypic expression. The α^+-thalassemia gene haplotype is characterized by a reduction in the output of α chains. This may be the result of a deletion of a single α gene on chromosome 16, which leaves the other α gene intact and able to function. Other types of α^+-thalassemia genes are caused by nondeletion mutants that affect the regulation of the α-chain synthesis. This is similar to the situation in the β thalassemias. A third type of α^+-thalassemia genetic background is associated with α-globin structural mutants. Overall, a minimum of 40 major genetic defects resulting in the α^+-thalassemia gene have been defined.[6] These different thalassemia genes result in different levels of α-chain output. For example, the nondeletion regulatory type of defect, also called $\alpha\alpha^T$ and found in Saudi Arabia, is more severe than the single gene deletion type of defect, also called $-\alpha$ and commonly found throughout the Mediterranean, Middle East, Indian subcontinent, Southeast Asia, Africa, and Malaysia.

Clinical Expression of the Different Gene Combinations

α Thalassemia can be divided into four clinical categories, depending on the severity of the disease. The most severe expression of α thalassemia is the hemoglobin Bart's hydrops fetalis syndrome, which is caused by homozygosity of the α^0-thalassemia gene haplotype. This is a lethal disease, and infants with hemoglobin Bart's hydrops fetalis die either in utero or soon after birth. They produce no α chain, and the only hemoglobins found are hemoglobin Bart's (γ_4) and hemoglobin Portland ($\zeta_2\gamma_2$). Because hemoglobin Bart's is useless as an oxygen carrier, survival of these fetuses into the third trimester or until birth is entirely due to the presence of hemoglobin Portland. This condition is quite common in Southeast Asia and is found sporadically in the Mediterranean area.

The second most severe clinical expression of a tha-

lassemia is hemoglobin H disease. In this entity only one α gene out of four is functioning. This is usually the result of a double heterozygosity of an α^0-thalassemia haplotype with an α^+-thalassemia haplotype but is also found in Saudi Arabia as the result of homozygosity of the more severe form of the α^+-thalassemia haplotype, the nondeleted $\alpha\alpha^T$ haplotype. Clinically, hemoglobin H disease is characterized by a variable degree of microcytic, hypochromic anemia, which is classified as thalassemia intermedia. Hemolytic crises may occur with infections. Adults with hemoglobin H disease will have from 5% to 40% hemoglobin H; the remainder is mostly hemoglobin A with a small amount of hemoglobin A_2 and hemoglobin Bart's. Infants who later develop hemoglobin H disease usually have between 19% and 27% hemoglobin Bart's at birth, with the remainder composed of hemoglobin F and hemoglobin A. Hemoglobin H and hemoglobin Bart's can easily be identified by hemoglobin electrophoresis, because they migrate anodally at pH 6.5 to 7.0 (Fig. 12–6). In addition, hemoglobin H shows a characteristic appearance of multiple ragged inclusions in many red cells after incubation with brilliant cresyl blue, the so-called golfball appearance (Fig. 12–7).

The α^0-thalassemia trait, also called α-*thalassemia 1 trait*, is caused by the defect of two of the four α genes. This is usually the result of heterozygosity for the α^0-thalassemia haplotype but could also be the result of homozygosity for the α^+-thalassemia haplotype. The condition is characterized by the presence at birth of 5% to 15% hemoglobin Bart's, which disappears with development and is not replaced by hemoglobin H. There is a minimal amount of anemia with slight hypochromia and microcytosis present. The mean corpuscular volume (MCV) is usually between 70 and 75 fL. After hemoglobin Bart's disappears, the hemoglobin electrophoretic pattern becomes normal. This condition exists in 3% of African Americans and may be confused with iron deficiency.

The last category of α thalassemia is the α^+-thalassemia trait, also called α-*thalassemia 2 trait*. This is the result of a defect in one of the four α-globin genes and is characterized by the presence of a very small amount (up to 2%) of hemoglobin Bart's at birth; after the disappearance of hemoglobin Bart's during development, no recognizable hematologic abnormality is present, except for a borderline low MCV (78 to 80 fL). This condition is found in up to 30% of African Americans.

Table 12–2 summarizes the different genetic backgrounds associated with the four different clinical expressions of a thalassemia.

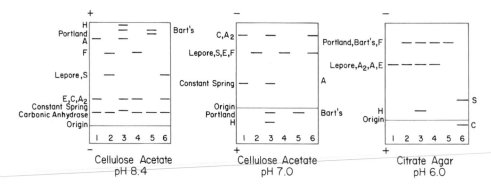

➤ **FIGURE 12–6** Diagram of the migration of the different hemoglobins at different pH: (*1*) normal adult (AA$_2$); (*2*) homozygous Hb Lepore (F, Lepore); (*3*) HbH/Constant Spring disease $\alpha^{CS}\alpha$/(Constant Spring, A$_2$, A, Bart's H); (*4*) double heterozygous HbE/β-thalassemia (E, F); (*5*) Hb Bart's hydrops fetalis syndrome (Portland, Bart's); (*6*) HbS/C disease (S, C).

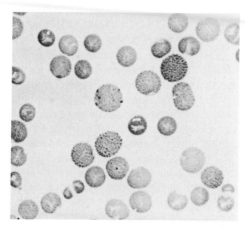

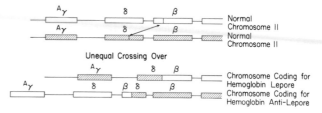

➤ **FIGURE 12–7** Hemoglobin H inclusions (supravital stain). (From Bell, A: Hematology. In: Listen, Look and Learn. Health and Education Resources, Inc., Bethesda, MD, with permission.)

➤ **FIGURE 12–8** Hemoglobin Lepore formation. An abnormal crossing over between β and δ genes gives rise to hemoglobin Lepore and to hemoglobin anti-Lepore.

Delta-Beta Thalassemia and Hemoglobin Lepore Syndrome

Delta-beta (δβ) thalassemias are a diverse group of thalassemias characterized by a combined defect in δ- and β-chain synthesis. They can be described as demonstrating a normal level of hemoglobin A_2 and an unusually high level of hemoglobin F in the heterozygote, and absent hemoglobin A and A_2 in the homozygote. The δβ thalassemias can be subdivided into two groups according to the type of hemoglobin F produced. If both $^G\gamma$ and $^A\gamma$ chains are produced—that is, if both γ genes are active—this variety is then called $^G\gamma^A\gamma\delta\beta$ thalassemia. If only $^G\gamma$ chains are produced, which means that the $^A\gamma$ gene as well as the δ and the β genes are inactive, this variety is then called $^G\gamma\delta\beta$ thalassemia. Another syndrome of δβ chain abnormality involves the production of an abnormal hemoglobin. This abnormal hemoglobin, called hemoglobin Lepore after the name of the family in which it was first found, has been shown to be a fusion of the δ and β chains, which is the product of a fusion gene formed by an unequal crossing over.

Figure 12–8 indicates diagrammatically the production of hemoglobin Lepore by this unequal crossing over. At least three different hemoglobin Lepores have been described, varying in the exact location of the unequal crossing over.

All δβ thalassemias studied thus far have been shown to be the result of a deletion. They can be described at the genetic level as three different entities, depending on the amount of DNA lost: hemoglobin Lepore syndrome results from a partial deletion of the δ and β genes, $^G\gamma^A\gamma\delta\beta$ thalassemia from a complete deletion of the δ and β genes, and $^G\gamma\delta\beta$ thalassemia from a deletion of the $^A\gamma$ gene in addition to the deletion of the δ and β genes. δβ Thalassemias are less common than β thalassemias and have been found sporadically in Greeks, American blacks, Italians, and Arabs.

The γ-chain synthesis in δβ thalassemia is usually more efficient than in β thalassemia, and in general the former results in a milder clinical disease than the latter. Patients with homozygous δβ thalassemia have a clinical course usually described as thalassemia intermedia. This is also true of the double heterozygous δβ and β thalassemia. However, the homozygous state for hemoglobin Lepore appears to be somewhat more severe and closer to the clinical state of homozygous β thalassemia. Most patients with homozygous hemoglobin Lepore are transfusion-dependent. Double heterozygosity for β thalassemia and hemoglobin Lepore also causes a clinical disorder similar to homozygous β thalassemia.

Heterozygosity for δβ thalassemia and hemoglobin Lepore results in a mild form of anemia that is clinically described as thalassemia minor and is similar to the condition of patients with heterozygous β thalassemia.

Hereditary Persistence of Fetal Hemoglobin

Hereditary persistence of fetal hemoglobin (HPFH) comprises a group of conditions characterized by the persis-

➤ **Table 12-2**
GENETIC BACKGROUND OF ALPHA-THALASSEMIA CLINICAL SYNDROMES (MATING COMBINATIONS)

Chromosome →	Normal	α^+			α^0
Genes ↓ →	αα	−α	$\alpha^{CS}\alpha$	$\alpha\alpha^T$	—
αα	N	α thal 2	α thal 2	α thal 2	α thal 1
−α	α thal 2	α thal 1	α thal 1	α thal 1	H
$\alpha^{CS}\alpha$	α thal 2	α thal 1	α thal 1	α thal 1	H
$\alpha\alpha^T$	α thal 2	α thal 1	α thal 1	H	H
—	α thal 1	H	H	H	Bart's

Abbreviations: αα = normal haplotype; −α = deletion of one alpha gene; $\alpha^{CS}\alpha$ = Hb Constant Spring: $\alpha\alpha^T$ = nondeletion alpha thalassemia gene; — = deletion of both alpha genes (Note: the clinical phenotype resulting from the combination of these haplotypes is found at the intersection of the corresponding column and row); N = normal clinical phenotype; α thal 1 = α^0 trait, 5%–15% Hb Bart's at birth, mild anemia; α thal 2 = α^+ trait, 0%–2% Hb Bart's at birth, minimal hematologic changes; H = hemoglobin H disease; Bart's = hemoglobin Bart's hydrops fetalis.

tence of fetal hemoglobin synthesis into adult life. These conditions can be classified into two different categories according to the distribution of hemoglobin F among the red cells. Fetal hemoglobin is more resistant than adult hemoglobin to elution at acid pH and can be demonstrated on a peripheral smear by the acid elution test of Kleihauer and Betke. Using this stain, the HPFH conditions can be divided into a pancellular form, in which hemoglobin F is uniformly distributed among the red cells, and a heterocellular form, in which hemoglobin F is found in only a small percentage of the cells (Fig. 12–9 and Color Plate 114). In the normal adult, cells containing hemoglobin F can occasionally be found, but the amount is always less than 2% and is usually less than 1%. These cells are called F cells.

Heterocellular HPFH appears to be an inherited condition in which the number of F cells is increased without concurrent abnormalities in δ- and β-chain production. Its most common form is the Swiss type, in which individuals have up to 3% hemoglobin F but are otherwise hematologically normal. At the DNA level, there appear to be no gross abnormalities of the δ or β genes.

On the other hand, pancellular HPFH appears to be a form of δβ thalassemia in which the γ genes were not switched off and are able to compensate fully for the lack of δ- and β-chain production. The most common form of pancellular HPFH is the African type, in which there is a deletion of the β- and δ-globin genes that is associated with synthesis of $^{G}\gamma$ and $^{A}\gamma$ chains, which almost compensates for the lack of production of δ and β chains. Hemoglobin F constitutes 100% of the hemoglobin in the homozygous state and 15% to 30% of the hemoglobin in the heterozygous state. The hemoglobin F is homogeneously distributed among the red cells and consists of a mixture of $^{G}\gamma$ and $^{A}\gamma$ chains. Clinically, the homozygotes will demonstrate features of thalassemia minor and the heterozygotes will be hematologically normal.

Another form of pancellular HPFH is the Greek type, in which about 15% hemoglobin F is present in the heterozygous state. This hemoglobin F is also found uniformly distributed among the red cells but is only of the $^{A}\gamma$ type. The homozygous state for this type of pancellular HPFH has not been described. In general, heterozygous or homozygous HPFH causes no significant clinical abnormalities.

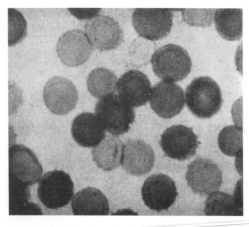

➤ FIGURE 12–9 Betke-Kleihauer stain of blood from a patient with hereditary persistence of fetal hemoglobin (HPFH). Note that all red cells stain red, owing to the varying amounts of hemoglobin F. (From Bell, A: Hematology. In Listen, Look and Learn. Health and Education Resources, Inc., Bethesda, MD, with permission.)

Thalassemia Associated with Hemoglobin Variants

The molecular basis of all hemoglobinopathies can be broadly divided into two groups. In the first group the genetic defect involves the synthesis of the β chain; this group includes β thalassemia, hemoglobin S, hemoglobin C, and hemoglobin E. In the second group the genetic defect involves the α-chain synthesis; the α thalassemias are included in this group. Homozygosity or double heterozygosity for defective genes within the same group usually results in severe disease that is often lethal. Double heterozygosity with one gene from one group and a second gene from the other group usually shows no interaction. A defective gene in one group may even result in a clinical improvement of the condition of a patient who is homozygous for a defective gene in the other group. Although thalassemia has been described in association with a large number of hemoglobin structural variants, the following discussion considers only the interactions with the more common hemoglobin variants (i.e., β thalassemia with hemoglobin S, hemoglobin C, and hemoglobin E, and α thalassemia with hemoglobin S).

β Thalassemia with Hemoglobin S

This condition was first recognized in individuals who had inherited a single hemoglobin S gene and who demonstrated about 65% hemoglobin S and 35% hemoglobin A, which is the reverse of the proportions found in patients with sickle cell trait. This condition is the result of the inheritance of a hemoglobin S gene from one parent and a β-thalassemia gene from the other. β Thalassemia with hemoglobin S (also called the β-thalassemia sickle cell syndrome) has been widely seen in Africa, the Mediterranean area, the Middle East, and the West Indies, as well as in African Americans. There is great variety in the clinical severity of this syndrome, depending mostly on the type of β-thalassemia gene inherited. If the β-thalassemia gene is the β^0 type, no hemoglobin A is produced and the clinical condition is indistinguishable from classic sickle cell anemia, characterized by severe anemia presenting in early childhood and recurrent sickling crises. If the β-thalassemia gene is β^+ type 1, a small amount of hemoglobin A is produced, possibly representing up to 15% of the total hemoglobin. Patients in this group have severe anemia with a hemoglobin level in the 7 to 8 g/dL range and experience less frequent and less severe sickling crises than those in the β^0 group. If the β-thalassemia gene is β^+ type 2, as found in most African Americans, a greater amount of hemoglobin A is produced, representing up to 30% of the total hemoglobin. Patients in this group have a very mild anemia with hemoglobin in the 11 g/dL range and are usually asymptomatic, the condition being diagnosed later in life or during the course of a family study. These patients, as a rule, do not experience any sickling crisis except under the most severe hypoxic conditions.

β Thalassemia with Hemoglobin C

The β thalassemia with hemoglobin C syndrome demonstrates great variability in clinical and hematologic manifestations, which is directly related to the type of β-thalassemia gene that interacts with the hemoglobin C gene; however, the great majority of patients with this syndrome are West Africans and African Americans. In this racial group the more common β-thalassemia gene is β^+ type 2. In this case the β thalassemia with hemoglobin C syndrome is characterized by a mild degree of usually asymptomatic anemia, in which the clinical and hematologic findings are very similar to those found in heterozygous β thalassemia.

β Thalassemia with Hemoglobin E

Double heterozygosity for β thalassemia and hemoglobin E is unusual because it results in a clinical disorder that is much more severe than homozygous hemoglobin E disease. Patients with this syndrome are distributed widely throughout the Far East. The condition follows a clinical course very similar to that of homozygous β thalassemia, with a very severe anemia occurring in early childhood and the development of the characteristic features of thalassemia major if the patient is not started on a regular blood transfusion program.

α Thalassemia with Sickle Cell Anemia

The occurrence of α thalassemia in conjunction with sickle cell anemia has a positive influence on the clinical expression of the disease. Patients with such a genetic background have an increased percentage of hemoglobin F, which is thought to result in a decreased severity of the sickling process. Of interest is the fact that the amount of hemoglobin F present is roughly proportional to the number of α genes affected. Patients with the α^0-thalassemia trait have an average of 16% hemoglobin F, and those with the α^+-thalassemia trait have an average of 8% hemoglobin F.[8]

► CLINICAL COURSE AND THERAPY

The clinical course and therapy of patients with thalassemia can be broadly subdivided into three categories: thalassemia major, thalassemia intermedia, and thalassemia minor. A fourth category, termed thalassemia minima, is applied to healthy silent carriers who show no clinical symptoms and minimal to no hematologic abnormalities. Table 12–3 summarizes the different genetic backgrounds that result in each of these clinical outcomes.

Hemoglobin Bart's Hydrops Fetalis

Hemoglobin Bart's hydrops fetalis is the result of homozygosity for the complete deletion of both α-globin genes. The affected infants are either stillborn or die within a few days after birth. At delivery, these infants are severely anemic and edematous, and demonstrate ascites, marked hepatomegaly, and splenomegaly. No therapy is available for this condition. The clinical significance of this entity is related to the obstetric problems that may arise in the affected infants' mothers. Pregnancy is often complicated by toxemia, obstructed labor, and postpartum hemorrhage, which may result in severe morbidity and mortality. Clinical emphasis for this entity is on the prevention of the disease through early antenatal diagnosis, which should result in termination of pregnancy for the protection of the mother's health.

Thalassemia Major

Thalassemia major is the most severe clinical expression of thalassemia and characteristically occurs in patients with homozygous β^0 or β^+ thalassemia or with double heterozygous β^0 and β^+ thalassemia, as well as in patients with homozygous hemoglobin Lepore, double heterozygous β thalassemia with hemoglobin Lepore, and double heterozygous β thalassemia with hemoglobin E.

Infants with thalassemia major usually present within the first year of life with failure to thrive, pallor, a variable degree of jaundice, and abdominal enlargement, with hemoglobin levels from 4 to 8 g/dL. This severe chronic anemia starting so early in life is a strong stimulus for erythropoiesis. This causes marked expansion of the marrow space and characteristic skeletal changes of the skull, long bones, and hand bones. The skull radiographs show widening of the diploid space and characteristic radiating striations giving the typical "hair-on-end" appearance (Fig. 12–10). The marrow expansion of the facial bones produces a characteristic facial appearance with hypertrophy of the maxilla causing forward protrusion of the upper teeth and overbite, a relatively sunken nose, widely spaced eyes, and prominent cheek bones, resulting in a Mongoloid facies (Fig. 12–11). The long bones of the hands and feet have cortical thinning with porosity of the medullary space. These changes are not a specific feature of thalassemia and are found in other severe, chronic congenital anemias, but they are most prominent in β thalassemia major.

Without careful medical supervision and a therapeutic pro-

► Table 12-3
GENETIC BACKGROUND OF THE DIFFERENT CLINICAL COURSES OF THALASSEMIA

Major	Intermedia	Minor	Minima
Homozygous β^0 thal	Homozygous β^0 or β^+ thal or double heterozygous	Heterozygous β^0 thal	Heterozygous β^+ thal (type 3)
Homozygous β^+ thal (type 1)	β^0/β^+ thal in association with α thal	Heterozygous β^+ thal (type 1 or type 2)	
Double heterozygous β^0/β^+ thal	Homozygous β^+ thal (type 2 or type 3)	Heterozygous δβ thal	
Homozygous Hb Lepore (some)	Homozygous Hb Lepore (some)	Heterozygous Hb Lepore	
Double heterozygous Hb Lepore/β^0 or β^+ thal	Double heterozygous δβ thal/β thal	Double heterozygous β thal/HPFH	Homozygous HPFH Heterozygous HPFH
Double heterozygous HbE/β^0 or β^+ thal	Double heterozygous Hb Lepore/δβ thal		
	Hemoglobin H disease	α Thalassemia 1	α Thalassemia 2

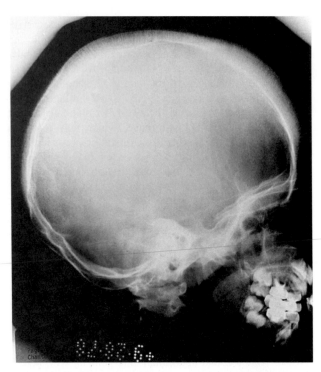

> **FIGURE 12–10**   Skull x-ray of 5-year-old child with homozygous β-thalassemia. Note the dilation of the diploic space and the typical "hair-on-end" appearance caused by subperiosteal bone growth in radiating striations.

gram, including blood transfusions, iron chelation, and early treatment of infection, these children will have numerous complications, which include massive hepatosplenomegaly, recurrent infections, spontaneous fractures, leg ulcers, dental and orthodontic problems, and compression syndromes caused by tumor masses from extramedullary hematopoiesis. If the condition is left untreated, these children will usually die in early childhood.

Survival of these patients is dependent on a lifelong chronic blood transfusion program. It is now clear that a high

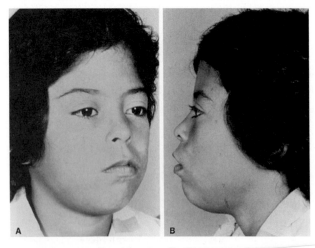

> **FIGURE 12–11**   Face (A) and profile (B) of an 11-year-old child with homozygous β thalassemia who is receiving hypertransfusion. The characteristic facial changes are not as prominent as those in an untransfused child, but are still present. Note the bossing of the skull, hypertrophy of the maxilla with prominent malar eminences, depression of the bridge of the nose, and mongoloid slant of the eyes.

transfusion program (hypertransfusion) that maintains the hemoglobin level at 11.5 g/dL on the average is better than an intermittent program that allows the hemoglobin level to drop to a point at which the child becomes severely symptomatic. Hypertransfusion allows for better development, suppresses ineffective erythropoiesis (thus preventing the serious bony deformities), and provides for an overall better quality of life. This, however, draws on considerable blood resources and may not be available in the very countries where thalassemia major is a main public health concern.

In the presence of splenomegaly, splenectomy plays a clear role in decreasing the blood transfusion requirement. However, it should preferably not be performed until the child has reached at least 5 years of age, to decrease the risk of overwhelming infection, particularly of pneumococcal origin.

With regular blood transfusion, these children survive but develop severe iron overload owing to increased iron absorption and to the loading of iron from the blood transfusions. This iron overload results in hemochromatosis, and these patients die in their second or third decade, usually of cardiac failure. They develop multiple organ damage, with lack of pubertal development probably caused by iron toxicity to the pituitary gland, cirrhosis of the liver (which may be the result of either hemochromatosis or posttransfusion hepatitis), and diabetes resulting from iron toxicity to the pancreas. This iron overload may be improved with the early introduction of iron chelation therapy. Subcutaneous iron chelation therapy with deferoxamine may result in an adequate iron balance, promoting a longer survival. However it is an expensive and difficult regimen that is often not available or rigorously followed by patients. Newer oral iron chelation therapies currently being developed may offer a better alternative worldwide.[9]

Alternate modes of therapy for thalassemia major in the future may be found in the areas of bone marrow transplantation,[10] genetic engineering, and pharmacologic manipulations, such as hydroxyurea or azacitinidine, that may induce the "switching back on" of the γ-globin gene.[11,12] The current optimal therapy for thalassemia major relies on intensive use of a fairly sophisticated level of health care. This cannot be achieved in most of the countries where thalassemia major is a serious problem without shunting the major thrust of the health resources in that direction.

Another approach to this problem at the health planning level is to decrease the number of births of infants with thalassemia major. This has been successful in certain countries, particularly Cyprus, with the implementation of mass population screening for the detection of heterozygous carriers, genetic counseling, and antenatal diagnosis for couples at risk. Reliable antenatal diagnosis, using DNA hybridization techniques in association with chorionic villus sampling, enable physicians to make a diagnosis during the first trimester of pregnancy, thus making early termination of pregnancy much more widely available and acceptable.

Thalassemia Intermedia

Thalassemia intermedia covers a broad spectrum of clinical expression of thalassemia, bridging the gap between the severe, lethal form of thalassemia major and the mild, often asymptomatic anemic state of thalassemia minor. The definition of thalassemia intermedia is relative, because the clinical state of patients in this group varies from a mild disability to severe incapacitation without transfusion. Thalassemia intermedia could be defined as a form of thalassemia in which patients have variable degrees of symptomatic anemia, jaundice, splenomegaly, and many of the complications of thalassemia major, but survive into adulthood without a large blood transfusion requirement.

The genetic background of thalassemia intermedia is also extremely varied. Worldwide, most of these patients have hemoglobin H disease and are of Asian origin. This clinical expression also includes patients with homozygosity for the less severe forms of the β-thalassemia gene (such as β^+ type 2 and β^+ type 3 thalassemia), homozygous $\delta\beta$ thalassemia, double heterozygous $\delta\beta$ thalassemia with β thalassemia, and patients who are homozygous for β thalassemia but who have also inherited a gene for α thalassemia or who have the ability to synthesize the γ chains more efficiently. The exact definition of the genetic background of a patient with thalassemia intermedia requires a careful and extensive family study.

Patients with thalassemia intermedia usually present at a somewhat older age—generally after the age of 2—and with a slightly higher level of hemoglobin (between 6 and 10 g/dL) than patients with thalassemia major. There is great overlap between the two conditions at presentation; however, it is very important to differentiate between them, as the only therapy for thalassemia major is regular blood transfusion in conjunction with iron chelation, whereas the management of thalassemia intermedia involves mostly supportive therapy with only occasional blood transfusion under special circumstances.

The serum bilirubin level is significantly more elevated in patients with thalassemia intermedia than in those with thalassemia major. These patients may develop the physical and bony characteristics of thalassemia major, as well as splenomegaly and hepatomegaly; however, they survive into adulthood without regular blood transfusion. The anemia usually becomes worse with infections, pregnancy, and folic acid deficiency states. These patients are susceptible to frequent, sometimes severe, infections, and gallbladder problems owing to the formation of gallstones. Children usually have an acceptable level of growth and development (although puberty may be delayed by a few years), and they reach adulthood if infections are controlled and if they enjoy good nutrition with particular emphasis on prevention of folic acid deficiency. They may become transfusion-dependent if severe hypersplenism occurs. This usually requires splenectomy. Women with thalassemia intermedia may become pregnant and may require blood transfusions as well as folic acid supplementation throughout pregnancy. In spite of the lack of transfusion, patients with thalassemia intermedia develop iron overload as a result of increased gastrointestinal absorption. This is a much slower process than that experienced by patients with thalassemia major, and the complications resulting from iron overload occur much later in life.[13] However complications from iron overload occur at a lower ferritin level owing to the smaller ferrihydrite form of iron deposition in contrast with the larger goethite form present in patients with transfusion-dependant thalassemia major.[14]

Thalassemia Minor

Thalassemia minor is a clinical entity in which the genetic defects of thalassemia are expressed as a mild microcytic, hypochromic anemia, usually in the 9 to 11 g/dL range. Patients are asymptomatic except during periods of stress such as pregnancy, infection, or folic acid deficiency. Most patients with thalassemia minor are heterozygous for the β^+-thalassemia gene, the β^0-thalassemia gene, or the α^0-thalassemia gene. The genetic background of thalassemia minor also includes heterozygosity for hemoglobin Lepore and for $\delta\beta$ thalassemia. Patients with thalassemia minor are usually diagnosed incidental to a family study of an index case with thalassemia major or by population screening. They usually require no therapy if they maintain good nutrition. It is important that they not be misdiagnosed as having iron-deficiency anemia.

➤ BLOOD TRANSFUSION IN THALASSEMIA

Three main concerns need to be addressed regarding patients with thalassemia major who will be receiving a regular blood transfusion program: (1) the development of iron overload, (2) the development of alloimmunization, and (3) the risk of transfusion-transmitted diseases. The problem of iron overload can be approached from two directions—by increasing the iron excretion or by decreasing the amount of iron transfused. This latter option can be performed by increasing the length of survival of the transfused red cells, which requires selection of younger red cells (also called neocytes) for transfusion. Young red cells and reticulocytes have a lower specific gravity than old red cells, and by using a differential centrifugation technique, the blood unit can be separated so that the upper layer of cells is collected. These red cells will have a longer life expectancy and can decrease the transfusion requirement of a patient by lengthening the interval of the blood transfusion schedule.

Alloimmunization is a recurrent problem of all chronically transfused patients. These patients often develop antibodies to white cell as well as to red cell antigens. Antibodies to white cell antigens cause febrile nonhemolytic transfusion reactions that are uncomfortable. These reactions can be avoided by routinely transfusing leukocyte-reduced red cells. Alloimmunization to red cell antigens is a more serious problem, because this can cause acute or delayed hemolytic transfusion reactions and may seriously affect the availability of compatible blood. It is recommended that a complete phenotype of the patient's red cells be obtained before embarking on a regular transfusion program.

Transfusion-transmitted diseases are a common complication in multitransfused patients. In the past, patients with thalassemia major often developed hepatitis. This risk has been significantly decreased in many areas of the world with the introduction of testing for hepatitis C. Some patients may develop a chronic form of hepatitis that, in conjunction with the toxicity of iron overload, may result in cirrhosis of the liver.

➤ LABORATORY DIAGNOSIS OF THALASSEMIA

The hallmark of thalassemia is the finding of a microcytic, hypochromic anemia. Although more sophisticated laboratory procedures are needed to define exactly the type of thalassemia, the original diagnosis of thalassemia can be made or strongly suspected on the basis of the results of routine hematology procedures.

Routine Hematology Procedures
Automated Blood Cell Analyzer (see Chap. 29)

The thalassemias in general are characterized by a decrease in hemoglobin level, hematocrit, mean corpuscular volume (MCV), and mean corpuscular hemoglobin (MCH) in conjunction with a normal-to-increased red blood cell (RBC) count, a normal to mildly decreased mean corpuscular hemoglobin concentration (MCHC), and a normal red cell volume distribution width (RDW). The only exception is thalassemia major, in which the degree of anisocytosis is such that the RDW is increased. The decrease in MCV is usually striking and disproportionate to the decrease in hemoglobin and hematocrit. This fact, in conjunction with the relatively high RBC count and the normal RDW, offers a useful discrimination index between heterozygous α or β thalassemia and iron deficiency.[15] In iron deficiency, the RDW is increased and the decrease in MCV is less striking and only observed when the anemia is more severe. In heterozygous thalassemia, the MCH is usually below 22 pg and the MCV below 70 fL, whereas the hemoglobin level is in the 9 to 11 g/dL range.

Peripheral Smear Examination

The careful examination of a well-prepared peripheral smear is essential to the diagnosis of thalassemia.

Wright's Stain

In homozygous β and double heterozygous non–α thalassemia, the peripheral smear demonstrates extreme anisocytosis and poikilocytosis with bizarre shapes, target cells, ovalocytes, and large numbers of nucleated red cells (see Fig. 12–4 and Color Plate 112). There is marked hypochromia and microcytosis. In heterozygous β thalassemia, the cells are hypochromic and microcytic with a mild to moderate degree of anisocytosis and poikilocytosis. Target cells are frequent, and basophilic stippling is often seen (see Fig. 12–5 and Color Plate 113). The peripheral smear of a patient with the sickle cell thalassemia syndrome can be differentiated from that of a patient with pure sickle cell anemia by the presence of hypochromia, microcytosis, numerous target cells, and only an occasional sickled cell.

In hemoglobin H disease, the peripheral smear demonstrates hypochromia with microcytosis, target cells, and mild to moderate anisopoikilocytosis. Patients with heterozygous α^0 thalassemia usually demonstrate a mild hypochromia and microcytosis, whereas those with heterozygous α^+ thalassemia usually have a perfectly normal peripheral smear.

Supravital Stains

The reticulocyte count is usually elevated up to 10% in hemoglobin H disease and up to 5% in homozygous β thalassemia but is disproportionately low in relation to the degree of anemia in the latter condition.

In hemoglobin H disease, incubation of the red cells with brilliant cresyl blue stain causes in vitro precipitation of hemoglobin H owing to the redox action of the dye. This results in a characteristic appearance of the majority of the red cells, which display multiple discrete inclusions, the appearance of which has often been compared to that of a golf ball (see Fig. 12–7). Occasionally, and after extensive searching, such cells containing hemoglobin H inclusions can be found in the α^0-thalassemia carrier.

In patients with homozygous β thalassemia or hemoglobin H disease who have undergone splenectomy, incubation of the blood with methyl violet stain can demonstrate Heinz body–like inclusions, which represent in vivo precipitation of the abnormal hemoglobin.

Acid Elution Stain (see Chap. 28)

The acid elution technique, originally described by Kleihauer and Betke, is based on the fact that at an acid pH of about 3.3, hemoglobin A is eluted from an air-dried, alcohol-fixed blood smear, whereas hemoglobin F is resistant to elution. After such treatment and subsequent staining with eosin or erythrosin, normal adult red cells appear as very faint ghosts. Red cells containing hemoglobin F demonstrate a variable amount of stain, depending on the amount of hemoglobin F present. A controlled preparation containing a mixture of adult and cord cells must also be stained and examined in parallel to check the quality of the technique, as this technique is very sensitive to many variables.

This stain is very useful in demonstrating the distribution of hemoglobin F and can be used to differentiate between pancellular and heterocellular HPFH. It is also useful in differentiating heterozygous δβ thalassemia from heterozygous pancellular HPFH, because the former usually has a heterocellular distribution of hemoglobin F.

Osmotic Fragility

The red cells of patients with homozygous or heterozygous β thalassemia, hemoglobin H disease, and α^0-thalassemia trait have a decreased osmotic fragility. This fact is not very useful for diagnostic purposes in a specific patient, but it is the basis of a simple, inexpensive method of screening for the thalassemia carrier state in large populations.

Hemoglobin Electrophoresis

Hemoglobin electrophoresis plays an important role in the diagnosis of thalassemia by allowing the detection of increased levels of hemoglobin A_2 and hemoglobin F as well as the presence of abnormal hemoglobins, such as hemoglobin H, hemoglobin Bart's, hemoglobin Lepore, hemoglobin Constant Spring, or other structurally abnormal hemoglobins that can be found in association with thalassemia (hemoglobin S, hemoglobin C, hemoglobin E). Table 12–4 contains a summary of the different patterns of the hemoglobins present in the non–α thalassemia syndromes.

Routine hemoglobin electrophoresis to confirm the diagnosis of thalassemia is performed at an alkaline pH around 8.4 on cellulose acetate or starch gel. At that pH, the hemoglobins migrate from the most cathodal to the most anodal in the following order: first hemoglobin Constant Spring, then hemoglobins A_2, C, and E migrate in the same band; next hemoglobins S and Lepore, again in the same band; then hemoglobin F, followed by hemoglobin A, hemoglobin Portland, hemoglobin Bart's, and finally, hemoglobin H. The different patterns of migration of these hemoglobins is illustrated in Figure 12–6. Cellulose acetate or starch gel electrophoresis can be performed at low to neutral pH to detect hemoglobin H and hemoglobin Bart's easily, as they migrate anodally (i.e., in the direction opposite to the other hemoglobins) at this pH.

Cellulose Acetate

Cellulose acetate electrophoresis is becoming more popular and has replaced starch gel electrophoresis in many lab-

> **Table 12-4**
LEVELS OF HEMOGLOBINS A, A₂, AND F IN THE DIFFERENT NON-α THALASSEMIAS

	HbA (%)	HbA₂ (%)	HbF (%)
Homozygous β^0 thal	0	2–5	95–98
Homozygous β^+ or double heterozygous β^+/β^0 thal	5–35	2–5	60–95
Homozygous δβ thal	0	0	100
Homozygous Hb Lepore	0	0	75 (25% Hb Lepore)
Heterozygous β thal	90–95	3.5–7	2–5
Heterozygous δβ thal	80–92	1–2.5	5–20
Heterozygous Hb Lepore	75–85	2	1–6 (7–15% Hb Lepore)
Homozygous HPFH	0	0	100
Heterozygous HPFH (African type)	65–85	1–2.5	15–35
Heterozygous HPFH (Greek type)	75–85	1.5–2.5	15–25
Normal	95–97	2–3	1–2

oratories, owing to its simple, rapid method. It uses a smaller sample than starch gel electrophoresis, and minor components such as hemoglobin Constant Spring and small amounts of hemoglobin A₂ may be overlooked. Small amounts of hemoglobin A in the presence of mostly hemoglobin F also can be difficult to detect.

Other Gels
Starch gel electrophoresis is a little more cumbersome and time-consuming. The results of the starch gel electrophoresis are similar to those of the cellulose acetate procedure. Electrophoresis with starch gel is better at defining the presence of hemoglobin Constant Spring and should always be used if such a variant is suspected.

Citrate agar gel electrophoresis, which is performed at an acid pH between 5.9 and 6.2, has a minor role in the diagnosis of the thalassemias.

Hemoglobin Quantitation
Although an experienced observer can detect an increased level in hemoglobin A₂ or hemoglobin F on cellulose acetate or starch gel electrophoresis, actual quantitation is necessary to truly establish the diagnosis of thalassemia.

Hemoglobin A₂ Quantitation
The elevation of hemoglobin A₂ is an excellent tool for the detection of a heterozygote carrier of β thalassemia. It is characteristic of heterozygous β thalassemia and has high specificity with no overlap values between heterozygous carriers and normal individuals. The level of hemoglobin A₂ ranges between 3.5% and 7% in heterozygous β thalassemia, whereas normal values are always less than 3.5%. A few rare variants of β thalassemia with normal A₂, which are called normal A₂ β thalassemia, do exist, and can only be distinguished in the carrier state from heterozygous α thalassemia by globin-chain synthesis. Also, in an iron-deficient patient with β thalassemia minor, hemoglobin A₂ may be reduced to normal levels. The percentage of hemoglobin A₂ can be quantified by elution following cellulose acetate electrophoresis, microcolumn chromatography, or high-performance liquid chromatography.[16]

Hemoglobin F Quantitation
The hemoglobin F levels are useful in the definition of the type of thalassemia involved, and a summary of the levels of hemoglobin F corresponding to the different types of thalassemia can be found in Table 12–4. The hemoglobin F level is normally below 2%. Approximately half of the β-thalassemia carriers have a mildly elevated level of hemoglobin F, usually below 5%.

Routine Chemistry
The indirect bilirubin level is elevated in thalassemia major and intermedia, ranging from 1 to 6 mg/dL. It is characteristically more elevated in thalassemia intermedia than in thalassemia major.

The assessment of the iron status of the patient by the determination of the serum iron level, total iron-binding capacity (TIBC), and serum ferritin level is useful in the differentiation of a thalassemia carrier from a patient with iron-deficiency anemia, as well as in the assessment of the iron load in a patient with thalassemia major or intermedia. The serum iron and serum ferritin levels are low and the TIBC increased in patients with iron deficiency. These values are normal in patients with thalassemia minor, unless they have concurrent iron deficiency. Patients with thalassemia major who have been transfused have increased levels of serum iron that approach 100% saturation of the TIBC. The serum ferritin level is elevated and indicates the amount of iron deposited in the tissues.

➤ DIFFERENTIAL DIAGNOSIS OF MICROCYTIC, HYPOCHROMIC ANEMIA
The differential diagnosis of microcytic hypochromic anemia includes iron deficiency, α thalassemia, β thalassemia, anemia of chronic disease, hemoglobin E disease, sideroblastic anemia, and lead poisoning. Evaluation of the clinical history, hemoglobin level, and red cell indices (in particular, MCV and MCH), and examination of the peripheral smear usually narrow the diagnosis. The sometimes difficult differentiation of the thalassemia carrier from the iron-deficiency state can be achieved by evaluating the serum

> ## Table 12-5
> ## DIFFERENTIAL DIAGNOSIS OF MICROCYTIC HYPOCHROMIC ANEMIA

	RDW	Serum Iron	TIBC	Serum Ferritin	FEP	A$_2$ Level
Iron deficiency	↑	↓	↑	↓	↑	nl
α Thalassemia	nl	nl	nl	nl	nl	nl
β Thalassemia	nl	nl	nl	nl	nl	↑
Hemoglobin E disease	nl	nl	nl	nl	nl	nl
Anemia of chronic disease	nl	↓	↓	↑	↑	nl
Sideroblastic anemia	↑	↑	nl	↑	↓	nl
Lead poisoning	nl	nl	nl	nl	↑	nl

Abbreviations: RDW = red cell distribution width; TIBC = total iron-binding capacity; FEP = free erythrocyte protoporphyrin; nl = normal.

iron and ferritin levels and the TIBC. A markedly elevated free erythrocyte protoporphyrin (FEP) identifies a child with lead poisoning. Cellulose acetate electrophoresis usually allows differentiation between a β-thalassemia carrier, an α-thalassemia carrier, or the presence of hemoglobin E. The differentiation between these diseases is summarized in Table 12–5.

> ## ➤ CASE STUDY

A 25-year-old man of Chinese extraction was evaluated because he was found to be anemic when he attempted to donate blood. He otherwise had no complaints. He stated that he is active in sports and feels healthy. A complete blood count gave the following results: RBC, 5.76 million; Hgb, 10.4 g/dL; Hct, 35.9%; MCV, 62 fL; MCH, 18.1 pg; MCHC, 29%; RDW, 13.5%. The peripheral blood smear showed hypochromic, microcytic erythrocytes with a mild anisocytosis, occasional target cells, but no basophilic stippling.

Questions

1. What diagnoses should be considered at this time?
2. What laboratory tests are most useful to diagnose the cause of the patient's anemia?

Further evaluation reveals the following findings: serum iron is 95 mg/dL (normal is 60 to 150 mg/dL); TIBC, 305 mg/dL (normal is 260 to 360 mg/dL); and ferritin level, 175 μg/dL (normal is 30 to 300 μg/dL). Cellulose acetate electrophoresis shows an increased amount of hemoglobins F and A$_2$, which are quantitated to 4.5% and 5%, respectively.

3. What is your diagnosis now, and what is the significance of this diagnosis for this patient?

Answers

1. On clinical history alone, the possibilities of anemia of chronic disease and lead poisoning can be ruled out in a healthy young man. This leaves the possibility of iron deficiency, a β-thalassemia carrier, an α-thalassemia carrier, sideroblastic anemia, and hemoglobin E disease (which should be considered in a person of Chinese extraction).

2. A serum iron level, TIBC, serum ferritin level, and cellulose acetate electrophoresis are appropriate tests that may differentiate among these conditions.

3. Sideroblastic anemia and iron deficiency can be ruled out by the normal iron level, TIBC, and ferritin level. Although hemoglobin E migrates in the same area as hemoglobin A$_2$, on cellulose acetate electrophoresis, a patient with heterozygous or homozygous hemoglobin E would have a much larger amount of hemoglobin in that band; thus, hemoglobin E disease is ruled out. An α-thalassemia carrier would have a normal hemoglobin electrophoresis pattern; therefore, the diagnosis in this patient is heterozygous β thalassemia. Making the diagnosis of β-thalassemia heterozygosity in this patient is important for two reasons. Firstly, the patient must be reassured that this level of hemoglobin and hematocrit is normal for him, and he should not be placed on iron therapy, which could be harmful. Secondly, the patient needs to be educated regarding the possibility of his having a child with a severe congenital anemia and its therapeutic implications if he marries someone who is a carrier of β thalassemia, hemoglobin E, or hemoglobin S. His spouse should be screened for the presence of these genes and genetic counseling such as antenatal diagnosis offered if she is a carrier.

QUESTIONS

1. What is the hemoglobin defect found in thalassemia syndromes?
   a. Abnormal incorporation of iron molecule
   b. Defective production of the globin portion
   c. Excessive production of porphyrins
   d. Amino acid substitution

2. What type of globin chains and hemoglobin are characteristics of α thalassemia?
   a. Two α chains and two β chains (HbA)
   b. Two α chains and two δ chains (HbA$_2$)
   c. Four β chains (HbH) or four γ chains (Hb Bart's)
   d. Two α chains and two γ chains (HbF)

3. Which type of thalassemia has primarily hemoglobin Bart's and shows the following clinical expressions: infants die in utero or soon after birth, severe anemia, marked hepatomegaly and splenomegaly, and ascites?
   a. Homozygous α thalassemia
   b. Homozygous β thalassemia
   c. Thalassemia minor
   d. α-Thalassemia trait

4. What is the term for the clinical course of homozygous thalassemias resulting from defects in δ- and β-chain synthesis?
   a. Thalassemia minor
   b. Thalassemia major
   c. Thalassemia trait
   d. Thalassemia intermedia

5. Hereditary persistence of fetal hemoglobin (HPFH) is characterized by the persistence of fetal hemoglobin into adult life. What are the clinical manifestations of this condition?
   a. Chronic anemia with skeletal abnormalities caused by excessive erythropoiesis
   b. Asymptomatic except during pregnancy or stressful situations
   c. Hydrops fetalis syndrome
   d. No significant abnormalities for heterozygous; minor symptoms for homozygous

6. What is the clinical manifestation of α thalassemia with sickle cell anemia?
   a. Severe, life-threatening anemia
   b. Relatively asymptomatic until placed in an oxygen-deprived environment
   c. Less severe than sickle cell anemia alone
   d. Skeletal abnormality, but milder anemia than sickle cell anemia

7. What is the primary risk to thalassemia major patients who are on a high-transfusion (hypertransfusion) program?
   a. Hyperviscosity of blood
   b. Iron overload
   c. Citrate toxicity
   d. Electrolyte imbalance

8. What routine hematologic finding is indicative of thalassemia?
   a. Microcytic, hypochromic anemia
   b. Macrocytic, hypochromic anemia
   c. Normocytic, normochromic anemia
   d. Macrocytic, normochromic anemia

9. How can iron deficiency be distinguished from heterozygous α or β thalassemia?
   a. Heterozygous thalassemia: decreased RDW, with increased MCH and MCV and Hgb in the 10 to 14 g/dL range; iron deficiency: increased RDW, MCH, and MCV
   b. Heterozygous thalassemia: normal RDW, with decreased MCH and MCV and Hgb in the 9 to 11 g/dL range; iron deficiency: increased RDW, with decreased MCV and MCH only in severe anemia
   c. Heterozygous thalassemia: increased RDW, with decreased MCH and MCV and Hgb in the 5 to 9 g/dL range; iron deficiency: normal RDW, with normal MCV and MCH
   d. Heterozygous thalassemia: normal RDW, MCH, and MCV; iron deficiency: RDW, MCH, and MCV all increased

10. Which of the following cells are not found in a patient with homozygous β thalassemia?
    a. Target cells
    b. Ovalocytes
    c. Sickle cells
    d. Nucleated red cells

11. Which test is useful in demonstrating the distribution of hemoglobin F and in differentiating pancellular HPFH, heterocellular HPFH, and heterozygous $\delta\beta$ thalassemia?
    a. Osmotic fragility
    b. Kleihauer-Betke acid elution test
    c. Serum ferritin level
    d. Complete blood count

12. Which of the following findings would be indicative of heterozygous β thalassemia?
    a. Hemoglobin A_2 level of 3.5% to 7%
    b. Hemoglobin F level less than 2%
    c. Hemoglobin A level of 65% to 85%
    d. Hemoglobin A_2 level less than 3.5%

SUMMARY CHART

➤ Thalassemia syndromes result from an abnormality in the rate of synthesis of one of the globin chains.

➤ Two main types of thalassemia exist: alpha (α) thalassemia and beta (β) thalassemia.

➤ In thalassemia, there is a decrease in the amount of normal physiologic hemoglobin produced, resulting in a microcytic, hypochromic anemia.

➤ There are three types of β thalassemia: type 1 β^+, found throughout the Mediterranean region; type 2 β^+, found in blacks of North America and West Africa; and type 3 β^+, found sporadically in Italy, Greece, and the Middle East.

➤ The homozygous form of thalassemia is severe and called *thalassemia major*, with the exception of homozygous type 2 or type 3 β^+ thalassemia, which is a milder form called *thalassemia intermedia*.

➤ The heterozygous form of thalassemia is mild and called *thalassemia minor*.

➤ α Thalassemia can be divided into four clinical categories depending on the severity of the disease: hemoglobin Bart's (hydrops fetalis syndrome), which is lethal; hemoglobin H disease; α^0-thalassemia trait (also called α-thalassemia 1 trait); and α^+-thalassemia trait also called α-thalassemia 2 trait.

➤ Delta-beta ($\delta\beta$) thalassemia is called hemoglobin Lepore syndrome.

➤ Hereditary persistence of fetal hemoglobin (HPFH) comprises a group of conditions characterized by the persistence of fetal hemoglobin synthesis into adult life.

➤ Thalassemia has been associated with a number of hemoglobin structural variants, including hemoglobin S, hemoglobin C, and hemoglobin E.

➤ The thalassemias are generally characterized by a decrease in hemoglobin level, hematocrit, mean corpuscular volume (MCV), and mean corpuscular hemoglobin (MCH), in conjunction with a normal-to-increased red cell count.

➤ Hemoglobin electrophoresis aids in the diagnosis of thalassemia by detecting increased levels of hemoglobin A_2 and hemoglobin F, as well as other abnormal hemoglobins.

References

1. Cooley, TB, and Lee, P: A series of cases with splenomegaly in children with anemia and peculiar bone changes. Trans Am Ped Soc 37:29, 1925.
2. Nagel, RL, and Roth, EF: Malaria and red cell genetic defects. Blood 74:1213, 1989.
3. Liebhaber, SA, et al: Human α-globin gene expression. The dominant role of the α2-locus in mRNA and protein synthesis. J Biol Chem 261:15327, 1986.
4. Liebhaber, SA, et al: Homology and concerted evolution at the α1 and α2 loci of human α-globin. Nature 290:26, 1981.
5. Ho, PJ: The regulation of β-globin gene expression in β thalassemia. Pathology 31:315, 1999.
6. Huisman, THJ, et al: A syllabus of thalassemia mutations. The Sickle Cell Anemia Foundation. Augusta, GA, 1997. Available: http://globin.csp.psu.edu/globin/html/huisman/thals/contents.html.
7. Tang, WT, et al: Immunocytological test to detect adult carriers of ($^{-SER}$/) deletional α-thalassemia. Lancet 342:1145, 1993.
8. Emburg, SH, et al: Concurrent sickle-cell anemia and α-thalassemia. Effect on severity of anemia. N Engl J Med 306:270, 1982.
9. Wonke, B, et al: Combined therapy with deferiprone and desferrioxamine. BMJ 103:361, 1999.
10. Lucarelli, G, et al: Marrow transplantation in patients with thalassemia responsive to iron chelation therapy. N Engl J Med 329:840, 1993.
11. Goldberg, MA, et al: Treatment of sickle cell anemia with hydroxyurea and erythropoietin. N Engl J Med 323:366, 1990.
12. Lowrey, CH, and Nienhuis, AW: Brief report: Treatment with azacitidine of patients with end-stage β-thalassemia. N Engl J Med 329:845, 1993.
13. Chen FE, et al.: Genetic and clinical features of hemoglobin H disease in Chinese patients. N Engl J Med 343: 544, 2000.
14. St. Pierre TG, et al.: The form of iron oxide deposits in thalassemic tissues varies between different groups of patients: A comparison between Thai β-thalassemia/hemoglobin E patients and Australian β-thalassemia patients. Biochim Biophys Acta 1407:51, 1998
15. Johnson, CS, et al: Thalassemia minor: Routine erythrocyte measurements and differentiation from iron deficiency. Am J Clin Pathol 80:31, 1982.
16. Tan, GB, et al: Evaluation of high performance liquid chromatography for routine estimation of haemoglobins A_2 and F. J Clin Pathol 46:852, 1993.

See the Bibliography for this chapter at the back of the book.

13 Hemolytic Anemias

Extracorpuscular Defects and Acquired Intracorpuscular Defects

V Paroxysmal Nocturnal Hemoglobinuria

LOUANN W. LAWRENCE, DRPH, MT(ASCP)SH, CLSPH(NCA)
DENISE M. HARMENING, PHD, MT(ASCP), CLS(NCA)
RALPH GREEN, BAPPSCI(MLS), FAIMLS

EXTRACORPUSCULAR DEFECTS
Immune Hemolytic Anemia
Nonimmune Hemolytic Anemia

ACQUIRED INTRACORPUSCULAR DEFECTS
Paroxysmal Nocturnal Hemoglobinuria

CASE STUDY 1

CASE STUDY 2

CASE STUDY 3

CASE STUDY 4

OBJECTIVES

At the end of this chapter, the learner should be able to:

1. List mechanisms of immune hemolysis.
2. Define alloimmune hemolytic anemia.
3. Characterize immediate hemolytic transfusion reactions.
4. Characterize delayed hemolytic transfusion reactions.
5. Describe the causes of hemolytic disease of the newborn.
6. Define autoimmune hemolytic anemia.
7. Characterize warm autoimmune hemolytic anemia.
8. List features of cold agglutinin syndrome.
9. Describe the principle of the Donath-Landsteiner test used for paroxysmal cold hemoglobinuria.
10. List mechanisms for drug-induced immune hemolytic anemia.
11. List classifications for nonimmune hemolytic anemias.
12. Define paroxysmal nocturnal hemoglobinuria.
13. Describe the red cell membrane abnormality associated with paroxysmal nocturnal hemoglobinuria.
14. List clinical features of paroxysmal nocturnal hemoglobinuria.
15. List laboratory findings characteristic of paroxysmal nocturnal hemoglobinuria (PNH).
16. Describe the sugar water test (sucrose hemolysis test).
17. Describe HAM's test.
18. Outline how immunophenotyping is used in diagnosis of PNH.

➤ EXTRACORPUSCULAR DEFECTS

Immune Hemolytic Anemia

Definition

The term *immune hemolytic anemia* describes a process in which erythrocytes are destroyed prematurely by an immune-mediated process. Hemolysis resulting from antibodies or complement, or both, attached to the red blood cell membrane is confirmed by a positive direct antiglobulin test (DAT).

Role of Complement

Complement is a group of serum proteins that interact with each other to bring about, among other events, complement-dependent cell-mediated lysis. Complement can be activated by two different routes, the classical or the alternate (properdin) pathway.[1]

Classical Pathway

Activation of the classical pathway is initiated by immune complexes containing immunoglobulin G (IgG1, IgG2, IgG3) or IgM. The first complement component, C1, consists of three subunits—C1q, C1r, and C1s—as well as calcium (recognition unit). Clq initiates the complement cascade by interacting with the Fc (crystallizable fragment) portion of the immunoglobulin (Fig. 13–1). Clq then causes the activation of Clr, which then activates Cls. (A bar across the top of a complement component denotes its active form as shown in Figs. 13–1 and 13–2.) C4 is the second complement protein to be activated. This occurs when $C\overline{1s}$ cleaves C4 into its activated components, $C\overline{4a}$, which remains in the plasma, and $C\overline{4b}$, of which a small number of molecules attach to the cell membrane with the rest remaining in the plasma, in the inactive form. C2 attaches to $C\overline{4b}$ in the presence of magnesium and is then cleaved by $C\overline{1s}$ into the a and b subunits. $C\overline{2a}$ combines with $C\overline{4b}$ and forms the enzyme C3 convertase ($C\overline{4b2a}$), and $C\overline{2b}$ is released into the plasma.

Amplification of complement activity occurs now with the action of C3 convertase on C3. This enzyme ($C\overline{4b2a}$) cleaves C3 into its active components, $C\overline{3a}$ and $C\overline{3b}$, and is able to cleave hundreds of C3 molecules. $C\overline{3a}$ is released into the plasma and acts as an anaphylatoxin. $C\overline{3b}$ binds to the cell membrane and combines with $C\overline{4b2a}$ to form another enzyme, C5 convertase ($C\overline{4b2a3b}$). Some of the $C\overline{3b}$ molecules attach to other sites on the cell, are inactivated (iC3b), or are cleaved by C3 inactivator to C3c, which is released into the plasma, and to C3d, an inactive subunit that remains attached to the cell. The components C4, C2, and C3, are referred to as the *enzyme activation unit*.

C5 convertase ($C\overline{4b2a3b}$) cleaves C5 into the components $C\overline{5a}$, which is released into the plasma and acts as an anaphylatoxin and a chemotactic agent, and $C\overline{5b}$, which binds C6 and C7 to the cell membrane. Membrane-bound $C\overline{5b67}$ causes binding of C8, resulting in immediate ion flux into the cell and the beginning of cell lysis. The $C\overline{5b678}$ complex can bind up to six C9 molecules, together forming the membrane attack unit, $C\overline{5b6789}$, which causes cell lysis and accelerated movement of ions into the cell. With the binding of C9, the rate of cell lysis is greatly accelerated (see Fig. 13–1).

Complement activity is regulated by certain inhibitors (Cls inhibitor, C3b inactivator, C4 inactivator) and by the instability of certain components ($C\overline{4b2a}$, and $C\overline{4b2a3b}$).[1]

Alternate (Properdin) Pathway

The alternate, or properdin, pathway of complement activation also results in cell lysis, but by a different mechanism and group of proteins. The alternate pathway bypasses the complement components C1, C2, and C4 and enters at C3. This pathway consists of a distinct group of proteins: complement component C3; factor B, which is enzymatically cleaved into fragments Bb (biologically active) and Ba; factor D, which cleaves factor B; properdin (P), a serum protein that stabilizes the C3bBb complex; and factor H (C3b inactivator accelerator), which aids in controlling activation of the alternate pathway[2] (Fig. 13–2).

The alternate pathway may be triggered by certain microorganisms, polysaccharides, liposaccharides, aggregates of IgA, and cells or particles even in the absence of specific antibody. Present in the plasma are small amounts of a "priming" C3 convertase (C3bBb). The priming C3 convertase is

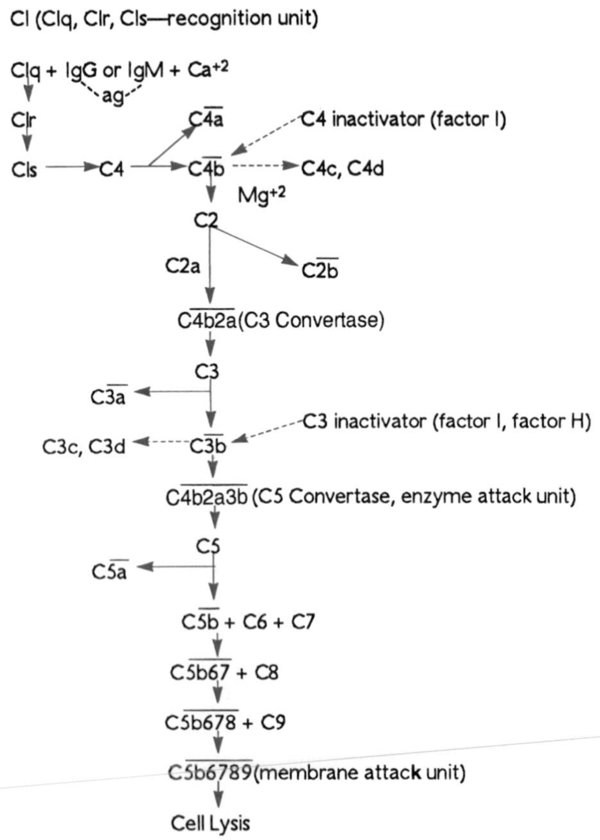

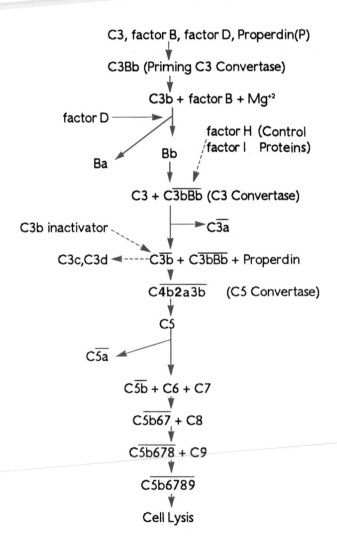

FIGURE 13–1 Classical pathway of complement activation.

FIGURE 13–2 Alternate pathway of complement activation.

produced continuously, owing to spontaneous interaction of intact C3, factor B, factor D, and properdin, an event not requiring activating substances. This results in the formation of small amounts of C3b. C3b binds to the cell surface and, under appropriate conditions and in the presence of magnesium, causes the attachment of factor B. The bound factor B is cleaved by factor D, releasing the Ba fragment and uncovering the C3 cleaving site on the Bb fragment. The C3bBb complex can rapidly lose activity or disassociate unless properdin is present. Properdin binds to the C3b part of the complex and stabilizes it. The C3bBb fragment (C3 convertase) then cleaves more C3, resulting in C3a and C3b fragments. A complex of C3bBbP3b (C5 convertase) forms and cleaves C5 into its fragments, C5a, and C5b. C5b along with C6, C7, C8, and C9 form the membrane attack unit, the same way as in the classical pathway, which results in cell lysis (see Fig. 13–2).

Control mechanisms also exist in the alternate pathway, just as they do in the classical pathway. Spontaneous dissolution of C3bBb may occur, or factor H with factor I protein may compete with factor B, as may Bb for the C3b fragment, then blocking the formation of C3 convertase (C3bBb). Factor H may increase the susceptibility of C3b to be destroyed by C3b inactivator.[2]

Mechanisms of Immune Hemolysis

Intravascular Hemolysis

Intravascular hemolysis, as the name implies occurs within the vascular system and results from activation of the classical complement pathway via IgG or IgM antibodies (see Chap. 20 for an explanation of immunoglobulins). Intravascular hemolysis occurs when antibodies that bind to antigenic determinants on red cells activate complement to completion (i.e., lysis). This occurs only when the activation process is intense enough to overwhelm the natural regulatory process that inactivates complement. IgM is a very efficient activator of complement because of its pentameric structure. A single molecule of IgM is capable of initiating complement activation by the classical pathway.[3,4] The ability of IgG antibodies to activate complement is dependent on several factors:

1. The IgG subclass; IgG3 is the most efficient at activating complement, followed by IgG1 then IgG2. IgG4 is not capable of complement activation.[5] The biologic properties of the IgG subclasses are summarized in Table 13–1.

2. The number and location of IgG molecules on the red cell surface; at least two IgG molecules must be in close enough proximity to allow cross-linking of complement receptors, which initiates complement activation.[3,5]
3. The physical location of the red cell antigens influences the binding of IgG.
4. The ability of the immunoglobulin to remain attached to the red cell surface (avidity) is important as well.

ANTIBODY-DEPENDENT CELLULAR CYTOTOXICITY (ADCC)

Another possible mechanism of direct (intravascular) lysis of immunoglobulin-coated red cells is antibody-dependent cellular cytotoxicity (ADCC). Many white cell lines (macrophages/monocytes, neutrophils, and natural killer lymphocytes [NK cells]) have receptors on their membranes that bind immunoglobulins and complement degradation products.[6] The cells with such receptors are collectively referred to as effector cells. The effector cell receptors specific for IgG1 or IgG3 are called Fc receptors (FcR). They are called FcR because they bind the Fc (Fragment, constant) of these immunoglobulins (see Chap. 20 for a review of immunoglobulin structure). The effector cells also have receptors for complement degradation products, C3b and iC3b. These receptors are called CR1 and CR3, respectively. ADCC results when the immunoprotein (IgG3, IgG1, C3b, or iC3b) is bound to its respective FcR (or CR) of the effector cell. This interaction causes the release of lytic enzymes.[7,8] It should be noted that not all IgG1 and IgG3 immunoglobulins are capable of mediating lysis.[9] The role of complement receptors in ADCC is not well established. It is very likely that complement degradation products work synergistically with IgG3 or IgG1, or both, to enhance ADCC.[7,10,11]

LABORATORY FINDINGS

Hemoglobin is released into the blood when red cells are destroyed intravascularly. This condition of free hemoglobin liberation in the blood is called hemoglobinemia. Free hemoglobin is filtered through the kidneys, resulting in hemoglobinuria (free hemoglobin in the urine). Hemoglobinuria may be confused with hematuria (intact red cells in the urine), especially when the urine is red. It is important to distinguish between the two because hemoglobinuria is an indicator of hemolysis whereas hematuria is not related to hemolysis. Microscopic examination of the urine may be helpful in differentiating the presence of intact red cells from hemoglobin.

Within hours of intravascular hemolysis, haptoglobin is depleted. As little as 5 mL of lysed red cells can bind all of the available haptoglobin. However, haptoglobin, which is synthesized in the liver, can return to normal levels within 24 hours (see Chap. 3 under Erythrocyte Senescence). Because haptoglobin is an acute phase reactant protein, concentrations may vary considerably, depending on several factors, such as underlying disease processes. Consequently, care must be taken when interpreting haptoglobin levels as an indicator of hemolysis. It is advisable to have a "baseline" haptoglobin level to compare to the haptoglobin level following suspected hemolysis. See Figure 13–3 for the sequence of laboratory findings.

Other laboratory findings that may be associated with intravascular hemolysis include elevated serum bilirubin (pri-

> ### ➤ Table 13–1
> ### BIOLOGIC PROPERTIES OF IgG ISOTYPES

Characteristic	IgG1	IgG2	IgG3	IgG4
% Total serum IgG	65–70	23–28	4–7	3–4
Complement fixation (classic pathway)	Yes	Yes	Yes	No
Binding to macrophage Fc receptors	Yes	No	Yes	No
Placental transfer	Yes	Yes	Yes	Yes
Biologic half-life (days)	21	21	7–8	21

INTRAVASCULAR HEMOLYTIC EVENT

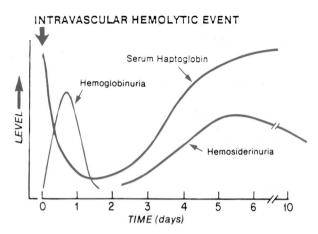

> **FIGURE 13–3** Indicators of acute intravascular hemolysis. Within a few hours of an acute hemolytic event, free hemoglobin is cleared from plasma and the serum haptoglobin falls to undetectable levels; hemoglobinuria ceases soon after. If no further hemolysis occurs, the serum haptoglobin level recovers, and methemalbumin disappears within several days. The urinary hemosiderin can provide more lasting evidence of the hemolytic event.

marily indirect); elevated lactate dehydrogenase (LD), an enzyme of red cell metabolism; and possible reticulocytosis. Table 13–2 summarizes the laboratory findings. (For a review of hemoglobin catabolism, see Chap. 3, Erythrocyte Senescence).

Extravascular Hemolysis

Extravascular hemolysis is the phagocytosis of red cells by fixed phagocytes within the mononuclear phagocyte system (MPS), formerly called the reticuloendothelial system. The two major organs of the MPS are the spleen and the liver. In the red pulp region of the spleen, macrophages with Fc receptors (see ADCC, earlier) line the splenic cords. Antibody-coated red cells interact with the Fc receptors, resulting in complete or partial phagocytosis. In the case of partial phagocytosis, part of the red cell membrane is removed. If the cell membrane is able to repair itself, a dense, sphere-shaped red cell called a spherocyte is formed. Spherocytes lack deformability and become physically trapped in the spleen; those that do escape the spleen can be seen in the pe-

ripheral blood and their presence is indicative of immune-mediated hemolysis (Fig. 13–4; see also Color Plate 115).

As previously mentioned, both IgG and IgM antibodies are capable of activating complement. However, the activation process does not always go to completion (C1 through C9). In most cases, complement activation is stopped by an inhibitory factor (control mechanism) at the C3b stage. C3b is cleaved to form iC3b. If activation is stopped, iC3b is further broken down into C3dg, which then remains attached to the red cell membrane.[8]

Red cells coated with IgG1 or IgG3 are preferentially removed in the spleen[6] rather than the liver, because blood passing through the spleen becomes hemoconcentrated, altering the ratio between free IgG in the plasma and cell-bound IgG. Free IgG can bind to Fc receptors, blocking their ability to bind the IgG that is attached to red cells. The condition of hemoconcentration in the spleen shifts the ratio of free IgG to red cell–bound IgG in favor of the red cell–bound IgG. The activated form of complement (C3b) or its inactivated form (iC3b) are not present in the free form in plasma; therefore, the hemoconcentration of blood in the spleen does not contribute significantly to the destruction of complement-coated red cells.[10] However, cells coated with both IgG and C3b/iC3b are phagocytized more

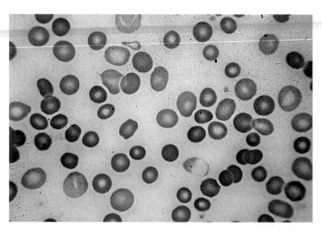

> **FIGURE 13–4** Autoimmune hemolytic anemia (peripheral blood). Note spherocytes and polychromasia.

> ### Table 13–2
> ## MECHANISMS OF IMMUNE HEMOLYSIS

	Intravascular	Extravascular
Mechanisms	IgM or IgG3, IgG1, IgG2 (two IgG molecules within close proximity of each other) activate complement to completion	IgM and/or IgG sensitization with/without iC3b (inactivated complement) Cell-mediated phagocytosis
	Antibody-dependent cellular cytotoxicity (ADCC)	
Organ	Occurs within blood vessels	Spleen: IgG alone or IgG + iC3b-coated cells
		Liver: iC3b alone or IgG + iCb-coated cells
Laboratory findings	Hemoglobinemia	Spherocytosis
	Hemoglobinuria	Serum haptoglobin: decreased
	Serum haptoglobin: decreased	
	Indirect bilirubin: elevated	Indirect bilirubin: elevated
	Lactate dehydrogenase (LD): elevated	Positive direct antiglobulin test

efficiently in the spleen than if they are sensitized by IgG alone.[10]

The liver has the largest concentration of macrophages with receptors specific for immune complexes; thus, the liver is the major site of removal for red cells coated with complement or heavily coated with IgG.[4,8] There is very little removal of red cells coated with small amounts of IgG in the liver, because of the high concentration of free IgG located there. Cells sensitized with both IgG and iC3b/C3d are removed in the liver and spleen.

LABORATORY FINDINGS

Spherocytes or spherocytosis may be seen on the peripheral blood smear when extravascular hemolysis has occurred. Serum bilirubin (indirect) may be elevated and urobilinogen may be increased in urine and stool specimens. The direct antiglobulin test (DAT) may be positive as well as the indirect antiglobulin test (antibody screening test). Table 13–2 provides a summary of laboratory findings. Table 13–3 lists the factors that influence immune hemolysis.

Classification of Immune Hemolytic Anemia

Numerous classifications of immune hemolytic anemias have been proposed; however, three broad categories are usually used:

1. *Alloimmune:* patient produces alloantibodies to foreign red cell antigens introduced through transfusions, pregnancy, or organ transplantation.
2. *Autoimmune:* control mechanism for autoreactive antibodies is lost and antibodies directed against the patient's own red cells develop.
3. *Drug-induced:* patient produces antibodies directed at a particular drug, its metabolites, or red cells coated with the drug.

Alloimmune Hemolytic Anemia

Alloimmunization is the process in which the immune system of an individual is stimulated by a foreign antigen and produces the corresponding antibody. The antibody produced by this immune response is termed an *alloantibody*. The antibody coats the foreign red cells introduced into the circulation, resulting in shortened red cell survival. Alloantibody production may result from (1) transfusion of blood (exposure to foreign donor red cell antigens), (2) pregnancy (foreign antigens on fetal cells released into the maternal circulation), and (3) organ transplantation (exposure to foreign antigens on "passenger cells" that may be released into the recipient).

Alloimmune hemolytic anemia is usually associated with blood transfusions. An antibody present in the recipient is directed against a foreign red cell antigen located on the transfused cells. Basically there are two types of transfusion reactions: acute hemolytic and delayed hemolytic.

Acute Hemolytic Transfusion Reactions

Acute hemolytic transfusion reactions (HTRs) are characterized by acute intravascular hemolysis and are associated with the ABO blood group antibodies. The immunoglobulins associated with the ABO blood group are IgM or both IgM and IgG. In individuals who have both types (IgM and IgG), the majority of antibody is IgM with a minor amount of IgG.[12] Ordinarily, an individual possesses antibodies directed toward the A or B antigens absent from his or her own red cells. As previously stated, IgM antibodies are efficient activators of complement, which results in immediate destruction of the transfused cells.

Symptoms of acute HTRs are variable. Typical symptoms are fever, shaking, chills, and pain or a burning sensation along the infusion site. Other symptoms include nausea, vomiting, lower back pain, hypotension, and chest pain. See Table 13–4 for a list of clinical features. An incoherent, unconscious, or anesthetized patient cannot verbalize his or her symptoms and therefore is at risk of receiving more than one unit of incompatible blood.

The laboratory findings in HTRs are those associated with intravascular hemolysis (see Table 13–2).

The treatment of HTR focuses on prompt termination of the transfusion. As stated in the discussion of intravascular hemolysis, free hemoglobin is filtered through the kidneys. Red cell stroma can clog and damage renal glomeruli; thus,

---

> **Table 13–3**
> ### FACTORS INFLUENCING THE PRESENCE AND EXTENT OF IMMUNE HEMOLYSIS

Antibody

Immunoglobulin class and subclass

Concentration

Avidity

Thermal reactivity (determined by the nature of the predominant noncovalent bonds formed at the time of the antigen-antibody reaction)

Antigen

Number and density

Cellular distribution

Presence of soluble antigen

Complement

Concentration of complement factors

Concentration and activity of regulating factors

Mononuclear Phagocyte System

Activity of phagocytic cells (influenced by underlying disease processes, generation and activity of lymphokines and interleukins, and any concurrent drug therapy)

> **Table 13-4**
> ### CLINICAL FEATURES OF ACUTE HEMOLYTIC TRANSFUSION REACTIONS

Fever	Hemoglobinuria
Chills	Shock
Chest pains	Generalized bleeding
Hypotension	Oliguria
Nausea	Anuria
Flushing	Back pain
Dyspnea	Pain at infusion site

Delayed Hemolytic Transfusion Reactions

Delayed hemolytic transfusion reactions (DHTRs) are associated with antibodies to blood groups other than the ABO blood group. Antibodies implicated in DHTR are usually IgG, which may activate complement, causing sensitization of the red cells with C3 but seldom leads to intravascular hemolysis. DHTRs are the most common type of transfusion reactions. They are caused by an anamnestic or secondary response to the transfused red cells. This occurs in previously immunized patients whose alloantibody level (after the initial stimulation) has dropped to serologically undetectable levels. As a result, the initial antibody screening and compatibility tests on the patient's pretransfusion sample are negative. Once re-exposed (transfused) to the foreign red cell antigen, an anamnestic response is mounted by the recipient. The titer rises and antibody may be detected in the posttransfusion sample as early as 48 hours after the transfusion. This type of reaction is termed *delayed,* because it takes time for the patient to produce sufficient antibody to destroy the transfused cells. Characteristically the reaction may occur anywhere from 2 to 10 days following transfusion.[13]

The symptoms of DHTRs are usually mild and nonspecific; therefore, DHTRs may not be recognized by clinicians.[14] Symptoms include mild fever, mild jaundice, and an unexpected fall in hemoglobin (or conversely, lack of expected rise in hemoglobin after transfusion). Laboratory findings are those associated with extravascular hemolysis, but most cases are subclinical and only discovered serologically (through direct antiglobulin test, antibody screening, and compatibility tests).[14]

Treatment is rarely necessary, and investigation focuses on accurately identifying the antibody to ensure that blood for future transfusions will be negative for the foreign antigen that corresponds to the patient's antibody. Table 13–5 lists the antibodies most commonly implicated in DHTRs, and Table 13–6 summarizes the laboratory findings.

Hemolytic Disease of the Newborn

Hemolytic disease of the newborn (HDN) is an immune hemolytic disorder caused by maternal-fetal blood group incompatibility (maternal IgG antibodies destroy antigen containing fetal red cells). The transport mechanism for maternal immunoglobulins is selective in that only IgG antibodies can cross the placenta.

Pregnant women can become immunized to foreign fetal red cell antigens when an exchange of fetal blood occurs during pregnancy and at delivery (fetal-maternal hemorrhage). The amount of whole blood exchanged is normally only 1 mL. There is some evidence that as little as 0.03 mL of red cells can stimulate an immune response.[15,16] Thus, it is possible to become immunized from miscarriages and abortions. Blood transfusions can also stimulate an immune response, as mentioned earlier, in alloimmune hemolytic anemia. If a pregnant woman has been previously immunized to a foreign red cell antigen and that antigen is present on the red cells of the fetus, the exchange of blood that occurs early in the pregnancy will be sufficient to stimulate an anamnestic response in the mother. The mother can produce increasing amounts of antibody directed against the fetal red cells.[17] The fetal red cells will become coated with maternal antibodies and destroyed by extravascular hemolysis. Responding to this increased red cell destruction, fetal hematopoietic tissue increases erythrocyte production. The fetal bone marrow may not be able to keep up with the increased need for red cells. Extramedullary hematopoiesis then occurs, causing liver and splenic enlargement. The fetus may not be able to compensate for the hemolysis, and an anemia characterized by increased numbers of erythroblasts may result. Hence, the term *erythroblastosis fetalis* has been used to describe HDN. There are two major forms of HDN: that associated with ABO, and that associated with Rh(D) or other blood groups. Table 13–7 lists the frequencies of the various types of HDN. Table 13–8 provides a comparison of ABO and Rh(D) HDN. (For further information on hemolytic disease of the newborn, see Harmening, DM: Modern Blood Banking and Transfusion Practices, ed 4. Philadelphia, FA Davis, 1999).

Autoimmune Hemolytic Anemia

Autoimmune hemolytic anemia (AIHA) represents an abnormality within the immune system whereby the ability for self-recognition of an individual's own red cell antigens is lost. Recent experiments support that recognition of self occurs during embryogenesis by inactivation of autoreactive B and T lymphocytes. Under certain conditions (e.g., bacterial or viral infections), these autoreactive B and T lymphocytes escape the mechanism for tolerance of self.[18] As a result, patients produce antibodies that bind to their own red cells (autoantibody). AIHA can be broadly divided into warm or cold types. The warm type (WAIHA) is the most common, accounting for approximately 70% of all cases.[19,20] This type involves autoantibodies whose serologic reactivity is optimal at 37°C. Cold AIHA involves autoantibodies whose serologic reactivity is optimal at 4°C but that also react at temperatures between 25°C and 31°C. Two types of cold AIHA have been described: (1) cold agglutinin syndrome (CAS) and (2) paroxysmal cold hemoglobinuria (PCH).

Some drugs may induce the formation of autoantibodies that may be difficult to distinguish from other cases of AIHA. Drug-induced immune hemolytic anemia is the third type of AIHA, representing approximately 12% of cases in various studies.[20] Table 13–9 lists the frequency of the various types of AIHA.

> **Table 13-5**
ANTIBODIES MOST COMMONLY IMPLICATED IN DHTRs

Antibody	Blood Group System
Anti-Jk^a	Kidd
Anti-K	Kell
Anti-c	Rh
Anti-E	Rh
Anti-Fy^a	Duffy
Anti-Jk^b	Kidd
Anti-C	Rh
Anti-e	Rh

➤ **Table 13-6**
DIFFERENTIAL DIAGNOSIS OF HEMOLYTIC ANEMIA

Parameter/Analyte	Extravascular	Intravascular
Serial hemoglobin and hematocrit	Decreased	Decreased
Reticulocyte count*	> 1%	> 1%
RBC morphology	Spherocytes	
Serum bilirubin (indirect)	Increased	Increased
Serum haptoglobin†	Decreased†	Decreased
Serum LD (isoenzyme LD1)	Increased†	Increased
Hemoglobinemia	Absent	Present
Hemoglobinuria	Absent	Present

*May not show increase immediately.
†Important to compare with a prehemolysis "baseline" value.
†More likely to be present with intravascular hemolysis.
Abbreviation: LD = lactate dehydrogenase.

DAT-Negative AIHA

Occasionally the DAT result is repeatedly negative in a patient who has clear evidence of hemolysis with no other apparent cause. These patients represent a small group that is referred to as having DAT-negative AIHA.[21] More sensitive techniques for the detection of IgG or C3d, or both, on red cells have shown that many of these patients have increased levels of these immunoproteins on their cells. The routine laboratory direct antiglobulin test (DAT) can detect immunoglobulin sensitization of as little as 200 molecules of IgG per red cell.[20] More sensitive techniques are capable of detecting as few as 20 IgG molecules.[22] When interpreting DAT results, it is important to remember that a positive DAT is not indicative of immune hemolysis, but if hemolysis is present or suspected, it could be the result of immune mechanisms. The DAT result can be positive in up to 8% of hospitalized patients who have no signs or symptoms of hemolysis.[19,20] In most of these patients, the positive result is a result of complement sensitization, probably secondary to the disease process from which the patient is suffering.

Warm Autoimmune Hemolytic Anemia

The incidence of warm autoimmune hemolytic anemia (WAIHA) is very rare (1 in 80,000)[23,24] with a slightly higher frequency of the disease in women than in men.[23] The majority of individuals who develop WAIHA are more than 40 years of age.[20]

Warm autoimmune hemolytic anemia may be idiopathic, with no underlying disease process (50% to 70% of cases), or it may be secondary to a pathologic disorder (30% to 50% of cases).[25] Table 13–10 lists the disorders reported to be associated with WAIHA. Signs and symptoms usually do not appear until a significant anemia has developed. Pal-

lor, weakness, dizziness, dyspnea, jaundice, and unexplained fever occasionally are presenting complaints. Hemolysis is usually extravascular and occurs predominantly in the spleen. The degree of hemolysis can be acute (hemoglobin less than 7.0 g/dL) or mild. The onset of WAIHA is usually gradual and may be precipitated by a variety of factors, such as infection, trauma, surgery, pregnancy, or psychological stress.

SEROLOGIC EVALUATION

Evaluation with a polyspecific antiglobulin reagent reveals a positive DAT. On further analysis with monospecific antiglobulin reagents, the DAT result is positive for both IgG and C3d in 67% of cases. The remaining cases are positive for IgG (20%) or C3d (13%) alone.[4]

The serum of a patient with WAIHA usually demonstrates evidence of free autoantibody at low titer (e.g., weak reactivity). In 80% of the cases, the immunoglobulin is IgG alone or together with IgA, IgM, and/or C3.[20] Complement proteins act synergistically with immunoglobulins to cause red cell hemolysis. In fact, the severity of hemolysis is correlated with the presence of complement in addition to IgG.[26,27] Although it is not performed in routine diagnostic testing, the presence of IgA or IgM, or both, may be found in addition to IgG if appropriate antisera are used.[20] WAIHA can present several difficult problems in serologic testing. The serologic problems of WAIHA are twofold:

1. The patient's red cells are strongly coated with autoantibody, which interferes with phenotyping.
2. Autoantibody present in the serum may mask an underlying alloantibody.

Autoantibody Specificity. The autoantibodies produced in WAIHA usually react with all cells tested. Serologic studies have suggested that some autoantibodies are directed at Rh blood group antigens because of their lack of reactivity (apparent compatibility) with Rh_{null} cells, which lack all Rh blood group antigens.[18] Further analysis of these autoantibodies with apparent Rh specificity have demonstrated that the reactivity was directed at a red cell membrane protein (which is also lacking in Rh_{null} cells).[28] On rare occasions, other specificities have also been reported.[4,18,20]

➤ **Table 13-7**
FREQUENCY OF TYPES OF HDN

ABO HDN	65%
Rh HDN	33%
Other	2%

> **Table 13-8**
> **COMPARISON OF ABO AND Rh HDN**

	ABO	Rh
Severity	Mild	Severe
Child affected	First-born (40%–50% of cases)	Usually second or subsequent births (first-born: 5% of cases)
Blood groups	Mother: O	Mother: Rh negative
	Child: A or B	Child: Rh positive
Anemia	Uncommon, mild	Severe
Stillbirths/hydrops fetalis	Rare	Frequent
Jaundice	Mild	Severe
Spherocytes on peripheral blood smear	Usually present	None
Direct Coombs' test result	Negative or weakly positive	Positive
Maternal antibodies	Inconsistent, inconclusive	Always present
Antenatal diagnosis	Unnecessary	Necessary
Treatment (dependent on severity)	Phototherapy (common)	Exchange transfusion (common newborn treatment)
	Exchange transfusion (rare)	Intrauterine (common antenatal treatment)
Types of antibody	IgG (immune)	IgG (immune)
Prophylaxis	None	RhIG
		Antenatal RhIG

LABORATORY DIAGNOSIS

Typically, patients with WAIHA exhibit a moderate to severe normocytic, normochromic anemia. The blood smear can display classic signs of extravascular hemolysis, polychromasia reflecting reticulocytosis (see Fig. 13–4 and Color Plate 115), spherocytosis, and red cell fragmentation. Occasionally, nucleated red blood cells may be seen. On rare occasions, WAIHA is associated with reticulocytopenia. Reticulocytopenia at the time of intense hemolysis indicates that the bone marrow is not responding by producing more red blood cells and is associated with a high patient mortality rate.

Evidence of hemolysis can be seen on laboratory analysis; bilirubin (particularly the unconjugated, indirect fraction) and urinary urobilinogen may be elevated. In severe cases, depleted serum haptoglobin, hemoglobinemia, hemoglobinuria, and increased LD may be demonstrated.

TREATMENT

The prognosis for patients with WAIHA is generally poor. Therapy is usually aimed at treating the primary disease if one is present. Measures to support cardiovascular function are important in patients who are severely anemic. Trans-

fusion is usually avoided, if possible, as this may only accelerate the hemolysis instead of ameliorating the anemia. However, transfusion should be used in life-threatening situations.

As all donor blood is invariably incompatible, it is general practice to use donor blood that is least reactive in the crossmatch and that is antigen negative for any clinically significant alloantibodies that may be present in the patient's serum. Blood is transfused slowly, in small volumes (100 mL), and the patient observed closely for any adverse reactions.[29] Some hematologists advocate the use of phenotypically similar blood irrespective of its degree of incompatibility in the crossmatch. The rationale for this approach is that patients with autoimmune antibodies may be more likely to produce alloimmune antibodies, which can

> **Table 13-9**
> **PERCENTAGE OF REPORTED CASES OF AIHA**

Warm AIHA	70%
Cold agglutinin syndrome	16%
Paroxysmal cold hemoglobinuria	1%–2%
Drug-induced	12%

> **Table 13-10**
> **DISORDERS REPORTED TO BE ASSOCIATED WITH WAIHA**

Lymphoproliferative disorders such as chronic lymphocytic leukemia, Hodgkin's disease, non-Hodgkin's lymphoma, multiple myeloma, and Waldenström's macroglobulinemia

Autoimmune disorders such as systemic lupus erythematosis, rheumatoid arthritis, scleroderma, and pernicious anemia

Neoplastic disorders, including solid tumors of the ovary, breast, lung, colon, pancreas, thymus, kidney, and uterus

Viral infections, including hepatitis B and hepatitis A

Chronic inflammatory disorders including ulcerative colitis

be masked by the autoantibodies. A recent study indicates that the incidence of alloimmunization or adverse hemolytic transfusion reactions in patients with WAIHA is no greater than the incidence found in other multitransfused patient populations.[30]

Treatment with corticosteroids is usually the first line of treatment. Corticosteroids such as prednisone produce their effect by several proposed mechanisms: (1) reduction of antibody synthesis,[31] (2) altered antibody avidity,[31] and (3) depression of macrophage activity,[32] which reduces the clearance of antibody-coated red cells.[20] Splenectomy is usually considered as the next step if corticosteroid therapy is ineffective. Splenectomy decreases the production of antibody and removes a potent site of red cell damage and destruction.[20] Only patients with Ig-coated cells respond to this treatment, because the spleen is the primary site of destruction of IgG antibody–coated cells. Immunosupressive drugs, intravenous immunoglobulin, antilymphocyte globulin, or plasma exchange may be used in patients who do not respond to conventional therapy. The success rate of these alternative therapies is variable, and they are used only in selected cases.[25,33,34]

Normal Cold Autoagglutinins

Cold reacting autoantibodies (autoagglutinins) are present in all normal human sera.[35–37] The specificity of these cold autoantibodies include anti-I, anti-H, and anti-IH. Practically all adults have I and H antigens present on their red cells. Generally, most examples of anti-I, anti-H, and anti-IH have no clinical significance, and these autoantibodies are often too weak to be detected by routine serologic testing. This is primarily owing to their low concentration in the serum and their narrow thermal range (4°C to 22°C).[36] Table 13–11 compares the characteristics of normal cold autoantibodies found in healthy adults with those of pathologic cold autoantibodies. The benign autoagglutinins differ in many ways from the pathologic cold autoagglutinins that produce cold agglutinin syndrome (or cold AIHA). The fundamental characteristic that differentiates benign autoagglutinins from pathologic autoagglutinins is the thermal range. Pathologic cold autoagglutinins may react at or above 30°C.[38]

Pathologic Cold Autoantibodies

Pathologic cold autoantibodies can be divided into (1) primary (idiopathic) cold agglutinin syndrome (primary CAS), (2) cold agglutinin syndrome secondary to infection (secondary CAS), and (3) paroxysmal cold hemoglobinuria (PCH).

COLD AGGLUTININ SYNDROME (PRIMARY CAS)

Cold agglutinin syndrome, also called cold hemagglutinin disease (CHD) or idiopathic cold AIHA, represents approximately 16% of the cases of AIHA.[20] Primary CAS is a chronic condition and occurs predominantly in older individuals, with a peak incidence after 50 years of age.[20] It is found in all racial groups, affecting both men and women. Although the disease is often called idiopathic, a careful evaluation of the patient may reveal the presence of a lymphoproliferative disorder.[18] Because of this association, it is prudent to investigate patients for possible malignancy when they present with a pathologic cold autoantibody and no other obvious cause, such as infection.

CAS is a hemolytic anemia produced by a cold autoantibody that optimally reacts at 4°C, but also reacts at temperatures greater than 30°C (i.e., wide thermal range).[20,39,40] The antibody is usually an IgM immunoglobulin, which quite efficiently activates complement.[35] Antibody specificity in this disorder is almost always anti-I,[35–37] less commonly anti-i, and rarely anti-Pr.[37]

CAS is rarely severe and usually seasonal, as the winter cold months often precipitate the signs and symptoms of a chronic hemolytic anemia. Acrocyanosis, also called Raynaud's phenomenon[35] (symptoms of cold intolerance, such as pain and a bluish tinge in the fingertips and toes, owing to vasospasm), is frequently the patient's main complaint, along with a sense of numbness in the extremities when exposed to the cold. These symptoms occur because the cold autoantibody agglutinates the individual's red cells in the capillaries of the skin, causing local blood stasis.[35] During cold weather, the temperature of an individual's skin and exposed extremities can fall to as low as 28°C, activating the cold autoantibody. This activated cold antibody agglutinates red cells and fixes complement as the erythrocytes flow through the capillaries of the skin. When the erythrocytes return to the body core (where the temperature is 37°C) the cold agglutinin elutes off the red cells, leaving ac-

> ### ► Table 13–11
> ## COMPARISON OF CHARACTERISTICS OF NORMAL AND PATHOLOGIC COLD AUTOANTIBODY

Characteristic	Benign	Pathologic
Thermal amplitude	< 22°C	Broad: up to 32°C
Spontaneous autoagglutination	None	Significant degree that disperses on warming to 37°C
Titer	< 64 at 4°C	> 1000 at 4°C
Albumin enhancement	None	Reactivity enhanced
Clonality of antibody	Polyclonal	Idiopathic = monoclonal
		Secondary to infection = polyclonal
Clinical significance	None	Causes cold AIHA
Usual antibody specificity	Anti-I	Anti-I
Direct antiglobulin test (DAT)	Negative or weak positive with polyspecific antiglobulin reagent	2 to 3+ with polyspecific antiglobulin reagent

tivated complement behind. Hemolysis occurs from the completion of the complement cascade or by removal of red cells sensitized with C3b/iC3b by macrophages in the liver (see the earlier section on Intravascular Hemolysis for a review). If any red cells coated with C3b/iC3b escape destruction in the liver, their complement proteins are further degraded to C3d, for which there are no receptors on macrophages.[7] The patient's DAT result will be positive with monospecific anti-C3d antiglobulin reagents.

This hemolytic episode is not associated with fever, chills, or acute renal insufficiency, characteristic of patients with PCH (see later discussion). Hemoglobinemia and less frequently hemoglobinuria may be detected after exposure to the cold. Patients also display weakness, pallor, and weight loss, which are characteristic symptoms of chronic anemia. CAS usually remains quite stable, and when it does progress, it intensifies gradually. Other clinical features of CAS may include jaundice and splenomegaly.

Laboratory Findings. Most patients with CAS present with reticulocytosis and a positive DAT result (C3d only). In some cases autoagglutination of anticoagulated whole blood samples occurs as the blood cools to room temperature. As a result of this autoagglutination, performance of blood counts and preparation of blood smears may be difficult. The patient's mean corpuscular volume (MCV) from an automated cell counter will be erroneously high and the red blood cell count erroneously low due to clumping of red blood cells. This causes unrealistic values in other calculated parameters, such as mean corpuscular hemoglobin (MCH), mean corpuscular hemoglobin concentration (MCHC), and hematocrit. The blood sample should be warmed to 37°C and rerun on the automated cell counter to obtain accurate values.

The tendency for spontaneous autoagglutination of red cells from these patients dictates that serum samples must be maintained and separated at 37°C to obtain accurate results for the antibody titer and thermal amplitude studies.[41] Similarly, samples for the determination of DAT results must be collected into ethylene diaminetetraacetic acid (EDTA) to inhibit any in vitro attachment of complement to the cells following collection.

A simple serum screening procedure can be performed by testing the ability of the patient's serum to agglutinate normal saline-suspended red cells at 20°C and 4°C. If this test result is positive, further steps must be taken to determine the titer and thermal amplitude of the cold autoantibody; if negative, the diagnosis of CAS is unlikely.[39]

The peripheral blood smear in patients with CAS may show rouleaux (red cells appear stacked on top of one another like a roll of coins) and autoagglutination (physical clumping of cells). (Fig. 13–5 and Color Plate 116). Table 13–12 summarizes the clinical criteria for diagnosis of CAS.

CAS SECONDARY TO INFECTIONS

Cold agglutinin syndrome can also occur as a transient disorder that is secondary to infections. Episodes of cold autoimmune hemolytic anemia often occur following upper respiratory infections. Approximately 50% of patients suffering from pneumonia caused by *Mycoplasma pneumoniae* have elevated titers (greater than 64) of cold autoagglutinins.[20,39,40] Secondary CAS develops in the second or third week of the patient's illness, and a rapid onset of hemolysis with symptoms of pallor and jaundice is usually

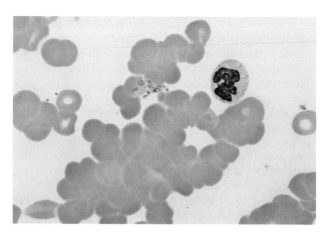

➤ **FIGURE 13–5** Cold hemagglutinin disease (peripheral blood). Note the autoagglutination of red cells.

found. Resolution of the episode usually occurs in 2 to 3 weeks, as the hemolysis is self-limiting.[35] The offending cold autoantibody is an IgM immunoglobulin with characteristic anti-I specificity. Very high titers of the cold autoagglutinnin are seen almost exclusively in patients with mycoplasmal pneumonia. It has been reported that the cold agglutinin produced in this infection is an immunologic response to the mycoplasmal antigens, and these antibodies cross-react with the red cell I antigen.[42,43]

Both the antibodies produced in primary CAS and CAS secondary to mycoplasma pneumonia have anti-I specificity. They differ in that the autoantibody in primary CAS is invariably monoclonal (IgM-kappa [κ] light chain),[44] whereas the autoantibody produced secondary to infection is polyclonal (IgM with both κ and lambda [λ] light chain types).[45] The monoclonality of the autoantibody in primary CAS suggests a possible underlying lymphoproliferative disorder.

Infectious Mononucleosis. Infectious mononucleosis may also be associated with a hemolytic anemia resulting from a cold autoagglutinin. Many studies have reported an association of anti-i production in infectious mononucleosis. The percentages of patients with infectious mononucleosis who developed anti-i varies from 8%,[46] 50%,[47] to 68%.[48] The antibody is usually a low titer, IgM cold agglutinin with a narrow thermal range. A small number (1%) of these pa-

> ### Table 13-12
> ### CLINICAL CRITERIA FOR THE DIAGNOSIS OF COLD AGGLUTININ SYNDROME

- Clinical signs of an acquired hemolytic anemia, with a history (which may or may not be present) of acrocyanosis and hemoglobinuria upon exposure to cold

- A positive DAT result using polyspecific antisera

- A positive DAT result using monospecific C3 antisera

- A negative DAT result using monospecific IgG antisera

- The presence of reactivity in the patient's serum owing to a cold autoantibody

- A cold agglutinin titer of 1000 or greater in saline at 4°C with visible autoagglutination of anticoagulated blood at room temperature

tients who develop anti-i produce a high titer, IgM cold agglutinin with a wide thermal range,[49] which causes in vivo hemolysis. Acute illness with sore throat and high fever, followed by weakness, anemia, and jaundice, are characteristic features of infectious mononucleosis. For a review of infectious mononucleosis, see Chapter 15. Table 13–13 lists the cold autoantibody specificity most commonly found in the various infections that cause secondary CAS.

Treatment. Treatment of primary CAS, secondary CAS and the anemia associated with infectious mononucleosis is the same. Most patients require no treatment and are instructed to avoid the cold, keep warm, or move to a milder climate.[25] One ingenious physician contacted the National Aeronautics and Space Administration (NASA) for an environmentally controlled space suit so his patient would not have to remain indoors during the acute phase of the disease.[50] Corticosteroids have been used, but have limited success.[34] Plasma exchange has been used in acute cases to provide temporary removal of antibodies.[33,34] Splenectomy is ineffective because extravascular hemolysis resulting from complement sensitization occurs predominantly in the liver.

Transfusion is rarely required. If blood is needed, the blood should be ABO/Rh compatible and lack any antigens for which the patient has an alloantibody. Blood should be warmed using a blood warmer and transfused slowly, with constant monitoring of the patient for adverse reactions.[35]

PAROXYSMAL COLD HEMOGLOBINURIA

PCH is the least common type of AIHA, with an incidence of only 1% to 7%.[20] It occurs almost exclusively in children in association with viral disorders such as measles, mumps, chickenpox, infectious mononucleosis, and the ill-defined flu syndrome.[51] Although PCH is transient and self-limiting, severe hemolysis may occur.

Originally, PCH was described in association with syphilis, in which an autoantibody was formed in response to *Treponema pallidum* organism, the causative agent of the disease.[52] However, with the discovery and use of antibiotics, PCH is no longer a commonly reported disorder related to syphilis.

Red cell destruction is the result of a cold-reacting, IgG autoantibody termed an *autohemolysin*. This autohemolysin binds to the patient's red cells at lower temperatures and fixes complement. Hemolysis occurs when the red cells return to the body core (where the temperature rises to 37°C) and the sensitized cells undergo complement-mediated intravascular hemolysis.[51] This autoagglutinin only attaches to red cells at cooler temperatures and then activates complement in warmer temperatures. Thus, the antibody produced in PCH is called a biphasic hemolysin. This antibody is also called the Donath-Landsteiner antibody, and its specificity is anti-P.[36]

As the name of PCH implies, paroxysmal or intermittent episodes of hemoglobinuria occur upon exposure to the cold. These acute attacks may be characterized by a sudden onset of fever, shaking chills, malaise, abdominal cramps, and back pains.[51] All the signs of intravascular hemolysis are evident, including hemoglobinemia, hemoglobinuria, and bilirubinemia (see Fig. 13–3). This results in a severe and rapidly progressive anemia. Polychromasia, nucleated red blood cells, and poikilocytosis are demonstrated in the peripheral blood smear. The symptoms of fever, chills, pain, and hemoglobinuria may resolve in a few hours or persist for days. Splenomegaly, hyperbilirubinemia, and renal insufficiency may also develop. Table 13–14 compares and contrasts PCH and cold agglutinin syndrome.

Donath-Landsteiner Test. There is one classic diagnostic test for PCH. This test was developed by the two physicians for whom the test is named. A blood sample drawn from the patient is split into two aliquots maintained at different temperatures. One aliquot, used as the control, is kept at 37°C for 60 minutes. The other aliquot is cooled at 4°C for 30 minutes and then incubated at 37°C for another 30 minutes. Both samples are then centrifuged and observed for hemolysis. A positive test result is hemolysis in the sample placed at 4°C and then at 37°C, and no hemolysis in the control sample. Table 13–15 summarizes the Donath-Landsteiner test.

Treatment. Protection from cold exposure is the only useful therapy. The hemolysis usually terminates spontaneously following resolution of the infectious process.[53] If anemia is severe, transfusions may be required. The same transfusion protocol as in CAS applies. Table 13–16 reviews and compares characteristics of warm and cold autoimmune hemolytic anemias.

Mixed Autoimmune Hemolytic Anemia

In the past two decades, a number of reports have drawn attention to the occurrence of mixed AIHA, in which patients exhibit autoantibodies having the characteristics of both warm and cold autoantibodies.[54–56] Less than 10% of cases of AIHA are considered mixed.[33] Patients with mixed-type AIHA usually present with an extremely acute condition.[57] They may exhibit signs of extravascular hemolysis from IgG antibodies and intravascular hemolysis from IgM or complement activation. This situation of both warm and cold autoantibodies may be expected when one realizes that a number of the lymphoproliferative and collagen diseases may be associated with either form of autoantibody.[4,57] Approximately half of the cases of mixed AIHA are idiopathic and the remainder are associated with collagen autoimmune diseases such as systemic lupus erythematosis.[33,34]

Drug-Induced Immune Hemolytic Anemia

The administration of drugs may lead to the development of a wide variety of hematologic abnormalities, including immune hemolytic anemia. Drug-induced immune hemolytic anemia represents approximately 12% of cases in various studies.[20,58] Historically, three mechanisms have been described that lead to the development of drug-induced immune hemolytic anemia, and a fourth mechanism that leads to the development of a positive DAT but is not associated with hemolysis. Sufficient new data have emerged to perhaps reclassify these mechanisms. Nevertheless, it is instructive to review the traditional mechanisms.

➤ Table 13–13
SECONDARY COLD AIHA

Type of Infection	Cold Autoantibody Specificity
Mycoplasma pneumonia	Anti-I
Infectious mononucleosis	Anti-i
Lymphoproliferative disorder	Anti-I, i, or Pr

> ## Table 13-14
> ## COMPARISON OF PCH AND COLD AGGLUTININ SYNDROME

	PCH	Cold Agglutinin Syndrome
Patient population	Children or young adults	Elderly or middle-aged
Pathogenesis	Following viral infection	Idiopathic, lymphoproliferative disorder following *Mycoplasma pneumoniae* infection
Clinical features	Hemoglobinuria: acute attacks upon exposure to cold (symptoms resolve in hours or days)	Acrocyanosis, autoagglutination of blood at room temperature
Severity of hemolysis	Acute and rapid	Chronic and rarely severe
Hemolysis	Intravascular	Extravascular, intravascular
Autoantibody	IgG (anti-P specificity) (biphasic hemolysin)	IgM (anti-I/i) (monophasic)
DAT	3+ (polyspecific Coombs' sera)/neg IgG/3–4+ C3 monospecific Coombs' sera	3+ (polyspecific Coombs' sera)/neg IgG/3–4+ C3 monospecific Coomb' sera
Thermal range	Moderate (< 20°C)	High (up to 30–31°C)
Titer (4°C)	Moderate (< 64)	High (> 1000)
Donath-Landsteiner test	Positive	Negative
Treatment	Supportive (disorder terminates when underlying illness resolves)	Avoid the cold

AIHA acute immune hemolytic anemia

Methyldopa-Induced (Autoimmune) Mechanism

This represents the most common drug-induced immune hemolytic anemia, accounting for approximately 70% of all cases.[59] The antibodies produced by this mechanism are considered "true autoantibodies," because they are reacting against intrinsic red blood cell antigens, not the drug or the drug-erythrocyte complex. The drugs implicated in this response include the antihypertensive drug α-methyldopa (Aldomet) and related drugs (L-dopa, procainamide)[60] (Table 13–17). Drug-induced AIHA by this mechanism is difficult to diagnose because it mimics WAIHA. It has been suggested that the autoantibodies produced in response to these drugs are the result of altered red cell antigens that are not recognized as self; however, the exact mechanism is still unknown.[61] A positive DAT develops in approximately 12% to 15% of the patients receiving α-methyldopa, and 1% to 3% of these patients go on to develop AIHA. The antibodies produced by patients suffering from this disorder react weakly with all cells tested or demonstrate specificities similar to those found in WAIHA. Hemolysis is extravascular and the DAT result is strongly positive with anti-IgG, and negative with anti-C3. Patients may continue to have a positive DAT result for up to 2 years after discontinuation of the drug.

Drug Adsorption (Hapten) Mechanism

This is the second most common mechanism of drug induced hemolytic anemia. The drugs implicated in this response include the penicillins and the cephalosporins.[59] This mechanism requires two components (Fig. 13–6). Firstly, the drug is nonspecifically adsorbed to the patient's red cells and remains firmly attached. Secondly, once adsorbed, the drug must be able to elicit an antibody response. The drug antibody is usually IgG and reacts only with drug-treated red cells. Large doses of intravenous penicillin (10 million units daily) are needed to produce an immune response.[20] Approximately 3% of patients on high-dose intravenous penicillin develop drug antibodies causing a positive DAT, but only 5% of these patients have actual clinical hemolysis.[20]

Laboratory findings include signs of extravascular hemolysis. The disorder develops over a period of 7 to 10 days. The DAT results are strongly positive with anti-IgG and negative with anti-C3.

Immune Complex Mechanism

The immune complex mechanism is the least common drug mechanism in drug-induced hemolytic anemia. The most common drug involved in this response is quinidine.[59] Table 13–17 lists other drugs associated with the immune complex mechanism. The patient responds to these drugs by producing an antibody (IgG or IgM, or both) against the drug that binds to the drug, forming an antibody-drug immune complex (Fig. 13–7). The antibody-drug complex then adsorbs onto the patient's red cells, and complement is activated. The antibody-drug immune complex is merely adsorbed onto the red cell membrane (not bound to it) and

> ## Table 13-15
> ## DONATH-LANDSTEINER TEST

	Whole Blood Control	Whole Blood Test
Procedure		
1. 30 min	37°C	4°C
2. 30 min	37°C	37°C
3. Centrifuge and observe		
Results		
Positive	No hemolysis	Hemolysis
Negative	No hemolysis	No hemolysis
Inconclusive	Hemolysis	Hemolysis

> **Table 13–16**
COMPARISON OF WARM AND COLD AUTOIMMUNE HEMOLYTIC ANEMIAS

	WAIHA	Cold AIHA
Optimal reactivity	> 32°C	< 30°C
Immunoglobulin class	IgG	IgM (exception: PCH-IgG)
Complement activation	May bind complement	Binds complement
Hemolysis	Usually extravascular (no cell lysis)	Usually intravascular (cell lysis)
Frequency	70%–75% of cases	16% of cases (PCH: 1%–2%)
Specificity	Frequently Rh	Ii system (PCH: anti-P)

> **Table 13–17**
PARTIAL LIST OF DRUGS ASSOCIATED WITH POSITIVE DAT OR HEMOLYTIC ANEMIA BY MECHANISM

Methyldopa-Induced (Autoimmune) Mechanism

α-Methyldopa

Ceftriaxone

Chlorpromazine

Ibuprofen

Levodopa

Mefenamic acid

Nomifensine

Procainamide

Thioridazine

Drug Absorption Mechanism

Cephalosporins

Diclofenac

Penicillins

Immune Complex Mechanism

Acetaminophen

Antihistamines

Cephalosporins

Chlorpromazine

Diclofenac

Isoniazid

Quinidine

Quinine

Rifampin

Streptomycin

Sulfonamides

Stibophen

Tetracycline

Membrane Modification Mechanism (Protein Adsorption)

Cephalosporins

Note: Some drugs may act by more than one mechanism.

easily disassociates, leaving activated complement behind. Only a small amount of the drug is necessary to produce this response.

Laboratory findings include evidence of intravascular hemolysis with hemoglobinemia and hemoglobinuria. The DAT result is positive with complement components only, because the immune complex has disassociated. In vitro agglutination reactions are generally observed during serologic testing only when the drug is added to the patient's serum and test red cell mixture.

Treatment is aimed at stopping the use of the drug if the

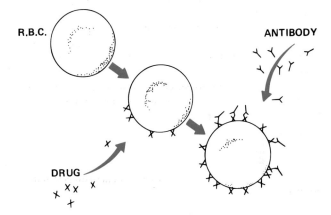

> **FIGURE 13–6** Drug adsorption mechanism. (From Petz, LD, and Garratty, G (eds): Acquired Immune Hemolytic Anemias. Churchill Livingstone, New York, 1980, with permission.)

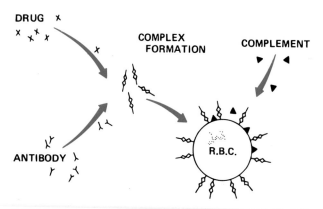

> **FIGURE 13–7** Immune complex mechanism. (From Petz, LD, and Garratty, G (eds): Acquired Immune Hemolytic Anemias. Churchill Livingstone, New York, 1980, with permission.)

patient is anemic because of active hemolysis. Steroid treatment may also be given.

An interesting note is that some of the drugs producing hemolysis by this mechanism are also associated with the development of drug-induced immune thrombocytopenia (ITP). The antidrug immune complex adsorbs onto the platelets.[62] However, it is rare to find a patient with simultaneous hemolysis and thrombocytopenia caused by antibodies to a single drug.

Membrane Modification Mechanism (Protein Adsorption)

As the name implies, the drug modifies the red cell membrane so that normal plasma proteins are nonspecifically adsorbed onto the patient's red cells (Fig. 13–8). Cephalosporins are the drugs implicated in this response.[63] The red cells become coated with numerous plasma proteins such as albumin, fibrinogen, and globulins. Approximately 3% of patients receiving the drug develop a positive DAT result owing to the nonspecific protein adsorption by the red cells. Hemolytic anemia has not been reported in association with this mechanism of drug-induced positive DAT.

The preceding classification used for the drug-induced immune hemolytic anemias provides a convenient mechanistic approach as to how drugs may be incriminated in immune hemolysis. Recent reports have demonstrated immune hemolytic anemia from certain drugs with more than one mechanism. More recently it has been suggested that only a single mechanism may be responsible for all drug-related immune hemolysis (unifying theory).[61,64] Table 13–18 compares the four mechanisms of drug-related anemia. Table 13–19 contrasts the antibody characteristics of the various types of autoimmune hemolytic anemias.

Nonimmune Hemolytic Anemia

Acquired nonimmune hemolytic anemias represent a diverse group of conditions that lead to the shortened survival of red cells by various mechanisms. Often a number of mechanisms are operative at the same time; for example, malaria leads to mechanical destruction of red cells and, in addition, immunologic factors play a role in shortened red cell survival. Classifications may be made along either causative or mechanistic lines. Table 13–20 provides a classification incorporating both approaches.

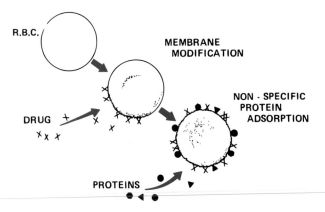

➤ FIGURE 13–8   Membrane modification mechanism. (From Petz, LD, and Garratty, G (eds): Acquired Immune Hemolytic Anemias. Churchill Livingstone, New York, 1980, with permission.)

Intracellular Infections

Malaria

Malaria is the most common protozoal infection in humans. It has a high incidence in the tropical and subtropical regions of the world, accounting for a fair percentage of the anemia in those regions. It has been estimated that more than 400 million people suffer from the disease, resulting in the deaths of more than 1.5 million annually. Most fatalities occur in nonimmune children; those who survive a childhood infection invariably suffer from an ongoing debilitating disease. Over the past 20 years control measures have significantly reduced the incidence of the disease, but recently, the incidence of the disease has risen to epidemic proportions. The increased incidence of infections has resulted from (1) the organism becoming resistant to many of the antimalarial drugs (e.g., chloroquine), and (2) the mosquito vector having become resistant to insecticides.[65] There are four species of malaria that can infect humans: *Plasmodium vivax, P. falciparum, P. ovale,* and *P. malariae. Plasmodium vivax* and *P. falciparum* are responsible for most infections producing disease in humans. In the case of *P. falciparum,* the disease can have a rapid and often fatal course. *Plasmodium malariae* and *P. ovale* infections are uncommon. *Plasmodium ovale* infections are confined to certain areas of Africa.

The number of patients presenting with malaria is also increasing in countries such as the United States, Europe, and Australia because of increased travel to endemic tropical and subtropical regions. It is estimated that from 10,000 to 30,000 travelers from industrialized countries contract malaria each year.[66]

LIFE CYCLE

The malarial parasite has a complex life cycle. The insect vector is the *Anopheles* mosquito, of which numerous species can transmit the parasite. Figure 13–9 illustrates the malarial life cycle.

CLINICAL PRESENTATION

The most commonly reported symptoms are fever, malaise, headache, chills, and sweats. Some patients show classic periodic episodes of fever and chills, correlating with rupture of infected erythrocytes. Nausea, vomiting, and diarrhea may be present. Quite often classic periodic episodes of fever and chills are absent, and these symptoms are mistakenly attributed to a viral infection, allowing malaria to go untreated and resulting in fatality. It is always advisable to inquire if the patient has been overseas and which countries have been visited.

Splenomegaly is present in 40% to 50% of patients with acute malaria. It is present in virtually all patients with chronic malaria, accounting for the high incidence of splenomegaly in the tropics.[67]

LABORATORY DIAGNOSIS

Anemia associated with *Plasmodium* is normochromic and normocytic. Leukopenia is present in many cases, as is thrombocytopenia (particularly in individuals with *P. falciparum* infections). Diagnosis of malaria is made by examination of a peripheral blood smear. Blood should be taken just prior to the onset of fever because the parasitemia is greatest at this time. However, this is only possible if clas-

> **Table 13-18**

MECHANISM LEADING TO DEVELOPMENT OF DRUG-RELATED ANTIBODIES

Mechanism	Prototype Drugs	Immunoglobulin Class	DAT	Biologic Results	Frequency of Hemolysis
Immune complex formation (innocent bystander)	Quinidine	IgM or IgG	Positive (often to complement fragments only; however, IgG may be present)	Eluate often negative	Small doses of drug may cause acute intravascular hemolysis with hemoglobinemia and hemoglobinuria; renal failure is common
Drug adsorption	Penicillins Cephalosporins	IgG	Positive (strongly) due to IgG sensitization	Eluate often negative	3%–4% of patients on large doses (10 million units) daily of penicillin, which is one of the most common causes of drug-induced immune hemolysis, usually extravascular in nature
Membrane modification (nonimmunologic protein adsorption)	Cephalosporins	Numerous plasma proteins (nonimmunologic sensitization)	Positive due to a variety of serum proteins	Eluate negative	No hemolysis; however, 3% of patients receiving the drug develop a positive DAT
Autoimmunity	Methyldopa (Aldomet)	IgG	Strongly positive (due to IgG sensitization)	Eluate positive (warm autoantibody identical to antibody found in WAIHA)	0.8% develop a hemolytic anemia that mimics a WAIHA (depends on the dose of the drug); 15% of patients receiving Aldomet develop a positive DAT

sic periodic episodes of fever and chills are present. It is best to make blood smears from a fingerstick. If anticoagulated blood must be used, smears should be made as soon as possible to prevent changes in erythrocyte and parasite morphology.[68] Examination of an unfixed Giemsa- or Wright-stained blood smear (thick preparation) is performed to ascertain the presence of malarial parasites. Staining is usually performed at a pH of 7.2 to enhance the blue staining of the parasites' cytoplasm. Determination of the species of parasite may be made on this smear if schizonts are present (by the number of merozoites within the schizont). If only trophozoites are present, the examination of a thin blood smear is necessary. Often more than one parasite is present in a single cell (Fig. 13–10 and Color Plate 117). *Plasmodium falciparum* gametocytes have a characteristic sausage or crescent shape, assisting in the identification. Occasionally it is possible to see irregular purple inclusions called Maurer's dots in the red cell cytoplasm, which are probably breakdown products of hemoglobin. *Plasmodium vivax* gametocytes are round, ameboid forms that expand and distort the red cell. Bluish purple inclusions called Schüffner's dots

are often seen in red cells infected with *P. vivax* and *P. ovale* (Fig. 13–11 and Color Plate 118). Table 13–21 summarizes the features of the different malarial parasites infecting humans.

Immunoassays are being introduced to help screen large numbers of patients for the presence of infection. Flow cytometry has also been used with some success to show the presence of malarial parasites in red cells.

Babesiosis

Infection by the organism *Babesia* represents a zoonotic infection, as humans are not natural hosts for the parasite. The disease is carried by ticks (*Ixodes* species) and normally infects cattle, deer, and rodents.[69] The disease is usually tick-borne in humans, but has apparently also been transmitted by blood transfusion.[70,71] In the United States, cases have been reported mostly in Massachusetts, Rhode Island, and New York owing to the presence of infected ticks and their hosts.[72] Infection tends to be self-limiting, although in some high-risk patients it can follow an acute course and be fatal. One study showed advanced age to be the most im-

> **Table 13–19**
SUMMARY OF ANTIBODY CHARACTERISTICS IN AIHA

	Warm Reactive Autoantibody	Cold Reactive Autoantibody	PCH	Drug-Related Autoantibody
Immunoglobulin characteristics	Polyclonal IgG, IgM, and IgA may also be present; rarely IgA alone	Polyclonal IgM-infection Monoclonal κ chain IgM in cold agglutinin disease	Polyclonal IgG	Polyclonal IgG
Complement activation	Variable	Always	Always	Depends on mechanism of drug, antibody, and RBC interaction
Thermal reactivity	20°C–37°C; optimum 37°C	4°C–32°C occasionally to 37°C; optimum 4°C	4°C–20°C; biphasic hemolysin	20°C–37°C; optimum 37°C
Titer of free antibody	Low (< 32) May only be detectable using enzyme-treated cells	High (> 1000 at 4°C)	Moderate to low (< 64)	Depends on mechanism of drug, antibody, and RBC interaction
Reactivity of eluate with antibody screening cells	Usually panreactive	Nonreactive	Nonreactive	Panreactive with Aldomet-type antibody. Nonreactive in all other circumstances
Most common specificity	Anti-Rh precursor -common Rh -LW -Enᵃ/Wrᵇ -U	-I -i -Pr	Anti-P	Anti-e–like; Aldomet, antidrug
Site of RBC destruction	Predominantly spleen with some liver involvement	Predominantly liver, rarely intravascular	Intravascular	Intravascular and spleen

portant risk factor for the disease, followed by absence of a spleen, and immunodeficiency.[72] Patients usually present with a history of malaise, headache, and fever, sometimes associated with vomiting and diarrhea. In splenectomized patients this condition can progress to rigors, acute intravascular hemolysis with associated hemoglobinemia, hemoglobinuria, jaundice, and renal failure.

LABORATORY DIAGNOSIS
Diagnosis of the disease is made by examination of the peripheral blood, where parasites very similar to *P. falciparum* are seen in the red cells (Fig. 13–12 and Color Plate 119). Features that distinguish babesiosis from malaria are the formation of tetrads of merozoites (Maltese cross), absence of pigment granules in infected erythrocytes, and the presence of extracellular merozoites.[72] A history of possible exposure to ticks and a lack of recent travel to areas where malaria is endemic help in making the correct diagnosis. Serologic tests for antibodies to *Babesia* by immunofluorescent assay or testing for deoxyribonucleic acid (DNA) by polymerase chain reaction have been described.[72,73]

Extracellular Infections

Bartonellosis (Oroya Fever)
This disease is restricted to northern areas of South America, including Peru, Ecuador, and Columbia. The name Oroya fever derives from the city of Oroya in the Peruvian Andes, where many railroad construction workers were affected by the disease in the late 1800s. It is also referred to as Carrion's disease,[74] named after the medical student who

died as a result of a self-experiment designed to determine the nature of the infection.

Bartonellosis has a high fatality rate in nonimmune patients and is caused by the organism *Bartonella bacilliformis*. Infection is transmitted by the sand fly (*Phlebotomus*), and there does not appear to be any intermediate host. The organisms adhere to the red cell surface and appear as gram-negative rods in the acute phase of the disease. In the recovery phase, they assume a coccoid appearance.

The disease has two clinical phases. The first is the hemolytic phase (Oroya fever), which may not occur in all patients. When it does occur, there is a rapid onset with marked intravascular hemolysis. Red cells are also sequestered in the spleen and liver.[75] The anemia can be quite severe, and blood smears show many nucleated red cells and a reticulocytosis.[75] Antibiotic therapy, including penicillin, streptomycin, and tetracyclines, is effective in treating patients in this stage of the infection.[67] The second stage of the disease (verruca peruviana) is nonhematologic and involves the development of verrucous nodes (warty tumors) over the patient's face and extremities.

Clostridium perfringens (welchii)
This organism is a gram-positive, spore-forming bacillus that is responsible for the development of gas gangrene. Infections with this organism are generally located in deep tissues where anaerobic conditions required for the organism's survival exist. The organism is normally present in the environment and may infect tissues exposed by trauma and surgical procedures. There is a high incidence of the infection in septic abortions.[76] The organism is responsible

➤ **Table 13–20**

CLASSIFICATION OF NONIMMUNE ACQUIRED HEMOLYTIC ANEMIAS

Cause	Examples	Mechanisms
Infections		
Intracellular	Malaria	Physical disruption and immune
	Babesiosis	Physical disruption
Extracellular	Bartonella	Direct action on RBC membrane and MPS sequestration
	Clostridia	Enzymatic action on RBC membrane
	Bacterial sepsis: meningococcal, pneumococcal	Physical disruption secondary to DIC
	Viral	Unknown
Mechanical		
Macroangiopathic	Cardiac prosthesis	Physical disruption because of shear stress
	March hemoglobinuria	Physical disruption
Microangiopathic	Hemolytic uremic syndrome (HUS)	Physical disruption
	Thrombotic thrombocytopenic purpura (TTP)	Physical disruption
Chemicals and physical agents		
Oxidative agents	Dapsone at high dosage	Direct oxidation of RBC membrane components
Nonoxidative agents	Lead	Alteration of RBC membrane components
	Venoms	Possible direct effect on RBC membrane by enzymes
Osmotic effect	Water (drowning or water irrigation during surgery)	Osmotic lysis
	Burns	Localized dehydration
Acquired membrane disorders	Vitamin E deficiency; abetalipo-proteinemia	RBC membrane oxidation; lack of membrane deformability
	Liver disease	Lipid abnormalities of RBC membrane lead to decrease in deformability
	Renal disease	Retained metabolic products cause membrane changes, leading to a decrease in deformability
Hypersplenism		Sequestration of normal cells

Abbreviations: DIC = disseminated intravascular coagulation; MPS = mononuclear phagocyte system.

for extensive tissue damage resulting from the release of enzymes and toxins. Septicemia caused by *C. perfringens* may produce an acute intravascular hemolytic process resulting from the release of an alpha (α) toxin or lecithinase. This process, combined with phospholipases and possibly proteinases also produced by the organism, acts on the red cell membrane to cause its destruction and subsequent lysis of the cell.[77] Hemolysis is often severe, with marked hemoglobinemia and hemoglobinuria. Acute renal failure may develop quite rapidly, and the prognosis is generally poor.[78] Microspherocytes are a common finding in the peripheral blood smear. Leukocytosis with a shift to the left and thrombocytopenia are present in most cases.

Improvements in the maintenance of aseptic conditions during and following surgery and the decrease in criminal abortions have caused this form of hemolytic anemia to become quite uncommon.

Table 13–22 lists other organisms that have been associated with hemolytic anemia.

Mechanical Etiologies

The passage of red cells through the vascular system subjects the cell to a wide range of environmental conditions. As red cells travel around the body, shear forces are highly variable and are influenced by (1) the surface conditions of the blood vessel, (2) the size of the vessel lumen, (3) the rate at which the cell is moving, and (4) the number of other cells present at the same time. Other environmental conditions the cell must contend with in its travels include changes in pH, electrolytes, and protein concentration. The result of this mechanical rupturing of the cell membrane is intravascular hemolysis accompanied by the presence of red cell fragments or schistocytes (Fig. 13–13 and Color Plate 120).

Cardiac Prosthesis

Historically, hemolytic anemia associated with prosthetic heart valves was a frequent complication of cardiac corrective surgery. Innovative changes in design and composition

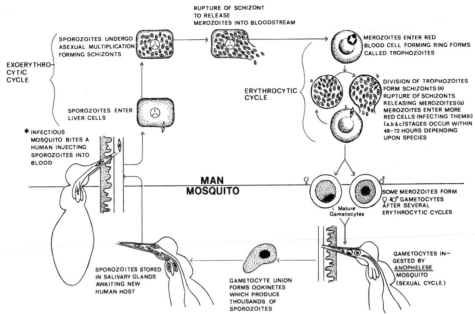

➤ **FIGURE 13–9**　Malarial life cycle in humans and mosquitoes. Beginning of cycle is indicated by an asterisk.

of valves has reduced the incidence to a rare and minor complication.[79]

The primary cause of hemolysis is mechanical trauma to red blood cells, resulting from turbulence of flow through the prosthesis.[80] The severity of the anemia is highly variable in patients with heart valve prostheses. Mild, compensated hemolysis is common; overt anemia is unusual, and rarely is the anemia severe enough to require transfusion.[79]

The peripheral blood smear shows many fragmented cells (schistocytes), helmet cells, and occasional spherocytes (Fig. 13–14 and Color Plate 121). The reticulocyte count and serum LD level are usually elevated.[80] Leukocytes are usually normal, and platelets are often reduced because of their interaction with the abnormal surface.[81] Decreased haptoglobin, mild hemoglobinemia, mild hemosiderinuria,[82] and occasionally hemoglobinuria are present (depending on the amount of red cell destruction).

Treatment of cardiac hemolysis can range from supportive therapy, which may include iron supplementation and transfusion,[83] to surgically correcting the faulty valve or vessel.

March Hemoglobinuria

This form of hemolytic anemia was first described in the late 1800s in a young German soldier who demonstrated frank hemoglobinuria following a field marching exercise.[84] The anemia has been described in individuals involved in strenuous and sustained physical activity.[85] Similar traumatic red cell destruction has been reported in a practitioner of karate[86] and a conga drum player.[87] The cause of the anemia is complex, involving (1) direct physical disruption of red cells as they flow through the capillaries of the feet or hands, (2) iron loss in sweat, and (3) adaptation to a right-shifted oxygen dissociation curve.[88]

Patients with march hemoglobinuria usually demonstrate a normal hemoglobin, although there may be an increase in the reticulocyte count. Hemoglobinemia and hemoglobinuria are episodic and present only following exercise. This obvious association with exercise is helpful in distinguishing the hemoglobinuria from other causes (such as paroxysmal nocturnal hemoglobinuria, discussed later in this chapter). Fragmented red cells are not a feature of this condition.

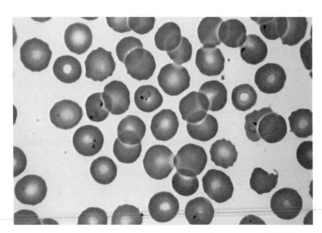

➤ **FIGURE 13–10**　Ringed forms of *Plasmodium falciparum* in red blood cells (RBCs). Note that the same RBCs may be infected with more than one ring.

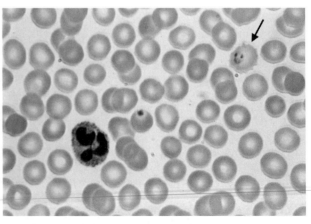

➤ **FIGURE 13–11**　Late stages of *Plasmodium vivax* malaria, Schüffner's dots. Note and contrast the platelet on the RBC *(center)* with the ring form of malaria toward the periphery *(arrow)*.

➤ **Table 13-21**
CHARACTERISTICS OF MALARIAL PARASITES INFECTING HUMANS

	P. falciparum	P. vivax	P. malariae	P. ovale
Incubation period (days)	6–10	10–12	13–16	10–12
Asexual life cycle (h)	48	48	72	48
RBCs infected	All	Reticulocytes	Senescent	Reticulocytes
Secondary exoerythro-cytic development	No	Yes	Yes	Yes
Duration of relapses in untreated patients	Not applicable	3–5 yr	up to 40 yr	3–5 yr
Level of parasitemia	50%–60%	2%–5%	2%–3%	2%–3%
Ring form	Small, delicate may have two chromatin dots, often on edge of RBC Maurer's dots	Large irregular, poor outline One chromatin dot Schüffner's dots	Large thick, promi-nent chromatin dot	Large irregular, poor outline One chromatin dot Schüffner's dots
Schizonts	Rarely seen in peripheral blood 8–32 merozoites	Large, about same size as RBC 12–25 merozoites	Small "daisy-head" 6–16 merozoites	Irregular arrangement 4–16 merozoites
Gametocytes	Crescent or sausage shape	Round and expand RBC	Round, same size as RBC	

Treatment involves wearing cushion-soled shoes or running on softer surfaces.

Microangiopathic Hemolytic Anemia

Microangiopathic hemolytic anemia (MAHA) refers to a group of clinical disorders that are characterized by fragmentation of the red cells as they pass through abnormal arterioles, resulting in intravascular hemolysis.[89] Most often the abnormalities in the microcirculation are caused by the deposition of fibrin strands resulting from intravascular activation of the coagulation system (see the discussion of disseminated intravascular coagulation [DIC] in Chap. 26).

In MAHA the mechanical process leading to fragmentation of the red cells occurs as the blood flow forces the cells to negotiate a blood vessel whose lumen is restricted by microthrombi.[90] The red cells are physically torn as they are forced along the narrow confines of the blood vessel. Schistocytes and other poikilocytes are seen on the peripheral blood smear, as well as decreased platelets in some cases. The degree of hemolysis correlates with the amount of thrombosis present.[91] In addition to the intravascular destruction of the red cells, the fragments produced lack deformability leading to an increase in extravascular hemolysis.

In addition to DIC, MAHA may be associated with invasive carcinoma, complications of pregnancy, and kidney or liver transplantation.[92] Manifestations of MAHA are also prominent in two related clinical entities: hemolytic uremic syndrome (HUS) and thrombotic thrombocytopenic purpura (TTP) (see Chap. 24).

Chemical and Physical Agents

Oxidative Hemolysis

Oxidative stress on the red cell resulting from either drugs or chemicals may affect either the globin chains or the heme group of the hemoglobin molecule. Most oxidizing agents affect the hemoglobin molecule by denaturing the globin chains, producing Heinz bodies, or by oxidizing the heme group, producing methemoglobinemia (see Chap. 10).

Nonoxidative Hemolysis

ARSENIC

Industrial processes involving the action of acids and metals may give rise to the production of arsenic gas. Continued exposure to the gas gives rise to intravascular hemolysis with anemia and hemoglobinuria.[93] Marked methemalbumin formation causes the serum of affected patients to turn a characteristic brown and often masks the presence of any red cells. Current federal Occupational Safety and Health Administration (OSHA) requirements have minimized this hazard in the workplace.

LEAD

The anemia produced by lead exposure is caused by decreased synthesis and not by direct hemolysis.[94] The red cells

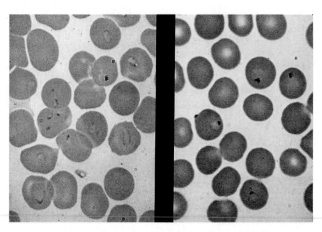

➤ FIGURE 13–12 Comparison of babesiosis (*left*) and parasitemia malaria (*right*).

> **Table 13–22**
ORGANISMS ASSOCIATED WITH HEMOLYTIC ANEMIA

Bacteria	Viruses	Protozoa	Fungi
Bartonella bacilliformis	Coxsackie	*Babesia microti*	*Aspergillus*
Clostridium perfringens	Cytomegalovirus	*B. divergens*	
Escherichia coli	Epstein-Barr	*Plasmodium falciparum*	
Haemophilus influenzae	Herpes simplex	*P. malariae*	
Mycobacteria tuberculosis	Influenza A	*P. ovale*	
Mycoplasma pneumoniae	Rubeola	*P. vivax*	
Neisseria meningitidis	Varicella	*Toxoplasma*	
Salmonella sp.			
Shigella sp.			
Streptococcus sp.			
Vibrio cholera			
Yersinia enterocolitica			

of patients exposed to lead have a shortened survival.[95] Lead poisoning is usually a problem of young children who have been eating materials painted with lead-based paints. Children affected by lead poisoning may show a normocytic to microcytic, hypochromic blood picture, with classic punctate basophilic stippling (Fig. 13–15 and Color Plate 122).

COPPER
Very high levels of copper ions have been associated with intravascular hemolysis. These levels may occur as a result of suicide attempts in which copper sulphate solution is ingested[96] or in Wilson's disease.[97] The hemolytic process is unknown, although it has been shown that high levels of copper ions can affect a number of intracellular enzymes (e.g., pyruvate kinase and hexokinase).[98] The anemia may be associated with the presence of spherocytes.

VENOMS
A number of venoms, particularly those from some spiders, contain potent enzymes capable of directly acting on the red cell membrane to produce lysis of the cell. Bee stings in some

people may produce a hemolytic process. Snake venoms, although hemolytic in vitro, rarely cause hemolysis in vivo.

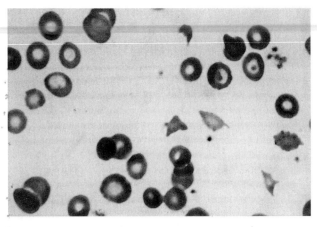

> FIGURE 13–14   RBC fragmentation in microangiopathic hemolysis from a patient with a prosthetic cardiac valve (mechanical hemolysis); note the presence of schistocytes.

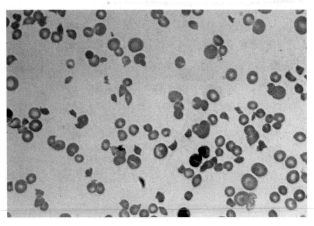

> FIGURE 13–13   Peripheral blood showing red cell fragmentation with thrombocytopenia and nucleated RBCs from a patient with thrombotic thrombocytopenia purpura (TTP) (magnification ×40).

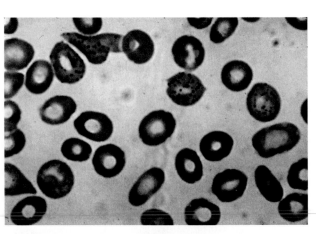

> FIGURE 13–15   Peripheral blood from a patient with lead poisoning. Note the normocytic, hypochromic red cells, with the classic punctate basophilic stippling.

Osmotic Effects

BURNS

Patients who have suffered severe burns to more than 15% of their body generally show evidence of intravascular hemolysis.[99] The hemolytic process is thought to result from the direct effect of the heat on the red cells in the affected area. Red cells that are heated to temperatures in excess of 47°C undergo changes, including fragmentation, budding, and microspherocyte formation; blood collected within 24 hours of such heating shows evidence of these changes[100] (Fig. 13–16 and Color Plate 123). Because the cells are osmotically and mechanically fragile, they are rapidly removed from the circulation, and blood collected after that time is often normal in appearance.

Acquired Membrane Disorders

A number of mechanisms can be implicated in producing changes to red cell membranes, which can result in the shortened life span of the cell. Any change that compromises the cell's deformability or its resistance to oxidative stress can potentially contribute to a hemolytic process. For example, spur-cell anemia, observed primarily in patients with alcoholic cirrhosis, is a condition in which the red cells assume a characteristic shape with a number of fine, finger-like spike projections (acanthocytes) (Fig. 13–17 and Color Plate 124). Lipid disorders can also result in a loss of red cell deformability. A congenital red cell abnormality seen in abetalipoproteinemia may contribute to the diagnosis of the condition as the cells assume the classic shape of acanthocytes (Fig. 13–18 and Color Plate 125). In end-stage renal disease, many of the cells take on the appearance of burr cells or echinocytes (Fig. 13–19 and Color Plate 126), which have numerous small spines over their entire surface. Other conditions in which echinocytes are seen include pyruvate kinase deficiency and bleeding stages associated with peptic ulcers.

➤ ACQUIRED INTRACORPUSCULAR DEFECTS

Paroxysmal Nocturnal Hemoglobinuria

Definition and History

Paroxysmal nocturnal hemoglobinuria (PNH) is an acquired hemolytic anemia that results from an abnormality in the red cell membrane, causing the red cells to be highly sensitive to

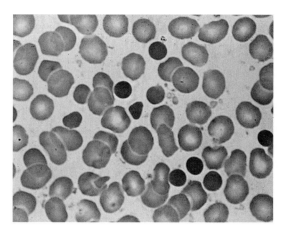

➤ FIGURE 13–16 Peripheral blood from a patient with extensive burns. Note the typical microspherocytes and membranous fragments. (From Bell, A: Hematology. In: Listen, Look and Learn. Health and Education Resources, Inc., Bethesda, MD, with permission.)

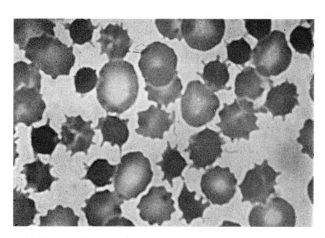

➤ FIGURE 13–18 Acanthocytosis from a patient with abetaliproteinemia. (From Hyun, BH, et al: Practical Hematology. A Laboratory Guide with Accompanying Filmstrip. WB Saunders, Philadelphia, 1975, with permission.)

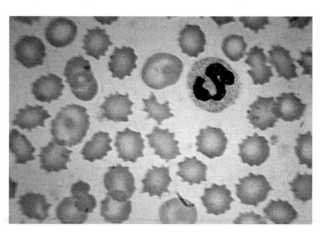

➤ FIGURE 13–17 Spur-cell anemia (acanthocytosis) associated with severe liver disease.

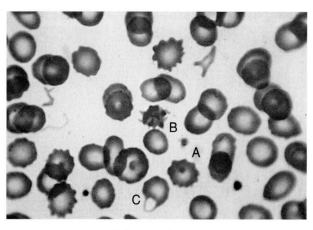

➤ FIGURE 13–19 Renal disease (peripheral blood). Note the presence of *(A)* burr cells, *(B)* thorn cell, and *(C)* blister cell. (From Bell, A: Hematology. In: Listen, Look and Learn. Health and Education Resources, Inc., Bethesda, MD, with permssion.)

the hemolytic action of complement. The membrane defect present in the blood cells is caused by a somatic mutation at the level of the multipotential stem cell, resulting in abnormalities in leukocytes and platelets, as well as erythrocytes.[101] In classic cases, hemolysis is intermittent (paroxysmal) and worsens during sleep (nocturnal), resulting in hemoglobinuria that is most noticeable in the first morning urine specimen. However, many cases exhibit a chronic hemolysis that is not associated with sleep, nor do these patients have hemoglobinuria.

In 1866, William Gull published a report of the first case of PNH.[102] He described an anemic patient with "hematuria" that varied throughout the day but was the worst in the morning. He recognized that the urinary pigment was caused by some breakdown product of the red cells. Other clinical investigators confirmed that hematuria was most pronounced in the morning and demonstrated that PNH erythrocytes underwent lysis when serum and cells were exposed to carbonic acid.[103]

In 1930, Thomas H. Ham observed that these cells had an increased sensitivity to some serum hemolytic protein (complement) that caused the cell to lyse when acidified. He used this observation to devise the Ham's test, which is still commonly performed to aid in the diagnosis of PNH. Ham also demonstrated that some patients with PNH, presenting with chronic hemolysis, had positive acidified serum lysis test results but did not have hemoglobinuria.[104,105]

Although PNH is fairly rare, much progress and research have increased our understanding of the mechanism of hemolysis, the role of complement, and causes of the defects.

Etiology and Pathophysiology

Paroxysmal nocturnal hemoglobinuria is an acquired intracorpuscular defect caused by an abnormality in the hematopoietic cell membranes. This abnormality causes the cells, especially the erythrocytes, to be more sensitive than normal to lytic action of complement (Fig. 13–20). Complement plays a major role in the pathogenesis of PNH and was discussed in detail at the beginning of this chapter. In PNH, the erythrocytes react abnormally with complement components C3 and C5 to C9. Because of a somatic mutation in the multipotent hematopoietic stem cell, the progeny cell membranes are missing at least nine cell surface proteins that are composed of complement-regulating proteins, membrane enzymes, and immune function proteins[106] (Table 13–23). These proteins are normally bound to the cell surface by a glycosyl phosphatidylinositol (GPI) anchor. In PNH, the GPI anchor is not synthesized by the cells (Figs. 13–21 and 13–22). Deficiency of the complement regulatory proteins decay-accelerating factor (DAF), or CD55; homologous restriction factor (HRF), or C8-binding protein; and the membrane inhibitor of reactive lysis (MIRL), or CD59, play the largest role in the complement sensitivity that is seen in PNH.[107–109] DAF is an integral membrane protein that accelerates the spontaneous decay of the C3 convertase enzyme for the classic and alternate complement activation pathways. The role of MIRL is to protect the membrane from attack by the C5-C9 complex. HRF regulates the activation of the terminal stages of complement, which causes cell lysis by binding C8.[110]

The deficiency of DAF, MIRL, and HRF expression resulting from a deficiency of GPI-anchored cell membrane proteins is the molecular explanation for the underlying clonal abnormality that affects granulocytes, monocytes, and platelets, as well as the erythrocytes, in patients with PNH. Recently the genetic mutation responsible for the defect has been located on the phosphatidylinositol glycan class A (*PIG-A*) gene on the short arm of the X chromosome. More than 100 different mutations have been reported, all resulting in complete or partial deficiency of GPI-anchored proteins.[111] The cause of the somatic mutation is unknown, but it sometimes appears after an episode of marrow damage such as severe hypoplasia. The abnormal clone of cells appears to have a proliferative advantage over normal cells that is not fully understood. It may relate to a resistance of triggers of apoptosis (programmed cell death) in normal hematopoietic cells.[110]

The PNH erythrocytes have been classified into three categories based on their sensitivity to complement lysis. In

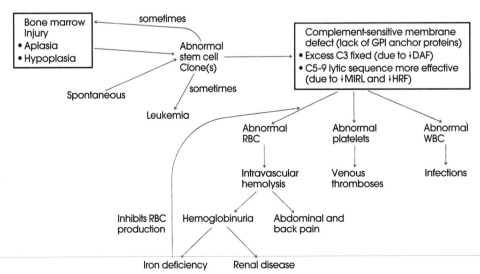

➤ **FIGURE 13–20** Pathophysiology of paroxysmal nocturnal hemoglobinuria (PNH) (GPI = glycosyl phosphatidylinositol; DAF = decay-accelerating factor; MIRL = membrane inhibitor of reactive lysis; HRF = homologous restriction factor) (Adapted from Beck, WS: Hematology, ed 5. MIT Press, Cambridge, 1991, with permission.)

> **Table 13-23**
> ## GPI-ANCHORED PROTEINS ABSENT FROM THE CELL MEMBRANE IN PNH

Complement-Regulating Proteins

Decay-accelerating factor (DAF), (CD55)

Membrane inhibitor of reactive lysis (MIRL), protectin, (CD59)

Homologous restriction factor (HRF), C8-binding protein (C8bp)

Membrane Enzymes

Erythrocyte acetylcholinesterase

Leukocyte alkaline phosphatase

Lymphocyte 5′-ectonucleotidase, (CD73)

Immune Function Proteins

Lymphocyte function antigen 3 (LFA-3), (CD58)

Neutrophil Fcγ III receptor, (CD16)

Monocyte antigen (CD14)

Abbreviation: GPI = glycosyl phosphatidylinositol.

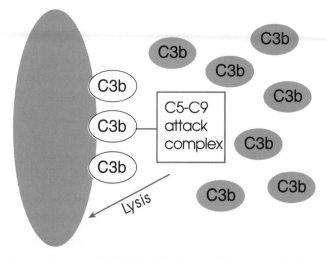

> ► **FIGURE 13–22** The PNH cell is not protected from C3b molecules; thus, lysis will occur. (From Leach, AP, and Gaumer, HR: Diagnosis and detection of PNH using GPI anchored proteins. Clin Lab Sci. 9:193, 1996, with permission.)

PNH I, erythrocytes react normally with complement and are thought to represent residual normal cells because they are similar to normal erythrocytes in all respects.[112] The PNH II erythrocytes have moderate sensitivity to complement and appear to have low levels of MIRL and varying levels of DAF. PNH III erythrocytes are the cells most sensitive to complement and are completely or partially deficient in DAF and completely deficient in MIRL.[111] Most studies indicate that deficiency of MIRL plays the most critical role in cell lysis.[110]

Patients with PNH usually have variable combinations of the three different types of PNH erythrocytes. Eighty percent of all patients with PNH have the combination of PNH I and PNH II cells, whereas the other 20% have variable combinations of PNH I, PNH II, and PNH III cells.[112] The degree of hemolysis depends on the proportion of abnormal

cells and the severity of the cellular membrane defects. The proportion of abnormal cells varies from patient to patient, and the intensity of the clinical symptoms is related to the percentage of PNH III cells present.

Clinical Features

Diverse clinical presentations of PNH are common. The disease most often occurs in middle-aged adults but occasionally occurs in children and the elderly. Both genders are equally affected. Most patients with PNH present with symptoms of anemia that may be mild to severe and are a result of the chronic hemolysis.

In addition to chronic hemolysis, the disease is characterized by periodic acute hemolytic episodes; bone marrow hypoplasia, causing cytopenias of varying severity; and a tendency to develop thrombosis. The classic presentation of hemoglobinuria in the first morning specimen, caused by significant intravascular hemolysis, actually occurs in only about 25% of cases.[112] However, irregular episodes of intravascular hemolysis with hemoglobinuria may be triggered by infections (most commonly viruses), surgery, menstruation, administration of iron, and a variety of drugs.

In contrast to hemoglobinuria, hemosiderinuria is present in most patients. Recurrent hemolysis results in loss of body iron into the urine. This iron is derived from plasma hemoglobin that is absorbed and catabolized in the renal tubules. Iron-laden tubular cells appear in the urine and can be stained for hemosiderin. Prolonged loss of iron can lead to iron-deficiency anemia, which may mask the diagnosis of PNH.

Patients commonly present with infections, abdominal pain, headaches, and back pain—symptoms thought to be caused by intravascular thrombi. One of the major complications of PNH is the formation of venous thromboses of the hepatic, abdominal, cerebral, or subdermal veins. Formation of these thrombi may be attributed to the activation of complement-sensitive platelets by the complement component C3.[113] Also, during the thrombotic episodes, features of DIC may appear (see Chap. 26).

Aplastic anemia may precede or coexist with PNH.[113] In such cases, pancytopenia and marrow hypoplasia are pres-

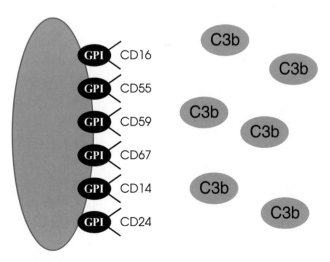

> ► **FIGURE 13–21** The normal cell is protected from C3b because CD55- and CD59-anchored proteins are present. (From Leach, AP, and Gaumer, HR: Diagnosis and detection of PNH using GPI anchored proteins. Clin Lab Sci. 9:193, 1996, with permission.)

ent. Complement-sensitive erythrocytes occur transiently and in small numbers in certain patients with aplastic anemia. A recent study showed up to 52% of patients with aplastic anemia have GPI-deficient blood cells at some stage of the disease.[110] In a few patients, complement-sensitive erythrocytes are increased in number and persist, making these rare cases of aplastic anemia indistinguishable from PNH.

Laboratory Evaluation

Characteristic laboratory findings in PNH are anemia, leukopenia, and thrombocytopenia.[110] The anemia may be mild to severe, depending on the number and type of PNH erythrocytes present. Hemoglobin levels may vary from normal to less than 6 g/dL. No characteristic red blood cell morphological abnormalities are observed in the peripheral blood; in fact, patients most commonly present with a normocytic, normochromic anemia. Slight macrocytosis and polychromasia, resulting from increased numbers of reticulocytes in the peripheral blood, may be seen (Fig. 13–23 and Color Plate 127). This reticulocytosis is a compensatory mechanism for the hemolytic process, and although the reticulocyte count is usually elevated (5% to 10%), the absolute reticulocyte count may be low with respect to the degree of anemia present. This discrepancy is attributed to the presence of iron deficiency or to the bone marrow stem cell defect itself.[114] With associated iron deficiency, the erythrocytes appear microcytic and hypochromic. During an exacerbation of hemolysis, nucleated red blood cells may be seen in the peripheral blood smear. Spherocytes, although present in other types of hemolytic anemias, are generally not seen. Schistocytes or fragmented red blood cells are occasionally seen with acute hemolysis and may suggest the presence of an intravascular thrombosis.[112]

Also present in PNH erythrocytes is decreased membrane acetylcholinesterase, a finding that is most apparent in the reticulocytes.[115] The severity of the decrease in acetylcholinesterase activity parallels the severity of the disease.

Granulocytes and platelets, similar to the red cells, have the same membrane defects that render them more sensitive to the lytic action of complement and to antibodies.[116] When observed by light microscopy and with routine staining, granulocytes appear to have no characteristic morphological abnormality. Leukopenia, primarily caused by a decrease in granulocytes, is often observed. The granulocytes have decreased leukocyte alkaline phosphatase (LAP) activity ranging from zero to low normal (Fig. 13–24 and Color Plate 128). The LAP score can aid in distinguishing PNH from aplastic anemia because in the latter, the LAP score is normal to elevated. Platelet counts vary in PNH. Moderate thrombocytopenia is present, with counts ranging from 50 to 100×10^9/L. Although platelets are decreased, venous thromboses (a severe complication) are common.

As expected, the bone marrow shows erythroid hyperplasia (Fig. 13–25 and Color Plate 129). This is the result of increased erythropoiesis subsequent to chronic hemolysis. The increased erythropoiesis is usually normoblastic, although some megaloblastic changes may be noted. Occasionally, a hypoplastic or even aplastic marrow is seen. The bone marrow usually reveals adequate numbers of myeloid and platelet precursors, except after an aplastic episode when the myeloid and platelet precursors are decreased. Bone marrow iron stains often reveal decreased iron stores.

Because almost all patients with PNH have hemosiderin in their urine, testing for urinary hemosiderin aids in confirming the diagnosis. A random urine sample is centrifuged and the sediment stained with potassium ferrocyanide (Prussian blue), which will detect the presence of hemosiderin. If present, the hemosiderin granules stain blue.[117]

Hemoglobinuria, when present, must be differentiated

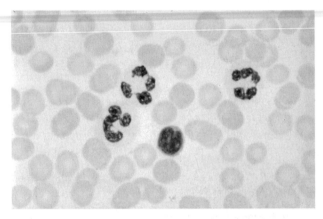

► FIGURE 13–24 Leukocyte alkaline phosphatase (LAP) stain of peripheral blood showing little or no activity in chronic myelocytic leukemia (CML).

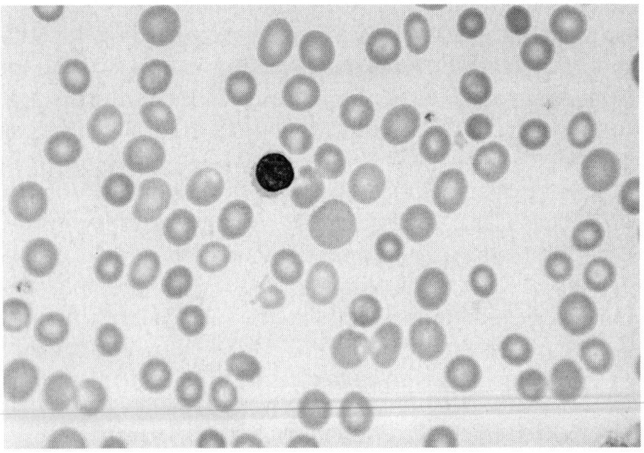

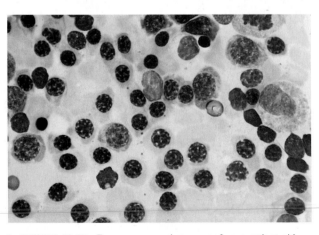

► FIGURE 13–25 Bone marrow aspirate smear from a patient with paroxysmal nocturnal hemoglobinuria demonstrating erythroid hyperplasia (magnification ×500).

► FIGURE 13–23 Peripheral blood smear from a patient with PNH (magnification ×600).

from hematuria. This may be accomplished by performing a routine urinalysis with microscopic examination to look for the absence of intact red cells and the presence of a positive blood result on the dipstick. Hemoglobinuria can lead to the formation of hemoglobin casts in the renal tubules and, eventually, can cause renal failure.

Other laboratory procedures that aid in diagnosing PNH are nonspecific tests for intravascular and extravascular hemolysis, including indirect bilirubin (increased), plasma hemoglobin (increased), haptoglobin (decreased), and direct antiglobulin test (negative).

Diagnostic Tests

Sugar Water Test (Sucrose Hemolysis Test)

The sugar water test (Fig. 13–26 and Color Plate 130) is used as a screening procedure when the diagnosis of PNH is considered. The sucrose provides a medium of low ionic strength that promotes the binding of complement, especially C3, to the red cell membranes. The low ionic strength solution used in the sugar water test activates complement via the classic or alternate pathway. The complement-sensitive PNH red cells are lysed, whereas normal cells will be unaffected.

To perform the sugar water test, the patient's cells are first washed, then mixed with ABO/Rh-compatible serum and "sugar water." The tubes are incubated at room temperature for 30 minutes and then centrifuged. The percent hemolysis is then determined. Ten to eighty percent red cell lysis is seen in PNH (see Fig. 13–26 and Color Plate 130). Less than 5% red cell lysis is usually considered negative for PNH. A small amount of lysis (less than 5%) has been observed in patients with megaloblastic anemia, autoimmune hemolytic anemia, and leukemia. False-negative results occasionally occur if the serum lacks complement or if an unbuffered sucrose solution is used. However, a definitive diagnosis of PNH depends of the results obtained with Ham's test.

Ham's Test (Acidified Serum Lysis Test)

Ham's test, or the acidified serum lysis test, is used to confirm the diagnosis of PNH (Fig. 13–27 and Color Plate 131). Serum is acidified, which activates complement via the alternate pathway and enhances the binding of C3 to the cell membrane. The PNH erythrocytes lyse because they are deficient in the membrane GPI-anchor proteins, rendering them more sensitive to lysis by complement. Normal erythrocytes are unaffected. To confirm a positive Ham's test result, the following characteristics must be demonstrated: (1) hemolysis occurs with the patient's cells and not with control cells, and (2) hemolysis is enhanced by acidified serum and does not occur with the heat-inactivated serum[114] (heating serum to 56°C for 30 minutes inactivates complement activity). For the interpretation of the Ham's test results, refer to Table 13–24. This test is specific for PNH when it is shown that the patient's own serum is capable of lysing his or her own cells.[118]

A positive Ham's test result is seen in the rare disorder congenital dyserythropoietic anemia (CDA) type II, or HEMPAS. In this disorder, lysis does not occur with the patient's own serum; lysis in this case is caused by an unusual red cell antigen that reacts with IgM, a complement-activating antibody present in many normal sera.[119] The sugar water test for this disorder also yields a negative result. Spherocytes also lyse in acidified serum because of the decreased pH; therefore, they will lyse in the tube containing the complement-inactivated serum.[119]

Immunophenotyping

The use of flow cytometry for immunophenotyping blood cells to assess the presence of GPI-anchoring proteins for diagnosis of PNH is increasing. This method is more sensitive and specific, and less time consuming than Ham's test. A panel of monoclonal antibodies against GPI-anchored proteins is run by immunofluorescence. GPI-anchored antigens are present on normal cells and lacking on PNH cells. Monoclonal antibodies to a series of GPI-anchored antigens, such as CD14, CD16, CD24, CD48, CD55, CD59, and CD73, may be used. This method is a simple, reliable assay for diagnosis of PNH and can also quantify the proportion of affected cells in each PNH group.[111,120,121]

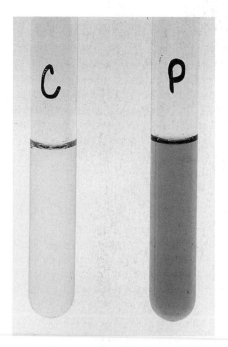

> ► **FIGURE 13–26** Sugar water test. The tube on the left represents the control *(C)* and the tube on the right represents the patient *(P)* with a positive sugar water test. Ten to 80% hemolysis is seen in PNH.

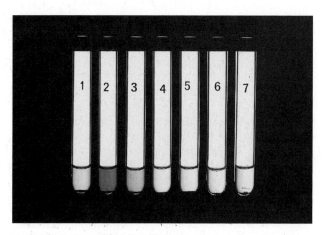

> ► **FIGURE 13–27** Ham's test. Positive results occur in patients with PNH. A positive test is reported when hemolysis occurs in tube number 1, containing fresh normal serum and patient cells; tube number 2, containing acidified normal serum and patient cells; and tube number 3, containing acidified patient serum and patient cells.

> **Table 13-24**
ACIDIFIED SERUM LYSIS TEST

Tube	1	2	3	4	5	6	7
Fresh normal serum	0.5 mL	0.5 mL			0.5 mL	0.5 mL	
Patient's serum			0.5 mL				
Heat-inactivated normal serum				0.5 mL			0.5 mL
0.2 N HCl		0.05 mL	0.05 mL	0.05 mL		0.05 mL	0.05 mL
50% patient's red cells	0.05 mL	0.05 mL	0.05 mL	0.05 mL			
50% normal red cells					0.05 mL	0.05 mL	0.05 mL
Pattern of lysis in positive test	Trace	+++	++	—	—	—	—

Source: Adapted from Dacie, JC, and Lewis, SM: Paroxysmal nocturnal hemoglobinuria, clinical manifestations, hematology, and nature of the disease. Sernin Haematol 5:3, 1972, and Nelson, D: Clinical Diagnosis and Management by Laboratory Methods, ed 17. WB Saunders, Philadelphia, 1984, p 673.

Therapy

No specific therapeutic regimen is employed in the treatment of PNH. Treatment is usually directed toward the complications that arise from infections, anemia, and thromboses. In uncomplicated mild cases, therapy is not needed.

Certain patients with PNH have such severe bone marrow hypoplasia that bone marrow transplantation may be indicated. Successful transplantation has been reported in some severe cases, but it carries significant risks.[110] After successful transplantation, the abnormal clone of cells may be eliminated and replaced by a normal cell population.

Clinical Course and Prognosis

PNH is a chronic disease. Patients have survived 20 to 43 years after diagnosis, although the average survival is 10 years.[119] The most common cause of death is thromboembolism. Patients with bone marrow hypoplasia often die from infections or hemorrhage.[112] In a minority of patients, the disease may decrease in severity or completely disappear with time. Some patients have complete clinical remissions with persisting laboratory abnormalities. Occasionally, acute myelogenous leukemia develops in patients with PNH.[122,123] PNH has also been classified as a preleukemic or myelodysplastic syndrome.[110]

> ### CASE STUDY 1

A 26-year-old white woman diagnosed with rheumatoid arthritis came to the emergency department with complaints of weakness and shortness of breath. Laboratory findings revealed the patient was severely anemic. The patient had received many red cell transfusions over the past 8 years, but had not received any transfusions in over a year. The peripheral blood smear demonstrated a mild spherocytosis and moderate polychromasia. The crossmatch and antibody screen tests were weakly positive at the antiglobulin phase. On further testing, the patient's direct antiglobulin test (DAT) was also weakly positive, with IgG immunoglobulin coating her red cells. The effort to obtain compatible blood for transfusion was complicated because the patient's serum reacted weakly with all cells tested.

1. What is the most likely diagnosis?
2. What type of hemolysis is characteristic of this type of disorder?
3. What other laboratory tests may be requested to aid in the diagnosis and what are expected results?

Answers
1. Warm autoimmune hemolytic anemia, secondary to rheumatoid arthritis.
2. Extravascular hemolysis.
3. Indirect bilirubin (increased), urine urobilinogen (increased), reticulocyte count (increased).

> ### CASE STUDY 2

A 38-year-old man was diagnosed with pneumonia 3 weeks previously. He returned to the hospital because he was experiencing severe weakness and shortness of breath on slight exertion. The patient was pale and jaundiced. Laboratory findings revealed severe anemia. The peripheral blood smear demonstrated marked aggregation of erythrocytes. The crossmatch and antibody screen tests were both strongly positive at the room temperature phase (20°C). On further testing, the patient's DAT was also strongly positive, with complement proteins. The Donath-Landsteiner test was negative. Thermal amplitude studies revealed immunoglobulin reactivity up to 34°C.

Questions
1. What is the most likely diagnosis?
2. What other laboratory test values may be affected by the agglutination of RBCs? What is the remedy?
3. What is the treatment for this patient?

Answers
1. Cold agglutinin syndrome, secondary to pneumonia infection.
2. Certain complete blood count (CBC) values from an automated instrument will be erroneous because of

the agglutination of RBCs at room temperature (see p. 210). The blood should be warmed to 37°C and rerun through the instrument.
3. The patient should be kept warm until the primary infection subsides.

➤ CASE STUDY 3

A 50-year-old African-American man had recently returned from a trip to Africa to visit relatives. He complained of headaches, fatigue, and general malaise over the past 2 weeks. The patient then developed a high fever followed by severe chills, which persisted for approximately a day. The fever and chills subsided, and the patient thought he was getting better until last night when he experienced another bout of fever and chills. Laboratory findings revealed the patient was anemic and slightly leukopenic. The laboratory noted that odd, blue, "crescent moon" inclusions were seen in approximately 10% of his red cells. On further testing the DAT was negative. The crossmatch and antibody screening tests were also negative.

Questions
1. What is the most likely diagnosis?
2. What other laboratory tests should be requested to aid in the diagnosis?
3. What is the vector for this disease? What are the reasons for a recent increased incidence of this disease?

Answers
1. *Plasmodium falciparum.*
2. Thick smear preparation, stained with Giemsa or Wright's stain; it is best to use fingerstick blood rather than anticoagulated blood.
3. The vector is the *Anopheles* mosquito. The incidence of malaria is increasing because the parasite has developed resistance to antimalarial drugs, and the mosquito vector has developed resistance to some insecticides.

➤ CASE STUDY 4

A 43-year-old man presented to his physician with complaints of lower back pain, fatigue, easy bruising, and a sudden onset of dark urine on arising in the morning. Laboratory studies and a bone marrow aspirate were ordered by his physician. The CBC revealed an anemia (hematocrit, 28%), leukopenia (white blood cell [WBC] count, 3300/μL), and thrombocytopenia (platelets, 76,000/μL). The reticulocyte count was 5.1%, (3.2% corrected). The RBCs showed moderate polychromasia, slight anisocytosis, and poikilocytosis, and 1 nucleated RBC per 100 WBCs (see Fig. 13–23 and Color Plate 127). The chemistry profile was normal except for an increased LD value

and an increased indirect bilirubin. The bone marrow analysis revealed a hypercellular marrow with relative erythroid hyperplasia. There were adequate numbers of myeloid and platelet precursors (see Fig. 13–25 and Color Plate 129).

Further studies were performed after initial test results were evaluated. The urinary hemosiderin, sugar water test, and the Ham's test were all positive.

Questions
1. What is the most likely diagnosis?
2. What type of hemolysis is evident in this patient?
3. If the granulocytes in this patient were scored for LAP activity, what would you expect the result to be?
4. What alternative testing may be performed instead of Ham's test?

Answers
1. Paroxysmal nocturnal hemoglobinuria.
2. Intravascular hemolysis.
3. LAP would be expected to be decreased.
4. Immunophenotyping by flow cytometry may be performed to check for the absence of GPI-anchored proteins.

QUESTIONS

1. What are the mechanisms of immune hemolysis?
   a. IgG or IgM antibodies that activate the classical complement pathway
   b. Antibody-dependent cellular cytotoxicity (ADCC) mediated by NK cells, monocytes/macrophages, and granulocytes
   c. Complete or partial phagocytosis of antibody-coated erythrocytes
   d. All of the above

2. Which would best distinguish hemolytic anemia caused by immune mechanisms from other hemolytic anemias?
   a. Presence of spherocytes on peripheral blood film
   b. Increased reticulocyte count
   c. Enlarged spleen
   d. Positive DAT

3. Which is true concerning autoimmune hemolytic anemia?
   a. Majority of cases are of the "cold" type
   b. May be seen in transfusion reaction
   c. Is demonstrated in hemolytic disease of the newborn
   d. Antibodies are produced against one's own erythrocyte antigens

4. What is the process in which the immune system produces antibodies to foreign red cell antigens introduced into their circulation through transfusion, pregnancy, or organ transplantation?
   a. Alloimmune hemolytic anemia

b. Autoimmune hemolytic anemia

c. Drug-induced immune hemolytic anemia

d. None of the above

5. What causes hemolytic disease of the newborn (HDN)?

a. Maternal IgG antibodies, formed as a result of a previous blood exposure or pregnancy, cross the placenta and attach to fetal cells

b. Fetal IgG antibodies cross the placenta and attach to maternal red cells

c. Maternal IgM antibodies, formed as a result of a previous blood exposure or pregnancy, cross the placenta and attach to fetal cells

d. Fetal IgM antibodies attach to fetal red cells and cross the placenta to enter the mother's circulation

6. Which is not a characteristic of warm autoimmune hemolytic anemia?

a. Variable anemia

b. Reticulocytosis and spherocytosis

c. Positive result for Donath-Landsteiner test

d. DAT result usually positive for both IgG and C3d

7. What are features of cold agglutinin syndrome?

a. Usually an IgM antibody

b. Reticulocytosis and positive DAT

c. Tendency for spontaneous autoagglutination of RBC samples

d. All of the above

8. What is the principle of the Donath-Landsteiner test?

a. Antibody binds red cells at 37°C and causes lysis at 4°C

b. Antibody binds red cells at 4°C and causes lysis at 37°C

c. Antibody binds red cells at 4°C or 37°C and causes immediate lysis

d. Antibody binds red cells at 4°C or 37°C but causes lysis only at 4°C

9. What are causes for nonimmune hemolytic anemia?

a. Infections

b. Mechanical, chemical, and physical agents

c. Acquired membrane disorders

d. All of the above

10. Which of the following organisms is (are) associated with hemolytic anemia?

a. *Mycoplasma pneumoniae*

b. *Clostridium perfringens*

c. *Babesia microti*

d. All of the above

11. Which of the following, as measured by an automated hematology instrument, would most likely be affected by a cold agglutinin?

a. Hemoglobin

b. Hematocrit

c. Platelet count

d. Leukocyte count

12. Which of the following is a hemolytic anemia caused by an acquired somatic mutation in a hematopoietic stem cell?

a. Warm autoimmune hemolytic anemia (WAIHA)

b. Paroxysmal cold hemoglobinuria (PCH)

c. Paroxysmal nocturnal hemoglobinuria (PNH)

d. Drug-induced hemolytic anemia

13. Which statement best describes paroxysmal nocturnal hemoglobinuria?

a. Acquired hemolytic anemia associated with cellular membrane abnormalities

b. Congenital hemolytic anemia associated with the inflammatory response

c. Acquired or congenital hemolytic anemia associated with enzyme deficiencies

d. Hemolytic anemia of unknown origin associated with autoantibodies

14. What causes the red cell defect of PNH?

a. Rare red cell antigens

b. Lack of GPI-anchored proteins on the erythrocyte membrane

c. Excessive amounts of complement components C5 to C9

d. Glucose-6-phosphate-dehydrogenase enzyme deficiency

15. Which of the following is a correct description of the sugar water test (sucrose hemolysis test)?

a. PNH cells are lysed by complement after exposure to low-ionic-strength sugar water

b. PNH cells are lysed by antibody and complement after heating to 56°C in sugar water solution (5%)

c. Patient's serum is acidified to enhance complement binding and lysis of patient cells

d. Patient's serum is heat-inactivated and treated with HCl; complement is added; patient cell lysis occurs

16. What is a correct description of Ham's test (acidified serum lysis test)?

a. PNH cells are lysed by complement after exposure to low-ionic-strength sugar water

b. PNH cells are lysed by antibody and complement after heating to 56°C in sugar water solution (5%)

c. Patient's serum is acidified to enhance complement binding and lysis of patient cells

d. Patient's serum is heat-inactivated and treated with HCl; complement is added; patient cell lysis occurs

17. Which of the following drugs causes a hemolytic anemia resulting from production of "true autoantibodies" rather than antibodies to the drug or to the drug-erythrocyte complex?

a. Penicillin

b. Cephalosporin

c. Aldomet

d. Quinidine

SUMMARY CHART

➤ Complement is a group of serum proteins that interact with each other to bring about complement-dependent cell-mediated lysis.

➤ Intravascular hemolysis occurs when antibodies bind to antigenic determinants on red cells and activate the classical complement pathway.

➤ Antibody-dependent cellular cytotoxicity (ADCC) is a form of direct (intravascular) lysis of immunoglobulin-coated cells; effector cells contain receptors for IgG1 and IgG3, and complement proteins C3b and iC3b, which facilitate cell lysis.

➤ Hemoglobinemia, hemoglobinuria, and decreased haptoglobin levels are common findings in intravascular hemolysis.

➤ Extravascular hemolysis is the phagocytosis of red cells by fixed phagocytes within the mononuclear phagocyte system (MPS); the two major organs of the MPS are the spleen and liver.

➤ Common laboratory findings in extravascular hemolysis may include the presence of spherocytes, increased serum indirect bilirubin, and urine urobilinogen.

➤ In alloimmune hemolytic anemia, patients produce alloantibodies to foreign red cell antigens introduced through transfusions, pregnancy, or organ transplantation.

➤ In autoimmune hemolytic anemia (AIHA), patients develop antibodies to their own red cell antigens.

➤ In drug-induced hemolytic anemia, patients produce antibodies directed at a particular drug, its metabolites, or red cells coated with the drug; the four major drug-induced mechanisms include immune complex, drug adsorption, membrane modification, and methyldopa-induced mechanism.

➤ Acute hemolytic transfusion reactions are characterized by acute intravascular hemolysis and associated with the ABO blood group antibodies.

➤ A delayed hemolytic transfusion reaction is characterized by exposure to red cell antigens other than the ABO blood group; the reaction may occur from 2 to 10 days following transfusion and is generally the result of an anamnestic response to transfused red cells.

➤ Hemolytic disease of the newborn (HDN) is an immune hemolytic disorder caused by maternal-fetal blood group incompatibility; maternal IgG antibodies with ABO, Rh, or other blood group specificity cross the placenta and destroy antigen-containing fetal red cells.

➤ Warm autoimmune hemolytic anemia (WAIHA) accounts for 70% of autoimmune hemolytic anemias, and the DAT is positive for both IgG and C3d in 67% of cases, in 20% with IgG alone, and in 13% with C3d alone.

➤ The specificity of normal cold autoantibodies includes anti-I, anti-H, and anti-IH, which react at temperatures from 4°C to 22°C.

➤ Cold agglutinin syndrome (CAS) represents 16% of autoimmune hemolytic anemias; it occurs at a wide thermal range (4°C to more than 30°C); antibody specificity is an IgM toward anti-I, anti-i, and anti-Pr.

➤ Secondary CAS, caused by infections to *Mycoplasma pneumoniae* and infectious mononucleosis, has antibody specificity toward anti-I and anti-i, respectively.

➤ Paroxysmal cold hemoglobinuria (PCH) is the least common type of AIHA, with an incidence of only 1% to 7%. Red cell destruction is caused by an IgG autoantibody termed an *autohemolysin*, which binds to patient cells at lower temperatures and fixes complement at warmer temperatures, causing intravascular hemolysis.

➤ The Donath-Landsteiner test is the classic diagnostic test for PCH.

➤ The four species of malaria that can infect humans through the mosquito vector are *Plasmodium falciparum, P. vivax, P. ovale,* and *P. malariae; P. falciparum* demonstrates an often fatal course.

➤ Bartonellosis is caused by the organism *Bartonella bacilliformis* and is transmitted by the sand fly; the disease is characterized by a hemolytic phase and a tumor phase.

➤ *Microangiopathic hemolytic anemia* refers to a group of disorders that are characterized by fragmentation of the red cells as they pass through abnormal arterioles, resulting in intravascular hemolysis.

➤ Spur-cell anemia is a condition in which the red cells assume a characteristic shape, with a number of fine, fingerlike spike projections resembling acanthocytes; it is frequently caused by alcoholic cirrhosis.

➤ Paroxysmal nocturnal hemoglobinuria is an acquired hemolytic anemia resulting from an abnormality in the red cell membrane that causes the red cells to be sensitive to the hemolytic action of complement. Diagnostic tests include the sugar water test and Ham's test.

References

1. Roitt, I, et al: Immunology, ed. 5. Mosby, Philadelphia, 1998, pp 45–52.
2. Fearson, ST, and Austin, KF: The alternate pathway of complement—A system of host resistance to microbial infections. N Engl J Med 303:259, 1980.
3. Frank MM: Mechanisms of cell destruction in immunohemolytic anemia. In Bell, CA (ed): Laboratory Management of Hemolysis. AABB, Arlington, VA, 1979.
4. Garratty, G: Autoimmune hemolytic anemia. In Garratty, G (ed): Immunobiology of Transfusion Medicine. Marcel Decker, New York, 1994.
5. Devine, DV: Complement. In Anderson, KC, and Ness, PM (eds): Scientific Basis of Transfusion Medicine: Implications for Clinical Practice. WB Saunders, Philadelphia, 1994.
6. Garratty, G: Factors affecting the pathogenicity of red cell auto and alloantibodies. In Nance, SJ (ed): Immune Destruction of Red Blood Cells. AABB, Arlington, VA, 1989.
7. Zupanska, B: Cellular immunoassays and their use for predicting the clinical significance of antibodies. In Garratty, G (eds): Immunobiology of Transfusion Medicine. Marcel Decker, New York, 1994.
8. Anderson, DR, and Kelton, JG: Mechanisms of intravascular and extravascular cell destruction. In Nance, SJ (ed): Immune Destruction of Red Blood Cells. AABB, Arlington, VA, 1989.
9. Rozsnyay, X, et al: Distinctive role of IgG1 and IgG3 isotypes in FcγR-mediated function. Immunology 66:491, 1989.
10. Horsewood, P, and Kelton, JG: Macrophage-mediated cell destruction. In Garratty, G (ed): Immunobiology of Transfusion Medicine. Marcel Decker, New York, 1994.
11. Freedman, J, and Semple, JW: Complement in transfusion medicine. In Garratty, G (ed): Immunobiology of Transfusion Medicine. Marcel Decker, New York, 1994.

12. Walker, RH (ed): Technical Manual, ed 11. AABB, Bethesda, MD, 1993.
13. Mollison, PL, et al: Blood Transfusions in Clinical Medicine, ed 9. Blackwell, Oxford, 1993.
14. Ness PM, et al: The differentiation of delayed serologic and delayed hemolytic transfusion reactions: Incidence, long-term serologic findings, and clinical significance. Transfusion 30:688, 1990.
15. Mollison, PL: Some aspects of Rh hemolytic disease and its prevention. In: Garratty, G (ed): Hemolytic Disease of the Newborn. AABB, Arlington, VA, 1984.
16. Jakobowicz, R, et al: Immunization of Rh negative volunteers by repeated injections of very small amounts of Rh positive blood. Vox Sang 23:376, 1972.
17. Keith, LG, and Berger, GS: The risk of Rh immunization associated with abortion, spontaneous and induced. In Frigoletto, FD, et al (eds): Rh Hemolytic Disease: New Strategy for Eradication. GK Hall, Boston, 1982.
18. Siegel, DL, and Silberstein, LE: Red blood cell autoantibodies. In Anderson, KC, and Ness, PM (eds): Scientific Basis of Transfusion Medicine: Implications for Clinical Practice. WB Saunders, Philadelphia, 1994.
19. Dacie, JV, and Worlledge, SM: Auto-immune hemolytic anemias. Progr Hematol 6:82, 1969.
20. Petz, LD, and Garratty, G: Acquired immune hemolytic anemias. Churchill Livingstone, New York, 1980.
21. Gilliland, BC, et al: Red cell antibodies in acquired hemolytic anemia with negative antiglobulin serum tests. N Engl J Med 285:252, 1971.
22. Rowe, GP, and Davies, H: A study using an enzyme linked antiglobulin test on patients with a positive direct antiglobulin test (absract). Book of Abstracts from the ISBT/AABB Joint Congress. AABB, Arlington, VA, 1990, p 87.
23. Pirofsky, B: Autoimmunization and the autoimmune hemolytic anemias. Williams & Wilkins, Baltimore, 1969, p 63.
24. Bottiger, LE, and Westerholm, B: Acquired haemolytic anaemia. Acta Med Scand 193:223, 1973.
25. Domen, RE: An overview of immune hemolytic anemias. Cleveland Clin J Med 65:89, 1998.
26. Hsu, TCS, et al: Instrumented PVP-augmented antiglobulin tests. Vox Sang 26:305, 1974.
27. Sokol, RJ, et al: Red cell autoantibodies, multiple immunoglobulin classes and autoimmune hemolysis. Transfusion 30:417, 1990.
28. Victoria, EJ, et al: IgG red blood cell autoantibodies in autoimmune hemolytic anemia bind to epitopes on red cell membrane band 3 glycoprotein. J Lab Clin Med 115:74, 1990.
29. Kruskall, MS: Clinical management of transfusions to patients with red cell antibodies. In Nance, SJ (ed): Immune Destruction of Red Blood Cells. AABB, Arlington, VA, 1989.
30. Salama, A, et al: Red blood cell transfusion in warm-type autoimmune haemolytic anaemia. Lancet 340:1515, 1992.
31. Rosse, JF: Quantitative immunology of immune hemolytic anemia. II. The relationship of cell-bound antibody to hemolysis and the effect of treatment. J Clin Invest 50:734, 1971.
32. Kay, NE, and Douglas, SD: Monocyte-erythrocyte interaction in vitro in immune hemolytic anemias. Blood 50:889, 1977.
33. Smith, LA: Autoimmune hemolytic anemias: Characteristics and classification. Clin Lab Sci 12:110, 1999.
34. Hashimoto, C: Autoimmune hemolytic anemia. Clin Rev Allergy Immunol 16:285, 1998.
35. Beck, ML: The I blood group collection. In Moulds, JM, and Woods, LL (eds): Blood Groups: P, I, Sd^a and Pr. AABB, Arlington, VA, 1991.
36. Issitt, PD: Applied Blood Group Serology, ed 3. Montgomery Scientific, Miami, FL, 1985.
37. Issitt, PD: Cold-reacting autoantibodies outside the I and P blood groups. In Moulds, JM, and Woods, LL (eds): Blood Groups: P, I, Sd^a and Pr. AABB, Arlington, VA, 1991.
38. Garratty, G, et al: The correlation of cold agglutinin titrations in saline and albumin with haemolytic anaemia. Br J Haematol 35:587, 1977.
39. Mougey, R: Cold autoimmune hemolytic anemia: A review of clinical and laboratory considerations. Immunohematology 1:1, 1984.
40. Judd, WJ: Investigation and management of immune hemolysis-autoantibodies and drugs. In Wallace, ME, and Lievitt, JS (eds): Current Applications and Interpretation of the Direct Antiglobulin Test. AABB, Arlington, VA, 1988.
41. Shirey, RS, and Barrasso, C: Cold agglutinins. In: Continuing Education Slide Presentation. Organon Teknika, 1993.
42. Janney, FA, et al: Cold hemagglutinin cross-reactivity with Mycoplasma pneumoniae. Infec Immun 22:29, 1978.
43. Costea, N, et al: Inhibition of cold agglutinins (anti-I) by M. pneumoniae antigens. Proc Soc Exp Biol (NY) 139:476, 1972.
44. Capra, JP, et al: Light chain sequences of human IgM cold agglutinins. Proc Natl Acad Sci Wash 69:40, 1972.
45. Harbo, M, and Lind, K: Light chain type of transiently occurring cold haemagglutinins. Scand J Haematol 3:269, 1966.
46. Jenkins, WJ, et al: Infectious mononucleosis: An unsuspected source of anti-i. Br J Haematol 11:480, 1965.
47. Wolledge, SM, and Dacie, JV: Haemolytic and other anaemias in infectious mononucleosis. In Carter, HG, and Penman, RL (eds): Infectious Mononucleosis. Blackwell Scientific, Oxford, 1969.
48. Rosenfield, RE, et al: Anti-i, a frequent cold agglutinin in infectious mononucleosis. Vox Sang 10:631, 1965.
49. Horwitz, CA, et al: Cold agglutinins in infectious mononucleosis and heterophile-antibody-negative mononucleosis like syndromes. Blood 50:195, 1977.
50. Bell, WR, et al: Cold agglutinin hemolytic anemia: Management with an environmental suit. Ann Intern Med 106:243, 1987.
51. Anstall, HB, and Blaylock, RC: The P blood group system: Biochemistry, genetics and clinical significance. In Moulds, JM, and Woods, LL (eds): Blood Groups: P, I, Sd^a and Pr. AABB, Arlington, VA, 1991.
52. Donath, J, and Landsteiner, K: Über kälte häemoglobinurie. Ergebn Hyg Bakt 7:184, 1925.
53. Levine, P, et al: The specificity of the antibody in paroxysmal cold hemoglobinuria (PCH). Transfusion 3:278, 1963.
54. McCann, EL, et al: IgM autoagglutinins in warm autoimmune hemolytic anemia: A poor prognostic feature. Acta Haematol 88:120, 1992.
55. Shirey, RS, et al: Fatal immune hemolytic anemia and hepatic failure associated with a warm-reacting IgM autoantibody. Vox Sang 52:219, 1987.
56. Sokol, RJ, et al: Autoimmune haemolysis: An 18 year study of 865 cases referred to a regional transfusion center. BMJ 282:2023, 1981.
57. Shulman, IA, et al: Autoimmune hemolytic anemia with both cold and warm autoantibodies. JAMA 253:1746, 1985.
58. Worlledge, SM: Immune drug induced haemolytic anaemias. In Girdwood, RH (ed): Blood Disorders Due to Drugs and Other Agents. Excerpta Medica, Amsterdam, 1973, p 11.
59. Garratty, G, and Petz, LD: Drug-induced immune hemolytic anemia. Am J Med 58:398, 1975.
60. Garratty, G, et al: The effect of methyldopa and procainamide on supressor cell activity in relation to red cell autoantibody production. Br J Haematol 84:310, 1993.
61. Mueller-Eckhardt, C, and Salama, A: Drug-induced immune cytopenias: A unifying pathogenic concept with special emphasis on the role of drug metabolites. Trans Med Rev 4:69, 1990.
62. Ackroyd, JF: The immunological basis of purpura due to drug hypersensitivity. Proc R Soc Med 55:30, 1962.
63. Jamin, D, et al: An explanation for nonimmunologic adsorption of proteins onto red blood cells. Blood 67:993, 1986.
64. Garratty, G: Review: Immune hemolytic anemia and/or positive direct antiglobulin tests caused by drugs. Immunohematology 12:41 1994.
65. Krogstad, DJ: Malaria as a reemerging disease. Epidemiol Rev 18:77, 1996.
66. Kain, KC, and Keystone, JS: Malaria in travelers. Infect Dis Clin North Am 12:267, 1998.
67. Buetler, E: Hemolytic anemia due to infections with microorganisms. In Beutler, E, et al (eds): Williams Hematology, ed 5. McGraw-Hill, New York, 1995.
68. Warhurst, DC, and Williams, JE: Laboratory diagnosis of malaria. J Clin Pathol. 49:33, 1996.
69. Ruebush, TK II, et al: Human babesiosis on Nantucket island. Ann Intern Med 86:6, 1977.
70. Jacoby, GA, et al: Treatment of transfusion-transmitted babesiosis by exchange transfusion. N Engl J Med 303:1098, 1980.
71. Smith, RP, et al: Transfusion-acquired babesiosis and failure of antibiotic treatment. JAMA 256:2726, 1986.
72. Boustani, MR, and Gelfand, JA: Babesiosis. Clin Infect Dis 22:611, 1996.
73. Chisholm, ES, et al: Indirect immunofluorescence test for human Babesia microti infection: Antigenic specificity. Am J Trop Med Hyg 35:921, 1985.
74. Ricketts, WE: Bartonella bacilliformis anemia (Oroya fever). A study of thirty cases. Blood 3:1025, 1948.
75. Reynafarje, C, and Ramos, J: The hemolytic anemia of bartonellosis. Blood 17:562, 1961.
76. Clancy, MT, and O'Brian, S: Fatal Clostridium welchii septicaemia following acute cholecystitis. Br J Surg 62:518, 1975.
77. Simpkins, H, et al: Structural and compositional changes in the red cell membrane during Clostridium welchii infection. Br J Haem 21:173, 1971.
78. Mahn, HE, and Dantuono, LM: Postabortal septicotoxemia due to Clostridium welchii. J Obstet Gynecol 70:604, 1955.
79. Erslev, AJ: Traumatic cardiac hemolytic anemia. In Beutler, E, et al (eds): Williams Hematology, ed 5. McGraw-Hill, New York, 1995.
80. Maraj, R, et al: Evaluation of hemolysis in patients with prosthetic heart valves. Clin Cardiol 21:387, 1998.
81. Harker, LA, and Slichter, SJ: Studies of platelet and fibrinogen kinetics in patients with prosthetic heart valves. N Engl J Med 283:1302, 1970.
82. Slater, SD, et al: Renal function in chronic intravascular haemolysis associated with prosthetic cardiac valves. Clin Sci 44:511, 1973.
83. Kornowski, R, et al: Erythropoietin therapy obviates the need for recurrent transfusion in a patient with severe hemolysis due to prosthetic valves. Chest 102:315, 1992.
84. Fleischer, R: Über eine neute form von hämoglobinurie beim menschen. Berlin Klin Wochenschr 18:691, 1881.
85. Gilligan, DR, et al: Psychologic intravascular hemolysis of exercise: Hemoglobinemia and hemoglobinuria following cross-country runs. J Clin Invest 22:859, 1943.
86. Streeton, JA: Traumatic hemoglobinuria caused by karate exercises. Lancet 2:191, 1967.
87. Furie, B, and Penn, AS. Pigmenturia from conga drumming: Hemoglobinuria and myoglobinuria. Ann Intern Med 80:727, 1974.
88. Erslev, AJ: March hemoglobinuria and sports anemia. In Beutler, E, et al (eds): Williams Hematology, ed 5. McGraw-Hill, New York, 1995.
89. Bull, BS, et al: Microangiopathic haemolytic anaemia: Mechanisms of red cell fragmentation: in vitro studies. Br J Haematol 14:643, 1968.
90. Kwaan, HC: Clinicopathologic features of thrombotic thrombocytopenia purpura. Semin Hematol 24:71, 1987.
91. Rubenberg, ML, et al: Microangiopathic haemolytic anaemia: The experimen-

tal production of haemolysis and red cell fragmentation by defibrination in vivo. Br J Haematol 14:627, 1968.

92. Martinez, J: Microangiopathic hemolytic anemia. In: Beutler, E, et al (eds): Williams Hematology, ed 5. McGraw-Hill, New York, 1995.

93. Jenkins, GC, et al: Arsenic poisoning: Massive haemolysis with minimal impairment of renal function. Br Med J 2:78, 1965.

94. Beutler, E: Hemolytic anemia due to chemical and physical agents. In: Beutler, E, et al (eds): Williams Hematology, ed 5. McGraw-Hill, New York, 1995.

95. Waldron, HA: The anemia of lead poisoning: A review. Br J Ind Med 23:83, 1966.

96. Klein, WJ Jr, et al: Acute copper intoxication: A hazard of hemodialysis. Arch Intern Med 129:578, 1972.

97. Hansen, PB: Wilson's disease presenting with severe haemolytic anaemia. Ugeskr Laeger 150:1229, 1988.

98. Boulard, M, et al: The effect of copper on red cell enzyme activities. J Clin Invest 51:459,1972.

99. Shen, SC, et al: Studies on the destruction of red blood cells. III. Mechanism and complications of hemoglobinuria in patients with thermal burns: Spherocytosis and increased osmotic fragility of red blood cells. N Engl J Med 229:701, 1943.

100. Wagner, HN Jr, et al: Removal of erythrocytes from the circulation. Arch Intern Med 110:90, 1962.

101. Beutler, E: Paroxysmal nocturnal hemoglobinuria. In: Beutler, E, et al (eds): Williams Hematology, ed 5. McGraw-Hill, New York, 1995.

102. Gull, WP: A case of intermittent hematuria, with remarks. Guys Hosp Rep 12:381, 1866.

103. Rosse, WF: Evolution of clinical understanding: Paroxysmal nocturnal hemoglobinuria as a paradigm. Am J Hematol 42:122, 1993.

104. Ham, TH, and Dingle, JH: Studies on destruction of red blood cells—II. Chronic hemolytic anemia with paroxysmal nocturnal hemoglobinuria—Certain immunological aspects of the hemolytic mechanism with special reference to serum complement. J Clin Invest 18:657, 1939.

105. Ham, TH: Chronic hemolytic anemia with paroxysmal nocturnal hemoglobinuria—A study of the mechanism of hemolysis in relation to acid base equilibrium. N Engl J Med 217:915, 1937.

106. Rosse, WF: Phosphatidylinositol-linked proteins and paroxysmal nocturnal hemoglobinuria. Blood 75:1595, 1990.

107. Nicholson-Weller, A, et al: Deficiency of the complement regulatory protein, "decay accelerating factor" on membranes of granulocytes, monocytes and platelets in paroxysmal nocturnal hemoglobinuria. N Engl J Med 312:1091, 1985.

108. Rosse, WF: Paroxysmal nocturnal hemoglobinuria and decay accelerating factor. Annu Rev Med 41:431, 1990.

109. Zalman, LS, et al: Deficiency of the homologous factor in paroxysmal nocturnal hemoglobinuria. J Exp Med 165:572, 1987.

110. Bessler, M, and Hillmen P: Somatic mutation and clonal selection in the pathogenesis and in the control of paroxysmal nocturnal hemoglobinuria. Sem Hematol 35:149, 1998.

111. Jarva, H, and Meri, S: Paroxysmal nocturnal hemoglobinuria: The disease and a hypothesis for a new treatment. Scand J Immunol 49:119, 1999.

112. Wintrobe, ME, et al: Clinical Hematology, ed 8. Lea & Febiger, Philadelphia, 1981, p 978.

113. Rosse, WF: Paroxysmal nocturnal hemoglobinuria in aplastic anemia. Clin Haematol 7:541, 1978.

114. Kjeldsberg, C, et al: Hematologic Disease, Practical Diagnosis, ed 2. ASCP Press, Chicago, 1989, p 162.

115. Chow, FL, Telen, MJ, and Rosse, WF: The acetylcholinesterase defect in paroxysmal nocturnal hemoglobinuria; Evidence that the enzyme is absent from the cell membrane. Blood 66:940, 1986.

116. Okuda, K, et al: Membrane expression of decay accelerating factor on neutrophils from normal individuals and patients with paroxysmal nocturnal hemoglobinuria. Blood 75:1186, 1990.

117. Brunzel, NA: Fundamentals of Urine and Body Fluid Analysis. WB Saunders, Philadelphia, 1994, p 257.

118. Hoffbrand, AV, and Lewis, SM: Post Graduate Hematology, ed 2. Appleton-Century Crofts, New York, 1981, p 232.

119. Dacie, JV, and Lewis, SM: Paroxysmal nocturnal hemoglobinuria, clinical manifestations, hematology and nature of the disease. Sem Haematol 5:3, 1972.

120. Leach, AP, and Gaumer, HR: Diagnosis and detection of PNH using GPI anchored proteins. Clin Lab Sci, 9:191, 1996.

121. Schubert, J, et al: Diagnosis of paroxysmal nocturnal haemoglobinuria using immunophenotyping of peripheral blood cells. Br J Haematol 79:487, 1991.

122. Crowell, DE, et al: Paroxysmal nocturnal hemoglobinuria terminating as acute leukemia. Cancer 43:1914, 1979.

123. Krause, JR: Paroxysmal nocturnal hemoglobinuria and acute nonlymphoblastic leukemia. Cancer 51:2078, 1983.

14 Anemia Associated with Other Disorders

Carmen J. Julius, MD
Sandra Gwaltney-Krause, MA, MT(ASCP)

OBJECTIVES

At the end of this chapter, the learner should be able to:

1. Describe the anemia of inflammation.
2. List the many causes of the anemia of inflammation.
3. Identify laboratory findings characteristic of the anemia of inflammation.
4. List the cytokines important in inducing the anemia of inflammation.
5. Describe the treatment for anemia of inflammation.
6. List the three categories of causes of the anemia associated with malignancy and some causes under each category.
7. Name the major cause of the anemia associated with renal disease and renal failure.
8. Discuss the many causes of the anemia associated with liver disease.
9. Describe the characteristics of the red blood cells in anemia associated with liver disease.
10. Describe the etiology of the anemia associated with alcoholism.

Anemias produced by inflammation and systemic diseases are perhaps the most common hematologic abnormalities encountered in the laboratory. It is important for the clinician and the medical technologist to recognize the characteristics of these anemias in patients with systemic diseases and to understand the hematologic assays that can differentiate them from other causes of anemia. Anemia without other clinical symptoms at the initial evaluation of a patient may be the first indication of a systemic disease (e.g., an occult malignancy). Likewise, a sudden change in the complete blood count (CBC) of a patient who has been diagnosed with an inflammatory or systemic disease may indicate a new complication.

Many disease entities are outlined in the following pages. All have a common theme that forms the basis of this chapter, that is, the effects of systemic disorders (i.e., nonhematologic disorders) on bone marrow and red blood cell production.

➤ ANEMIA ASSOCIATED WITH CHRONIC DISORDERS AND INFLAMMATION

Anemia associated with chronic disorders (ACD) is the term formerly used to describe the anemia associated with chronic infections and other states of chronic inflammation. Because these disorders are common, this is one of the most frequently encountered anemias.[1] Recent research has demonstrated a mechanism involved in the inflammatory response to tissue injury, rendering the term ACD obsolete. Anemia of inflammation (AOI) has been suggested as a more appropriate term because it more definitely describes the mechanism of the disorder.[2,3] Therefore, this term is used throughout this chapter.

The Inflammatory Response and Body Defense Mechanisms

The General Inflammatory Response (First Line of Defense)

Inflammation is one of the body's responses to tissue injury from physical agents, foreign organisms, and immune reactions in the host. Inflammatory and hemostatic responses occur simultaneously to control any damage at the injured area (see Chaps. 26 and 27). The coagulation cascade and the complement, fibrinolytic, and kinin systems interact to modulate inflammation (see Chaps. 23, 26, and 27).

During the inflammatory process, complement can be activated directly by microorganisms via the alternative pathway or the antibody-induced classical pathway. The presence of C3a, C5a, and other chemotaxins attracts phagocytes to the site of injury, where they recognize and phagocytize foreign substances or organisms. Neutrophilic granulocytes, monocytes, and macrophages possess receptors for complement that can induce exocytosis of granules containing proteolytic enzymes, free ion radicals, and other inflammatory metabolites and endocytosis of complement-coated foreign substances.

Inflammation will continue as long as injury and damage continue. When the source of inflammation is persistent and the condition is chronic, mediators from the humoral and cell-mediated immune responses contribute to the onset of anemia. (Fig. 14–1). Table 14–1 lists the functions of the various types of T-cell lymphocytes in cell-mediated immunity.

Etiology and Pathophysiology

Evidence does not uphold one single cause for AOI, but rather several overlapping mechanisms, all induced by the inflammatory process. Possible causes include (1) de-

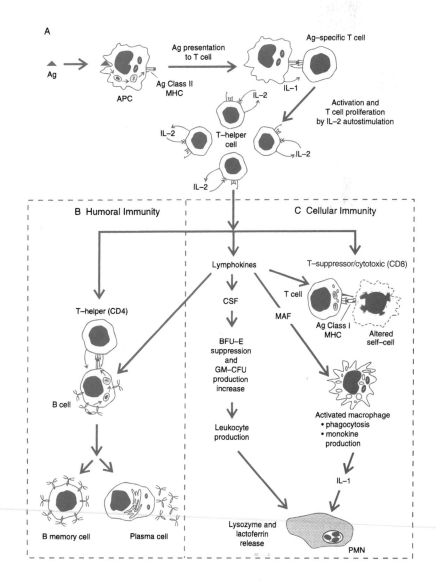

➤ **FIGURE 14–1** The mechanism of humoral and cellular immunity. *A.* The antigen phagocytized by the APC is digested, and small antigenic fragments or epitopes are associated with the class II MHC and presented to a T cell with a receptor specific for the antigen. Formation of the antigen-receptor complex between the two cells and IL-1 secreted by the APC provide the signals for the T cell to be activated and secrete IL-2 for its autostimulation and proliferation to effector T-helper cells. *B.* Humoral immunity. The T-helper effector cell (CD4) and some of its lymphokines provide the necessary signals for the B cell with the same antigen specificity to be activated and proliferate to B memory and antibody-producing plasma cells. *C.* Cellular immunity. Some of the lymphokines from the activated CD4 cells and the complex formed between antigens associated with class I MHC on altered self-cell and T-cytotoxic cell (CD8) receptors cause the activation of the CD8 cells, which mediate the cytotoxic killing of the altered self-cells. Some of the other lymphokines produced also play significant roles in hematopoiesis and activation of phagocytic cells. (Ag = antigen; APC = antigen-presenting cell; MHC = major histocompatibility complex; IL-1 = interleukin-1; IL-2 = interleukin-2; CSF = colony-stimulating factor; BFU-E = burst-forming unit–erythroid; GM-CFU = granulocyte/macrophage–colony-forming units; PMN = polymorphonuclear neutrophils; MAF = macrophage-activating factor.)

> ## Table 14-1
> ### THYMUS-DERIVED LYMPHOCYTES
>
> **Helper (Inducer) T Cells**
>
> Aid B-cell maturation in bone marrow
>
> Supply activating (permissive) signals to B cells
>
> Activate the generation of different antibody classes
>
> Activate effector T cells
>
> **Effector T cells**
>
> Two types, producing delayed hypersensitivity and cytotoxic effects. Responsible for:
>
> 1. Immunologic surveillance for malignant cells
>
> 2. Eradication of established viral and fungal infection
>
> 3. Eradication of intracellular bacterial infection
>
> 4. Destruction of parasites
>
> **Suppressor (Immunoregulatory) T Cells**
>
> Control inflammation produced by T cells
>
> Control antibody production
>
> Balance ratio of immunoglobulin classes
>
> Block activation of T- and B-cell clones reactive to "self"

Source: From Dwyer, JM: The Cell-Mediated Immune System. Cutter Biologicals, Emeryville, CA, 1982, p. 3, with permission.

creased red blood cell (RBC) life span, (2) impaired iron metabolism from faulty iron release from reticuloendothelial (RE) stores, (3) decreased erythropoietin levels, and (4) suppression of erythropoiesis by cytokines from activated macrophages and lymphocytes because of the underlying disease and inflammation. Each of these possibilities contributes to AOI.[4] Table 14–2 lists the cytokines that contribute to inflammation and Table 14–3 summarizes the functions of macrophages.

Decreased Red Blood Cell Survival and Life Span

Decreased life span of RBCs is seen in patients with AOI.[4] Mean survival of RBCs in some cases is 90 days, compared with 120 days in healthy persons.[4] The mechanism for this decrease is unclear, but it may be because of the extracorpuscular effects of activated macrophage-monocytes of the reticuloendothelial system.[5,6] Activated macrophages clear minimally damaged erythrocytes from the circulation more rapidly, including red cells damaged by the infectious process. These cells have increased phagocytic capabilities in patients with inflammatory processes and may be responsible for the shortened erythrocyte survival.

Reticuloendothelial Iron Block

Anemia from reticuloendothelial iron block is another possible contributor to AOI. Although there is a decrease in intestinal iron absorption[4] and impaired iron reutilization by the hepatocytes in these patients,[4] there is an abundance of iron transported to the reticuloendothelial system stores.[7] Iron in the reticuloendothelial system stores is normally available to the plasma by both slow and quick release mechanisms.[8] In AOI, there is increased apoferritin synthesis.[9] Surplus apoferritin binds a larger amount of iron en-

tering the cell.[9] Therefore, the rapid release mechanism or pool of iron is markedly decreased.

Macrophages of the reticuloendothelial system demonstrate large coarse aggregates of iron despite the low serum iron. The iron appears trapped within the reticuloendothelial system and is unable to be fully utilized in erythropoiesis. Ferritin is increased because of the increased reticuloendothelial system iron stores (see Chap. 6). This results in the paradoxic ferrokinetics typical of AOI (i.e., a sideropenic or functionally iron-deficient state). The resulting hypoferremia sets off a "domino effect" of decreased transferrin saturation, which limits the supply of iron to the marrow and increases the amount of free erythrocyte protoporphyrin (FEP)—that is, a porphyrin ring without iron.[6] Thus there is decreased heme production.

Decreased Erythropoietin Levels

One of the controversies regarding AOI is whether or not patients have an ineffective level of erythropoietin.[10,11] Numerous investigators have reported that AOI is characterized by a blunted erythropoietin response; that is, for any given decrease in hemoglobin or hematocrit, the increase in serum or plasma erythropoietin is less than would be found in an equally anemic patient with iron deficiency.[12–14] From this information it appears that the patient attempts to counteract the anemia with increased erythropoietin production by the kidneys, but that the response is not adequate for compensation of the anemia. The response of the bone marrow to erythropoietin is much less than expected for the amount of erythropoietin secreted.[15] This is most likely the major problem and perhaps one of the major reasons for the development of AOI.[16]

Suppression of Erythropoiesis and the Role of Cytokines

One of the newest keys to understanding anemia of inflammation is the suppressor-inhibitor effects of erythropoiesis by interleukin-1 (IL-1), tumor necrosis factor–alpha (TNF-α) and interferon gamma (IFN-γ).[16] Sera from patients with chronic inflammatory disorders (e.g., rheumatoid arthritis, systemic lupus erythematosus, and juvenile chronic arthritis) have been shown to inhibit erythropoiesis in vitro.[17,18] The inhibition of early erythrocytic progenitors, burst-forming unit–erythroid (BFU-E) and colony-forming unit–erythroid (CFU-E), corresponds with the severity of the anemia and indicators of inflammation such as the presence of acute phase reactants. Research now indicates that cytokines may be the key signal regulating hematopoiesis in inflammatory disease states.[16]

IL-1 has been examined for its potential hematopoietic suppressive capabilities because of its mediation of various facets of the acute phase reaction. There is also a close correlation between the severity of anemia and the severity of inflammatory activity.

Evidence also suggests that TNF-α, another cytokine from activated macrophages, may be involved in the pathogenesis of AOI.[19] Very low concentrations of TNF-α were shown to inhibit erythroid progenitor growth in normal bone marrow cultures. This was demonstrated at concentrations similar to those found in affected patients.[16]

It is becoming increasingly evident that what was originally regarded by early investigators as a "simple anemia" is far from simple. The effect of monokines and lymphokines

> **Table 14-2**
CYTOKINES THAT CONTRIBUTE TO INFLAMMATION

Cytokine	Target Cell	Activity
IL-1	T cells, B cells, macrophages, and tissue cells	Lymphocyte activation, macrophage activation, acute-phase reaction
IL-2	T lymphocytes	Stimulates proliferation of activated T cells
IL-3 (multilineage colony-stimulating factor)	Stem cells	Stimulates differentiation of bone marrow stem cells
IL-4 (B-cell growth factor)	B lymphocytes	B-cell proliferation
IL-5	B lymphocytes, eosinophils, precursor cells	B-cell growth and differentiation, eosinophil differentiation
IL-6	B lymphocytes, hepatocytes	Stimulates antibody production and acute-phase reactants
Migration inhibition factor (MIF)	Macrophages	Inhibits migration
Macrophage activation factor (MAF)	Macrophages	Activates macrophages and enhances their functions
Leukocyte chemotaxis factor (LCF)	Phagocytes	Promotes chemotaxis to site of injury
Leukocyte inhibition factor (LIF)	Phagocytes	Inhibits migration
GM-CSF	Stem cells	Stimulates differentiation of granulocyte-monocyte precursor cells
M-CSF	Stem cells	Stimulates differentiation of monocytes
G-CSF	Stem cells	Stimulates differentiation of granulocytes
Interferon gamma (INF-γ)	Macrophages	Activates macrophages for cytotoxic functions; induces MHC II molecules on APCs
Tumor necrosis factor-alpha (TNF-α)	Macrophages, granulocytes	Activates macrophages, granulocytes, and cytotoxic cells

Abbreviations: MHC = major histocompatibility complex; GM-CSF = granulocyte/macrophage–colony-stimulating factor; M-CSF = monocyte–colony-stimulating factor; G-CSF = granulocyte–colony-stimulating factor; APC = antigen-processing cell.

on granulocyte, macrophage, and other hematopoietic progenitor cells appears to be responsible for AOI. Indeed, mechanisms responsible for host protection against infection and tissue injury become detrimental to the host indirectly. Although the exact mechanism is still being researched, IL-1 and TNF-α (products of activated macrophages) have emerged as key pathogenic factors.[15] Synergy among many cytokines has also been postulated.[4,20] Theoretically, any disease that involves tissue injury and inflammation can, over a period of 1 to 2 months, result in anemia.

Characteristics

Anemia of inflammation is a hypoproliferative, mild anemia that is usually normocytic and normochromic. There is very little reticulocytosis for the severity or degree of anemia. It may be hypochromic if the disease increases in severity.

Anemia of inflammation is characterized by a normal or low mean corpuscular hemoglobin concentration (MCHC), mean corpuscular volume (MCV), a low serum iron level, decreased total iron-binding capacity (TIBC), and a low iron transferrin saturation, despite normal to increased iron stores in reticuloendothelial cells. The fact that iron stores can be elevated in bone marrow aspirates in AOI is helpful in differentiating this anemia from iron-deficiency anemia. Indeed, bone marrow iron stores are increased, yet RBC

iron is decreased. Sideroblast (iron-laden nucleated RBC precursors) counts approach 0%. Normal range is at least 15% to 20% of all nucleated RBC precursors. This is in contrast to iron-deficiency anemia, in which both storage and sideroblast iron are markedly decreased or absent.

Serum ferritin levels are usually increased in AOI—another useful aid in differentiating it from iron-deficiency anemia (Table 14–4). Transferrin saturation generally falls between 5% and 16%. Free erythrocyte protoporphyrins are elevated because no iron is available to the red cell precursors for incorporation into the porphyrin ring. Thus the RBC cannot complete production of the heme moiety for production of the hemoglobin molecule.

Slight decreases can be seen in hematocrit (Hct), hemoglobin (Hgb), MCV, and MCHC, with a corresponding increase in RBC distribution width (RDW).[21] The anemia can become fully developed within 1 to 2 months after the onset of the illness or inflammatory stimulus and usually worsens as the underlying disease becomes aggravated or more severe.

Several other biochemical changes occur in patients with anemia of inflammation. Acute-phase reactants appear in the serum, including fibrinogen, C-reactive protein, amyloid A protein, ceruloplasmin, haptoglobin, and C3.[3] The increase in fibrinogen contributes to the accelerated eryth-

> **Table 14-3**
FUNCTIONS OF MACROPHAGES

Production of IL-1

Fever

Neutrophil activation

Release of acute-phase reactants

Lymphocyte activation and proliferation

    Lymphokine production

    Antibody production

Antigen Processing and Presentation

Tumor Destruction

Production of TNF

Cytotoxic action

Toxic factors

Phagocytic Activities

Fc and C3 receptors

Microcidal and bacteriostatic activities

Protection from parasites

Removal of particulate substances and damaged cells

Lymphokine receptors (MAF, MIF)

Inflammation and Tissue Alterations

Fibroblast activation

    Collagenase synthesis

Synthesis and secretion of factors

Lysozyme, plasminogen activators, elastase,
    complement components

Abbreviations: TNF = tumor necrosis factor; MAF = macrophage-activating factor; MIF = macrophage inhibitory factor.

rocyte sedimentation rate (ESR) seen in patients with infections and chronic inflammatory conditions. Some have called the persistent acute phase response of AOI a "chronic" acute-phase response.[3] If vitamin B_{12}, folate, or iron deficiency also occurs during AOI (because of loss or decreased intake), it can change the parameters of the otherwise normocytic, normochromic anemia. Macrocytosis and megaloblastosis are present with vitamin B_{12}–folate deficiency, whereas microcytosis is seen in iron deficiency (see Chaps. 6 and 7). This is true in any subcategory of anemia associated with systemic disorders.

Treatment

The degree of anemia seen in patients with AOI correlates with the severity of the inflammatory disease. Severity of inflammation is usually measured by ESR and the presence of other acute-phase reactants. The anemia seen with inflammatory processes is generally mild and usually does not require intervention. When the underlying disorder is treated, the CBC (hemogram) results return to normal. If the inflammatory process is treated with long-term anti-inflammatory medications, acute-phase reactants decrease, Hgb levels increase, and erythropoietin levels decrease to normal level.[10] When an inflammatory disorder becomes exacerbated, or remains severe for a long time, the anemia is more severe and may necessitate treatment.

Despite the low serum iron levels, there is not a true iron deficiency. Instead, there is a lack of iron availability. Treatment of this anemia with iron is ineffective and, in some cases, can actually be harmful. An excess of iron could increase the virulence of an infecting organism and exacerbate an underlying infection. Transfusion may be another possibility, depending on the Hgb and Hct levels in a given patient.[4] In patients with severe anemia and no sign of remission in their disease, this may be a viable alternative, but only after a proper evaluation of body iron stores, possibly including a bone marrow evaluation, has taken place.

In the past few years, recombinant human erythropoietin (rHuEpo) has offered a new treatment alternative. Clinical trials have indicated that rHuEpo may improve erythropoiesis in most patients with anemia of renal failure.[22] More recently, rHuEpo has been approved by the Food and Drug Administration (FDA) to treat the severe anemia in patients with acquired immunodeficiency syndrome (AIDS) who are receiving azidothymidine (AZT) and in patients with rheumatoid arthritis.[23] Although AOI is not entirely caused by an erythropoietin deficiency, high concentrations of this hormone were able to counteract the suppressive effects of IL-1.[4,24]

> **Table 14-4**
COMPARISON OF AOI WITH IRON-DEFICIENCY ANEMIA

	Normal	AOI	IDA
Serum iron (µg/dL)	50–150	↓	↓
TIBC (µg/dL)	300–360	↓	↑
Ferritin (µg/dL)	20–250	↑	↓
Transferrin saturation (%)	20–45	↓	↓
FEPs (µg/dL of RBCs)	15–80	↑	↑
RE marrow iron deposits	2–3+	↑	↓
Sideroblasts (%)	40–60	↓	↓
Reticulocytes (%)	0.5–2.0	↓	↓

Abbreviations: IDA = iron-deficiency anemia; FEPs = free erythrocyte protoporphyrins.

► ANEMIA ASSOCIATED WITH INFECTION

Anemia is frequently seen with chronic infections. In essence, it is a subset of AOI. This type of anemia is usually brought on by inflammatory mediators. It, too, is a sideropenic anemia; that is to say, a "functional" iron deficiency. It can develop gradually and will remain until the infection is successfully treated. Although most infections can now be treated effectively with antibiotic therapy, a number of chronic infections still remain that can produce anemia.

Bacterial, Fungal, and Viral Infection

In general, any bacterium or fungus that is capable of persisting for more than 2 weeks can cause anemia. Figures 14–2 to 14–5 and Color Plates 132 to 135 are examples of AOI. The severity of the anemia correlates with the intensity of fever and, thus, the presence of inflammatory products (acute-phase reactants). Some examples of infections and causative agents giving rise to this form of anemia are listed in Table 14–5. All of these infections tend to be chronic and may result in weight loss and inflammation. Other lingering infections, such as leprosy, typhoid fever, tularemia, brucellosis, and Lyme disease, can also produce this type of anemia.[25]

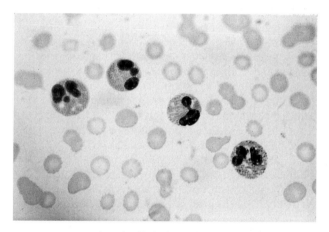

► **FIGURE 14–2** Anemia of infection (AOI). Peripheral blood of a patient with septicemia (bacterial infection in the blood). Note the increase in neutrophils with vacuolization and toxic granulation.

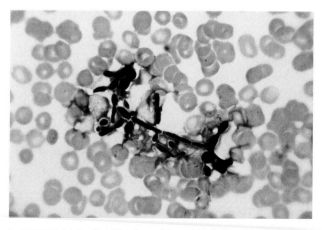

► **FIGURE 14–3** Candidemia, peripheral blood. *Candida albicans* is seen in the peripheral blood in hyphae, pseudohyphae, and yeast forms. Note that some of the organism has broken out of the cytoplasm of disintegrating monocytes, of which nuclear remnants are still visible.

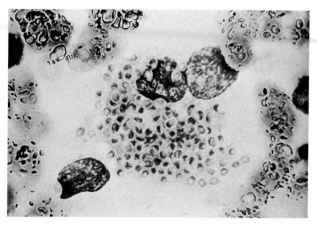

► **FIGURE 14–4** *Histoplasma capsulatum* (peripheral blood).

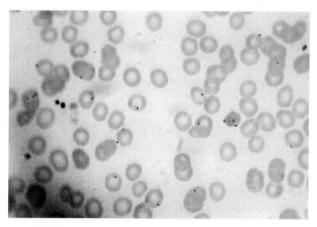

► **FIGURE 14–5** Malaria infection—*Plasmodium* species (peripheral blood).

Anemia may also result from infection with organisms and various induced processes, such as hemorrhage caused by toxins and parasite invasion (see Figs. 13–10 through 13–12, and Color Plates 117–119), virus-induced autoimmune hemolytic anemias (see Chap. 13), and virus-induced aplastic anemias[26] (see Chap. 8).

Parvovirus B19 is an interesting virus in that it has specific tropism for erythroid precursors.[27] Infection with this parvovirus can cause bone marrow erythroid hypoplasia[28] and absolute reticulocytopenia[29]—in essence, an RBC aplastic "crisis."[30,31]

Viral Infection: Human Immunodeficiency Virus Infection and the Acquired Immunodeficiency Syndrome

Viral infections are usually not associated with AOI and are caused by many different mechanisms. One notable exception is the anemia associated with human immunodeficiency virus (HIV) infection and AIDS. HIV infection is a devastating condition caused by direct destruction of CD4 T lymphocytes (helper-inducer cells) by HIV. By reducing the CD4 T-cell count, HIV renders the host immunocompromised and susceptible to many opportunistic pathogens. Most HIV-infected patients may develop pancytopenia or one or more of the cytopenias during the course of the disease.[32]

> ## Table 14-5
EXAMPLES OF CHRONIC BACTERIAL AND FUNGAL INFECTIONS THAT COMMONLY CAUSE ANEMIA

Infection	Common Causative Agents
Chronic meningitis	*Mycobacterium tuberculosis, Cryptococcus neoformans, Coccidioides immitis*
Malignant otitis externa	*Pseudomonas aeruginosa*
Empyema	Anaerobic bacteria, *Staphylococcus aureus*, aerobic gram-negative bacilli
Cavitary pulmonary disease	*M. tuberculosis, Histoplasma capsulatim, Nocardia asteroides, Actinomyces israelii,* anaerobic bacteria, *Aspergillus niger, Blastomyces dermatitidis, Pseudomonas pseudomallei*
Endocarditis	Staphylococci and streptococci, *Candida albicans*
Intra-abdominal abscess (hepatic, splenic, renal, and so on)	Anaerobic bacteria, streptococci, aerobic gram-negative bacilli
Chronic peritonitis	*M. tuberculosis*
Chronic osteomyelitis	*Staphylococcus aureus*, anaerobic bacteria, aerobic gram-negative bacilli, *Blastomyces dermatitidis*
Chronic arthritis	*M. tuberculosis*

Source: From Strausbaugh, LJ: Hematologic manifestations of bacterial and fungal infections. In Bagby, GC (ed): Hematologic Aspects of Systemic Disease, Hematol Oncol Clin North Am, WB Saunders, Philadelphia, 1987, with permission.

Anemia develops early and becomes more severe as the disease progresses. Approximately 85% of patients with AIDS are anemic.[33] Anemia has been noted in preliminary findings of HIV-infected individuals before secondary infections ensue and medications are started.[32] Infections with *Mycobacterium avium, M. intracellulare,* herpes simplex virus, *Pneumocystis carinii,* and cytomegalovirus (CMV) contribute to the state of chronic infection and chronic inflammation.[33,34] The anemia associated with HIV infection can be worsened by a concurrent condition, such as one or more opportunistic infections, as HIV infection persists and progresses.

Pathophysiology and Characteristics

The hematologic picture seen in HIV-positive patients is a normocytic, hypoproliferative anemia with a decreased reticulocyte count. Bone marrow aspirates demonstrate dysplastic features,[32,34–36] an increase in marrow reticulin, and progressive aplasia. The direct infection of bone marrow cells has been implicated as the main pathogenic factor in the thrombocytopenia of HIV infection.[37,38] A direct effect on RBC precursors has also been postulated.[34] Decreased production of RBCs can be attributed to several possible mechanisms, which are outlined in Table 14–6.

Because of the already documented effects of IL-1 and TNF-α on erythropoiesis, current theory suggests that the inflammatory process is predominantly responsible for the anemia associated with AIDS. The normocytic, normochromic anemia is thus similar to AOI but can be slightly more severe in degree. Indeed, AIDS patients demonstrate a reticuloendothelial system iron blockade[32] and iron studies similar to AOI.[35] For the most part, the anemia of HIV infection and AIDS is a subset of AOI.

Treatment

Treatment in HIV infections includes antibiotics (prophylactic or with infections), supportive care, and AZT therapy, if applicable. Anemia in the HIV-positive patient can be exacerbated by the use of AZT; however, AZT inhibits HIV replication and has helped to prolong life in many AIDS patients. Anemia and granulocytopenia are the major adverse effects associated with AZT.[39] Patients with less advanced infection at the initiation of AZT therapy are less likely to develop severe anemia and granulocytopenia.

AZT therapy can cause a macrocytosis that can somewhat change the features of the anemia of AIDS.[40] It does this because it is a deoxyribonucleotide synthesis inhibitor acting at a similar point in the deoxyribonucleic acid (DNA) synthetic pathway as would a vitamin B_{12} or folate deficiency. It has also been associated with a worsening of the reticuloendothelial system iron blockade seen in HIV infection and AIDS.[32] Just as in any AOI, when the hematologic pic-

> ## Table 14-6
PATHOPHYSIOLOGY OF ANEMIA IN HIV-POSITIVE INDIVIDUALS

- Suppression of erythropoiesis caused by cytokines IL-1 and TNF-α
- Phagocytosis of erythroblastic cells by bone marrow histiocytes
- Antibodies to HIV, which circulate in bone marrow and destroy red cell precursors
- Production of complement protein, C3, and IgG, which form immune complexes on red cell membranes, causing hemolysis
- Infections of red cell precursors by parvovirus B19 and *Mycobacterium*, halting the maturation process in the bone marrow
- Inhibitory serum protein, which results in a decrease in BFU-E not present in normal individuals
- Defective erythropoietin response to anemia
- Treatment with AZT, which inhibits DNA synthesis of blood cells and results in a macrocytic anemia

ture changes, one should suspect complicating factors. In AZT treatment, this means the emergence of macrocytosis in an otherwise normocytic, normochromic AOI.[40]

When AZT therapy is stopped, increases in Hct and reticulocyte counts are observed. To treat this severe anemia, AZT therapy often must be discontinued or the drug dosage reduced. Recently, the FDA has approved the use of rHuEpo to treat severe anemia in patients with AIDS.[22,41,42] Recombinant Epo may reduce or eliminate the need for red cell transfusions in AIDS patients receiving AZT therapy.

➤ ANEMIA ASSOCIATED WITH CONNECTIVE TISSUE (COLLAGEN) DISORDERS

All of the chronic, systemic connective tissue (collagen) disorders have the ability to produce AOI because they are, by nature, inflammatory diseases. Indeed, the anemia of connective tissue disorders is a subset of AOI. Anemia is the most common hematologic abnormality seen in patients with rheumatoid arthritis (RA), systemic lupus erythematosus (SLE), mixed connective tissue disease (MCTD), scleroderma, dermatomyositis, and Sjögren's syndrome.[43] Figure 14–6 shows a lupus erythematosus (LE) cell from a patient with active SLE.

Etiology and Pathophysiology

As in all other types of AOI, there is a direct correlation among acute-phase reactants, disease severity, and the presence or absence of anemia.[44] Production of altered transferrin molecules has been demonstrated in RA with anemia.[45] This could lead to different affinity for iron in these altered transferrin molecules. Furthermore, some authors have reported decreased serum erythropoietin levels in patients with RA,[46] as well as decreased marrow response to erythropoietin.[47] This is in addition to suppression of marrow by cytokines, lactoferrin release,[48] and iron binding similar to AOI[47] and acute-phase reactant inhibition of transferrin iron uptake.[49] Indeed, there are many mechanisms that cause AOI in RA.[47] In SLE, serum inhibitors against myeloid and erythroid colony formation have been found.[50,51]

Other factors may complicate the picture of this anemia.

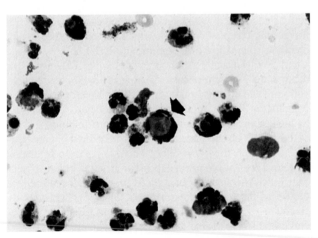

➤ FIGURE 14–6 Pleural fluid from an individual with systemic lupus erythematosus (SLE). The predominant cell is a polymorphonuclear leukocyte (PMN). A PMN that has phagocytized nuclear material (LE cell) is seen *(arrow).*

Iron-deficiency anemia may develop from gastrointestinal blood loss from the ingestion of aspirin or other anti-inflammatory drugs. Gastrointestinal blood loss can occur as a consequence of ulcer disease, which may represent "stress ulcers" from disease activity or ulcers in response to medication administered for the primary disease.

Some collagen diseases (e.g., SLE, RA, and scleroderma) are also associated with the production of autoantibodies (see the discussion of warm autoimmune hemolytic anemia in Chap. 13). This response can lead to a spherocytic and microcytic anemia in addition to or as opposed to the normocytic anemia of AOI, which is typical of an otherwise uncomplicated collagen disorder.

Renal disease is yet another complication of certain disorders such as SLE. The development of chronic renal disease, superimposed on AOI, can change the hematologic picture (see Anemia Associated with Renal Disease and Renal Failure, later in this chapter).

Characteristics

These patients exhibit the laboratory features typical of AOI. The anemia is usually normocytic, normochromic, and mild, and its severity reflects the activity and severity of the primary disease process. The reticulocyte count is depressed or low. Bone marrow findings are nonspecific in regard to myeloid, erythroid, and megakaryocytic cell lines.[52] Plasmacytosis is commonly seen. This most likely represents a response to chronic antigen stimulation in the background of these chronic autoimmune disorders.[52] Table 14–7 summarizes characteristics of RA and SLE.

Treatment

The AOI seen in collagen disorders is treated similarly to the other disorders in this category. If the underlying disease can be treated effectively to decrease the inflammatory process, the anemia should improve. Severe disease is associated with a more profound anemia. As stated earlier, the anemia, similar to other AOIs, is refractory to iron therapy.[4]

The use of rHuEpo has become an attractive alternative to transfusion to increase hematopoiesis in the anemic patient. This therapy has been used and approved for individuals with RA.[53,54]

➤ ANEMIA ASSOCIATED WITH MALIGNANCY

Hematologic abnormalities are very common in patients with both hematologic and nonhematologic malignancies (Fig. 14–7). Their type and their presence or absence depend on a multitude of factors, including the type of cancer, the site or sites involved by the malignancy in the body, the patient's therapy protocol, and the extent of the primary disease's involvement of the hematopoietic tissues (bone marrow) (Table 14–8). Anemia may be a presenting symptom of an otherwise occult malignancy. It can be caused by decreased RBC production, increased red blood cell destruction, and the toxic effects of the treatment of the malignancy.

Etiology and Pathophysiology

Direct Effects

When the bone marrow is infiltrated by a malignant tumor (myelophthisis), it can lead to anemia (myelophthisic ane-

> **Table 14-7**
CHARACTERISTICS OF RHEUMATOID ARTHRITIS AND SYSTEMIC LUPUS ERYTHEMATOSUS

	RA	SLE
Classification	N/N	N/N
Pathophysiology of anemia	Suppression of bone marrow by cytokines	Antibodies to myeloid and erythroid cells
Pancytopenia	Present	Present
LE cells	Absent	Present
RDW	↑	Normal
Sideroblasts	↓	↓ or nl
FEP	↑	↑ or nl
TIBC	↓	↓ or nl
Ferritin	↑	Variable
ESR	↑	↑
IL-6	↑	↑
TNF-α	↑	↑
C' activation	Yes	Yes
Antibodies	IgA, IgM, IgG	Anti-DNA
Respond to rHuEpo	Yes	No

Abbreviations: RA = rheumatoid arthritis, SLE = systemic lupus erythematosus, RDW = red cell distribution width, FEP = free erythrocyte protoporyphrin, TIBC = total iron-binding capacity, ESR= erythrocyte sedimentation rate, IL-6 = interleukin-6, rHuEpo = recombinant human erythropoietin, C' = complement, nl = normal, N/N = normocytic/normochromic.

mia). Leukoerythroblastosis (the presence of both immature WBC and RBC precursors) can frequently be seen on the peripheral blood smear (Fig. 14–8 and Color Plate 136). Although leukoerythroblastosis can be seen in reactive and congenital conditions in approximately one-third of cases,[55] it is a result of the myelophthisis in the balance of cases. Indeed, most individuals would reserve the term *leukoerythroblastosis* for the myelophthisic variant, only; most often the term refers to marrow fibrosis.

Leukoerythroblastosis with "teardrop" RBCs is often a clue to marrow infiltration by the tumor and associated bone marrow fibrosis (Fig. 14–9) as opposed to a reactive process that usually demonstrates leukoerythroblastosis and normal RBC morphology (Fig. 14–10). Marrow fibrosis for any rea-

son can lead to "teardrop"-shaped RBCs and leukoerythroblastosis. This includes metastatic tumor to the bone marrow. Marrow invasion can occur with solid tumors, particularly oat cell carcinoma; carcinoma of the lung; breast carcinoma; prostate cancer; gastrointestinal tumors; and, in some instances, lymphoma.[56–58] Extensive marrow invasion can eventually lead to pancytopenia. The anemia usually improves, but only if there is a response to treatment for the malignancy.

Blood loss can be another major cause of anemia in patients with malignancies. Chronic blood loss results in a hypochromic anemia more consistent with iron-deficiency anemia. Renal cell carcinoma and transitional cell carcinoma are two tumors that produce significant blood loss through hematuria.[59] Metastatic mucin-producing tumors (e.g., adenocarcinoma of stomach and adenocarcinoma of the prostate) can be associated with chronic or acute disseminated intravascular coagulation (DIC), which can be associated with bleeding (blood loss) or nonimmune RBC hemolysis (see Chap. 26). Metastatic carcinoma with high cell "turnover" or death and significant release of tissue factor can lead to activation of the coagulation system, depletion of platelets and coagulation factors, and bleeding tendencies. Microangiopathic hemolytic anemia is one of the more common sources of the hemolytic anemia seen in widespread disseminated carcinoma. Again, this is a result of activation of the coagulation system. This leads to fibrin deposition in small blood vessels, causing mechanical "shear-induced" trauma to the red cells as they pass through the vessel (see Chap. 26). Schistocytes, fragmented cells, and helmet cells can be seen on the peripheral blood smear (Table 14–9). Refer to Chapter 5.

Indirect Effects

Malignant tumors elicit a chronic inflammatory response that is not related to necrosis or infection. The production

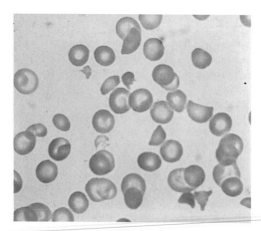

> **FIGURE 14–7** Peripheral blood from a patient with disseminated carcinoma. Note presence of schistocytes and helmet cells. (From Bell, A: Hematology. In: Listen, Look, and Learn. Health and Education Resources, Inc., Bethesda, MD, with permission.)

➤ Table 14-8
MECHANISMS OF ANEMIA IN MALIGNANCY

1. Direct Effects

Replacement of marrow by malignant cells

  Primary hematologic malignancy

    Ineffective erythroid production

    Qualitative reduction in erythropoiesis

  Metastatic marrow infiltration

    Quantitative reduction in erythropoiesis

Replacement of marrow by fibrosis

Acute and chronic blood loss

2. Indirect Effects

"Anemia of malignant disease"

Anemia of associated organ failure (e.g., renal, hepatic)

Malnutrition and vitamin deficiency

Microangiopathic hemolytic anemia

Immune hemolytic anemia

3. Treatment-Associated Anemia

Immediate

  Chemotherapy

  Radiation therapy

Late

  Secondary myelodysplasia or leukemia

  Idiopathic

  ?Depleted marrow reserve

  Microangiopathic hemolytic anemia (postmitomycin)

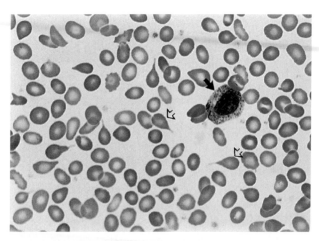

➤ FIGURE 14–9 Peripheral blood smear from an individual with myelophthisic anemia. Note left-shifted granulocyte precursors (*solid arrow*). Teardrop-shaped red blood cells (*open arrow*) are indicative of marrow fibrosis in this type of leukoerythroblastic reaction. Nucleated red blood cell precursors were seen in other fields.

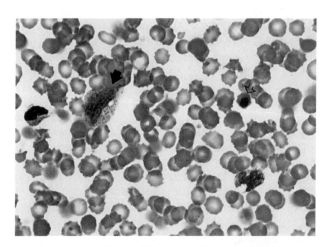

➤ FIGURE 14–10 Peripheral blood smear from a neonate with leukoerythroblastosis caused by severe blood loss associated with birth (a reactive condition). Left-shifted granulocyte precursors (*solid arrow*) and nucleated red blood cell precursors (*open arrow*) are seen. Although some "burr" cells are seen, no teardrop-shaped red blood cells are identified.

and release of IL-1 and TNF-α by macrophages is responsible for the inflammatory process seen in malignancies. The consequence of the process is the alteration of normal red cell production, resulting in anemia. In other words, any malignant neoplasm that persists for more than a few weeks may result in AOI.

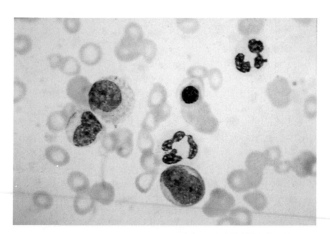

➤ FIGURE 14–8 Leukoerythroblastosis, a peripheral blood picture that often accompanies marrow infiltration by tumors (myelophthisic anemia). Note the presence of immature red and white cells.

➤ Table 14–9
RBC MORPHOLOGY IN ANEMIA OF MALIGNANCIES

Morphology	Pathophysiology
Leukoerythroblastosis	Myelophthisis, marrow fibrosis
Teardrop RBC	Marrow fibrosis
Schistocytes*	Microangiopathic hemolytic anemia
Helmet cells*	Microangiopathic hemolytic anemia
Burr cells*	Microangiopathic hemolytic anemia
Fibrosis	Myelophthisis
Hypochromia	Chronic blood loss, ↓ Fe

*Disseminated carcinomas.

The anemia seen in malignancies is similar to other AOIs in that there is a correlation between the degree of anemia and the extent of the underlying disease. Erythropoietin levels and response are blunted, and bone marrow is impaired in its response to endogenous erythropoietin.[60] Severe anemia is usually seen in patients with metastatic cancer. The development of this type of anemia does not require or imply the invasion of the bone marrow by the tumor.

Treatment-Associated Anemia

Transient pancytopenia is expected in any patient undergoing aggressive treatment for hematologic or nonhematologic malignancies. Most combination chemotherapy protocols use one or more of the alkylating agents, which are directly toxic to rapidly dividing cells. When given frequently by intervals, alkylating agents can cause a dramatic decrease in the peripheral blood cell counts. Radiation therapy can also be toxic to bone marrow stem cells. The sequence of recovery in bone marrow is quite variable. Both erythroid and granulocytic regeneration usually precede megakaryocyte regeneration.[61] The half-life of RBCs is considerably longer than the half-lives of the other two cell lines; therefore, RBC recovery in the peripheral blood lags behind white blood cell and platelet recovery. In addition, persistent anemia can result because of the need for multiple nutrients (e.g., folate, vitamin B_{12}).

Characteristics

The anemia of malignancy is usually classified as normocytic and normochromic. As stated earlier, many other processes can occur to change the severity or morphology of the anemia. The most important changes would be leukoerythroblastosis with "teardrop"-shaped RBCs, indicating marrow fibrosis and a poor prognosis because of metastasis. Another change would be schistocytes, indicating DIC and, most likely, widely disseminated carcinoma.

Treatment

In most cases, the anemia associated with malignancy is AOI. It is mild and requires little intervention.

➤ ANEMIA ASSOCIATED WITH RENAL DISEASE AND RENAL FAILURE

Renal disease is associated with a wide variety of hematologic abnormalities. These include anemia, abnormal platelet function, abnormal white blood cell function,[62] and coagulopathy. The latter two are usually the result of the effects of uremia on platelet function and coagulation factor function. Anemia is a well-documented feature of acute and chronic renal failure.

Etiology and Pathophysiology

The major cause of the anemia of renal failure is decreased production of erythropoietin by damaged kidneys. The serum erythropoietin level in patients with renal failure does not increase in response to the developing anemia, which is the primary cause of inadequate erythropoiesis. The normocytic, normochromic anemia develops in chronic renal failure when the glomerular filtration rate drops below 20 to 30 mL/min.[63] Through studies that employ the use of Epoetin (recombinant Epo) to correct the anemia, the response of hematopoietic progenitor cells is not diminished in renal failure. However,

the efficacy of Epoetin is affected by reduced iron availability, inadequate dialysis, infection, and hyperparathyroidism, secondary to renal failure.[64] Some renal diseases (e.g., renal cell carcinoma and polycystic kidney disease) are usually associated with erythrocytosis because of increased erythropoietin production and release from the neoplastic or altered renal tissue. However, that is not always the case, as some patients may develop anemia (Table 14–10).

Inhibitory properties on erythropoiesis have been demonstrated in the plasma of patients with chronic renal failure, but identity of the inhibitor is unclear. One group of investigators showed that colony formation by colony-forming units–erythroid (CFU-E) was inhibited in uremic patients with inflammatory disease. The inhibitory factors were identified as interferon gamma (IFN-γ) and TNF-α.[65]

Mild hemolysis and decreased red cell survival also contribute to this anemia. Hemolysis is in part caused by acquired defects in the erythrocyte membrane sodium-potassium ATPase and pentose phosphate shunt. The latter defect leaves the cell susceptible to oxidants (sulfonamides and dialysis tapwater) and can induce Heinz body (denatured Hgb) formation and hemolysis. Hypersplenism in patients receiving chronic hemodialysis also contributes to shortened red cell survival. Coagulopathy develops in some patients with renal failure (see Chap. 26).

Iron-deficiency anemia may develop in patients with renal failure because of blood loss during dialysis. Occult gastrointestinal blood loss from "stress" ulcers or uremic bleeding because of poor platelet function can also account for chronic iron loss.

Characteristics

In general, patients with renal failure are anemic primarily because of an inadequate quantity of circulating erythro-

> **Table 14–10**
> **MECHANISMS INVOLVED IN ANEMIA OF RENAL DISEASE**

Hypoproliferative Anemia

↓ Erthropoietin- ↓ Erythroid committed precursors

Suppressive effects of uremic toxins on erythroid precursors

Folate deficiency (hemodialysis)

Hemolytic Anemia

Unfavorable chemical environment

Uremic toxins

Dilutional Anemia

Abnormal fluid retention

Blood Loss Anemia

Gastrointestinal bleeding

Blood drawn for laboratory tests

Hemodialysis

Chronic iron deficiency

Hypersplenism

Chronic renal dialysis–associated splenomegaly

poietin and suppression of bone marrow response to the anemia. In most cases, the anemia is hypoproliferative, normocytic, and normochromic. Electrolyte disturbances as part of uremia can lead to the development of "burr" cells (Fig. 14–11). Renal failure patients with severe metabolic or electrolyte derangements (increasing creatinine and blood urea nitrogen [BUN] paralleling worsening disease) demonstrate these anomalies in peripheral blood smears of freshly drawn samples.

There is usually good compensation for the degree and severity of anemia. Other characteristics, including schistocytes and microcytes (Table 14–11 and Chap. 5), can be seen because the anemia may evolve into other forms as a result of disease-related complications (e.g., DIC or iron loss because of chronic blood loss).

Treatment

Until the advent of rHuEpo, there was no completely satisfactory treatment of the anemia associated with renal disease. Most patients treated with rHuEpo are able to become transfusion-independent.[63] Anemia and morbidity are reduced with rHuEpo therapy.[66] Major side effects have included iron deficiency (treated with iron supplements)[67] and an increase in blood pressure that can be treated with antihypertensive medications.[68]

Recombinant Epo has been used in dialysis and predialysis patients with renal disease with good efficacy.[69–71]

➤ ANEMIA ASSOCIATED WITH LIVER DISEASE

A wide array of hematologic disorders is encountered in patients with liver disease. The morphology and degree of anemia, however, differ somewhat depending on the nature, acuity, or chronicity of the liver disease and on other associated effects (Table 14–12). Most cases of anemia associated with liver disease are seen in patients with chronic liver disease.

Etiology and Pathophysiology

In chronic liver disease, the anemia may appear marked but does not correlate with the degree of hepatocellular failure or severity of disease. Target cells and acanthocytes may be

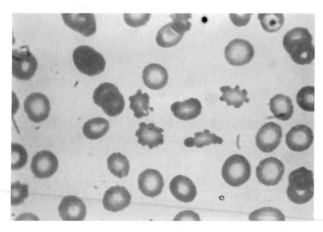

➤ FIGURE 14–11 Peripheral blood from a patient with renal disease. Note the burr cells. (From Bell, A: Hematology. In: Listen, Look, and Learn. Health and Education Resources, Inc., Bethesda, MD, with permission.)

➤ **Table 14–11**
RBC MORPHOLOGY IN RENAL DISEASE

Morphology	Pathophysiology
Heinz bodies	Oxidative stress
Burr cells	Electrolyte imbalance
Schistocytes	DIC
Microcytes	Chronic blood loss, ↓ Fe

seen on the peripheral blood smear and are considered a consequence of the altered lipid production (Fig. 14–12 and Chap. 3). Macrocytosis can also be seen (Table 14–13). Hemolytic anemia may occur with the presence of macrocytes and acanthocytes ("spur cells") because of the RBC membrane's rigidity or lack of permeability.[72]

A microcytic, hypochromic anemia may develop as a result of acute or, usually, chronic blood loss. Patients with liver disease or liver failure because of end-stage cirrhosis have decreased synthetic capacity for the production of coagulation factors, especially the vitamin K–dependent factors (see Chaps. 23 and 25). This may be a cause of chronic blood loss or severe bleeding associated with hemostatic challenges (i.e., surgery). Patients may also have hyposplenism. Hypersplenism may be found in 15% to 20% of patients with cirrhosis and advanced liver disease.[73] This condition can be a cause of platelet sequestration leading to thrombocytopenia and chronic bleeding tendencies, especially gastrointestinal and mucosal surface bleeding. Hypersplenism can also lead to decreased red cell survival as abnormal RBCs are trapped in this major reticuloendothelial system organ.

➤ **Table 14–12**
MECHANISMS OF ANEMIA IN LIVER DISEASE

Direct Effects

Toxic effects of ethanol

Vacuolization of marrow hematopoietic precursor cells

   Decreased marrow cellularity

   Megaloblastic changes unassociated with folate deficiency

Acute and chronic blood loss

   Gastrointestinal bleeding (alcoholism)

   Liver disease–associated coagulopathies

Viral suppression of erythropoiesis

Indirect Effects

Dilutional anemia

Hypersplenism, erythrocyte sequestration

Hemolytic anemia

   Spur-cell anemia (acanthocytosis)

   RE macrophage activity

Malnutrition

   Protein, folate, iron, and vitamin deficiencies

Anemia of inflammation

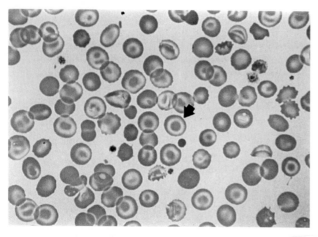

➤ FIGURE 14–12   Peripheral blood smear from an individual with liver disease. Target cells *(solid arrow)* are caused by altered lipid metabolism with subsequent effects on red cell membrane.

Characteristics

Macrocytosis can be seen in patients with cirrhosis, obstructive jaundice, and other types of liver disease. These macrocytes are round, slightly flattened RBCs with a slight increase in size and volume. The RBC MCV in liver disease is usually between 100 and 110 femtoliters (fL). These macrocytes are not, however, the macro-ovalocytes seen in megaloblastic anemia (see Fig. 7–4). Bone marrow examination shows macronormoblastic RBC precursors but no megaloblastic changes such as giant band forms, or hypersegmented neutrophils typical of a true megaloblastic anemia. The survival of these red cells is decreased owing to increased membrane lipids and lack of good deformability. This type of macrocytosis does not respond to vitamin B$_{12}$ or folate therapy, and usually resolves only after improvement in liver function.

Megaloblastic macrocytes caused by folate deficiency may be seen in some patients with liver disease. This abnormality is caused by poor nutrition, usually as a result of chronic alcohol intake. Chronic alcohol intake is a significant cause of end-stage liver disease.

The anemia of chronic liver failure is often complicated by portal hypertension, hypersplenism, and increased plasma volume seen in splenomegaly. RBC mass is "pooled" in the venous system, sequestered in the spleen, or diluted in an increased plasma volume. These factors can yield a falsely decreased hematocrit, which may cause difficulty in evaluating the anemia. Therefore, anemia associated with chronic liver disease is initially considered normocytic and normochromic, with variable RBC morphology and variable numbers of

➤ Table 14-13
RBC MORPHOLOGY IN LIVER DISEASE

Morphology	Pathophysiology
Target cells	↑ Membrane lipids
Spur cells	↑ Membrane lipids
Macrocytosis	↓ Folate, ↑ membrane lipids
Reticulocytosis	Anemia
Macronormoblasts*	↑ Membrane lipids

*Bone marrow erythroblasts.

macrocytes, but it can be complicated by the simultaneous effects of iron deficiency (from blood loss) or folate deficiency (from poor dietary habits). Reticulocytosis is present depending on the degree of anemia. Serum ferritin is increased, reflecting a "chronic" acute-phase response. Decreased plasma iron may represent an element of AOI.

Treatment

Correction of dietary deficiencies (lack of iron or folate) can help the anemia. However, resolution of the liver disease corrects the macrocytosis, acanthocytosis, and anemia. In most instances, advanced liver disease and hypersplenism are present and irreversible. In these cases, dietary supplementation (iron, vitamin B$_{12}$, and folate) can be efficacious in preventing hematologic sequelae; however, bizarre red cell morphology and low-grade anemia may persist.

➤ ANEMIA ASSOCIATED WITH ALCOHOLISM

One of the most common forms of liver disease is the result of chronic alcohol ingestion (Table 14–12). One of the widest arrays of hematologic abnormalities occurs in complications of acute and chronic alcoholism.

Etiology and Pathophysiology

Ethanol has direct toxic effects on precursor cells, marrow cellularity, and red cell morphology.[74] Vacuolization of erythroblasts in the bone marrow can be observed in alcoholic patients.[74] Heavy and prolonged alcohol abuse will also result in decreased bone marrow cellularity. Alcohol and its metabolites are suppressants of hematopoietic-progenitor cell production.[75]

Macrocytosis is very common in chronic alcoholics and may not be caused by megaloblastic anemia.[76] In alcoholics who are not malnourished or have mild liver disease, there is still a macrocytosis that is not accompanied by any megaloblastic changes in the bone marrow or neutrophilic hypersegmentation in the peripheral blood. The mechanism of macrocytosis in alcoholism is unknown.

Characteristics

The anemia associated with alcoholism is usually macrocytic. This change in cell size remains until the patient stops consuming ethanol. The MCV remains elevated for 1 to 4 months afterward.[77] The anemia of liver disease may be present if advanced liver damage or disease is present.

Iron deficiency because of chronic blood loss (i.e., gastrointestinal bleeding such as bleeding from esophageal varices formed as a consequence of cirrhosis) or poor nutrition may also be present with folate deficiency, demonstrating a dimorphic blood picture on the peripheral blood smear. In this case, the MCV may be normal, but it will be a result of the average of two widely disparate "peaks," representing two populations of RBCs. Evaluation of the MCV histogram from an automated hematology instrument will demonstrate this fact. The RDW will be increased. This can also serve as a clue to the presence of these two nutritional deficiencies when they occur simultaneously.

"Spur-cell" anemia because of acanthocytosis is mostly associated with severe alcoholic liver disease.[72] Spur cells have an increase in cholesterol, which decreases the deformability of the cell as it passes through the spleen.

Treatment

Treatment of the underlying liver disease is essential to the reversal of the anemia. Abstinence from alcohol will reverse the direct toxic effects on the bone marrow, and in a few months the MCV and RBC morphology should return to normal.

➤ ANEMIA ASSOCIATED WITH ENDOCRINE DISEASE AND DISORDERS

The spectrum of endocrine disease is wide, and its effect on metabolism is far-reaching and varied. Many hormones are involved in the regulation of hematopoiesis. Diseases of the pituitary, adrenal, thyroid glands, and gonads are most often involved in the development of anemia (Table 14–14).[78–81]

The subject matter in this chapter is both wide and diverse. However, the anemias discussed in this chapter have a common theme. They are associated with systemic diseases. As a group, they are probably the most frequently encountered of the anemias. All of the diseases discussed can lead to an anemia that is secondary to or associated with mechanisms causing the underlying disease state. Some of these disorders are linked by dysfunction or abnormalities in ferrokinetics and the mechanism of inflammation.

The anemia seen in these diseases is normochromic and normocytic. Other complicating factors can induce anisocytosis or poikilocytosis, which changes the characteristics of the RBC and the anemia.

These anemias are treated differently from other forms of anemia. The primary disease state deserves the most attention because it is the correction of this state that usually allows for the correction of the anemia. It should be noted that not every systemic disease demonstrates anemia.

This chapter discusses the characteristic features of the anemias associated with many systemic, nonhematologic disorders. Anemia may be the first sign of a previously undetected systemic disease. Changing RBC parameters may indicate new, complicating factors in an otherwise stable anemia associated with a systemic disease.

These are anemias the health-care worker should be familiar with due to their frequency in all patient groups seeking medical care.

➤ CASE STUDY 1

A 22-year-old woman was admitted from the emergency department for tests. She had fever, dysuria, and lower back pain. Immediate laboratory results revealed the following:

Urinalysis	CBC
4+ urine protein	WBC: 11.8×10^9/L
1+ Hgb	RBC: 2.9×10^{12}/L
Many bacteria	Hgb: 8.3 g/dL
Moderate blood	Hct: 25%
Moderate WBCs	MCV: 88 fL
Casts: few hyaline, few granular	MCH: 29 pg
Chemistry:	MCHC: 300 g/L or 30%
BUN: 113 mg/dL	RDW: 14.7%
Creatinine: 7.7 mg/dL	1+ aniso
	1+ poik
	1+ crenated RBCs

Blood cultures were drawn and eventually produced coagulase-negative *Staphylococcus*. Blood was still present in the patient's urine after 2 days, and bleeding was noted from intravenous infusion sites. Coagulation tests were ordered before the patient was to go to surgery for kidney biopsy.

Platelet count: 296×10^9/L

PT: 11.7 seconds (control: 10.0–12.9 seconds)

continued

➤ Table 14–14
ENDOCRINE DISORDERS/DISEASES[78–81]

Endocrine Disorder/Disease	Type of Anemia	Pathogenesis (cause of)	Treatment
Pituitary dysfunction	N/N	Hypopituitarism	Exogenous replacement of thyroid hormone
			Androgens and/or estrogens
			Administration of corticosteroids
Adrenal insufficiency	N/N	Idiopathic (unknown cause)	Exogenous source of corticosteroids
Addison's disease		Destructive autoantibodies directed against parenchymal cells of the organs (autoimmune)	
Thyroid disease	N/N	Hyperthyroidism	Exogenous thyroid hormone
	Mild macrocytic	Hypothyroidism	
Hypogonadism	N/N	Defective internal secretion of the gonads	Androgens

Abbreviation: N/N = normocytic/normochromic.

APTT: 32 seconds (control: 23–35 seconds)

Bleeding time: > 20 seconds

FDP: > 40 µg/mL

(APTT is activated partial thromboplastin time; FDP means fibrin/fibrinogen degradation products.)

This patient was suffering from bacterial sepsis and renal failure. The admitting CBC demonstrated a mild anemia with some created red cell morphology typical of renal disease. The patient had received several units of packed red cells with no noticeable difference in her hematocrit (Hct). The anemia could be the product of several mechanisms. First, there was blood loss from her abnormal platelets (see Chap. 23) and from the DIC that she later developed. Her presenting anemia was most likely a result of the anemia of inflammation. Chronic and acute infections can produce this form of anemia. The anemia of renal disease was also present in this patient and was seen in conjunction with other causes of anemia.

Questions

1. Classify the anemia with regard to RBC indices.
2. Explain the significance of the RDW value in this case.
3. List the laboratory parameters in this case that coincide with anemia associated with renal disease.
4. What is the major cause of renal failure associated with anemia?
5. Why would chronic iron loss be a concern in this patient?

➤ CASE STUDY 2

A 42-year-old woman presented to her physician with pain in both of her wrists and in the proximal joints of both of her hands. She had also recently begun experiencing right knee pain. Her laboratory results revealed the following:

WBC: 10.0×10^9/L

Hgb: 8.5 g/dL

Hct: 25%

MCV: 90 fL

RDW: 12.5% (normal 11%–14%)

Erythrocyte sedimentation rate (ESR): 100 mm/h (normal 0–10 mm/h)

Rheumatoid factor: Positive

Questions

1. What is the patient's diagnosis?
2. What could cause the increase in ESR?
3. Why was the patient anemic?

The patient's physician placed her on enteric-coated aspirin to protect her gastric lining for 3 months. She then reported no pain in her joints, wrists, or hands. Her ESR remained at 10 mm/h and her hemoglobin remained at 8.5 g/dL. Her physician decided to continue her on enteric-coated aspirin, since she had completed her course of iron supplements. She still reported feeling tired. Her physician also decided to start her on erythropoietin (rHuEpo) in an attempt to correct the anemia. After 4 weeks of rHuEpo therapy, the patient's Hgb was 12.8 g/dL and her Hct was 38%.

Her laboratory values were:

WBC: 10.0×10^9/L

Hgb: 12.8 g/dL

Hct: 0.38 L/L (or 38%)

MCV: 90 fL

RDW: 2.5% (normal, 11%–14%)

➤ CASE STUDY 3

A 29-year-old woman with cholecystitis (inflammation of the gallbladder) was taken to elective surgery, where she underwent a cholecystectomy. Her preoperative laboratory values revealed:

WBC: 10.0×10^9/L

Hgb: 1.25 g/dL

Hct: 38%

Platelets: 150×10^9/L

The patient was transported to the recovery room where, over 2 hours, her blood pressure was noted to be unstable. She was also noted to have a distended, tender abdomen. Laboratory tests revealed:

WBC: 10.0×10^9/L

Hgb: 1.24 g/dL

Hct: 38%

Platelets: 150×10^9/L

She was given 3 to 4 L of 0.9% saline, which stabilized her blood pressure enough to allow her to be transferred back to surgery. Laboratory tests revealed:

WBC: 6.0×10^9/L

Hgb: 7.5 g/dL

Hct: 20%

Platelets: 100×10^9/L

The evening shift medical technologist noted a significant change in the patient's hemoglobin level over the course of 1 to 2 hours in the recovery room by the use of a delta check (i.e., a significant change in laboratory values). The technologist called the recovery room to report the now lower value and to ask about proper specimen collection. The call was transferred to the operating room, where the patient was now undergoing an emergency laparotomy. The technologist reported the value to the physician (surgeon), who explained that the patient's abdomen was now full of blood (approximately 2 L) because of a damaged artery that was not "tied off" during surgery. The surgeon had just sutured the artery and was closing the abdominal wound after evacuating and suctioning the blood from the cavity.

Questions
1. Why was the patient's hemoglobin level normal when she had a distended abdomen full of blood?
2. What caused the hemoglobin value to decrease?
3. What other tests would be abnormal in this patient?

QUESTIONS

1. Which of the following lists of laboratory findings would be most characteristic of the anemia of inflammation?
   a. Normocytic, hypochromic red blood cell; high serum iron level; increased TIBC; decreased ferritin levels; decreases in hemoglobin and hematocrit
   b. Normocytic, normochromic red blood cell; low serum iron level; decreased TIBC; increased ferritin levels; decreases in hemoglobin and hematocrit
   c. Microcytic, hypochromic red blood cell; normal serum iron level; decreased TIBC; normal ferritin levels; decreases in hemoglobin and hematocrit
   d. Macrocytic, normochromic red blood cell; low serum iron level; decreased TIBC; decreased ferritin levels; decreases in hemoglobin and hematocrit

2. Which of the following are causes for the anemia of inflammation?
   a. Increased destruction of red blood cells
   b. Impaired iron metabolism
   c. Suppression of erythropoiesis by cytokines
   d. All of the above

3. What are the main immune processes responsible for reducing hematopoiesis and inducing nutritional immunity?
   a. Cytokines from macrophages and lymphokines
   b. Antibodies from B lymphocytes
   c. Erythropoietin from the kidney
   d. Hepatocellular factors from the liver

4. What is the treatment for anemia of inflammation?
   a. Blood transfusion
   b. Iron therapy
   c. Treatment of the inflammation
   d. Human recombinant IL-1

5. Which are causes of anemia not associated with inflammation?
   a. Malignancy and neoplastic processes
   b. Connective tissue disorders
   c. Bacterial and fungal infections
   d. Endocrine, kidney, and liver disease

6. Leukoerythroblastosis with teardrop-shaped red blood cells is indicative of:
   a. Bone marrow fibrosis
   b. Bone marrow stress
   c. Abnormal lipid metabolism
   d. Renal disease

7. Macrocytosis in liver disease is caused by all of the following except:
   a. Abnormal lipid metabolism
   b. Direct effects of alcohol
   c. Iron deficiency
   d. Vitamin B_{12} and folate deficiency

8. What are the typical hematologic findings associated with anemia from endocrine dysfunction?
   a. Mild normocytic, normochromic anemia
   b. Anemia, abnormal platelets, and coagulopathy
   c. Target cells, macrocytes, and acanthocytes
   d. Marked anisocytosis and poikilocytosis, and dysfunctional leukocytes

9. What is the primary cause of anemia associated with renal disorders and renal failure?
   a. Blood loss from dialysis
   b. Decreased Epo production
   c. Hemolytic processes
   d. Vitamin B_{12} and folate deficiencies

10. What is the typical appearance of anemia associated with liver disease?
    a. Normal red blood cell morphology
    b. Hypochromic, microcytic
    c. Macrocytic, normoblastic
    d. Macrocytic, megaloblastic

SUMMARY CHART

➤ Anemias produced by inflammation and systemic diseases are perhaps the most common hematologic abnormalities encountered in the clinical laboratory.
➤ The four major systems that serve to mediate the inflammatory response include the coagulation, complement, fibrinolytic, and kinin systems.
➤ Possible etiologies for the anemia of inflammation (AOI) include decreased red blood cell (RBC) life span, impaired iron metabolism from faulty iron release from reticuloendothelial (RE) stores, decreased erythropoietin levels, and suppression of erythropoiesis by cytokines from activated macrophages and lymphocytes resulting from the underlying disease.
➤ Cytokines that have been reported to inhibit erythropoiesis in AOI include: interleukin-1 (IL-1), tumor necrosis factor-alpha (TNF-α), and interferon gamma (INF-γ).
➤ AOI is characterized by a normocytic, normochromic anemia with a normal or low mean corpuscular hemoglobin (MCHC), mean corpuscular volume (MCV), low serum iron, decreased total iron-binding capacity (TIBC), and low iron transferrin saturation; the RBC distribution width (RDW) and erythrocyte sedimentation rate (ESR) are usually increased.
➤ Anemia caused by infections increases in severity

in the presence of fever and acute-phase reactants; infection with parvovirus B19 results in bone marrow erythroid hypoplasia and absolute reticulocytopenia.

➤ Anemia associated with HIV infection is characterized as a normocytic, normochromic, hypoproliferative anemia with a decreased reticulocyte count and dysplastic bone marrow features; 85% of patients with acquired immunodeficiency syndrome (AIDS) are anemic.

➤ Diseases associated with connective tissue disorders may include rheumatoid arthritis, systemic lupus erythematosus, mixed connective tissue disease, dermatomyositis, and Sjögren's syndrome.

➤ Anemia associated with connective tissue disorders is characterized as normocytic and normochromic, with a low reticulocyte count; the bone marrow reflects a plasmacytosis in association with autoimmune disorders.

➤ Anemia seen in malignancies is dependent on the type of cancer, the site of infiltration, the patient's therapy, and the extent of bone marrow involvement.

➤ Myelophthisis refers to infiltration of the bone marrow by a malignant tumor; the most characteristic RBC morphology associated with myelophthisis is leukoerythroblastosis with teardrop-shaped red cells.

➤ Chemotherapy agents result in a transient pancytopenia resulting from alkylating agents that are directly toxic to rapidly dividing cells.

➤ Renal disease may be associated with anemia, abnormal platelet and white blood cell function, and coagulopathy.

➤ The major cause for the anemia seen in renal disease is decreased production of Epo by damaged kidneys; the anemia is characterized as hypoproliferative, normocytic, and normochromic, with the presence of burr cells, schistocytes, and microcytes resulting from blood loss.

➤ The RBC morphology seen in chronic liver disease may include macrocytosis, target cells, acanthocytes, and thrombocytopenia if hypersplenism is present; a microcytic, hypochromic anemia is evident in the presence of chronic blood loss.

➤ The bone marrow picture in chronic liver disease reflects a macronormoblastic stage in RBC precursors with decreased survival because of increased membrane lipids and lack of deformability.

➤ Anemia caused by alcoholism is the result of ethanol toxicity on precursor cells in the bone marrow; macrocytosis, vacuolization of erythroblasts in the bone marrow, and spur cells are usually seen.

➤ A dimorphic blood picture may be seen in anemia of alcoholism because of iron deficiency caused by chronic blood loss; the MCV is normal and the RDW, increased.

➤ Anemia associated with endocrine disease is

usually normocytic and normochromic and may be caused by pituitary dysfunction, adrenal insufficiency, Addison's disease, thyroid disease, and hypogonadism.

References

1. Krantz, SB: Pathogenesis and treatment of the anemia of chronic disease. Am J Med Sci 307:353, 1994.
2. Schilling, RF: Anemia of chronic disease: A misnomer (editorial). Ann Intern Med 115:572, 1991.
3. Kushner, I: Letter to the editor. Ann Intern Med 116:521, 1992.
4. Damon, LE: Anemias of chronic disease in the aged: Diagnosis and treatment. Geriatrics 47:47, 1992.
5. Means RT: The anemia of chronic disorders. In Lee, GR, et al: Wintrobe's Clinical Hematology, ed 10. Lippincott, Williams & Wilkins, Baltimore, 1998.
6. Cartwright, GE, and Lee, GR: The anemia of chronic disorders. Br J Haematol 21:147, 1971.
7. Denz, H, et al: Altered iron metabolism and the anemia of chronic disease: A role of immune activation (letter to the editor). Blood 79:2797, 1992.
8. Konijn, AM: Iron metabolism in inflammation. Baillieres Clin Haematol 7:829, 1994.
9. Weiss, G: Iron and anemia of chronic disease. Kidney Int Suppl 69:S12, 1999.
10. Jongen-Lavrencic, M, et al: Elevated levels of inflammatory cytokines in bone marrow of patients with rheumatoid arthritis and anemia of chronic disease. J Rheumatol 24:1504, 1997.
11. Leng, HM, and Folb, PI: Erythropoiesis and erythropoietin synthesis during aseptic acute inflammation. Inflamm Res 45:541, 1996.
12. Means, RT: Erythropoietin in the treatment of anemia in chronic infectious, inflammatory, and malignant disease. Curr Opin Hematol 2:210, 1995.
13. Jelkmann, W: Proinflammatory cytokines lowering erythropoietin production. J Interferon Cytokine Res 18:555, 1998.
14. Chambers, JK: Epoetin alfa: Focus on inflammation and infection. Case study of the anemia patient. ANNA J 25:353, 1998.
15. Greendyke, RM, et al: Serum levels of erythropoietin and selected other cytokines in patients with anemia of chronic disease. Am J Clin Pathol 101:338, 1994.
16. Means, RT, and Krantz, SB: Progress in understanding the pathogenesis of the anemia of chronic disease. Blood 80:1639, 1992.
17. Liu, H, et al: Suppression of haematopoiesis by IgG autoantibodies from patients with systemic lupus erythematosus (SLE). Clin Exp Immunol 100:480, 1995.
18. Allen, DA, et al: Inhibition of CFU-E colony formation in uremic patients with inflammatory disease: Role of IFN-gamma and TNF-alpha. J Investig Med 47:204, 1999.
19. Bertero, MT, and Caligaris-Cappio, F: Anemia of chronic disorders in systemic autoimmune diseases. Haematologica 82:375, 1997.
20. Yucel-Lindberg, T, et al: Signal transduction pathways involved in the synergistic stimulation of prostaglandin production by interleukin-1 beta and tumor necrosis factor alpha in human gingival fibroblasts. J Dent Res 78:61, 1999.
21. Means, RT: Advances in the anemia of chronic disease. Int J Hematol 70:7, 1999.
22. Moudgil, A, and Bagga, A: Evaluation and treatment of chronic renal disease. Indian J Pediatr 66:241, 1999.
23. Henry, DH: Experience with epoetin alfa and acquired immunodeficiency syndrome anemia. Semin Oncol 25:64, 1998.
24. Schreiber, S, et al: Recombinant erythropoietin for the treatment of anemia in inflammatory bowel disease. N Engl J Med 334:619, 1996.
25. Hardalo, CJ, et al: Human granulocytic ehrlichiosis in Connecticut: Report of a fatal case. Clin Infect Dis 21:910, 1995.
26. Crespo, J, et al: Hepatitis G virus infection as a possible causative agent of community-acquired hepatitis and associated aplastic anemia. Postgrad Med J 75:159, 1999.
27. Crook, TW: Unusual bone marrow manifestations of parvovirus B19 infection in immunocompromised patients. Hum Pathol 31:161, 2000.
28. Pamidi, S, et al: Human parvovirus B19 infection presenting as persistent anemia in renal transplant recipients. Transplantation 69:2666, 2000.
29. Wong, TY, et al: Parvovirus B19 infection causing red cell aplasia in renal transplantation on tacrolimus. Am J Kidney Dis 34:1132, 1999.
30. Sabella, C, and Goldfarb, J: Parvovirus B19 infections. Am Fam Physician 60:1455, 1999.
31. Rugolotto, S, et al: Intrauterine anemia due to parvovirus B19: Successful treatment with intravenous immunoglobulins. Haematologica 84:668, 1999.
32. Harris, CE, et al: Peripheral blood and bone marrow findings in patients with acquired immune deficiency syndrome. Pathology 22:206, 1990.
33. Cosby, C, et al: Hematological complications and quality of life in hospitalized AIDS patients. AIDS Patient Care STDS 14:269, 2000.
34. Bodey, GP: Community respiratory viral infections in the immunocompromised host: Past, present, and future directions. Am J Med 102:77, 1997.
35. Kuritzkes, DR: Neutropenia, neutrophil dysfunction, and bacterial infection in patients with human immunodeficiency virus disease: The role of granulocyte colony stimulating factor. Clin Infect Dis 30:256, 2000.
36. Corti, M, et al: Bone marrow involvement by Pneumocystis carinii in an AIDS patient. Enferm Infec Microbiol Clin 17:420, 1999.
37. Sato, T, et al: HIV infection of megakaryocytic cell lines. Leuk Lymphoma 36:397, 2000.

38. Sutor, GC, et al: Thrombotic microangiopathies and HIV infection: Report of two typical cases, features of HUS and TTP, and review of the literature. Infection 27:12, 1999.

39. Krown, SE, et al: Phase II, randomized, open-label, community-based trial to compare the safety and activity of combination therapy with recombinant interferon-alpha2b and zidovudine versus zidovudine alone in patients with asymptomatic to mildly symptomatic HIV infection. HIV Protocol C91–253 Study Team. J Acquir Immune Defic Syndr Hum Retrovirol 20:245, 1999.

40. Snower, DP, and Weil, SC: Changing etiology of macrocytosis. Zidovudine as a frequent causative factor. Am J Clin Pathol 99:57, 1993.

41. Glaspy, JA, and Chap, L: The clinical application of recombinant erythropoietin in the HIV-infected patient. In Spivak, JL (ed): Hematol Oncol Clin North Am 8:945, 1994.

42. Phair, JP, et al: Recombinant human erythropoietin treatment: Investigational new drug protocol for the anemia of the acquired immunodeficiency syndrome. Overall results. Arch Intern Med 153:2669, 1993.

43. Rodriguez-Cuartero, A, et al: Sjogren's syndrome and pernicious anemia. Scand J Rheumatol 27:83, 1998.

44. Rosenthal, NS, and Farhi, DC: Bone marrow findings in connective tissue disease. Am J Clin Pathol 92:650, 1989.

45. Noe, G, et al: Serum erythropoietin and transferrin receptor levels in patients with rheumatoid arthritis. Clin Exp Rheumatol 13:445, 1995.

46. Bertero, MT, and Caligaris-Cappio, F: Anemia of chronic disorders in systemic autoimmune disease. Haematologica 82:375, 1997.

47. Krantz, SB: Erythropoietin and the anemia of chronic disease. Nephrol Dial Transplant 2:10, 1995.

48. Baveye, S, et al: Lactoferrin: A multifunctional glycoprotein involved in the modulation of the inflammatory process. Clin Chem Lab Med 37:281, 1999.

49. Graziadei, I, et al: The acute-phase protein alpha 1-antitrypsin inhibits growth and proliferation of human early erythroid progenitor cells (burst forming units–erythroid) and of human erythroleukemia cells (K562) in vitro by interfering with transferrin iron uptake. Blood 83:260, 1994.

50. Voulgarelis, M, et al: Anaemia in systemic lupus erythematosus: Aetiological profile and the role of erythropoietin. Ann Rheum Dis 59:217, 2000.

51. Iqbal, S, et al: Diversity in presenting manifestations of systemic lupus erythematosus in children. J Pediatr 135:500, 1999.

52. Pereira, RM, et al: Bone marrow findings in systemic lupus erythematosus patients with peripheral cytopenias. Clin Rheumatol 17(3):219, 1998.

53. Tanaka, N, et al: Autologous blood transfusion with recombinant erythropoietin treatment in anemic patients with rheumatoid arthritis. Clin Rheumatol 18:293, 1999.

54. Peeters, HR, et al: Recombinant human erythropoietin improves health-related quality of life in patients with rheumatoid arthritis and anemia of chronic disease; utility measures correlate strongly with disease activity measures. Rheumatol Int 18:201, 1999.

55. Shamdas, GJ, et al: Leukoerythroblastic anemia in metastatic prostate cancer. Clinical and prognostic significance in patients with hormone-refractory disease. Cancer 71:3594, 1993.

56. Wong, KF, et al: Solid tumor with initial presentation in the bone marrow—A clinicopathologic study of 25 adult cases. Hematol Oncol 11:35, 1993.

57. Lebtahi, N, et al: Evaluating bone marrow metastasis of neuroblastoma with iodine-123-MIBG scintigraphy and MRI. J Nucl Med 38:1389, 1997.

58. Broll, R, et al: Tumor cell dissemination in bone marrow and peritoneal cavity. An immunocytochemical study of patients with stomach or colorectal carcinoma. Langenbecks Arch Chir 381:51, 1996.

59. Ou, JH: Transitional cell carcinoma in dialysis patients. Eur Urol 37:90, 2000.

60. Ozguroglu, M, et al: Serum erythropoietin level in anemic cancer patients. Med Oncol 17:29, 2000.

61. Foucar, K: Effects of therapy, transplantation and detection of minimal residual disease. In Foucar, K (ed): Bone Marrow Pathology. American Society of Clinical Pathologist Press, Chicago, 1995.

62. Zachee, P, et al: Hematologic aspects of end-stage renal failure. Ann Hematol 69:33, 1994.

63. Eckardt, KU: Pathophysiology of renal anemia. Clin Nephrol 53:S2, 2000.

64. Gallieni, M, et al: Hyperparathyroidism and anemia in renal failure. Am J Nephrol 20:89, 2000.

65. Allen, DA, et al: Inhibition of CFU-E colony formation in uremic patients with inflammatory disease: Role of IFN-gamma and TNF-alpha. J Investig Med 47:204, 1999.

66. Kausz, AT, et al: Intraperitoneal erythropoietin in children on peritoneal dialysis: A study of pharmacokinetics and efficacy. Am J Kid Dis, Oct 34(4):651, 1999.

67. Sanders, HN, et al: Nutritional implications of recombinant human erythropoietin therapy in renal disease. J Am Diabet Assoc 94(9):1023, 1994.

68. Wada, Y, et al: Erythropoietin impairs endothelium-dependent vasorelaxation through cyclooxygenase-dependent mechanisms in humans. Am J Hypertens 12:980, 1999.

69. Hayashi, T, et al: Cardiovascular effect of normalizing the hematocrit level during erythropoietin therapy in predialysis patients with chronic renal failure. Am J Kidney Dis 35:250, 2000.

70. Muirhead, N: Erythropoietin and renal transplantation. Kidney Int Suppl 69:S86, 1999.

71. Silverberg, DS, et al: Intravenous iron for the treatment of predialysis anemia. Kidney Int Suppl 69:S79, 1999.

72. Allen, DW, and Manning, N: Cholesterol-loading of membranes of normal erythrocytes inhibits phospholipid repair and arachidonoyl-CoA:1-palmitoyl-sn-glycero-3-phosphocholine acyl transferase. A model of spur cell anemia. Blood 87:3489, 1996.

73. O'Reilly, RA: Splenomegaly at a United States County Hospital: Diagnostic evaluation of 170 patients. Am J Med Sci 312:160, 1996.

74. Zima, T: Ethanol metabolism and pathobiochemistry of organ damage—1992. IV. Ethanol in relation to the cardiovascular system. Hematologic, immunologic, endocrine disorders and muscle and bone damage caused by ethanol. Fetal alcohol syndrome. Sb Lek 94:303, 1993.

75. Seppa, K, et al: Evaluation of macrocytosis by general practitioners. J Stud Alcohol 57:97, 1996.

76. Seppa, K, et al: Macrocytosis as a consequence of alcohol abuse among patients in general practice. Alcoholism 15:871, 1991.

77. Seppa, K: Intervention in alcohol abuse among macrocytic patients in general practice. Scand J Prim Health Care 10:217, 1992.

78. Sikole, A: Pathogenesis of anemia in hyperparathyroidism. Med Hypotheses 54:236, 2000.

79. Zitzmann, M, and Nieschlag, E: Hormone substitution in male hypogonadism. Mol Cell Endocrinol 30:161, 2000.

80. Sohmiya, M, and Kato, Y: Effect of long-term treatment with recombinant human growth hormone on erythropoietin secretion in an anemic patient with panhypopituitarism. J Endocrinol Invest 23:31, 2000.

81. Antonijevic, N, et al: Anemia in hypothyroidism. Med Pregl 52:136, 1999.

See the Bibliography for this chapter at the back of the book.

White Blood Cell Disorders

15 Cell Biology, Disorders of Neutrophils, Infectious Mononucleosis, and Reactive Lymphocytosis

DEIRDRE DESANTIS PARSONS MS, MT(ASCP), SBB
JOE MARTY, MS, MT(ASCP)
RONALD G. STRAUSS, MD

OBJECTIVES

At the end of this chapter, the learner should be able to:

1. Characterize the changes in neutrophil count and morphology that develop in response to bacterial infection.
2. Define the three modes of neutrophilic migration.
3. Describe the changes in migration pattern and appearance that occur in a neutrophil as a result of chemoattractant stimulation.
4. Characterize the sequence of events that occur during phagocytosis.
5. Define neutropenia.
6. Identify three causes of acquired neutropenia.
7. Describe the classic clinical features of Chédiak-Higashi syndrome and the associated changes in neutrophil morphology.
8. Describe the inheritance of and molecular basis for chronic granulomatous disease.
9. Compare and contrast three white cell anomalies in regard to morphology.
10. Define lymphocytosis.
11. List several disorders that present with lymphocytosis.
12. Distinguish between absolute and relative lymphocytosis.
13. Distinguish between benign and malignant lymphocytosis.
14. Recognize morphological features of infectious mononucleosis and other reactive lymphocytoses.
15. List clinical features of infectious mononucleosis.
16. Describe how the Epstein-Barr virus effects the B- and T-lymphocyte populations.
17. Utilize laboratory results for distinguishing infectious mononucleosis from other lymphocytoses.

➤ NEUTROPHILS

Granulocytes may be divided into three subsets—neutrophils, eosinophils, and basophils—based on morphology by light and electron microscopy and on the staining characteristics and contents of cytoplasmic granules. Neutrophils are the most numerous leukocytes found in peripheral blood, accounting for 50% to 70% of all circulating white blood cells in the adult. Similar to monocytes, neutrophils function as phagocytes that are capable of ameboid movement into the tissues to engulf and destroy bacteria or fungus; they are the first phagocytic cells to mobilize at a site of infection. Neutrophils also play a role in mediating inflammatory processes.

Circulating Kinetics and Morphology of Neutrophils

Mature neutrophils (or polymorphonuclear leukocytes) are easily recognized on blood smears prepared with Wright's stain by their dense multilobed nucleus and pinkish-tan cytoplasm, which is peppered with pinkish-purple granules. They are smaller than their myeloid precursors, but more mobile and deformable. Two types of cytoplasmic granules, primary (azurophilic or nonspecific) and secondary (specific), are present in the mature neutrophil, although only the secondary granules are visible with light microscopy. Recently, a third type of granule (tertiary) has been identified using electron microscopy.[1,2] The contents of these the primary, secondary, and tertiary granules are enzymes, most of which are involved in the killing and digestion of bacteria and fungi (Table 15–1).

Neutrophils are considered to be one of the most mobile cell lines in humans.[3] Once in the bloodstream, mature neutrophils are equally divided into marginating and circulating pools between which there is a constant exchange of cells. The marginating pool consists of cells adhering to vessel endothelium within the vascular spaces. Marginating cells are described as rolling along vessel endothelium in search of an area of injury or inflammation where, by diapedesis, they enter the tissues for action. Neutrophils in the circulating pool leave the blood by random migration after a half-life of approximately 7 hours and do not return to the bloodstream from tissues. Little is known of the kinetics of neutrophils after having entered the tissues; they are believed to remain in tissues for 2 to 5 days, where, if not used in an inflammatory process, they die or are destroyed by other phagocytic cells. The bone marrow quickly replaces the neutrophils that have exited the bloodstream with cells from the bone marrow storage pool. The daily production of neutrophils is approximately 1×10^{11}/L in adults with 20% remaining in circulation.[2]

Neutrophil Counts in Bone Marrow and Peripheral Blood

Variations in the number and morphology of leukocytes in the bloodstream and bone marrow have long been used as clinical guides for the diagnosis of many diseases. These variations reflect the response of normal leukocytes to an underlying disease, or indicate a primary disorder intrinsic to leukocytes, such as leukemia. A thorough knowledge of established normal values and morphological characteristics of all cellular elements is important for recognizing and interpreting unexpected findings.

Marrow Counts

Although leukocytes are generally regarded to be residents of peripheral circulation, blood serves as a route of transportation from sites of production in the bone marrow to sites of function in the tissues. Granulocytes, lymphocytes, and monocytes are formed in the bone marrow for release into the bloodstream. In addition, lymphocytes proliferate in extramedullary lymphoid tissue such as the thymus. Values for the various cell types, as determined by differential cell counting of bone marrow samples from healthy individuals, are presented in Table 15–2.

Values are fairly constant except during infancy, when they vary according to age.[2] Erythrocyte precursors decrease in number shortly after birth and remain sparse until active erythropoiesis resumes during the second to third month of life. The percentage of myelocytic precursors (predominately neutrophils) falls dramatically during the first month of life owing to a decrease in mature forms. Values are stable during infancy and increase during later childhood to adult levels. The number of lymphocytes increases markedly during the first month of life, and this cell becomes the most numerous in the marrow throughout infancy. Plasma cells are virtually absent until approximately 6 months of age. In older children and adults, myelocytic precursors outnumber erythroid by about 4:1 in the bone marrow with the postmitotic neutrophil forms (metamyelocytes, bands, and polymorphonuclear neutrophils) predominating to form the neutrophil storage pool. During bacterial infections the myeloid-to-erythroid (M:E) ratio may increase further owing to increased granulocyte production.

Peripheral Blood Counts

Complete blood cell counting (the CBC) is accomplished routinely by automated methods on electronic analyzers based on electrical impedance and laser technologies. These whole blood analyzers determine white cell, red cell, and platelet counts in addition to differentiating leukocytes ac-

---

➤ **Table 15–1**

ABRIDGED LISTING OF THE CONTENTS OF NEUTROPHIL GRANULES

Primary Granules

Lysozyme

Myeloperoxidase

Acid phosphatase

Elastase

Secondary Granules

Lysozyme

NADPH oxidase

Cytochrome b

Lactoferrin

Tertiary Granules

Plasminogen activator

Alkaline phosphatase

Gelatinase

> ## Table 15-2
> ### PERCENTAGES OF PRECURSOR CELL TYPES IN THE BONE MARROW

Cell Type	Birth	1 mo	3 mo	12 mo	Adult
Erythrocytes	7–21	3–12	8–19	4–12	18–30
Granulocytes	54–72	27–33	25–50	25–44	50–70
early:late	1:12	1:9	1:9	1:10	1:5
Lymphocytes	8–20	35–55	32–56	32–58	3–17
Plasma cells	0	0	0	0–1	0–2

cording to the percentage of granulocytes, lymphocytes, and monocytes present. White blood cell counts vary considerably with age; the established normal range for white cell counts is provided in Table 15–3. Generally, mature, polymorphonuclear neutrophils predominate in the peripheral blood of healthy persons, with an occasional neutrophilic band noted. Because of the high number of cells evaluated by automated instruments, an occasional immature form can be seen; a single unexpected leukocyte should not be interpreted as abnormal unless other clinical or laboratory findings suggest the presence of disease.

A wide range in expected white blood cell number exists at birth in healthy infants, with the neutrophil presenting as the predominant cell.[4] Although not apparent in Table 15–3, significant changes in the differential white blood cell count occur during the first few days of life. At birth, the mean neutrophil count is about 8.0×10^9/L. This count rises rapidly to a peak value of about 13.0×10^9/L at 12 hours of age but then drops to a mean of about 5.0×10^9/L by 72 hours of age. Thereafter, the neutrophil count slowly decreases so that the lymphocyte becomes the predominant cell by the age of 2 to 3 weeks (4.0×10^9/L). During the first few days of life, an increased number of slightly immature neutrophils such as metamyelocytes and bands may be observed transiently in circulation. This early release of metamyelocytes and bands from the bone marrow reserve into the bloodstream is referred to as a "shift to the left."

In neonatal populations, the activity of neutrophils is reported to be diminished. Studies in healthy newborns show reduced neutrophil mobility, deformability, and adherence, whereas stressed neonates show an additional decrease in phagocytic and bactericidal activity.[5] The compromised activity of neutrophils in the neonate predisposes this population to septicemia and should be considered if the expected

shift to the left persists and is accompanied by a relatively low white blood cell count (less than 3.0×10^9/L, with 70% neutrophils and immature forms such as metamyelocytes and bands).[1,6] Newborns are particularly likely to develop severe neutropenia during bacterial infections as a result of depletion of the neutrophil storage pool in the bone marrow.

Response to Infections

Neutrophils play a central role in removing infectious and inflammatory agents that challenge host immunity. Within minutes, neutrophils are stimulated to migrate from circulation through junctions between endothelial cells to the site of infection or inflammation. The classic response to infectious and inflammatory processes is an increase in the relative number of neutrophils, termed *neutrophilia*. The accelerated release of neutrophils from the bone marrow reserve is accompanied by a shift to the left that is defined as an increased number of metamyelocyte and band forms observed in the circulating pool. The increase in circulating neutrophil number and immaturity is similarly observed in the early stages of neoplastic conditions, such as chronic myelocytic leukemia, and in myeloproliferative disorders. The major distinction is that the myelocytic precursors released during the infectious response are more limited to the metamyelocyte and band, whereas in neoplastic processes, earlier precursor cells such as myelocytes, promyelocytes, and blasts are also present. The cytochemical staining technique, leukocyte alkaline phosphatase, is useful for differentiating neutrophilic response to infection (leukemoid reaction) from chronic myelocytic leukemia (see Chap. 31). The kinetics of circulating neutrophils vary greatly depending on the type, duration, and intensity of the infection. The immediate response to infection is transient neutropenia, resulting from increased margination and accelerated delivery of neutrophils to the infected site. Within an hour, neutrophils are released from the bone marrow reserve into the bloodstream. In the early phases of infection, the circulating half-life of neutrophils is shortened and cell turnover is accelerated.[7] Later, the circulating half-life returns to normal.

In addition to changes in neutrophil number, reactive changes in neutrophil morphology can be observed in the forms of toxic granulation, Döhle bodies, and cytoplasmic vacuolization (Figs. 15–1 to 15–3; see also Color Plates 137 to 139 and Chap. 5). Toxic granulation is frequently associated with severe infection in which the cytoplasmic granules enlarge and take on darker staining properties than normal. The toxic granules have been identified as primary granules that are peroxidase positive. Toxic granulation can be accompanied by the presence of pale blue inclusions in the pe-

> ## Table 15-3
> ### RANGE OF BLOOD LEUKOCYTE COUNTS (ABSOLUTE NUMBER $\times\ 10^9$/L)

Cell Type	Birth	6 mo	4 yr	Adult
Total leukocytes	4–40	5–24	5–15	4–11
Neutrophils	2–20	0.5–10	1.5–7.5	1.5–7.5
Lymphocytes	1–9	1.5–22	1.5–8.5	1–4.5
Monocytes	0–2	0–2.5	0–1	0–1
Eosinophils	0–1.5	0–2.5	0–1	0–0.5
Basophils	0–0.3	0–0.4	0–0.2	0–0.2

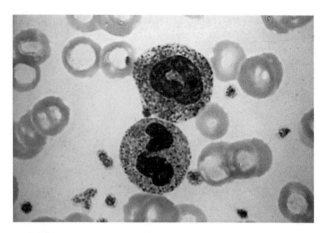

➤ FIGURE 15–1   Toxic granulation (peripheral blood). Note the prominent dark-staining granules.

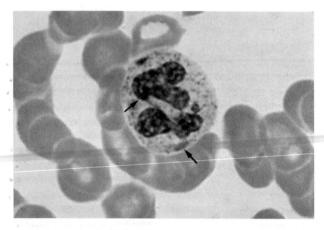

➤ FIGURE 15–2   Döhle bodies (*arrows*). Note the large bluish bodies in the periphery of the cytoplasm.

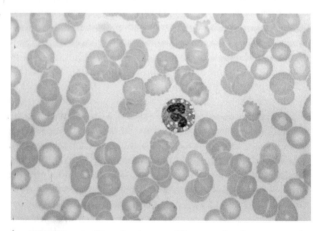

➤ FIGURE 15–3   Vacuolated neutrophils suggesting the presence of infection or a severe inflammation.

riphery of the cytoplasm, which are referred to as Döhle bodies. They consist of a few strands of rough endoplasmic reticulum that have aggregated. Döhle bodies are similar, but not identical, to the inclusions found in the hereditary leukocyte and platelet disorder known as the May-Hegglin anomaly (see Fig. 15–4 and Color Plate 140). Lastly, in response to infection, the cytoplasm may become vacuolated and, occasionally, contain ingested microorganisms. The presence of

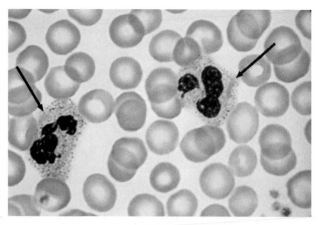

➤ FIGURE 15–4   May-Hegglin anomaly. Note the Döhle body present in each neutrophil (*arrows*). Not shown in the slide but associated with May-Hegglin anomaly is the presence of giant platelets. (From Dutcher, T: Hematology. In Listen, Look, and Learn. Health and Education Resources, Inc., Bethesda, MD, with permission.)

one or more of these reactive changes suggests progression toward sepsis.[8] Although these morphological features are viewed to be a clinically sensitive tool for predicting severe infection, they are not specific to infection.[9] All have occasionally been observed during uncomplicated pregnancy, massive trauma, inflammatory processes, drug reactions, and other toxic states. Furthermore, all three morphological features are commonly observed, with toxic granulation being reported as the most common morphological change in response to bacterial infection, followed by Döhle bodies and cytoplasmic vacuolization.[8] Table 15–4 summarizes the possible quantitative and qualitative changes in neutrophils during infection.

The function of circulating neutrophils, as well as their number and appearance, can be affected by infection. Both enhanced and impaired functions have been reported when compared with normal values in studies performed during infections.[10] Despite the fact that exceptions exist, it is generally accepted that mild infections enhance neutrophil function,[11] whereas severe infections impair neutrophil function. The role that these acquired functional abnormalities play in the course of infections is unknown.

Neutrophil Function

The main function of the neutrophil is the internalization of microorganisms for destruction; a process referred to as phagocytosis. Once bacteria infiltrate the tissues, neutrophils are stimulated for immediate action. For the purposes of discussion, phagocytosis is described as occurring in

> ## Table 15–4
> ## QUALITATIVE AND QUANTITATIVE NEUTROPHIL CHANGES NOTED IN RESPONSES TO INFECTION

- Neutrophilia
- Shift to the left
- Toxic granulation
- Döhle bodies
- Vacuolization

three distinct phases: migration and diapedesis; opsonization and recognition; and ingestion, killing, and digestion (Fig. 15–5).

Migration and Diapedesis

Neutrophils in the marginating pool roll along vessel endothelium in a random and nondirectional pattern called locomotion until a site of injury or infection is encountered. Bacteria and sites of inflammation in the host send out signals in the form of chemoattractants (Table 15–5), which stimulate changes in morphology and migration pattern.[12] The chemoattractant forms a concentration gradient, with the neutrophil migrating toward the area of highest concentration. A re-engineering of the plasma membrane occurs that transforms the neutrophil shape from smooth and round to ruffled and flat, with pseudopods and a tail (Fig. 15–6). Under the stimulus of chemoattractants, the activated neutrophil migrates in a repetitive, wavelike motion to the site of infection. The process of directional migration under the guidance of chemoattractants is known as chemotaxis. The neutrophil adheres to endothelial receptors and, by diapedesis, penetrates through narrow junctions between endothelial cells into the tissues. In diapedesis, the neutrophil is briefly retained by the vascular basement membrane but then enters the tissues by passing through small openings in this membrane. Chemoattractants further accelerate the rate of neutrophil migration by a process known as chemokinesis. With neutrophils being the first phagocytes to migrate to the site of infection, the lag time between microorganism invasion and timely neutrophil migration is crucial for limiting the spread of infection or even preventing infection.[1] All three modes of neutrophil migration contribute to the efficient mobilization of neutrophils to the site of injury (Table 15–6).

Opsonization and Recognition

Migrating neutrophils cannot efficiently recognize and attach to most microorganisms. A mechanism referred to as opsonization facilitates recognition and attachment by marking the organism for ingestion. The term *opsonin* is of Greek origin and literally means "to prepare for dining."[2] Although

Table 15-5
CHEMICAL FACTORS THAT SIGNAL NEUTROPHIL ACTIVATION

Chemoattractants	Source
N-formyl oligopeptides	Bacteria
C5a, C3b, and C3bi factors	Complement
Interleukin-8	Monocyte
Leukotriene B$_4$	Membrane phospholipid
Platelet-activating factor	Endothelium

chemotaxis is taking place, circulating immunoglobulin and activated complement components coat the surface of the bacteria. The marked bacteria, referred to as an opsonin, is readily recognized and ingested by the neutrophil. Ingestion will not take place without the presence of membrane-bound immunoglobulin. The plasma membrane of the neutrophil carries receptors for the Fc fragment of immunoglobulin G (IgG) molecules and activated complement only. Proteins that most effectively mark bacteria for recognition and attachment are IgG1, IgG3, C3b, and C3bi.[13]

Phagocytosis: Ingestion, Killing, and Digestion

The ingestion of the opsonized microbe begins as soon as the membrane surface receptor of the neutrophil and microbe bind together. Membrane pseudopods extend around and envelop the microbe, forming an isolated vacuole within the neutrophil cytoplasm known as a phagosome. Simultaneously, cytoplasmic granules migrate to and fuse with the membrane of the phagosome, forming a phagolysosome (Fig. 15–7). Once fusion is complete, the cytoplasmic granules undergo degranulation, whereby their contents are released into the phagolysosome. Studies performed in vitro suggest an orderly sequence of events for phagolysosome formation, with the degranulation of secondary granules preceding that of the primary granules.[14] The ingested organism is exposed to the lytic activity of granular enzymes within the phagolysosome that leads to eventual killing and digestion.

Microorganism destruction (killing) is accomplished by oxygen-dependent and non–oxygen-dependent mechanisms. The non–oxygen-dependent mode of killing the internalized particle is represented by an alteration in pH and the release of the lysosomal and proteolytic enzymes into the phagolysosome.[15] The lytic enzymes possess bactericidal activity that cleaves segments of the bacterial cell wall. Alternately,

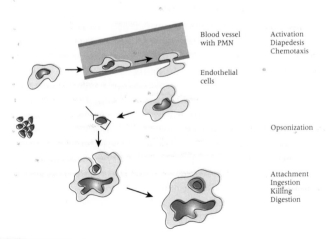

Blood vessel with PMN

Activation
Diapedesis
Chemotaxis

Endothelial cells

Opsonization

Attachment
Ingestion
Killing
Digestion

► **FIGURE 15–5** Illustration of the phases of neutrophilic phagocytosis, which include activation, diapedesis, chemotaxis, opsonization, ingestion, killing, and digestion. PMN = polymorphonuclear neutrophil. (From Abramson, JS, and Wheeler, JG: The Natural Immune System—The Neutrophil. Oxford University Press, Oxford, 1993, p 110, with permission.)

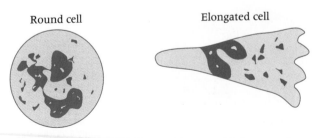

Round cell

Elongated cell

► **FIGURE 15–6** The shape change of the neutrophil, from smooth and round to ruffled and flat with pseudopods, is a result of stimulation by chemoattractants. (Adapted from Kaplan, S, and Brams, CA: Testing for Neutrophil Function. Advance, 7(1), 1995, p 8, with permission.)

> ## Table 15-6
> ### THREE MODES OF NEUTROPHIL MIGRATION

Mode of Migration	Characteristics
Locomotion (random)	Nondirectional
Chemokinesis	Nondirectional acceleration of migration speed
Chemotaxis	Directional

oxygen-dependent killing involves the release of nictinomide adenine dinuleotide phosphatase (NADPH) oxidase, which mediates the production of the active oxygen metabolites, superoxide and hydrogen peroxide, during a process known as the respiratory burst. These active oxygen metabolites are capable of microorganism injury. To further enhance the antibacterial activity, superoxide and hydrogen peroxide react with other products of phagocytosis such as myeloperoxidase (in primary granules of neutrophils and monocytes) to produce highly toxic agents such as hypochlorous acid (household bleach).[16]

Disorders of Neutrophils

Disorders of the neutrophil cell line predispose an individual to recurrent bacterial infections that are resistant to treatment. Neutrophil disorders are classified as quantitative and qualitative, reflecting changes in neutrophil number and function, respectively. Quantitative disorders present a significant decrease in the absolute neutrophil number and are referred to as neutropenia. Inadequate neutrophil number limits the potential for effective mobilization and killing at the site of microbial invasion. Alternately, qualitative disorders are marked by neutrophil dysfunction as a result of impaired migration or altered bactericidal activity. As noted, phagocytosis occurs in a complex sequence of events ranging from activation, migration, and diapedesis to the recognition, ingestion, and killing of an opsonized particle. A deficiency or dysfunction in any one or a combination of these processes modifies neutrophil function.

Quantitative Disorders—The Neutropenias

Neutropenia is defined as an absolute decrease in the number of circulating neutrophils and is suspected when patients present with absolute neutrophil counts of less than 1.5×10^9/L. Absolute counts can be obtained by multiplying the total white blood cell count by the percentage of neutrophils (and bands) seen in the differential cell count. The low neutrophil count is not the sole indicator of disease and should be correlated with patient history and clinical and laboratory findings. The normal level of circulating neutrophils varies with age and race, and refers to mature polymorphonuclear and band forms, only. Recurrent bacterial infections are the hallmark of persistent neutropenia, with the clinical severity being reflected by the absolute neutrophil count as well as the frequency and duration of neutropenic episodes. Neutropenia can range from mild, with absolute counts from 1.0 to 1.5×10^9/L, to moderate, with counts from 0.5 to 1.0×10^9/L, to severe, with counts less than 0.5×10^9/L.[8] Life-threatening infections are not generally observed until blood counts fall below 0.2×10^9/L.

Infections in the neutropenic patient are most commonly caused by endogenous normal flora such as *Staphylococcus aureus, Streptococcus viridans,* and gram-negative enteric organisms.[17] Although neutropenia increases host susceptibility to bacterial infection, the risk of viral, fungal, and parasitic infection is not increased. Most infections in the neutropenic individual occur in the cutaneous and soft tissues. The major concern for these infections is the spread of the organism from the localized site into the bloodstream, resulting in a superinfection such as septicemia.

Neutropenic disorders are described as acquired or congenital. Persistent cases of neutropenia are generally attributed to an intrinsic problem of the hematopoietic system whereas transient conditions are linked to factors extrinsic to the bone marrow. The absolute reduction in the circulating number of neutrophils is attributed to decreased production, impaired marrow release, or increased destruction. Identification of the cause is important for selecting appropriate therapy, monitoring prognosis, and counseling family members in congenital cases.

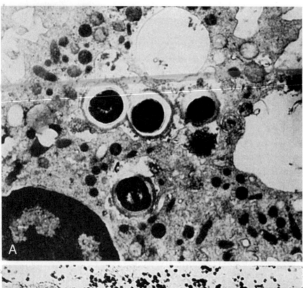

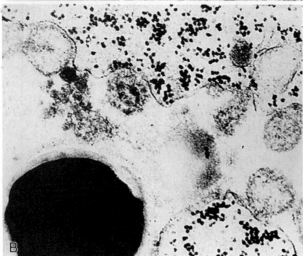

> ► FIGURE 15-7   Electron microscopy of phagolysosome formation. (*Left*) Staphylococci lie within phagocytic vesicles limited by sacs formed from inverted pieces of the neutrophil membrane. Cytoplasmic granules are approaching the phagocytic vesicles. (*Right*) Higher magnification shows degranulation with the discharge of granule contents into the vicinity of the staphylococcus.

Acquired Neutropenia

Most acquired neutropenias occur as transient conditions caused by factors extrinsic to the bone marrow. In order of frequency, concomitant viral infection, the ingestion of certain medications, and alloantibody or autoantibody activity are all reported to be causes (Tables 15–7 and 15–8). Neutropenia can also be acquired as a secondary condition to processes such as aplastic anemia, malignancy of the bone marrow, and dietary B_{12} and folate deficiency.

Infection

Viral infections are recognized to be the most common cause of acquired neutropenia especially in children under the age of six. The neutropenia appears during the first few days of illness, when the peak level of virus is reached and lymphocytosis develops. Viruses implicated in inducing neutropenia include influenza A and B, rubella, rubeola, herpes simplex, hepatitis A and B, and respiratory syncytial virus. The accompanying neutropenia appears within 24 to 48 hours of viral infection onset and can persist for the period of acute viremia.[8]

Immune-Mediated Neutropenia

Neutropenia can result from the activity of antineutrophil antibodies that mediate the removal of opsonized neutrophils from circulation. Immune-mediated neutropenia can be caused by either alloantibody or autoantibody when patients present with absolute neutrophil counts less than 0.5×10^9/L and recurrent infections of mild to moderate severity. Alloimmune neonatal neutropenia has been described as being analogous to red cell hemolytic disease of the newborn. The neutropenia develops after maternal sensitization to fetal neutrophil antigens. The antigens are shared by the fetus and the father, but are absent in the mother. During pregnancy, antineutrophil antibody production is stimulated in the maternal immune system, and these IgG antibodies cross the placenta and destroy fetal neutrophils. The antineutrophil antibodies are directed against neutrophil-specific antigens, such as NA1, NA2, and NB1, or HLA antigens that are shared by neutrophils and other nucleated cells. Alloimmune neutropenia is encountered in approximately 3% of all live births[18]; the condition is more common in firstborn children. Severe neutropenia can persist for an average of 7 weeks or until the antineutrophil antibodies are cleared from neonatal circulation. After this time, the neutrophil count returns to the normal range expected for this age group. Alloimmune neonatal neutropenia can be accompanied by cutaneous infections and infrequently progresses into respiratory infection and life-threatening sepsis. Therapy is usually supportive and consists of antibiotics when infections occur.

> ### Table 15-7
> ### FACTORS ASSOCIATED WITH ACQUIRED NEUTROPENIA

Infection, especially viral

Drug ingestion

Alloantibodies

Autoantibodies

Secondary to underlying disease

> ### Table 15-8
> ### DRUGS ASSOCIATED WITH CAUSING NEUTROPENIA

Drug Class	Drug Prototype
Antibiotics	Penicillin
	Chloramphenicol
Anti-inflammatory	Ibuprofen
Anticonvulsants	Phenytoin
Antithyroid	Propylthiouracil
Cardiovascular	Procainamide
Hypoglycemic	Chlorpropamide
Tranquilizer	Phenothiazine

Autoantibodies directed against neutrophils have also been detected in the serum of some patients with neutropenia. Survival studies utilizing radiolabeled techniques demonstrate that neutrophils coated by autoantibody exhibit a shortened half-life in circulation.[19] Clinically, the condition is classified as primary autoimmune neutropenia of idiopathic origin, or as secondary to disease states such as Felty's syndrome, rheumatoid arthritis, systemic lupus erythematosus, and chronic hepatitis. The antineutrophil autoantibodies can be of the IgG, IgM, or IgA immunoglobulin class, with the NA1 specificity being observed most often. Autoimmune neutropenia has been identified in both adults and children, although it is observed more frequently as the cause of chronic benign neutropenia of childhood.[20] Although no standard treatment has been established, antibiotics are used to treat specific bacterial infections and prednisone to limit the autoimmune response.

Congenital Neutropenias

Congenital or chronic neutropenias occur as persistent or intermittent disorders arising from an inherited abnormality in cells of the myeloid line or those involving hematopoietic regulation (Table 15–9). The defective or deficient production is intrinsic to the bone marrow microenvironment. Consequences of these defects result in decreased or arrested cell production, or impaired release by the bone marrow. These disorders are not caused by factors extrinsic to the bone marrow such as infection, drug ingestion, or antibodies. Most are extremely rare and genetically heterogeneous.

> ### Table 15-9
> ### DISORDERS OF CONGENITAL NEUTROPENIA

Chronic benign neutropenia

Severe congenital neutropenia (Kostman's)

Myelokathexis

Cyclic neutropenia

Reticular dysgenesis

Fanconi's anemia

Dyskeratosis congenita

Shwachman-Diamond syndrome

Clinical presentation varies from little, if any, increased risk of infection as seen in chronic benign neutropenia to the overwhelming, recurrent infections in severe congenital neutropenia that result in death within the first year of life. In severe congenital cases, clinical benefits have been seen with the administration of granulocyte–colony-stimulating factor (G-CSF) in terms of neutrophil increment and infection prophylaxis.[21]

Qualitative Disorders of Neutrophils

Qualitative disorders of neutrophil function are characterized by bacterial infections that are caused by hereditary abnormalities in function. The occurrence of most qualitative conditions is extremely rare; many are familial and stem from a general metabolic defect. The exact pathophysiology of nearly all qualitative neutrophil disorders is unknown. Neutropenia commonly accompanies these disorders. The qualitative disorders are classified according to the major defect expressed—cytoplasmic granules, disturbances of the respiratory burst, and chemotaxis; however, multiple abnormalities (including neutropenia) can be observed in some patients (Table 15–10). For practical purposes, the most clearly understood qualitative disorders are addressed here.

Chédiak-Higashi Syndrome

Chédiak-Higashi syndrome (CHS) is a rare autosomal-recessive condition featuring recurrent bacterial infections, partial albinism, and the presence of giant lysosomal granules in cells such as granulocytes, monocytes, lymphocytes, melanocytes, tissue macrophages, and platelets. Mild bleeding tendencies are frequently observed (Figs. 15–8 and 15–9 and Color Plates 141 and 142). Progressive neurologic complications develop during childhood, with moderate neutropenia accompanying nearly all cases. Many of these patients die as a result of infection during early childhood. Those who survive early childhood enter an accelerated phase that progresses through pancytopenia, lymphoma-like cell infiltration, organomegaly, systemic infections, and eventually death. *Staphylococcus aureus* accounts for the majority of infections.

In addition to the neutropenia, inefficient and prolonged

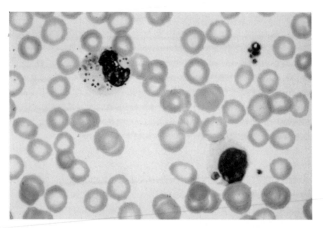

> FIGURE 15–8   Peripheral blood from a patient with Chédiak-Higashi syndrome. (*Right*) Lymphocyte. (*Left*) Neutrophil. (From Dutcher, T: Hematology. In Listen, Look, and Learn. Health and Education Resources, Inc., Bethesda, MD, with permission.)

bacterial killing has been identified as a key dysfunction in phagocytic activity. The release of lysosomal enzymes is impaired by the abnormal granule membrane fusion that results in the characteristic giant lysosomal granules. These abnormal granules develop during early myelopoiesis because of an initial aggregation of primary granules followed by fusion with the secondary granules (see Fig. 15–8 and Color Plate 141). The giant lysosomal granules are more evident in cells of the bone marrow than in peripheral white cells. In circulation, the most striking granules can be seen in natural killer cells (NK subset of lymphocytes). The granules stain from dark red to deep purple with Wright's stain and are strongly positive for peroxidase.

Management of CHS, before the onset of the accelerated phase, includes prophylactic antimicrobial therapy and high daily doses of ascorbic acid.[8] In the case of infection, aggressive intravenous treatment is required. The Epstein-Barr virus (EBV) is believed to trigger the accelerated phase of CHS, so immunization against EBV may be beneficial.[8] Bone marrow transplantation holds the only hope for cure, with success being reported in a small number of patients. Optimally, bone marrow transplantation should be performed before the onset of the accelerated phase.[22]

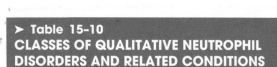

> ### Table 15–10
> ### CLASSES OF QUALITATIVE NEUTROPHIL DISORDERS AND RELATED CONDITIONS

Cytoplasmic Granules

Chédiak-Higashi syndrome

Myeloperoxidase deficiency

Specific granule deficiency

Biochemical Disturbance of Respiratory Burst

Chronic granulomatous disease

Glucose-6-phosphate dehydrogenase deficiency

Glutathione deficiency

Chemotaxis

Lazy leukocyte syndrome

Monosomy

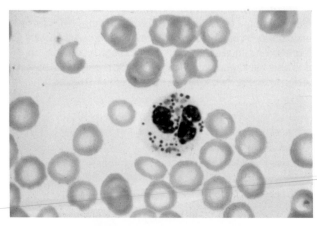

> FIGURE 15–9   Neutrophil from a patient with Chédiak-Higashi syndrome. The cytoplasm is filled with strikingly large primary (azurophilic) granules. (From Dutcher, T: Hematology. In Listen, Look, and Learn. Health and Education Resources, Inc., Bethesda, MD, with permission.)

Chronic Granulomatous Disease

Chronic granulomatous disease (CGD) is a familial, heterogeneous disorder of the neutrophil that can be chronic or intermittent. CGD is the best-understood disorder of neutrophils. It is seen in 1 out of every 500,000 individuals who exhibit recurrent bacterial and fungal infections, generally during the first year of life. The congenital abnormality is attributable to a failure in the activation of the respiratory burst that results in little or no superoxide production. The characteristic clinical picture of these patients is of lymphadenitis, deep tissue infections such as osteomyelitis, and visceral and hepatic abscesses, recurrent pulmonary infections, organomegaly, and infected eczematoid rash. CGD patients exhibit neutrophilia rather than neutropenia. The hallmark of CGD is the formation of granulomas during chronic inflammatory reactions that keep the organisms localized. Life-threatening infections are often caused by *Aspergillus, S. aureus,* and enteric organisms.

The first cases of CGD were observed in boys presenting with severe bacterial infections by the first year of life, and were believed to be inherited as a sex-linked recessive disorder. Most of these patients died of septicemia or chronic pulmonary disease in early childhood. Additional cases of CGD were identified in girls who exhibited separate but genetically similar defects. It is now recognized that CGD can be inherited in a sex-linked–recessive or autosomal-recessive pattern, depending on the subunit of NADPH oxidase affected[23] (Table 15–11).

Chronic granulomatous disease results from one of four single gene mutations in NADPH oxidase, which is composed of oxidase components known as phagocytic oxidase subunits, or *phox*. The interaction of these subunits results in the formation of superoxide during the respiratory burst. Each *phox* subunit is identified as a glycoprotein (gp) or a protein (p). Two of the subunits, gp91-*phox* and p22-*phox*, are located in the plasma membrane and together form the enzyme cytochrome b. The other subunits, p47-*phox*, p67-*phox*, and p40-*phox*, reside in the cytosol. Stimulation of NADPH oxidase leads to the migration of the cytosol subunits to the plasma membrane. With the help of secondary mediators, the *phox* subunits assemble into the active oxidant, superoxide.[23] The classic X-linked form demonstrates a total absence of cytochrome b whereas most autosomal-recessive cases present with deficiencies in one of the cytosol subunits (see Table 15–11). Regardless of the subunit defect, superoxide cannot be produced, and, in turn, bacterial killing is ineffective. Ingestion of bacteria, degranulation, and phagolysosome formation are normal.

Diagnosis is established by demonstrating a bactericidal defect resulting from the absence of the oxidative burst on the nitroblue tetrazolium test (NBT), a luminol-enhanced assay, or by measuring respiratory burst activity with flow cytometry. The X-linked–recessive inheritance may be confirmed by studying the family history. Indicators of CGD include the presence of disease in male members of the maternal family and intermediate to low neutrophil activity in the mothers and sisters of affected boys. In most cases, the female relatives are clinically well, but occasionally they present with an increased susceptibility to infections or a syndrome resembling systemic lupus erythematosus.

Progress has been made in modalities of treatment and the prognosis is improving. Aggressive prophylactic antibiotic therapy should be initiated as soon as a diagnosis is made. Gamma (γ) interferon has been effective in limiting the frequency of infections, and granulocyte transfusions are useful in patients who respond poorly.[24] Bone marrow transplantation has proved to be beneficial when performed in children, even during ongoing infection; however, the rate of success is dependent on the HLA-match and supportive therapy with both G-CSF and granulocyte infusions. In vitro studies of gene correction for CGD have been carried out using peripheral blood progenitor cells, making the prospect of a cure most encouraging.[25,26]

White Blood Cell Anomalies

Several hereditary abnormalities in neutrophil morphology are observed in patients without the involvement of infection, neutrophil dysfunction, or altered neutrophil number. Such abnormalities in neutrophil morphology are collectively referred to as white blood cell anomalies. Hypersegmentation and hyposegmentation of the nucleus are white cell anomalies that reflect the number of segmented lobes demonstrated in the mature neutrophil. Hypersegmentation describes larger-than-normal neutrophils with six or more nuclear lobes present (see Chap. 7). A similar hypersegmentation of eosinophils has been reported, with five or more nuclear lobes present. Hypersegmentation in the granulocytes may be an indicator of megaloblastic anemia or of a benign autosomal-dominant condition known as hereditary hypersegmentation of neutrophils.

Hyposegmentation of the nucleus is characteristic of Pelger-Huët anomaly, a condition in which the nucleus is found to be bilobed or to have no lobulation whatsoever. Moreover, nuclear chromatin is exceptionally coarse and condensed. In the heterozygous state, predominantly bilobed neutrophil forms are present that are described as having a "dumbbell" or "pince-nez" appearance with two symmetric lobes being joined by a filament. In the homozygous state, no segmentation is evident, and the nucleus takes on a round or oval appearance (Fig. 15–10 and Color Plate 143). "True" Pelger-Huët anomaly is inherited in an autosomal-dominant manner and is reported to be a benign familial condition that is observed in 1 out of 6000 individuals.[8] Acquired Pelger-Huët can be induced by drug ingestion or occur secondary to conditions such as leukemia. Acquired forms, in which 10% of the neutrophils are trilobed, are often referred to as pseudo-Pelger-Huët. Care must be taken to distinguish Pelger-Huët cells from a "shift to the left," in which an increase in metamyelocytes and bands is observed during severe infection. Generally the nuclear chromatin is more condensed and coarse in Pelger-Huët neutrophils than in bands and metamyelocytes. Furthermore, in Pelger-Huët anomaly, more than 70% to 90% of all neutrophils are affected.

> **Table 15–11**

MOLECULAR BASIS OF CHRONIC GRANULOMATOUS DISEASE

Cytochrome b Subunit Affected	Mode of Inheritance	Neutrophil Structure Involved
p47-*phox*	Autosomal	Cytosol
p67-*phox*	Autosomal	Cytosol
gp91-*phox*	X-linked	Plasma membrane
p22-*phox*	Autosomal	Plasma membrane

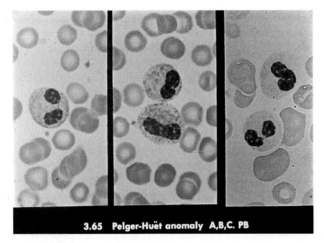

3.65   Pelger-Huët anomaly A,B,C. PB

➤ **FIGURE 15–10**   Pelger-Huët anomaly (peripheral blood). (From Hyun, BH, et al: Practical Hematology. A Laboratory Guide with Accompanying Filmstrip. WB Saunders, Philadelphia, 1975, with permission.)

Morphological changes may also be noted in the neutrophilic cytoplasm. The presence of prominent, dark-staining, coarse cytoplasmic granules in neutrophils, eosinophils, basophils, monocytes, and occasionally lymphocytes is known as Alder's anomaly or Alder-Reilly inclusions (Fig. 15–11 and Color Plate 144). In some patients only one cell line is affected. These cytoplasmic inclusions are composed of precipitated mucopolysaccharide and are seen in association with inherited disorders of mucopolysaccharidosis such as Hunter's and Hurler's syndromes. These prominent granules are similar to those in toxic granulation, with the exceptions that they are larger, stain positive with metachromatic stains, and are a permanent morphological characteristic of the neutrophils.

Toxic granulation is a transient change in morphology caused by infectious or toxic agents. Granulocytes in the hereditary May-Hegglin anomaly demonstrate larger, blue-staining cytoplasmic inclusions that resemble Döhle bodies except that they are larger (see Fig. 15–4). Under electron microscopy these neutrophils are shown to have large, granule-free areas in the cytoplasm that contain fibrils of ri-

bonucleic acid. These Döhle-like inclusions are also seen in monocytes. In addition to this morphological feature of the neutrophil, thrombocytopenia is reported along with giant platelets (see Chap. 23).

➤ LYMPHOCYTES

Definition of Lymphocytosis

Lymphocytosis is present when there is an excess of lymphocytes in the peripheral blood. Absolute lymphocyte counts decrease with age. In infants and young children, lymphocyte counts greater than $10.0 \times 10^9/L$ represent lymphocytosis. In adults, a finding of more than $4.0 \times 10^9/L$ lymphocytes is defined as lymphocytosis. The absolute lymphocyte count is determined by multiplying the percentage of lymphocytes (obtained from the peripheral blood differential) by the total leukocyte count (obtained from the CBC).

Relative lymphocytosis refers to an increase in the percentage of lymphocytes when the absolute lymphocyte count is within normal range. This situation may occur when other hematopoietic elements are decreased; that is, in neutropenia in which lymphocytes are not affected.

The term *reactive lymphocytes* is used to describe transformed or benign lymphocytes. The term *atypical* should *not* be used interchangeably with reactive because, in pathology, atypical is used to describe malignant-appearing cells. Other terms that have been used to describe the spectrum of reactive lymphocytes include immunocytes, transformed lymphocytes, immunoblasts, plasmacytoid lymphocytes, Turk cells, and Downey cells. Reactive lymphocytes occur in normal patients, but usually account for less than 10% of the total lymphocytes present. In order to maintain consistency with laboratory reporting, laboratories should have criteria and normal ranges for reactive lymphocytes in their procedure manual. Control slides with reactive lymphocytes should be reviewed on a regular basis with staff to ensure uniformity in the reporting of reactive lymphocytes.

Lymphocyte Morphology

Reactive lymphocytes and normal lymphocytes (Table 15–12) vary in size, shape, and immunophenotypic markers (polyclonal). The cells do *not* originate from one precursor cell or clone. In contrast, lymphocytes in malignant disorders are similar with regard to size, shape, (monomorphous), and immunophenotype, because they originate from the same malignant clone (monoclonal). Lymphomas may vary in size depending on the particular malignancy. However, for any one malignancy, the size and appearance tend to be constant.

Reactive lymphocytes range in size from 9 to 30 μm. Figure 15–12 and Color Plate 145 illustrate the size variation that can be seen with reactive lymphocytes. Resting small lymphocytes tend to be much smaller than reactive lymphocytes, ranging in size from 8 to 12 μm, and are similar in size to the top right lymphocyte in Figure 15–12 (right arrow).

The ratio of the nuclear area to the visible cytoplasmic rim (N:C ratio) varies with reactive lymphocytes. One of the most important features in distinguishing reactive lymphocytes is the abundant amounts of cytoplasm present when compared with smaller resting lymphocytes. Resting small lymphocytes have relatively little cytoplasm whereas

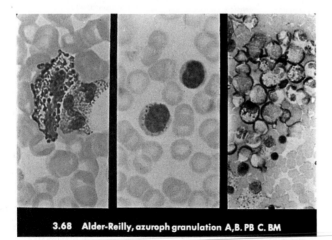

3.68   Alder-Reilly, azuroph granulation A,B. PB C. BM

➤ **FIGURE 15–11**   Alder-Reilly anomaly. (*Left and middle*) Note azurophilic granulation in cells from peripheral blood. (*Right*) Bone marrow. (From Dutcher, T: Hematology. In Listen, Look, and Learn. Health and Education Resources, Inc., Bethesda, MD, with permission.)

> **Table 15-12**
> **LYMPHOCYTE MORPHOLOGIES**

	Reactive Lymphocyte	Resting Small Lymphocyte*
Size	Large (9–30 μm)	Small (8–12 μm)
N:C Ratio†	Low to moderate	High to moderate
Cytoplasm	Abundant	Scant
	Colorless to dark blue	Colorless to light blue
Nucleus	Round to irregular	Round
Chromatin	Coarse to moderately fine†	Coarse
Nucleoli	Absent to distinct	Absent
Typing	Polyclonal	Polyclonal

*Normal peripheral blood may contain a few medium-sized natural killer cells that are larger than resting small lymphocytes but smaller than large reactive lymphocytes.
†The N:C ratio is the ratio of the nuclear area to the visible cytoplasmic rim.
†The chromatin is not as fine as that seen in blast cells.

NK cells may have moderate amounts of cytoplasm. In Figure 15–12 and Color Plate 145, three lymphocytes are present. In the center of the field is a large reactive lymphocyte with abundant cytoplasm (large arrow). The cytoplasm is usually pale blue, with occasional azurophilic granules. A significant morphological feature of reactive lymphocytes is the uneven staining of the cytoplasm. In reactive lymphocytes, peripheral portions of the cytoplasm often stain darker blue than areas of the cytoplasm closer to the nucleus. Also, the cytoplasmic border is usually round with an occasional indentation.

The nucleus in reactive lymphocytes may be round, indented, or lobulated (Fig. 15–13 and Color Plate 146). In reactive conditions, the appearance of the nuclear chromatin in the lymphocyte population is variable and not monotonous. Generally, the nuclear chromatin is coarse or clumped, and prominent clumping or coarseness of the chromatin similar to plasma cells may occur. Figure 15–14 and Color Plate 147 illustrate a small "plasmacytoid" lymphocyte with prominent chromatin clumping, perinuclear halo, and an eccentric nucleus similar in appearance to a

plasma cell. The nucleus in resting small lymphocytes is round and less variable. The chromatin may vary in coarseness but not to the extent seen with reactive lymphocytes.

Nucleoli may be present in reactive lymphocytes. Such reactive lymphocytes can be differentiated from lymphoblasts or myeloblasts by having more abundant cytoplasm

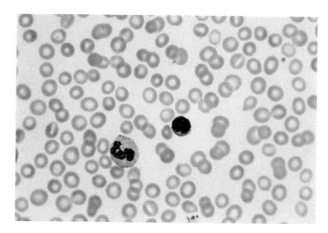

> **FIGURE 15–13**   Lymphocyte with nuclear indentation.

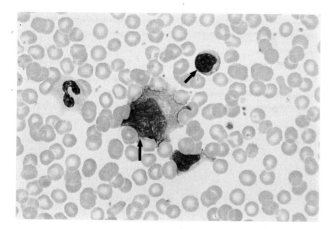

> **FIGURE 15–12**   Three lymphocytes are present, one with abundant cytoplasm (low N:C ratio) and two with moderate amounts of cytoplasm, from a patient with infectious mononucleosis. Note the variation in the chromatin coarseness. The larger or reactive-appearing lymphocyte has prominent cytoplasm indentations (*center arrows*).

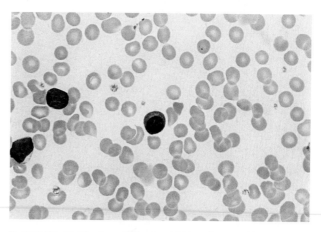

> **FIGURE 15–14**   A small plasmacytoid lymphocyte with coarse chromatin and an eccentric nucleus.

and a clumped chromatin pattern. Figure 15–15 and Color Plate 148 illustrate a reactive lymphocyte with a prominent nucleolus, often referred to as an "immunoblast." *Immunoblast* is a descriptive morphological term and has no bearing on the lymphocyte type. Nucleoli are not present in resting small lymphocytes.

A few granules may be seen in the cytoplasm of lymphocytes (Fig. 15–16 and Color Plate 149). These granules are azurophilic, appear lilac or purple, and are larger than the fine, pink, secondary granules present in neutrophils. When there are many lymphocytes with azurophilic granules and abundant cytoplasm, "large granular lymphocytosis" must be considered (Fig. 15–17 and Color Plate 150). In contrast, the cytoplasm of monocytes contains many small granules and has a "ground-glass" appearance. Auer rods are never seen in lymphocytes.

In order to make a correct morphological evaluation, blood smears need to be made from a fingerstick or fresh tube of ethylene diaminetetraacetic acid (EDTA)-anticoagulated blood. The cells need to be well stained, and the observer should look at areas of the smear that are neither too thick nor too thin. Improper pH of the Wright's stain buffer makes it difficult to evaluate nuclear and cytoplasmic features by altering the staining characteristics of these structures.

Morphological criteria alone usually enable one to dis-

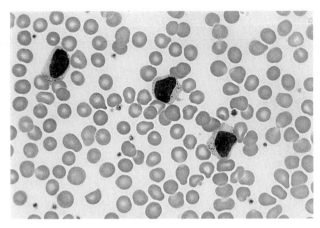

➤ FIGURE 15–17   Reactive-appearing lymphocytes with prominent granulation from a patient with large granular lymphocytosis.

tinguish reactive lymphocytosis from malignant disorders. When there is ambiguity, clinical history, cell typing, and serologic findings help. If necessary, a bone marrow or lymph node biopsy may lead to the correct diagnosis. The most common causes of reactive lymphocytosis are shown in Table 15–13. Malignant conditions that may be confused with reactive lymphocytosis are listed in Table 15–14.

Causes of Reactive Lymphocytosis

Infectious Mononucleosis

History

In 1907, Turk described clinical symptoms in several patients who probably suffered from infectious mononucleosis caused by EBV infection.[27] Reactive lymphocyte morphology and clinical symptoms were correlated in 1920 by Sprunt, who named the syndrome "infectious mononucleosis."[28] Downey, in 1923, described in further detail the unusual lymphocyte morphology associated with infectious mononucleosis.[29] Although morphology is still important, Downey's descriptive terminology of morphology is seldom used today. *Infectious mononucleosis* is a historical term. We now know that the large mononuclear cells originally described in infectious mononucleosis are lymphocytes and not monocytes.

Later, in 1932, Paul noticed that serum from patients with infectious mononucleosis contained antibodies against sheep erythrocytes.[30] This discovery was the basis for the Monospot test (Ortho Pharmaceuticals). This contemporary test is the most popular and the simplest method available for measuring IgM heterophile antibodies. Heterophile antibodies are antibodies that also react with cells of other species. In particular, the IgM antibodies react with sheep and horse erythrocytes. The antibodies are not absorbed by guinea pig kidney in the Monospot test and, thus, if present, agglutinate horse erythrocytes.

The deoxyribonucleic acid (DNA) virus responsible for infectious mononucleosis was first observed in lymphoblasts cultured from patients with Burkitt's lymphoma[31] (see Chap. 21). This virus is now known as the Epstein-Barr virus (EBV). In addition to Burkitt's lymphoma, EBV has been associated with other malignancies, including B-cell lymphoproliferative syndromes, nasopharyngeal carcinoma, Hodgkin's disease, and gastric carcinoma.[32] The

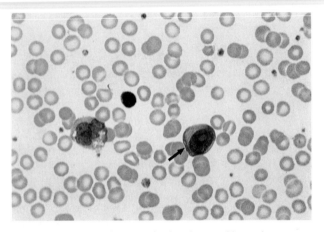

➤ FIGURE 15–15   A large reactive lymphocyte with prominent nucleolus (immunoblast).

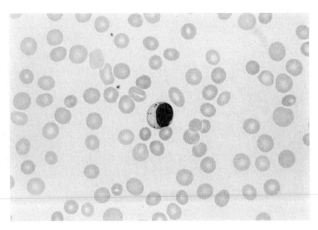

➤ FIGURE 15–16   A small, mature-appearing lymphocyte with azurophilic granules.

> **Table 15-13**
> ## CAUSES OF REACTIVE LYMPHOCYTOSIS

Viral

Adenovirus

Chickenpox

Cytomegalovirus

EBV (infectious mononucleosis)

Hepatitis

Herpes simplex

Herpes zoster

Human immunodeficiency virus (HIV)

Influenza

Paramyxovirus (mumps)

Rubella (measles)

Bacterial

Brucellosis

Paratyphoid fever

Pertussis (whooping cough)

Tuberculosis

Typhoid fever

Drug Reactions

During recovery from acute infections (especially in children)

Miscellaneous

Acute infectious lymphocytosis

Allergic reactions

Autoimmune diseases

Hyperthyroidism

Malnutrition

Rickets

Syphilis

Toxoplasmosis

> **Table 15-14**
> ## MALIGNANT CONDITIONS THAT MAY BE CONFUSED WITH REACTIVE LYMPHOCYTOSIS

Acute Lymphocytic Leukemias

L1

L2

L3

Acute Myelocytic Leukemias

M3m

M5a

Chronic Leukemias

Chronic lymphocytic leukemia (CLL)

Hairy-cell leukemia

Lymphocytosis of large granular lymphocytes

Prolymphocytic leukemia

Leukemic Phase of Lymphoma

Follicular lymphoma (typically small cleaved cell)

Mantle cell lymphoma

Other non-Hodgkin's lymphomas (e.g., large cell)

Miscellaneous

Adult T-cell leukemia/lymphoma (ATL/L)

Mycosis fungoides, Sézary syndrome

Plasma cell leukemia

malignancies appear to occur after the virus has been dormant in the host for years.

In regard to acute viral illness, EBV was first linked as the causative agent for infectious mononucleosis by Henle in 1967.[33] He was able to establish a lymphocyte cell line from the blood of a laboratory worker who was infected with EBV and managed to show by serologic studies that EBV was responsible for infectious mononucleosis. Additional evidence supporting the role of EBV in infectious mononucleosis has been provided by the detection of EBV nucleic acid sequences using polymerase chain reaction on lymphoid tissue from patients with infectious mononucleosis.[34,35] Unlike EBV-associated malignant conditions, infectious mononucleosis results from primary infection.

Humans can be infected by one of two strains of EBV, type A or B, which are widespread in North America and can coinfect the same individual.[36] EBV primarily infects B lymphocytes and epithelial cells of the pharynx and cervical lymph nodes, which all share the CD21 receptor.[37] Interestingly, the majority of atypical lymphocytes associated with infectious mononucleosis have been identified to be T lymphocytes of the cytotoxic-suppressor subset, although T helper cells and NK cells are also present.[38] Initial stimulation of the T cells appears to be nonspecific; this is later followed by direct stimulation from EBV-infected B lymphocytes.[39] The direct stimulation results in such rapid T-lymphocyte proliferation that the lymph nodes enlarge and the cells released are reactive in appearance.

Clinical Manifestations

Infectious mononucleosis is more commonly present in young individuals, with the peak incidence between 17 and 25 years of age. The virus enters the body orally through the lymphoid tissue in the pharynx and, in turn, infects B lymphocytes. The onset is generally abrupt, the most consistent initial symptoms being sore throat, lymphadenopathy, fever, dysphagia, general malaise, and excessive fatigue that can persist for 2 to 3 weeks. The severity of the sore throat pain leads to difficulty in swallowing and anorexia. Other commonly observed symptoms include nausea, headache, myalgia, sweats, and chills. Infrequently, individuals present with mild autoimmune hemolytic anemia because of cold-reacting antibodies (agglutinins) specific for the "i" red cell antigen (see Chap. 13), and immune thrombocytopenia caused by increased splenic activity.

Multiple organ involvement with related symptoms may be present in infectious mononucleosis. Enlargement of the anterior cervical lymph nodes is another physical finding during the first week. Following a week or two, the swelling usually subsides. The nodes are firm but not tender or warm. At least one-half of patients demonstrate a palpable spleen during the course of infection and, rarely, splenic rupture may occur. Hypersplenism can contribute to mild anemia or immune thrombocytopenia, or both. Hepatomegaly may be detected in up to 25% of patients with infectious mononucleosis. Liver enzymes and bilirubin levels may be elevated because of liver involvement.

Infectious mononucleosis is uncommon in older adults and, therefore, the differential diagnosis of lymphocytosis is influenced by the age of the patient. For example, in a 50-year-old patient with increasing numbers of benign-looking lymphocytes, the diagnosis of chronic lymphocytic leukemia (CLL) is more likely than infectious mononucleosis; however, in a child or young adult, CLL is extremely rare.

Differential Diagnosis

The differential diagnosis for infectious mononucleosis includes a variety of entities listed in Tables 15–13 and 15–14. The differential may be narrowed considerably by evaluation of a blood smear and serologic findings. The skilled morphologist should be able to readily differentiate the reactive lymphocytes seen in infectious mononucleosis from malignant cells seen in leukemia or lymphoma. Cytomegalovirus, rubella, hepatitis, and other viral illnesses may have reactive lymphocytes and may require additional serologic findings to distinguish them from EBV infection. Acute streptococcal pharyngitis, diphtheria, and other bacterial infections are identifiable by culture, and the lymphocytes usually do not have the typical morphology seen in viral infections. Classical reactive lymphocytes and definitive serologic findings may not always be present and, therefore, it may be difficult in some instances to distinguish between infectious mononucleosis and other processes. In those rare cases, additional studies, such as lymph node biopsy may be indicated.

Treatment, Clinical Course, and Prognosis

Treatment of infectious mononucleosis is mostly symptomatic, with some patients requiring bed rest. Acetaminophen or ibuprofen products are often taken to relieve muscle pain and headache. Little progress has been made in decreasing the duration of illness, with antiviral therapies showing few benefits.[40] In the few patients with severe or persistent cases, corticosteroids have been indicated to treat associated hemolytic anemia and progressive neurologic problems. Intravenous γ globulin is frequently administered to treat infectious mononucleosis–associated immune thrombocytopenia,[41] and limited success has been seen using γ interferon to treat complications such as pneumonia or encephalitis.[42]

Antibiotics are not useful unless there are complications such as streptococcal pharyngitis. The fatality rate of infectious mononucleosis is approximately 1 in 3000 cases.[43] In acute cases, complete recovery usually occurs within 2 months, and recurrences are extremely rare. It should be noted that not all children who have acquired immunity had a prior history or clinical symptoms of infectious mononucleosis. EBV infections in immunocompromised patients may be life threatening. In view of the increasing incidence of patients with immunodeficencies, the morbidity rate is likely to increase.

Cytomegalovirus Infection

Cytomegalovirus (CMV) belongs to the herpesvirus family and is endemic worldwide. The virus may be transmitted by oral, respiratory, and sexual means or by blood transfusion and organ transplantation. Patients with CMV infection may have recurrent or reactivation of a latent infection such as is seen in herpes simplex infection, or patients may be reinfected with a different CMV strain. CMV infection is the most common cause of heterophile-negative infectious mononucleosis. The diagnosis is made by demonstrating the presence of IgM antibodies to CMV or by shell vial tissue cultures.

Clinical Manifestations

In the majority of immunocompetent individuals, CMV infection is usually asymptomatic. The clinical manifestations reflect the organ(s) of involvement. When CMV infection occurs in previously healthy individuals, the symptoms mimic EBV infection. Symptoms include fever, sore throat, splenomegaly, lymphadenopathy, and myalgia. Morphological changes in lymphocytes are indistinguishable from those seen in EBV infection. Because of liver involvement, mild to moderate elevation of liver function tests is common.

In immunocompromised individuals, CMV infection can be life threatening. Because CMV infection is endemic, parenterally acquired infection from transfusions is a concern, especially with the increase in the numbers of individuals who are immunocompromised from chemotherapy, immunosuppressive drugs, or human immunodeficiency virus (HIV) infection.

Other Viral Infections

Any viral infection has the potential to elicit an immune response, resulting in absolute lymphocytosis. Lymphocytes that appear "stimulated" or reactive may be seen in CMV and infectious hepatitis, in addition to infectious mononucleosis. With a negative Monospot test, other viral infections—for example, rubella, HIV,[44,45] herpesvirus-6,[46] and the adenoviruses—should be considered.

Bacterial Infections

Lymphocytosis in bacterial infections occurs more commonly in chronic infections and during the recovery period following acute infections. The organisms most often responsible include *Brucella, Mycobacterium tuberculosis,* and spirochetes. Marked lymphocytosis with mature-appearing lymphocytes is seen in children with pertussis (whooping cough), and absolute lymphocyte counts exceeding 50×10^9/L can be seen in 4% of patients.[47] Morphologically, these cells appear similar to those seen in CLL and small lymphocytic lymphoma (SLL). In pertussis, immunologic marker studies reveal that the lymphocytes are predominantly helper T cells.[48] Prominent lymphadenopathy, which may be present in lymphoma or EBV infection, is also unusual in children with pertussis or infectious lymphocytosis.

Malignant Conditions

Table 15–14 lists malignant disorders that may be confused with reactive lymphocytosis. In general, the malignant cells in leukemia and lymphomas are monotonous in appearance and, therefore, are morphologically different from the reactive lymphocytes seen in benign conditions. Malignant cells in leukemias and lymphomas are monoclonal when immunophenotypically analyzed.

The morphology of lymphoblasts seen in acute lymphoblastic leukemia (ALL) is different from that of reactive lymphocytes. ALL is morphologically classified as L1, L2, or L3, depending on the morphology of the cells (see Chap. 16). In contrast to reactive lymphocytes, blast cells in L2 leukemia have fine chromatin and prominent nucleoli (Fig. 15–18 and Color Plate 151). The cells in L1 leukemia are monotonous in appearance and do not have as much cytoplasm as do reactive lymphocytes (Fig. 15–19 and Color Plate 152). The N:C ratio is much higher in L1 leukemia cells than in reactive lymphocytes. In L3 leukemias (Fig. 15–20 and Color Plate 153), abundant cytoplasmic vacuoles are present which are lacking in reactive lymphocytes. The cells present in prolymphocytic leukemia (PLL) may also be confused with reactive lymphocytes. Figure 15–21 and Color Plate 154 show the prominent, usually single, nucleoli that are present in PLL. Reactive lymphocytes have more abundant cytoplasm and less prominent nucleoli than prolymphocytes.

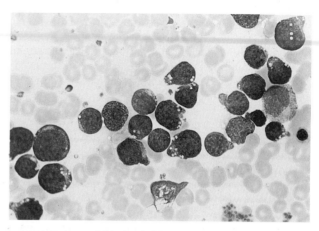

➤ **FIGURE 15–20** L3 leukemia. Note the abundant cytoplasmic vacuoles and clumped chromatin.

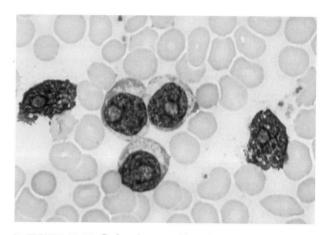

➤ **FIGURE 15–21** Prolymphocytes with moderate amounts of cytoplasm and prominent nucleoli.

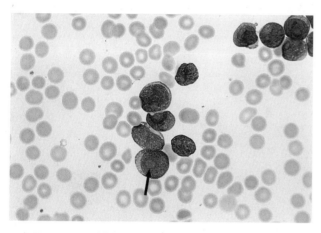

➤ **FIGURE 15–18** L2 leukemia. The L2 lymphoblasts have fine chromatin with a moderate amount of cytoplasm and nucleoli. Note the prominent nucleolus in one of the lymphoblasts (*arrow*).

Severe cytopenias that occur in acute leukemias are infrequent in benign lymphocytosis. With anemia or severe thrombocytopenia, the diagnosis of leukemia must be considered.

Patients with lymphoma may have a leukemic phase with circulating malignant cells. Except for the large-cell lymphomas, circulating lymphoma cells may be easily distinguished from reactive lymphocytes. Figure 15–22 and Color

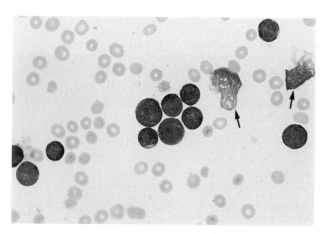

➤ **FIGURE 15–19** L1 leukemia. These L1 lymphoblasts have a high N:C ratio (scant cytoplasm), fine chromatin, and indistinct nucleoli. Except for the fine chromatin, note the similarity to mature lymphocytes. These cells should not be confused with reactive lymphocytes. Note the large "smudge cells" (*arrows*).

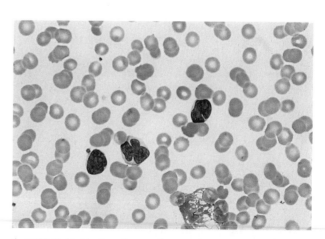

➤ **FIGURE 15–22** Lymphocytes from a patient with follicular small cleaved-cell lymphoma. Note the prominent nuclear clefting.

Plate 155 show the nuclear clefting seen in the leukemic phase of follicular small cleaved-cell lymphoma. Fortunately, in large-cell lymphoma, malignant cells in the peripheral blood are rare. Prominent generalized lymphadenopathy is unusual in infectious mononucleosis but may occur in non-Hodgkin's lymphoma and Hodgkin's disease.

Laboratory Examination

A variety of laboratory procedures may help in the correct diagnosis of patients with absolute lymphocytosis. CBC, serology, and microbiologic culture are often performed. Of these procedures, a CBC with differential and serologic studies are the most useful.

Proper evaluation of the peripheral blood smear is crucial for the correct differential diagnosis in patients with absolute lymphocytosis. Especially in infectious mononucleosis, reactive lymphocytes are prominent and should easily be identified by the experienced observer. Figure 15–12 and Color Plate 145 shows a reactive lymphocyte with abundant cytoplasm (low N:C ratio) and indented cytoplasmic borders (large arrow). The less experienced observer may mistake these unusual-appearing reactive lymphocytes for monocytes or blasts. However, as seen in Figure 15–23 and Color Plate 156, monocytes typically have linear condensation of chromatin whereas blasts (see Fig. 15–18 and Color Plate 151) have chromatin strands that are finer and evenly dispersed.

The lymphoblasts in L2 leukemia or monoblasts in M5a leukemia, a category of acute myelocytic leukemia, may also be mistaken for reactive lymphocytes. Figure 15–24 and Color Plate 157 illustrates M5a, monoblastic leukemia. Monoblasts have a low N:C ratio but fine chromatin is present as well as prominent nucleoli. Figure 15–18 and Color Plate 151 show the fine chromatin and prominent nucleoli (arrow) present in an L2 lymphoblast. With reactive lymphocytes, a careful review of the cell morphology will reveal that overall, the chromatin is not fine enough for the cells to be classified as blasts and that the overall morphology is variable and *not* monotonous as seen in leukemias.

Serologic tests play a critical role in establishing the diagnosis in patients with absolute lymphocytosis. In the proper clinical setting, a positive Monospot (heterophile antibody) test with reactive lymphocytes in the peripheral blood (see Fig. 15–12 and Color Plate 145) is diagnostic of infectious mononucleosis. A variety of antibodies formed by humoral responses may be measured when it is necessary to further elucidate the etiology of lymphocytosis in difficult cases or in cases in which the Monospot test is negative[49] (Table 15–15).

In the first week of viral infections, IgM antibodies are formed against viral capsid antigens. During the second

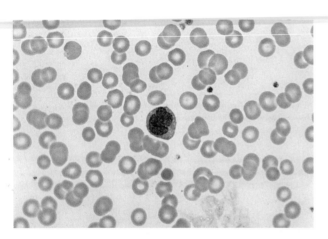

➤ FIGURE 15–23   This monocyte has very fine granular cytoplasm, cerebriform nucleus, linear condensation of chromatin, and no nucleolus.

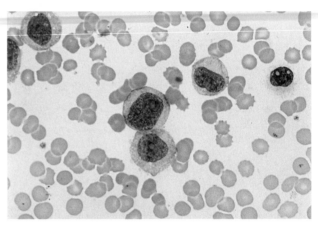

➤ FIGURE 15–24   M5a leukemia. These monoblasts have abundant cytoplasm (low N:C ratio), fine chromatin with some chromatin clumping, and prominent nucleoli.

➤ **Table 15–15**

SUMMARY OF ANTIBODY TESTS USEFUL IN THE DIFFERENTIAL DIAGNOSIS OF INFECTIOUS MONONUCLEOSIS

Antigen	Test Used	Description	Clinical Significance
Heterophile	Monospot	Antibodies to a variety of antigens	Appears late in the first week; detected with Monospot test; transient
EBV-VCM (IgM)	ELISA	IgM antibody to viral capsid antigen	Detectable in first week of infection; earliest detectable antibody; declines rapidly after second week
EBV-VCA (IgG)	ELISA	IgG antibody to viral capsid antigen	Detectable approximately 7 days after exposure; levels persist for life; responsible for immunity
EBNA	ELISA	Antibody to EBV nuclear antigen	Appears late in first month of infection and persists for life; may indicate past infection
EBV-EA	ELISA	Antibody to EBV early antigen complex	Seen in < 5% of normal, healthy subjects; may indicate EBV-carrier state

week, as the immunologic response matures, IgG antibodies are formed. Figure 15–25 illustrates the pattern of the immunologic response and lymphocytosis that is expected in patients with infectious mononucleosis. A rise in titer should be demonstrated by comparing serum obtained during acute and convalescent phases. Also, by using enzyme-linked immunosorbent assay (ELISA) techniques, antibodies to CMV and hepatitis can be measured. Finally, viral cultures may be performed.

The Monospot test is most frequently used for infectious

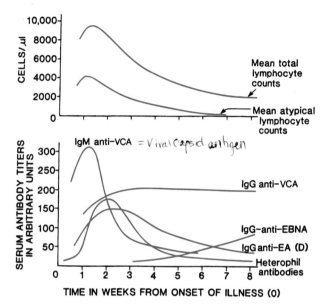

FIGURE 15–25 Time-course relationship between heterophile antibodies, various anti-Epstein-Barr antibodies, and the mean total and reactive lymphocyte counts. VCA = viral capsid antigen, EBNA = Epstein-Barr nuclear antigen, EA = early antigen, D = diffuse component. (From Lee, RG, et al: Wintrobe's Clinical Hematology, ed 9. Lea & Febiger, Philadelphia, 1993, p 1658, with permission.)

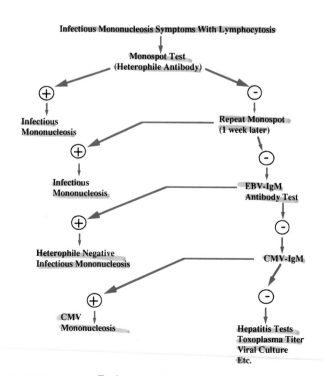

FIGURE 15–26 Testing strategies for infectious mononucleosis differential diagnosis.

mononucleosis because the rise in titer of heterophile antibodies parallels the rise in titer of the more specific EBV antibodies. The Monospot test is much quicker, easier to use, and less expensive than measuring viral-specific antibodies. If the Monospot test is initially negative, it should be repeated in 1 week if infectious mononucleosis is suspected. Serum may be analyzed for antibodies to specific EBV antigens; antibodies to CMV and hepatitis may be measured, and viral cultures may be performed. Figure 15–26 diagrams some of the possible testing strategies.

In cases where malignancy is being considered, lymphocytes may be further characterized by immunophenotype. With leukemias and lymphomas, typing usually reveals a monoclonal cell population. As previously noted, it is the B cell that is infected by the EBV, with most of the reactive lymphocytes seen in infectious mononucleosis being polyclonal T cells.

➤ CASE STUDY 1

History of Present Illness

A 3-year-old boy was admitted with a diagnosis of liver abscess after ultrasound examination. He had been ill with many infections since the age of 1 month. Types of infections included recurrent episodes of pneumonia and ear infection, perirectal abscess, osteomyelitis of the metacarpals, suppurative lymphadenitis, and mastoiditis. Organisms that were recovered from these sites of infection were *Staphylococcus aureus* and *Aspergillus*. Despite these episodes of infection, he experienced normal growth and development. The family medical history was remarkable in that an older brother and a cousin (a son of a maternal aunt) had suffered similar chronic infections, and one had died of chronic pneumonia caused by a gram-positive organism. On physical examination, the boy appeared to be generally well. The skin was covered with scattered areas of crusted scabs described as an infected eczematoid rash. A Gram stain of the rash revealed gram-positive cocci in clusters (*Staphylococcus*). Lymph nodes and liver were enlarged.

Laboratory Data

The hemoglobin level was determined to be 9 g/dL, and the erythrocyte morphology was normal with slight hypochromia. The total white blood cell count (WBC) was 33.0×10^9/L (28.0×10^9/L neutrophils). The neutrophils contained moderate toxic granulation and vacuoles. The platelet count was 427×10^9/L. Concentrations of serum immunoglobulins and complement components were all increased moderately. Neutrophilia was consistently found on several occasions when earlier laboratory data were reviewed. Neutropenia was never documented. Studies of neutrophil migration and phagocytosis were normal. Oxidative metabolism in response to neutrophil stimulation was completely absent. Specifically, there was no postphagocytic increase in oxygen consumption, and superoxide anion and hydrogen peroxide were not formed.

continued

Finally, neutrophils were unable to oxidize and kill *Staphylococcus* that had been phagocytized. Neutrophils from the mother were studied and on some assays performed at about 50% of normal capacity.

Discussion

This patient exhibits characteristic features of the X-linked recessive form of chronic granulomatous disease of childhood, with severe and persistent infections caused by *Staphylococcus* organisms. Anemia and persistent neutrophilia are seen even when these patients are relatively free of infection. Neutrophils from these children are numerous; they migrate normally; they are capable of phagocytosis; and they form phagocytic vesicles. The neutrophils of these patients, however, are unable to kill the phagocytized microorganisms because they are unable to generate active oxygen metabolites such as superoxide anion and hydrogen peroxide. In some families, the X-linked nature of the inheritance pattern may be established by finding disease in male members of the maternal family and by finding moderate defects in the mother.

► CASE STUDY 2

History of Present Illness

A 13-year-old girl went to her physician because of sore throat, general malaise, and fever. On questioning, she explained that she had been feeling fatigued for about a week, with some nausea and difficulty in drinking fluids. Physical examination revealed bilateral enlarged, firm cervical lymph nodes, mild splenomegaly, and hepatomegaly.

Laboratory Data

The laboratory data revealed a WBC count of 15.0×10^9/L; hematocrit, 42%; platelets, 4.5×10^9/L; and reticulocytes, 2.0%. A differential count of the peripheral blood revealed 65% lymphocytes, 25% granulocytes, and 10% monocytes. The differential report noted that 36% of the lymphocytes were reactive (see Fig. 15–12). Chemistry results showed that liver enzymes and bilirubin levels were slightly increased. No other abnormalities were noted.

After the physical examination, additional laboratory work was ordered. The throat culture for streptococci was negative. A Monospot test was then performed and found to be positive. No further laboratory work was ordered. After a few days of rest at home, the patient was allowed to return to school. No further problems were noted.

Discussion

The differential diagnosis in this case includes EBV infectious mononucleosis, viral pharyngitis, diphtheria, and streptococcal pharyngitis. The clinical history and clinical presentation is not consistent with other infections or malignancy. If the Monospot test had been negative, the differential diagnosis would need to be expanded.

With a negative Monospot test, further testing should first include an ELISA for EBV-VCA (IgM) and possibly a repeat Monospot in a week. If infectious mononucleosis as a diagnosis is ruled out, then other laboratory procedures need to be performed. These would include further cultures, serologic tests, and possibly lymph node and bone marrow biopsies. In this case, the liver enzymes were elevated; up to 25% of individuals with infectious mononucleosis can have liver involvement.

QUESTIONS

1. The enzymatic contents of primary (azurophilic) granules include:
   a. NADPH oxidase and hydrogen peroxide
   b. Cytochrome b and collagenase
   c. Myeloperoxidase and lysozyme
   d. Alkaline phosphatase and gelatinase

2. Directional migration toward a gradient stimulated by a chemoattractant is referred to as:
   a. Chemotaxis
   b. Random mobility
   c. Opsonization
   d. Chemokinesis

3. The marking of an invading microbe with IgG and complement to facilitate recognition is referred to as:
   a. Chemokinesis
   b. Opsonization
   c. Phagolysosome fusion
   d. Signal transduction

4. Which sequence reflects the correct order for phagocytosis?
   a. Release of cytoplasmic granules; binding of particle; ingestion; fusion of phagolysosome
   b. Ingestion; binding of particles; fusion of phagolysosome; release of cytoplasmic granules
   c. Binding of particle; ingestion; fusion of phagolysosome; release of cytoplasmic granules
   d. Fusion of phagolysosome; binding of particle; release of cytoplasmic granules; ingestion

5. In oxygen-dependent killing, the enzyme responsible for mediating the production of active oxygen metabolites during the respiratory burst is:
   a. Myeloperoxidase
   b. Lysozyme
   c. Lactoferrin
   d. NADPH oxidase

6. The two most important biochemical products of the respiratory burst that are involved with particle digestion during active phagocytosis are:

a. Lactoferrin and gelatinase
b. Superoxide dismutase and catalase
c. Glutathione peroxidase and copper-zinc enzymes
d. Superoxide anion and hydrogen peroxide

7. The morphological characteristic(s) associated with Chédiak-Higashi syndrome is (are):
   a. Giant lysosomal granules
   b. Hypersegmented agranular neutrophils with vacuolization
   c. Prominent dark-staining granules and pyknotic nuclei
   d. Pale blue inclusions in cytoplasm of neutrophils and giant platelets

8. The defect in chronic granulomatous disease is attributed to:
   a. Delayed degranulation
   b. Inefficient ingestion of microbes
   c. Defective bacterial killing
   d. Abnormal phagolysosome formation

9. Identify the disease characteristic(s) associated with Chédiak-Higashi syndrome.
   a. Partial albinism, recurrent infections, and mild bleeding tendencies
   b. Granulomas, osteomyelitis, and hepatic abscesses
   c. Hypopigmentation of skin and chronic, swollen lymph nodes
   d. Periodic pneumonia that may result in lesions called pneumatoceles

10. Pelger-Huët anomaly may be described by:
    a. Large neutrophils and hypersegmentation of the nucleus with greater than six lobes
    b. Dark-staining, coarse granules in cytoplasm of neutrophils, eosinophils, basophils, and monocytes
    c. Pale blue inclusions of the cytoplasm of neutrophils and giant platelets
    d. Hyposegmentation of the nucleus with the majority of neutrophils being bilobed or monolobed

11. Reactive lymphocytes may best be distinguished from blasts by the presence of which of the following morphological features?
    a. Prominent nucleoli
    b. Fine chromatin
    c. Heterogeneous cell population
    d. High N:C ratio

12. Which of the following antigens is detectable first by ELISA?
    a. EBNA
    b. EBV-VCA (IgM)
    c. EBV-VCA (IgG)
    d. Heterophile

13. The Epstein-Barr virus infects which of the following cells?
    a. Helper T lymphocytes
    b. Cytotoxic T lymphocytes
    c. B lymphocytes
    d. NK cells

14. What is the most frequent cause of a heterophile (Monospot) negative mononucleosis-like syndrome?
    a. HIV
    b. CMV
    c. Hepatitis C
    d. *Toxoplasma gondii*

15. In which of the following conditions are reactive lymphocytes found?
    a. Infectious mononucleosis
    b. CMV infection
    c. Rubella
    d. All of the above

16. Absolute lymphocytosis is best described as:
    a. Greater than 70% lymphocytes on differential
    b. Presence of nucleoli in lymphocytes
    c. Monoclonal population of lymphocytes
    d. Greater than 4.0×10^9 lymphocytes per liter in an adult

17. Which of the following features are seen in reactive lymphocytes?
    a. Low N:C ratio
    b. Blue cytoplasm
    c. Indented cytoplasmic borders
    d. All of the above

18. Which of the following clinical manifestations would be unexpected in infectious mononucleosis?
    a. Skin rash
    b. Sore throat
    c. Fatigue
    d. Fever

19. Which of the following features best differentiates malignant lymphomas from infectious mononucleosis?
    a. Clonality
    b. Monotony
    c. Pattern of lymphadenopathy
    d. All of the above

20. Which of the following viral agents causes infectious mononucleosis?
    a. Heterophile virus
    b. Human herpes-6 virus
    c. EBV
    d. HIV

SUMMARY CHART

➤ Neutrophils are capable of amoeboid movement into the tissues to engulf and destroy bacteria and fungus.
➤ Phagocytosis occurs in three distinct phases: migration and diapedesis; opsonization and recognition; and ingestion, killing, and digestion.
➤ The three modes of migration that contribute to

efficient neutrophil mobilization to a site of injury are random locomotion, directional chemotaxis, and accelerated chemokinesis.

➤ A *shift to the left* is defined as the early release of bands and metamyelocytes from the bone marrow into circulation in response to infection or inflammation.

➤ Neutrophilia is known as an increase in the number of circulating neutrophils.

➤ In response to bacterial infection, reactive changes in neutrophil morphology can be observed in the forms of toxic granulation, Döhle bodies, and vacuolization.

➤ *Neutropenia,* which can be acquired or congenital, is defined as an absolute decrease in the number of circulating neutrophils below $1.5 \times 10^9/L$.

➤ Chédiak-Higashi syndrome is a rare disorder of neutrophil function that is characterized by recurrent bacterial infections, partial albinism, and the presence of giant lysosomal granules in nucleated cells.

➤ Chronic granulomatous disease, the best understood disorder of neutrophil function, is a defect that is attributed to one of four mutations in NADPH oxidase, resulting in ineffective bacterial killing.

➤ In Pelger-Huët anomaly, more than 70% to 90% of neutrophils have a bilobed nucleus or no nuclear segmentation at all.

➤ In Alder's anomaly, prominent, dark-staining, coarse cytoplasmic granules are observed in neutrophils.

➤ Individuals with May-Hegglin anomaly demonstrate large, dark blue–staining cytoplasmic inclusions in granulocytes; thrombocytopenia; and giant platelets.

➤ Lymphocytosis is known as an increase in the number of circulating lymphocytes.

➤ The term *reactive lymphocytes* is used to describe transformed or benign lymphocytes, which usually account for less than 10% of the total lymphocytes present.

➤ An absolute lymphocyte count is determined by multiplying the percentage of lymphocytes (from the peripheral blood differential) by the total leukocyte count (from the complete blood count).

➤ Reactive changes in lymphocyte morphology are heterogeneous and include a low N:C ratio; round, indented, or lobulated nucleus; abundant, uneven-staining cytoplasm with a round or indented cytoplasmic border; and the possible presence of nucleoli.

➤ Malignant cells in leukemia and lymphoma can be distinguished morphologically from reactive lymphocytes in as much as malignant cells are monotonous in appearance, similar in size and shape, as they originate from a single clone.

➤ Reactive changes in lymphocytes commonly accompany infectious mononucleosis, cytomegalovirus (CMV), rubella, hepatitis, and other viral infections.

➤ Caused by the Epstein-Barr virus (EBV), infectious mononucleosis is characterized by sore throat, fatigue, fever, headache, difficulty swallowing, and generalized malaise in teenagers and young adults.

References

1. Abramson, JS, and Wheeler, JG: The Natural Immune System—The Neutrophil. Oxford University Press, Oxford, 1993.
2. Nathan, DG, and Oski, FA: Hematology of Infancy and Childhood, ed 4. WB Saunders, Philadelphia, 1993, pp 882–951.
3. Krause, KH, and Lew, D: Bacterial toxins and neutrophil activation. Semin Hematol 25:2, 1988.
4. Manroe, BL, et al: The neonatal blood count in health and disease: I. Reference values for neutrophilic cells. J Pediatr 95:89, 1979.
5. Christensen, RD, et al: The leukocyte left shift in clinical and experimental neonatal sepsis. J Pediatr 98:101, 1981.
6. Christensen, RD, et al: Granulocyte transfusion in neonates with bacterial infection, neutropenia, and depletion of mature marrow neutrophils. Pediatrics 70:1, 1982.
7. Walker, RI, and Willemze, R: Neutrophil kinetics and the regulation of granulopoiesis. Rev Infect Dis 2:282, 1980.
8. Lee, RG, et al: Wintrobe's Clinical Hematology, ed 10. Williams & Wilkins, Baltimore, 1999, pp 1836–1902.
9. Seebach, JG, et al: The diagnostic value of the neutrophil left shift in predicting inflammatory and infectious disease. Am J Clin Pathol 107:582, 1997.
10. McCall, CE, et al: Human toxic neutrophils: III. Metabolic characteristics. J Infect Dis 127:26, 1973.
11. Hill, HR, et al: Hyperactivity of neutrophil leukotactic responses during active bacterial infection. J Clin Invest 53:996, 1974.
12. O'Flaherty, IT, and Ward, PA: Chemotactic factors and the neutrophil. Semin Hematol 16:163, 1979.
13. Scribner, DJ, and Farhney, D: Neutrophil receptors for IgG and complement: Their roles in the attachment and ingestion phases of phagocytosis. J Immunol 116:892, 1976.
14. Bainton, DF: Sequential degranulation of the two types of polymorphonuclear leukocyte granules during phagocytosis of microorganisms. J Cell Biol 58:249, 1973.
15. Jacques, YV, and Bainton, DF: Changes in pH within the phagocytic vacuoles of human neutrophils and monocytes. Lab Invest 39:179, 1978.
16. Nauseef, WM: Insights into myeloperoxidase biosyntheses from its inherited deficiency. J Mol Med 76:661, 1998.
17. Oppenheim, BA: The changing pattern of infection in neutropenic patients. J Antimicrob Chemother 41(Suppl D):7, 1998.
18. Stroncek, DF, et al: Alloimmune neonatal sepsis due to an antibody to the neutrophil Fc-gamma receptor III with maternal deficiency of CD16 antigen. Blood 77:1572, 1991.
19. Conway, LT, et al: Natural history of primary autoimmune neutropenia in infancy. Pediatrics 79:728, 1987.
20. Bauduer, F: G-CSF: a very efficient therapy for chronic autoimmune neutropenia. A brief review of the literature. Hematol Cell Ther 40:189, 1998.
21. Welte, K, and Boxer, LA: Severe chronic neutropenia: Pathophysiology and therapy. Semin Hematol 34:267, 1997.
22. Haddad, E, et al: Treatment of Chédiak-Higashi syndrome by allogenic bone marrow transplantation: Report on 10 cases. Blood 85:3328, 1995.
23. Meischl, C, and Roos, D: The molecular basis of chronic granulomatous disease. Semin Immunopathol 19:417, 1998.
24. Ozahin, H, et al: Successful treatment of invasive aspergillosis in chronic granulomatous disease by bone marrow transplantation, granulocyte colony-stimulating factor-mobilize granulocytes, and liposomal amphotericin-B. Blood 92:2719, 1998.
25. Weil, WM, et al: Genetic correction of p67phox deficient chronic granulomatous disease using peripheral blood progenitor cells as a target for retrovirus mediated gene transfer. Blood 89:1754, 1997.
26. Becker, S, et al: Correction for respiratory burst activity in X-linked chronic granulomatous cells to therapeutically relevant levels after gene transfer into bone marrow CD34+ cells. Hum Gene Ther 9:1561, 1998.
27. Turk, W: Septische Erkrankungen bei Verkummerung des Granulozylensystems. Wien Klin Wochenschr 20:157, 1907.
28. Sprunt, TP, and Evans, FA: Mononuclear leukocytosis in reaction to acute infections ("infectious mononucleosis"). Bull Johns Hopkins Hosp 31:410, 1920.
29. Downey, H, and McKinlay, CA: Acute lymphadenosis compared with acute lymphatic leukemia. Arch Intern Med 32:82, 1923.
30. Paul, JR, and Bunnell, WW: The presence of heterophile antibodies in infectious mononucleosis. Am J Med Sci 183:90, 1932.
31. Epstein, MA, et al: Virus particles in cultured lymphoblasts from Burkitt's lymphoma. Lancet 1:702, 1964.
32. Pagano, JS: Epstein-Barr virus: The first human tumor virus and its role in cancer. Proc Assoc Am Phys 111:6, 1999.
33. Henle, G, et al: Relation of Burkitt's tumor-associated herpes-type virus to infectious mononucleosis. Proc Natl Acad Sci USA 59:94, 1968.
34. Weiss, LM, and Movahed, LA: In situ demonstration of EBV genomes in viral-associated B cell lymphoproliferations. Am J Pathol 134:651, 1989.
35. Larouche, C, et al: Measurement by the polymerase chain reaction of the Epstein-Barr virus load in infectious mononucleosis and AIDS-related non-Hodgkin's lymphomas. J Med Virol 46:66, 1995.
36. Sixby, JW, et al: Detection of a second widespread strain of EBV virus. Lancet 2:761, 1989.
37. Anagnostopoulos, I, et al: Morphology, immunophenotype and distribution of latently and/or productively Epstein-Barr virus-infected cells in acute infectious mononucleosis: Implications for the interindividual infection route of Epstein-Barr virus. Blood 85:744, 1995.

38. Tosato, G, et al: Epstein-Barr virus as an agent of hematological disease. Baillieres Clin Haematol 8:165, 1995.

39. Klein, G: Epstein-Barr virus strategy in normal and neoplastic B cells. Cell 77:791, 1993.

40. Tynell, E, et al: Acyclovir and prednisone treatment of acute infectious mononucleosis: A multicenter double-blind, placebo controlled study. J Infect Dis 174:324, 1996.

41. Cyran, EM, et al: Intravenous gammaglobulin treatment for immune thrombocytopenia associated with infectious mononucleosis. Am J Hematol 38:124, 1991.

42. Andersson, J: EBV, everybody's virus: The management of Epstein-Barr virus infections. Herpes 3:55, 1996.

43. Penman, HG: Fatal infectious mononucleosis: A critical review. J Clin Pathol 23:765, 1970.

44. Rosenberg, ES, et al: Acute HIV infection among patients tested for mononucleosis [letter]. N Engl J Med 340:12, 1999.

45. Steeper, TA, et al: Heterophile-negative mononucleosis-like illnesses with reactive lymphocytosis in patients undergoing seroconversions to the human immunodeficiency virus. Am J Clin Pathol 90:169, 1988.

46. Steeper, TA, et al: The spectrum of clinical and laboratory findings resulting from human herpesvirus-6 (HHV-6) in patients with mononucleosis-like illnesses not resulting from Epstein-Barr virus or cytomegalovirus. Am J Clin Pathol 93:776, 1990.

47. Lagergren, JE: The white blood cell count and the erythrocyte sedimentation rate in pertussis. Acta Paediat 52:405, 1963.

48. De Martino, M, et al: Preferential increase of a T-cell subset as a cause of lymphocytosis in children with whooping cough. Boll Ist Sieroter Milan 63:479, 1984.

49. Hodge, AM: Simultaneous detection of heterophile-positive and heterophile-negative mononucleosis-like syndrome in the routine laboratory. Am Clin Lab 18:6, 1999.

16 Introduction to Leukemia and the Acute Leukemias

Teresa M. Launder, MD
Lyle C. Lawnicki, MD
Mary L. Perkins, MS, MT(ASCP)SH

OBJECTIVES

At the end of this chapter, the learner should be able to:

1. Define leukemia.
2. Compare and contrast acute and chronic leukemia.
3. Compare and contrast acute myeloid and acute lymphocytic leukemia.
4. List and describe each of the FAB subtypes of acute lymphocytic and acute myeloid leukemia.
5. Interpret characteristic morphology and cytochemical staining patterns for each of the FAB subtypes of acute myeloid leukemia.
6. List the criteria for immunologic classification of acute lymphocytic leukemia, including early pre-B, pre-B, B-cell, and T-cell leukemias.
7. Describe the role of cytogenetic analysis of newly diagnosed leukemia.
8. Identify the common chromosome abnormalities associated with acute promyelocytic leukemia (M3 and M3m) and acute myelomonocytic leukemia with eosinophilia (M4Eo).

➤ INTRODUCTION TO LEUKEMIA

Definition

Leukemia is a malignant disease of hematopoietic tissue, characterized by replacement of normal bone marrow elements with abnormal (neoplastic) blood cells. These leukemic cells are frequently (but not always) present in the peripheral blood and commonly invade reticuloendothelial tissue, including the spleen, liver, and lymph nodes. They may also invade other tissues, infiltrating any organ of the body. If left untreated, leukemia eventually causes death.

Historic Perspective

The initial description of leukemia as a clinical entity was made by John Bennett in Scotland and Rudolf Virchow in Germany, who independently published their findings in 1845. They described a series of autopsy studies of victims of a progressive chronic disorder of unknown origin, in which enlarged spleens and purulent-appearing blood were found. The blood, when examined microscopically, revealed an astounding increase in "colorless" corpuscles. Bennett initially suggested that the marked increase in white blood cells was the result of an inflammatory process.

Virchow chose the term *Weisses Blut* (white blood), which was later translated into Greek as *leukemia*. He proposed that leukemia was caused by a neoplastic proliferation, or hyperplasia, of white blood cells. The ensuing debate between Bennett and Virchow continued for several years, but eventually even Bennett rejected inflammation as the etiology of leukemia.[1]

Virchow continued his study of leukemia, and defined two groups characterized either by predominantly splenic or nodal involvement. Today these are recognized as chronic myelogenous leukemia and chronic lymphocytic leukemia, respectively.

In 1857 Friedreich gave a classic account of a rapidly progressive form of leukemia, to which Epstein applied the term *acute* in 1889. Further classification was made possible in 1877 by Paul Ehrlich's discovery of a triacid stain that permitted the morphological characterization of blood cells. It was readily shown that acute leukemia was associated with primitive cells whereas chronic leukemia was associated with mature, well-differentiated cells. At the turn of the century, Naegeli described the myeloblast and divided the acute leukemias into myeloblastic and lymphoblastic forms. A decade later, Shilling described a monoblastic variant. Thus, the main morphological variants of acute and chronic leukemia were well established by 1930. Since that time classification of leukemia has been refined, and clinically distinct subgroups have been characterized.

Today the clinical laboratory plays an important role in the diagnosis and classification of leukemia. The standard morphological analysis of leukemia is now augmented by cytochemical, cytogenetic, immunologic, and molecular techniques. Together these methods are used to delineate specific categories of leukemia for which distinct treatment protocols are used.

Certainly the most significant application of the biologic understanding of leukemia has been in the area of treatment. Complex therapeutic protocols using cytotoxic drugs, radiation, and, in some cases, bone marrow transplantation have improved the survival of many patients with leukemia, and especially those with acute forms. This is most notable for children with acute lymphoblastic leukemia (ALL). Before the 1960s, childhood ALL was universally fatal, but with modern combined regimens the majority of children with ALL achieve long-term remission and are potentially cured.

Classification

Leukemia is classified according to cell type—with regard to both cell maturity and cell lineage. Cell maturity is used to distinguish between acute and chronic forms of leukemia. When the malignant cells are immature (stem cells, blasts, or other immature precursors), the leukemia is classified as acute; when the cells are predominantly mature, it is described as chronic. In general these two groups correspond to a rapid (acute) or slow (chronic) clinical course. Leukemias are further defined according to cell lineage as lymphoid or myeloid. The term *myeloid* (from *myelo*, Greek for marrow, and *eidos*, form) encompasses granulocytic, monocytic, megakaryocytic, and erythrocytic leukemias. Thus, utilizing cell maturity and cell lineage, leukemia is divided into four broad categories: acute lymphoblastic leukemia (ALL), acute myeloid leukemia (AML; also known as acute nonlymphoblastic leukemia, ANLL), chronic lymphocytic leukemia (CLL), and chronic

myelogenous leukemia (CML). The term *myeloid* is employed in this chapter for AML; other synonyms include "nonlymphoblastic," "myelogenous," "myeloblastic," and "granulocytic." The acute leukemias are further defined by specific cell type, as outlined in Table 16–1. For example, ALL is either B- or T-cell derived. AML is subdivided into acute myeloid, promyelocytic, myelomonocytic, monocytic, erythroleukemic, and megakaryoblastic forms.

Etiology and Risk Factors

The origin of leukemia at the genetic level in most cases appears to be related to mutation and altered expression of oncogenes and tumor suppressor genes. Most oncogenes regulate cell proliferation and differentiation. Abnormal oncogene or tumor suppressor gene expression induced by translocation and genetic fusion or mutation often results in unregulated cellular proliferation. Although the events that lead to this are not entirely understood, a number of host and environmental factors have been identified that are associated with increased risk of leukemic transformation. The epidemiologic aspects of acute leukemia have been recently reviewed[2]; a few salient points are summarized next.

Host Factors

Heredity
Leukemia does not appear to be inherited, although some individuals have an increased predisposition for acquiring it. There is an increased incidence of leukemia in family members of leukemic patients. An identical twin of a patient with acute leukemia possesses a markedly increased relative risk of developing leukemia. These findings do not rule out shared environmental factors; in fact, recent molecular data have shown that the shared risk in twins may be owing to shared placental circulation (and possible in utero exposures) rather than to an inherited genetic mutation.

Congenital Chromosomal Abnormalities
Leukemia occurs with increased frequency in patients with congenital disorders that have an inherited tendency for chromosomal fragility (e.g., Bloom's syndrome and Fanconi's anemia) or with an abnormal chromosome constitution (e.g., Down syndrome, Klinefelter's syndrome, and Turner's syndrome). A 10- to 20-fold increased incidence of acute leukemia is seen in children with Down syndrome. This risk may be partially explained by the discovery that the *AML1* gene, associated with some cases of AML, has been identified on chromosome 21 in a region believed to be responsible for the Down syndrome phenotype.

Immunodeficiency
An unusually high incidence of lymphoproliferative disease (lymphoid leukemia and lymphoma) has been noted in patients with hereditary immunodeficiency states, such as ataxia-telangiectasia and sex-linked agammaglobulinemia.

Chronic Marrow Dysfunction
Patients with chronic marrow dysfunction syndromes have an increased risk of acute leukemic transformation. Examples include the myelodysplastic syndromes, myeloproliferative disorders, aplastic anemia, and paroxysmal nocturnal hemoglobinuria.

> ## Table 16-1
> ## CLASSIFICATION OF LEUKEMIA

Type of Leukemia	Abbreviation	FAB*	Alternate Names
Acute Myeloid			Acute nonlymphoblastic (ANLL)
Acute myeloblastic leukemia	AML		
without cytologic maturation		M0	
with minimal maturation		M1	
with maturation		M2	
Acute promyelocytic leukemia	APL	M3	Hypergranular promyelocytic
Acute myelomonocytic leukemia	AMML	M4	Naegeli-type leukemia
Acute monocytic leukemia	AMoL	M5	Schilling-type leukemia
Erythroleukemia	AEL	M6	Di Guglielmo's syndrome, erythremic myelosis
Acute megakaryoblastic leukemia	AMegL	M7	
Acute Lymphoblastic	ALL		
Precursor B-cell ALL			
Early-Pre-B-cell ALL		L1, L2	Common ALL
Pre-B-cell ALL		L1, L2	Common ALL
B-cell ALL		L3	Burkitt's leukemia
T-cell ALL		L1, L2	
Chronic Myeloid			
Chronic myelogenous leukemia	CML		Chronic granulocytic leukemia
Chronic eosinophilic leukemia	CEL		
Chronic basophilic leukemia	CBL		
Chronic Lymphoid			
Chronic lymphocytic leukemia	CLL		
B-cell CLL			
T-cell CLL			
Prolymphocytic leukemia	PLL		
Hairy cell leukemia	HCL		Leukemic reticuloendotheliosis
Plasma cell leukemia			Multiple myeloma, leukemic phase
Sézary syndrome			Mycosis fungoides, leukemic phase

*French-American-British classification of acute leukemia.

Environmental Factors

Ionizing Radiation

Leukemia is associated with exposure to ionizing radiation; this fact is dramatically illustrated in data collected in populations exposed to the use of nuclear weapons in Hiroshima and Nagasaki (Fig. 16–1). The occurrence of leukemia in this population is many times that of individuals not exposed to ionizing radiation, and it is highest in those survivors with the greatest exposure. Both acute and chronic forms of leukemia were reported, including AML, ALL, and CML. The role of exposure to electromagnetic radiation in causation of leukemia is controversial.

Chemicals and Drugs

Many chemicals and drugs have been associated with development of leukemia. In humans, benzene is the most frequently documented chemical toxin. Pharmacologic agents include chloramphenicol and phenylbutazone. Certain cytotoxic chemotherapeutic agents, especially alkylating drugs, are also associated with leukemic transformation, and the risk in patients receiving alkylating agents is increased by the use of therapeutic radiation. This has been noted particularly in patients treated with combined chemoradiotherapy for Hodgkin's disease. Secondary AML following chemotherapy in adults accounts for 10% to 20% of all AML cases. Secondary AML cases related to prior treatment with epipodophyllotoxins and other topoisomerase inhibitors are often associated with 11q23 abnormalities and a poor prognosis.[3]

Smoking has been implicated as a risk factor (albeit slight) for AML in adults. Results of studies on maternal smoking have been inconclusive in childhood acute leukemias. Some studies have shown increased risk of childhood AML with maternal alcohol consumption during pregnancy.

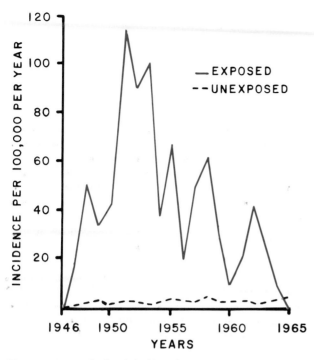

> **FIGURE 16–1** Leukemia incidence in Hiroshima, 1946–1965, in individuals exposed and nonexposed to atomic radiation. (From Gunz, FW: In Wintrobe, MM (ed): Blood, Pure and Eloquent. McGraw-Hill, New York, 1980, p 528, with permission.)

Viruses

The human T-cell leukemia/lymphoma virus-1 (HTLV-1) has been implicated as the causative agent of adult T-cell leukemia/lymphoma (ATL). This rare form of leukemia has a mature helper-inducer T-cell phenotype. ATL is endemic to southwestern Japan, the Caribbean basin, Africa, the southeastern United States, and several other geographic regions.[4] Another related virus, HTLV-2, has been isolated from patients with atypical hairy-cell leukemia (a chronic lymphoid leukemia). The Epstein-Barr virus has been linked to malignancies, including African Burkitt's lymphoma, a high-grade B-cell lymphoma that may have leukemic manifestations.[5]

Incidence

The overall incidence of leukemia in the United States is 8 to 10 new cases per 100,000 individuals per year. In 1998 approximately 28,700 new cases were reported, about half of which were acute and half, chronic.[6] The incidence increases exponentially with age, and the median age at diagnosis of AML (acute myeloid leukemia) in the United States is currently 63 years.[7] As the elderly population continues to increase, leukemia will strike many more adults than children. Currently, the ratio of adult cases to childhood cases is 10:1 and males have a slightly increased incidence compared to females (1–2:1).

Acute leukemia occurs at all ages, but ALL is more common in children and AML is more common in adults. Seventy-five percent of childhood leukemias are classified as ALL whereas nearly 80% of AML cases occur in adults.

Chronic leukemia is generally considered to be a disease of adults. CLL is extremely rare in children and is unusual before the age of 40. CML may be seen at any age, but its peak incidence is between 30 and 50 years of age. The disease is rare in children, but a distinct juvenile variant is recognized—jCML.

Comparison of Acute and Chronic Leukemia

The clinical and laboratory features of acute and chronic leukemia differ in a number of respects, as summarized in Table 16–2. Patients with acute leukemia usually present with a sudden onset of symptoms, and if left untreated, the disease runs a rapidly fatal course of 6 months or less. In contrast, patients with chronic leukemia tend to have an insidious onset and a more indolent clinical course, usually lasting 2 to 6 years.

Patients with acute and chronic leukemia also show differences in their hematologic parameters. In general, bone marrow failure and its sequelae are much more prominent in the initial presentation of acute leukemia than in that of the chronic form. Anemia is consistently observed in the acute leukemic patient, although its severity is variable. Thrombocytopenia is common. The white blood cell count may be markedly elevated with numerous blasts; it may be normal or, in some cases, even decreased. Typically the various normal circulating white blood cells are diminished in number. In chronic leukemic patients, anemia is often mild at presentation. The platelet count is usually normal, but it may actually be increased in CML. Chronic leukemias almost always present with elevated white blood cell counts, which are often striking.

Both acute and chronic leukemic patients can display enlargement of the spleen, liver, or lymph nodes, but this is more consistently seen in patients with chronic leukemia, in whom organomegaly tends to be more prominent and can occasionally be massive.

➤ INTRODUCTION TO ACUTE LEUKEMIA

Clinical Features

The majority of patients with acute leukemia display clinically abrupt onset of signs and symptoms of only a few weeks duration. Patients often seek medical attention because of weakness, bleeding abnormalities, or flulike symptoms. These abnormalities reflect the failure of the bone marrow to produce adequate numbers of normal cells and are caused by the proliferation and accumulation of leukemic cells in the marrow. Leukemic replacement

> **Table 16-2**
> **COMPARISON OF ACUTE AND CHRONIC LEUKEMIA**

	Acute	Chronic
Age	All ages ~ 63	Adults
Clinical onset	Sudden	Insidious
Course (untreated)	< 6 mo	2–6 yr
Leukemic cells	Immature	Mature
Anemia	Mild to severe	Mild
Thrombocytopenia	Mild to severe	Mild
White blood cell count	Variable	Increased
Organomegaly	Mild	Prominent

eventually results in marrow failure and the resultant life-threatening complications of anemia, thrombocytopenia, granulocytopenia, and their sequelae. Anemia, the most consistent presenting feature, is associated with fatigue, malaise, and pallor. Hemorrhagic complications related to thrombocytopenia and, in some cases, to disseminated intravascular coagulation (DIC) are also common. These may be mild and restricted to easy bruising, petechiae, and mucosal bleeding; or they may be more severe, involving gastrointestinal tract, genitourinary tract, or central nervous system hemorrhage. Infections result from severe granulocytopenia. Bacterial infections are common (e.g., *Staphylococcus, Pseudomonas, Escherichia coli,* and *Klebsiella*) but fungal infections also occur (e.g., *Candida* and *Aspergillus*). Viral infections are less frequent.

Infiltration of other tissues, especially organs that play a role in fetal hematopoiesis, is often manifested by hepatosplenomegaly or lymphadenopathy, particularly in ALL and the acute monoblastic leukemia (AMoL) subtype of AML. A mediastinal mass resulting from thymic involvement is a hallmark of T-cell ALL. Gingival hypertrophy and oral lesions are primarily seen in AMoL. Bone or joint pain, caused by pressure of the expanding leukemic cell population in the marrow cavity, commonly accompanies the acute leukemias. Leukemic infiltration of the central nervous system, an ominous feature infrequently observed at initial presentation, is associated with signs and symptoms of increased intracranial pressure (nausea, vomiting, headache, papilledema) or cranial nerve palsies. These clinical features and their relationship to pathophysiology are summarized in Table 16–3.

Between 5% and 10% of cases of AML are preceded by a recognizable "preleukemic" (myelodysplastic) syndrome. The myelodysplastic syndromes are more common in patients over the age of 50 years and are associated with unexplained and persistent anemia, leukopenia, thrombocytopenia, and monocytosis, alone or in combination. The myelodysplastic syndromes are discussed in more detail in Chapter 19.

Laboratory Evaluation of Acute Leukemia

When acute leukemia is suspected, a series of laboratory tests is required to confirm the diagnosis and to classify the disease. The distinction between AML and ALL is particularly important; major features of this distinction are outlined in Table 16–4.

Preliminary evaluation should include a complete blood count (CBC), platelet count, white cell differential, and peripheral blood smear examination. Anemia, which may be mild to severe and is usually normochromic and normocytic, is the most consistent finding. Typically the platelets are decreased, although they may be normal in number. The white blood cell count is highly variable, ranging from decreased to markedly elevated. The blood smear usually reveals blasts or other immature cells, but they may be rare or absent ("aleukemic" leukemia). Circulating nucleated red blood cells are occasionally seen. Myelodysplastic features are sometimes present, including pseudo-Pelger-Huët cells and hypogranular neutrophils. These are more common in elderly patients with acute myeloid leukemia.

Once the diagnosis of leukemia is suggested by the clinical history, physical examination, CBC, and peripheral blood smear findings, a bone marrow aspirate and biopsy is usually obtained. Morphological examination of the bone marrow is usually required to establish the diagnosis. The most widely accepted classification system, called the French-American-British (FAB) system, requires a blast count of 30% in bone marrow aspirate smears for confirmation of the diagnosis of acute leukemia.[8,9] A subsequent and widely adopted recommendation by a workshop of the National Cancer Institute also permits diagnosis of acute leukemia when blasts in peripheral blood are 30% or more.[10] Although a diagnosis of acute leukemia may be established by a peripheral blood examination, well-prepared smears of bone marrow aspirate material are still the specimen of choice for classification of leukemia by morphological and cytochemical criteria.

A systematic approach to the classification of leukemia begins with a review of cellular morphology, which provides important clues about cell lineage and guides further studies required to make a definitive diagnosis. Morphological evaluation should be followed by cytochemical staining and immunologic cell marker studies. A battery of cytochemical stains that define granulocytic and monocytic differentiation is used to distinguish AML from ALL. When positive, cytochemical studies permit subclassification of most cases of AML and exclude ALL. An additional useful marker in initial evaluation is the nuclear enzyme terminal deoxynucleotidyl transferase (TdT), which is present in most cases of ALL and is less commonly expressed in AML. Other immunologic cell marker studies are routinely used for confirmation of myeloid or lymphoid lineage and for further subclassification.

Other laboratory studies used to evaluate acute leukemia include chromosome analysis, molecular genetic studies, deoxyribonucleic acid (DNA) flow cytometry and electron microscopy. Chromosome analysis is a valuable tool in identifying prognostically important subgroups of patients, and providing baseline data that may be useful in monitoring patients. Molecular diagnostic studies are playing an emerging role in primary diagnosis and detection of minimal residual disease, and DNA flow cytometry yields prognostic information in patients with ALL. Electron microscopy is very

> **Table 16–3**
CLINICAL FEATURES OF ACUTE LEUKEMIA

Pathogenesis	Clinical Manifestations
Bone Marrow Failure	
Anemia	Fatigue, malaise, pallor
Thrombocytopenia	Bruising, bleeding
Granulocytopenia	Fever, infections
Organ Infiltration	
Marrow expansion	Bone or joint pain
Spleen	Splenomegaly
Liver	Hepatomegaly
Lymph nodes	Lymphadenopathy
Central nervous system	Neurologic symptoms
Gums, mouth	Gingival hypertrophy, oral lesions

➤ **Table 16-4**
COMPARISON OF ACUTE MYELOBLASTIC AND ACUTE LYMPHOBLASTIC LEUKEMIA

Factor	AML	ALL
Age	Common in adults, rare in children	Common in children, rare in adults
Blood	Anemia, neutropenia, thrombocytopenia; myeloblasts and promyelocytes	Anemia, neutropenia, thrombocytopenia; lymphoblasts and prolymphocytes
Morphology	Medium-to-large blasts, more cytoplasm than lymphoblasts, cytoplasmic granules, Auer rods; fine nuclear chromatin and distinct nucleoli	Small or medium blasts, scarce cytoplasm, no granules; fine nuclear chromatin and indistinct nucleoli
Cytochemistry	Positive peroxidase and Sudan black; negative TdT	Negative peroxidase and Sudan black; positive TdT
Extramedullary and focal disease	Common in spleen and liver; less common in lymph nodes and CNS	Common in lymph nodes, spleen, liver, CNS, and gonads

Abbreviations: AML = acute myeloblastic leukemia; ALL = acute lymphoblastic leukemia; TdT = terminal deoxynucleotidyl transferase; CNS = central nervous system

Source: From Kjeldsberg, CR (ed): Practical Diagnosis of Hematologic Disorders. ASCP Press, Chicago, 1989, p 349, with permission.

rarely utilized, except in evaluation of poorly differentiated leukemia or acute megakaryoblastic leukemia.

The purpose and principles of these laboratory methods are discussed in the following pages; detailed procedures are outlined in Chapter 28.

Specimens

At the outset, care must be taken to ensure that an adequate specimen is obtained and that it is properly handled. Lack of technical excellence may obscure or complicate an otherwise straightforward diagnosis; an inadequate or improperly handled specimen is a common cause of diagnostic error.

Ideally, evaluation of the peripheral blood cell morphology should be performed on nonanticoagulated fingerstick smears. Anticoagulant (ethylene diaminetetraacetic acid; EDTA) causes subtle morphological artifacts of nucleated cells and platelets. A specimen left in EDTA for over 30 minutes may show artifactual vacuolation of monocytes and neutrophils, nuclear shape changes and swelling, as well as degranulation of platelets.[11,12] These possible alterations should be kept in mind if only a routine EDTA-anticoagulated peripheral blood smear is available for review.

Before a bone marrow specimen is collected, arrangements for any special studies, including cytochemistry and flow cytometric immunophenotyping, should be made, and any special handling procedures should be noted; such procedures are also of importance to cytogenetic and ultrastructural studies. During the bone marrow procedure, the aspirate is collected first and smears are made immediately to avoid clotting. As the aspirate smears are pulled, the presence of bone marrow spicules should be confirmed. If spicules are not present, another aspiration may be necessary. For immunophenotyping or cytogenetic studies, the marrow aspirate is anticoagulated by aspirating directly into a syringe coated with heparin. After sufficient aspirate material is collected, the biopsy is obtained. The biopsy should be used, before fixation, to make touch preparations by gently touching or rolling the biopsy along a glass slide. The biopsy should be blotted prior to making the touch preparations, because excess blood will obscure morphological detail. Touch preparations are especially important when the aspirate produces a "dry" tap. Further details of the bone marrow procedure are discussed in Chapter 2.

Evaluation of Morphology

Cellular morphology is evaluated on a Romanowsky (Wright-Giemsa)-stained blood or bone marrow smear in carefully chosen areas in which cells are not distorted by overcrowding. In the hands of an experienced morphologist, the leukemic cell type may be correctly identified; however, additional testing is always necessary to confirm the diagnosis.

Several cytologic features (outlined in Table 16–5) are helpful in distinguishing lymphoblasts from myeloblasts. These include the size of the blast, amount of cytoplasm, nuclear chromatin pattern, and the presence of nucleoli. The typical myeloblast (Fig. 16–2 and Color Plate 158) is a large cell (15 to 20 μm in diameter) with a moderate amount of cytoplasm. Its nucleus has a fine, reticulated chromatin pattern, and multiple distinct nucleoli are often present. The typical lymphoblast (Fig. 16–3 and Color Plate 159) is a smaller cell with scant cytoplasm. The nuclear chromatin often appears denser than in the myeloblast, and nucleoli are usually indistinct when present. For a review of morphological descriptions of the blast stage, see Chapter 1.

Granulocytic differentiation is suggested by the presence of azurophilic granules. A very helpful morphological feature is the Auer rod, the presence of which excludes ALL. Auer rods are cytoplasmic inclusions that result from an abnormal fusion of primary granules and are pathognomonic for a myeloproliferative process, particularly AML (and rarely chronic myelocytic leukemia or CML in myeloid blast crisis); they have also been described in myelodysplastic syndromes in transformation to AML.[13] On Romanowsky-stained smears, Auer rods appear as pink- or purple-staining rods or splinter-shaped inclusions (see Fig. 16–2 and Color Plate 158). They are present in up to 60% of patients with AML,[14] but it may take a long, careful review of the blood or marrow smear to find them; given their diagnostic importance, this search is well worth the effort. In acute promyelocytic leukemia, Auer rods are easy to find, some cells having "bundles" of cigar-shaped rods.

Cytochemistry

Special stains are used to identify chemical components of cells such as enzymes or lipids. These cytochemical stains are an important aid in the classification of acute leukemia be-

> **Table 16–5**

CYTOLOGIC FEATURES OF BLASTS IN ACUTE MYELOID AND ACUTE LYMPHOBLASTIC LEUKEMIAS

Feature	AML	ALL
Blast size	Larger, usually uniform	Variable, small to medium size
Nuclear chromatin	Usually finely dispersed	Coarse to fine
Nucleoli	1–4, often prominent	Absent or 1 or 2, often indistinct
Cytoplasm	Moderately abundant, fine granules often present	Usually scant, coarse granules sometimes present (~7%)
Auer rods	Present in 60%–70% of cases	Not present
Other cell types	Often dysplastic changes in maturing myeloid cells	Myeloid cells not dysplastic

From Kjeldsberg, CR (ed): Practical Diagnosis of Hematologic Disorders, ed 2. ASCP Press, Chicago, 1995, p 381, with permission.

cause they identify cellular components that are associated with specific cell lines. For example, a positive myeloperoxidase or Sudan black B stain indicates myeloid differentiation, and a positive nonspecific esterase stain indicates monocytic differentiation. When any of these stains is positive, lymphoid origin is ruled out, with rare exceptions. Thus, the cytochemical stains help distinguish between ALL and AML. They are also used to subclassify AML.

The cytochemical reactions are performed by applying staining techniques to peripheral blood smears, bone marrow smears, or touch preparations. Fresh preparations are preferred, especially for enzyme reactions. Control smears can be fixed in the appropriate fixative, allowed to air-dry and stored at −20°C for future staining. Caution should be taken when interpreting cytochemical stains. It is the leukemic cell population whose identity (cell lineage) is in question; therefore, a positive reaction is determined by finding positive staining in the leukemic blasts rather than in mature cells. Table 16–6 summarizes the cytochemical reactions that are useful in the classification of acute leukemia.

Myeloperoxidase

Peroxidase is present in the primary granules of myeloid cells (Fig. 16–4 and Color Plate 160). These granules first appear in the early promyelocyte (late blast) and persist through subsequent stages of cell maturation. Monocytes have variable staining with peroxidase and are most often only weakly positive. This enzyme is not present in lymphocytes or their precursors and is, therefore, useful in differentiating AML from ALL. It is more specific for granulocytic differentiation than the Sudan black B stain.

Smears are incubated in a buffered solution of hydrogen peroxide with an appropriate substrate, such as 3-amino-9-ethylcarbazole (AEC) or benzidine. In the presence of the enzyme peroxidase, the hydrogen peroxide oxidizes the substrate, resulting in precipitation of a colored product at the site of enzyme activity. Effort should be made to use fresh smears when staining for peroxidase because the enzyme is labile.

Sudan Black B

Phospholipids, neutral fats, and sterols are stained by Sudan black B (SBB) (Fig. 16–5 and Color Plate 161). This reaction is thought to be a result of the solubility of the dye in the lipid particles. Phospholipids occur both in primary and secondary granules of granulocytic cells and, to a lesser extent, in monocytic lysosomal granules.

The SBB is the most sensitive stain for granulocytic precursors, with a staining pattern that generally parallels the myeloperoxidase stain. As with the peroxidase stain, the SBB is used to differentiate AML from ALL. Positivity seldom occurs in lymphoid cells, but rare cases of SBB-positive ALL are observed.[15] The SBB stain, whose reactivity does not diminish with time, is particularly useful for specimens that are not fresh.

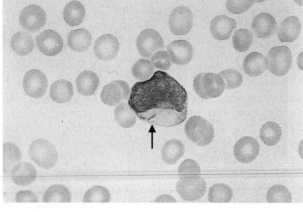

> **FIGURE 16–2**   Myeloblast (note the Auer rod).

> **FIGURE 16–3**   Lymphoblasts (peripheral blood).

> ► **Table 16-6**

SUMMARY OF CYTOCHEMICAL REACTIONS USEFUL IN DIAGNOSING ACUTE LEUKEMIA

Special Stain	Site of Action	Cells Stained	Comment
Myeloperoxidase	Mainly primary granules; Auer rods	Late myeloblasts, granulocytes; monocytes less intensely	Valuable in that the primary granules are not always visible; separates AML (+) from ALL (−)
Sudan black B	Phospholipids: sterols, neutral fats	Late myeloblasts, granulocytes; monocytes less intensely	Parallels peroxidase, but smears do not need to be fresh
Specific esterase (Naphthol AS-D chloroacetate)	Cytoplasm	Neutrophilic granulocytes; mast cells	Parallels peroxidase, but less sensitive; useful on paraffin-embedded tissues
Nonspecific esterase Alpha-naphthyl acetate (ANAE) and butyrate	Cytoplasm	Monocytes; focal staining in T cells; ANAE also + in megakaryocytes	Useful for determing degree of monocytic differentiation; separates mono (+) from myelo (−) blasts
Periodic acid–Schiff	Glycogen and related substances	Lymphocytes, granulocytes, megakaryocytes	Helpful in supporting diagnosis of erythroleukemia

Specific Esterase (Naphthol AS-D Chloroacetate)

The specific esterase stain (Fig. 16–6 and Color Plate 162), commonly referred to as chloroacetate esterase (CAE), roughly parallels the peroxidase and SBB stains, although it is not as sensitive, and it is negative in eosinophils and monocytes. Its most important use is in demonstrating myeloid differentiation in paraffin-embedded tissue sections.

Smears or hydrated paraffin tissue sections are incubated in a buffered solution containing the substrate naphthol AS-D chloroacetate and a diazo salt (pararosaniline). The esterase enzyme within neutrophils, basophils, mast cells, and their precursors hydrolyzes the chloroacetate. This hydrolyzed substrate rapidly couples with the diazo salt, causing dye to precipitate at the site of enzymatic activity.

Nonspecific Esterase (Alpha-Naphthyl Acetate or Butyrate)

The nonspecific esterase (NSE) stain (Fig. 16–7 and Color Plate 163) is used to identify monocytic cells. It is diffusely positive in these cells and negative in granulocytic cells. Lymphoid cells are negative, except for T lymphocytes,

which can demonstrate a focal dotlike cytoplasmic staining pattern.

Just as with the specific esterase stain, the NSE stain is performed by incubating fixed smears in a buffered solution containing a substrate and diazo salt. The difference in

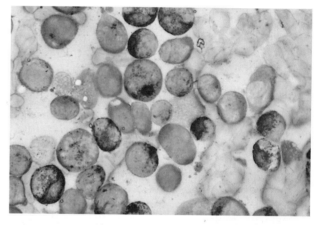

> ► **FIGURE 16–5** Sudan black B positivity in acute myeloblastic leukemia (AML), M2.

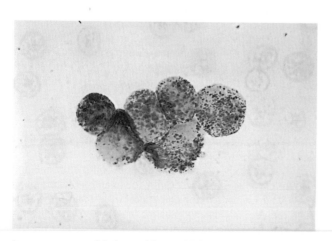

> ► **FIGURE 16–4** Myeloperoxidase positivity in acute promyelocytic leukemia.

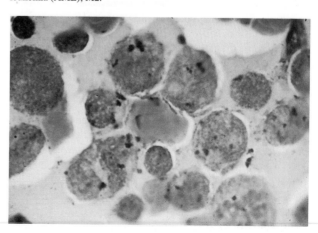

> ► **FIGURE 16–6** Specific esterase (naphthol AS-D chloroacetate) positivity in AML, M2.

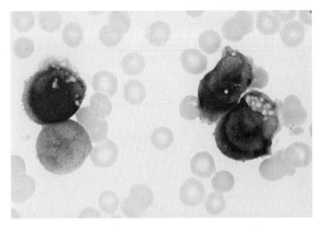

➤ **FIGURE 16–7**   Nonspecific esterase (alpha-naphthyl butyrate) positivity in acute monocytic leukemia (M5).

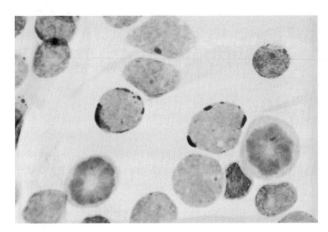

➤ **FIGURE 16–8**   Periodic acid–Schiff positivity in acute lymphoblastic leukemia (ALL). Note the "block" staining pattern.

staining specificity lies in the naphthol derivative used for the substrate and in the pH and time of incubation. Different substrates are available for use in the NSE stain. Alpha-naphthyl butyrate is the most specific for monocyte differentiation, whereas alpha-naphthyl acetate is more sensitive. Both are positive in monocytes and their precursors as well as in macrophages. The alpha-naphthyl acetate, but not the butyrate, is also positive in megakaryocytes and platelets. Another substrate, naphthol AS-D acetate (NASDA), is less specific and stains both monocytes and granulocytes. NASDA must be used in conjunction with a sodium fluoride inhibition step, which renders monocytic cells negative and thus differentiates them from granulocytic cells, which remain positive. The NASDA staining pattern gave the "nonspecific" esterase its name.

Periodic Acid–Schiff

The periodic acid–Schiff (PAS) reaction stains for glycogen and related compounds, including mucoproteins, glycoproteins, glycolipids, and polysaccharides. Periodic acid (HIO_4) oxidizes glycols to aldehydes. The resulting aldehydes react with Schiff's reagent (fuchsin-sulfurous acid) to form a magenta color. Lymphocytes, granulocytes, monocytes, and megakaryocytes may be positive, having either a diffuse or sometimes granular staining pattern. Normal erythroid precursors are negative.

The PAS reaction is not very useful for characterizing acute leukemia, and it is no longer commonly used for classification. The typical block positivity (Fig. 16–8 and Color Plate 164) associated with lymphoblastic leukemia may also occur in acute myeloid leukemia, especially the acute monocytic type.[16,17] Burkitt's type ALL (L3) is negative. The PAS stain should not be used to distinguish AML from ALL.

The PAS reaction may sometimes be helpful in supporting the diagnosis of erythroleukemia when strong PAS positivity may be present in normoblasts. When present, this feature is helpful for differentiating erythroleukemia from pernicious anemia in which the PAS reaction is negative except in rare cases. Normoblasts may also be positive in iron deficiency, thalassemia, severe hemolytic anemias, and some of the myelodysplastic syndromes.

Immunologic Marker Studies

A number of immunologic methods have proved to be indispensable to the diagnosis and classification of acute leukemia, especially of ALL. Antibodies are used to detect markers associated with cell lineage and maturation stage. Depending on the location of these cell markers (cell surface, cytoplasm, or nucleus), different methods are used to detect them. The following paragraphs briefly introduce the immunologic cell marker procedures. Their utility in the evaluation of acute leukemia is discussed in the individual sections on AML and ALL.

Cell Surface Markers

Cell surface markers are proteins on the cell membrane that can be detected with immunologic reagents. Different proteins are expressed at different stages of maturation; some are present early in development whereas others do not appear until much later. Still other proteins may appear, disappear, and then reappear at a later stage of development. This unique expression of proteins enables them to be used as markers of both cell lineage and maturation stage.

Although some surface markers can be detected with polyclonal antisera, many can only be detected with monoclonal antibodies. Table 16–7 lists some antibodies that are commonly used to evaluate leukemias and other lymphoproliferative and myeloproliferative disorders.

Surface marker studies are performed on cell suspensions derived either from bone marrow aspirates or peripheral blood. It is important to have fresh specimens with viable cells; nonviable cells lead to nonspecific staining, which may make interpretation impossible. An immunofluorescent method (direct or indirect) is used to stain the cells, and a flow cytometer is used to analyze them. (See Chap. 30 for a review of flow cytometry.) Figure 16–9 and Color Plate 165 show the surface-staining pattern, as observed with a fluorescent microscope, that is typical of a strongly positive reaction.

Cytoplasmic Markers

Cell marker studies can also be directed at cytoplasmic antigens. The cells to be analyzed are fixed and permeabilized to allow antibody to enter through the cell membrane and into the cytoplasmic space. Often the quantity of antigen on the cell surface and in the cytoplasm varies, and some antigens are exclusively cytoplasmic. Plasma cell neoplasms, for example, often have very weak surface and strong cytoplasmic immunoglobulin staining intensity.

Cytoplasmic markers are very useful in assessing cell

> ## ➤ Table 16-7
> ## MONOCLONAL ANTIBODIES USED FOR STUDY OF LEUKEMIA AND LYMPHOMA

Cluster Designation	Specific Antibodies	Major Hematopoietic Reactivity
CD1a	T6, Leu-6	Thymic and Langerhans' cells
CD2	T11, Leu-5	E-Rosette–forming T cells
CD3	T3, Leu-4	Mature T cells
CD4	T4, Leu-3	Helper-inducer T-cell subset
CD5	T1, Leu-1	Pan-T and some B cells
CD7	Leu-9	Pan-T, early thymocytes
CD8	T8, Leu-2	Suppressor-cytotoxic T-cell subset
CD10	J5, CALLA	B-cell pre, some thymocytes, grans and ALL
CD11b	Mo1, Leu-15	Monos and grans, C3bi receptor
CD11c	Leu-M5	Monos, myeloid precursors, HCL
CD13	My7	Most grans, minority of monos, and other
CD14	My 4, Leu-M3	Monos, minority of grans, and DRC
CD15	Leu-M1	Myeloid cells, RS
CD19	B4, Leu-12	B cells, early B-cell precursors
CD20	B1, Leu-16	B cells, midstage B-cell precursors
CD21	B2	C3d receptor on B cells and DRC
CD22	Leu-14	B cells, ALL, HCL
CD23	B6	B cells, EBV-transformed B lymphoblasts
CD25	IL-2R1, IL-2R	IL-2 receptor on T cells and other, HCL, NHL
CD30	Ber-H2	Activated B and T cells, RS, ALCL
CD33	My 9	Myeloid progenitors
CD34	My 10, HPCA	Hematopoietic progenitor-stem cells
CD38	T10, Leu-17	Plasma cells, ALL, AML
CD41	J15	Plts and megakaryocytes (GPIIb/IIIa), AML M7
CD42b	AN51	Plts and megakaryocytes (GPIb), AML M7
CD43	DF-T1	T cells, myeloid cells
CD45	T200, HLe, LCA	Leukocytes
CD56	Leu-19	NK cells, T-cell subset
CD57	Leu-7	T cells, NK cells
CD61	gpIIIa	Plts, AML (M7)
CD75	LN-1	B cells, follicular center cells
CD79a	MB-1	B cells, ALL
CD103	HML-1	Intraepithelial lymphocytes, HCL
	HLA-DR, Ia	B cells, activated T cells, and monos

Abbreviations: CD = cluster designation; B cells = B lymphocyte; T cell = T lymphocyte; Pan = reactivity with many leukocyte populations; ALL = acute lymphoblastic leukemia; AML = acute myeloid leukemia; DRC = dendritic reticulum cells; grans = granulocytes; monos = monocytes; Plts = platelets; RS = Reed Sternberg cells; HCL = hairy cell leukemia; ALCL = anaplastic large cell lymphoma; NK = natural killer cells

lineage in ALL. Cytoplasmic CD3 is present early in T-cell development, and strong expression is seen in most cases of precursor T-cell ALL. Likewise, the presence of cytoplasmic CD22 and CD79a aids in defining B-cell lineage in ALL.

The presence of cytoplasmic IgM heavy chain (μ) is a defining characteristic of pre-B cells; the earlier precursor B cells are cytoplasmic μ negative. Pre-B-cell ALL has traditionally been associated with a worse prognosis than early-pre-B-cell ALL. However, the poor prognosis is now known to be more closely linked to the frequently associated t(1;19) in pre-B-cell ALL than to pre-B-cell phenotype.[18] Accordingly, cytoplasmic μ staining is no longer routinely performed in many laboratories.

Another helpful cytoplasmic marker used in immunophenotyping acute leukemias is cytoplasmic myeloperoxidase.

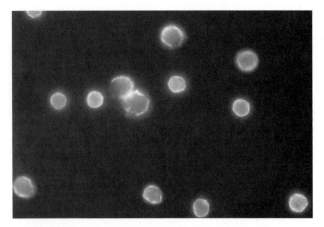

➤ **FIGURE 16–9**   Surface immunoglobulin (sIg)–positive cells in B-cell ALL, L3.

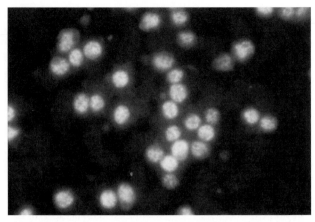

➤ **FIGURE 16–10**   TdT positivity in ALL using immunofluorescence method.

This myeloid marker is often used as part of a flow cytometric panel, in addition to the traditional myeloid markers, CD13 and CD33. Immunohistochemical stains for cytoplasmic myeloperoxidase can also been performed on formalin-fixed, paraffin-embedded sections. However, immunohistochemical staining with currently available antibodies does not seem to be as specific for myeloid lineage as either the traditional cytochemical method or flow cytometry.

Terminal Deoxynucleotidyl Transferase (TdT)

Antibodies can also be directed at nuclear antigens using the same cell membrane permealization procedure. Terminal deoxynucleotidyl transferase (TdT) is a unique nuclear enzyme (DNA polymerase) present in stem cells and precursor B- and T-lymphoid cells.[19] High levels are found in the majority (90%) of the lymphoblastic leukemias, including both B- and T-lineage ALL. TdT, although not lineage-specific, provides information useful in the distinction of ALL from AML. Detectable levels of this enzyme have been noted in 5% to 10% of cases of AML,[20] although the level is usually lower than in lymphoblasts. TdT is also present in most cases of lymphoblastic lymphoma and in approximately one-third of cases of chronic myeloid leukemia in blast crisis (CML-BC).[21]

TdT can be detected by a number of immunologic methods, including flow cytometry and immunohistochemical methods. TdT can be routinely used as part of a flow cytometry leukemia panel. Immunohistochemical methods for TdT can be performed on paraffin sections of the biopsy core or clot, and only nuclear staining is considered a positive reaction. TdT can also be detected by a variety of other immunologic techniques (immunocytochemical or immunofluorescent), using fresh smears, touch preparations, or cytopreparations. When heparinized specimens are to be studied, the sample must be washed to remove heparin, which causes false-negative staining. A positive reaction, as in the immunohistochemical method, is indicated by a nuclear staining pattern (Fig. 16–10 and Color Plate 166).

Cytogenetics

Cytogenetic analysis of leukemic cells is a critically important adjunct to the standard classification of acute leukemia. It is currently considered to be an essential component in the evaluation of the newly diagnosed leukemic patient, playing a major role in diagnosis, subclassification, selection of appropriate therapy, and monitoring the effects of therapy. A number of chromosomal abnormalities have been associated with distinct forms of leukemia (see the following discussion of molecular genetics). Classic examples of this are the Philadelphia chromosome (t[9;22]) associated with CML, and the translocation t(15;17) consistently observed in acute promyelocytic leukemia. The clinical significance of cytogenetic studies in AML has been the subject of a recent review.[22] In addition to cytogenetic evaluation, flow cytometric analysis for DNA ploidy status may provide information useful to the evaluation of ALL.[23]

Cytogenetic studies are performed by evaluating stained chromosome metaphase preparations to detect numeric and structural karyotype (from *karyon,* Greek for nucleus, plus *typos,* meaning mark) abnormalities. Normal human cells have 46 chromosomes and are said to be diploid (*diplous,* double, plus *eidos,* form); that is, they have two haploid sets of chromosomes. An aneuploid population can be either hypodiploid or hyperdiploid, and can be identified as such by DNA flow cytometry as well as by cytogenetic examination.

Structural rearrangements include translocations, inversions, deletions, duplications, and isochromosomes. Of particular importance to the study of acute leukemia are the translocations that result from the movement of a DNA segment from one chromosome to another and that are often associated with oncogene rearrangement, genetic fusion, and abnormal gene expression. Usually these translocations result from a reciprocal interchange of portions of two nonhomologous chromosomes.

Chromosomal abnormalities (both numeric and structural) are found in the majority of patients with acute leukemia and seen in over 60% of patients with AML and in over 65% of patients with ALL. The most common structural abnormalities are translocations. A number of these have been associated with distinct subgroups of AML or ALL, with prognostic significance (see the discussion that follows). For example, patients with acute myelomonocytic leukemia (AML, M4) who exhibit an inversion or deletion of the long arm of chromosome 16 (inv[16q] or del[16q]) have a longer median survival than patients with other types of AML. Table 16–8 lists common cytogenetic abnormalities associated with acute leukemia.

The recent development of fluorescently labeled chromosome painting probes and automated differential color analysis (automated spectral karyotyping) should greatly enhance the sensitivity and accuracy of karyotypic analy-

> ## Table 16-8
> ### COMMON CHROMOSOME ABNORMALITIES AND MOLECULAR CORRELATES ASSOCIATED WITH ACUTE LEUKEMIA

Chromosome Abnormality	Associated Disorder	Involved Genes on Respective Chromosomes	Method
t(6;9)	AML (M2) and AMML (M4) with marrow basophilia	DEK/CAN	RT-PCR
t(8;21)	AML with myelocytic maturation (M2) (associated with a favorable prognosis and good response to therapy)	ETO/AML1	Southern blot RT-PCR
t(15;17)	Unique to APL (M3 and M3m) (associated with a favorable prognosis)	PML/RARα	RT-PCR
t(11;17)	APL variants; not ATRA responsive	PLZF/RARα	
t(5;17)		NuMa/RARα	
16q abnormality: inv(16) and del(16)	AMML with abnormal eosinophilia (M4Eo) (associated with a favorable prognosis)	CBFβ/MYH11	RT-PCR
t(9;22)	Most common in CML; occasionally found in AML and ALL (early pre-B, pre-B cell, and T cell) (very poor prognosis in ALL)	ABL/BCR	RT-PCR
11q23 reciprocal translocations	Poor prognosis in pediatric ALL and AML	MLL	RT-PCR
t(9;11)	AMoL, especially poorly differentiated (M5a); other types of AML, e.g., AMML (M4)	AF9/MLL	
t(4;11)	Mixed lineage leukemia with lymphoblastic (early pre-B) or monocytic features; common in infants	AF4/MLL	
t(11;19)	Precursor B-cell ALL	ENL/MLL	
t(12;21)	ALL, precursor B cell (favorable prognosis)	TEL/AML1	RT-PCR
T(1;19)	ALL, pre-B-cell phenotype (30% incidence in this group; associated with a very poor prognosis)	PBX1/E2A	RT-PCR
t(8;14), t(2;8) and t(8;22)	ALL, B-cell phenotype (Burkitt's lymphoma); c-myc translocated to chromosome Ig heavy or light-chain gene	cMYC/IgH	
t(1;14)	ALL, T-cell phenotype (common thymocyte)	TAL1/TCRαδ	

Abbreviations: t = translocation; inv = inversion; del = deletion; RT-PCR = reverse transcriptase polymerase chain reaction

sis. This technique holds great promise for the identification of additional chromosomal abnormalities in leukemic patients, who frequently have complex karyotypes.[24]

Molecular Genetics

The molecular genetic basis for many of the acute leukemias has been elucidated in recent years. Extensive studies of the immunoglobulin and T-cell antigen receptor genes have been carried out, and other genes involved in many of the recurrent cytogenetic abnormalities described in the preceding section have been cloned and characterized. DNA probes and polymerase chain reaction (PCR)-based primers are available for rapid and precise detection of many specific cytogenetic abnormalities at the molecular level. Molecular diagnostic studies are primarily used for confirmation of the presence of a suspected chromosomal abnormality not detected by conventional cytogenetics, for the analysis of specimens that are not suitable for conventional cytogenetics, and for the monitoring of minimal residual disease following therapy.

These methods permit detection of residual leukemic disease at extremely low levels, and clinical applications of these techniques are still being developed. The sensitivity of molecular techniques enables detection of leukemic subpopulations that are not identifiable by conventional morphology or other methods; therefore, patients who are in clinical remission may be observed to possess minimal residual disease when PCR-based techniques are employed. The significance and clinical applications of this capability are not clearly defined at present. The molecular correlations of some of the most common chromosomal abnormalities in acute leukemia are listed in Table 16–8 and some specific examples are discussed next.

t(12;21)—TEL/AML1

In most series, this is now the most common translocation in precursor B-cell ALL in children, occurring in 16% to 28% of unselected cases. It is virtually never found in adults. The translocation results in fusion of the *TEL* gene on chromosome 12 and the *AML1* gene on chromosome 21q. *AML1* is part of a transcription factor complex. This translocation is more commonly detectable by reverse transcriptase (RT)-PCR than by routine cytogenetic analysis and identifies a subgroup of pediatric ALL patients with an excellent prognosis.[18,25,26]

t(1;19)—PBX1/E2A

This translocation results in the fusion of the *PBX1* gene on chromosome 1 with the *E2A* gene on chromosome 19, and the formation of an abnormal fusion protein.[27–29] Detectable by RT-PCR methods, it is associated with a very poor prognosis in pediatric ALL.[30,31]

t(8;21)—ETO/AML1

This translocation occurs in AML, often of the FAB-M2 type, and results in the fusion of the *ETO* gene on chromosome 8 with the *AML1* gene on chromosome 21.[29] Southern blot and RT-PCR assays for this abnormality are quite reliable.[32,33] The t(8;21) is associated with a favorable prognosis and good response to therapy.[34]

t(9;22)—BCR/ABL

The t(9;22) is associated with high-risk B-lineage ALL (as well as CML). This form of ALL is almost uniformly fatal in all age groups. The translocation results in fusion of the *ABL* oncogene on chromosome 9 with the *BCR* gene on chromosome 22, and production of a fusion protein with strong transforming activity. This abnormality may be detected by RT-PCR methods.[35]

t(4;11)—AF4/MLL

This translocation is seen in the most common form of ALL in infancy and involves fusion of the *AF4* gene into the *MLL* gene (also called *ALL1* and *HRX*) on chromosome 11q23. MLL is a transcription factor.[36,37] The t(4;11) may be detected by RT-PCR method.[38] Another translocation, t(11;19) is closely related. These 11q23 abnormalities may also be seen in secondary AML in adults. In both pediatric ALL and in AML, 11q23 abnormalities are associated with a poor prognosis.[26,39]

t(15;17)—PML/RARα

This translocation is associated with acute promyelocytic leukemia (APL, FAB-M3), a type of acute leukemia that has a favorable prognosis. The translocation results in the fusion of a transcription factor called PML on chromosome 15 with the alpha (α)-retinoic acid receptor gene (RARα) on chromosome 17.[40] The specific characteristics of this translocation may correlate with responsiveness to all transretinoic acid (ATRA), a therapy targeted specifically for this type of leukemia, which induces cellular differentiation.[41,42] RT-PCR methods are available for detection of minimal residual disease.[43] Variant translocations, including t(11;17) and t(5;17), may occur in cases that are morphologically and immunologically similar to classic APL. The translocations also involve the RARα gene. It is important to identify these patients, because they are not responsive to ATRA.[25]

inv(16)—CBFβ/MYH11

Pericentric inversion of chromosome 16 is associated with another type of AML that has a favorable prognosis, acute myelomonocytic leukemia with marrow eosinophilia (FAB-M4Eo). The inv(16) results in the fusion of the *CBFβ* gene

on 16q22 with the *MYH11* gene on 16p13.[44] The inversion may lead to transcriptional alterations, and detection of the hybrid transcript is closely associated with the finding of abnormal bone marrow eosinophils. RT-PCR assays for detection of this abnormality are available.[45]

Treatment of Acute Leukemia

Treatment of leukemia has two principal objectives: to eradicate the leukemic cell mass (cytoreduction) and to give supportive care. Cures are infrequently realized except in children with common ALL; however, induction of complete remission is a realistic goal for most patients with acute leukemia. Complete remission is defined as the absence of leukemia-related signs and symptoms, absence of demonstrable disease, and return of marrow and blood granulocyte, platelet, and red cell values to normal ranges.

Three forms of antileukemic therapy are commonly employed: cytoreductive chemotherapy, radiotherapy, and bone marrow transplantation. Chemotherapy is the mainstay of treatment, although bone marrow transplantation is being used more frequently. Radiotherapy is used as an adjunct to chemotherapy in patients who have localized tissue involvement that may be targeted with irradiation, and has been used for central nervous system (CNS) prophylaxis.

The treatment of patients is administered in different phases, including an induction and postremission phase. Induction therapy, the most intense phase of treatment, is designed to attain complete remission as quickly as possible; its success is the best predictor of long-term disease-free survival. The approach to postremission treatment differs depending on the type of leukemia being treated. In children with ALL, postremission therapy includes intensification, CNS prophylaxis, consolidation, and maintenance therapy. In patients with AML, postremission chemotherapy is more controversial and contributes less to long-term survival.

A number of different cytotoxic chemotherapeutic agents are used to treat acute leukemia. Their modes of action differ but, in general, they poison dividing cells, usually by blocking DNA or RNA synthesis. Combinations of drugs, each with different modes of action, are used. This approach helps to overcome leukemic cell drug resistance. Prednisone, vincristine, and asparaginase are used in most induction regimens for treatment of childhood ALL. CNS prophylaxis, an aspect of therapy given to prevent CNS relapse, has been essential to the improved survival of pediatric patients with ALL in recent decades. Patients with AML are usually treated with a combination of cytarabine and daunorubicin, among other agents. The drugs are given in dosages that have substantial marrow toxicity. The most common complications in patients undergoing chemotherapy arise from marrow hypoplasia and the resulting cytopenias. The use of hematopoietic growth factors such as granulocyte-macrophage/monocyte colony-stimulating factor (GM-CSF) or granulocyte colony-stimulating factor (G-CSF) may potentially improve the status of supportive care in these patients.

Allogeneic bone marrow transplantation has emerged as an important treatment modality, especially for patients with AML, as well as ALL refractory to standard therapy. The patient's bone marrow is completely eradicated with intensive chemotherapy and total body radiation. This is followed by rescuing the patient with donor bone marrow cells collected from an HLA-compatible donor (or from the treated leukemic patient in complete remission, in the case of an autologous transplant) by repeated bone marrow aspirates. The donor cells are processed and then infused into the recipient intravenously. The infused cells travel to the recipient's "empty" marrow, where they engraft, multiply, and repopulate the patient's marrow with healthy hematopoietic tissue. Engraftment takes 3 to 4 weeks, and hematologic values return to normal in 2 to 3 months. The complications of bone marrow transplantation, including infections, hemorrhage, and graft-versus-host disease, are numerous and can be fatal; it is not suitable therapy for all patients with leukemia. But for some, it offers a chance for long-term survival and a potential cure.

➤ ACUTE MYELOID LEUKEMIA

FAB Classification of AML

The need for uniform nomenclature and classification of acute leukemia prompted a group of French, American, and British hematologists to propose a morphological classification scheme for leukemia in 1976.[46] This scheme, the FAB Classification, proved to be useful in standardizing the morphological classification of both acute myeloid and lymphoid leukemias. In the years since it was first introduced, the FAB cooperative group has made several modifications, striving to make the classification as objective and unambiguous as possible.[9] Although there are still some areas of ambiguity, the FAB system has gained wide acceptance, and it will likely form the basis for subsequent leukemia classifications.

The acute myeloid leukemias are divided into the following groups:

M0: Myeloid without cytologic maturation

M1: Myeloid with minimal maturation

M2: Myeloid with maturation

M3: Promyelocytic

M4: Myelomonocytic

M5: Monocytic (a) well and (b) poorly differentiated

M6: Erythroid

M7: Megakaryoblastic

These groups are defined according to the predominant cell type observed on Romanowsky and cytochemically stained blood and bone marrow aspirate smears (Table 16–9). Additional specialized studies are required to confirm the diagnosis of M0 (AML without cytologic maturation) and M7 (acute megakaryocytic leukemia). A summary of the cytochemical reactions in each type of AML is found in Table 16–10.

AML, especially M6 type (erythroleukemia), is sometimes difficult to distinguish from certain myelodysplastic syndromes (refractory anemia with excess blasts [RAEB] and RAEB in transformation). To address this problem, the FAB cooperative group proposed revised criteria for the classification of AML, including a stepwise evaluation of the bone marrow aspirate (Fig. 16–11).[9] A differential count is done of all nucleated cells (ANC) and of only nonerythroid cells (NEC). The ANC differential is used to determine the percentage of erythroblasts (all nucleated erythroid precursors): those cases with greater than 50% erythroblasts are further evaluated to differentiate between M6 (blasts greater than 30% of NEC) and myelodysplastic syndrome (MDS; blasts less than 30% of NEC); those cases with less than 50% erythroblasts are evaluated to differentiate between AML, types M1 to M5, (blasts greater than 30% of ANC) and MDS (blasts less than 30% of ANC). The final classification of AML (M1 to M5) is based on characterization of the NEC fraction. The FAB subgroups are discussed in more detail later in this chapter.

The FAB classification system has improved diagnostic

➤ Table 16-9
FAB CLASSIFICATION OF ACUTE MYELOBLASTIC LEUKEMIA

Type	Characteristics
M0	*Myeloid without cytologic maturation:* Morphologically undifferentiated leukemic blasts with myeloid immunophenotype
M1	*Myeloid without maturation:* Marrow leukemia cells are primarily myeloblasts with no azurophilic granules
M2	*Myeloid with maturation:* Leukemia cells show prominent maturation beyond myeloblast stage
M3	*Promyelocytic:* Abnormal, hypergranular promyelocytes dominate; Auer rods easily found; increased incidence of DIC
M3m	*Microgranular variant of M3:* Indistinct granules; nucleus often reniform or bilobed; increased incidence of DIC
M4	*Myelomonocytic:* Both monocytic (monocytes and promonocytes) and myeloid differentiation (maturation beyond myeloblast stage)
M4Eo	*M4 with bone marrow eosinophilia:* Similar to M4 with marrow eosinophilia (abnormal and immature); associated with abnormal 16q karyotype
M5a	*Monocytic, poorly differentiated:* Monoblasts predominate, typically with abundant cytoplasm and single distinct nucleoli
M5b	*Monocytic, well differentiated:* Predominantly promonocytes in marrow and more pronounced maturation in blood
M6	*Erythroleukemia:* Dysplastic erythroblasts with multinucleation, cytoplasmic budding, vacuolation, and megaloblastoid changes
M7	*Megakaryoblastic:* Wide range of morphology; cytoplasmic projections sometimes present; electron microscopy or immunocytochemical stains necessary for diagnosis

> **Table 16-10**
CYTOCHEMICAL REACTIONS IN ACUTE MYELOBLASTIC LEUKEMIA

	FAB CLASSIFICATION							
	M0	M1	M2	M3	M4	M5	M6	M7
Peroxidase or Sudan black	< 3%	> 3%	> 50%	~100%	20%–80%	Var	> 3%	< 3%
Nonspecific esterase	< 20%	< 20%	< 20%	Var	20%–80%	> 80%	Var	Var

Abbreviation: Var = variable

(handwritten annotations: "often -ve" pointing to M5 Peroxidase; "often -ve" pointing to M3 Nonspecific esterase; "NSE" pointing to Nonspecific esterase)

accuracy and uniformity. It is useful for the student and laboratory technician as an aid to recognizing the wide morphological variations possible in leukemic cells. However, the FAB classification system has largely failed to define groups of patients with AML that have distinct clinical outcomes. These patients generally have similar clinical courses, regardless of their FAB subtype. Exceptions to this are patients having AML with monocytic differentiation (M4 and M5b), who tend to have a lower rate of complete remission and a lower rate of survival,[14] and those with acute promyelocytic leukemia (M3), which is associated with a longer average survival rate.[47] Because of the limitations of morphological and cytochemical classification in prediction of biologic behavior in AML, immunologic and cytogenetic techniques are used to augment the FAB classification; these methods provide additional data that are useful in determining appropriate patient management.

The World Health Organization (WHO) is developing a revised classification scheme for hematologic malignancies, including the acute leukemias. The WHO classification will retain the basic nomenclature, and morphological and cytochemical criteria of the FAB classification, but it will also incorporate clinical, immunophenotypic, and genotypic data.

The classification will likely reduce the percentage of marrow blasts required for a diagnosis of acute leukemia from 30% to 20% and formally recognize additional subtypes of acute leukemia and those associated with certain cytogenetic abnormalities.[7,25] Because the new classification has yet to be finalized and accepted for general clinical use and because it builds on the basics of the FAB classification, the discussion to follow will be based on the FAB system.

Surface Marker Analysis of AML

The availability of myeloid-specific monoclonal antibodies has permitted surface marker analysis of AML. The rationale for this is based on the notion that AML is a clonal disorder derived from a myeloid stem line, which displays the surface membrane antigens expressed in normal myeloid differentiation pathways. A schematic representation of surface antigen expression in normal myeloid differentiation is shown in Figure 16–12.

Surface marker analysis has begun to replace conventional cytochemical methods for lineage determination in acute leukemia. Surface marker studies are used to distinguish AML from ALL, particularly when the leukemic cells are poorly differentiated, with negative or equivocal cytochemical stains (FAB-M0 or M1).

When surface marker analysis is performed to distinguish AML from ALL, it is important to choose a panel of markers that includes antibodies to several myeloid-associated antigens (e.g., CD33 [My9], CD13 [My7], CD14 [My4], CD41a [platelet GP IIb/IIIa]), as well as B- and T-lymphoid antigens. Multiple myeloid lineage-specific markers are necessary because no single marker defines all forms of AML.

The surface phenotypes expressed in cases of AML do not correlate well with the FAB classification or with specific genetic alterations, although certain trends exist.[1] For example, cases of AML with monocytic differentiation (M4 and M5) may express monocyte-related surface markers (CD14), and cases of acute promyelocytic leukemia (M3) tend to express a promyelocytic phenotype (CD13 and CD33 positive, CD34 negative). Other AML subgroups exhibit widely variable phenotypes. Occasionally, mixed lineage phenotypes are encountered, with coexpression of myeloid and lymphoid markers. These biphenotypic or bilineage leukemias may reflect origination of the malignant cell line from an early progenitor capable of both myeloid and lymphoid differentiation.

Acute Myeloid Leukemia without Cytologic Maturation (M0)

Certain cases of acute myeloid leukemia are encountered that show no definitive myeloid differentiation by conventional morphological and cytochemical analysis. These cases are

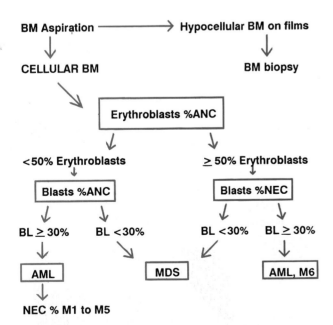

> **FIGURE 16–11** Suggested steps in the analysis of a bone marrow (BM) aspirate to reach a diagnosis of acute myeloid leukemia (AML, M1 to M6) or myelodysplastic syndrome (MDS). BL = blast cells; ANC = all nucleated bone marrow cells; NEC = nonerythroid cells, bone marrow cells excluding erythroblasts. (From Bennett, JM, et al: Proposed revised criteria for the classification of acute myeloid leukemia. Ann Intern Med 103:626, 1985, with permission.)

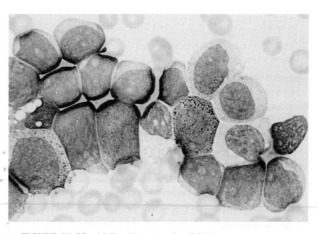

(Figure 16–12 diagram showing lineage from CFU-GM to Monocyte, Promonocyte, Monoblast on left and Myeloblast, Promyelocyte, Myelocyte, PMN on right, with antigen distribution bars for (CD14) My4, (CD11b) Mo1, (CD33) My9, (CD13) My7, and HLA-DR)

➤ **FIGURE 16–12** Distribution of myeloid and monocytic surface antigens. PMN = polymorphonuclear neutrophil; CFU-GM = colony-forming unit granulocyte macrophage/monocyte.

characterized by the presence of primitive leukemic blasts that show no distinctive myeloid morphological features, and lack reactivity with the conventional battery of cytochemical stains (myeloperoxidase, Sudan black B, NSE). However, they exhibit immunologic reactivity for at least one myeloid lineage-specific antigen (CD33, CD13, CD14) in the absence of lymphoid antigens. Such reactivity is required for classification as FAB-M0. Accordingly, surface marker flow cytometry or another form of immunophenotyping is required for the diagnosis. If a case fulfilling these criteria also shows positivity for ultrastructural platelet peroxidase or platelet-specific antigens (CD41a, factor VIII), it is classified as acute megakaryoblastic leukemia (FAB- M7).[48–50]

Acute Myeloid Leukemia with Minimal Maturation (M1)

The leukemic cells seen in cases of AML-M1 subtype are predominantly poorly differentiated myeloblasts (Figs. 16–13 and 16–14 and Color Plates 167 and 168). The nucleus typically has a fine, lacy chromatin pattern and distinct nucleoli. The quantity of cytoplasm is usually moderate, though this varies. In AML-M1, FAB criteria require less than 10% of the NEC to be differentiating granulocytic or monocytic cells. The peroxidase or Sudan black reactions must demonstrate at least 3% positivity in the blast population to document myeloid differentiation. The NSE reaction is positive in less than 20% of the cells.

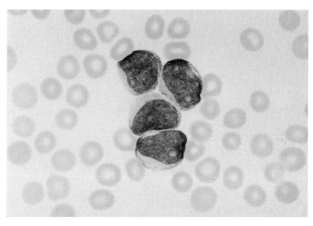

➤ **FIGURE 16–14** AML, M1, peripheral blood.

Acute Myeloid Leukemia with Maturation (M2)

In cases of AML-M2 subtype, the leukemic marrow infiltrate resembles M1 except evidence of maturation to or beyond the promyelocyte stage is present (Figs. 16–15 to 16–17 and Color Plates 169 to 171). Romanowsky-stained bone marrow smears show that promyelocytes and later granulocytic forms make up more than 10% of the NEC. At least 3% of the leukemic cells are peroxidase or Sudan black positive, and usually the percentage is much higher. The NSE activity does not exceed 20%.

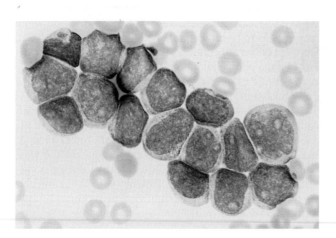

➤ **FIGURE 16–13** Acute myeloblastic leukemia (AML) without maturation, M1, bone marrow.

➤ **FIGURE 16–15** AML with maturation, M2, bone marrow.

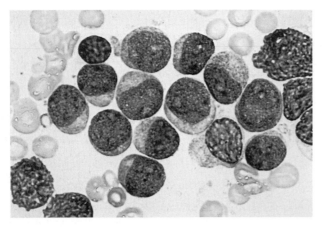

> FIGURE 16–16   AML, M2.

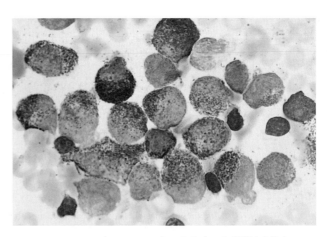

> FIGURE 16–18   Acute promyelocytic leukemia (APL), M3, bone marrow.

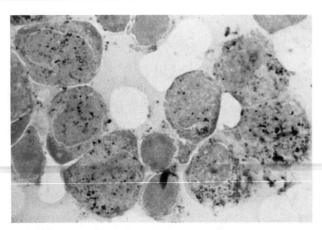

> FIGURE 16–17   AML, M2 (myeloperoxidase stain).

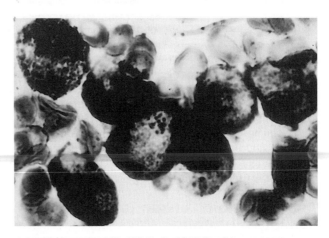

> FIGURE 16–19   APL, M3 (Sudan black B stain).

The acute myeloblastic leukemias (M1 and M2 combined) are the most common types of AML. Together, M1 and M2 account for approximately 50% of cases of AML. Aside from their morphology and cytochemistry, they do not have unique features that set them apart from other myeloid subgroups. Although a translocation of chromosomes 8 and 21 (t[8;21]) has been identified in approximately 18% of patients with AML-M2,[50] this chromosome abnormality has also been found, albeit less frequently, in other FAB groups of AML. As described earlier, it is associated with the fusion gene *ETO/AML1* and with a favorable prognosis, high rates of remission, and relatively long median survivals.

Acute Promyelocytic Leukemia (M3)

The FAB classification defines APL solely by morphological criteria. The leukemic infiltrate is composed of abnormal promyelocytes with heavy granulation, sometimes obscuring the nucleus, and, often, abundant cytoplasm (Figs. 16–18 and 16–19, and Color Plates 172 and 173). Auer rods are frequently seen, and some cells may contain bundles or stacks of Auer rods ("faggot cells"). The nucleus varies in size and shape and is often reniform (kidney-shaped) or bilobed. These cells are strongly positive with the peroxidase stain and are usually negative with the NSE stain, but cases with positive NSE activity have been reported.[51]

APL is associated with distinctive clinical, molecular, and immunophenotypic characteristics as compared with other forms of AML.[52] APL is associated with a high incidence of DIC. The abnormal promyelocytes are rich in thromboplastic substances that, if released, trigger DIC. The majority (80%) of patients with APL present with hemorrhagic manifestations, including petechiae, small ecchymoses, hematuria, and bleeding from venipuncture and bone marrow sites. These presenting signs and symptoms may precede the diagnosis by several weeks. The most consistent coagulation abnormalities include a prolonged prothrombin time and thrombin time, elevated fibrin degradation products, and decreased amounts of plasma fibrinogen. Thrombocytopenia, which tends to be more severe than in other types of AML, is almost universally present. Schistocytes are sometimes evident on the peripheral blood smear. Because of the hemorrhagic complications associated with DIC, it is important to distinguish APL from other forms of AML.

A unique feature of APL is the occurrence of a translocation involving chromosomes 15 and 17 t(15;17).[53] This abnormality has not been reported in any other type of leukemia. It is associated with the hybrid gene *PML/RARα*, which forms the basis of a specifically targeted form of differentiation therapy, ATRA. Patients with APL are best treated with combined ATRA and intensive chemotherapy; recent randomized trials have shown complete remission rates of 93%.[52]

A second form of APL is the microgranular variant (M3m). The leukemic cells of M3m have primary granules that are not readily visible on Romanowsky-stained smears (Fig. 16–20 and Color Plate 174). These granules can, however, be demonstrated with peroxidase and Sudan black staining or by transmission electron microscopy.[54] The disease has a high incidence of DIC, and it is, therefore, important to recognize it for therapeutic considerations. Patients with the microgranular variant tend to have a higher white blood cell count than patients with typical APL and may have a shorter survival.[14]

Morphologically, microgranular APL can be mistaken for acute myelomonocytic or monocytic leukemia. The leukemic cells appear monocytoid with prominent nuclear folding and abundant cytoplasm. The nucleus of most cells in the peripheral blood is reniform or bilobed. Granulation of these cells is scant or absent, although occasional cells with heavy granulation are almost always present. The bone marrow aspirate may reveal a morphological pattern that more closely resembles typical APL.[55]

The diagnosis of M3m can be confirmed with cytochemical studies, including peroxidase or Sudan black stain, which are strongly positive. The NSE reaction is usually negative, but can be positive.[51] Cytogenetic studies of microgranular APL reveal the same abnormal karyotype [t(15;17)] that is found in the hypergranular form.

Although the FAB classification defines APL solely by morphological criteria, in clinical practice the demonstration of t(15;17) by cytogenetic or molecular methods is required for confirmation of diagnosis. Only cases that are positive for the t(15;17) respond to ATRA.[25]

Acute Myelomonocytic Leukemia (M4)

Acute myelomonocytic leukemia (M4) is one of the most commonly diagnosed forms of AML, second only to the M2 group.[14] The leukemic cells of M4 are characterized by both granulocytic and monocytic differentiation (Figs. 16–21 and 16–22, and Color Plates 175 and 176). On a Romanowsky-stained smear it is usually easy to find cells with primary granules (granulocytic differentiation) as well as cells with folded nuclei and moderate to abundant cytoplasm (monocytic differentiation). Both the peroxidase (or Sudan black) and NSE reactions are positive in 20% to 80% of the cells. When morphological and cytochemical similarities make the distinction between M4 and M2 difficult, the diagnosis of

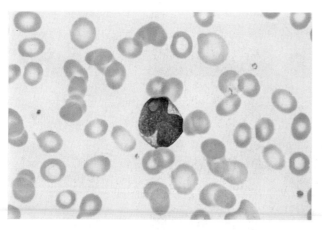

➤ FIGURE 16–20 Acute "microgranular" promyelocytic leukemia, M3m, peripheral blood.

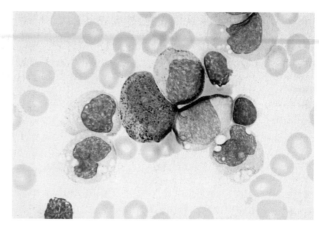

➤ FIGURE 16–21 Acute myelomonocytic leukemia (AMML), M4, bone marrow.

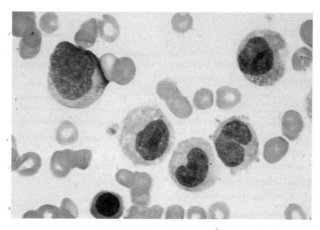

➤ FIGURE 16–22 AMML, M4, peripheral blood.

M4 can be supported by finding a serum lysozyme level exceeding three times the normal level and a peripheral blood monocyte count of greater than 5×10^9/L.[9]

Some cases of M4 are associated with eosinophilia (usually 5% or more of the NEC). The eosinophils appear immature and may have large basophilic-staining granules. Unlike normal eosinophils, these cells stain positive with chloroacetate esterase (specific esterase) and with the PAS reaction.

This M4 variant (M4Eo)[9] is closely associated with an abnormal chromosome 16 including either a deletion[56] or inversion of the long arm (16q).[57] Patients with the 16q abnormality and bone marrow eosinophilia have a longer median survival than patients with typical M4. The molecular genetic correlate is the hybrid gene *CBFβ/MYH11*.

Acute Monocytic Leukemia (M5)

The FAB classification system divides acute monocytic leukemia (M5) into two subtypes: poorly differentiated (M5a) and well differentiated (M5b). M5a is characterized by a predominance of monoblasts, which typically are large with abundant cytoplasm and distinct nucleoli (Fig. 16–23 and Color Plate 177). M5b is characterized by a spectrum of monocytic differentiation, including promonocytes and monocytes. The peripheral blood usually has more monocytes than the bone marrow, where the predominant cell is the promonocyte. This cell has abundant cytoplasm, its nu-

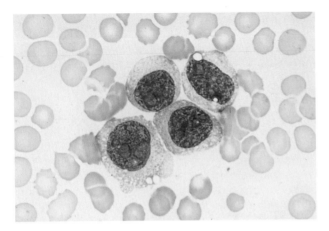

> **FIGURE 16–23**   Acute monocytic leukemia (AMoL), poorly differentiated, M5a, peripheral blood.

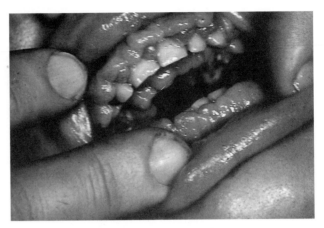

> **FIGURE 16–25**   Gum hypertrophy: A clinical manifestation of acute leukemia.

cleus shows delicate folding or lobulation, and nucleoli may be seen (Fig. 16–24 and Color Plate 178). Both subtypes of M5 show greater than 80% positivity with the NSE stain. The peroxidase and Sudan black stains are negative or only weakly positive.

Acute monocytic leukemia (AMoL) has distinctive clinical manifestations associated with the monocyte's propensity to migrate to extramedullary sites. Skin and gum involvement (Fig. 16–25 and Color Plate 179) are particularly characteristic. Lymphadenopathy frequently occurs, and sometimes the spleen and liver are markedly enlarged. CNS involvement also has an increased incidence in these patients.

The white blood cell count is frequently elevated in patients with AMoL; the median value of 60×10^9/L was reported in one study.[58] Markedly elevated leukocyte counts in AMoL patients have been shown to have a significant correlation with increased lysozyme levels, renal failure, and hypokalemia.[59] DIC is relatively common in patients with AMoL, especially following therapy, although hemorrhagic features are not as prominent as in patients with acute promyelocytic leukemia.

Serum and urine lysozyme levels (muramidase) are often elevated in cases of AML that have a significant monocytic component, including AML types M4 and M5. Lysozyme is a hydrolytic enzyme found in mature monocytes and to a lesser extent in granulocytes. Serum and urine levels of this enzyme are elevated when there is rapid cell turnover. Such

elevations are most striking in the monocytic leukemias and are directly proportional to the amount of monocytic differentiation[60]; they are more elevated in cases of M5b than M5a. Those patients who have heavy urinary excretion of lysozyme may develop renal dysfunction resulting in hypokalemia, hypocalcemia, and azotemia.

Abnormalities involving the long arm of chromosome 11 (11q) have been found in about 35% of all M5 AML and in an even higher percentage of patients with M5a. The 11q abnormality appears to be particularly associated with children with M5a.[50]

Erythroleukemia (M6)

Acute erythroleukemia is characterized by an abnormal proliferation of erythroid and myeloid precursors. Patients with erythroleukemia have hypercellular bone marrows with marked erythroid hyperplasia (greater than 50% of ANC) associated with abnormal erythroid forms. Megaloblastoid changes can be seen in the erythroblasts along with other dysplastic features, including bizarre multinucleation, markedly vacuolated cytoplasm of erythroblasts, and cytoplasmic budding (Figs. 16–26 and 16–27, and Color Plates 180 and 181). Cytoplasmic PAS-positive staining in the neoplastic erythroblasts is consistent with the diagnosis of erythroleukemia but is not absolutely specific, and negative staining does not rule it out. Myeloblasts and promyelocytes are present in increased numbers (greater than 30% of

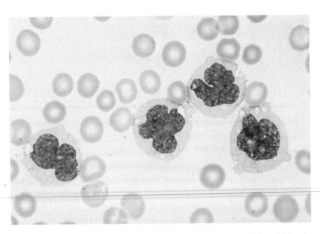

> **FIGURE 16–24**   AMoL, well-differentiated, M5b, peripheral blood.

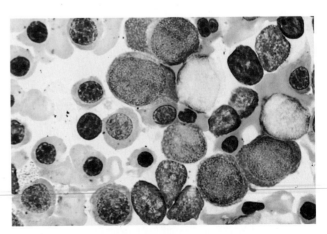

> **FIGURE 16–26**   Erythroleukemia, M6, bone marrow.

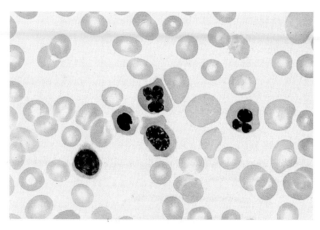

➤ **FIGURE 16–27**   Erythroleukemia, M6, peripheral blood.

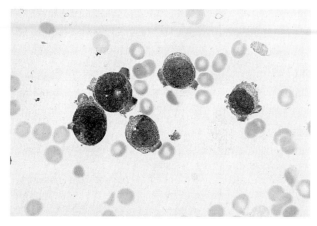

➤ **FIGURE 16–28**   Acute megakaryoblastic leukemia (AMegL), M7.

NEC), and Auer rods may be seen. Abnormal megakaryocytes may also be present.

Many cases that fulfill strict criteria for FAB-M6 (M6A) evolve into a leukemic stage indistinguishable from AML, M1, M2, or M4 type,[46] in effect behaving as myelodysplastic or "preleukemic" states. Although not addressed in the original FAB description of M6, cases in which pronormoblasts alone exceed 30% are now recognized as FAB-M6B, or pure erythroleukemia. The subclassification of this group of leukemias is still somewhat controversial.[61]

Anemia is invariably present in patients with erythroleukemia and is often more pronounced than in patients with other types of AML. Reticulocytopenia is common and is a result of ineffective erythropoiesis. Frequently the peripheral blood exhibits nucleated red blood cells and myeloblasts, but it is possible to see patients who are anerythremic (no NRBCs) or aleukemic (no blasts).

Caution must be taken when the diagnosis of erythroleukemia is considered. The possibility of megaloblastic anemia resulting from vitamin B_{12} or folic acid deficiency, congenital dyserythropoietic anemia, or the myelodysplastic syndromes must be excluded. These disorders may, at times, mimic erythroleukemia.

Acute Megakaryoblastic Leukemia (M7)

Acute megakaryoblastic leukemia (AMegL) is a relatively uncommon form of leukemia characterized by neoplastic proliferation of megakaryoblasts and atypical megakaryocytes. Recognition of this entity was aided by the use of platelet peroxidase (PPO) ultrastructural studies. PPO, which is distinct from myeloperoxidase, is specific for the megakaryocytic cell line.[62]

AMegL was not initially included in the FAB classification of AML because it could not be identified by conventional morphological and cytochemical studies; however, in 1985 increased recognition of this entity prompted the FAB cooperative group to add AMegL to the classification (M7).[63]

The blasts observed in AMegL display a wide range of morphology, from small cells with scant cytoplasm and dense chromatin to large cells with a moderate amount of cytoplasm and a fine reticulated chromatin pattern. Cytoplasmic projections are sometimes present (Fig. 16–28 and Color Plate 182), and in some cases azurophilic granules resembling early granular megakaryocytes can be seen. The

presence of megakaryocytic fragments in the peripheral blood is also suggestive of AMegL.

Conventional cytochemistry can suggest the diagnosis of AMegL but is not definitive. The myeloperoxidase and Sudan black reactions are negative, whereas acid phosphatase, PAS, and alpha-naphthyl acetate esterase (ANAE) are usually positive. The combination of a positive ANAE and a negative alpha-naphthyl butyrate esterase rules out monocytic leukemia and is highly suggestive of megakaryoblastic lineage.[64]

Electron microscopy for platelet peroxidase may be performed, but the diagnosis of AMegL is usually made by using an immunocytochemical demonstration of platelet-specific antigens. Antibodies against factor VIII–related antigen and platelet surface glycoprotein IIb/IIIa (fibrinogen receptor, CD41a) are the most sensitive and specific immunologic markers of AMegL.

AMegL may arise in the context of myelodysplasia or de novo. It has been observed as a transformation of existing hematologic disorders such as myelodysplastic syndromes and chronic myeloproliferative disorders, including chronic myelocytic leukemia, and agnogenic myeloid metaplasia. AMegL has also been associated with acute myelofibrosis, which is characterized by diffuse marrow fibrosis, pancytopenia, and bone marrow megakaryoblast proliferation, but which usually lacks the splenomegaly and characteristic red cell morphological changes of chronic myelofibrosis. It has been suggested that acute myelofibrosis may be synonymous with AMegL, and may be related to neoplastic elaboration of platelet-derived growth factor (PDGF).[65]

Secondary AML and AML in the Elderly

AML may occur de novo, or secondary to chemotherapy, radiotherapy, or environmental and occupational exposures. It has been observed that AML in older individuals shares biologic and cytogenetic features with cases of secondary leukemia and that both types of leukemia have a poor prognosis. Recent studies show that the multidrug resistance gene (*MDR1*) is frequently expressed in these leukemias. The gene encodes a protein that mediates drug efflux out of leukemic cells. Thus, the leukemic cells in these patients may be inherently resistant to chemotherapeutic agents, accounting in part for the poor prognosis.[25]

► CASE STUDY 1

A 42-year-old woman presented with a 2-month history of fatigue and weakness and a 2-week history of a sore throat. She reported a 15-pound weight loss over the past month or two. One week prior to admission she started antibiotics for her sore throat, but she reported little improvement; she subsequently developed a peritonsillar abscess. On admission to the hospital she was found to have an elevated white blood cell count with a large number of circulating blasts.

The physical examination of the patient showed an anxious, middle-aged woman whose vital signs were normal, aside from a slightly elevated temperature (37.6°C). Her right tonsil was enlarged and erythematous. She had no adenopathy, and her liver and spleen were not palpable.

Laboratory studies were ordered, and the following results were reported: hematocrit, 19.5%; hemoglobin, 6.3 g/dL; platelets, 64×10^9/L; and white blood cell (WBC) count, 79.2×10^9/L. The differential included 80% blasts. The majority of these cells were relatively large (15 to 20 μm) with a moderate amount of cytoplasm. The nuclei varied in shape from round to oval, and some were indented or folded; most had several distinct small nucleoli. An occasional blast had azurophilic granules, but this was the exception. A bone marrow aspirate and biopsy were obtained, which both showed virtually total replacement of normal elements with sheets of poorly differentiated cells (Fig. 16–29 and Color Plate 183). The biopsy specimen was hypercellular, approaching 100% cellularity in some areas. The morphology of the aspirated cells was similar to those seen in the peripheral blood except that fewer of the cells had folded nuclei, and, in general, the nuclear-to-cytoplasmic (N:C) ratio was higher. Most of these cells showed very little differentiation, although occasional cells with granulation were noted. Rare Auer rods were also observed. Cytochemical studies of the aspirate smears were positive: the myeloperoxidase stain was positive in approximately 30% of the blasts and the NSE (alpha-naphthyl butyrate) was positive in occasional cells (less than 10%).

Diagnosis: Acute myeloid leukemia, FAB-M1.

Follow-up: HLA matching was performed on the patient's brother and sister, but neither had a compatible tissue type. The possibility of bone marrow transplantation was subsequently ruled out. The patient was placed on a standard protocol for acute myeloid leukemia. During her induction chemotherapy she developed anemia, thrombocytopenia, and leukopenia. She required platelets and packed red blood cell transfusions. She also required broad-spectrum antibiotics for fever resulting from neutropenia, although no specific pathogen could be identified. Three weeks after her induction chemotherapy, a repeat bone marrow biopsy showed no residual leukemia. She remained in complete remission for 11 months, but then relapsed. Attempts to induce a second remission were unsuccessful. She developed progressive hepatomegaly, jaundice, and persistent neutropenia. She also developed multiple infections and was unable to recover.

This case illustrates a typical course of acute myeloid leukemia. Although the patient was not cured, she did achieve and maintain a complete remission for nearly a full year.

► ACUTE LYMPHOBLASTIC LEUKEMIA

FAB Classification of ALL

The FAB classification system separates ALL into three morphological groups (Table 16–11):

L1: Small, uniform lymphoblasts

L2: Large, pleomorphic lymphoblasts

L3: Burkitt's type (vacuolated and deeply basophilic cytoplasm)

The morphology of these groups is evaluated on a bone marrow aspirate smear rather than peripheral blood. L1 ALL (Fig. 16–30 and Color Plate 184) exhibits a uniform population of small blasts with scant cytoplasm, a homogeneous chromatin pattern, and inconspicuous nucleoli. The nuclear shape is regular, but occasional clefting may be present. L2 ALL (Figs. 16–31 and 16–32, and Color Plates 185 and 186) is characterized by cellular heterogeneity. Some blasts may exhibit L1 features, whereas others are larger and have more abundant cytoplasm, a variable chromatin pattern, and prominent nucleoli. Nuclear clefting and indentation are characteristic. This type may be difficult or impossible to distinguish morphologically from AML-M1. L3 ALL (Fig. 16–33 and Color Plate 187) is composed of a uniform population of relatively large blasts that are characterized by moderate to abundant, deeply basophilic, vacuolated cytoplasm. The nucleus has a round to oval contour without indentations. L3 ALL is referred to as "Burkitt's type" because its morphology is that seen in Burkitt's leukemia/lymphoma.

The distinction between L1 and L2 ALL is not always clear. Because of this the FAB cooperative group proposed a simple scoring system based on cytologic features.[66] Other groups have modified this system, assessing each case on a cell-by-cell basis to determine the percentage of L1 and L2 cells. Individual L1 and L2 lymphoblasts can be differentiated most reliably by evaluating the N:C ratio (high in L1, low in L2) and the absence (L1) or presence (L2) of nucleoli. Cases of "pure L1" ALL (more than 90% L1 blasts) have

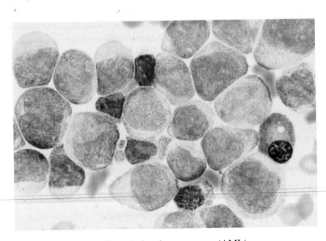

► **FIGURE 16–29**   Case study—bone marrow (AML).

> ## Table 16-11
> ## FAB CLASSIFICATION OF ACUTE LYMPHOBLASTIC LEUKEMIA

Cytologic Features	L1	L2	L3
Cell size	Predominantly small	Large, heterogeneous	Large, homogeneous
Nuclear chromatin	Homogeneous in any one case	Heterogeneous	Finely stippled, and homogeneous
Nuclear shape	Regular, occasional clefting	Irregular, clefting and indentation common	Regular (round to oval)
Nucleoli*	Inconspicuous	One or more, often large	One or more, prominent
Cytoplasm*	Scanty	Variable; often moderately abundant	Moderately abundant; strongly basophilic
Cytoplasmic vacuolation	Variable	Variable	Prominent

*The most useful cytologic features in separating L1 from L2 lymphoblasts are quantity of cytoplasm and presence and prominence of nucleoli.
Adapted from Bennett, JM, et al: Minimally differentiated AML (FAB M0). Br J Haematol 78:325, 1991.

the best prognosis, cases of "pure L2" ALL (more than 50% L2 blasts) have a worse prognosis, and those cases with mixed cell types have an intermediate prognosis. L3 morphology is associated with the worst prognosis.[67] Regardless of the morphological classification described here, immunologic and cytogenetic techniques serve a critical function in determining modern therapeutic approaches to ALL. In fact, many treatment centers have completely abandoned the FAB classification system of ALL and rely strictly on im-munophenotypic, cytogenetic, and molecular findings for therapeutic decisions. The upcoming WHO classification of acute leukemia will likely altogether drop the L1 and L2 morphological distinction for purposes of classification.

Immunologic Classification of ALL

The immunologic classification of ALL is based on the stages of lymphocyte development, whose phenotypes are summarized in Table 16–12. Lymphoblasts are phenotyped

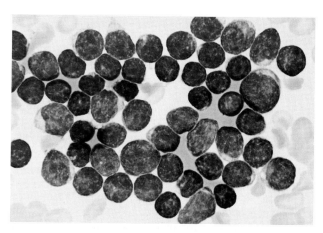

> **FIGURE 16–30**   ALL, L1, bone marrow.

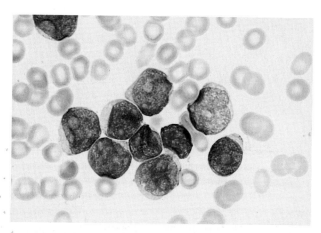

> **FIGURE 16–32**   ALL, L2, peripheral blood.

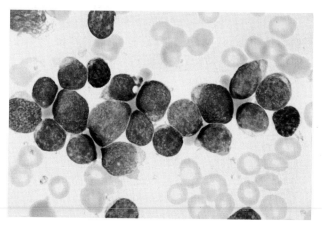

> **FIGURE 16–31**   ALL, L2, bone marrow.

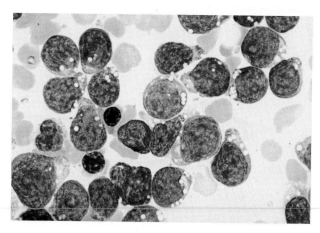

> **FIGURE 16–33**   ALL, L3, bone marrow.

> **Table 16-12**
> ## IMMUNOLOGIC CLASSIFICATION OF ACUTE LYMPHOBLASTIC LEUKEMIA

Subtype	Phenotype
Precursor-B cell	HLA-DR, CD34, TdT, CD19, CD20 (±), CD10
Pre-B ALL	HLA-DR, TdT (±), CD19, CD20 (±), CD10, cIgM
B-ALL	HLA-DR, CD19, CD20, CD22, CD10 (±), sIg
LL	HLA-DR (±), CD1, CD2, cCD3, dual CD4/CD8, CD5, CD7 (±), CD10 (±), CD34 (±), TdT

using monoclonal antibodies (see Table 16–7). The nuclear enzyme TdT, which is found in immature lymphoid cells (both B and T lineage), is also utilized.

To fully appreciate the immunologic classification of ALL and other lymphoproliferative disorders (e.g., CLL, lymphoma, and multiple myeloma), it is important to understand lymphocyte ontogeny. These processes result from clonal proliferation of lymphoid cells—cells that have been "frozen" at a given stage of maturation, retaining some features of their normally differentiated counterparts. In the case of ALL, the malignant clone is arrested at an early stage of lymphocytic differentiation.

Lymphocyte Ontogeny

Lymphocytes originate from pluripotent stem cells (see Fig. 1–2) that are present in the yolk sac, fetal liver, spleen, and bone marrow. At birth and into adulthood, the stem cells are normally found only in the bone marrow, where they respond to specific growth factors (hormone-like substances) that trigger their commitment toward B- or T-lymphocyte differentiation. The microenvironment of these developing cells plays a critical role in their maturation: B cells develop in the bone marrow (bursa-equivalent tissue) whereas T cells develop in the thymus (from committed stem cells that have migrated there). Lymphocyte maturation in these organs is antigen-independent. After the lymphocytes have matured they migrate to the peripheral lymphoid organs, including the lymph nodes, spleen, and other lymphoid tissues. In these organs the lymphocytes remain in a resting state until they are stimulated to undergo antigen-dependent development.

B-Lymphocyte Development

Early B-cell maturation (antigen-independent), is divided into three stages: early pre-B cell, pre-B cell, and mature B cell (Fig. 16–34). These stages are identified by their expression of TdT, surface markers (HLA-DR, CD10 [CALLA], CD19, CD20), and immunoglobulin (cytoplasmic or surface Ig). The early pre-B cell is TdT positive and expresses HLA-DR, CD19, and usually CALLA (CD10). HLA-DR, a histocompatibility-related antigen, is expressed first, followed by CD19 and then CD10. CD19 is the most sensitive and specific surface marker for early B cells. During this stage the immunoglobulin genes begin to undergo structural rearrangement (see later discussion), followed by the production of cytoplasmic mu (Cμ)-heavy chain. The presence of cytoplasmic μ distinguishes the pre-B cell from its predecessor, which otherwise has a similar phenotype. As the cell continues to mature, immunoglobulin light chains are produced, and IgM is assembled and inserted into the plasma membrane. This surface Ig (sIg) is the hallmark of the mature B cell, which no longer expresses TdT. Each B cell expresses only one type of Ig light chain (kappa [κ] or lambda [λ]), a feature that is extremely helpful in identifying monoclonal proliferations of mature B cells.

Immunoglobulin genes are rearranged in a unique process that is normally limited to cells committed to B-cell differentiation. The Ig genes are composed of discontinuous segments of minigene families that, when productively rearranged, encode for the heavy chain and the κ or λ light chains. The heavy chain gene (on chromosome 14) is composed of four minigene families including the variable (VH), diversity (DH), joining (JH), and constant (CH) regions. The CH region has separate DNA sequences that encode for the different Ig isotypes including μ (Cμ), delta (δ), gamma (γ), alpha (α), and epsilon (ε). The V, D, and J regions are the first to undergo rearrangement forming a VDJ complex (Fig. 16–35). In this process, intervening sequences (introns) are excised and the V, D, and J regions are spliced together. Messenger RNA is transcribed from this VDJ complex along with DNA sequences downstream from it, including an intron and the Cμ region. The mRNA itself is then spliced to bring the VDJ complex adjacent to the Cμ region, creating a template for cytoplasmic μ-heavy chain synthesis. This process is closely followed by a similar rearrangement of the κ gene (on chromosome 2), which, if unsuccessful, is in turn followed by rearrangement of the λ gene (on chromosome 22). As B-cell development continues, the heavy chain may undergo additional rearrangements in the CH region, initiating an isotype switch from μ

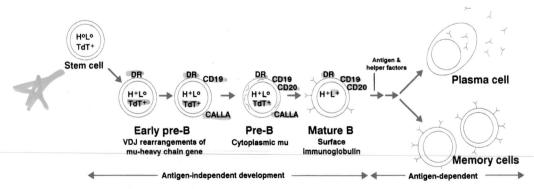

> **FIGURE 16–34**   B-cell development. Heavy chain (H) and light chain (L) are designated as H°, L° if in embryonic form, and H+, L+ if rearranged.

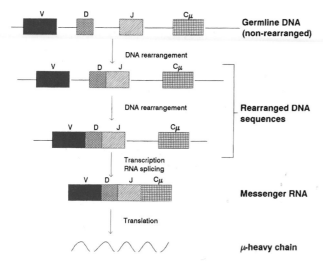

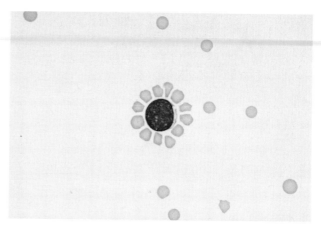

► **FIGURE 16-36**   E-rosette formation in T-cell ALL.

► **FIGURE 16-35**   Schematic of immunoglobulin μ-heavy chain gene rearrangement. The variable (V), diversity (D), and joining (J) regions of germline DNA are linked through rearrangement and loss of intervening sequences. The VDJ complex, more intervening sequences, and a constant (Cμ) region are then transcribed. The resulting RNA is spliced, linking the VDJ and Cμ regions and creating a template for the Ig μ-heavy chain.

to δ. Both IgM and IgD are expressed on the surface of the majority of mature B cells.

After maturation in the bone marrow, B cells circulate through the blood to the peripheral lymphoid organs, where they remain in a resting state until stimulated by specific antigens to undergo further development. Activated B cells undergo clonal expansion, producing daughter cells that retain the same antibody idiotype (antigen-binding region). Some daughter cells become memory cells and regain the small mature B-cell morphology and phenotype, whereas others continue development toward a short-lived antibody-secreting cell—the plasma cell. During this final development, the Ig heavy chain may undergo another isotype switch, to IgG, IgA, or IgE. The plasma cell produces large quantities of Ig and is characterized by a high concentration of cytoplasmic Ig. It does not express SIg, CD19, nor CD20, although other antigens are sometimes expressed (e.g., PCA-1, PC-1).

T-Lymphocyte Development

In the past, T cells were identified by incubating lymphocytes with sheep red blood cells and observing for E-rosette formation (Fig. 16–36 and Color Plate 188). Now, with the availability of monoclonal antibodies, T cells are identified and subclassified using immunologic reagents. T-cell development (antigen-independent) in the thymus is divided into three main stages: stage I, early thymocyte; stage II, common thymocyte; and stage III, mature thymocyte. Stages I and II occur in the thymic cortex, and the last stage occurs in the thymic medulla. Similar to early B cells, thymocytes express TdT and unique surface markers (Fig. 16–37). CD7, which is present on early thymocytes, is one of the earliest T-cell markers to be expressed; it is also the most sensitive marker for T-cell ALL. Its expression is followed by that of CD2 and CD5. As the thymocytes move into stage II of thymic development, they express CD1, a marker of common thymocytes, along with both CD4 and CD8. CD3 is the next marker to be expressed; it is usually absent or only weakly expressed

at stage II, but it is fully expressed in the mature thymocyte (stage III). At this stage CD1 and CD4 or CD8 are lost, giving the mature thymocyte a helper (CD4+) or suppressor (CD8+) phenotype.

During thymic maturation, the T-cell synthesizes an antigen-receptor molecule called the T-cell receptor (TCR), which is closely associated with the CD3 molecule on the plasma membrane. Two TCR isotypes have been discovered, TCR-αβ and TCR-γδ. The genes that encode for the α, β, γ, and δ polypeptides undergo rearrangement in a manner that parallels Ig gene rearrangements in the B cell. The TCR-β gene (on chromosome 7) rearrangements precede TCR-α (on chromosome 14) rearrangements. Less is known about the γ and δ genes or about the function of the TCR-γδ, but it is clear that rearrangement of the γ gene precedes that of the α and β genes. The majority of mature T cells express the TCR-αβ isotype.

Precursor B-Cell ALL (Early Pre-B and Pre-B)

Precursor B-cell ALL, including both early pre-B and pre-B-cell types, is the most frequently encountered form of lymphoblastic leukemia. It is predominantly seen in the pediatric age group although it may occur at any age. Its peak incidence is between the ages of 3 and 5 years, and it is characterized in most childhood cases by L1 morphology. In adults L2 morphology is more common. Early pre-B-cell ALL expresses HLA-DR and CD19. Pre-B-cell ALL has the same surface phenotype but also expresses Cμ. Most of these precursor B-cell leukemias have CALLA (CD10) on their surface and are referred to as "common ALL." Some of these, particularly pre-B-cell ALL, also express CD20, a pan-B-cell marker that first appears during the midstage of B-cell development.

Patients with precursor B-cell ALL usually present with disease predominantly localized to the blood and bone marrow. Prominent splenomegaly, hepatomegaly, and lymphadenopathy are infrequently seen at presentation. It is also uncommon for these patients to exhibit a markedly elevated white blood cell count (greater than 100×10^9/L).

In children, pre-B-cell ALL (Cμ present) is associated with a poorer outcome than early pre-B ALL (Cμ absent). Both groups have a high rate of achieving complete remission; however, patients with pre-B-cell ALL appear to have a shorter duration of remission.[68] Twenty to thirty percent

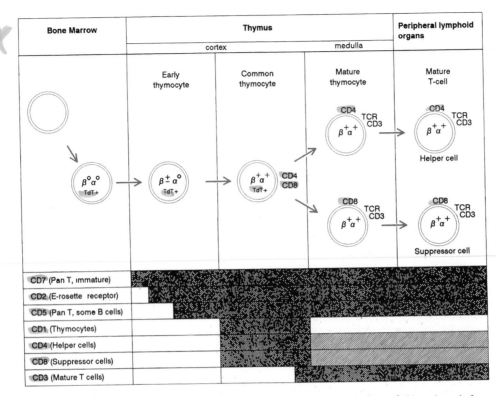

> ➤ FIGURE 16–37   T-cell maturation. T-cell receptor (TCR) β- and α-chain genes are designated as β° and α° if in embryonic form, and β+ and α+ if rearranged.

of these patients have a translocation of chromosome one and nineteen (t[1;19]).[69] This rearrangement is not generally found in cases of early pre-B-cell ALL. In adults, approximately 30% of pre-B-cell ALL is associated with the Philadelphia chromosome (t[9;22]).

B-Cell ALL (Burkitt's Leukemia/Lymphoma)

B-cell ALL is a homogeneous group that accounts for only a small portion (2% to 5%) of all cases of ALL. It is the only phenotype that can be reliably predicted on the basis of morphology alone; L3 morphology is consistently observed, with a mature B-cell phenotype characterized by a high concentration of surface immunoglobulin (usually sIgM) and monoclonal light-chain restriction. CD19, CD20, and HLA-DR are positive; TdT is negative; and most cases do not express CD10. It is likely that these cells are derived from a transformed or stimulated B cell. Virtually all cases have a characteristic translocation involving a rearrangement of the c-*myc* oncogene on chromosome 8 with the immunoglobulin heavy-chain gene on chromosome 14 or the light-chain genes on chromosomes 2 or 22 (t[8;14], t[2;8], or t[8;22]).[70,71]

The lymphoblasts found in cases of B-cell ALL are indistinguishable by cytologic, cytochemical, and immunologic criteria from tumor cells found in cases of Burkitt's lymphoma.[72] It is likely that B-cell ALL represents a leukemic phase of Burkitt's lymphoma (non-African type).

The prognosis for patients with B-cell ALL is poor. They respond poorly to current chemotherapy regimens and rarely achieve remission.[73]

T-Cell ALL

T-cell markers are found in approximately 15% to 25% of all patients with ALL. These cases can be further catego-

rized into one of the three stages of thymocyte development. CD7 is the most reliable marker of T-cell ALL, but CD2 and CD5 are also expressed in many cases. CD4 and CD8 are occasionally coexpressed and may be accompanied by the presence of CD3; approximately 10% express CALLA. The blasts of T-cell ALL are TdT positive and are associated with both L1 and L2 morphology.

Patients with T-cell ALL often present with a mediastinal mass, a high white blood cell count (greater than $100 \times 10^9/L$ in 50% of cases), hepatosplenomegaly, and early meningeal involvement. Males are affected more often than females, and the disease occurs more often in older children. These patients generally have a poorer prognosis than those with common ALL. Features that most consistently correlate with a better response to therapy include a low white blood cell level, younger age (less than 15 years), and L1 morphology. There is also some evidence that certain surface markers may be associated with a better (CD5) or worse (CD3) prognosis.[74,75]

When patients present with a mediastinal mass, it may be difficult to distinguish T-cell ALL from lymphoblastic lymphoma. The cytologic features of this type of lymphoma are similar to those of ALL, although the lymphoma is generally associated with a more mature immunophenotype.[76] After a variable time, patients with lymphoblastic lymphoma almost always develop bone marrow involvement, which renders their condition indistinguishable from T-cell ALL. This distinction is generally based on clinical criteria. Patients who first present with prominent marrow and peripheral blood involvement are usually diagnosed with T-cell ALL.

Acute Leukemia—Mixed-Lineage or Unclassified

With the advent of immunophenotyping and other forms of biologic assessment of acute leukemia, subsets of acute leukemia that do not follow clear lineage definitions are being described more frequently. A significant number of patients are found to have features of both cell lines, using immunologic, molecular, or biochemical techniques. The lymphoid and myeloid antigens may be coexpressed by a single population of leukemic cells, or there may be biphasic populations with distinct lineage-specific phenotypes. A sequential transformation may occur from one cell lineage to another. The significance of these forms of mixed-lineage expression are unclear at present. Studies on the prognostic significance of mixed-lineage expression have yielded conflicting results, in part because of nonuniform terminology and a failure to recognize that most antigens are lineage-associated rather than lineage-specific. The most important lineage-specific antigens are CD22, CD3, and myeloperoxidase for B, T, and myeloid lineages, respectively. A scoring system for acute biphenotypic (mixed-lineage) leukemia has been proposed to facilitate more uniform diagnosis and prospective studies to determine the possible prognostic significance of these phenotypes.[77,78] Currently, most mixed-lineage leukemias are classified and treated on the basis of traditional morphological and cytochemical criteria.

With the routine use of flow cytometric immunophenotyping of acute leukemia, fewer than 1% of cases remain unclassified. Typical unclassified or undifferentiated leukemia is HLA-DR+ and CD34+ with no lineage-specific markers. Most are treated as AML if the morphology and cytochemistry suggest undifferentiated leukemia.[10]

Childhood versus Adult ALL

The incidence of ALL differs markedly with age. For this reason and because of the generally poorer prognosis in adults, ALL may be considered in the broad context of childhood and adult ALL. The childhood group generally consists of those patients who present with ALL at 15 years of age or earlier.

L1 morphology occurs most frequently in the pediatric age group, whereas the L2 type tends to be seen in adults. The incidence of L3 ALL does not differ significantly in children and adults.

B- and T-lineage ALL occurs at similar rates in children and adults, but differences in phenotypes are observed. For example, a relatively high proportion of adults with early pre-B-cell ALL do not express CD10 (formerly termed "null-cell" ALL).

Prognostic indicators are especially important in cases of childhood ALL. Most of these patients are able to achieve a complete remission, and many are potentially cured. Unfortunately, some children relapse, and some of these eventually succumb to their disease. The therapy used to achieve a cure has potentially toxic effects that are a special concern in growing children. To select those patients who will have an optimal response to less aggressive therapy, investigators have identified prognostic factors and defined clinical risk categories. These tools allow the type and intensity of therapy to be focused to each child's level of clinical risk of relapse and death. Indicators of a poor prognosis include older age (later than 13 years), a high white blood cell count (more than 20×10^9/L), T-cell or mature B-cell phenotypes, L2- and L3-type morphology, and structural chromosome abnormalities. Children with an early pre-B-cell phenotype, with hyperdiploid lymphoblasts (more than 50 chromosomes), a low white blood cell count, and without a structural chromosome abnormality have a very good prognosis.

> **CASE STUDY 2**

T.J. was 4 years old when he first presented to his family doctor with a 3-week history of fatigue, weakness, and a persistent sore throat. On physical examination he had a palpable spleen but no evidence of lymphadenopathy. He appeared pale and had multiple bruises over his lower extremities. A CBC, platelet count, and differential were carried out, with the following results:

CBC

WBC 2.40×10^9/L		MCV	87.0 fL
RBC 2.41×10^{12}/L		MCH	29.0 pg
Hct 21.0%		MCHC	33.3 g/dL
Hgb 7.0 g/dL		Platelets	6.7×10^9/L

Differential

PMN	3%
Blasts	97%

A bone marrow examination was performed that revealed sheets of small blasts having scant cytoplasm and indistinct nucleoli (see Fig. 16–30). Cytochemical and cell marker studies of the bone marrow aspirate gave the following results:

Cytochemistry

Peroxidase: Negative
NSE: Negative
TdT: Strongly positive

Surface Markers

CD3	Negative	CD10	100%
CD5	Negative	CD19	98%
CD7	Negative	CD20	Negative
Cμ	Negative		

Diagnosis: Acute lymphoblastic leukemia, common ALL (early pre-B; L1 type).

Follow-up: This patient was placed on a protocol for ALL to which he responded very well. His physical examination 2 months after induction chemotherapy was unremarkable except for some hair loss. His CBC was entirely normal, although his white blood cell count was low-normal. A bone marrow examination at this time was also normal. He was continued on therapy, including one reintensification phase followed by maintenance therapy. Eight years later, he is free of any signs of leukemia and is living a normal life.

QUESTIONS

1. A 4-year-old boy presents with bruising, fever, and coughing. His white blood cell count is 15×10^9/L; hematocrit, 23%; and platelets, 53×10^9/L. A bone marrow aspirate is obtained that reveals sheets of

immature cells. Cytochemical studies for peroxidase and NSE are negative; the TdT is positive. Surface markers studies are done that show the following phenotype: HLA-DR+; CD19+; CD10+; Cµ−; sIg−; CD7−. What is the diagnosis?

a. B-cell ALL
b. Early pre-B-cell ALL
c. Pre-B-cell ALL
d. T-cell ALL

2. The white blood cell count is 50 x 10⁹/L with 80% blasts, 15% segmented neutrophils, and 5% lymphocytes. The bone marrow reveals sheets of immature cells. Cytochemical studies of these show that they are peroxidase-positive (20%) and the nonspecific esterase is negative. What is the diagnosis?

a. AML, M1 type
b. AML, M2 type
c. AML, M4 type
d. AML, M5 type

3. The white blood cell count is 15 × 10⁹/L with 90% blasts, 6% segmented neutrophils, and 4% monocytes. The blasts are relatively large and have abundant cytoplasm. Over 90% of them are positive with the nonspecific esterase stain, and an occasional blast is positive with Sudan black. What is the diagnosis?

a. AML, M2 type
b. AML, M3 type
c. AML, M4 type
d. AML, M5 type

4. Cytochemical stains were performed on bone marrow smears from an acute leukemia patient. All blasts were TdT negative. The majority of the blasts showed varying amounts of Sudan black B positivity. Fifty percent of them stained positive for nonspecific esterase. What type of leukemia is indicated?

a. Acute myeloblastic leukemia
b. Acute lymphoblastic leukemia
c. Acute myelomonocytic leukemia
d. Acute erythroleukemia

5. Bone marrow examination reveals a hypercellular marrow with lymphoblasts that react with antisera specific for CD7 and TdT; however, the lymphoblasts are negative for sIg (surface immunoglobulins), and CD10 (CALLA). The diagnosis is:

a. ALL, B-cell type
b. ALL, early pre-B-cell type
c. ALL, pre-B-cell type
d. ALL, T-cell type

6. A 49-year-old woman was admitted to the hospital for easy bruising and menorrhagia. She had evidence of disseminated intravascular coagulation. Her white blood cell count is 3 × 10⁹/L with 95% large, atypical mononuclear cells. Many of these cells are packed with large, purple-staining granules; some have

multiple Auer rods; and all are strongly peroxidase-positive. What is the diagnosis?

a. AML, M2 type
b. AML, M3 type
c. AML, M4 type
d. AML, M5 type

7. A 21-year-old patient's bone marrow is classified morphologically by the FAB system as an L3 acute lymphoblastic leukemia. Which of the following results best support this diagnosis?

a. Expression of CD19
b. Presence of Cµ
c. Presence of sIg
d. Nuclear TdT reactivity

SUMMARY CHART

➤ Acute leukemia tends to present with a sudden clinical onset and a rapidly fatal course if untreated.
➤ Chronic leukemia has a more insidious onset and an indolent clinical course.
➤ The neoplastic cells in acute leukemia are immature (blasts, early myeloid cells), whereas the neoplastic cells in chronic leukemias are more mature.
➤ A diagnosis of acute leukemia is made using current FAB criteria by the presence of more than 30% blast cells in bone marrow aspirate smears.
➤ Acute leukemia is divided into two basic categories based on cell lineage: myeloid and lymphoid.
➤ The distinction is critically important because the treatment and prognosis are different.
➤ Myeloblasts are usually large in size and have fine chromatin and prominent nucleoli. Lineage is confirmed by cytochemical staining and immunophenotyping.
➤ Lymphoblasts tend to be small- to medium-sized blasts with dense chromatin and less distinctive nucleoli. Lineage is confirmed by cytochemical staining and immunophenotyping.
➤ Auer rods are pathognomonic for a myeloproliferative process, which is usually acute myeloblastic leukemia (AML).
➤ Using cytochemical stains, myeloblasts are positive for myeloperoxidase and Sudan black B.
➤ Lymphoblasts are positive for terminal deoxynucleotidyl transferase (TdT) by immunologic methods and usually negative for myeloperoxidase and Sudan black B.
➤ Nonspecific esterase (NSE) is positive in blasts with monocytic differentiation.
➤ Flow cytometry is an extremely useful tool for analyzing cell surface and cytoplasmic antigen expression in leukemic blasts and can be effective in monitoring residual disease.
➤ Cytogenetic analyses of leukemic cells can often

identify chromosomal abnormalities, which can be critical in directing therapeutic decisions.

➤ Molecular diagnostic studies are becoming increasingly important and are used to confirm a suspected chromosomal abnormality or to monitor minimal residual disease following treatment or bone marrow transplantation.

References

1. Gunz, FW: The dread leukemias and the lymphomas: Their nature and their prospects. In Wintrobe, MM (ed): Blood, Pure and Eloquent: A Story of Discovery, of People, and of Ideas. McGraw-Hill, New York, 1980, p 511.
2. Sandler, DP, and Ross, JA: Epidemiology of Acute Leukemia in Children and Adults. Semin Oncol 24:3, 1997.
3. Karp, JE, and Smith, MA: The molecular pathogenesis of treatment-induced (secondary) leukemias: Foundations for treatment and prevention. Semin Oncol 24:103, 1997.
4. Blattner, WA, et al: Epidemiology of human T-cell leukemia/lymphoma virus. J Infect Dis 147:406, 1983.
5. Weiss, LM, and Chang, KM.: Association of the Epstein-Barr virus with hematolymphoid neoplasia. Adv Anat Pathol 3:1, 1996.
6. Cancer Facts & Figures—1998. American Cancer Society, Atlanta GA, 1998.
7. Brunning, R : Proposed World Health Organization (WHO) classification of acute leukemia and myelodysplastic syndromes [abstract]. Mod Pathol 12:102, 1999.
8. Bennett, JM, et al: Proposals for the classification of myelodysplastic syndromes. Br J Haematol 51:189, 1982.
9. Bennett, JM, et al: Proposed revised criteria for the classification of acute myeloid leukemia. Ann Intern Med 103:626, 1985.
10. Cheson, BD, et al: Report of the National Cancer Institute–sponsored workshop on definitions of diagnosis and response in acute myeloid leukemia. J Clin Oncol 8:813, 1990.
11. Shafer, JA: Blood and marrow morphology in acute leukemia patients receiving chemotherapy: A photo-essay. AM J Med Technol 49:77, 1983.
12. Shafer, JA: Artifactual alterations in phagocytes in the blood smear. Am J Med Technol 48:507, 1982.
13. Seigneurin, D, and Audhuy, B: Auer rods in refractory anemia with excess blasts: Presence and significance. Am J Clin Pathol 80:359, 1983.
14. Stanley, M, et al: Classification of 358 cases AML by FAB criteria: Analysis of clinical and morphologic features. In Bloomfield CD (ed): Chronic and Acute Leukemias in Adults. Martinus Nijhoff Publishers, Boston, 1985, pp 147–178.
15. Stass, SA, et al: Sudan black B positive acute lymphoblastic leukemia. Br J Haematol 57:413, 1984.
16. Hayhoe, FGJ, and Quaglino, D: Haematological Cytochemistry. Churchill Livingstone, Edinburgh, 1980, pp 130, 243, 265.
17. Bennett, JM, and Reed, CE: Acute leukemia cytochemical profile: Diagnostic and clinical implications. Blood Cells 1:101, 1975.
18. Jennings, CD, and Foon, KA: Recent advances in flow cytometry: Application to the diagnosis of hematologic malignancy. Blood 90:2863, 1997.
19. Bearman, RM, et al: Terminal deoxynucleotidyl transferase activity in neoplastic and non-neoplastic hematopoietic cells. Am J Clin Pathol 75:794, 1981.
20. Casoli, C, et al: Ph1-positive acute myelocytic leukemia with high TdT levels. Cancer 52:1210, 1983.
21. Kung, PC, et al: TdT in the diagnosis of leukemia and malignant lymphoma. Am J Med 64:788, 1978.
22. Mrozek, K, et al: Clinical significance of cytogenetics in acute myeloid leukemia. Semin Oncol 24:17, 1997.
23. Look, AT: The emerging genetics of acute lymphoblastic leukemia: Clinical and biologic implications. Semin Oncol 12:92, 1985.
24. Veldman, T, et al. Hidden chromosome abnormalities in hematological malignancies detected by multicolor spectral karyotyping. Nat Genet 15:406, 1997.
25. Willman, CL: Acute leukemias: A paradigm for the integration of new technologies in diagnosis and classification. Mod Pathol 12:218, 1999.
26. Thandla, S, and Aplan, PD: Molecular biology of acute lymphoblastic leukemia. Semin Oncol 24:45, 1997.
27. Borowitz, MJ, et al: Predictability of the t(1;19)(q23;p13) from surface antigen phenotype: Implications for screening cases of childhood ALL for molecular analysis. A Pediatric Oncology Group study. Blood 82:1086, 1993.
28. Nourse, J, et al. Chromosomal translocation t(1;19) results in synthesis of a homeobox fusion mRNA that codes for a potential chimeric transcription factor. Cell 60:535, 1990.
29. Downing, JR, et al: An AML-1-ETO fusion transcript is consistently detected by RNA-based polymerase chain reaction in AML containing the (8;21)(9q22;q22) translocation. Blood 81:2860, 1993.
30. Crist, WM, et al. Poor prognosis of children with pre-B acute lymphoblastic leukemia is associated with the t(1;19)(q23;913). A Pediatric Oncology Group study. Blood 76:117, 1990.
31. Izraeli, S, et al: Detection and clinical relevance of genetic abnormalities in pediatric ALL: A comparison between cytogenetic and PCR analyses. Leukemia 7:671, 1993.
32. Maseki, N, et al: The 8;21 chromosome translocation in AML is always detectable by molecular analysis using AML1. Blood 81:1573, 1993.
33. Nucifora, G, et al: Detection of DNA rearrangements in the AML1 and ETO loci and an AML-1/ETO fusion mRNA in patients with t(8;21) AML. Blood 81:883, 1993.
34. Nucifora, G, et al: Persistence of the 8;21 translocation in patients with AML type M2 in long term remission. Blood 82:712, 1993.
35. Crist, W, et al: Philadelphia chromosome positive acute lymphoblastic leukemia: Clinical and cytogenetic characteristics and treatment outcome. A Pediatric Oncology Group study. Blood 76:489, 1990.
36. Hunger, SP, et al: HRX involvement in de novo and secondary leukemias with diverse 11q23 abnormalities. Blood 81:3197, 1993.
37. Thirman, MJ, et al: Rearrangement of the MLL gene in ALL and AML with11q23 chromosomal translocations. N Engl J Med 329:909, 1993.
38. Hilden, JM, et al: Heterogeneity in MLL/AF4 fusion messenger RNA detected by PCR in t(4;11) acute leukemia. Cancer Res 53:3853, 1993.
39. Caligiuri, MA, et al: Molecular biology of acute myeloid leukemia. Semin Oncol 24:32, 1997.
40. Biondi, A, et al: RARA gene rearrangements as a genetic marker for diagnosis and monitoring in acute promyelocytic leukemia. Blood 77:1418, 1991.
41. Castaigne, S, et al: All-trans retinoic acid as a differentiation therapy for acute promyelocytic leukemia. Blood 76:263, 1990.
42. Warrell, RP, et al: Differentiation therapy of acute promyelocytic leukemia with tretinoin (all trans retinoic acid). N Engl J Med 324:1385, 1991.
43. Miller, WH, et al: Detection of minimal residual disease in APL by a reverse-transcription PCR assay for the PML/RARA fusion mRNA. Blood 82:1689, 1993.
44. Liu, P, et al: Fusion between transcription factor CBFB/PEBP2B and a myosin heavy chain in acute myeloid leukemia. Science 261:1041, 1993.
45. Hebert, J, et al: Detection of minimal residual disease in acute myelomonocytic leukemia with abnormal marrow eosinophils by nested polymerase chain reaction with allele specific amplification. Blood 84:2291, 1994.
46. Bennett, JM, et al: Proposals for the classification of acute leukemia. Br J Haematol 33:451, 1976.
47. Cunningham, I, et al: Acute promyelocytic leukemia: Treatment results during a decade at Memorial Hospital. Blood 73:116, 1989.
48. Sultan, C, et al: Distribution of 250 cases of acute myeloid leukemia according to the FAB classification and response to therapy. Br J Haematol 47:545, 1981.
49. Bennett, JM, et al: Minimally differentiated AML (FAB M0). Br J Haematol 78:325, 1991.
50. Bitter, MA, et al: Associations between morphology, karyotype, and clinical features in myeloid leukemias. Hum Pathol 18:211, 1987.
51. Tomonaga, M, et al: Cytochemistry of acute promyelocytic leukemia (M3): Leukemic promyelocytes exhibit heterogeneous patterns in cellular differentiation. Blood 66:350, 1985.
52. Fenaux, P, et al: Acute promyelocytic leukemia: Biology and treatment. Semin Oncol 24:92, 1997.
53. Rowley, JD, et al: 15/17 translocation. A consistent chromosomal change in acute promyelocytic leukemia. Lancet 1:549, 1977.
54. Goulomb, HM, et al: "Microgranular" acute promyelocytic leukemia: A distinct clinical, ultrastructural, and cytogenetic entity. Blood 55:253, 1980.
55. Bennett, JM, et al: Correspondence: A variant form of hypergranular promyelocytic leukemia (M3). Br J Hematol 44:169, 1980.
56. Arthur, DC, and Bloomfield, CD: Partial deletion of the long arm of chromosome 16 and bone marrow eosinophilia in acute nonlymphocytic leukemia: A new association. Blood 61:994, 1983.
57. LeBeau, MM, et al: Association of an inversion of chromosome 16 with abnormal marrow eosinophils in acute myelomonocytic leukemia. N Engl J Med 309:630, 1983.
58. Tobelem, G, et al: Acute monoblastic leukemia: A clinical and biologic study of 74 cases. Blood 55:71, 1980.
59. Cuttner, J, et al: Association of monocytic leukemia in patients with extreme leukocytosis. Am J Med 60:555, 1980.
60. Catovsky, D, et al: Significance of cell differentiation in acute myeloid leukaemia. Blood Cells 1:201, 1975.
61. Mazzella, FM, et al: Acute erythroleukemia: Evaluation of 48 cases with reference to classification, cell proliferation, cytogenetics and prognosis. Am J Clin Pathol 110:590, 1998.
62. Breton-Gorius, J, et al: Megakaryoblastic acute leukemia: Identification by the ultrastructural demonstration of platelet peroxidase. Blood 51:45, 1978.
63. Bennett, JM, et al: Criteria for the diagnosis of acute leukemia of megakaryocyte lineage (M7). Ann Intern Med 103:460, 1985.
64. Koike, T: Megakaryoblastic leukemia: The characterization and identification of megakaryoblasts. Blood 64:683, 1984.
65. Bain, BJ, et al: Megakaryoblastic leukemia presenting as acute myelofibrosis: A study of four cases with the platelet-peroxidase reaction. Blood 58:206, 1981.
66. Bennett, JM, et al: The morphologic classification of acute lymphoblastic leukaemia: Concordance among observers and clinical correlations. Br J Heamatol 47:533, 1981.

67. Lilleyman, JS, et al: FAB morphological classification of childhood lymphoblastic leukemia and its clinical importance. J Clin Pathol 39:998, 1986.

68. Crist, W, et al: Prognostic importance of the pre-B-cell immunophenotype and other presenting features in B-lineage childhood acute lymphoblastic leukemia: A Pediatric Oncology Group study. Blood 74:1252, 1989.

69. Carroll, AJ, et al: Pre-B cell leukemia associated with chromosome translocation 1;19. Blood 63:721, 1984.

70. Taub, R, et al: Translocation of the c-myc gene into the immunoglobulin heavy chain locus in human Burkitt lymphoma and murine plasmacytoma cells. Proc Natl Acad Sci USA 79:7937, 1982.

71. Dalla-Favera, R, et al: Translocation and rearrangements of the c-myc oncogene locus in human undifferentiated B-cell lymphomas. Science 219:963, 1983.

72. Flandrin, G, et al: Acute leukemia with Burkitt's tumor cells: A study of six cases with special reference to lymphocyte surface markers. Blood 45:183, 1975.

73. Greaves, MF, et al: Immunologically defined subclasses of acute lymphoblastic leukaemia in children: Their relationship to presentation features and prognosis. Br J Haematol 48:179, 1981.

74. Pui, CH, et al: Heterogeneity of presenting features and their relation to treatment outcome in 120 children with T-cell acute lymphoblastic leukemia. Blood 75:174, 1990.

75. Shuster, JJ, et al: Prognostic factors in childhood T-cell acute lymphoblastic leukemia: A Pediatric Oncology Group study. Blood 75:166, 1990.

76. Roper, M, et al: Monoclonal antibody characterization of surface antigens in childhood T-cell lymphoid malignancies. Blood 61:830, 1983.

77. Catovsky, D, et al: A classification of acute leukaemia for the 1990s. Ann Hematol 62:16, 1991.

78. European Group for the Immunological Classification of Leukemias (EGIL), Bene, MC, et al: Proposals for the immunological classification of acute leukemias. Leukemia 9:1783, 1995.

17

Chronic Leukemia and Related Lymphoproliferative Disorders

Laurel D. Holmer, MEd, MT (ASCP) SH
Walid Hamoudi, MD, PhD
Carlos E. Bueso-Ramos, MD, PhD

CHRONIC LYMPHOCYTIC LEUKEMIA/SMALL LYMPHO-CYTIC LYMPHOMA

Etiology and Pathophysiology

Immunologic Features and Methods for Studying Lymphocytes

Clinical Features

Laboratory Features

Chromosomal Abnormalities

Clinical Course, Prognostic Factors, and Staging

Treatment

Differential Diagnosis

Case Study 1

CHRONIC MYELOGENOUS LEUKEMIA

Etiology and Pathophysiology

Clinical Features

Laboratory Features

Clinical Course and Prognostic Factors

Treatment

Differential Diagnosis

Case Study 2

OBJECTIVES

At the end of this chapter, the learner should be able to:

1. List general features of chronic lymphocytic leukemia.

2. Name laboratory methods used to study lymphocytes in lymphoproliferative disorders.

3. List diagnostic criteria of chronic lymphocytic leukemia.

4. Describe treatment for chronic lymphocytic leukemia.

5. Explain differential diagnostic criteria that are used to characterize lymphoproliferative disorders.

6. List general features of chronic myelogenous leukemia.

7. Name laboratory features characteristic of chronic myelogenous leukemia.

8. Describe treatment for chronic myelogenous leukemia.

9. Explain differential diagnostic criteria that are used to characterize chronic myelogenous leukemia.

10. Evaluate case studies and pertinent laboratory data.

Chronic lymphoproliferative disorders are clonal proliferations of morphologically and immunophenotypically mature B or T lymphocytes. Although the morphological and cytologic features of chronic lymphoproliferative disorders are critical to the subclassification of these disorders, the final diagnosis represents a synthesis of morphological, immunologic, cytogenetic, molecular, and clinical features. Disorders affecting bone marrow and peripheral blood are regarded as *leukemias*, whereas diseases affecting lymph nodes and other extramedullary sites are *lymphomas*. The chronic lymphoid leukemias may proceed through different phases: an early phase in which tumor cells are predominantly small in size, with a low proliferation rate and prolonged cell survival; and a transformation phase, with the frequent occurrence of extramedullary proliferation and an increase in large, immature cells.

During the past years, considerable progress has been made in our ability to diagnose and classify hematopoietic malignancies accurately. Through cytogenetics and molecular biology, it has been shown that many hematopoietic neoplasms are associated with a unique genotypic profile and that these genetic lesions often have a direct bearing on the pathogenesis of the disease and its clinical behavior. Similarly, the development of widely available monoclonal antibodies has allowed the identification of a unique immunophenotypic profile for most leukemias and lymphomas. Moreover, the use of these techniques enhances both diagnostic accuracy and reproducibility.

➤ CHRONIC LYMPHOCYTIC LEUKEMIA/SMALL LYMPHOCYTIC LYMPHOMA

Chronic lymphocytic leukemia (CLL)/small lymphocytic lymphoma is included in a general category of conditions known as the *lymphoproliferative disorders* (Table 17–1). Chronic lymphocytic leukemia is the most common type of leukemia in older adults and is most frequently a neoplasm of B lymphocytes (B-CLL). A malignant proliferation of T lymphocytes (T-CLL) can occur, but this is less common. The hematologic abnormalities of CLL are characterized by a peripheral blood and bone marrow lymphocytosis. In contrast, small lymphocytic lymphoma involves mainly lymph nodes and, to a lesser extent, peripheral blood and bone marrow. Morphologically, the lymphocytes are small or slightly larger than a normal lymphocyte and have a relatively mature, well-differentiated appearance with a hypercondensed, almost "soccer ball"-appearing nuclear chromatin pattern. Bare nuclei called *smudge cells* are common (Fig. 17–1; and Color Plate 189). Morphological heterogeneity in CLL does exist and has been addressed by the French-American-British (FAB) group.[1]

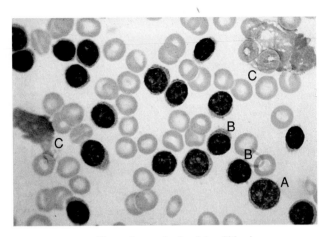

➤ **FIGURE 17–1**   Photomicrograph of peripheral blood smear from a patient with chronic lymphocytic leukemia (CLL). Note the characteristic mature-appearing lymphocyte morphology with hypercondensed nuclear chromatin creating a "soccer-ball" pattern. Two smudge cells are also seen. Note the lack of platelets in this thrombocytopenic patient. *A*, denotes lymphoblasts; *B*, lymphocytes; and *C*, smudge cells.

➤ **Table 17–1**
LYMPHOPROLIFERATIVE DISORDERS

Peripheral B-Cell Neoplasms

B-cell CLL/small lymphocytic lymphoma

Prolymphocytic leukemia

Lymphoplasmacytic lymphoma/immunocytoma

Mantle cell leukemia/lymphoma

Follicle center lymphoma, follicular lymphoma

Marginal zone B-cell lymphoma

Provisional entity: Splenic marginal zone lymphoma
(± villous lymphocytes)

Hairy-cell leukemia

T-Cell and Putative NK-Cell Neoplasms

T-cell CLL/prolymphocytic leukemia

   Large granular lymphocytic leukemia

      T-cell type

      NK-cell type

   Mycosis fungoides/Sézary syndrome

   Peripheral T-cell lymphoma, unspecified (multiple
   provisional variants)

   Adult T-cell lymphoma/leukemia

Abbreviation: NK = natural killer

  Source: Harris, NL, H, et al: A revised European-American classification of lymphoid neoplasms: A proposal from the International Lymphoma Study Group. Blood 84;1361, 1994.

The consequences of the accumulating lymphocyte mass in CLL include neutropenia, anemia, and thrombocytopenia. Lymphadenopathy, splenomegaly, or both may be present. The excessive lymphoid accumulation literally crowds out the normal bone marrow elements, and the marrow space is packed with malignant lymphocytes. In addition to the consequences of organ infiltration by malignant lymphocytes, altered humoral immunity in patients with CLL results from suppression of all classes of immunoglobulin (Ig), leading to hypogammaglobulinemia and a subsequent increase in susceptibility to infections. Another important complication of altered immunity that can develop in the patient with CLL is autoimmune disease. The production of autoantibodies may lead to idiopathic thrombocytopenic purpura (see Chap. 24), or autoimmune hemolytic anemia (see Chap. 13) to further compromise the patient's hematologic status.

Patients with CLL are typically older than 50 years at the time of diagnosis and frequently have a prolonged survival. Although some patients may die within a few years of diagnosis, more often they succumb to an unrelated disorder associated with the elderly. Generally, 50% of patients with CLL are living 5 years after diagnosis, whereas 30% of patients can expect a survival of 10 years or more.

Etiology and Pathophysiology

Although ribonucleic acid (RNA) tumor viruses (retroviruses) are a common cause of leukemia in animals, and exposure to certain agents such as radiation may lead to other chronic leukemias, namely chronic myeloid leukemia (CML), no specific etiologic agent or cause of CLL is currently known. A possible viral etiology has been investigated ever since the isolation of human T-lymphotropic virus type 1 (HTLV-1), a type C retrovirus from the leukemic cells of patients with T-cell malignancies.[2-4] The B-CLL cells from some patients appear to be a malignant transformation of an antigen-committed B cell responding to the HTLV-1 infection, suggesting an indirect role for this retrovirus in leukemogenesis.[5] Infection with HTLV-1 has preceded the development of CLL in some patients.[6]

In its classic form, this neoplastic disorder is characterized by the gradual accumulation of small mature B cells, most of which are in G_0/G_1 phase of the cell cycle and are long-lived, nonproliferating, immunologically dysfunctional lymphocytes in the peripheral blood and bone marrow.[7] B-CLL represents the quintessential example of a malignancy caused by failed programmed cell death (PCD), also called *apoptosis,* as opposed to altered cell-cycle regulation.[8] In essentially all self-renewing tissues, new cell production is normally offset by a commensurate amount of cell destruction through PCD. Imbalances in the activities of opposing genes that either promote or block physiologic apoptosis can, therefore, slow or halt the rate of cell turnover, creating a selective survival advantage for a particular clone that permits expansion at the expense of its normal neighbors.[8]

Most B-CLL cells have been reported to contain high levels of the antiapoptotic protein.[9] The mechanisms responsible for the high amounts of *BCL2* observed in more than 80% of B-CLL cells remain unknown, but only rarely do they involve rearrangements of the *BCL2* gene as a result of chromosomal translocations.[10]

Additional infiltration of the lymph nodes and spleen by the malignant lymphocytes occurs in 50% of patients, whereas cutaneous invasion occurs in 5% of patients.[11] As the bone marrow becomes more extensively infiltrated by the leukemic clone, marrow replacement results in anemia, thrombocytopenia, and neutropenia (Fig. 17–2 and Color Plate 190). Organ infiltration can lead to massive adenopathy with splenomegaly, hypersplenism, and subsequent peripheral cytopenias. An increased tendency for hemorrhage further contributes to anemia and compromises hemostasis.

Patients with CLL have significantly impaired immunologic activity. Hypogammaglobulinemia is found in approximately 50% of patients with CLL. The deficiency in Ig leads to infections with a variety of agents. Bacterial infections, especially of the respiratory tract, urinary tract, and skin, as well as viral infections such as herpes zoster and herpes simplex are common and dramatically contribute to patient morbidity and mortality (Fig. 17–3). Autoimmunity is a phenomenon that is frequently seen in CLL, with 15% to 35% of patients developing autoimmune hemolytic anemia at some time during the course of the disease.[11] Antibodies produced against red blood cells and detected with the direct antiglobulin (Coombs') test may precede, simultaneously occur with, or follow the development of CLL. Red cell aplasia is a rare occurrence.[12] Autoantibodies to platelets and neutrophils may

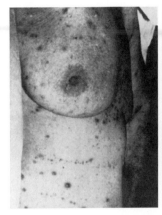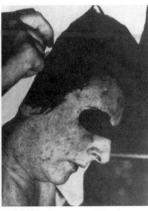

➤ **FIGURE 17–3** Severe generalized herpes zoster with a varicelliform rash in a patient with CLL. (From Henderson, ES: Diagnosis of leukemia. In Gunz, FW, and Henderson, ES (eds): Leukemia, ed 4. Grune & Stratton, New York, 1983, p 409, with permission.)

also develop and lead to immune thrombocytopenic purpura (ITP) and neutropenia. The production of autoantibodies coupled with marrow crowding and hypersplenism can lead to strikingly low peripheral platelet and neutrophil counts. Although the leukemic clonal B cells from CLL patients often are the source of pathogenic autoantibodies that may react with antigens present on red blood cells or platelets, or both, it is the nonmalignant polyclonal bystander B cells that have been shown to produce autoantibodies that contribute even more significantly to autoimmune disease.[13] Interestingly, the relatives of patients with CLL have also been shown to have an increased risk of autoimmune diseases. Immune paresis in some patients may include the production of paraproteins. Bence Jones paraproteinemia has been reported in up to 51% of patients with B-CLL,[14] and heavy-chain paraproteins, either IgM or IgG, can be detected. Figure 17–4 summarizes the pathophysiology of CLL.

Immunologic Features and Methods for Studying Lymphocytes

In normal adult peripheral blood, up to 20% of the circulating lymphocytes have surface Ig (sIg) and are B cells, 61% to 89% are T cells, and up to 22.3% are natural killer (NK) cells. On the basis of morphological features alone, it is not possible to distinguish B cells from T cells. When a lymphoproliferative process exists, it is important to be able to characterize the nature of the lymphocytes involved. A number of methods are available to study lymphocytes in lymphoproliferative disorders such as CLL and are listed in Table 17–2.

For the most part, CLL can be diagnosed morphologically. An immunophenotypic characterization of the neoplasm as either B cell or T cell using the monoclonal antibodies (mAb) available for detecting differentiation antigens, (cluster differentiation CD antigens), as shown in Table 17–3, confirms the diagnosis. Monoclonal antibodies are homogeneous populations of antibody molecules that are generally produced by somatic cell hybrids (hybridomas) between activated normal B cells and a plasmacytoma cell line. A list of current CD designations and some basic information concerning the molecules defined by these antibodies has been established by the Sixth International Workshop and Conference on Human Leukocyte Differentiation Antigens.[15] Monoclonal antibody technology is possible because as lymphocytes ma-

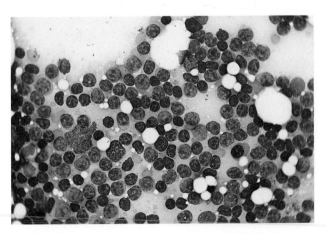

➤ **FIGURE 17–2** Photomicrograph of bone marrow aspirate smear from a patient with CLL. Note monotonous appearance of mature-appearing lymphocytes with condensed nuclear chromatin.

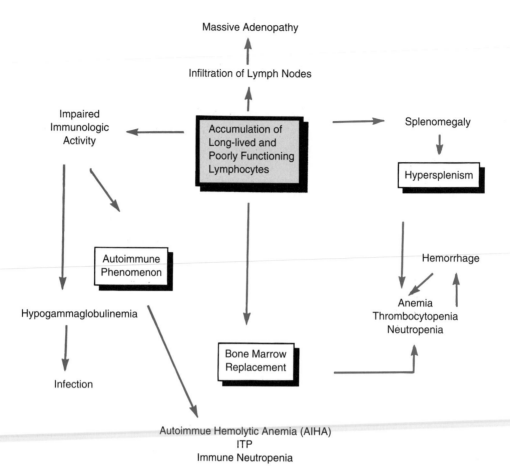

> **FIGURE 17–4**   The pathophysiology of CLL. The three major processes that typically interact are marrow replacement by long-lived lymphocytes, hypersplenism, and autoimmunity. ITP = immune thrombocytopenic purpura.

ture from pluripotent stem cells and migrate to lymphoid tissue, they acquire a variety of developmental markers that are helpful in identifying lymphocyte subpopulations.

Immunophenotypic marker expression and gene re-

arrangement during normal B-cell ontogeny is shown in Figure 17–5. The malignant B lymphocytes of CLL do not progress normally to the final stages of B-cell development, namely the formation of plasma cells, but rather appear to be

> **Table 17–2**
METHODS USED TO STUDY LYMPHOCYTES IN LYMPHOPROLIFERATIVE DISORDERS

Method	Marker Detected or Feature Demonstrated
Immunofluorescence	Surface and cytoplasmic immunoglobulin on mature B cells
	TdT on immature B and T lymphoblasts
Molecular probes	Rearrangements of the B-cell Ig and T-cell receptor genes
Cytochemistry	Absence of myeloperoxidase, Sudan black, and esterase positivity in lymphoblasts
	Tartrate-resistant isoenzyme 5 of acid phosphatase in hairy cells
	Localized alpha-naphthol acetate esterase positivity in Golgi area of T cells, i.e., T-ALL, Sézary cell, T-CLL
Cytogenetics	Consistent chromosomal abnormalities such as t (8;14)—B-ALL, Burkitt's lymphoma; t (14;18)—follicular lymphoma; trisomy 12—CLL, SLL; t (11;14)—mantle cell lymphoma; t (4;11)—ALL-L2
Electron microscopy	Nuclear and cytoplasmic ultrastructure such as nuclear whorls in Sézary cells and ribosomal lamellar cytoplasmic aggregates in hairy cells
Immunoperoxidase and flow cytometry	Various differentiation antigens on B cells and/or T cells using monoclonal antibodies (see Table 17–3)

Abbreviations: T-ALL = T-lineage acute lymphoblastic leukemia; B-ALL = B-lineage acute lymphoblastic leukemia; SLL = small lymphocytic leukemia

> **Table 17-3**
CLUSTER DIFFERENTIATION (CD) MARKERS AND PROLIFERATION

Markers (CD Designation)	Monoclonal Antibodies	Clinical Application
B Cells		
CD5	T1, T101, Leu1	B-CLL, some NHL, T lymphomas
CD9	BA-2 (p24)	Pre-B
CD10	J5, BA-3 (CALLA)	Lymph progenitor, CALL, some NHL
CD19	B4, Leu12	CALL, B-CLL, B-PLL, HCL
CD20	B1, Leu16	CALL, B-CLL, B-PLL, HCL
CD22	B3, Leu14	Late B cells, hairy cells
CD23	CD23.1 (BU38), Leu20	B-CLL, activated B cell
CD24	BA-1	Most B cells
CD25	TAC (IL-2 receptor)	HCL
CD43	Leu22	B-CLL, mantle cell lymphoma
CD79	CD79	B cells
CD103	HML-1	Hairy cells
T Cells		
CD1	T6	Some T-CLL, T-PLL, T-ALL
CD2	T11, Leu5, 9.6 (E rosette)	T-CLL, T-PLL, Sézary cells, LGL, ATLL
CD3	T3, Leu4	T-CELL, T-PLL, Sézary cells, IM
CD4	T4, Leu3	T-PLL, Sézary cells, IM, ATLL
CD5	T1, Leu1, 10.2	T-CLL, T-PLL, Sézary cells, ATLL
CD7	3A1, Leu9	T-PLL
CD8	T8, Leu2	T-CLL, some LGL, IM
CD25	Tac (IL-2 receptor)	ATLL
CD57	Leu7 (HNK1)	LGL
Other Cells		
CD38	T10, Leu17	Plasma cells, germinal center B cells, cortical thymocytes
CD52	CAMPATH-1H	All lymphoid cells and monocytes

Abbreviations: B-CLL = B-lineage chronic lymphocytic leukemia; NHL = non-Hodgkin's lymphoma; CALL = common acute lymphocytic leukemia; B-PLL = B-lineage prolymphocytic leukemia; HCL = hairy-cell leukemia; T-ALL = T-lineage acute lymphoblastic leukemia; LGL = large granular lymphocytosis (T-gamma lymphocytosis); ATLL = adult T-cell leukemia/lymphoma; IM = infectious mononucleosis; HNK = human natural killer

developmentally arrested at an earlier B-lymphocyte stage of differentiation. Studies have shown, however, that under certain in vitro conditions such as stimulation with phorbol ester, typical CLL cells can undergo transformation to more mature levels of B-cell development.[16,17] Genetic recombination in pre-B cells in the bone marrow generates an immature B cell that expresses a functional Ig on the surface, IgM or IgM and IgD, which then exits the bone marrow as a virgin (mature) B cell (antigen-independent phase) and migrates to the secondary lymphoid tissues. The normal B cell may undergo stimulation by antigen (antigen-dependent phase) and enter the lymphoid follicle. At this point in differentiation, the somatic hypermutation mechanism is activated, introducing point mutations into the variable (V) region genes. In the presence of limiting antigen, there will be subsequent selection of V gene sequences that provide increased affinity for antigen. After antigen-driven B-cell proliferation, B cells can initiate two pathways of maturation.

Some B cells revert back to small lymphocytes to generate memory B cells, whereas others undergo terminal differentiation into long-lived plasma cells.[18,19] The postulated normal B-cell development is shown in Figure 17–6.

The level of somatic mutation in CLL is low.[20] This has led to the conclusion that the cell of origin has not encountered antigen. The subset that remains unmutated, perhaps derived from naive B cells, appears prone to accumulate the trisomy 12 abnormality. In contrast, the mutated subset of CLL, perhaps derived from more mature B cells, appears more prone to abnormalities of 13q14.[20]

The characteristic immunophenotype for B-CLL is expression of faint or low-density sIg with kappa (κ) or lambda (λ) light-chain restriction and expression of B-cell–associated antigens (CD19, CD20, CD79a), CD5, CD23, CD43, and faint CD11c (Table 17–4). A typical example of a B-CLL immunophenotype is shown in Figure 17–7.

Of particular interest is the unique expression of CD5 in

B-Cell Ontogeny

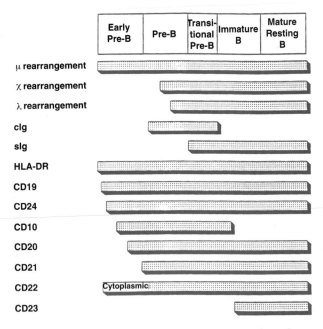

	Early Pre-B	Pre-B	Transitional Pre-B	Immature B	Mature Resting B
μ rearrangement					
χ rearrangement					
λ rearrangement					
cIg					
sIg					
HLA-DR					
CD19					
CD24					
CD10					
CD20					
CD21					
CD22	Cytoplasmic				
CD23					

➤ **FIGURE 17–5** Hypothetical scheme of marker expression and gene rearrangement during normal B-cell ontogeny. cIg = cytoplasmic immunoglobulin; sIg = surface immunoglobulin. (From Pui, CH, et al: Blood 82(2):344, July 1993, with permission.)

B-CLL. Expression of CD5 is normally seen on T lymphocytes and on the majority of B cells of early ontogeny such as cord blood cells; however, normally less than 20% of B cells in adult human peripheral blood express CD5. Although CD5-negative B-CLL does exist,[21,22] it accounts for less than 10% of all B-CLL cases. The precise functional role of the CD5 molecule is unknown. CD5 has been shown

to physically associate with the antigen-specific receptor complex present on both T and B lymphocytes.[15] Studies are ongoing to determine whether differences in antigen expression and gene rearrangement are associated with variation in clinical course.[22–25] As mentioned earlier, T-CLL/T prolymphocytic leukemia is rare but can be distinguished from B-CLL on the basis of differentiation antigens. Immunophenotypic marker expression and gene rearrangement during normal T-cell ontogeny is shown in Figure 17–8.

The demonstration of sIg in B-CLL was mentioned earlier and is, in fact, the classic marker for B cells. The detection of a predominance of either κ or λ light chains by the B cells indicates monoclonality.[26,27] In contrast, no immunophenotypic markers for T-cell clonality are available, and molecular studies are necessary. Aberrant loss of T-cell–associated antigens, such as CD3, CD5, and CD7 on CD3, or the predominance of specific T-cell subsets, either CD3+CD4+, CD3+CD8+, or CD3+CD4+CD8+, in blood or bone marrow suggests the need for T-cell receptor molecular studies. A typical example of a T-CLL/T-PLL immunophenotype is shown in Figure 17–9.

When the conventional immunophenotypic techniques fail to reveal the nature of the lymphoid neoplasm, molecular probe technology using DNA probes can often contribute to the diagnosis and classification of malignancy by detecting gene rearrangements that occur in lymphocytes. On a molecular level, Ig heavy and light chains are rearranged. The rearrangement of heavy-chain Ig genes occurs first and is followed by rearrangement of light-chain genes. The order of this rearrangement proceeds from mu (μ) to κ to λ and is the earliest detectable commitment to B-cell development.[27] Monoclonality rather than polyclonality (the presence of a mixture of κ- and λ-bearing B lymphocytes) is a feature of many malignancies, including CLL; however, it is not, per se, indicative of malignancy. Analogous to the detection of Ig gene rearrangements in B

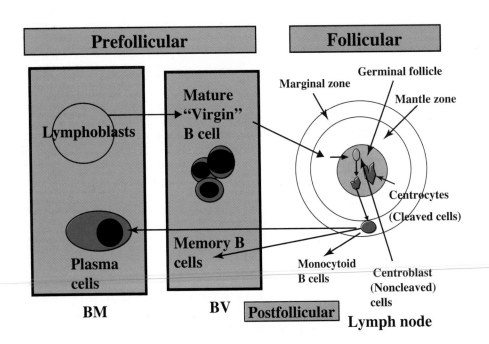

➤ **FIGURE 17–6** Postulated B-lymphocyte development scheme. Lymphoblasts undergo several maturation steps in the microenvironment of the bone marrow (BM), giving rise to mature (virgin or naive) lymphocytes. Naive B lymphocytes enter blood vessels (BV) to reach lymph nodes and populate the mantle zone of the lymphoid follicles. These cells differentiate into centroblasts (large, noncleaved follicular center cells) in the dark zone of the germinal center. Centroblasts undergo rearranged-immunoglobulin gene hypermutation and develop into centrocytes (cleaved follicular center cells). Centrocytes that bind antigen on the surface of the follicular dendritic cells survive, whereas those that fail to bind die by apoptosis. Surviving centrocytes in the light zone of the germinal center may differentiate into monocytoid B cells, which populate the marginal zone of the lymphoid follicle, and plasma cells, which reenter the bone marrow and memory cells. Memory cells actively recirculate between the blood, lymph, and lymphoid organs.

> **Table 17-4**

IMMUNOPHENOTYPIC FEATURES AND GENETIC ABNORMALITIES OF B-LYMPHOPROLIFERATIVE DISORDERS

Disorder	Common Phenotype	Comments/Variations	Associated Genetic Abnormalities
Chronic lymphocytic leukemia/small lymphocytic lymphoma	CD19, CD20, CD5, CD22(−), CD23, CD10(−), CD11c−/+, CD43, clonal sIgM and sIgD weak	CD20 dim *BCL2* overexpressed Bright SIg, CD20, FMC7	Abnormalities of 13q, 14q, 11q Trisomy 12
Prolymphocytic leukemia	CD19, CD20, CD5(−/+) CD22, CD23(−), CD10(−), bright clonal sIg	CD20 and FMC7 bright	No consistent alteration
Mantle cell lymphoma	CD19, CD20, CD5, CD22, CD23(−) CD10(−), CD43, moderate clonal sIg (IgM > IgD)	Cyclin D1 (*BCL1*) overexpressed	t(11;14)
Follicular lymphoma	CD19, CD20, CD5(−), CD22, CD10, CD11c(−), CD43(−), CD23(−/+), bright clonal sIg	CD10 negative < 20% *BCL2* overexpressed Clonal evolution	t(14;18) del(17p)
Marginal zone and associated lymphomas	CD19, CD20, CD5(−), CD22, CD23(−), CD10(−), CD11c, CD25(−), CD103(−), moderate clonal sIg		Trisomy 3
Hairy-cell leukemia	CD19, CD20, CD5(−), CD22, CD23(−), CD10(−), CD11c, CD25, CD103, moderate clonal sIg	Bright CD22, CD22, and CD11c, and CD103	No consistent alteration
Plasma cell dyscrasias	DR(−), CD19(−), CD20(−), CD22(−), CD38, CD45, clonal cIg	Two-color bright CD38 and dim CD45-sensitive marker	Add(14) (q32), total loss chromosome 13, 3q27, 17q24–25, and 20q11

Abbreviations: +/− = variable, more often positive; −/+ = variable, more often negative; (−) = negative; DR = HLA-DR; sIg = surface Ig; cIg = cytoplasmic Ig, *BCL2* gene expression

cells is the ability of molecular probes to detect rearrangement patterns of the genes coding for the T-cell receptor (TCR), the antigen-specific surface molecule characteristic of T cells.[28] With the use of Ig and TCR gene probes to detect gene rearrangements, the unusual case of CLL that cannot be diagnosed and classified by morphology and cell markers can now be characterized. It must be stressed that it is extremely important that the final diagnosis of any lymphoproliferative disorder be made as a result of composite information from clinical data in addition to morphological, histologic, and immunologic analysis.

Although CLL is generally characterized by an elevated white blood cell count in which there are abundant lymphocytes to analyze, if the number of neoplastic cells is low, a technique for amplifying a specific segment of deoxyribonucleic acid (DNA), called the polymerase chain reaction (PCR), can be applied to improve sensitivity. The PCR method involves denaturation, primer annealing, and polymerization to yield millions of copies of the original scarce sequence of DNA.[29] This technique is valuable for detecting minimal residual disease in patients who have previously been treated for CLL (or other leukemias or lymphomas) but who currently lack histopathologic evidence of relapse.[30,31] The purpose of using PCR is to identify as early as possible those patients who will subsequently have a relapse but who currently have only 1% to 5% malignant cells present or have gene rearrangements present in malignant clones that require amplification in order to be detected.

Clinical Features

CLL occurs mainly in older adults, with 90% of all cases occurring in persons older than 50 years. In patients younger than 40 years of age CLL is rare; however, CLL has been described in young adults.[32] As with most other leukemias and myeloproliferative disorders, CLL is found in twice as many males as females. Unlike acute leukemia, the signs and symptoms of CLL develop gradually, and the onset of the disease is difficult to pinpoint. In fact, it is not unusual for the disease to be accidentally discovered during the course of a routine visit to a physician. The duration of a relatively asymptomatic phase of CLL is extremely variable. Unexplained absolute and persistent lymphocytosis; cervical, supraclavicular, or axillary lymphadenopathy; and splenomegaly are the earliest signs of CLL. The clinical course is indolent, but as the disease progresses, chronic fatigue, recurrent or persistent infections, and easy bruising are the consequences of anemia, neutropenia, B-cell immunologic dysfunction, and thrombocytopenia. Hepatomegaly may accompany splenomegaly. Dermatologic manifestations such as nodular and diffuse skin infiltrations, erythroderma, exfoliative dermatitis, and secondary skin infections may occur. Leukemic lymphocytes may invade unusual locations such as the scalp, orbits, subconjunctivae, gums, pharynx, pleura and lung parenchyma, gastrointestinal tract, prostate, and gonads.[33] CLL has also been reported to occur simultaneously with acute myeloblastic leukemia (AML).[34] In general, CLL is not considered curable with available therapy.

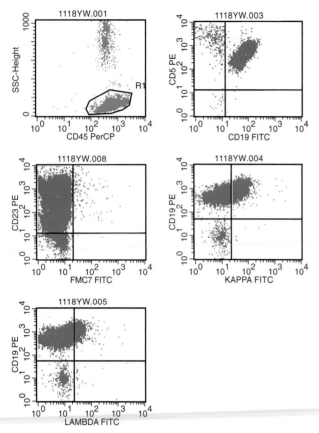

T-Cell Ontogeny

	Prothymic Cell	Early Thymocyte	Intermediate Thymocyte	Mature Thymocyte	Circulating T-Cell
TCR δ rearrangement	?				
TCR γ rearrangement	?				
TCR β rearrangement	?				
TCR α rearrangement					
CD7					
CD5					
CD2					
CD1					
CD4					
CD8					
CD3	Cytoplasmic				
TCR (α β or γ δ)		Cytoplasmic			

➤ **FIGURE 17–8** Hypothetical scheme of marker expression and gene rearrangement during T-cell ontogeny. TCR = T-cell receptor. (From Pui, CH, et al: Blood 82(2):344, July 1993, with permission.)

➤ **FIGURE 17–7** Flow cytometric analysis of chronic lymphocytic leukemia. Leukemic bone marrow lymphocytes are gated by CD45-scattered analysis. The plot of CD5 versus CD19 is used to demonstrate dual-positive neoplastic lymphocytes with weak CD19 fluorescence intensity. The plot of CD23 versus FMC7 illustrates positive staining of the cells for CD23 but no staining of FMC7. The cells are then plotted for both CD19 versus kappa and CD19 versus lambda, showing kappa light-chain clonality with a 15:1 ratio of kappa to lambda for the dual CD19+, CD5+ cells.

Laboratory Features

The requirements for the diagnosis of CLL have undergone revision since earlier criteria were established by Rai and colleagues[35] in 1975 and Binet and colleagues in 1981.[36,37] The International Workshop on Chronic Lymphocytic Leukemia[38] recommends a minimum peripheral blood B-cell lymphocytosis of 5000 cells/μL (5 × 10^9 cells/L) along with a 30% lymphocytosis of the bone marrow, consisting of morphologically mature-appearing lymphocytes. This guideline is similar to an earlier set of criteria established by the National Cancer Institute–sponsored working group.[39] A new classification and terminology for the lymphocytic neoplasms, including CLL, has recently been proposed by the International Lymphoma Study Group.[40]

Anemia, when it occurs, is usually normochromic and normocytic, with a normal or low reticulocyte count. Autoimmune hemolytic anemia may precede, accompany, or follow the development of CLL and be characterized by a secondary reticulocytosis, a positive direct antiglobulin test, and an elevated indirect serum bilirubin level. A decreased platelet count is not uncommon in CLL and is related to bone marrow replacement by leukemic cells, hypersplenism, and platelet antibodies.

The lymphocytes of CLL may be morphologically indis-

tinguishable from normal mature lymphocytes when examined with Wright's stain. Alternatively, the leukemic lymphocytes may have exaggerated nuclear chromatin clumping with numerous dark-staining chromatin aggregates separated by light-staining areas of parachromatin. The staining pattern that results from the contrast between the nuclear chromatin and parachromatin resembles the surface pattern of a soccer ball, which may be a helpful image to recall in distinguishing the lymphocytes of CLL from those of other lymphoproliferative disorders. The morphology of peripheral blood lymphocytes in CLL is duplicated in the bone marrow aspiration and biopsy specimens (see Fig. 17–2 and Color Plate 190). The extent of marrow infiltration varies from patchy accumulations of lymphocytes to diffuse sheets that involve the entire marrow space. The pattern of bone marrow involvement is categorized into three types; nodular, interstitial, and diffuse, but combinations of these types also occur. The nodular pattern (Fig. 17–10 and Color Plate 191) is characterized by distinct, randomly distributed aggregates of small lymphocytes. In the interstitial pattern, the lymphocytes infiltrate the interstitium to a greater or lesser degree without displacement of fat cells. The nodular and interstitial patterns are usually accompanied by preservation of normal hematopoiesis. In the diffuse pattern (Fig. 17–11 and Color Plate 192), the entire bone marrow space between bone trabeculae is replaced by small lymphocytes. The life expectancy is significantly longer in patients with a nodular or an interstitial pattern than in those with a diffuse pattern.

Although the morphological characteristics of the lymphocytes involved in most cases of CLL are quite distinctive, the membrane phenotype of the neoplastic cells must be determined for a definitive diagnosis.[40] Immunologic features and methods used to characterize lymphocytes as B cells or T cells were discussed earlier in the section entitled Immunologic Features and Methods for Studying Lymphocytes.

Immune dysfunction within the proliferating B cells is indicated by the presence of hypogammaglobulinemia or hypergammaglobulinemia and monoclonal gammopathy. The frequent expression of autoantibodies in CLL contributes to a variety of autoimmune phenomena, including those leading to anemia and thrombocytopenia.

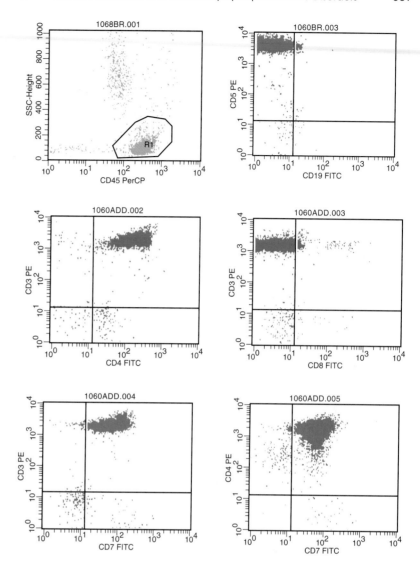

➤ **FIGURE 17–9** Flow cytometric analysis of T-prolymphocytic leukemia (T-PLL). Leukemic peripheral blood lymphocytes are gated by CD45–side scattered analysis. Comparison of CD5 versus CD19 shows a predominance of CD5-positive cells *(upper panel)*. Comparisons of CD3 versus CD4 and CD3 versus CD8 demonstrate a predominance of CD4+ T lymphocytes *(middle panel)*. CD4+ T lymphocytes also express CD7 antigen *(lower panel)*.

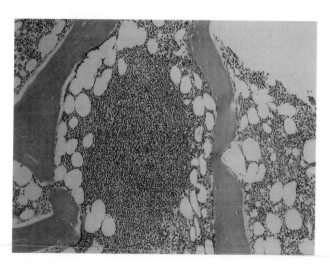

➤ **FIGURE 17–10** Photomicrograph of bone marrow biopsy section showing involvement by CLL, nodular pattern, characterized by distinct, randomly distributed aggregates of small lymphocytes.

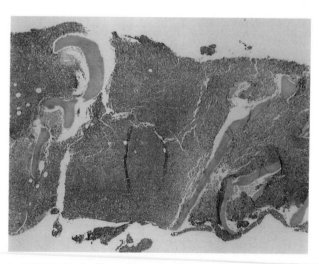

➤ **FIGURE 17–11** Photomicrograph of bone marrow biopsy section showing involvement by CLL, diffuse pattern. The entire bone marrow space between bone trabeculae is replaced by small lymphocytes.

Chromosomal Abnormalities

The most common chromosomal abnormality in B-CLL is an extra chromosome 12, called trisomy 12 (in 15% to 20% of cases)[41-43] which may occur alone or together with deletions or translocations of chromosome 13q14 (in 25% of cases).[44] The 13q14 deletions represent early clonal aberrations and suggest the presence of a tumor suppressor gene whose loss or inactivation may be crucial to development of CLL. Most of the 13q14 deletions are undetectable at the cytogenetic level but are detectable in more than 50% of the CLL cases with the use of molecular probes for the 13q14 region.[44]

Genetic abnormalities, including the most common chromosomal abnormalities and gene rearrangements, are listed in Table 17-4.[41-52] The presence of multiple chromosomal abnormalities in B-CLL have been implicated as poor prognostic indicators. None of the proto-oncogenes involved in the pathogenesis of other mature B-cell malignancies, including *BCL2, BCL6, PAX5,* and c-*MYC,* show primary alterations in CLL.[45]

Clinical Course, Prognostic Factors, and Staging

The overall median survival for CLL is currently 4 to 5 years; 50% of patients are living 5 years after diagnosis, whereas 30% have a 10-year survival. CLL can be an indolent disease with an asymptomatic presentation and may not require any treatment until progressive lymphocytosis of the peripheral blood and marrow, lymphadenopathy, splenomegaly, anemia, neutropenia, thrombocytopenia, autoimmune phenomena, and infection develop. This may be as late as 10 to 15 years after the initial diagnosis. In contrast to those with an indolent course of disease, approximately 20% of patients with CLL have a very aggressive clinical course that progresses rapidly from initial diagnosis and results in death

within 1 to 2 years. The wide variation seen among patients is not fully understood, but clinical and pathologic data have been used to try to predict the CLL patient's prognosis and identify various stages and risk groups.

The Rai system,[35] the Binet system,[36,37] and the International Workshop on CLL system[38] are the three major staging systems developed for CLL; however, only the Rai system is widely used in the United States. The Rai and Binet staging systems, along with median survival for each system by stage, are shown in Table 17-5. Staging systems for CLL do not consistently predict whether a patient's clinical course is more likely to be indolent or progressive. The most reliable predicting factors for indolent CLL are blood lymphocyte doubling time (LDT) greater than 12 months[53] and a nondiffuse pattern of bone marrow lymphocyte infiltration,[54] along with a Rai stage of 0, I, or II. A short LDT (less than 12 months), a diffuse lymphocyte infiltration of the bone marrow, a Rai stage of III or IV, an elevated level of serum β_2 microglobulin, elevated level of soluble CD23 in serum, and the presence of chromosomal abnormalities are associated with a more progressive clinical course and shorter survival duration.[55,56]

Several types of transformation in B-CLL have been described: prolymphocytoid transformation, which is relatively low grade and slowly progressive; Richter's syndrome (diffuse large-cell lymphoma), which is rapidly progressive and accounts for about 5% of all deaths in CLL[57]; and acute leukemia. Transformation to acute leukemia is unusual in CLL, unlike the blast cell transformation, which is responsible for almost all deaths in chronic myeloid leukemia. Most patients with CLL die with residual leukemia and usually succumb to infection or a cause totally unrelated to their CLL, such as cardiovascular disease.[58] The onset of the terminal transformation of CLL is suggested when there is a proliferation of a new population of lymphoid cells, namely, larger cells with immature-appearing morphological features, a

> **Table 17-5**
> **STAGING SYSTEMS FOR CHRONIC LYMPHOCYTIC LEUKEMIA**

STAGE			
Original Rai System	**Modified Rai System**	**Clinical Features**	**Median Survival (Years)**
0	Low	Lymphocytosis in PB and BM ($\geq 5 \times 10^9$ lymphs/L in PB, $\geq 30\%$ lymphs in BM)	> 12.5
I	Intermediate	Lymphocytosis + enlarged lymph nodes	8.5
II	Intermediate	Lymphocytosis, + splenomegaly, +/– lymphadenopathy	6
III	High splenomegaly	Lymphocytosis + anemia (Hgb < 11 g/dL) +/– lymphadenopathy or	1.5
IV	High	Lymphocytosis + thrombocytopenia (platelets $< 100 \times 10^9$/L) +/– anemia +/– organomegaly	1.5
Binet System			
A		Two or fewer node-bearing regions, * > 10 + no anemia or thrombocytopenia (Hgb ≥ 10 g/dL, platelets $> 100 \times 10^9$/L)	†
B		Three or more node-bearing regions + no anemia or thrombocytopenia	5
C		Anemia and/or thrombocytopenia independent of regions involved	2

*Cervical, axillary, inguinal, palpable spleen and liver.
†Survival equivalent to that of age- and sex-matched (French) population.
Abbreviations: PB = peripheral blood; BM = bone marrow; Hgb = hemoglobin

finer nuclear chromatin pattern, and a prominent nucleolus. This morphological transformation is often accompanied by the appearance of complex chromosomal changes that were not present earlier or are in addition to the commonly present trisomy 12. The proliferation of a more malignant clone of cells is accompanied by an increasing resistance to therapy and an exceptionally poor prognosis.[55,56]

A variety of techniques is available to help determine whether the transformation represents a clonal evolution of the original CLL or an independent disease; these include cytogenetic analysis, immunoglobulin gene rearrangement by Southern blot analysis and anti-idiotypic antibodies.[58] Molecular studies have shown that the development of Richter's syndrome in CLL may represent either the identical clone of cells present in the preceding CLL or a different malignant clone.[59] Additionally, *p53*, a tumor suppressor gene that is frequently mutated in a variety of human cancers, has been discovered in 15% of CLL patients and in 40% of patients with Richter's syndrome.[60–64] The close association of *p53* with transformation of CLL into a very aggressive lymphoma may also be a prognostic indicator for resistance to chemotherapy by interference with normal programmed cell death (apoptotic) pathways in tumor cells.[63,64]

Treatment

Some patients diagnosed with CLL do not require immediate treatment; however, when the signs and symptoms of progressive disease appear, it is time to begin therapeutic intervention. Major physical and clinical signs and symptoms identify advancing disease. These include progressive marrow failure with resulting anemia; thrombocytopenia and neutropenia; progressive lymphocytosis; progressive lymphadenopathy; enlarging spleen; autoimmunity (autoimmune hemolytic anemia or ITP); and increased susceptibility to infection and persistent constitutional symptoms such as night sweats, fever, and weight loss. There is currently no curative therapy for CLL; therefore, the goal of treatment is to reduce the signs and symptoms of disease with minimal discomfort or risk to the patient.

Conventional treatment for CLL is chemotherapy. Combinations of chemotherapeutic agents are used for patients with disease that is refractory to conventional therapy or those with advanced disease.[55,65–68] Table 17–6 summarizes the initial management of patients with CLL according to Rai staging groups.

Radiation therapy is an alternative or adjunctive therapeutic approach in treating CLL.[69] Leukemic masses in enlarged lymph nodes and in the spleen may respond to focused, local irradiation to relieve discomfort or eliminate obstruction. As with chemotherapy, irradiation also has its detrimental effects, especially in terms of causing life-threatening neutropenia.

Splenectomy is recommended in patients with massive splenomegaly and autoimmune hemolytic anemia or autoimmune thrombocytopenia resulting from splenic pooling that is uncontrollable by chemotherapy.[70]

In addition to chemotherapeutic intervention, the use of high-dose intravenous gammaglobulin therapy prevents major bacterial infections,[71,72] and the immunosuppressant cyclosporine, a fungal metabolite, aids in the prevention or treatment of red cell aplasia, both of which can be management problems in patients with CLL.

Experimental therapies are also being studied. They include not only new drugs but also the use of the monoclonal antibodies and biologic mediators.[55,73–79]

Bone marrow transplantation (autologous and allogeneic) is being explored as a possible curative therapy for patients with aggressive CLL, especially in patients younger than 50 years of age.[55,79–83]

Differential Diagnosis

As previously outlined in Table 17–1, CLL is a lymphoproliferative disorder that must be differentiated from other malignant or reactive lymphoid proliferations. The differential diagnosis includes acute lymphoblastic leukemia (ALL); prolymphocytic leukemia (PLL); non-Hodgkin's lymphomas in leukemic phase, especially mantle cell lymphoma (MCL), small cleaved-cell lymphoma (SCCL); hairy cell leukemia (HCL); Sézary syndrome; T-cell large granular lymphocytic leukemia; and reactive lymphocytosis (Fig. 17–12 and Color Plate 193). The morphological and immunologic characteristics of these lymphoproliferative disorders are shown in Table 17–7. In addition to these disorders, other hematologic malignancies may be confused with CLL. These include adult T-cell leukemia/lymphoma (ATLL)[84,85] (see Chap. 21) and Waldenström's macroglobulinemia[86] (see Chap. 20).

The diagnosis of CLL requires a sustained absolute lymphocytosis of mature-appearing lymphocytes in the absence of other causes. The diagnosis of CLL is established when the peripheral blood lymphocyte count is 10×10^9 or more cells/L (which is typically the case), lymphocyte infiltration of the bone marrow is more than 30% lymphocytes of all nucleated cells, and the circulating lymphocytes have a B-CLL immunophenotype. When lymphocyte counts are between 5×10^9 and 10×10^9 cells/L, the presence of both bone

> **Table 17–6**
TREATMENT OPTIONS FOR CHRONIC LYMPHOCYTIC LEUKEMIA

Rai System Risk Group	Treatment Options
Low (stages 0–I)	Observation only if asymptomatic, every 1–3 months
Intermediate (stage II)	Observation only if asymptomatic; fludarabine, cytoxan, prednisone, chlorambucil, or radiation if symptomatic or progressive disease
High (stages III and IV)	Combination chemotherapy: fludarabine, prednisone with chlorambucil
	or
	Intensive regimens: CHOP (cyclophosphamide, doxorubicin, oncovin, vincristine, prednisone); anti-CD20, anti-CD52 antibody therapy, other nucleoside analogs (experimental)

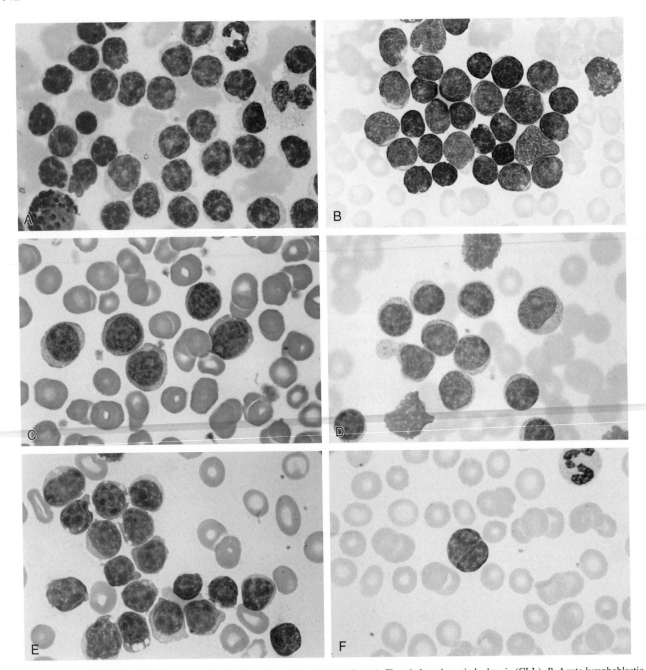

➤ **FIGURE 17–12** Peripheral blood smears of various lymphoproliferative disorders. *A.* Chronic lymphocytic leukemia (CLL). *B.* Acute lymphoblastic leukemia (ALL). *C.* Prolymphocytic leukemia (PLL). *D.* CLL with occasional prolymphocyte. *E.* Small lymphocytic lymphoma (SLL) in leukemic phase. *F.* Small cleaved-cell lymphoma (SCCL). (*continued*)

marrow infiltration of more than 30% lymphocytes and B-CLL immunophenotype (dim CD20+, CD19+/CD5+, CD23+, FMC7−, and weak surface intensity Ig) is necessary for the diagnosis of CLL.

The distinction between CLL and ALL is easily made in most instances based on morphological differences of the proliferating cell population (see Fig. 17–12*A* to *L*). The difference between the smoother nuclear chromatin pattern of the lymphoblast in ALL and the heavy condensation of nuclear chromatin in the CLL lymphocyte is readily appreciated when examining an appropriate monolayer area or feather-like edge of a well-stained blood smear. Lymphoblasts show positive expression of the nuclear enzyme terminal deoxynucleotidyl transferase (TdT). B-CLL cells are TdT-negative. The age of the patient is also helpful. CLL is typically seen in

patients older than 50 years and is only rarely reported in childhood,[87] whereas ALL is the most common form of childhood leukemia. The dramatic prognostic and therapeutic implications of misdiagnosing a chronic leukemia for an acute leukemia or vice versa cannot be overstated.

B-Prolymphocytic leukemia (B-PLL) is characterized by a predominance of circulating prolymphocytes (greater than 55%, usually greater than 70%). Prolymphocytes are larger, less mature-appearing cells than the typical lymphocytes seen in CLL, with moderately condensed nuclear chromatin and a prominent vesicular nucleolus (see Fig. 17–12*C*). The clinical and laboratory features that make PLL a distinct lymphoproliferative disorder include extreme leukocytosis (often greater than 100×10^9 cells/L) and prominent splenomegaly without lymphadenopathy.[84–86] As in all disorders accompa-

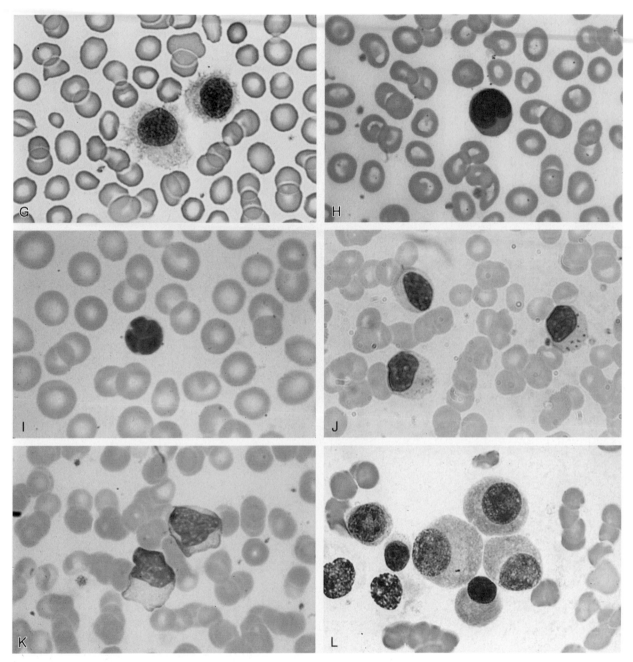

➤ **FIGURE 17–12** *(CONTINUED) G.* Hairy-cell leukemia (HCL). *H.* Sézary syndrome. *I.* Adult T-cell leukemia/lymphoma. *J.* T-gamma lymphocytosis with large granular lymphocytes. *K.* Infectious mononucleosis with atypical lymphocytes. *L.* Plasma cell dyscrasia.

nied by leukocytosis, morphological detail of the predominating cell may not be appreciated unless appropriate areas of well-stained blood and bone marrow smears are examined. Prolymphocytes may be seen in patients with CLL but account for less than 10% of the circulating cells (see Fig. 17–12*D*). When 11% to 55% prolymphocytes are present, a mixed-cell type of CLL, designated CLL/PLL is diagnosed.[87] This category includes patients with prolymphoid transformation.[88] Most cases of PLL are B cell in nature (B-PLL) as demonstrated by strong CD20 and sIg (in contrast to weak CD20/sIg in CLL), and reactivity with the B-cell markers CD19 and CD22.[89]

For cases of T-cell CLL or PLL, in addition to immunophenotype two cytochemical techniques are helpful in distinguishing T cells from B cells, namely, the alpha-

naphthol acetate esterase (ANAE) stain and the acid phosphatase (AP) reaction.[90] The typical T-lymphocyte pattern with ANAE and AP is one large, localized dot of reaction product positivity (Fig. 17–13 and Color Plate 194).

Small lymphocytic lymphoma (SLL) is the nodal counterpart of B-CLL.[40] It is a diffuse non-Hodgkin's lymphoma characterized by neoplastic transformation of small B lymphocytes (Fig. 17–14 and Color Plate 195). When SLL progresses to a leukemic phase, the circulating cells cannot be morphologically differentiated from those of CLL (see Fig. 17–12*E*).

Mantle cell lymphoma arises from the centrocytes of the mantle zone of lymphoid follicles (see Fig. 17–6). In the lymph node, MCL usually exhibits a diffuse pattern with complete effacement of lymph node architecture.[40] It can also

> Table 17-7
MORPHOLOGICAL AND IMMUNOLOGIC CHARACTERISTICS OF LYMPHOPROLIFERATIVE DISORDERS

DISORDER

Identifying Characteristic	ALL	CLL	PLL	SCCL	HCL	Sézary Syndrome	T-Gamma Lymphocytosis	Infectious Mononucleosis
Predominating or significant cell type	Lymphoblast	"Mature" lymphocyte	Prolymphocyte	"Abnormal" lymphocyte	Hairy cell	Sézary cell	Large granular lymphocyte	Atypical lymphocyte
Nuclear chromatin pattern	Fine	Condensed; "soccer ball"	Moderately condensed	Condensed	Fine to moderately condensed	Dark-staining	Condensed	Varies but generally less condensed than normal lymphocyte
Nuclear shape	Varies; round/oval	Regular	Regular	Irregular with clefts, notches, folds	Regular to slightly irregular; may have some folding	Irregular; many folds	Regular	
Nucleoli	Prominent	Not prominent	Prominent	Not prominent	Not prominent	Not prominent	Not prominent	May be prominent
Cytoplasm	Scanty	Scanty	Scanty to moderate	Scanty	Moderate with hairlike projections	Scanty	Moderately abundant with prominent vacuoles and/or azurophilic granules	Abundant; may have azurophilic granules and/or vacuoles
Cell size	Varies; generally homogeneous population with some variation in size and age	Varies; homogeneous population	Varies; heterogeneous population	Varies	Varies	Varies	Large	Large
Immunologic marker profile	Common ALL (early B) (70%) HLA-DR TdT CD19 CD10 (CALLA) CD20 Early T-cell ALL (15%–20% of ALL is T-cell type)	B-cell CLL (98%) Weak sIg (IgM, IgD) HLA-DR CD5 CD19/20/24 T-cell CLL (2%) CD2 (E rosette) CD3 CD8	B-cell PL (80%) Strong sIg HLA-DR CD19/20/24 CD22 ±CD10 T-cell PLL (20%) CD2 (E rosette) CD3, CD4, CD5 CD7, ±CD8	B-cell Strong sIg HAL-DR CD19/20/24 ±CD10 (CALLA)	B-cell subset Strong sIg HLA-DR CD19/20/24 CD22 CD25 (IL-2 receptor, Tac)	T-cell Lymphoma E rosette CD2, CD3, CD4 CD5	T-cell CLL (LGL) Fc gamma receptor CD2 (E rosette) CD3 CD8 CD57 (HNK-1)	Reactive T cells CD3 CD8 or CD4

Abbreviations: ALL = acute lymphoblastic leukemia; CLL = chronic lymphocytic leukemia; PLL = prolymphocytic leukemia; SCLL = small cleaved-cell lymphoma; HCL = hairy-cell leukemia; HNK = human natural killer cell

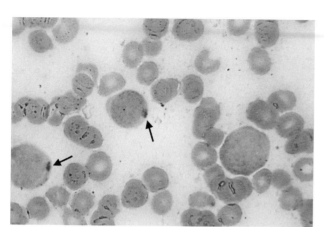

> ➤ **FIGURE 17–13** Alpha-naphthol acetate esterase (ANAE) stain showing localized "dotlike" positivity in two T lymphocytes.

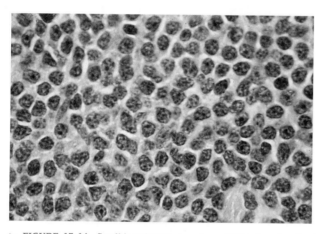

> ➤ **FIGURE 17–14** Small lymphocytic lymphoma (SLL), lymph node.

form a nodular or mantle zone pattern. MCL is composed of a homogeneous population of small- to intermediate-sized neoplastic lymphoid cells, usually slightly larger than normal lymphocytes. The nuclear characteristics and cytology of the cells are variable: round to clefted nuclear contour, and clumped to dispersed and blastoid chromatin.

MCL involves the peripheral blood in up to 25% of cases, and the peripheral blood count may exceed 200×10^9 cells/L. Under these circumstances, morphological recognition of MCL and its distinction from CLL/SLL are difficult. Identification of these two entities is important because MCL is considered to have a poor prognosis, with a median survival of 3 to 5 years. Bone marrow involvement may also occur with or without peripheral lymphadenopathy. MCL shows diffuse or focal bone marrow involvement (paratrabecular and nonparatrabecular).

Neoplastic lymphoid cells in MCL cells are exclusively of B-cell lineage. The common immunophenotype of this lymphoma is shown in Tables 17–4 and 17–7. In contrast to B-CLL, the cells in MCL lack expression of the CD23 surface antigen.[40,89] A typical example of the MCL immunophenotype is shown in Figure 17–15. The bright sIg expression and positivity for CD19, CD20, CD5, and FMC7 are characteristic. This immunophenotype also distinguishes MCL from SCCL, which is CD10-positive and CD5-negative (see Tables 17–4 and 17–7). In most cases, a distinctive chromosomal translocation t(11;14)(q13;q32) may occur.[91–94] It

involves the Ig heavy-chain locus on chromosome 14 and the *BCL1* locus on the long arm of chromosome 11. The hybrid gene is associated with overexpression of the cyclin D1 *(PRAD 1)* mRNA and protein. This chromosomal translocation can be detected in MCL (70%) by Southern blot analysis or (30% to 45%) by PCR. Unlike most other B-cell neoplasms, MCL is cyclin D1–positive (72% to 100%) as demonstrated using immunohistochemical staining on sections of formalin-fixed tissue.[95]

Small cleaved-cell lymphoma is also a non-Hodgkin's lymphoma consisting of B lymphocytes that may be nodular (follicular) or diffuse in distribution[40] (Fig. 17–16 and Color Plate 196) and can progress to a leukemic phase.[96] The circulating cells of SCCL are morphologically characterized by nuclei that are irregular in shape and that demonstrate irregular clefts, notches, or folds that may traverse the entire width of the nucleus (see Fig. 17–12*F*). These abnormal lymphocytes typically have very scanty cytoplasm and were formerly called "lymphosarcoma cells,"[97] a term that is no longer used. Compared with immunologic markers in B-CLL, SCCL shows strong sIg, CD22 positivity, CD5 negativity, and often CD10 positivity.[40,89]

Hairy-cell leukemia is another form of B lymphocyte–derived chronic leukemia and so named because of the fine, hairlike, irregular cytoplasmic projections that typify the disease (see Fig. 17–12*G*). Pancytopenia is common in HCL (unlike the other lymphoid disorders discussed in this chapter), along with splenomegaly and marrow fibrosis. A bone marrow aspirate is often difficult to obtain because of associated fibrosis (the so-called dry tap). Nevertheless bone marrow biopsy and biopsy touch imprints are essential for diagnosis. The bone marrow biopsy shows a loose interstitial lymphocytic infiltrate surrounded by a clear cytoplasm that separates one cell from another, creating a "fried-egg" appearance (Fig. 17–17 and Color Plate 197). The most characteristic cytochemical feature of HCL is a strong acid phosphatase reaction that is not inhibited by tartaric acid, known as the tartrate-resistant acid phosphatase stain (Fig. 17–18 and Color Plate 198); this enzyme corresponds to the isoenzyme 5, as demonstrated by polyacrylamide gel electrophoresis.[98] Immunologic markers that support the diagnosis of HCL are reactivity with B-cell–associated antigens (CD19, CD20, CD22, CD79a), CD11c, CD25 (the monoclonal antibody that recognizes the interleukin-2 receptor, Tac), FMC7, and CD103.[40,89] CD103 is the most useful marker for distinguishing HCL from other B-cell leukemias. A typical example of the HCL immunophenotype is shown in Figure 17–19.

A variant of HCL with splenomegaly and leukocytosis has been described,[99] as well as a splenic form of non-Hodgkin's lymphoma that resembles HCL, called splenic lymphoma with villous lymphocytes (SLVL).[40,100] SLVL has a distinct immunologic profile, underscoring the importance of using immunophenotyping to differentiate SLVL from CLL, HCL, and other lymphoproliferative disorders.[89,101]

Sézary syndrome is the leukemic phase of the most common cutaneous T-cell lymphoma, mycosis fungoides, and is characterized by abnormal circulating lymphocytes, called Sézary cells.[102] A Sézary cell is typically the size of a small lymphocyte and has a dark-staining and a hyperchromatic nuclear chromatin pattern with numerous folds and grooves that is referred to as cerebriform (see Fig. 17–12*H*). Nuclear folding is best appreciated at the ultrastructural level using

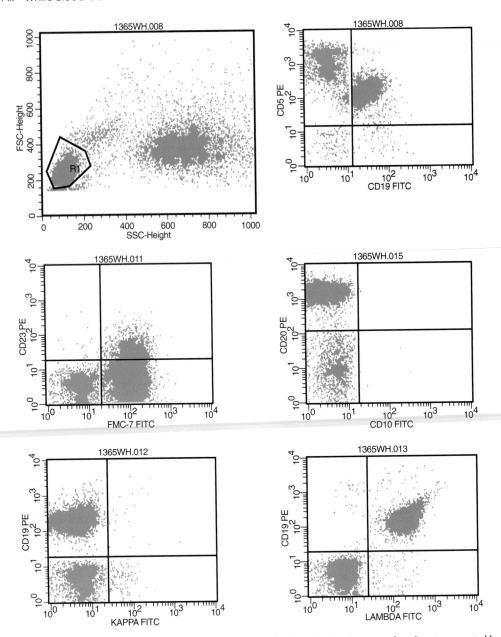

➤ **FIGURE 17–15** Flow cytometric analysis of mantle cell lymphoma in leukemia phase. Leukemic marrow lymphocytes are gated by CD45-scattered analysis. The plot of CD5 versus CD19 demonstrates dual positive neoplastic lymphocytes. In contrast to CLL, the neoplastic lymphocytes in mantle cell lymphoma show positive staining for FMC7 but no staining of CD23.

electron microscopy. A less common large cell variant of the Sézary cell is larger than a neutrophil and often larger than a monocyte, but has the same grooved nuclear chromatin pattern as the smaller Sézary cell. The bone marrow is infrequently involved. The diagnosis of Sézary syndrome is dependent on the primary diagnosis of the cutaneous T-cell lymphoma mycosis fungoides in the skin. The skin biopsy shows infiltration in the epidermis with an accumulation of atypical convoluted lymphocytes forming structures called Pautrier microabcesses (Fig. 17–20 and Color Plate 199). The nuclear folding of a Sézary cell may at first glance suggest a monocytic cell line; however, a monocyte gives a diffuse pattern of cytoplasmic positivity with the nonspecific esterase stain ANAE (mentioned earlier) as compared with a localized dotlike positivity pattern that identifies T cells. Immunologic marker studies of Sézary cells show a mature T-lymphocyte phenotype with reactiv-

ity for CD2, CD3, and CD4 (the monoclonal antibody that recognizes the helper/inducer subset of T lymphocytes). The detection and amplification of markers of T-cell clonality at the TCR and alpha-beta ($\alpha\beta$) and gamma-delta ($\gamma\delta$) loci by PCR can significantly improve the sensitivity in detecting a clonal T-lymphoid population.[103]

Adult T-cell leukemia/lymphoma, common in Japan and the Caribbean, is caused by human T-cell leukemia/ lymphoma virus-1 (HTLV-1). Although there is a large heterogeneity in the clinical manifestations of the disease, characteristic clinical features include generalized lymphadenopathy, hypercalcemia, bone and skin lesions, and 10% to 80% abnormal lymphoid cells in the blood and bone marrow.[104,105] The most outstanding feature of these abnormal lymphocytes is the highly convoluted nuclear shape, which often is "cloverleaf" in appearance (see Fig. 17–12*I*). There is marked variation in the size of the cells, ranging from that

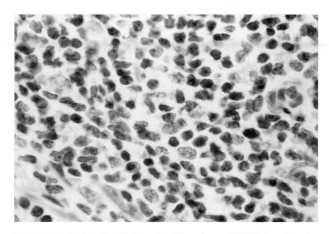

➤ **FIGURE 17–16** Small cleaved-cell lymphoma (SCCL), lymph node.

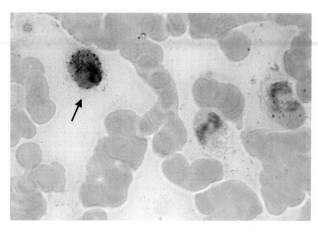

➤ **FIGURE 17–18** Tartrate-resistant acid phosphatase (TRAP) stain of peripheral blood showing positivity in hairy cell and no staining in neutrophilic.

of a small lymphocyte to that of a large monocyte. Nucleoli are typically inconspicuous but, when present, may be prominent and cause confusion with prolymphocytes. The clinical course of ATLL can be acute, with a high white cell count and survival less than 1 year; chronic, with a lower white cell count and survival of more than 1 year; or "smoldering," with a normal white cell count and low numbers of abnormal T lymphocytes. As seen in T-PLL and Sézary syndrome, ATLL cells show reactivity with T-cell–associated antigens (CD2, CD3, and CD5); most are CD4+, CD25+ but usually lack CD7. Rare CD8+ cases have been reported. Mutation in the tumor suppressor gene *p53* is seen in 30% to 50% of patients with ATLL.[106]

Chronic T-cell large granular lymphocytic leukemia (LGL) has the morphological distinction of persistent circulating lymphocytes that have abundant pale blue cytoplasm with azurophilic granules (see Fig. 17–12*J*). These granular lymphocytes usually constitute 50% to 95% of the circulating white cells. Large granular lymphocytic leukemia was first described in patients with CLL of T-cell origin[107] then subsequently in patients with chronic neutropenia.[108] Three distinct clinical syndromes are now described in patients with an increased number of circulating LGL cells.[109] When LGL carries a phenotype of T-LGL leukemia (a clonal proliferation of CD3+ LGL), then chronic neutropenia and autoimmunity, especially rheumatoid arthritis, are characteristic.[110–112]

Natural killer LGL leukemia is characterized by a clonal CD3−LGL proliferation with an aggressive clinical course and multiorgan involvement.[113] The majority of patients with increased numbers of CD3− cells do not have features of NK-LGL leukemia but rather demonstrate a more indolent clinical course.[112] Because quantitative abnormalities of LGL are fairly common and their presence in peripheral blood may represent a transient reactive phenomenon associated with viral infections, it is important to perform immunophenotyping and molecular studies, and to correlate these data with the clinical picture. Oral low-dose methotrexate has been shown to be an effective treatment for some patients with LGL.[114]

Reactive (atypical) lymphocytosis is self-limiting, rarely exceeds 5×10^9 cells/L, and is most commonly caused by a viral infection such as infectious mononucleosis, viral hepatitis, and cytomegalovirus in adults and *Bordetella* pertussis in children.[115] The large reactive lymphocytes that characterize viremia are polyclonal and T cell in origin. Abundant cytoplasm that may vary in degree of basophilia from very pale to deep blue is the most prominent feature of the reactive lymphocyte. These cells often have an irregular nuclear outline resembling a monocyte, and the nuclear chromatin is mostly coarse. Cytoplasmic vacuolization may be present (see Fig. 17–12*K*). Reactive B-cell lymphocytosis is rare. See Chapter 15, which discusses infectious mononucleosis and other causes of reactive lymphocytosis.

Plasma cell dyscrasias, namely Waldenström's macroglobulinemia, multiple myeloma, and plasma cell leukemia, may be associated with the presence of abnormal circulating plasma cells (see Fig. 17–12*L*). Plasma cells are characterized by abundant basophilic cytoplasm, an eccentric nucleus with clumped nuclear chromatin, and a prominent perinuclear clear zone. Plasma cells are end-stage B lymphocytes with the aforementioned characteristic morphology and distinctive immunologic markers, namely, the presence of monoclonal cytoplasmic Ig and expression of CD38. Plasma cell disorders are covered extensively in Chapter 20.

The significant clinical, morphological, and immunophenotypic features of CLL, as well as treatment, prognosis, and differential diagnosis, are shown in Table 17–8.

In summary, B-cell small lymphocytic disorders are clonal diseases that usually present in an indolent fashion in older patients. The diagnosis is often made incidentally from a persistent lymphocytosis. B-cell CLL is a clonal accumulation of mature-appearing B lymphocytes caused by failed apoptosis, exhibiting monoclonal sIg. An unusual

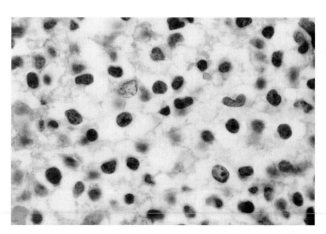

➤ **FIGURE 17–17** Hairy-cell leukemia (HCL), bone marrow aspirate.

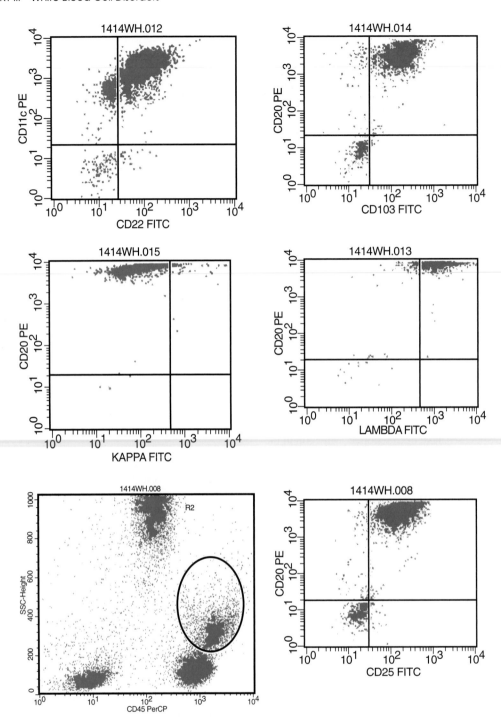

➤ **FIGURE 17–19** Flow cytometric analysis of hairy-cell leukemia. Large mononuclear cells in leukemic bone marrow are gated by CD45–side scattered analysis *(left lower panel)*. The plots of CD22 versus CD11c and CD20 versus CD103 demonstrate predominance of dual positive B cells *(upper panel)*. The plots for both CD20 and lambda show lambda light-chain clonality *(middle panel)*. The B cells are also reactive with anti-CD25 (anti–interleukin-2 receptor) *(lower right-sided histogram)*.

feature is expression of the CD5 membrane antigen seen on mature T lymphocytes. The B lymphocytes accumulate slowly in the bone marrow, blood, spleen, liver, and lymph nodes. About half of the patients with B-CLL exhibit hypogammaglobulinemia and an increased susceptibility to infection. Red cell aplasia, immune-mediated anemia, and thrombocytopenia are also common.

The course of CLL disease depends on the leukemia burden, which can be assessed by clinical staging systems.

Lymphoproliferative disorders caused by T lymphocytes are rare. T-prolymphocytic and ATLL are rapidly progressive diseases with more aggressive clinical courses. Morphological and immunophenotypic studies, and positive HTLV-1 serology, are helpful in characterizing these entities.

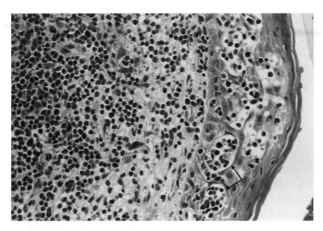

▶ FIGURE 17–20 Infiltration of the epidermis and upper dermis by lymphocytes, many with convoluted (cerebriform) nuclei, histiocytes, and formation of Pautrier microabscesses, characteristic of the cutaneous T-cell lymphoma mycosis fungoides.

▶ **Table 17–8**

TYPICAL FEATURES OF CHRONIC LYMPHOCYTIC LEUKEMIA

Clinical features	Patient > 50 years of age, lymphadenopathy, lymphocytosis
Morphology	Mature-appearing lymphocytes in blood and marrow, often showing hyperclumped nuclear chromatin pattern; smudge cells
Immunophenotype	Positive sIg, CD19, CD20, CD5, CD23, CD43
Treatment	Varies from no treatment to use of single or combination chemotherapeutic agents with or without radiation therapy
Prognosis	50% 5-year survival; 30% ≥ 10-year survival
Differential diagnosis	ALL, PLL, SLL, SCCL, HCL, Sézary syndrome, LGL, ATLL, Waldenström's macro-globulinemia, viral infection

Abbreviations: ALL = acute lymphoblastic leukemia; PLL = prolymphocytic leukemia; SLL = small lymphocytic lymphoma; SCCL = small cleaved-cell lymphoma; HCL = hairy-cell leukemia; LGL = large granular lymphocytosis; ATLL = adult T-cell leukemia/lymphoma

---

▶ **CASE STUDY 1**

A 74-year-old black woman was admitted to the hospital for confusion. Her past medical history revealed chronic obstructive pulmonary disease, hypertension, renal insufficiency, sickle-cell trait, and CLL. The CLL had been diagnosed 13 years ago and treated with chlorambucil, prednisone, vincristine, and bleomycin. A recent follow-up bone marrow analysis showed no lymphoid infiltrates. On the day before admission she was confused, minimally communicative, and weak. In the emergency de-

partment, she became gradually more unresponsive and appeared to be guarding her abdomen. Blood was found rectally and in the nasogastric tube that was placed in the patient during the initial examination. She was also found to be markedly acidotic, with a pH of 6.7. Her lactic acid level was 15.8 mg/dL with no acetone or ketones present, and her glucose level was less than 10 mg/dL. Coagulation studies revealed fibrinogen of 48 mg/dL, positive fibrinogen degradation products, and prolonged prothrombin and partial thromboplastin times. The patient was thought to be clinically septic and was started on clindamycin, gentamicin, and ampicillin therapy. Supportive care included fluid, blood products, sodium bicarbonate, and pressor agents. Blood and urine cultures were negative. X-rays showed an abdominal ileus, increased congestion in the lungs, and left lower lobe atelectasis. The patient had an episode of bradycardia and expired.

Autopsy findings were remarkable for a monomorphic lymphocytic infiltrate of the lymph nodes, liver, and spleen, which also showed the presence of sickled red blood cells. The pyloric region of the stomach showed a large ulcer, which contained adenocarcinoma, necrotic tissue, chronic inflammation, and colonization with fungus resembling *Candida*. Fungus was also found along the tracheal epithelium and invading the tracheal mucosa. Gomori methenamine silver stain showed no septation and branching of the hyphae consistent with *Candida*.

Note: This case illustrates how susceptibility to opportunistic infections and immunologic deficiency can contribute to morbidity and mortality in a patient with CLL. Although patients with CLL frequently have a prolonged survival and succumb to an unrelated disorder, the course of CLL varies widely in different patients.

▶ # CHRONIC MYELOGENOUS LEUKEMIA

Chronic myelogenous leukemia, also known as chronic granulocytic leukemia or chronic myeloid leukemia, is a clonal myeloproliferative disorder of the hematopoietic pluripotent stem cell that has undergone neoplastic transformation and is characterized by excessive production of granulocytes and their precursors.[116] Although CML was first described in 1845,[117–119] it was not until 1960 that the association with a consistent chromosomal abnormality was made. This chromosome was called the Philadelphia chromosome (Ph), because it was first identified at the University of Pennsylvania School of Medicine in Philadelphia.[120] This was the first report of a chromosomal abnormality associated with a malignancy; the abnormality was described as a small, deleted G group chromosome in the metaphases recovered from the bone marrow of patients with CML. Approximately 90% to 95% of patients with the typical characteristics of CML carry the Ph chromosome in their leukemic cells,[121] and consequently its presence is virtually diagnostic of the disease. Another hallmark of CML is found at the molecular level. The Ph chromosome results from the aberrant conjoining of the proto-oncogene c-*ABL* from chromosome 9 with the break-point cluster region (*BCR*) gene on chromosome 22. This new fusion protein *BCR/ABL* is considered essential in the pathogenesis of

CML.[122,123] In addition to the presence of the Ph chromosome, CML is characterized by marked leukocytosis with the presence of all stages of granulocytic maturation, organomegaly, especially splenomegaly, and low levels of leukocyte alkaline phosphatase (LAP). The clinical course may be characterized by three separate phases—(1) the chronic phase, which is generally controllable with chemotherapeutic agents and lasts 2 to 5 years; (2) the accelerated phase, which lasts approximately 6 to 18 months; and (3) the blastic acute leukemia-like phase, which lasts 3 to 4 months and is generally unresponsive to treatment, including those used for de novo acute leukemia[116]—or the course may be biphasic, in which case the chronic phase progresses directly to blast crisis.

CML is primarily considered an adult leukemia because it usually occurs in individuals between 30 and 50 years of age. However, the disease can strike any age group, including the elderly, infants, and toddlers. Although rare, when infants and toddlers are diagnosed, the disease is called juvenile CML and demonstrates marked hematopoietic, cytogenetic, and clinical differences from the adult form.[124] CML accounts for approximately 20% to 25% of all leukemia cases, and in western countries it is diagnosed in about 2 of every 100,000 people annually, resulting in an estimated 5000 new cases each year.[125] CML is slightly more predominant in men, and the median survival is 3 to 4 years once the diagnosis of CML is made.

Etiology and Pathophysiology

CML is a clonal stem cell disorder.[126] Although the majority of patients with CML have no history of excessive exposure to ionizing radiation or chemical leukemogens, the presumed role in leukemogenesis of a variety of agents is well documented. These leukemogens include exposure to ionizing radiation[127] (such as has been seen in radiologists prior to the use of safety shielding techniques, patients treated for ankylosing spondylitis, and survivors of nuclear explosions) and to cytotoxic drugs, especially alkylating agents, and biologically active chemicals such as benzene.[128] The cause in more than 95% of CML cases is unknown. CML is not an inherited disease but rather appears to be acquired, as suggested by the rarity of familial aggregations of CML[129] and the failure of the second member of pairs of identical twins to develop the chronic leukemia.[130] The Ph chromosome is not present in nonhematopoietic tissues, nor is it found in the parents or offspring of patients.

The Ph chromosome has been found in neutrophil, monocyte, erythrocyte, platelet, and basophil precursors from CML patients' blood and bone marrow.[131] This stem cell origin helps to define the translocation that produces the Ph chromosome as a clonal abnormality and provides the subsequent progeny with a growth advantage over normal cells. Giemsa-trypsin (G bands) or quinacrine fluorescent (Q bands) chromosomal banding analysis shows that the Ph chromosome is derived from the G-group chromosome 22 rather than chromosome 21 as originally thought.[132–134] The notation t(9;22) refers to the specific chromosomal translocation found in the majority of CML patients. In CML the main portion of the long arm of chromosome 22 is deleted and translocated, most often to the distal end of the long arm of chromosome 9 (or to another chromosome in variant translocations), resulting in an elongated chromosome 9 (9q+). A small part of chromosome 9 is reciprocally translocated to the broken end of the

deleted chromosome 22 (22q−). The unequal exchange of chromosomal material results in the tiny or "minute" chromosome 22, which is smaller than any normal chromosome and is easily recognized as the Ph chromosome under the microscope following appropriate cell culture, harvesting, chromosome preparation, and staining (Fig. 17–21). Thus, the notation for the most common translocation in CML is t(9;22)(q34.1;q11.1), frequently simply referred to as the 9/22 translocation.

Approximately 5% of CML patients have the deleted portion of chromosome 22 translocated to other chromosomes[135]; that is t(4;22), t(12;22), and t(19;22)—called simple variant Ph translocations—whereas other patients have complex variant Ph translocations involving more than one chromosome in addition to chromosome 22[136]; that is, t(9;11;22). Additionally it has been found that on occasion the Ph chromosome may be "masked" by the presence of chromatin material translocated to the deleted chromosome 22 from one of the other chromosomes involved in the rearrangement.[137] Nonrandom chromosomal abnormalities such as duplication of the Ph chromosome, trisomy 8, and isochromosome 17 are detected in at least 50% of patients in the accelerated phase of CML and in up to 80% of those in the blastic phase.[138]

Changes at the gene level in proliferating leukemic cells appear to endow clonal advantage on the cell because of gene deregulation or because qualitatively altered gene products are produced. Some of the genes involved in chromosomal alterations have been identified as cellular protooncogenes. Proto-oncogenes are normal cellular genes that, when activated by a molecular process such as mutations, deletions, and insertions of DNA sequences, can be converted to an oncogene, a gene that can cause malignant transformation. Human transforming DNA sequences have been found to be homologous to various viral oncogenes and are called *cellular oncogenes*.[139] The proto-oncogene c-*ABL* is the human counterpart to the Abelson murine leukemia virus and normally resides on chromosome 9 at band 9q34, the same location involved in the 9/22 translocation in CML. Because chromosome rearrangements have been shown to be associated with activated genes in appropriate cells,[140] it is possible that regulation of cell growth and differentiation may be expressed inappropriately as a result of chromosomal changes.

The designation *BCR* refers to the narrow 5.8-kilobase (kd) DNA fragment localized on chromosome 22. That

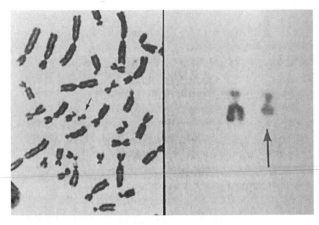

> FIGURE 17–21 Philadelphia chromosome A (*left*) and B (*right*).

fragment defines the chromosomal break associated with the Ph chromosome abnormality and is based on restriction enzyme patterns of DNA probes from normal subjects and those with CML.[141] In CML the balanced translocation between chromosomes 9 and 22 results in c-ABL shifting from 9q34 to the BCR gene at 22q11. The subsequent formation of a BCR/ABL hybrid gene product, a 210-kd protein possessing increased tyrosine kinase activity, provides an important mediator of oncogenesis in the pathophysiology of CML.[142–144] It has been shown that the BCR/ABL fusion protein expressed in CML acts as an antiapoptosis gene.[145] Apoptosis, also known as programmed cell death, is the major form of cell death associated with the action of chemotherapeutic agents on tumor cells. The susceptibility of CML cells to treatment-induced cell death may depend on the expression of genes that interfere with apoptosis, such as BCR/ABL.[145–147] Most patients with CML have both the Ph chromosome and the BCR/ABL gene, whereas some patients with clinically documented CML lack the Ph chromosome but have the BCR/ABL gene.[142] The gene rearrangement of the BCR region of chromosome 22 can be detected using DNA technology in Southern blots[123,142] or biotin-labeled gene probes.[148] Fluorescence in situ hybridization to detect BCR/ABL translocation[149,150] and a western blot method to detect the leukemia-causing proteins[151] have also been shown to be effective methods of monitoring the efficacy of therapy. The molecular basis of the Ph chromosome is summarized in Figure 17–22.

Another cellular oncogene, c-SIS, the homologue of the transforming gene of simian sarcoma virus, has been mapped to chromosome 22. In CML, c-SIS is translocated from chromosome 22 to a recipient chromosome, usually chromosome 9.[152] The c-SIS oncogene encodes sequences for the β chain of platelet-derived growth factor (PDGF),[153] which may play a role in the myelofibrosis that accompanies some cases of CML.

The category of Ph-negative CML has led to much discussion in the past.[154–156] Patients who were at one time diagnosed as having Ph-negative CML may, as a result of the development of criteria for the myelodysplastic syndromes (see Chap. 19) and other myeloproliferative disorders (see Chap. 18) be reclassified. The diseases that are characterized by the absence of the Ph chromosome and that are distinguishable from CML on clinical grounds include chronic neutrophilic leukemia[157] and the myelodysplastic syndrome chronic myelomonocytic leukemia (CMML).[158] Rarely, true Ph-negative CML does exist and is diagnosed by the same clinical and hematologic parameters, other than the presence of Ph chromosome, as classic CML.[159] However, in the majority of these patients the molecular defect, namely the juxtaposition of c-ABL and BCR genes as seen in typical CML, can be demonstrated even though there is no cytogenetic evidence of the Ph chromosome. Occasionally, patients are encountered who lack the Ph translocation, the BCR rearrangement and, a BCR/ABL gene product. Nevertheless, these patients have a disease phenotype at diagnosis that is a morphological facsimile of classic chronic-phase CML, with a clinical course that is not marked by increases in blast cells.[159]

Clinical Features

Patients with CML may be asymptomatic or symptomatic. Detecting CML in its early stages may be difficult, and it is not uncommon for the disease to be discovered accidentally during a routine physical examination or hematologic evaluation analogous to the incidental discovery of CLL. When symptoms do appear, the most common complaints of patients are general malaise; complaints attributable to anemia, such as weakness, fatigue, diminished exercise tolerance, dizziness, headache, fever, and irritability; complaints resulting from a hypermetabolic state, such as excessive perspiration, night sweats, and weight loss, bone tenderness, and aching due to marked marrow expansion; and fullness in the upper abdomen with accompanying easy satiation or loss of appetite resulting from hepatomegaly and splenomegaly. Ex-

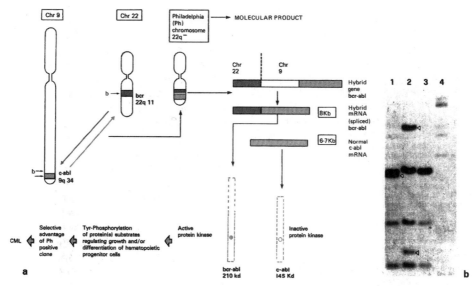

➤ FIGURE 17–22 Molecular basis of the Philadelphia (Ph) chromosome. (a) Sequence of molecular and biochemical events involved in generating the Ph chromosome and its phenotypic consequences. (b) Southern blot analysis of DNA from CML cells analyzed with a bcr probe to show clonal rearrangements in the bcr region. Lane 1: Ph-positive CML DNA showing one rearranged band; lane 2: Ph-positive CML as in lane 1 but with a different break point in the bcr region; lane 3: Ph-negative leukemic cell DNA showing no rearranged bcr; and lane 4: molecular weight markers. (From Greaves, MF: Cellular identification and markers. In Zucker-Franklin, D, et al. (eds): Atlas of Blood Cells. Lea & Febiger, Philadelphia/EE edi-ermes, Milano, Italy, 1988, p 43, with permission.)

cessive bleeding after a minor injury or surgical procedure, bleeding in the form of purpura, retinal hemorrhage or hematuria resulting from quantitative or qualitative platelet defects, or abnormal or unexplained bruising may also occur. Although less common, patients may experience an increase in infections, attacks of gouty arthritis caused by the accumulating uric acid from myeloid cell breakdown, ankle edema, menorrhagia, peripheral vascular insufficiency, and priapism. On rare occasions, the presenting sign of a patient with CML is a chloroma, an infiltrating skin tumor, so named because of the characteristic green color of the tumor mass. Table 17–9 summarizes the clinical signs and symptoms of CML.

Laboratory Features

The laboratory features of CML, similar to the clinical features, are predominantly caused by an excess of myeloid cells, which may be increased more than a hundredfold. The bone marrow produces and releases large numbers of cells, resulting in extreme leukocytosis, often in excess of 100×10^9cells/L. A spectrum of myeloid forms is seen in the peripheral blood, ranging from blast forms to mature neutrophils (Fig. 17–23 and Color Plate 200); however, the segmented neutrophil and the myelocyte are the most numerous forms in the differential count. The immaturity seen in the granulocytic series is referred to as a "left shift." Eosinophils, basophils, and platelets may be increased, and pelgeroid granulocytes may also be present at any phase of CML (Fig. 17–24 and Color Plate 201). As in other myeloproliferative disorders, the blood smears of patients with CML may demonstrate giant platelets or megakaryocytic fragments (Fig. 17–25), or both. A normocytic, normochromic anemia that varies in degree from patient to patient but is frequently associated with hemoglobin levels below 10 g/dL is typically present. Nucleated red blood cells may be present with varying degrees of anisocytosis, poikilocytosis, polychromasia, basophilic stippling, and reticulocytosis. As the disease progresses, the degree of anemia may worsen, thrombocytope-

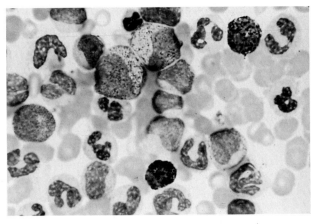

➤ FIGURE 17–23   Photomicrograph of peripheral blood from a patient with CML.

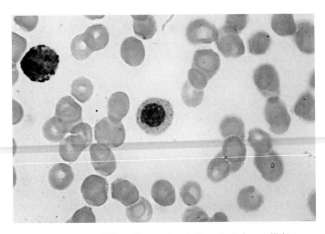

➤ FIGURE 17–24   Pelgeroid granulocyte (pseudo-Pelger cell) in a patient with CML, peripheral blood. Note that the nucleus is round with condensed chromatin and should not be mistaken for a normal myelocyte or a nucleated red blood cell.

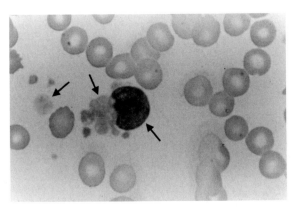

➤ FIGURE 17–25   Photomicrograph of peripheral blood from a patient with CML demonstrating giant platelets and a megakaryocytic fragment.

➤ Table 17–9 CLINICAL SIGNS AND SYMPTOMS OF CHRONIC MYELOCYTIC LEUKEMIA (CML)/CHRONIC GRANULOCYTIC LEUKEMIA (CGL)	
Symptoms related to hypermetabolism	Weight loss; anorexia; low-grade fever; warm, moist skin; night sweats; sternal tenderness (present in 2/3 of patients)
Splenomegaly	Present in more than 90% of patients, and frequently massive, associated discomfort, pain, and indigestion
Symptoms related to anemia	Pallor, dyspnea, tachycardia
Other physical signs or symptoms	Bruising or ecchymoses over the extremities, epitaxis, retinal hemorrhages, menorrhagia in women, or hemorrhage from other sites

nia develops, and there may be a shift toward the younger myeloid forms with increasing numbers of blasts.

The bone marrow is hypercellular with a marked myeloid hyperplasia. The myeloid-to-erythroid ratio is generally at least 10:1 instead of the normal 3:1 (Fig. 17–26 and Color Plate 202). A secondary myelofibrosis may accompany the

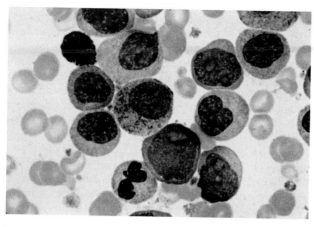

➤ **FIGURE 17-26** Photomicrograph of bone marrow aspirate from patient with CML. Note marked myeloid hyperplasia (magnification ×54).

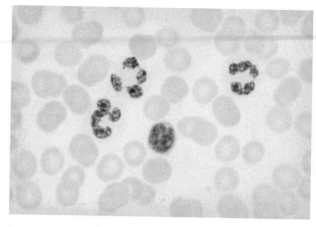

➤ **FIGURE 17-28** Leukocyte alkaline phosphates (LAP) stain of peripheral blood showing little or no activity in CML.

CML and is diagnosed by examining the bone marrow biopsy stained for reticulin or collagen fibers using a silver stain (Fig. 17-27 and Color Plate 203). Sea-blue histiocytosis, the appearance of storage cells with deep sea-blue pigmentation, may be seen scattered throughout the marrow of patients with CML. These contain accumulated glycolipids caused by the expanded membrane turnover of the myeloid cell pool[160] (see Color Plate 204).

As mentioned earlier, in 90% to 95% of CML patients, cytogenetic studies on the peripheral blood and bone marrow reveal the hallmark Ph chromosome t(9:22)(q34:q11).

Another characteristic laboratory finding in CML is low to absent LAP, also called neutrophilic alkaline phosphatase (Fig. 17-28 and Color Plate 205). This absent LAP activity in CML is in contrast to the increased activity in leukemoid reactions (Fig. 17-29 and Color Plate 206). During remission, LAP levels may increase as a reflection of enhanced maturation of normal granulocytes.[161] Although there is abnormal biochemical reactivity of LAP, not all bactericidal and phagocytic functions of the leukemic granulocytes are compromised; however, adhesion to marrow stroma and endothelial cells is altered.[162,163]

Other laboratory findings include elevated uric acid levels, elevated lactic dehydrogenase, and increased levels of serum vitamin B_{12}—findings resulting from the increased catabolism of large numbers of granulocytes that are common to the myeloproliferative disorders.

Clinical Course and Prognostic Factors

As mentioned earlier, CML can be divided into two or three phases: chronic, accelerated, and acute (blastic). The median survival from time of diagnosis is generally 3 to 4 years, and fewer than 30% of patients survive 5 years. Achieving a cytogenetic response with interferon-α therapy in patients with CML is independently associated with improved survival.[163] However, the transformation to the accelerated or blastic phase can occur at any time. In the majority of patients, transformation is associated with development of chromosomal abnormalities in addition to Ph positivity. The blood composition changes from predominantly myeloid cells with neutrophils and myelocytes to an increase in the number of blasts and promyelocytes. Systemic symptoms of fever, night sweats, or weight loss reappear or worsen as does hepatosplenomegaly and extramedullary disease in the lymph nodes, bone, skin, and soft tissue.[164,165] The median time from development of extramedullary disease to blastic crisis is 4 months, and median survival is 5 months. The acute blastic phase is the terminal event in CML and resembles acute leukemia in that the cells no longer differentiate to mature granulocytes and 30% or more blasts are present in the bone marrow. The

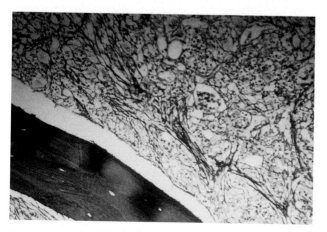

➤ **FIGURE 17-27** Silver stain for reticulin and collagen fibers on bone marrow biopsy sample from a patient with CML and secondary myelofibrosis.

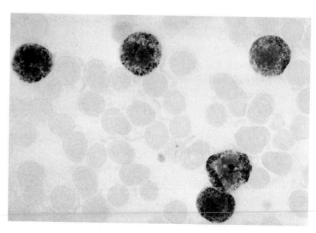

➤ **FIGURE 17-29** Leukemoid reaction; increased LAP activity.

term *maturation arrest* refers to the absence of cellular differentiation beyond the blast or promyelocyte stage. The blasts of the blastic phase are usually myeloid, as demonstrated by myeloperoxidase activity. However, approximately 25% of patients develop a lymphoid blast crisis, as demonstrated by immunophenotyping, TdT, and molecular studies. Fewer than 10% of patients develop megakaryocytic or erythroid blast crisis. Most patients die of complications arising during blast crisis, the most common of which are bleeding caused by thrombocytopenia, infection, therapy-related marrow aplasia, or aplasia exacerbated by progressive myelofibrosis.

The prognosis in CML can be predicted by several factors, present at the time of diagnosis, which are associated with early transformation to blast crisis. These poor risk factors include absence of the Ph chromosome or presence of other karyotypic abnormalities in addition to the Ph chromosome, enlarged spleen or liver, thrombocytopenia (less than 150×10^9 cells/L) or thrombocytosis (more than 500×10^9 cells/L), extreme leukocytosis (more than 100×10^9 cells/L), peripheral blood blasts above 1%, bone marrow blasts above 5%, and peripheral blood basophils above 15%.[116,164-166] CML in myeloid blast crisis is also considered a poor risk factor in contrast to lymphoid blast crisis, which traditionally is more responsive to chemotherapy. The morphological, cytochemical, and immunologic characteristics of blast cells in CML have been widely studied.[167,168]

The number and morphological characteristics of megakaryocytes in bone marrow sections have also been used to identify histologic types of CML and may have prognostic significance.[169] The presence of *p53*, a tumor suppressor gene, is altered in 20% to 30% of CML patients in blast crisis. Mutations in the *p53* gene may have prognostic significance, as these mutations could induce drug resistance by interfering with normal programmed cell death pathways in leukemic CML cells.

Treatment

The usual objectives of therapy for the chronic phase of CML are to reduce the proliferating myeloid mass; relieve the symptoms of hyperleukocytosis, thrombocytosis, and splenomegaly; and maintain the patient in a symptom-free condition without causing therapy-related complications. These objectives can be achieved by the conventional chemotherapeutic agents busulfan (Myeleran) and hydroxyurea (Hydrea); however, neither cytotoxic drug postpones, prevents, or controls blast crisis.[116,164,170,171] The only curative treatment for CML is bone marrow transplantation. Cure is defined as a persistence of Ph-negative and *BCR/ABL*-negative cells.

Interferons are naturally occurring proteins that exist in α, β, and γ forms, and have antitumor activity. Investigations of interferon-α therapy to treat CML have confirmed its efficacy as a single agent or as part of combined modality therapy to achieve hematologic remission.[116,170,172] Although its exact mechanism of action is unclear, interferon-α has been shown to prolong overall median survival, especially when there is a cytogenetic response.[116] Currently, the median survival in CML is about 60 to 65 months, with survival rates of 75% to 85% at 3 years and 50% to 60% at 5 years.

Bone marrow transplantation can be syngeneic (the donor is the patient's identical twin), allogeneic (the donor is genetically compatible, most often an HLA-identical sibling), or autologous (the patient's own marrow or peripheral blood is harvested during the chronic phase and stored until transplantation).[170-172] Syngeneic or HLA-identical allogeneic bone marrow transplantation following high-dose chemotherapy is capable of eradicating the Ph chromosome–containing leukemic clone. The procedure is recommended within 1 year of diagnosis for patients in the chronic phase who are younger than 40 years of age (or than 55 years, at some centers)[170,172] and for any child with juvenile CML as soon as possible after diagnosis and identification of a suitable donor. For patients without a suitable family donor, donor registries are being established to tally the names of volunteer unrelated allogeneic bone marrow donors. The importance of bone marrow transplantation in the chronic phase rather than in the accelerated or blast phase is emphasized when the survival data are considered. Earlier studies have shown that 49% to 64% of patients receiving allogeneic transplants while in the chronic phase have long-term survival in contrast to 15% to 30% for those receiving transplantation in the accelerated phase and approximately 10% for those receiving transplantation in the acute blastic phase.[170,173]

Although transplantation gives CML patients a hope for a cure, transplantation-related mortality is high (20% to 30%), with graft-versus-host disease (GVHD) being a major cause of death. The use of autologous bone marrow transplantation avoids the debilitating effects of GVHD. In one study, 56% of patients lived 5 years after undergoing autograft[174]; however, earlier studies have shown less than a 10% long-term survival, with treatment most often failing due to leukemic relapse.[175] The incidence of acute GVHD can be reduced by depleting the donor marrow of the cells responsible for the GVHD reaction, namely T lymphocytes, by using various methods including T-cell monoclonal antibodies, sheep erythrocytes (E)-rosetting, and soybean lectin agglutination. Additionally, many transplantation teams attempt to prevent GVHD using methotrexate with or without cyclosporine,[176] glucocorticoids, or a combination of these therapies. Unfortunately, the use of T-cell depletion for GVHD prophylaxis significantly increases the incidence of leukemic relapse,[177-179] suggesting that the graft-versus-leukemia effect mediated by T lymphocytes is important in the successful cure of CML. Research is ongoing to retain the graft-versus-leukemia effect despite T-cell depletion.[180] Several approaches are under investigation for purging contaminating leukemic cells from nonleukemic hematopoietic cells collected for autologous transplantations.[181,182] The ability to determine the success of bone marrow transplantation in terms of detecting minimal residual disease has been dramatically enhanced by the DNA amplification technique PCR described briefly in the CLL section of this chapter (under the heading Immunologic Features and Methods for Studying Lymphocytes).[183-185]

Adjunctive or alternative measures for treating CML include leukopheresis, splenic irradiation or splenectomy, intensive combination chemotherapy,[186] and immunotherapy; however, none of these approaches are guaranteed to prolong the duration of the chronic phase or improve overall survival.

The response to standard chemotherapeutic regimens is poor once the disease progresses to the accelerated or blast phase of CML. Standard AML therapy (cytosine arabinoside and thioguanine), when used in patients with myeloid blast crisis, rarely results in survival beyond 5 months, whereas patients with lymphoid blast crisis have a median survival of approximately 8 months when treated with standard ALL therapy (vincristine and prednisone).[170,172,186]

Differential Diagnosis

Chronic myeloid leukemia is a myeloproliferative disorder and must be distinguished from the other hematologic disorders in this group, including polycythemia vera, essential thrombocythemia, and agnogenic myeloid metaplasia (see Chap. 18). The presence of the Ph chromosome, *BCR* rearrangement, and low to absent LAP activity are virtually pathognomonic for CML and clearly distinguish it from the other myeloproliferative disorders. Reactive granulocytic leukocytosis, such as the leukemoid reaction or leukoerythroblastic blood characteristics that may accompany bacterial infection or acute hemolysis may be differentiated from CML mainly by lack of the Ph chromosome and absence of typical molecular aberrations of CML as well as their normal to high LAP levels. Table 17–10 summarizes the differential laboratory diagnosis between leukemoid reaction and CML. The typical features that characterize the significant clinical and diagnostic laboratory findings of CML, as well as treatment, prognosis, and differential diagnosis, are shown in Table 17–11.

Chronic myeloid leukemia originates with the acquisition of the t(9,22) chromosomal translocation that generates the Ph chromosome and the *BCR/ABL* chimeric gene. The *BCR/ABL* gene, present in about 95% of cases of CML, is necessary in the pathogenesis of the leukemia. Progression of disease to the accelerated phase and blast crisis is probably a result of further genetic changes.

The various positions of the breakpoints in *BCR* and *ABL* genes and the resulting *BCR/ABL* protein are implicated at various points in different signal transduction pathways, but the mechanism by which it causes CML remains enigmatic. Treatment options in CML have become complex in recent years. There is increasing support for the notion that interferon-α prolongs life in comparison with other agents. Interferon-α plus other agents may be better than interferon-α alone. Allografting can cure eligible patients, but the risk of transplantation-related mortality is still appreciable, especially in older patients and in recipients of marrow from donors other than HLA-identical siblings.

> ## Table 17–11
> ### TYPICAL FEATURES OF CHRONIC MYELOGENOUS LEUKEMIA

Clinical features	Any age group, but usually 30–50 years of age; splenomegaly; constitutional symptoms, i.e., fatigue, weight loss, night sweats
Morphology	"Left shift" of the granulocytic series, thrombocytosis, basophilia, and/or eosinophilia in blood and marrow
Cytogenetics	Ph chromosome–positive t(9:22) (q34;q11)
Molecular marker	*BCR* gene
Other laboratory findings	Decreased or absent LAP activity; increased uric acid, LDH, and serum B$_{12}$
Treatment	Chemotherapy/BMT
Prognosis	Median survival = about 5 years; 75%–85% 3-year survival; 50%–60% 5-year survival
Differential diagnosis	Leukemoid reaction; other myeloproliferative disorders, namely, polycythemia vera, essential thrombocythemia, and myelofibrosis

Abbreviations: LAP = leukocyte alkaline phosphatase; LDH = lactic dehydrogenase; BMT = bone marrow transplantation

> ## Table 17–10
> ### DIFFERENTIAL DIAGNOSIS BETWEEN LEUKEMOID REACTION AND CHRONIC MYELOID LEUKEMIA

	Leukemoid Reaction	CML
Toxic vacuoles	2–4+	0–1+
Toxic granules	2–4+	0–1+
Döhle bodies	Frequent	Rare
Eosinophilia	0	1–3+
Basophilia	0	1–3+
Pseudo–Pelger-Huët	0–1+	Occasional
Karyorrhexis	0–1+	1–2+
Giant bizarre nuclei	1–1+	1–3+
Leukemic hiatus	0	Occasional
LAP score	High	Low
Ph chromosome	Negative	Positive

Abbreviation: LAP = leukocyte alkaline phosphatase

> ## CASE STUDY 2

A 60-year-old white man initially sought medical attention because of fatigue and fever. At that time, his white blood cell count was 45×10^9 cells/L with a left shift; hemoglobin, 11.4 g/dL; hematocrit, 35%; platelet count, 500×10^9 cells/L; and LAP score, 0. His spleen was palpable 8 cm below the left costal margin. The patient's history was significant for multiple exposures to a variety of herbicides and insecticides as a result of his occupation as a farmer. A bone marrow examination and cytogenetic studies revealed hypercellularity with marked granulocytic hyperplasia, a myeloid-to-erythroid ratio greater than 10:1, and the presence of Ph chromosome t(9q+,22q−). Treatment with the alkylating agent busulfan (Myleran) was started, his white blood cell count began to drop within 2 weeks, and the symptoms of fatigue and fever subsided. Busulfan was continued at various intervals for the next 2 years. The patient continued to do well during the 2 years of busulfan treatment. Subsequently he again complained of chronic fatigue and was again found to have marked leukocytosis. He received hydroxyurea for the next 6 months, with minimal improvement of his white blood cell count. He was admitted to the hospital 1 month later for further evaluation, which included another bone marrow examination and cytogenetic studies. This bone marrow specimen showed hypercellularity with granulocytic hyperplasia, and a myeloid-to-erythroid ratio of 8:1, with foci of blasts. In addition to the Ph chromosome, an isochromosome of the long arm of chromosome 17 (i[17q]) was present. A complete blood count revealed a white blood cell count of 62×10^9 cells/L; hematocrit, 38%; hemoglobin, 12.8g/dL; platelet count, 269×10^9 cells/L; 36 neutrophils, 5 bands, 1 metamyelocyte, 3 myelocytes, 13 promyelocytes, 21 blasts, 13 basophils, 3 lymphocytes, and 5 monocytes; pelgeroid granulocytes were also noted.

The patient was once again started on busulfan. More aggressive therapy was considered and discussed; however, the patient refused further treatment and left the hospital against the advice of his physicians.

Questions

1. The cells of CLL are morphologically identical to those of:
   a. ALL
   b. Small lymphocytic lymphoma
   c. Infectious mononucleosis
   d. Sézary syndrome

2. Surface immunoglobulin is the most reliable surface marker for:
   a. T lymphocytes
   b. Plasma cells
   c. B lymphocytes
   d. Histiocytes

3. Cells that demonstrate a positive reaction with the tartrate-resistant acid phosphatase (TRAP) stain are most likely:
   a. T lymphoblasts of ALL
   b. Atypical lymphocytes of a viral infection
   c. Large granular lymphocytes of T-gamma lymphoproliferative disorder
   d. Hairy cells of hairy-cell leukemia

4. A mutated tumor suppressor gene found in a variety of human cancers, including CLL and CML, is:
   a. p53
   b. MDM2
   c. HLA-DR
   d. CD4

5. The translocation that results in formation of the Philadelphia chromosome involves chromosomes:
   a. 21 and 22
   b. 22 and 9
   c. 8 and 14
   d. 21 and 9

6. Blast crisis in CML is:
   a. Followed by the chronic phase and the accelerated phase

   b. Seen only in the juvenile form of CML
   c. The terminal phase of CML, characterized by increased numbers of blasts in the bone marrow and peripheral blood
   d. The first phase of a typical case of CML

7. Each of the following favors a diagnosis of CML rather than a leukemoid reaction except:
   a. Absence of eosinophils and basophils in the peripheral blood
   b. Low LAP score with myeloblasts through neutrophils in the peripheral blood
   c. Ph chromosome
   d. Enlarged spleen

8. The only curative treatment for CML is:
   a. Combination chemotherapy
   b. Total-body radiation
   c. Bone marrow transplantation
   d. There is no cure

9. At the molecular level, the aberrant conjoining of genetic material from chromosome 9 and chromosome 22 in patients with CML results in the formation of a new gene product called the:
   a. BCR/ABL gene
   b. BCL2 gene
   c. Multidrug resistance gene
   d. Blast crisis gene

10. The immunophenotype that best describes mantle cell lymphoma is:
    a. CD5+, CD191+, CD23+, FMC7+, cyclin D1+
    b. CD5+, CD19+, CD23+, FMC7+, cyclin D1−
    c. CD5+, CD19+, CD23+, FMC7−, cyclin D1+
    d. CD5+, CD19+, CD23−, FMC7+, cyclin D1+
    e. CD5−, CD19+, CD23+, FMC7+, cyclin D1+

11. In chronic lymphocytic leukemia:
    a. The absolute lymphocyte count is usually equal to or exceeds 5000×10^9 cells/L
    b. Hemoglobin level, platelet count, and absolute number of neutrophils may be normal or elevated
    c. The neoplastic lymphocytes in the blood or bone marrow are large with fine chromatin and prominent nucleoli

Directions: Each item below contains one or more correct answers. Use the following letters to answer questions 12 through 16.
   a. If **1, 2,** and **3** are correct
   b. If **1** and **3** are correct
   c. If **2** and **4** are correct
   d. If **4** is correct
   e. If **1, 2, 3,** and **4** are correct

12. Which of the following findings would point to a diagnosis of CLL?
    1. Clonal proliferations of B lymphocytes
    2. CD19+/CD5+, CD23−
    3. CD19+/CD51+, CD23+
    4. Ph chromosome–positive

13. Which of the following clinical and laboratory manifestations would point to a diagnosis of hairy-cell leukemia?
    1. Pancytopenia

2. Splenomegaly
3. CD20+, CD103+, CD25+
4. Prominent generalized lymphadenopathy
14. The poorest prognosis for patients with CLL is associated with which of the following features?
   1. Anemia
   2. Splenomegaly
   3. Thrombocytopenia
   4. White cell count greater than 15,000 cells/μL
15. The Philadelphia chromosome involves:
   1. t(9;22)
   2. The *BCR* and *c-ABL* genes
   3. A 210-kd protein possessing increased tyrosine kinase activity
   4. A 145-kd protein gene product
16. Which of the following laboratory procedures is likely to be useful in the diagnosis of CML?
   1. Southern blot
   2. Fluorescence in situ hybridization
   3. Western blot
   4. Reverse transcription-polymerase chain reaction (RT-PCR)

Case Study: A 64-year-old man with no significant past medical history was admitted to the hospital with mild upper abdominal pain, malaise, anorexia, weight loss, and low-grade fever of 1-month's duration. He denied having a cough, dyspnea, nausea, vomiting, jaundice, or recent viral infection. His vital signs were essentially unremarkable except for a mild fever of 37.8°C. Physical examination revealed marked splenomegaly with no hepatomegaly or peripheral lymphadenopathy. Radiologic examination, however, disclosed retroperitoneal lymphadenopathy. Laboratory workup showed marked leukocytosis (182×10^9 cells/L), thrombocytopenia (71×10^9 cells/L), and anemia (hemoglobin, 8.1 g/dL). Peripheral blood and bone marrow aspirate smears were performed. More than 60% of the leukocytes counted in the peripheral blood and 85% of all nucleated cells counted in the bone marrow specimen were described as "medium to large atypical cells with distinct rim of cytoplasm, round nuclear contour, dispersed nuclear chromatin, and a single prominent nucleolus."

Directions: Choose the one best answer:

17. The workup step(s) include:
   a. Cytochemical staining, including myeloperoxidase and nonspecific esterase, and TdT
   b. Immunohistochemical study of trephine biopsy sections
   c. Immunophenotypic study by flow cytometry
   d. Cytogenetic studies
   e. All of the above
18. Immunophenotypic study using flow cytometry shows negative T-cell markers. However, neoplastic cells express bright CD19, CD20, and weak CD5 and show monotypic κ light-chain restriction. These cells will also express:
   a. CD103
   b. Strong FMC7

c. CD23
d. Dim surface immunoglobulin
e. CD38
19. Cytochemical stains (myeloperoxidase, nonspecific esterase) and TdT performed on samples of bone marrow aspirate smear were negative. The most likely diagnosis is:
   a. Chronic myelocytic leukemia, accelerated phase
   b. Typical chronic lymphocytic leukemia
   c. Acute lymphoblastic leukemia
   d. Chronic lymphocytic leukemia/Prolymphocytic leukemia
   e. B-cell prolymphocytic leukemia

SUMMARY CHART

➤ Chronic lymphoproliferative disorders are clonal proliferations of morphologically and immunophenotypically mature B or T lymphocytes.
➤ Methods for studying lymphocytes include immunofluorescence, molecular probes, cytochemistry, cytogenetics, electron microscopy, immunoperoxidase, and flow cytometry.
➤ The Rai system, the Binet system, and the International Workshop on Chronic Lymphocytic Leukemia (CLL) are the three major staging systems developed for CLL; however, the Rai system is widely used in the United States.
➤ The clinical course of CLL is indolent, but as the disease progresses, chronic fatigue, recurrent or persistent infections, and easy bruising resulting from anemia, neutropenia, B-cell immunologic dysfunction, and thrombocytopenia may occur.
➤ Laboratory findings in CLL include normocytic, normochromic red cells. Lymphocytes are small or slightly larger than normal size and have a relatively mature, well-differentiated appearance. Autoimmune hemolytic anemia may precede, accompany, or follow the development of CLL and is characterized by secondary reticulocytosis, a positive direct antiglobulin test, and an elevated indirect serum bilirubin level.
➤ Differential diagnosis includes acute lymphoblastic leukemia (ALL), prolymphocytic leukemia (PLL), non-Hodgkin's lymphomas in leukemic phase, mantle cell lymphoma (MCL), small cleaved-cell lymphoma (SCCL), hairy-cell leukemia (HCL), Sézary syndrome, T-cell large granular lymphocytic leukemia, and reactive lymphocytosis.
➤ Currently there is no curative therapy for CLL. The goal of treatment is to reduce the signs and symptoms of disease with minimal discomfort to the patient. Forms of treatment may include chemotherapy, radiation therapy, splenectomy, intravenous gammaglobulin to prevent bacterial infections, and the immunosuppressant drug cyclosporine, which aids in prevention and treatment of red cell aplasia.
➤ The clinical course of chronic myelogenous

leukemia (CML) may be symptomatic or asymptomatic. Common complaints attributable to anemia include weakness, fatigue, dizziness, headache, fever, and irritability. Complaints resulting from hypermetabolic state include excessive perspiration, night sweats and weight loss, bone tenderness, and aching.

➤ Laboratory findings in CML may contain an excess of myeloid cells, extreme leukocytosis (more than 100, 000 cells/L), thrombocytosis, eosinophilia, basophilia, and giant platelets. Normocytic, normochromic anemia varies in degree but is frequently associated with hemoglobin levels below 10 g/dL.

➤ CML must be distinguished from polycythemia vera, essential thrombocythemia, and agnogenic myeloid metaplasia. The presence of the Philadelphia (Ph) chromosome or *BCR* rearrangement and low to absent lactic dehydrogenase (LAP) activity are pathognomonic for CML.

➤ Treatment for CML is to reduce the proliferating myeloid mass and relieve symptoms of hyperleukocytosis, thrombocytosis, and splenomegaly. The only curative treatment for CML is bone marrow transplantation. The cure is defined as a persistence of Ph-negative and *BCR/ABL*–negative cells.

References

1. Bennett, JM, et al: The French American British (FAB) Cooperative Group: Proposals for the classification of chronic (mature) B and T lymphoic malignancies. J Clin Pathol 42:567, 1989.
2. Gallo, RC, et al: Association of type C retrovirus with a subset of adult T-cell cancers. Cancer Res 43:3892, 1983.
3. Popovic, RC, et al: Isolation and transmission of human retrovirus. Science 219:856, 1983.
4. Poisez, BJ, et al: Detection and isolation of type C-retrovirus particles from fresh and cultured lymphocytes with cutaneous T-cell lymphoma. Proc Natl Acad Sci USA 77:7415, 1980.
5. Garver, FA, et al: Characterization of a human retrovirus from cultured chronic lymphocytic leukemia B-cells [abstract]. Blood 64:202, 1984.
6. Mann, DL, et al: HTLV-I associated B-cell CLL: Indirect role for retrovirus in leukemogenesis. Science 236:1103, 1987.
7. O'Brien, S, et al: Advances in the biology and treatment of B-cell chronic lymphocytic leukemia. Blood 85:307, 1995.
8. Korsmeyer, SJ: BCL-2 gene family and the regulators of programmed cell death. Cancer Res 59:1693, 1999.
9. McConkey, DJ, et al: Apoptosis sensitivity in chronic lymphocytic leukemia is determined by endogenous endonuclease content and related expression of BCL-2 and BAX. J Immunol 156:2624, 1996.
10. Raghobier, S, et al: Oncogene rearrangements in chronic B-cell leukemia. Blood 77:1560, 1991.
11. Rozman, C, and Montserrat, E: Chronic lymphocytic leukemia. N Engl J Med 333:1052, 1995.
12. Chikkappa, G, et al: Pure red cell aplasia in patients with chronic lymphocytic leukemia. Medicine 65:339, 1986.
13. Kipps, TJ, Carson, DA: Autoantibodies in CLL and related systemic autoimmune diseases. Blood 81:2475, 1993.
14. Melo, JV, et al: Splenic B cell lymphoma with circulating villous lymphocytes: Differential diagnosis of B cell leukaemias with large spleens. J Clin Pathol 40:642, 1987.
15. Kishimoto, T, and Kikutani, H: B-cell antigens. In Kishimoto, T (ed): Leukocyte Typing VI: White Cell Differentiation Antigens. Garland Publishing, New York, 1998, p 125.
16. Conley, CL, et al: Genetic factors predisposing to chronic lymphocytic leukemia and to autoimmune disease. Medicine 5:323, 1980.
17. Caligaris-Cappio, F, et al: Lineage relationship of chronic lymphocytic leukemia and hairy cell leukemia with TPA. Leuk Res 8:567, 1984.
18. Berek, C, and Milstein, C: Mutation drift and repertoire shift in the maturation of the immune response. Immunol Rev 96:23, 1997.
19. Gray, D: Immunological memory. Ann Rev Immunol 11:49, 1993.
20. Oscier, DG, et al: Differential rates of somatic hypermutation in V_H genes
21. Ikematsu, W, et al: Surface phenotype and Ig heavy-chain gene usage in chronic B-cell leukemias and expression of myelomonocytic markers in CD5⁻ chronic B-cell leukemia. Blood 83:2602, 1994.
22. Shapiro, JL, et al: CD5⁻ B-cell lymphoproliferative disorder presenting in blood and bone marrow. Am J Clin Pathol 111:477, 1999.
23. Newman, R, et al: Phenotypic markers and bcl-1 gene rearrangement in B-cell chronic lymphocytic leukemia: A cancer and leukemia group B study. Blood 82:1239, 1993.
24. Rouby, SE, et al: p53 Gene mutation in B-cell chronic lymphocytic leukemia is associated with drug resistance and is independent of MDR1/MDR3 gene expression. Blood 82:3452, 1993.
25. Molica, S, et al: CD11$_C$ expression in B cell CLL. Blood 81:2466, 1993.
26. Knowles, DM: Lymphoid cell markers, Am J Clin Pathol 9:85, 1985.
27. Korsmeyer, SJ: Antigen receptor genes as molecular markers of lymphoid neoplasms. J Clin Invest 79:1291, 1987.
28. Foroni, L, et al: Rearrangement of the T-cell receptor delta genes in human T-cell leukemias. Blood 73:559, 1989.
29. Dimond, P: About PCR. Diagnostics and clinical testing. Lab Med 27:12, 1989.
30. Stevenson, MS, et al: Detection of occult follicular lymphoma by specific DNA amplification. Blood 72:1822, 1988.
31. Crescenzi, M, et al: Thermostable DNA polymerase chain amplification of t(14;18) chromosome breakpoints and detection of minimal residual disease. Proc Natl Acad Sci USA 85:4869, 1988.
32. Spier, CM, et al: Chronic lymphocytic leukemia in young adults. Am J Clin Pathol 84:675, 1985.
33. Johnson, LE: Chronic lymphocytic leukemia. Am Fam Physician 38:167, 1988.
34. Conlan, MG, and Mosher, DF: Concomitant chronic lymphocytic leukemia, acute myeloid leukemia, and thrombosis with protein C deficiency. Cancer 63:1398, 1989.
35. Rai, KR, et al: Clinical staging of chronic lymphocytic leukemia. Blood 46:216, 1975.
36. Binet, JL, et al: A clinical staging system for chronic lymphocytic leukemia. Cancer 48:198, 1981.
37. Binet, JL, et al: Chronic lymphocytic leukemia: Proposals for a revised prognostic staging system. Br J Haematol 48:365, 1981.
38. Binet, JL, et al: Chronic lymphocytic leukemia: Recommendations for diagnosis, staging and response criteria, International workshop on CLL. Ann Intern Med 110:236, 1989.
39. Chenson, BD, et al: Revised guidelines for the diagnosis and treatment for CLL: Recommendations of the NCI-sponsored working group. Blood 87:4990, 1996.
40. Harris, N, et al: A revised European-American classification of lymphoid neoplasms: A proposal from the International Lymphoma Study Group. Blood 84:1361, 1994.
41. Rowley, JD, and Testa, JR: Chromosomal abnormalities in malignant hematologic diseases. Adv Cancer Res 36:103, 1982.
42. Knuutila, S, et al: Trisomy 12 in B cells of patients with B-cell chronic lymphocytic leukemia. N Engl J Med 314:865, 1986.
43. Que, TH, et al: Trisomy 12 in chronic lymphocytic leukemia detected by fluorescence in situ hybridization: Analysis by stage, immunophenotype and morphology. Blood 82:571, 1993.
44. Kalachikov, S, et al: Cloning and gene mapping of the chromosome 13q14 region detected in chronic lymphocytic leukemia. Genomics 42:369, 1997.
45. Gaidano, G, et al: Analysis of alterations of oncogenes and tumor suppressor genes in chronic lymphocytic leukemia. Am J Pathol 144:1312, 1994.
46. Croce, CM, and Kloin, G: Chromosome translocations and human cancer. Science 3:54, 1985.
47. Dohner, H, et al: Chromosome aberrations in B-cell chronic lymphocytic leukemia: Reassessment based on molecular genetic analysis. J Mol Med 77:266, 1999.
48. Athan, E, et al: Bcl-1 rearrangement: frequency and clinical significance among B cell chronic lymphocytic leukemia and non-Hodgkin's lymphoma. Am J Clin Pathol 138:501, 1991.
49. Dyer, MJS, et al: BC1–2 translocations in leukemias of mature B cells. Blood 83:3682, 1994.
50. Miyashita, T, and Reed, JC: BCL-2 oncoprotein blocks chemotherapy-induced apoptosis in a human leukemia cell line. Blood 81:151, 1993.
51. Campos, L, et al: Effects of bcl–2 antisense oligodeoxynucleotides on in vitro proliferation and survival of normal marrow progenitors and leukemic cells. Blood 84:595, 1994.
52. Korsmeyer, SJ: Immunoglobulin gene rearrangement and cell surface antigen expression in acute lymphocytic leukemias of T-cell and B-cell precursor origins. J Clin Invest 71:301, 1983.
53. Montserrat, E, et al: Lymphocyte doubling time in chronic lymphocytic leukaemia: Analysis of its prognostic significance. Br J Haematol 62:567, 1986.
54. Rozman, C, and Montserrat, E: Bone marrow histologic pattern-the single best prognostic parameter in chronic lymphocytic leukemia: A multivariate survival analysis of 329 cases. Blood 64:642, 1984.
55. Koller, CA, and Keating, MJ: New therapies for chronic lymphocytic leukemia. In Brenner, MK, and Hoffbrand, AV (eds): Recent Advances in Hematology, vol 8. Churchill Livingstone, New York, p 65, 1996.
56. Faguet, GB: Chronic lymphocytic leukemia: An updated review. J Clin Oncol 12:1974, 1994.

57. Galton, DA: Terminal transformation in B-cell chronic lymphocytic leukemia. Bone Marrow Transplant 4:156, 1989.
58. Foon, KA, et al: Transformation of chronic lymphocytic leukemia as a model. Ann Intern Med 119:63, 1993.
59. Matolcsky, A, et al: Molecular genetic demonstration of the diverse evolution of Richter's syndrome (chronic lymphocytic leukemia and subsequent large cell lymphoma). Blood 83:1363, 1994.
60. Imamura, J, et al: p53 in hematologic malignancies. Blood 84:2412, 1994.
61. Gaidano, G, et al: p53 mutation in human lymphoid malignancies associated with Burkitt's lymphoma and chronic lymphocytic leukemia. Proc Natl Acad Sci USA 88:5413, 1991.
62. Fenaux, P, et al: Mutations of the p53 gene in B-cell CLL. A report of 39 cases with cytogenetic analysis. Leukemia 6:246, 1993.
63. El Ronby, S, et al: p53 gene mutation in B-cell chronic lymphocytic leukemia is associated with drug resistance and is independent of MDR1/MDR3 gene expression. Blood 82:3452, 1993.
64. Wattel, E, et al: p53 mutations are associated with resistance to chemotherapy and short survival in hematological malignancies. Blood 84:3148, 1994.
65. Foon, KA, et al: Chronic lymphocytic leukemia: New insights into biology and therapy. Ann Intern Med 113:525, 1990.
66. Meloni, G, et al: Chronic lymphocytic leukemia: From palliative therapy to curative intent. Haematologica 83:660, 1998.
67. Hansen, MM, et al: CHOP versus prednisolone + chlorambucil in chronic lymphocytic leukemia (CLL): Preliminary results of a randomized multicenter study. Nouv Rev Fr Hematol 3:433, 1988.
68. O'Brien, S, et al: Results of fludarabine and prednisone therapy in 264 patients with CLL with multivariate analysis–derived prognostic model for response to treatment. Blood 82:1695, 1993.
69. Richards, F, et al: The control of chronic lymphocytic leukemia with mediastinal irradiation. Am J Med 64:947, 1978.
70. Yam, LT, and Crosby, WH: Early splenectomy in lymphoproliferative disorders. Arch Intern Med 133:270, 1974.
71. Cooperative Group for the Study of Immunoglobulin in CLL: Intravenous immunoglobulin for the prevention of infection in CLL. N Engl J Med 319:902, 1988.
72. Bunch, C: Immunoglobulin replacement in chronic lymphocytic leukemia. Nouv Rev Fr Hematol 30:419, 1988.
73. Grossbord, ML, et al: Serotherapy of B-cell neoplasms with anti-B4 blocked ricin: A phase I trial of daily bolus infusion. Blood 79:576, 1992.
74. Osterborg, A, et al: Phase II multicenter study of human CD52 antibody in previously treated chronic lymphocytic leukemia. European study group of CAMPATH-1H treatment in chronic lymphocytic leukemia. J Clin Oncol 15:1567, 1997.
75. Bowen, AL, et al: Subcutaneous CAMPATH-1H in fludarabine-resistant/relapsed chronic lymphocytic leukemia and B-prolymphocytic leukemia. Br J Haematol 96:617, 1997.
76. Pangalis, GA, and Griva, E: Recombinant alpha-2b-interferon therapy in untreated, stages A and B chronic lymphocytic leukemia. Cancer 61:869, 1988.
77. Rozman, C, et al: Recombinant α_2-interferon in the treatment of B chronic lymphocytic leukemia in early stages. Blood 71:1295, 1988.
78. Kay, NE, et al: Evidence for tumor reduction in refractory or relapsed B-CLL patients with infusional interleukin-2. Nouv Rev Fr Hematol 30:475, 1988.
79. Dighiero, G, et al: Chlorambucil in indolent chronic lymphocytic leukemia. N Engl J Med 338:1506, 1998.
80. Michallet, M, et al: HLA-identical sibling bone marrow transplantation in younger patients with chronic lymphocytic leukemia. European group for blood and marrow transplantation and the international bone marrow transplant registry. Ann Intern Med 124:311, 1996.
81. Khouri, IF, et al: Allogeneic blood and marrow transplantation for chronic lymphocytic leukemia: Timing of transplantation and effect of fludarabine on acute graft-versus-host disease. Br J Haematol 97:466, 1997.
82. Provan, D, et al: Eradication of polymerase chain reaction–detectable chronic lymphocytic leukemia cells is associated with improved outcome after bone marrow transplantation. Blood 88:2228, 1996.
83. Khouri, I, et al: Transplant-lite: Induction of graft-versus-malignancy using fludarabine-based nonablative chemotherapy and allogeneic blood-progenitor-cell transplantation as treatment for lymphoid malignancy. J Clin Oncol 16:2817, 1998.
84. Galton, DAG, et al: Prolymphocytic leukemia. Br J Haematol 27:7, 1974.
85. Katayama, I, et al: B-lineage prolymphocytic leukemia as a distinct clinical pathological entity. Am J Pathol 99:399, 1980.
86. Lampert, I, et al: Histopathology of prolymphocytic leukemia with particular reference to the spleen: A comparison with chronic lymphocytic leukemia. Histopathology 4:3, 1980.
87. Melo, JV, et al: The relationship between chronic lymphocytic leukemia and prolymphocytic leukemia. I. Clinical and laboratory features of 300 patients and characterization of an intermediate group. Br J Haematol 63:377, 1986.
88. Villalona-Calero, M, et al: Phenotypic characteristics of prolymphocytoid transformed (CLL/PLL) chronic lymphocytic leukemia (CLL) cells. Proc Am Soc Clin Oncol 10:230, 1991.
89. Jennings, CD, and Foon, KA: Recent advances in flow cytometry: Application to the diagnosis of hematologic malignancy. Blood 90:2863, 1997.
90. Catovsky, D, and Costello, C: Cytochemistry of normal and leukemic lymphocytes: A review. Basic Appl Histochem 23:255, 1979.
91. Swerdlow, SH, et al: Centrocytic lymphoma: A distinct clinico-pathologic and immunologic entity. Am J Pathol 113:181, 1983.
92. Medeiros, LJ, et al: Association of bcl-1 rearrangements with lymphocytic lymphoma of intermediate differentiation. Blood 76:2086, 1990.
93. Williams, ME, et al: Genotypic characterization of centrocytic lymphoma: Frequent rearrangement of chromosome 11 bcl-1 locus. Blood 76:1387, 1990.
94. Coiffier, B, et al: Mantle cell lymphoma: A therapeutic dilemma. Ann Oncol 6:208, 1995.
95. Swerdlow, SH, et al: Expression of cyclin D1 protein in centrocytic/mantle cell lymphomas with and without rearrangement of the BCL-1/cyclin D1 gene. Hum Pathol 26:999, 1995.
96. Lambrechts, AC, et al: Translocation (14;18)-positive cells are present in the circulation of the majority of patients with localized (stage I and II) follicular non-Hodgkin's lymphoma. Blood 82:2510, 1994.
97. Mintzer, DM, and Hauptman, SP: Lymphosarcoma cell leukemia and other non-Hodgkin's lymphoma in leukemic phase. Am J Med 75:110, 1983.
98. Yam, LT, et al: Tartrate-resistant acid phosphatase isoenzyme in the reticulum cells of leukemic reticuloendotheliosis. N Engl J Med 284:357, 1971.
99. Visser, L, et al: Monoclonal antibodies reactive with hairy cell leukemia. Blood 74:320, 1989.
100. Catovsky, D, et al: Hairy cell leukemia (HCL) variant: An intermediate between HCL and B-prolymphocytic leukemia. Semin Oncol 11:362, 1984.
101. Melo, JV, et al: Splenic B-cell lymphoma with circulating villous lymphocytes: Differential diagnosis of B-cell leukemias with large spleens. J Clin Pathol 40:642, 1987.
102. Matutes, E, et al: The immunophenotype of splenic lymphoma with villous lymphocytes and its relevance to the differential diagnosis with other B-cell disorders. Blood 83:1558, 1994.
103. Flandrin, G, and Brouet, JC: The Sezary cell: Cytologic, cytochemical and immunologic studies. Mayo Clin Proc 49:575, 1974.
104. Bottaro, M, et al: Heteroduplex analysis of T-cell receptor γ gene arrangements for diagnosis and monitoring of cutaneous T-cell lymphomas. Blood 83:3271, 1994.
105. Poiesz, BJ, et al: Detection and isolation of type C retrovirus particles from fresh and cultured lymphocytes of a patient with cutaneous T cell lymphoma. Proc Natl Acad Sci USA 77:7415, 1980.
106. Shimoyama, M, members of the Lymphoma Study Group (1984–87): Diagnostic criteria and classification of clinical subtypes of adult T-cell leukemialymphoma. Br J Haematol 79:428, 1991.
107. Sakashita, A, et al: Mutations of the p53 gene in adult T-cell leukemia. Blood 70:477, 1992.
108. Brouet, JC, et al: Chronic lymphocytic leukemia of T-cell origin: Immunological and clinical evaluation in eleven patients. Lancet 2:890, 1975.
109. McKenna, RE, et al: Chronic lymphoproliferative disorder with unusual clinical morphological, ultrastructural and membrane surface characteristics. Am J Med 62:588, 1977.
110. Loughran, TP: Clonal diseases of large granular lymphocytes. Blood 82:1, 1993.
111. Scott, CS, et al: Disorders of the large granular lymphocytes and natural killer-associated cells. Blood 83:301, 1994.
112. Kaushik, AS, and Logue, GL: Autoimmune neutropenia. Blood 8:1984, 1993.
113. Tefferi, A, et al: Chronic natural killer cell lymphocytosis: A descriptive clinical study. Blood 84:2721, 1994.
114. Loughran, TP, et al: Treatment of LGL leukemia with oral low dose methotrexate. Blood 84:2164, 1994.
115. Bennett, JM, et al: Proposals for the classification of chronic (mature) B and T lymphoid leukemias. J Clin Pathol 42:567, 1989.
116. Kantarjian, HM, et al: Chronic myelogenous leukemia: A concise update. Blood 82:691, 1993.
117. Bennett, JH: Case of hypertrophy of the spleen and liver, in which death took place from suppuration of the blood. Edinburgh Med Surg J 64:413, 1845.
118. Craigie, D: Case of disease of the spleen in which death took place in consequence of the presence of purulent matter in the blood. Edinburgh Med Surg J 64:400, 1854.
119. Virchow, R: Weisses blut. Froiep Notizen 36:151, 1845.
120. Nowell, PC, and Hungerford, DA: A minute chromosome in human chronic granulocytic leukemia. Science 132:1497, 1960.
121. Rowley, JD: Ph-positive leukemia, including chronic myelogenous leukemia. Clin Haematol 9:55, 1980.
122. Litz, CE, et al: Duplication of small segments with the major breakpoint cluster region in chronic myelogenous leukemia. Blood 81:1567, 1993.
123. Melo, JV, et al: The abl-bcr fusion gene is expressed in chronic myeloid leukemia. Blood 81:158, 1993.
124. Chi-Sing, NG, et al: Juvenile chronic myeloid leukemia. Am J Clin Pathol 90:575, 1988.
125. Bertino, JR, et al: Chronic Myelogenous Leukemia. Leukemia Society of America: Public education and information department booklet, Jan. 1988.
126. Fialkow, PJ, et al: Chronic myelocytic leukemia: Clonal origin in a stem cell common to the granulocytic, erythrocytic, platelet and monocyte/macrophage. Am J Med 63:125, 1977.
127. Gunz, FW: Ionizing radiation and human leukemia. In Gunz, FW, and Henderson, ES (eds): Leukemia, ed 4. Grune & Stratton, New York, 1983, p 359.
128. Askoy, M, et al: Leukemia in shoeworkers exposed chronically to benzene. Blood 44:837, 1974.
129. Baikie, AG, et al: Cytogenetic studies in familial leukemias. Austral Ann Med 18:7, 1969.

130. Jacobs, EM, et al: Chromosome abnormalities in human cancer: Report of a patient with chronic myelocytic leukemia and his nonleukemic monozygotic twin. Cancer 19:869, 1966.
131. Sandberg, AA: The Chromosomes in Human Cancer and Leukemia. Elsevier, New York, 1980.
132. Caspersson, T, et al: Identification of the Philadelphia chromosome on a number 22 by quinacrine mustard fluorescence analysis. Exp Cell Res 63:238, 1970.
133. Prieto, F, et al: Identification of the Philadelphia (Ph) chromosome. Blood 35:23, 1970.
134. Dickstein, JI, and Vardiman, JW: Hematopathologic findings in the myeloproliferative disorders. Semin Oncol 22:355, 1995.
135. Oshimura, M, et al: Variant Ph translocations in CML and their incidence, including two cases with sequential lymphoid and myeloid crises. Cancer Genet Cytogenet 5:187, 1982.
136. Cork, A: Chromosomal abnormalities in leukemia. Am J Med Technol 49:703, 1983.
137. London, B, et al: A new translocation in chronic myeloid leukemia—t(4;9;22)—resulting in a masked Philadelphia chromosome. Cancer Genet Cytogenet 20:5, 1986.
138. Kantarjian, HM, et al: Characteristics of accelerated disease in chronic myelogenous leukemia. Cancer 61:1441, 1988.
139. Bishop, MJ: Cellular oncogenes and retroviruses. Ann Rev Biochem 52:301, 1984.
140. Hunter, T: Oncogenes and protooncogenes: How do they differ? J Natl Cancer Inst 73:773, 1984.
141. Groffen, J, et al: Philadelphia chromosomal breakpoints are clustered within a limited region, bcr, on chromosome 22. Cell 36:93, 1984.
142. Kurzrock, R, et al: The molecular genetics of Philadelphia chromosome-positive leukemias. N Engl J Med 319: 990, 1988.
143. Lugo, TG, et al: Tyrosine kinase activity and transformation potency of bcr-abl oncogene products. Science 250:559, 1990.
144. Voncken, JW, et al: BCR-ABL P210 and P190 cause distinct leukemia in transgenic mice. Blood 86:4603, 1995.
145. McGahon, A, et al: Bcr-abl maintains resistance of chronic myelogenous leukemia cells to apoptotic cell death. Blood 83:1179, 1994.
146. Evans, CA, et al: Activation of the Abelson tyrosine kinase activity is associated with suppression of apoptosis in hematopoietic cells. Cancer Res 53:1735, 1993.
147. Amos, TA, et al: Apoptosis in chronic myeloid leukaemia: Normal responses by progenitor cells to growth factor deprivation, X-irradiation and glucocorticoids. Br J Haematol 91:387, 1995.
148. Telzer, LL, and Concepcion, EG: Detection of the gene rearrangement in chronic myelogenous leukemia with biotinylated gene probes. Am J Clin Pathol 91:464, 1989.
149. Bemtz, M, et al: Detection of chimeric bcr-abl genes on bone marrow samples and blood smears in chronic myeloid and acute lymphoblastic leukemia by in situ hybridization. Blood 83:1922, 1994.
150. Tkachuk, DC, et al: Detection of bcr-abl fusion in chronic myelogenous leukemia by in situ hybridization. Science 250:559, 1990.
151. Guo, JQ, et al: Comparison of bcr-abl protein expression and Philadelphia chromosome analyses in chronic myelogenous leukemia patients. Am J Clin Pathol 106:442, 1996.
152. Groffen, J, et al: C-sis is translocated from chromosome 22 to chromosome 9 in chronic myelocytic leukemia. J Exp Med 158:9, 1983.
153. Doolittle, RF, et al: Simian sarcoma virus gene, v-sis is derived from the gene (or genes) encoding a platelet-derived growth factor. Science 221:275, 1983.
154. Travis, LB, et al: Ph-negative chronic granulocytic leukemia: A nonentity. Am J Clin Pathol 85:186, 1986.
155. Fitzgerald, PH, and Beard, MEJ: Ph-negative chronic myeloid leukaemia. Br J Haematol 66:311, 1987.
156. Pugh, WC, et al: Philadelphia-negative chronic myelogenous leukemia: A morphological reassessment. Br J Haemat 60:457, 1985.
157. Pane, F, et al: Neutrophilic–chronic myeloid leukemia: A distinct disease with a specific molecular marker (bcr/abl with C3A2 junction). Blood 88:2410, 1996.
158. Bennet, JM, et al: The French-American-British (FAB) Cooperative Group. Proposals for the classification of the myelodysplastic syndromes. Br J Haematol 51:189, 1982.
159. Kurzrock, R, et al: Philadelphia-negative CML without bcr rearrangement: A chronic myeloid leukemia with a distinct clinical course [abstract]. Blood 74:102, 1989.
160. Ulirsch, R: Sea-blue histiocytosis in chronic myelocytic leukemia. American Society of Clinical Pathologists Tech Sample H-4, 1985.
161. Rosner, F, et al: Leukocyte alkaline phosphatase: Fluctuations with disease status in chronic granulocytic leukemia. Arch Intern Med 130:892, 1972.
162. Gordon, MY, et al: Adhesive defects in chronic myeloid leukemia. Curr Top Microbiol Immunol 149:151, 1989.
163. Bazzoni, G, at al: Bcr/Abl expression stimulates integrin function in hematopoietic cell lines. J Clin Invest 98:521, 1996.
164. Kantarjian, HM, et al: Prolonged survival in chronic myelogenous leukemia after cytogenetic response to interferon-α therapy. Ann Intern Med 122:254, 1995.
165. Terjanian, T, et al: Clinical and prognostic features of patients with Philadelphia chromosome–positive chronic myelogenous leukemia and extramedullary disease. Cancer 59:297, 1987.
166. Sokal, JE, et al: Prognostic discrimination in "good-risk" chronic granulocytic leukemia. Blood 63:789, 1984.
167. Polli, N, et al: Characterization of blast cells in chronic granulocytic leukaemia in transformation, acute myelofibrosis and undifferentiated leukaemia. I. Ultrastructural morphology and cytochemistry. Br J Haematol 59:277, 1985.
168. San Miguel, JF, et al: Characterization of blast cells in chronic granulocytic leukaemia in transformation, acute myelofibrosis and undifferentiated leukaemia. II. Studies with monoclonal antibodies and terminal transferase. Br J Haematol 59:297, 1985.
169. Lorand-Metze, IJ, et al: Histological and cytological heterogeneity of bone marrow in Philadelphia-positive chronic myelogenous leukaemia at diagnosis. Br J Haematol 67:45, 1987.
170. Kantarjian, HM, et al: Treatment of chronic myeloid leukemia: Current status and investigational options. Blood 87:3069, 1996.
171. Goldman, JM, et al: Treatment of chronic myeloid leukemia—some topical questions. Baillieres Clin Haematol 10405, 1997.
172. Sawyers, CL: Chronic myeloid leukemia. N Engl J Med 340:1330, 1999.
173. Borten, MM, et al: 1993 progress report from the International bone marrow registry. Bone Marrow Transplant 12:97, 1993.
174. Hoyle, C, et al: Autografting for patients with chronic myelocytic leukaemia in chronic phase: An update. Br J Haematol 85:76, 1994.
175. Butturini, MM, et al: Autotransplants in chronic myelogenous leukemia: Strategies and results. Lancet 335:1244, 1990.
176. Clift, RA, et al: Treatment of chronic myeloid leukemia by marrow transplantation. Blood 82:1954, 1993.
177. Santos, GW: Problems and strategies for bone marrow transplantation in acute leukemia and chronic myelogenous leukemia. Cancer Detect Prev 12:589, 1988.
178. Apperley, JF, et al: Bone marrow transplantation for chronic myeloid leukaemia in first chronic phase: Importance of a graft-versus-leukaemia effect. Br J Haematol 69:239, 1988.
179. Goldman, JM: Allogeneic bone marrow transplantation: state of the art and future directions. Bone Marrow Transplant 4:131, 1989.
180. Champlin, R, et al: Selective CD8 depletion of donor marrow: Retention of graft-versus-leukemia effect following bone marrow transplantation for chronic myelogenous leukemia [abstract]. Blood 74:95, 1989.
181. Leemhuis, T, et al: Identification of bcr-abl-negative primitive hematopoietic progenitor cells within chronic myeloid leukemia marrow. Blood 81:801, 1993.
182. Dekter, TM, and Chang, J: New strategies for the treatment of chronic myeloid leukemia. Blood 84:673, 1994.
183. Kohler, S, et al: Application of the polymerase chain reaction to the detection of minimal residual disease after bone marrow transplantation for patients with chronic myelogenous leukemia [abstract]. Blood 74:96, 1989.
184. Synder, DS, et al: Definition of remission based on the expression of bcr-abl RNA following bone marrow transplant for chronic myelogenous leukemia in chronic phase [abstract]. Blood 74:97, 1989.
185. Lee, M, et al: Clinical usage of polymerase chain reaction to analyze the bcr/abl splicing patterns and minimal residual disease in Philadelphia chromosome–positive chronic myelogenous leukemia [abstract]. Blood 74:745, 1989.
186. Clift, RA, et al: Marrow transplantation for chronic myeloid leukemia: A randomized study comparing cyclophosphamide and total body irradiation with busulfan and cyclophosphamide. Blood 84:2036, 1994.

18 Chronic Myeloproliferative Disorders

Barbara S. Caldwell, MS, MT(ASCP)SH

OBJECTIVES

At the end of this chapter, the learner should be able to:

1. Describe the origin of myeloproliferative disorders.
2. List characteristics for chronic myeloproliferative disorders.
3. Identify the predominant abnormal erythrocyte morphology associated with idiopathic myelofibrosis.
4. Select features for myelofibrosis that distinguish it from chronic myelogenous leukemia.
5. Name conditions that may cause an absolute erythrocytosis.
6. List laboratory findings for polycythemia vera.
7. Describe the therapeutic control of polycythemia vera.
8. Select features for secondary erythrocytosis and relative erythrocytosis that distinguish them from polycythemia vera.
9. State the diagnostic criteria for essential thrombocythemia.
10. List the most common cause of reactive thrombocytosis.

► INTRODUCTION TO MYELOPROLIFERATIVE DISORDERS

Historic Perspective

The term *myeloproliferative disorders* (*MPDs*) was proposed in 1951 by Dr. William Damashek[1] to describe a closely related group of acquired, malignant disorders that share several common clinical and hematologic features. He speculated on the presence of a common myelostimulatory factor that, under certain conditions, would cause excessive proliferation of both hematopoietic cells and fibroblasts in the bone marrow. According to Damashek, this factor also appeared to activate dormant embryonal hematopoietic tissue in the spleen and liver (extramedullary hematopoiesis). Although recent discoveries regarding hematopoiesis have necessitated certain modifications to the original hypothesis, the Damashek concept of myeloproliferative syndrome has been widely accepted.

Definition and Classification

Chronic MPDs are characterized by a hypercellular bone marrow with increased quantities of one or more cellular lineages, erythrocytes, leukocytes, and platelets in the peripheral blood. The physical hallmark feature in 60% to 100% of patients is splenomegaly.

The MPDs may be subdivided into two groups: acute and chronic. The former include all the variants of acute non-lymphocytic leukemia (ANLL) that are morphologically designated according to the predominant cell type. The ANLLs have been classified according to the French-American-British (FAB) system as M0 to M7, and all are characterized by excessive proliferation of immature cells (see Chap. 16 for complete discussion of these diseases). The chronic MPDs classically embrace the clinical entities of chronic myelocytic leukemia (CML, see Chap. 17), polycythemia vera (PV), idiopathic myelofibrosis (IMF), and essential thrombocythemia (ET). (Table 18–1).

These specific myeloproliferative disorders are distinguished by the predominant cell type involved. The most prominent feature of CML is excessive production of granulocytes; in PV, overproduction of erythrocytes; and in ET, overproduction of platelets. IMF is recognized by a prominence of marrow fibrosis and extramedullary hematopoiesis in the liver and spleen. The finding of a variable amount of fibrosis may complicate any of the chronic MPDs[2] (Fig. 18–1).

The evidence for the clonal and, therefore, neoplastic nature of the MPDs is derived from cytogenetic isoenzyme studies of glucose-6-phosphate dehydrogenase (G6PD) and clonogenic assays. These studies demonstrated that the hemopoietic abnormalities arise from a neoplastic transformation of a single multipotential stem cell, a progenitor cell that is committed to differentiation of myeloid cell lines (i.e., granulocytes, monocytes, platelets, and erythrocytes). The increased sensitivity of the precursor granulocyte-macrophage, megakaryocytic, and erythroid progenitor cells to small

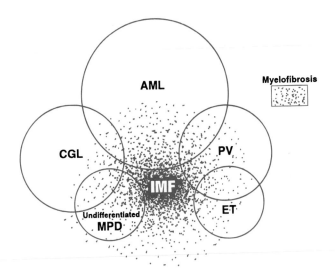

➤ FIGURE 18–1   Myelofibrosis in the myeloproliferative variants. Myelofibrosis occurs in a wide spectrum of myeloproliferative diseases, but is a predominant feature of idiopathic myelofibrosis (IMF). AML = acute myeloblastic leukemia; PV = polycythemia vera; ET = essential thrombocythemia; CGL = chronic granulocytic leukemia. (Adapted from Lewis, SM: Myelofibrosis, Pathology and Clinical Management, Hematology, vol 4. Marcel Dekker, New York, 1985, p 17.)

amounts of growth factor accounts for the variably programmed predisposition of the affected stem cells to undergo transformation into abnormal blast-forming cells, as well as the subsequent deranged production of a spectrum of mature cells. It is also conceivable that these stem cell disorders involve an inappropriate secretion of cytokines that induce abnormally low production of normal hematopoietic cells.

Marrow fibroblasts, however, do not share a common ancestry with the pluripotent hemopoietic precursor cell responsible for the hyperplasia and dysplasia that characterize each of the MPDs. Cell karyotypes and G6PD expression have both revealed the bone marrow fibroblasts to be polyclonally derived. Therefore, fibrosis is thought to reflect a reactive rather than an intrinsic neoplastic process.

There is a close qualitative and quantitative identity at the committed precursor cell level for IMF, PV, and ET, and as such, these diseases are discussed at length in this chapter. Cell culture studies have demonstrated a progression of increasing abnormality in the stem cells, from the least abnormal in PV to the intermediate abnormality in ET, to the most abnormal state in IMF. A genetic predisposition to a particular MPD is supported by the report of a family with IMF, PV, and ET in three siblings, with ET in the child of the sibling with IMF and in a cousin. The pathophysiology, clinical and laboratory findings, and therapy for each of these chronic MPD variants are reviewed in detail.

➤ COMMON CLINICAL AND HEMATOLOGIC FEATURES OF CHRONIC MYELOPROLIFERATIVE DISORDERS

All of the clinical variants of the chronic myeloproliferative disorders (CMPDs) may share, to varying extents, the following characteristics:

1. Predominantly affects middle-aged and older groups

➤ Table 18–1
MYELOPROLIFERATIVE DISORDERS (MPDs)

Acute MPDs

Acute nonlymphocytic leukemia

   Acute myeloblastic leukemia

   Acute promyelocytic leukemia

   Acute myelomonocytic leukemia

   Acute monocytic leukemia

   Erythroleukemia

Unusual variants

   Megakaryocytic leukemia

   Eosinophilic leukemia

   Basophilic leukemia

Chronic MPDs

   Chronic myelogenous leukemia

   Idiopathic myelofibrosis

   Polycythemia vera

   Essential or idiopathic thrombocythemia

2. Insidious, sometimes silent, asymptomatic onset
3. Panhyperplasia of bone marrow (granulocytic with or without monocytic, erythrocytic, and megakaryocytic elements)
4. Extramedullary hematopoiesis; myeloid metaplasia manifesting primarily in the spleen and less frequently in the liver, causing portal hypertension
5. Bone marrow fibroblastic proliferation and reticulin/collagen formation (see Fig. 18–1)
6. Frequent transitions between these disorders, with overlapping manifestations causing difficulty in classification (Fig. 18–2)
7. Increased propensity for terminating in acute leukemia
8. Bone marrow that may demonstrate large numbers of megakaryocytes, which are sometimes atypical in appearance
9. Elevation of platelet count; giant or bizarre platelets, or both
10. Hemorrhagic and thrombotic complications as a result of platelet dysfunction
11. Cytogenetic abnormalities: the most common, in decreasing order of frequency, are 20q−, +8, +9, 13q−, +6;9, +23p, +34q, and partial trisomy 1q7. (The Philadelphia chromosome +9;22 is present in about 90% of patients with CML.)
12. Molecular abnormalities: abnormal *p53* genes have been noted in the acute phase of *BCR/ABL*-negative CMPDs. Apoptosis (programmed cell death) is normally induced by the suppressor gene *p53*. In the presence of altered or absent *p53*, apoptosis does not occur, resulting in continued proliferation. Increased levels of mRNA and protein produced by the C-kit proto-oncogene (the stem cell growth factor receptor) are also noted in patients with MPDs that evolve into leukemia.

Although the CMPDs share clinical manifestations, each disorder is well defined in regard to important differences between the subtypes, pathophysiology, laboratory findings, clinical course, therapeutic options, and prognosis. A comparison of the type and amount of cellular proliferations and other specific findings in the CMPDs is provided in Table 18–2.

➤ IDIOPATHIC MYELOFIBROSIS

Definition and History

Within the family of myeloproliferative disorders, idiopathic myelofibrosis (IMF) is an important entity. The syndrome is characterized by the classic triad of findings of (1) fibrosis of the marrow, at first patchy and later widespread, that may or may not be accompanied by sclerosis; (2) extramedullary hematopoiesis or myeloid metaplasia of the spleen and liver, giving rise to moderate to marked splenomegaly and hepatomegaly; and (3) leukoerythoblastosis and teardrop poikilocytosis of the peripheral blood.

IMF was first reported in 1879 by Heuck[3], who described the case of a 24-year-old butcher who had been afflicted with severe fatigue for one year. On examination, severe anemia, leukocytosis with myeloid immaturity, and marked hepatosplenomegaly were noted. The patient survived for only 2 years and, on autopsy, was demonstrated to have severe osteosclerosis and extramedullary hematopoiesis. Heuck[3] thus concluded, based on the unique features of the case, that myelofibrosis with myeloid metaplasia was distinct from leukemia.

IMF is known by at least 20 synonyms. Some of the most frequently employed are agnogenic myeloid metaplasia, myelosclerosis, osteosclerosis, chronic erythroblastosis, aleukemic myelosis, and chronic or primary myelofibrosis. The term *idiopathic myelofibrosis with myeloid metaplasia* (*IMF/ MM*), or just *idiopathic myelofibrosis* (*IMF*) for brevity, highlights the essential features of fibrosis and extramedullary hematopoiesis.

Incidence, Epidemiology, and Etiology

There have been a limited number of epidemiologic studies in IMF. The overall annual incidence is 0.6 per 100,000 and the disease is approximately one-quarter as common as chronic myelocytic leukemia. Male-to-female ratio is approximately 2:1. The age distribution is generally between 50 and 70; therefore, as with other MPDs, most IMF cases occur in middle-aged and elderly people. Very few cases of this disorder have been reported in the below-30 age group. Certain racial factors of interest have been studied. IMF is said to be less common in individuals of African or Spanish descent. Familial CMPDs have been reported in several generations within the same family where no environmental causative agent was found. This finding suggests that a genetically inherited etiology is possible.

As the name implies, the etiology of the majority of patients with IMF is unknown. Exposure to ionizing radiation is a likely factor in the development of some cases, and myelofibrosis secondary to exposure to toxins such as benzene, toluene, arsenic, lead, and fluorine has been documented. Conditions associated with abnormal immunologic mechanisms have been implicated in the genesis of IMF, as evidenced by its development in patients with lupus erythematosus and the existence in a majority of IMF patients of a

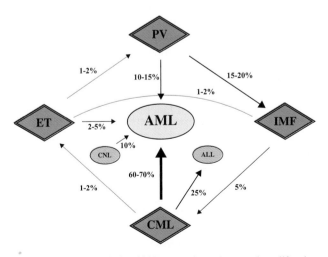

➤ **FIGURE 18–2** Relationship between the various myeloproliferative disorders. Frequencies of transitions between each of these bone marrow stem cell disorders are shown. AML = acute myeloblastic leukemia; PV = polycythemia vera; IMF = idiopathic myelofibrosis; CML= chronic myelogenous leukemia; ET = essential thrombocythemia; ALL = acute lymphoblastic leukemia; CNL = chronic neutrophilic leukemia. (A solid line indicates a strong relationship between disorders, a dashed line indicates a weak relationship.)

> **Table 18-2**
DIFFERENTIAL CHARACTERISTICS OF THE CHRONIC MYELOPROLIFERATIVE DISORDERS

	CML	Idiopathic Myelofibrosis	Polycythemia Vera	Essential Thrombocythemia
Hemoglobin	N–↓	↓	↑↑↑	N–↓
WBC count (× 10⁹/L)	> 50	Variable	12–25	Variable
Platelet count (× 10⁹/L)	Variable–↑	450–1000	450–800	600–2500
NRBCs	Common	Common	Rare	Rare
LAP	↓↓	N–↑↑	Usually ↑	N
Bone marrow	Marked myeloid hyperplasia	Fibrosis, dry tap	Hypercellular, ↑ iron stores	Hypercellular, ↑↑↑ megakaryo-cytes
Fibroblasts	None–↑	↑↑–↑↑↑	None–↑	None–↑↑
Splenomegaly (% patients)	60%–80%	80%–99%	80%	40%–50%
Blastic transformation	90%	5%–20%	10%–15%	5%
Special studies	Ph′ chromosome	Marrow imaging	RBC mass ↑, erythropoietin ↓	Abnormal platelet function tests

Abbreviations: WBC = white blood cell; NRBCs = nucleated red blood cells; LAP = leukocyte alkaline phosphatase
Reference range: WBC = 5–11 × 10⁹/L; platelets = 150–450 × 10⁹/L; N = normal; ↓ = slight decrease; ↓↓ = moderate decrease; ↑ = slight increase; ↑↑ = moderate increase; ↑↑↑ = marked increase.

high proportion of peripheral leukocytes containing immune complexes. Myelofibrosis has also occurred secondary to chronic infections, especially tuberculosis, histoplasmosis, and after myocardial infarction; however, the fibrosis seen in these disorders represents a secondary or reactive process.

Pathogenesis

Stem Cell Defect

The hemopoietic abnormalities in IMF arise from the mutation of a single multipotential stem cell, with bone marrow fibrosis occurring as a secondary, nonneoplastic process. The pathogenesis of the progenitor cell defect must be considered separately from that of the fibrosis.

The clonal proliferation of abnormal progenitor cells colony-forming unit–granulocyte/monocyte (CFU-GM) and colony-forming unit–megakaryocyte (CFU-MK) has been well documented by isoenzyme and cytogenetic studies. It has been shown that in women heterozygous for G6PD isoenzymes A and B, the bone marrow fibroblasts express both isoenzymes, but the blood cells express only one type. This finding, therefore, suggests that the blood cells are clonally derived, whereas the fibroblasts do not proliferate as a result of the malignant clone. The blood cells from an IMF patient have a consistent chromosomal abnormality, in comparison to bone marrow fibroblasts, which have abnormal karyotypes. Recently, evidence of N-ras mutation in all three hematopoietic lineages and studies using X-linked restriction length polymorphism have also confirmed that hematopoietic cells are monoclonal, whereas fibroblast proliferation is polyclonal. Thus, culture studies, isoenzyme and chromosomal analysis, and molecular diagnostic studies all clearly demonstrate that marrow fibroblasts do not share a common ancestry with hematopoietic cells.

Marrow Fibrosis

The pathogenesis of fibro-osteosclerotic changes characterizing IMF is related to an increased accumulation of mar-row collagen and the source of collagen synthesis is the fibroblasts. Hematopoietic cells, their products, or both, provide the provoking stimulus that activates the marrow collagen-producing cells, thus establishing the reactive nature of fibrosis.

A number of factors have been described that are capable of stimulating fibroblastic proliferation. There is current evidence that megakaryocytes are intimately involved in the pathway whereby increased collagen deposition takes place and as such are a prerequisite for osteosclerotic changes. Three megakaryocytic growth factors have been described that are capable of causing potent fibrotic stroma generation. The first, transforming growth factor–beta (TGF-β) recently was implicated as the most important cytokine involved in the pathogenesis of bone marrow fibrosis. TGF-β is secreted by monocytes and megakaryocytes and is capable of promoting secretion of type I and type III collagen from fibroblasts.

The second, platelet-derived growth factor (PDGF), is released from abnormal megakaryocytes and platelets undergoing intramedullary cell death. Both ineffective megakaryopoiesis and elevated levels of PDGF are found in all patients with IMF. PDGF stimulates fibroblasts to divide and secrete collagen (Fig. 18–3). Several reports postulate that immune complexes also interact with platelets to cause release of PDGF with subsequent activation of fibroblastic proliferation and collagen deposition. Studies have shown consistently impaired natural killer (NK) cells in patients with myelofibrosis. The CD16+ NK cells had detectable PDGF on their surface, and this finding correlates with significantly inhibited NK cytotoxicity.

The third megakaryocytic growth factor is basic fibroblast growth factor (bFGF), which is produced by stromal cells, megakaryocytes, and platelets. The higher the concentration of bFGF, the more advanced the phase of IMF. Basic FGF has been shown to affect megakaryocytopoiesis by modulating megakaryocyte–stromal cell interactions, leading to abnormal stimulation and proliferation of stromal cells.

The histologic course of IMF encompasses several phases.

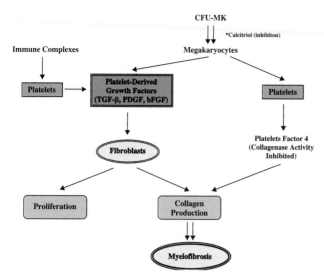

> ➤ **FIGURE 18–3** Schematic representation of possible relationships involved in collagen deposition in myelofibrosis. CFU-MF = colony-forming unit–megakaryocyte; TGF-β = transforming growth factor-beta; PDGF = platelet-derived growth factor; bFGF = basic fibroblast growth factor. * Calcitriol, $1,15(OH)_2D_3$ is the active metabolite of vitamin D_3.

In the so-called cellular phase of IMF, the bone marrow displays panhyperplasia with a predominance of megakaryocytes. As the disease progresses, there is deranged marrow architecture with an increase in reticulin (or a neutral soluble collagen type III) and a progressive change to and deposition of the type I collagen, which is insoluble and cross-linked. It is the type I collagen that occurs in osteosclerosis.

Vitamin D also appears to play a role in the regulation of collagen deposition in the marrow. Calcitriol (1,25-dihydroxyvitamin D_3), the active metabolite of vitamin D_3, inhibits collagen synthesis by suppressing megakaryocyte proliferation. A deficiency of this factor would allow abnormal accumulation of marrow collagen, hence leading to development of myelofibrosis (see Fig. 18–3). Furthermore, platelet factor 4, a cationic polypeptide synthesized by megakaryocytes and contained in platelet alpha (α) granules, inhibits collagenase activity, thereby offsetting the natural balance between marrow collagen production and degradation. This action conversely leads to enhancement of myelofibrosis.

The disturbance to the normal hemopoietic microenvironment is responsible for the hematologic abnormalities characteristic of IMF: increase in circulating stem cells, trilineage proliferation and dysplasia (particularly dysmegakaryocytopoiesis), and extravascular hematopoiesis.

Clinical Features

Myelofibrosis is a chronic progressive disorder with an insidious onset such that the patient may be symptom-free for many years. Athens and associates[4] reported a case in which a patient with a palpable spleen was known to have had the enlarged spleen for 15 years before diagnosis. In about one-third of the cases, diagnosis is made following routine physical examination and the incidental finding of unexplained splenomegaly or abnormal peripheral blood results, or both. As the myeloid metaplasia gradually increases, with eventual enlargement of the spleen and sometimes the liver, the patient presents with the customary sensation of splenomegaly.

This involves left or mid-abdominal fullness and distension and early satiety for food intake, resulting from decreased abdominal capacity due to splenic encroachment. With massive splenomegaly, urinary frequency and incontinence may be a problem. Splenomegaly is more pronounced in IMF than in almost any other disease (Fig. 18–4).

Patients also present with the signs and symptoms of anemia such as weakness, pallor, lethargy, and dyspnea on exertion. Approximately 10% of patients present with a serious bleeding diathesis secondary to thrombocytopenia or thrombocytosis, qualitative platelet defects, and coagulation abnormalities that may cause petechiae, ecchymoses, gastrointestinal or urogenital bleeding, and esophageal varices. Unusual masses of extramedullary hematopoietic tissue have been reported to occur in lymph nodes, lungs, gastrointestinal tract, kidneys, central nervous system, and skin. Severe, chronic bone pain may occur later in the disease process. Infection may ensue related to immune deficiency, even when neutropenia is absent.

The metabolic consequences of myelofibrosis often result in night sweats, fever, itching, anorexia, and weight loss. Gout may be a complication stemming from hyperuricemia and has been reported in about 15% of patients with massive splenomegaly. Although hepatomegaly is found in about 50% of patients, it is not generally excessive but may be accompanied by mild to moderate jaundice or ascites, or both.

Extramedullary Hematopoiesis

The most common location of extramedullary hematopoiesis is the liver and spleen (Fig. 18–5; see also Color Plate 207) with splenomegaly and hepatomegaly present to varying degrees. The spleen is mildly enlarged in one-third of patients, palpable 5 cm below the left costal margin in another third, and massively enlarged in the remaining third. The extraordinary splenic hyperplasia present in IMF is multifactorial in origin. The enlargement results from a combination of extramedullary hematopoiesis and fibrosis, as well as congestion from increased blood flow through the celiac axis. The exaggeration of red cell pooling is so pronounced that up to two-thirds of the red cell mass may be detained in transit through the splenic cords. Hematopoietic precursors evicted from the bone marrow find a hospitable surrogate microenvironment in the spleen and, to some extent, in the liver and

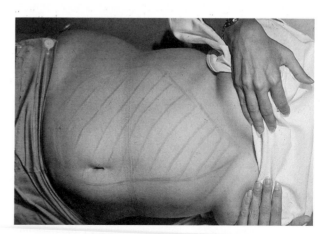

> ➤ **FIGURE 18–4** Hepatosplenomegaly, a characteristic finding in patients with idiopathic myelofibrosis with myeloid metaplasia (IMF/MM).

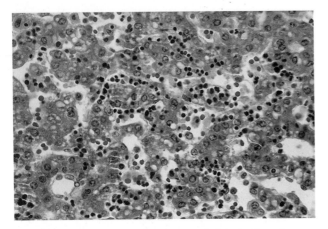

> **FIGURE 18–5** Extramedullary hematopoiesis in the liver of a patient with IMF.

lymph nodes. Stem cells capable of self-renewal give rise to neoplastic islands that may circulate via the splenic vein to other reticuloendothelial system organs. Extramedullary tumors may occasionally arise in the central nervous system, accounting for symptoms of speech impairment, semiblindness, partial paralysis, coma, and possibly death if the intracranial space has been invaded. Extramedullary hematopoiesis has also reportedly involved the thorax, breast, kidneys, heart, and adrenal glands.

Radiologic Features

Myelofibrosis is defined as an increase in fine fibers (reticular) in the marrow; *myelosclerosis* means an increase in coarse fibers (collagen), and *osteomyelosclerosis* refers to

new bone formation. Approximately 40% to 50% of patients demonstrate radiologic osteosclerosis using computed tomographic (CT) examination. The most readily recognizable pattern is a diffuse increase in bone density in the long bones, which is readily visible on chest x-ray examinations in most cases.

Hematologic Features

A normocytic, normochromic anemia is often found at presentation and becomes more severe as the myelofibrosis progresses. The anemia results from a complex reaction of factors representing the additive effects of bone marrow failure, ineffective or dyserythropoiesis, pooling of over 35% of the erythrocyte mass in the enlarged spleen (dilutional anemia), and an underlying hemolysis caused by hypersplenism.

The morphological changes become increasingly abnormal, and the classic leukoerythroblastic blood picture unfolds (Fig. 18–6). The characteristic findings are the appearance of abundant nucleated red cells, immature granulocytes, and teardrop poikilocytosis in the peripheral blood (Fig. 18–7). Improvement or even normalization of red cell morphology after splenectomy supports the concept of a causative relationship between splenic fibrosis and red cell changes. Marrow fibrosis in conjunction with splenic fibrosis presumably account for teardrop formation, as the erythrocytes assume the teardrop shape upon passage through narrow, fibrotic sinusoids of the bone marrow and spleen (Fig. 18–8).

In half of the anemic patients, there is shortened red cell survival, resulting from the ineffective erythropoiesis combined with hyperplasia. Severe hemolytic anemia develops in 15% of cases and is evidenced by marked reticulocytosis. It is generally antiglobulin (Coombs) test–negative,

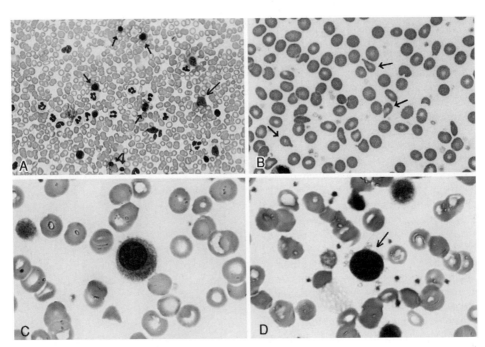

> **FIGURE 18–6** Leukoerythroblastosis, teardrop poikilocytosis, and abnormal platelet morphology associated with idiopathic myelofibrosis. *A.* Leukoerythroblastosis. Note the myeloblast at the large arrow and the numerous nucleated red blood cells at the small arrows. *B.* Teardrop poikilocytosis. *C.* Dwarf megakaryocyte (or micromegakaryocyte). This pathologic alteration of a megakaryocyte may be found in any of the myeloproliferative disorders. Although often difficult to distinguish from cells of other lineages, observation of the marked cytoplasmic granularity and further comparison of this cytoplasm to that of other platelets present on the peripheral smear will aid in identification. *D.* Dwarf megakaryocyte. The cell at the pointer displays cytoplasmic blebs or budding, which is another characteristic of a micromegakaryocyte. Also note the giant platelets present on this peripheral blood smear.

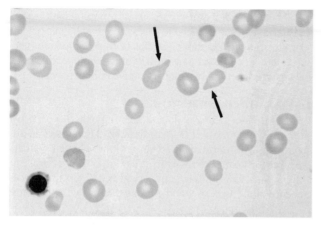

➤ FIGURE 18–7 Teardrop-shaped cells (*arrows*): peripheral blood in a patient with myelofibrosis.

however, in some cases of IMF the erythrocytes are mildly Coombs-positive. This is because of deposition of immunoglobulin G (IgG), IgM, or complement immune complexes on the erythrocyte surfaces. Occasionally patients develop a hypochromic, microcytic anemia secondary to gastrointestinal bleeding or peptic ulcer, and sometimes the hyperproliferative state induces folate deficiency and a concomitant megaloblastic macrocytosis.

The leukocyte count is variable in IMF. In about 50% of cases the white blood cell (WBC) count exceeds 10.0×10^9/L; in approximately 35%, the WBC count is normal; and in nearly 15%, the WBC count is below normal. As the disease evolves, the leukocyte level declines, with an increase of immature myeloid cells dominating the peripheral blood picture, but not to the degree seen in acute myelocytic leukemia. In rare cases in which the WBC count exceeds 100×10^9/L, the diagnosis of CML may be erroneously applied. The leukocyte alkaline phosphatase (LAP) score is typically normal or moderately increased. Serum levels of vitamin B_{12} are increased, but not to the degree found in untreated CML. Eosinophils and basophils may also be increased in number in many patients.

The platelet count may be normal, elevated, or decreased. In approximately 50% of IMF patients, platelet counts are increased to between 450 to 1000×10^9/L at time of diagnosis, and the concentration may be occasionally in excess of 1000×10^9/L. As the disease progresses, thrombocytopenia becomes increasingly prevalent. Giant dysplastic platelets are often conspicuous, and megakaryocytic fragments or even dwarf megakaryocytes may be present in the peripheral blood (see Fig. 18–6). These findings attest to malignant platelet physiology and support the correlation of platelet dysfunction found in up to 50% of patients. Platelet adhesiveness is often reduced and, conversely, spontaneous aggregation may occur, clinically resulting in increased risk of hemorrhage or thrombosis. The bleeding time (a measure of platelet number and function) is prolonged in up to 20% of patients, which is particularly important in relation to gastrointestinal or cerebral hemorrhage.

If a patient has undergone splenectomy, the amount of immature WBCs, bizarre red cells, and platelet morphology increases, because even infiltrated spleens help correct the marrow's mistakes.

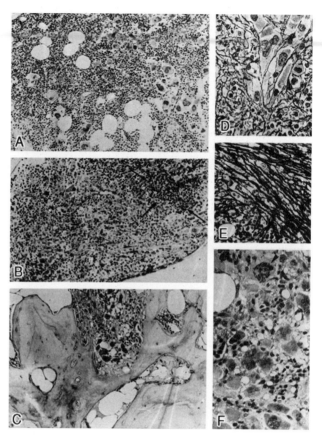

➤ FIGURE 18–8 Histopathology of the bone marrow in idiopathic myelofibrosis. *A.* Early hyperplastic state without fibrosis. *B.* Advanced stage with a conspicuous increase in reticulin fibers, a still hypercellular marrow, and a lymphoid infiltrate (*arrows*). *C.* Late osteosclerotic state with endophytic bone formation, a residual cluster of hematopoiesis, and large areas of fatty tissue. *D.* Moderate degree of reticulin fibers surrounding atypical megakaryocytes in early IMF. *E.* Coarse bundles of obvious collagen fibers encompassing a few hematopoietic elements in terminal stages of IMF. *F.* Clusters of pleomorphic megakaryocytes displaying an abnormal maturation and mitosis (*arrowhead*). *A–C,* magnification ×140; *D–F,* ×350. *A–C* and *F,* periodic acid–Schiff (PAS) stain; *D* and *E,* Gomori's silver impregnation. (From Thiele, J, et al. Primary myelofibrosis-osteosclerosis, agnogenic myeloid metaplasia. AntiCa Res 9:430, 1989, with permission.)

Bone Marrow Findings

Attempts at bone marrow aspirations are unsuccessful in nearly 90% of patients, resulting in the so-called dry tap of myelofibrosis. The reticulin and collagen fibrosis locks in the marrow contents, making a needle biopsy essential for a reliable diagnosis (see Fig. 18–8). Trilineage hyperplasia is found early in the disease, along with nonuniform fibrosis (Table 18–3). At later stages, there is decreasing number of hematopoietic islands, with residual foci consisting mainly of clumps of dysplastic megakaryocytes. Finally, marked hypocellularity is observed, and fibrotic features begin to predominate. Osteosclerosis (new bone deposition) is common, occurring in about 40% of patients. The bone marrow hypocellularity and peripheral blood pancytopenia prevail because the myeloid metaplasia does not compensate for the loss of bone marrow function resulting from the marrow fibrosis.

Coagulation Abnormalities

Platelet dysfunction (mentioned earlier) can cause troublesome hemostatic complications in IMF patients. Both hy-

> Table 18-3
HISTOLOGIC COURSE OF IDIOPATHIC MYELOFIBROSIS AS SEEN IN BONE MARROW

Cellular Phase

Diffusely hyperplastic; normal maturation of erythropoiesis and granulopoiesis

Megakaryocytes may predominate; some immature forms

Reticulin ± increase

Fibrotic Phase

Megakaryocytes still predominant; decreasing number of other hemopoietic cells

Altered sinus architecture

Reticulin ++

Collagen +

Sclerotic Phase

Grossly disturbed architecture

Markedly reduced hematopoiesis

Megakaryocyte and megakaryoblast clusters

Fibroblasts +++

Reticulin +++

Collagen +++

Osteosclerotic Phase

Fibroblasts +++

Collagen +++

Osteocyte proliferation with bone formation

Source: Lewis, SM: Myelofibrosis, Pathology and Clinical Management, Hematology, vol 4. Marcel Dekker, New York, 1985, p. 4, with permission.

poplatelet and hyperplatelet function has been reported, with hypofunction seen more often. In addition, patients in approximately half of the cases demonstrate prolonged prothrombin and thrombin times, as well as elevated levels of fibrin degradation products and reduced levels of factors V and VIII. These features suggest occult disseminated intravascular coagulation (DIC). Hepatic dysfunction is found in many patients in the later stages of the disease, setting the scene for coagulation factor deficiencies, chronic DIC, and fibrinolytic activation.

Miscellaneous Findings

Most patients possess some type of chromosome abnormality; particularly common are deletions of chromosomes 13q−, 20q−, 5q−, and 7q−. Monosomy, trisomy, and translocation abnormalities are also common, notably t(1;13). Patients in the blastic phase of IMF have been reported to have molecular aberrations of *p53* or *RAS* mutations.

Hyperuricemia and elevated liver enzymes are found in one-third of IMF patients. Circulating anti-Gal antibodies directed against a terminal galactosyl α(1,3) galactose molecules have been shown to increase in correlation with disease activity and may provide a future sensitive tool to detect IMF.

Monoclonal antibodies to epitopes of procollagen types I and III have been produced to assess active collagen synthesis in the tissue. A serum assay has been developed to measure the concentration of type III collagen propeptides. An increased concentration suggests active collagen synthesis.

Differential Diagnosis

Idiopathic myelofibrosis must be distinguished from other diseases within the spectrum of the CMPDs, as well as differentiated from fibrosis secondary to infiltrative disorders (see Tables 18–2 and 18–4).

The American Polycythemia Vera Study Group has defined myelofibrosis as encompassing the following features:

1. Splenomegaly
2. Fibrosis involving more than one-third of the sectional area of an adequate bone marrow biopsy specimen
3. A leukoerythroblastic blood picture
4. Absence of increased red cell mass
5. Absence of Philadelphia (Ph) chromosome
6. Exclusion of systemic disorders
7. A diagnosis of osteomyelosclerosis requiring the presence of sclerotic changes detected radiologically in axial skeleton long bones[5]

CML is the diagnosis considered most frequently in the differential diagnosis of IMF. In chronic cases of CML, there is marked leukocytosis, whereas in IMF the WBC

> Table 18-4
DIFFERENTIAL DIAGNOSIS OF MYELOFIBROSIS

Idiopathic Myelofibrosis

Other Chronic Myeloproliferative Disorders

Chronic myelogeneous leukemia

Polycythemia vera

Essential thrombocythemia

Transitional myeloproliferative disorders

Secondary to Infiltrative Disorders

Metastatic carcinoma

Hematologic malignancies involving bone marrow

Acute leukemia

Myelodysplastic syndromes (preleukemia)

Hairy-cell leukemia

Non-Hodgkin's lymphoma

Myeloma

Secondary to Nonmalignant Conditions

Granulomatous disorders	Osteoporosis
Sarcoidosis	Vitamin D deficiency
Tuberculosis	Systemic lupus erythematosus
Histoplasmosis	Systemic sclerosis
Toxic exposure to chemicals	
Hypo- and hyperparathyroidism	

count is usually less than 30×10^9/L. Red cell morphology in CML is generally normal or may show a slight amount of anisocytosis and poikilocytosis, compared with the significant teardrop poikilocytosis in IMF. The presence of the Ph and LAP score are the strongest differentiating features that distinguish CML from IMF. Ordinarily, differentiation from CML is not difficult. However, in atypical cases such as Ph-negative CML, it may be virtually impossible to characterize CML as a separate entity from IMF with leukocytosis and minimal fibrosis (the cellular phase of IMF).

Approximately 15% to 20% of patients with known PV undergo a transition to terminal myelofibrosis with marked anemia, bone marrow fibrosis and hypofunction, and progressive splenomegaly. An intermediate or transitional myeloproliferative disease has been described as occurring in a group of patients with polycythemic peripheral blood counts and concomitant features of myelofibrosis, including myeloid metaplasia, leukoerythroblastic blood picture, and extensive reticulin/collagen fibrosis of the marrow. This subset of transitional patients seems to remain in a steady state for several years, whereas patients in the terminal post-PV spent phase of myelofibrosis undergo a more aggressive course.

Idiopathic myelofibrosis must be differentiated from secondary causes of myelofibrosis. Metastatic carcinoma and lymphoma are frequent causes of fibrosis. Granulomatous disorders such as tuberculosis, histoplasmosis, or sarcoidosis of the marrow can cause myelofibrosis. Other hematologic diseases, including acute leukemia, hairy-cell leukemia, autoimmune diseases, and myelodysplastic syndromes, may induce secondary fibrosis (see Table 18–4). The cause of the infiltrative disorders can usually be established by careful scrutiny of the blood and bone marrow for evidence of abnormal cells that characterize the disease, by use of microbiologic cultures and other diagnostic tests such as chest x-rays or skin tests. In certain situations (such as when a patient has acute leukemia), techniques of cytochemistry, immunologic surface markers, electron microscopy studies, and chromosomal analysis may help to define the nature of the malignancy.

Treatment

The primary aim of treatment in IMF is to improve the quality of life, because few patients with IMF have been cured. Approximately 30% of patients will be asymptomatic at diagnosis. Experimental therapies to prevent the progression of myelofibrosis are being investigated. Eventually, most patients manifest symptoms caused by anemia, splenic enlargement, bleeding, bone pain, or hypermetabolism. Treatment for these complications is palliative, and invasive procedures should be limited.

One of the major problems requiring therapy is anemia. It has been estimated that 60% of IMF patients manifest signs of anemia during their clinical course. Transfusion dependence develops as the anemia becomes more severe. In most cases, the anemia is normochromic and normocytic, whereas 5% of patients develop iron-deficiency anemia, and rare patients demonstrate folate or vitamin B_{12} deficiency. When nutritional deficiencies are suspected, patients are treated with iron, folate, or pyridoxine as appropriate. If inefficient erythropoiesis is the predominant mechanism, androgen therapy is indicated. However, approximately 40% of anemic individuals respond to androgen therapy and should be given a trial of either oxymetholone (50 to 200 mg orally daily) or testos-

terone enanthate (400 mg intramuscularly every 3 to 4 weeks). Patients receiving oxymetholone require careful monitoring of liver function tests. Patients with thrombocytopenia may be treated with adrenal steroids. About 50% of patients respond to the combination of androgen and glucocorticoid therapy (prednisone, 30 mg daily). Long-term treatment may have annoying side effects, particularly fluid retention and hirsutism (excessive unusual growth of hair, especially in women).

The main aim of treatment in patients with progressive splenomegaly is to remove the spleen or reduce its size, thereby relieving the severe pain caused by pressure and ameliorating the constitutional symptoms of serious digestive disturbances, weight loss, and diarrhea. Although there is no general agreement on the indications and value of this invasive modality, splenectomy is important in the management of IMF patients with profoundly enlarged spleens. The main problem is that patients with symptoms that can be relieved by splenectomy are poor surgical risks. Timing for a splenectomy operation is difficult, and the postoperative complication rate is above average.

Four major life-threatening conditions have been espoused as situations warranting consideration of splenectomy[6]:

1. Painful splenic enlargement, unresponsive to irradiation
2. Severe refractory hemolytic or dilutional anemia sufficient to cause cardiopulmonary symptoms
3. Severe life-threatening thrombocytopenia
4. Portal hypertension with bleeding varices

Whenever splenectomy is contemplated, an extensive coagulation workup is necessary, because bleeding is a major hazard.

Because the spleen may become the major hematopoietic organ in patients whose marrow has been replaced by fibrosis, it is vital to ensure that splenectomy is considered only in patients when splenic hemopoiesis contributes a minor (less than 15% to 20%) proportion of total hematopoiesis. This situation can be quantified by bone imaging and measurement of transferrin-bound ^{52}Fe uptake. Mean survival following splenectomy is approximately 25 months. This procedure does not seem to alter the overall clinical course, and the mortality and morbidity, estimated at 10%, are mainly the result of bleeding, thromboembolism, and infection (the same causes as in patients who have not had splenectomy). After splenectomy, approximately 16% of patients develop a compensatory myeloid metaplasia of the liver, further increasing the amount of hepatomegaly.

Chemotherapy is an alternative to splenectomy, reducing spleen size and controlling thrombocytosis, but it has little or no beneficial effect on the anemia. The alkylating agents busulfan (2 to 4 mg daily) or chlorambucil (4 to 6 mg daily) and hydroxyurea (500 mg daily) have been used. Unfortunately, reports have confirmed the leukemogenic potential for hydroxyurea used in treatment of patients with MPDs. Other additional agents, such as radiophosphate and 6-thioguanine, have also been advocated. If antitumor therapy is used, the treatment must be strictly monitored by regular blood counts to avoid inducing dangerous cytopenias in the patient.

Radiation therapy is also considered in patients with massive mechanical splenomegaly, although, as with the use of chemotherapy, the duration of the reduction in splenic size is usually measured in months. In patients having acute splenic infarction, ascites demonstrating prominent megakaryocytosis, or focal, but severe bone pain, the use of radiation may produce gratifying effects.

Allogeneic marrow transplantation following ablative chemotherapy and radiotherapy has been attempted in a few patients and offers a rational means for curing myelofibrosis. However, it is controversial whether or not the application of this rigorous therapy to a chronic disease, generally limited to the elderly, is judicious. Disappearance of fibrosis and regeneration of normal medullary hematopoiesis has been achieved in responsive patients.

Another significant approach to the treatment of myelofibrosis is the utilization of antifibrosing agents such as penicillamine or colchicine. Biochemically, as myelofibrosis progresses, there is increasing conversion of soluble to insoluble collagen. Penicillamine interferes with the cross-linkage of collagen and, therefore, with its use, a decrease in fibrous tissue occurs. It is still unclear whether penicillamine has a significant effect on the natural course of this disease. Colchicine appears to cause its antifibrosing effect through two mechanisms: (1) it produces a decreased rate of procollagen, and (2) it increases the secretion of collagenases. New agents called lathyrogens, such as β-aminoproprionitrile, are being studied and show promise in blocking the cross-linking of collagen by inhibiting the copper-dependent enzyme important in collagen cross-linking.

Recently, interferon α has been used to prevent the progression of myelofibrosis to blastic transformation, allowing patients to maintain a remission status without allogenic bone marrow transplantation. Lastly, allopurinol therapy is warranted in almost all patients to prevent the hyperuricemia from progressing to gout or urate nephropathy.

Prognosis

Patients with IMF comprise extremely heterogeneous populations, and survival varies considerably. Median survival is approximately 5 years from the time of diagnosis; however, at least two major subpopulations have been identified. The first (low-risk) group is characterized by a benign or slowly progressive disease with a median survival of 10 years or longer and young age (less than 45). The second, less fortunate (high-risk) group is distinguished by a short-lived survival of 2 years and older age group (more than 45). Many patients in this subgroup die following acute blastic transformation.

Besides age, a number of prognostic indicators have been identified; the most important in regard to long survival include the following:

1. Lack of symptoms
2. Effective erythropoiesis, as evidenced by hemoglobin level greater than 10 g/dL, reticulocyte count greater than 2%, and bone marrow showing normal erythropoiesis
3. Platelet counts above 100×10^9/L
4. Absence of significant hepatosplenomegaly

Conversely, patients with severe, ineffective hematopoiesis and marrow failure, marked splenomegaly with plasma volume expansion and portal hypertension, anemia, or excessive hemolysis fair poorly, with an average survival of only 1 to 2 years. The major causes of death are acute myocardial infarction, congestive heart failure, gastrointestinal and cerebral hemorrhage, pneumonia, and infection.

Between 5% and 15% of cases have a terminal transformation to leukemia, acute myelogenous leukemia in most instances, with a rapidly progressive, fatal course. Rare patients die of liver or renal failure, and development of acute lymphocytic leukemia and erythroleukemia has been reported. IMF is infrequently found in children, but when discovered has a rapidly fatal course. It is associated with trisomy 21 and appears to be a variant of acute megakaryoblastic leukemia.

Major scientific advances and application of new knowledge have taken place in recent years. Relevant discoveries in the areas of collagen biochemistry and histochemistry, bone marrow ultrastructure, cell culture studies, and cell growth regulation have allowed a more in-depth understanding of the pathologic processes involved in the disease of myelofibrosis. As new, innovative strategies are applied to the treatment of this complex disease, it is hoped that there will be a significant improvement in both the survival and quality of life of patients with IMF.

► ERYTHROCYTOSIS

A number of diverse conditions may cause an elevation in the hematocrit (Hct). Initially, these disorders can be separated into two groups based on the determination of the red cell mass (Table 18–5). In the *absolute erythrocytosis* group, the red cell mass (or red cell volume) is elevated, implying a true increase in the number of circulating erythrocytes. By contrast, in *relative erythrocytosis,* there is an increased Hct in the absence of an elevation in red cell volume. This state is the result of an increase in the ratio of red cell mass to the plasma volume, as would occur with dehydration (in which the plasma volume was contracted or decreased).

Absolute erythrocytosis may be further divided into three distinct groups: (1) polycythemia vera, a chronic myeloproliferative disorder, arising as a clonal hematologic malignancy of the bone marrow; (2) secondary erythrocytosis, representing a physiologic response to abnormal stimulus (e.g., tissue hypoxia, increased erythropoietic activity); or (3) an idiopathic group for which neither a myeloproliferative nor secondary cause of sustained erythrocytosis can be implicated. An overall comparison of these three groups of polycythemia can be found in Table 18–6. Primary polycythemia vera is discussed in length first.

Polycythemia Vera: Description, History, and Pathogenesis

Polycythemia vera (PV) is a hematopoietic stem cell disorder predominantly characterized by accelerated erythropoiesis and, to varying degrees, excessive proliferation of myeloid and megakaryocytic elements of the bone marrow (Figs. 18–9 and 18–10, and Color Plates 208 and 209). As mentioned earlier, the absolute increase in red cell mass is an important finding for establishing the diagnosis of PV. A routine complete blood count (CBC) shows the following values: in women, the RBC count is increased to more than 5.9×10^{12}/L, and in men, to more than 6.6×10^{12}/L. In keeping with other myeloproliferative disorders, the manifestations of splenomegaly, myeloid metaplasia, and myelofibrosis are variably expressed at diagnosis and throughout the course of the disease. Most commonly at the time of initial presentation, the degree of extramedullary hematopoiesis is usually mild, and marrow fibrosis is most often minimal. However, 15% to 20% of

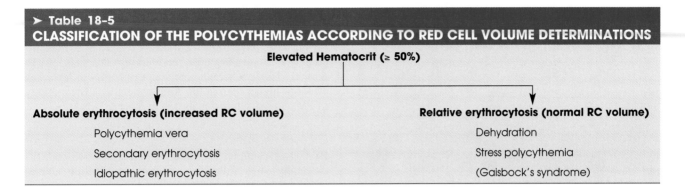

> **Table 18-5**
CLASSIFICATION OF THE POLYCYTHEMIAS ACCORDING TO RED CELL VOLUME DETERMINATIONS

Elevated Hematocrit (≥ 50%)

Absolute erythrocytosis (increased RC volume)	**Relative erythrocytosis (normal RC volume)**
Polycythemia vera	Dehydration
Secondary erythrocytosis	Stress polycythemia
Idiopathic erythrocytosis	(Gaisbock's syndrome)

patients transform to a spent phase with progressive anemia and increasing splenomegaly, this development being virtually indistinguishable from idiopathic myelofibrosis.

The nature of this disease has been controversial over the years. Hippocrates recognized "plethora vera,"[7] and Von Haller in 1730 associated thrombosis with the frequent occurrence of gangrene. Vasques,[8] Cabot, and, in 1903, Osler,[9] first characterized the disease as autonomous erythrocytosis, additionally noting the concurrent feature of splenomegaly. Turk[10] in 1904 described the leukoerythroblastic blood picture as well as documenting the finding of increased granulocytic and megakaryocytic activity. The replacement of normal marrow by fibrotic and sclerotic tissue was reported by Hirsch[11] in 1935, and by 1938, Rosenthal and Sessen[12] had delineated the natural history and cause of the disease. The concept of the myeloproliferative diseases was originally proposed in the 1950s by Dameshek,[1] and since that time the body of knowledge encompassing polycythemia has greatly expanded.

It has now been clearly established that the cell of origin in PV is an abnormal pluripotent stem cell. This has been demonstrated by studies of black women with PV who were heterozygous for the two different G6PD isoenzymes. In these women, only one of the isoenzymes was present in the progenitors and progeny of erythroid, granulocytic, monocytic, and megakaryocytic cell lines, whereas non-hematopoietic tissue displayed both isoenzymes A and B. In normal healthy women, equal amounts of both isoenzyme types were found in blood cells. These findings strongly suggested that abnormal hematopoietic cells arise from a single malignant clone. Furthermore, some patients eventually develop marrow fibrosis, and this occurrence is

> **Table 18-6**
FEATURES OF POLYCYTHEMIA VERA, SECONDARY (HYPOXIC) POLYCYTHEMIA, AND RELATIVE ERYTHROCYTOSIS

Manifestations	PV	Secondary Erythrocytosis	Relative Erythrocytosis
Clinical Features			
Cyanosis	Absent	Present	May be present
Heart or lung disease	Absent	Present	Absent
Splenomegaly	Present in 75%	Absent	Absent
Hepatomegaly	Present in 35%	Absent	Absent
Laboratory Features			
Red cell mass	Increased	Increased	Normal
Erythropoietin	Decreased (rarely normal)	Increased (rarely normal)	Normal
Arterial O_2 saturation	Normal	Decreased	Normal
Leukocyte	Increased in 80%	Normal	Normal
Platelet count	Increased in 50%	Normal	Normal
NRBCs, poikilocytes	Often present	Absent	Absent
LAP	Increased in 70%	Normal	Normal
Bone marrow	Hypercellular; increased erythropoiesis and myelopoiesis; increased megakaryocytes; fibrosis	Increased erythropoiesis	Normal
Serum vitamin B_{12}	Increased in 75%	Normal	Normal
Culture studies	Autonomous, erythroid proliferation	Epo-dependent colony formation	Not applicable

Abbreviations: NRBCs = nucleated red blood cells; EPO = erythropoietin

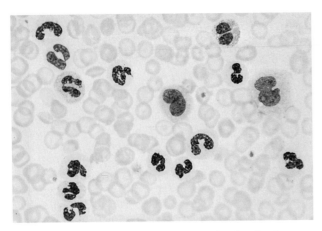

► FIGURE 18–9   Peripheral blood smear seen in polycythemia vera. Note hypochromia and increased cellularity (magnification ×400).

a reactive process. Just as in myelofibrosis, the excessive fibroblastic proliferation is a result of the release of certain growth factors from abnormal megakaryocytes.

When blood and bone marrow cells from patients with PV are cultured on semisolid media, erythroid colonies (colony-forming unit–erythroid [CFU-E] and burst-forming unit–erythroid, [BFU-E]) are formed without the addition of exogenous erythropoietin. This led to the original presumption that erythroid colonies grow spontaneously in PV, because in normal individuals, formation of erythroid colonies is dependent on erythropoietin, which acts on the committed erythroid cell line, causing increased proliferation. Erythroid progenitors are extremely sensitive to low levels of erythropoietin supplied by the serum that is inherently present in the basic culture medium. Cultures of erythroid precursor cells are one of the tests currently advocated in the differential diagnosis of PV versus secondary polycythemia.

Epidemiology

Polycythemia vera is a relatively rare disease of older adults with an annual incidence of approximately 2 cases per 100,000 population. The median age at diagnosis is 60 years, but onset may occur from adolescence to old age. Only nine cases of childhood PV have been documented. The disease has a slightly higher incidence in men than in

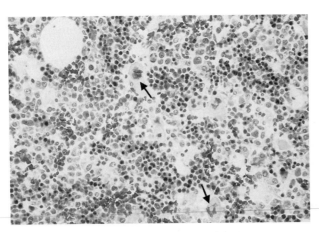

► FIGURE 18–10   Bone marrow showing panhyperplasia in polycythemia vera. Note increased number of megakaryocytes (arrows). Hematoxylin and eosin stain (low power).

women; however, in younger patients PV reportedly shows less of a male preponderance. Familial occurrences, although rare, have been reported. A cluster of MPDs, including PV cases, has been reported in Ashkenazi Jews in northern Israel, where the incidence of MPDs in Jews was 10 times higher than in the Arab population. The etiology of PV remains unknown, as it is in other MPDs.

Clinical Features

PV has an insidious onset and is often discovered quite incidentally when, following a routine examination, an elevated red blood cell (RBC) count, hemoglobin (Hgb), or Hct is discovered following routine examination. Although some patients are asymptomatic, others develop characteristic symptoms related to increased red cell volume or hyperviscosity (Fig. 18–11). Common complaints caused by cerebral circulatory disturbances and transient ischemic attacks include headaches, dizziness, weakness, vertigo, visual phenomena (blurred vision, diplopia, scotomata), tinnitus, and rarely, mild dementia. Vascular complications are manifested equally in arteries and veins. Thrombotic episodes, such as phlebitis, myocardial infarction, erythromelalgia (painful red extremities), paresthesia, and burning sensation, particularly in the feet, reflect impairment of blood flow to the peripheral circulation. The coexistent thrombocytosis acts in conjunction with the hyperviscosity and high blood volume to increase the incidence of thrombosis, thromboembolism, and hemorrhage in these patients. Incidence of morbidity and mortality from vessel wall disease is already high in this age group, and the concomitant high Hct adversely influences the outcome of occlusive events.

Hemorrhagic diathesis is often seen in patients with PV. Life-threatening hemorrhage may occur in association with trauma, surgery, or peptic ulcer. Spontaneous minor hemorrhages, in the form of epistaxis, gingival bleeding, and ecchymoses, are common events almost certainly caused by qualitative platelet abnormalities.

The presence of splenomegaly in about 80% of patients is a finding of significant differential importance. The splenic enlargement is usually mild to moderate and results from extramedullary hematopoiesis and not from the expanded blood volume per se (the spleen size does not diminish as blood volume is reduced by phlebotomy). Patients having moderate splenomegaly appear more likely to evolve to IMF at an early stage. Modest hepatomegaly is observed in one-third of patients at the time of initial presentation (see Table 18–6).

Portal hypertension may occur because of the excessive flow of blood from the spleen into the portal system. Gastrointestinal disorders associated with PV include peptic ulcers and, possibly, massive hemorrhage from varices in the esophagus, stomach, or bowel.

A common physical finding is ruddy cyanosis (reddish-purple color) of the face, nose, ears, and lips. This facial plethora results from conjunctival and mucosal blood vessel congestion. Patients have stated that the appearance of their ruddy complexion has prompted friends to comment that they "look wonderful."

Aquagenic pruritus (itching), occurring in about 50% of patients, is especially troublesome after a hot shower. The pathogenesis of this persistent itching and urticaria is related to elevated levels of histamine produced by basophils and other granulocytes.

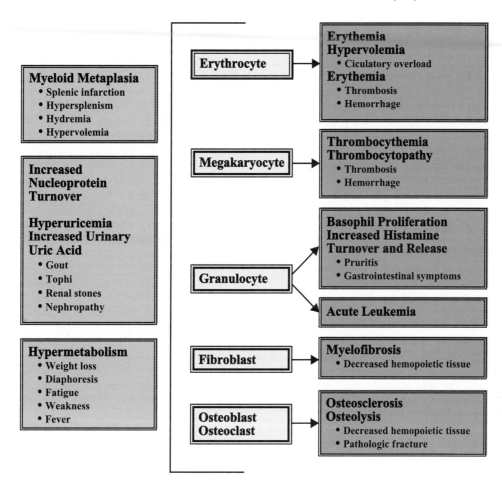

> ► FIGURE 18-11 Physiologic complications of polycythemia vera. The clinical features of this disorder are attributable to the excessive proliferation of the three main hematopoietic cell lines and reactive proliferation of bone marrow fibroblasts. (Adapted from Gilbert, HS: The spectrum of myeloproliferative disorders. Med Clin North Am 57:355–359, with permission.)

Fever, night (and day) sweats, and weight loss may occur as a result of the hypermetabolic state. Gout ascribed to increased nucleoprotein turnover occurs in 5% to 10% of patients. Uric acid calculi or urate nephropathy may arise from the increased uric acid excretion.

Laboratory Features

Elevation of the RBC count, Hgb, and Hct are the most important findings in PV. The Hct concentration is usually more than 58% in men and more than 52% in women. Because of the variation in plasma volume, the Hct gives only an approximate indication of the size of the red cell mass. Therefore, the diagnosis of PV, particularly in borderline cases in which the Hct is in the upper normal range, may require the direct measurement of total red cell mass. This is most often determined using the well-established ^{51}Cr dilution technique. Absolute erythrocytosis is present in men with values of at least 36 mL/kg and in women with at least 32 mL/kg.

Determination of serum erythropoietin allows for a cost-effective diagnostic workup for evaluation of erythrocytosis. Most values in PV are decreased, indicating autonomous production of red cells by the bone marrow; however, sometimes the result may be in the normal range. There is no significant rise in the levels of erythropoietin following phlebotomy and normalization of the Hgb and Hct.

Characteristically, at presentation there is increased red cell production in intramedullary sites. The erythrocytes are normochromic, normocytic, and have a normal life span. As the disease progresses, extramedullary ineffective hematopoiesis leads to an increasing anisocytosis and poikilocytosis, as well as shortened red cell life span secondary to splenic sequestration. Many patients demonstrate the microcytosis and hypochromia associated with iron deficiency, with low serum iron, decreased mean corpuscular volume (MCV) and mean corpuscular hemoglobin concentration (MCHC) occurring in about one-half of patients. This iron deficiency is attributed to consumption of iron resulting from the tremendous increase in erythropoiesis as well as possible occult gastrointestinal blood loss and defective platelet function. The reticulocyte count is usually normal, and only rarely are immature erythrocytes found in the peripheral blood.

Relative and absolute granulocytosis occurs in two-thirds of the patients. The elevation in the total WBC count is usually moderate, with counts in the range of 12 to 25 × 10⁹/L. Occasionally, basophilia and eosinophilia are apparent, and few metamyelocytes, myelocytes, and even more immature cells may be seen on examination of the peripheral smear.

Thrombocytosis is present at the time of diagnosis in about one-half of the patients with PV. The platelet count is most often moderately elevated, with counts between 450 and 800 × 10⁹/L, but in about 5% the platelet count exceeds 1000 × 10⁹/L. Platelet life span may be shortened in proportion to the extent of pooling in the spleen. Morphological alterations of platelets include the presence of giant platelets as well as deficient granulation. Studies show that most patients with PV form spontaneous megakaryocytic colonies analogous to the spontaneous erythroid colony formation seen in all myeloproliferative disorders. Platelets from most patients demonstrate some abnormality in aggregation studies, but the results of these laboratory tests correlate poorly with clinical thrombotic and hemorrhagic episodes. Also of interest is the fact that in the majority of patients, even those with bleeding diathesis, the bleeding time, which is the best measurement of in vivo platelet function, is nearly always normal.

The arterial oxygen saturation is normal in most patients with PV; however, infrequently the oxygen saturation may be slightly lowered (88% to 92%). This feature is helpful in excluding erythrocytosis secondary to pulmonary and cardiac abnormalities, wherein the oxygen saturation is routinely decreased.

The prothrombin time (PT), activated partial thromboplastin time (APTT), thrombin time (TT), and fibrinogen levels are generally normal in patients with PV. When performing coagulation tests on PV patients, the anticoagulant-to-blood ratio must be maintained at the 1:9 ratio. Sodium citrate functions as an anticoagulant by binding calcium in plasma. In the case of erythrocytosis, wherein the plasma volume is decreased, citrate is left in excess in the vacutainer tube. This residual citrate is then available to bind calcium in the test system, thus causing falsely prolonged clotting times. When the Hct is greater than 55%, the following adjustment for the volume of anticoagulant should be applied:

$$(0.00185)\,(V)\,(100 - Hct) = C$$

where V = volume of whole blood

C = anticoagulant, in mL

The LAP activity is increased in 70% of PV cases (Fig 18–12 and Color Plate 210). The determination of the LAP is not always the most helpful test in the differential diagnosis of erythrocytosis, because some patients with PV have a normal LAP score, as do the majority of patients with secondary erythrocytosis (in the absence of inflammation, infection, or hormonal therapy).

The bone marrow is hypercellular, with decreased fat

content in nearly all cases. Panhyperplasia is evident to a varying extent, in contrast to the exclusive erythroid hyperplasia seen in secondary erythrocytosis (see Fig. 18–10 and Color Plate 209). Besides the striking increase in the number of megakaryocytes, they are often increased in size. Marrow iron stores, demonstrated by Prussian blue staining, are reduced or absent. This decrease results from the increased utilization of iron in the process of excessive erythropoiesis and the subsequent expansion of red cell mass, in addition to the chronic occult blood loss. Early in the course of PV, fibrosis is a rare finding. If serial biopsies are performed, a progressive increase in reticulin deposits can often be demonstrated during the active phase of the disease and before the spent phase develops. As the disease runs its course, cellularity usually decreases, although megakaryocytosis may persist. The transition to frank myelofibrosis occurs in 15% to 20% of patients.

Autonomous or spontaneous erythroid colonies may be grown in culture medium without the addition of exogenous erythropoietin; this demonstrates that endogenous erythroid colony (EEC) formation can occur from culture of peripheral blood of PV patients. This finding is considered by many investigators to be of diagnostic value. The addition of both interleukin-3 (IL-3) or interferon α and subsequent increase in EEC has given an even better diagnostic discrimination between PV and secondary erythrocytosis patients.

Two of the three vitamin B_{12}–binding proteins, transcobalamin I and III, are frequently elevated in PV, as in other MPDs. Transcobalamin III is the binding protein most commonly elevated in PV, whereas transcobalamin I is predominantly increased in chronic myelogenous leukemia. These increased serum values are attributed to the excessive granulocyte turnover. Furthermore, the unsaturated B_{12}-binding capacity ($UB_{12}BC$) is increased in approximately 75% of patients.

Hyperuricemia and uricosuria are found in 40% of patients with PV at the time of presentation. This is a frequent finding in many hypoproliferative disorders in which increased synthesis and degradation of cellular nucleotides occur. Most patients remain asymptomatic, but uncommonly, clinical gout may develop.

Other relatively new parameters have been described in association with PV. The mean platelet distribution width (PDW, as measured by a Coulter counter analyzer) is a reflection of the average platelet size and is significantly increased in PV as compared with secondary erythrocytosis. The platelet nucleotide ratio (ATP:ADP as determined by a lumiaggregometer) may also be increased in PV as compared with values seen in secondary erythrocytosis.

A low-normal erythrocyte sedimentation rate (ESR) is commonly present in PV patients. The increased Hct, as well as the elevated ratio of red cell membrane to plasma fibrinogen and globulins, may account for this finding. Nonrandom chromosome abnormalities are seen in about 15% of patients, increasing to 50% with disease progression. The most common trisomies and deletions are trisomy 8, trisomy 9, and deletions of 20q, 5q, 6q, 7q, 11q, 13q, and 20q. These cytogenetic findings appear to correlate with disease stage and duration.

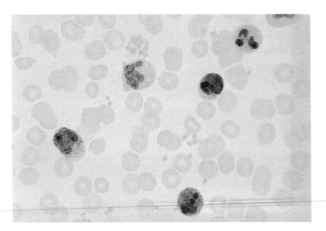

► FIGURE 18–12 Leukocyte alkaline phosphatase (LAP) stain of peripheral blood showing increased activity in polycythemia vera (red staining).

Differential Diagnosis

The diagnostic criteria for evaluating a patient with erythrocytosis should encompass procedures that systematically exclude the various causes of secondary and relative poly-cythemia (Table 18–7). In 1968 the Polycythemia Vera Study Group (PVSG) developed a set of criteria that indi-cate with a high degree of probability the establishment of the diagnosis of PV (Table 18–8). Because of the sensitiv-ity and specificity of these criteria, they have become the standard approach to this diagnostic problem worldwide. A recent revision to the PVSG's standard diagnostic criteria takes a more streamlined, cost-effective approach. The measurement of total red cell mass is now considered su-

> ## Table 18-7
> ### CLASSIFICATION OF THE DISORDERS ASSOCIATED WITH ABSOLUTE ERYTHROCYTOSIS

Primary Polycythemia

Polycythemia vera

Secondary Erythrocytosis

Appropriate increase in erythropoietin (tissue hypoxia)

   Chronic pulmonary disease

   Cyanotic congenital heart disease

   Cirrhosis

   Alveolar hypoventilation (obesity/sleep apnea, Pickwickian syndrome, instrinsic lung disease)

   High altitude

Inappropriate increase in erythropoietin

   Renal ischemia

      Renal tumors

      Renal cysts

      Renal transplantation rejection

      Renal artery stenosis

      Hydronephrosis

   Neoplasms

      Uterine fibroids

      Hepatoma

      Cerebellar hemangioblastoma

   Endocrine disorders

      Pheochromocytoma

      Conn's syndrome

      Ovarian tumors (androgen-secreting)

      Cushing's syndrome

Defective oxygen transport

   Smoking (carboxyhemoglobinemia)

   Methemoglobinemia

   High oxygen affinity hemoglobinopathies

   Defective oxidative metabolism (cobalt therapy)

Relative Erythrocytosis

Dehydration

Stress erythrocytosis (Gaisbock's snydrome)

> ## Table 18-8
> ### PVSG CRITERIA FOR DIAGNOSIS OF POLYCYTHEMIA VERA*

Category A (Major Criteria)

1. Elevated red cell mass

2. Normal arterial oxygen saturation

3. Splenomegaly

Category B (Minor Criteria)

1. Leukocytosis

2. Thrombocytosis

3. Elevated leukocyte alkaline phosphatase score

4. Increased serum vitamin B_{12} or vitamin B_{12}–binding proteins

*To establish a diagnosis of polycythemia vera, either all three diagnostic criteria from category A or an elevated red cell mass and normal arterial oxygen *saturation in addition to* two criteria from category B must be present.
Source: From Beck, WS: Hematology, ed 3. MIT Press, Cambridge, 1982, p 297, with permission.

perfluous if the Hct is greater than 60%, erythropoietin is decreased, and splenomegaly is present.

As always, a careful history and physical examination should preclude more extensive (and costly) diagnostic pro-cedures. Of particular importance are such elements as smoking, cardiopulmonary status, alcohol intake, family his-tory, and examination for evidence of hepatosplenomegaly.

A diagnostic algorithm to assist in the differential diag-nosis of (primary) PV versus secondary erythrocytosis is displayed in Figure 18–13. A serum erythropoietin assay is now considered most helpful in distinguishing between primary and secondary erythrocytosis. Most values in PV are decreased, whereas the erythropoietin levels are always increased in secondary erythrocytosis.

Normal arterial oxygen and oxygen saturation (at least 92%), along with a normal chest x-ray, can help to rule out chronic pulmonary or cardiac disease; both are causes of secondary erythrocytosis. Additionally, these patients have symptoms and other complications as a consequence of their primary underlying disorder.

If evidence of tissue hypoxia is lacking, investigation for the presence of an occult erythropoietin-secreting tumor or other cause of inappropriate erythropoietin production should be undertaken. Common procedures at this level of evalua-tion include an intravenous pyelogram, renal ultrasound, CT scan of the abdomen or head, or both, and a liver scan. Car-boxyhemoglobin levels should be measured in patients who smoke, because Hct levels above normal have been demon-strated in some of these patients.

Erythrocytosis in the absence of characteristic features of either PV or cardiopulmonary secondary erythrocytosis should prompt consideration of the possibility of inherited hemoglobin abnormality (high oxygen affinity hemoglo-bin). Hemoglobin electrophoresis is abnormal in the major-ity of these cases; however, the measurement of the oxygen affinity ($P_{50}O_2$) can help reveal the few cases in which the hemoglobin mutation is electrophoretically silent. Further-more, family history can be very useful, as the inheritance mode of these disorders is autosomal dominant. In difficult

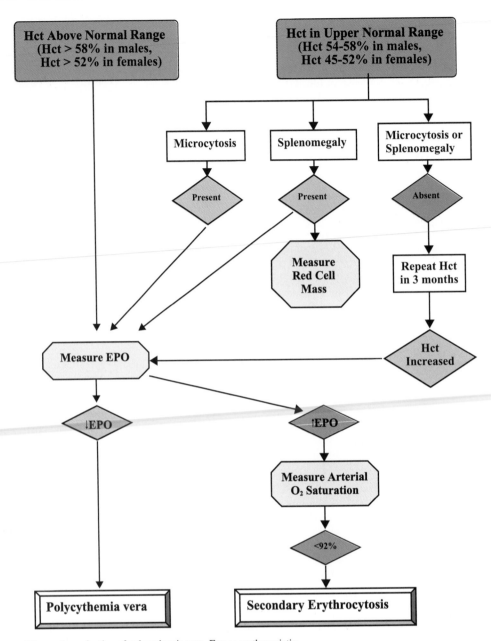

➤ **FIGURE 18–13**   Diagnostic evaluation of polycythemia vera. Epo = erythropoietin.

cases, culture studies of peripheral blood or bone marrow may identify autonomous producing erythroid colonies and, hence, verify a myeloproliferative disorder.

In summary, the most significant characteristic findings in PV are increased Hct, splenomegaly, pancytosis, and decreased erythropoietin. Occasionally a patient may present with a normal or near-normal Hgb, iron deficiency, splenomegaly, leukocytosis, and thrombocytosis; and the disease may, therefore, be difficult to distinguish from essential thrombocythemia. In this case, the presumed blood loss and iron deficiency is masking the erythrocytosis of the underlying PV, and a trial of iron administration is warranted to establish a definitive diagnosis. In PV, the Hgb and Hct can be expected to rise to polycythemic levels, thus clarifying the diagnosis. Conversely, the combination of heavy smoking and excessive alcohol consumption has led to false-positive diagnoses of PV. In this setting the smokers' erythrocytosis and alcoholic liver disease, manifested by

splenomegaly, elevated serum vitamin B_{12} levels, leukocytosis, and, in some cases, elevated LAP, has erroneously prompted diagnosis of PV. Again, measurement of carboxyhemoglobin levels, bone marrow examination for the presence of panhyperplasia, and erythropoietin assay (expected decrease) can help to rule in PV.

Treatment

Early descriptions indicated that the life expectancy of untreated PV patients postdiagnosis' averaged 6 to 36 months. Over the years, therapeutic modalities have been complex and controversial. Today, however, these patients can enjoy a relatively normal life span if their disease is adequately treated, controlled, and monitored by their physician. No treatment at present can completely eradicate this disease.

The major complications of PV are those of thrombotic events resulting from hyperviscosity and complications resulting from transition to an MPD (myelofibrosis, leukemia, or both). The primary objective of therapy is the reduction of the total red cell mass, thereby eliminating the distressing plethora of symptoms. The use of phlebotomy or cytotoxic myelosuppressive agents, or both, to control the malignant proliferative process is advocated. Apparently no single therapy is optimal for patients of all ages and stages of this disease; therefore, decisions as to the most effective approach must be based primarily on individual patient characteristics. The treatment of the erythrocytic phase may be divided into induction and maintenance therapy.

Induction

Rapid reduction of the blood volume to normal can be accomplished by phlebotomy, thereby relieving the patient of the characteristic painful symptoms of hyperviscosity. This is a safe and relatively inexpensive method of controlling the erythrocytosis and is the cornerstone of treatment in PV. Removal of 250 to 500 mL of blood may be done every 2 to 3 days until the Hct is reduced to 40% to 45%. Studies have demonstrated that the cerebral blood flow is significantly improved and mental alertness heightened if the Hct can be maintained within this range. Phlebotomies can then be performed on a bimonthly basis. In elderly patients or those with a history of cardiovascular disease, it is undesirable to remove more than 200 to 300 mL of blood at a time. Surgery in an untreated patient is hazardous owing to the increased risk of thrombohemorrhagic complications. In such emergency situations, intensive phlebotomy accompanied by plasma infusion is advisable to maintain intravascular volume.

Because removal of every unit of blood will cause a loss of approximately 250 mg of elemental iron, nearly all patients regularly treated by phlebotomy will develop iron deficiency with microcytic, hypochromic red cell changes. Development of this iron deficiency and concomitant disruption of normal erythropoiesis allows maintenance of the Hct at an acceptable level and a decreased frequency of phlebotomies. Most patients do not show the classic symptoms of glossitis, dysphagia, cheilosis, weight loss, and so on generally associated with iron deficiency; however, some patients have unexplained tiredness. Iron therapy is not usually required, but if iron is administered, the Hct must be carefully monitored as it may rise quickly, necessitating more frequent phlebotomies. The microhematocrit method is preferable over the automated cell counter method, as the Hct may be overestimated by up to 10% at low mean corpuscular hemoglobin (MCH) and MCHC values.

Management by phlebotomy alone is recommended for patients younger than age 40, particularly for women in the childbearing years, unless specific thrombosis-associated risk factors are present (i.e., high platelet counts, preexisting vascular disease). The major limitation of phlebotomy is that it has no suppressive effect on the abnormal bone marrow proliferation, particularly that of thrombocytosis. Also, phlebotomy further excites hematopoiesis, therefore increasing the rate of production of red cells. Additionally, it does not alleviate pruritus or control any symptoms related to splenomegaly. Myelosuppression is often advocated to repress these manifestations.

Maintenance

Long-term control of the peripheral blood counts is essential to minimize the risk of thrombotic complications. Although phlebotomy relieves the burden of erythrocytosis, the reduction is short term and all patients require close supervision by a physician to cope with the increased risk of thrombosis during the first years of treatment, especially those patients with elevated platelet counts.

Extensive data on the management of PV by use of phlebotomy alone or in combination with the various myelosuppressive modalities is now available thanks to the past 25 years of investigation by the PVSG. In a long-term study, 431 patients were randomized into three modes of treatment: phlebotomy alone, chlorambucil with phlebotomy as needed, and radioactive phosphorus ^{32}P and phlebotomy as needed.[13] An additional study examined the results of long-term control of PV with a nonalkylating agent, hydroxyurea (HU). Patients treated with phlebotomy alone exhibited an increased incidence of thrombotic complications, whereas significantly greater percentages of patients who were regulated by either radioactive phosphorous or an alkylating agent subsequently developed acute leukemia and other neoplasms.[14] The comparison studies also show that HU, supplemented by phlebotomy, is *not* accompanied by excessive thrombotic complications. As a result of these studies showing the leukemogenic potential of chlorambucil and ^{32}P, these agents are no longer used in treatment of PV, and HU has been advocated as the myelosuppressive drug of choice for PV. Other studies have demonstrated that patients treated with HU, which originally was not considered leukemogenic, have indeed shown an increased rate of development of acute leukemia. Because myelosuppressive treatment has not been shown to prolong survival in PV patients, the indications for the use of cytotoxic chemotherapy must outweigh the risk of inducing leukemia.

The following guidelines have been suggested to provide the best control of the disease:

1. In patients under age 40, the disease should be controlled with phlebotomy alone unless thrombosis-associated risk factors are demonstrated. Treatment with interferon α can also be considered, although it is still under investigation for use in young patients. If the requirement for phlebotomy is excessive or there is a history of a previous thrombotic episode, myelosuppression with HU may be cautiously used even in this young age group.

2. Because the role of myelosuppression is controversial in patients aged 40 to 70 years, phlebotomy alone can be used if no thrombosis-associated risks are present. If cardiovascular risk factors exist (coronary heart disease, hypertension, or history of smoking), HU may be used judiciously. Symptomatic hypersplenomegaly, resistant pruritus, bone pain, or poor veins may be other indications for the additive use of myelosuppression.

The average dose of 1 g/day of HU is sufficient to maintain a normal Hct and platelet count. Supplemental phlebotomies may be necessary. The initial response to HU treatment is positive, with between 80% and 90% of patients achieving good control of the disease and more than 60% retaining long-term control after 5 years. Weinfeld and co-workers[15] report that most transformations to acute leukemia take place during the first 4 years of treatment. In a high percentage of patients, HU also seems to have a beneficial effect on pruritus and splenomegaly. Possible side effects include rashes, drug fever, and megaloblastoid changes.

Besides phlebotomy and HU therapy, several other alternative techniques and therapies have been successfully employed to control PV. Plateletpheresis may be considered to keep the platelet count between 100 and 400×10^9/L. If HU treatment fails, anagrelide, a platelet-lowering agent, can be used to treat thrombosis-associated PV. As with IMF, interferon α has been shown to be effective in treating MPDs and even inducing remission of the disease. Specifically, this agent has been shown to be helpful in eliminating the need for phlebotomy in PV patients. However, interferon α is associated with considerable side effects.

Adjuvant therapy is often necessary to control hyperuricemia and hyperuricosuria. In addition to standard colchicine therapy, allopurinol (300 mg/day), an agent that blocks the formation of uric acid from its precursors, is used to prevent or control acute attacks of gout. In patients receiving myelosuppressive therapy, the need for allopurinol is diminished because of the decreased nucleic acid turnover effected by suppression of cellular proliferation. Allopurinol may be continued indefinitely in patients treated by phlebotomy alone.

Severe pruritus is a most distressing symptom in many cases. It is best managed by controlling the erythrocytosis; however, it may persist in some patients despite a normal Hct and physical examination findings. The antihistamines cyproheptadine and cimetidine may be of benefit. Cholestyramine, an anion exchange resin that functions by binding bile acids, has been reported to provide some relief of pruritus.

Course and Prognosis

The course of patients with PV is determined by the natural history of the disease and the development of complications that may or may not be related to the mode of therapy employed.

As previously mentioned, this disease progresses through several stages, each of variable duration. In the active erythrocytic phase, the red cell mass can be maintained at satisfactory levels with administration of treatment that is dictated by age and the presence of certain risk factors. Many patients eventually enter a period characterized by increasing anemia, and this spent phase is associated with transformation to frank myelofibrosis in 15% to 20% of cases. The appearance of teardrop RBCs on peripheral blood smear heralds the transition of PV to IMF. The progressive splenomegaly appears to be a manifestation of the natural course of the disease, but splenectomy carries a high incidence of morbidity and mortality in this group of patients. The treatment of this phase is predominantly supportive and may be very difficult. The cause of the anemia may be multifactorial, being a result of one or more of the following factors: (1) iron, folic acid, or vitamin B_{12} deficiency; (2) inefficient hematopoiesis; or (3) splenic sequestration and destruction of erythrocytes, leukocytes, and platelets. Treatment of the anemia may involve appropriate nutritional replacement or administration of steroids to help control the ineffective erythropoiesis. Ongoing transfusion of packed red cells is often required. Despite possible splenic sequestration, thrombocytosis and leukocytosis may persist. Myelosuppressive therapy may be indicated to control the myelofibrotic proliferation. Prognosis is poor for this phase of the disease and median survival is about 2 years.

Malignant transformation to acute leukemia, usually acute myeloblastic leukemia (AML), occurs in 10% to 15% of cases. This complication is almost universally fatal. As discussed earlier, the therapeutic modality affects the rate of leukemic transformation. In patients treated by phlebotomy alone, the incidence of transition to leukemia is only 1% to 2%, whereas those treated by chemotherapy have a risk approaching 15%. A few cases each have been documented of PV transforming into a myelodysplastic syndrome, myeloma, and also chronic lymphocytic leukemia.

Reported survival rates in PV range from 8 to 15 years. Thrombohemorrhagic incidents account for 40% of deaths, and acute leukemia and myeloid metaplasia each account for 15%. As the mean age of diagnosis is 60 years, many other patients die of additional unrelated reasons.

Continued research of the pathophysiologic abnormalities associated with this disease as well as the effects of various treatment modalities will undoubtedly lengthen the future life expectancy of patients with PV.

Secondary Erythrocytosis

Absolute erythrocytosis may have a wide variety of causes (see Table 18–7). Secondary erythrocytosis differs from PV in that autonomous bone marrow proliferation occurs in PV. Increased secretion of erythropoietin has been implicated as the responsible stimulus for all cases of secondary erythrocytosis (see Fig 18–13). The causes of secondary erythrocytosis can be separated into three groups: (1) those in which there is an appropriate, compensatory increase in erythropoietin in response to tissue hypoxia; (2) those resulting from an inappropriate or pathologic secretion of erythropoietin; and (3) those resulting from defective oxygen transport.

Appropriate Increase in Erythropoietin

In this group of disorders, the underlying mechanism is release of erythropoietin as part of a compensatory effect to minimize impending tissue hypoxia. The most common causes of secondary polycythemia are cardiac or respiratory diseases that lead to significant arterial oxygen desaturation. Of the lung diseases causing hypoxia and erythrocytosis, chronic obstructive pulmonary disease (COPD) is the most frequent offender. In COPD, the release of erythropoietin appears to be appropriately responsive to the level of hypoxia, with the degree of increase in the Hct being inversely proportional to the arterial oxygen saturation. Other intrinsic lung diseases that may involve significant hypoxia are pulmonary fibrosis, pulmonary aneurysms, and hereditary hemorrhagic telangiectasia with pathologic lung changes.

Right-to-left shunting in congenital heart disease is caused by a number of different anatomic defects and leads to profound arterial hypoxia and extreme erythrocytosis. Indeed, some of the highest Hct levels (75% to 80%) have been reported in these patients. The serum erythropoietin level is most often normal in congenital heart disease patients because the erythrocytosis usually compensates for the decreased arterial oxygen saturation. The erythrocytosis in these cardiac anomalies results from the shunting of poorly oxygenated venous blood into systemic circulations and necessitates surgical intervention. It is recommended that patients with particularly high Hct levels undergo phlebotomy to reduce the Hct to less than 65%.

Ascent to high altitudes causes tissue hypoxia because of the low atmospheric pressure. This leads to the release of erythropoietin, with subsequent increase in red cell production. Although tolerance to high altitude varies, most normal individuals experience no symptoms at altitudes of up to 7000 feet (2130 m). For the indigenous mountain inhabitants living higher than 16,440 feet (5000 m), hematocrits in the range of 60% to 70% are regularly seen. The physiologic adaptation of erythrocytosis allows most individuals to function normally, having life spans equivalent to their counterparts at sea level. The clinical and laboratory features of humans living at high altitudes include a ruddy cyanosis; venous and capillary engorgement of the conjunctiva, mucous membranes, and skin; emphysema; normocytic, normochromic erythrocytosis; increased reticulocyte count; and increased iron turnover. The syndrome of acute mountain sickness occurs in nonacclimatized persons who rapidly ascend to high altitudes. The manifestations of cerebral hypoxia are headaches, dizziness, insomnia, weakness, nausea, and vomiting.

The alveolar hypoventilation syndromes are characterized by impaired or inadequate ventilation. Intermittent alveolar hypoventilation has frequently been reported in normal men during sleep and, if severe, can cause hypoxia, cyanosis, apnea, and secondary polycythemia. This condition may also be seen in neuromuscular disorders, in the mechanical impairment of the chest wall, and in the colorful pickwickian syndrome (extreme obesity, somnolence, and associated erythrocytosis).

Methemoglobinemia can result from a hereditary deficiency of the enzyme NADH-methemoglobin reductase, from ingestion of various drugs or toxic substance exposure, or from hemoglobin M disease. Methemoglobin is formed when heme iron is oxidized to the ferric state. In this oxidized form, the heme moiety is incapable of carrying oxygen and cyanosis is clinically observed. Interestingly enough, even alarming degrees of cyanosis may be seen with arterial oxygen saturation still being normal (92% or higher). Mild, associated erythrocytosis is rare, but when it does occur, it is the result mostly of a shift to the left of the oxygen-dissociation curve (increased oxygen affinity).

Cases of familial secondary erythrocytosis have been demonstrated wherein the hemoglobin molecule itself is abnormal. Amino acid substitutions in these variants may interfere with release of oxygen to the tissues by preventing normal conformational changes required for deoxygenation. This extraordinarily avid oxygen affinity leads to tissue hypoxia and increased erythropoietin production. A left-shifted oxygen-dissociation curve is characteristic, and a compensatory erythrocytosis ensues. Approximately 30 different high-affinity hemoglobin variants have been described, including hemoglobins Chesapeake, Rainer, Yakima, Hiroshima, Little Rock, and San Diego. In many cases the aberrant hemoglobin is apparent on hemoglobin electrophoresis; however, in some patients the hemoglobin migrates along with hemoglobin A and is, therefore, undetectable. Determination of reduced oxygen affinity ($P_{50}O_2$) in patients with erythrocytosis of questionable origin is necessary to disclose these electrophoretically silent hemoglobins.

Inappropriate Increase in Erythropoietin

A wide range of disorders is associated with inappropriately increased erythropoietin production and resultant erythrocytosis, in spite of the absence of generalized tissue hypoxia. This secondary erythrocytosis confers no physiologic advantage, and the underlying disease accounts for most of the clinical features observed in the patient. The Hct and red cell mass are increased, but classically there is no accompanying increase in WBC or platelet counts. Because the kidneys predominantly produce erythropoietin, renal disease can cause anemia as a result of decreased production or erythrocytosis as a result of increased production. Benign and malignant tumors may promote excessive secretion of erythropoietin. Renal tumors account for about 50% of these patients. When these disorders are associated with thrombocytosis or granulocytosis, it may be difficult to establish a clear diagnosis. In this case, documentation of increased erythropoietin and the absence of splenomegaly can assist in ruling out primary PV.

Defective Oxygen Transport

Heavy cigarette smoking (20 to 30 cigarettes per day) can result in chronic carbon monoxide intoxication, with levels of up to 10%. When hemoglobin is bound to carbon monoxide, the resulting carboxyhemoglobin loses its capacity to carry oxygen. Tissue hypoxia results, the oxygen-dissociation curve is shifted to the left, and, because of the reduced oxygen delivery, the erythropoietin level increases, causing a mild erythrocytosis. The incidence of erythrocytosis secondary to smoking has been estimated to be approximately 600 to 1000 per 100,000 population, which contrasts with the prevalence of about 10 per 100,000 population of PV. It is of interest to note that the reduction in plasma volume that occurs in individuals who smoke heavily can be reversed by abstaining from smoking for 4 to 5 days, and this smoking cessation should decrease the Hct. Smokers with a concomitant lung disease or nocturnal hypoventilation most often have increased Hct levels.

Environmental pollution from industrial sources and vehicle exhaust emissions have also been associated with increased levels of carboxyhemoglobin and mild erythrocytosis. Although the increase in Hct is usually on the order of 2% to 4%, the Hct may still fall within normal limits.

Relative Erythrocytosis

Relative erythrocytosis may be seen in patients with an elevated Hct, normal red cell mass, and decreased plasma volume. Two groups can be clearly distinguished among patients with relative erythrocytosis: (1) those individuals suffering from dehydration, and (2) those with stress erythrocytosis. Relative erythrocytosis is most often clinically seen in the group of patients with depletion in circulating plasma volume caused by acute or subacute dehydration resulting from a number of conditions (such as burns). The second group of patients is characterized predominantly by asymptomatic middle-aged white men who are hypertensive, obese, and have a long history of heavy smoking. In 1905, Gaisbock[16] first described a condition of "polycythemia hypertonica" in several hypertensive patients who had increased red cell counts and plethora, but no accompanying splenomegaly. Today, this condition is variously termed *Gaisbock's syndrome, stress* or *benign erythrocytosis,* or *pseudopolycythemia.* It is well documented that excessive smoking causes mild to moderate erythrocytosis and a decreased plasma volume, hence the term *smokers' polycythemia,* as previously mentioned. Undoubtedly some patients with erythrocytosis merely represent the extreme physiologic range of Hct. The combined effect of a high-normal red cell mass and a low-normal plasma volume, resulting in a so-called spurious erythrocytosis, is not considered pathologic. Physical stress, extreme alcohol consumption, and diuretic therapy have also been documented as possible causes of plasma volume reduction.

This condition usually follows a benign course; however, a few patients may progress to an absolute erythrocytosis with an obvious underlying cause becoming apparent. There may be a few nonspecific symptoms reported in these patients such as headache, nausea, and dyspepsia. Hypertension, with possible increased risk of thromboembolic complications, is seen in approximately one-third of the patients. The Hct value is generally between 50% and 60%. Therapy indicated is in the form of encouragement of the cessation of smoking or alcohol intake, or both; reduction of obesity; treatment of hypertension; stress counseling; and discontinuance of diuretic therapy, where appropriate. Additionally, the Hct should be maintained below 50% by phlebotomy to decrease the risk of vascular occlusive episodes.

➤ ESSENTIAL THROMBOCYTHEMIA

Essential thrombocythemia (ET) is a rare, chronic myeloproliferative disorder characterized by marked thrombocytosis associated with abnormal platelet function. ET was the last of the MPDs to be identified as a distinct entity, owing to the fact that extreme thrombocytosis is also frequently observed in CML, IMF, and PV. Sex-linked G6PD cell marker studies established ET as a clonal disorder involving the multipotential stem cell, which supported the placement of ET within the MPD classification.

Diagnostic criteria that define ET were proposed by the PVSG in the mid-1970s. These guidelines include: (1) platelet count in excess of 600×10^9/L (and generally greater than 1000×10^9/L; (2) megakaryocytic hyperplasia in the marrow; (3) absence of identifiable causes of reactive thrombocytosis; (4) the absence of the Ph; (5) hemoglobin no higher than 13 g/dL or normal red cell mass; (6) absence of significant marrow fibrosis; and (7) presence of stainable iron in marrow or failure of iron trial.[17]

Synonyms for this condition include idiopathic thrombocythemia, primary thrombocythemia, and primary hemorrhagic thrombocythemia.

Epidemiology

The mean age at time of diagnosis is approximately 60 years, the majority of patients being older than 50. This disease has occasionally been described as a benign form devoid of hemorrhagic or thrombotic symptoms in the 20- to 40-year-old age group, and very rarely in patients younger than age 20. Most studies do not demonstrate a statistical difference between frequency of males and females affected. The incidence of the disease has been estimated at 7 per million population per year. The etiology of thrombocythemia remains unknown.

Clinical Features

With the introduction of automated instruments that routinely perform whole blood platelet counts, asymptomatic patients with coincidental high platelet counts are being discovered more frequently, especially in young patients. Approximately two-thirds of patients are asymptomatic at diagnosis, with the remaining one-third presenting with hemorrhagic or vaso-occlusive symptoms, or both. In most instances bleeding is mild and manifestations are primarily mucocutaneous (epistaxis and ecchymoses); however, life-threatening hemorrhage may occur following accidental trauma or, rarely, following surgery. Bleeding of the gastrointestinal tract as well as esophageal varices bleeding has also been reported. Hemorrhage has been attributed to several mechanisms: (1) platelet functional abnormalities; (2) thrombosis with infarction, ulceration of the infarction, and subsequent bleeding; (3) consumption of coagulation factors; and (4) increased numbers of circulating platelets, causing excessive production of prostacyclin (PGI_2) by endothelial cells (increased PGI_2 suppresses platelet granule release and aggregation).

Thrombosis is the other major manifestation of ET and is caused by intravascular clumping of sludged, hyperaggregable platelets. Vascular occlusive symptoms are usually related to small vessel obstruction (microvascular occlusion), although larger vessel occlusive events such as myocardial infarction and stroke may occur. Erythromelalgia of the toes, feet, and occasionally fingers (localized painful redness, burning, and "pins-and-needles" tingling sensation) is a characteristic vaso-occlusive symptom and may progress to cyanosis or necrosis of the extremities, or both. The involvement of the hands and feet may simulate a diabetic neuropathy. The erythromelalgia, just as in PV, is a source of continual torment and frustration for ET patients. The toxic effect of the metabolites of platelet arachidonic acid appears to be responsible for the erythromelalgia, and this may be relieved by decreasing the platelet count or by use of anti-inflammatory agents such as aspirin. Thrombotic complications are more common when the platelet count is greater than 2000×10^9/L.

Neurologic manifestations are usually of a transient ischemic nature and include visual disturbances, headaches, paresthesia, dizziness, transient ischemic attacks, and, rarely, seizures. Complete stroke is an uncommon occurrence. In older patients, underlying degenerative vascular disease in combination with thrombocytosis and platelet functional defects all contribute to the thrombohemorrhagic complications.

Other signs and symptoms that have been observed in this disease are recurrent abortions and fetal growth retardation, pruritus, gout, and priapism. Modest splenomegaly is present in approximately 40% of patients with ET. Splenic atrophy resulting from splenic vascular thrombosis and silent infarctions occur in up to 20% of patients.

Laboratory Features

The platelet count is always elevated, in the range 600 to 2500×10^9/L. Platelets are usually morphologically normal, although some degree of platelet anisocytosis may be apparent. When present, this correlates with an elevation of the platelet distribution width (PDW), as determined by automated Coulter instruments. Abnormal morphological findings may include giant platelets (megathrombocytes) as well as microthrombocytes, platelet aggregates, abnormally granulated platelets, and megakaryocytic cytoplasmic fragments (Fig. 18–14 and Color Plate 211).

A mild normocytic, normochromic anemia may be present in up to 50% of patients although the hemoglobin value is not usually less than 10 g/dL. Recurrent mucosal or gastrointestinal bleeding leads to iron-deficiency anemia, and MCV and MCHC are decreased, with a microcytic, hypochromic blood picture becoming apparent on examination of

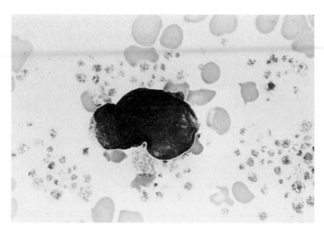

➤ **FIGURE 18–14** Essential thrombocythemia ET; peripheral blood megakaryocyte and numerous platelets. (From Hyun, BH: Morphology of Blood and Bone Marrow, American Society of Clinical Pathologists, Workshop 5121, Philadelphia, 1983, with permission.)

the peripheral smear. Erythrocyte morphological findings reflective of hyposplenism, which occurs in the occasional patient with splenic infarction and atrophy, include the presence of Howell-Jolly bodies, Pappenheimer bodies (siderotic granules), target cells, and acanthocytes.

Leukocytosis is present in about one-third of patients, with WBC counts rarely exceeding $50 \times 10^9/L$. Neutrophilia is observed in the majority of patients with elevated WBC counts, but a mild eosinophilia or basophilia, or both, may occasionally be seen. Rarely, nucleated red cells and immature granulocytes may also be evident. The LAP score is variable but most commonly is normal.

The bone marrow in patients with ET demonstrates trilineage hyperplasia with a marked increase in the megakaryocytic component. The megakaryocytes are typically larger than normal, multilobed, and may be dysplastic in appearance (Fig 18–15 and Color Plate 212). Stainable iron is normal to slightly decreased in most cases, and increased reticulin content is often seen. Marrow karyotype is generally normal; however the deletion of the long arm of chromosome 21 (21q−) has been reported in some patients.

Platelet function studies reveal a variety of abnormalities in some patients. Abnormal platelet aggregation to epi-

nephrine, collagen, adenosine diphosphate (ADP), and ristocetin are quite frequent. Studies have demonstrated both normal bleeding times (even in the case of patients with hemorrhagic tendencies) and prolonged bleeding times. Reduced platelet factor 3 (PF3), reduced platelet adhesion, low protein S levels, and nucleotide storage pool defects have all been reported in association with ET. Despite all of these identified abnormalities, there is poor correlation with any of these findings and the incidence of clinical thrombohemorrhagic manifestations.

Differential Diagnosis

Essential thrombocythemia must be differentiated from the various causes of reactive thrombocytosis (Table 18–9), from other chronic MPDs with associated thrombocytosis (Fig. 18–16), and from the myelodysplastic syndromes in which the platelet count is markedly elevated. This distinction is important because hemorrhagic complications are more common in ET than reactive thrombocytosis, and there is a considerable variation in prognosis and therapy in ET versus chronic MPDs.

Most cases of extreme thrombocytosis represent incidental findings in patients with a wide variety of inflammatory and trauma-associated conditions. Reactive thrombocytosis, even when persistently present for weeks or months, is usually well tolerated in these patients and is not generally associated with thrombosis or hemorrhage. Bone marrow examination, virtually always performed in patients suspected of having an MPD, is rarely done in instances of reactive thrombocytosis. The platelet count in secondary thrombocytosis seldom exceeds $1000 \times 10^9/L$, and commonly falls in the range of 500 to $750 \times 10^9/L$. Platelet morphology and function are generally normal in chronic reactive states compared to the variety of abnormalities seen in MPDs.

When the platelet count is persistently greater than $600 \times 10^9/L$ and the bone marrow demonstrates predominant megakaryocytic hyperplasia, the diagnosis of ET should be investigated (see Fig. 18–16). Because there are no unique clinical, hematologic, or histopathologic findings in this disease, it is by nature a diagnosis of exclusion. At presentation, the hemoglobin should be less than 13 g/dL and the red cell mass should be normal in order to shift the diagnosis from PV with thrombocytosis (one-third of PV cases) to ET. To ensure that masked PV has not been overlooked in those patients having a normal or decreased red

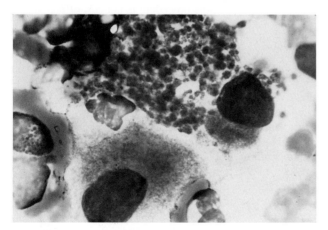

➤ **FIGURE 18–15** Essential thrombocythemia, bone marrow. Note increased megakaryocytes. (From Hyun, BH: Morphology of Blood and Bone Marrow, American Society of Clinical Pathologists, Workshop 5121, Philadelphia, 1983, with permission.)

➤ **Table 18-9**
CAUSES OF REACTIVE THROMBOCYTOSIS

Acute hemorrhage	Trauma
Postsplenectomy and hyposplenism	Hemolytic anemia
Postoperative	Myelodysplastic diseases
Malignancy	Graft-versus-host disease
Chronic inflammatory disorders	Vitamin E deficiency
Chronic infection	Hyperadrenalism
Iron-deficiency anemia	Rebound recovery from thrombocytopenia
Drug-induced	Exercise

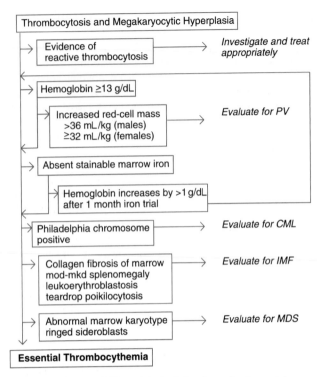

```
┌─────────────────────────────────────────────┐
│ Thrombocytosis and Megakaryocytic Hyperplasia │
└─────────────────────────────────────────────┘
    ┌───────────────────────┐
 →  │ Evidence of           │ ──────→  Investigate and treat
    │ reactive thrombocytosis│          appropriately
    └───────────────────────┘
    ┌───────────────────────┐
 →  │ Hemoglobin ≥13 g/dL   │
    └───────────────────────┘
       ┌──────────────────────┐
    →  │ Increased red-cell mass│ ────→  Evaluate for PV
       │ >36 mL/kg (males)     │
       │ ≥32 mL/kg (females)   │
       └──────────────────────┘
    ┌─────────────────────────┐
 →  │ Absent stainable marrow iron│
    └─────────────────────────┘
       ┌───────────────────────────┐
    →  │ Hemoglobin increases by >1 g/dL│
       │ after 1 month iron trial   │
       └───────────────────────────┘
    ┌───────────────────────┐
 →  │ Philadelphia chromosome│ ────→  Evaluate for CML
    │ positive              │
    └───────────────────────┘
    ┌───────────────────────┐
 →  │ Collagen fibrosis of marrow│ ──→  Evaluate for IMF
    │ mod-mkd splenomegaly   │
    │ leukoerythroblastosis  │
    │ teardrop poikilocytosis│
    └───────────────────────┘
    ┌───────────────────────┐
 →  │ Abnormal marrow karyotype│ ──→  Evaluate for MDS
    │ ringed sideroblasts    │
    └───────────────────────┘
    ┌───────────────────────┐
    │ Essential Thrombocythemia│
    └───────────────────────┘
```

➤ **FIGURE 18–16**   Differential criteria for diagnosis of essential thrombocythemia. PV = polycythemia vera; CML = chronic myelogenous leukemia; IMF = idiopathic myelofibrosis; MDS = myelodysplastic syndrome; mod = moderate; mkd = marked. (Adapted from Iland, HJ, et al: Essential thrombocythemia: Clinical and laboratory characteristics at presentation. Trans Assoc Am Physicians 96:165, 1983, with permission.)

cell mass as a result of iron deficiency, the establishment of the absence of marrow iron stores helps to exclude the diagnosis of ET. Additionally, if the clinical situation permits, a 1-month trial of iron therapy should be administered. The response to iron therapy should be carefully monitored, and if a rise in the Hct level and red cell volume is observed, the patient should be evaluated for evidence of PV, evidence of blood loss, or both.

Chromosomal analysis of the bone marrow should be performed to ensure that the Ph′ chromosome is not present. In those approximately 15% of patients with CML and thrombocytosis that are Ph′ chromosome–negative, the findings of profound myeloid metaplasia, low LAP score, *bcl* and *abl* gene abnormalities and moderate to marked splenomegaly are important for supporting the diagnosis of CML.

Early IMF is often associated with extreme thrombocytosis. However, there is usually marked splenomegaly, a leukoerythroblastic blood picture, teardrop poikilocytosis, and the characteristic myelofibrotic involvement of the bone marrow (increased reticulin and collagen fibrosis). In ET, less than one-third of the biopsy area demonstrates fibrosis. Additionally, the platelet morphology in ET has been described as nondysplastic, in comparison to the abundance of bizarre and atypical platelets seen in IMF.

Plasma levels of interleukin-6 (IL-6), which is primarily produced by monocytes, are increased during acute phase response, such as the reactive thrombocytosis that may accompany acute and chronic inflammatory states. Increased IL-6 levels have been reported in 60% of patients with reactive thrombocytosis, whereas IL-6 levels were not detected in all patients with ET. Plasma fibrinogen and C-reactive protein (CRP) levels also are both increased with reactive thrombocytosis but are normal with ET.

Myelodysplastic syndromes associated with thrombocytosis usually present with a more severe degree of anemia that is often macrocytic in appearance as compared with that seen in patients with ET. Additionally, the presence of either the 5q− syndrome or of ringed sideroblasts in the bone marrow denotes a myelodysplastic syndrome as the cause of associated thrombocytosis rather than essential thrombocythemia.

Cell cultures analyzing BFU-E colonies show that most patients with ET develop spontaneous erythroid colonies without the addition of erythropoietin. Because no patients with reactive thrombocytosis develop this growth pattern, this increased BFU-E activity always indicates a myeloproliferative rather than reactive cause.

Treatment

The therapeutic approach to ET depends on a number of factors, including the patient's age and childbearing potential, the elevation of the platelet count, and, most importantly, the presence and duration of symptoms. Careful monitoring, without therapy specifically aimed at lowering the platelet count, is generally advocated for asymptomatic patients with extreme thrombocytosis. Young patients with few or no symptoms do not require treatment unless surgery is indicated or childbirth is imminent. In these cases, plateletpheresis is useful in controlling the elevated platelet count. Additionally, a young patient with vaso-occlusive manifestations may respond to aspirin therapy alone.

Treatment in patients older than age 50 who are symptomatic is divided into control of hemorrhage and manifestation of vascular occlusion, and control of the progressive megakaryocyte proliferation. Thrombotic events have been reported to occur more often than hemorrhagic events. It is interesting to note that the degree of thrombocytosis does not correlate with the risk of thrombosis. There may be an even greater incidence of occlusive ischemic complications in the presence of cardiovascular risk factors, particularly smoking. Acute hemorrhage and occlusive events, which occur in approximately 30% of patients, indicate the necessity for immediate therapy. Plateletpheresis achieves a dramatic reduction in the platelet count in a matter of hours; however, this reduction is transient and therefore inadequate for long-term control. In addition, the procedure is not cost-effective and involves a difficult process if done 4 to 5 times per week.

Chemotherapy should be initiated in addition to plateletpheresis whenever thrombohemorrhagic complications develop, age is greater than 60, and the platelet count is more than 1.5×10^9/L. A number of effective myelosuppressive agents have been administered, but their use has been associated with an increased potential for induction of acute leukemia. The antimetabolite HU is generally considered to be the drug of choice because of its efficacy. HU administration should be continued daily at a dosage of 15 mg/kg of body weight, with adjustment according to response. In 90% of patients, the platelet count will be decreased to less than 600×10^9/L in 2 to 6 weeks. A lower continuous dosage is required to maintain disease control, because once this treatment is halted the platelet count rises again. The only common side effects are dose-related, reversible leukopenia, macrocytic red cell changes, and low-grade fever.

Platelet antiaggregating agents, aspirin (300 mg daily) and dipyridamole (50 mg three times a day) have been shown to reverse incipient gangrene in patients with limb ischemia, provide long-lasting relief of symptoms of erythromelalgia, and improve the neurologic manifestations in ET. An important role for aspirin may be found in patients with recurrent miscarriages, because this treatment does not carry the risk of teratogenicity of the other treatment options. However, continuous use of aspirin once symptoms have abated or myelosuppression has controlled the platelet count, or both, is not advisable because of the significant risk of hemorrhage, particularly from the gastrointestinal tract.

The drug anagrelide is now being used to treat thrombocytosis. It is considered an excellent drug for long-term use, because it does not have mutagenic or leukemogenic potential. However, 15% of patients experience intolerable side effects, including cardiovascular (congestive heart failure), neurologic, and gastrointestinal disorders. For the 85% of patients without these side effects, however, it is an excellent alternative to conventional therapies.

Interferon α has also been advocated for treatment in ET. This agent exerts an inhibitory effect on the growth of megakaryocyte progenitors that correlates clinically with a marked decrease in platelet count following treatment with interferon. Interferon α treatments of 1 to 5 million units/day exert a dose-dependent inhibitory effect on thrombocytopoiesis. However, the treatment also causes moderate depression in granulate levels and is associated with significant side effects. Considering the expense, toxicity, and inconvenience of parenteral therapy, interferon α shows the most promise for use as an alternative to failed chemotherapy.

If surgery is indicated, the platelet count should be controlled preoperatively by use of plateletpheresis or myelosuppression, or both. Platelet concentrates may be needed to provide normal functional platelets.

Course and Prognosis

ET is associated with a better overall prognosis than other MPDs. Recent follow-up studies by the PVSG and others suggest that survival time in ET is lengthy. Eighty percent of patients survive 5 years, and the prognosis been particularly good for younger patients. Acute leukemia transformation and MDS have been reported following treatment of ET with HU, but the incidence of transitions is less common compared with that occurring in other MPDs.

➤ CASE STUDY 1

A 74-year-old man presented with complaints of increasing weakness, night sweats, shortness of breath, easy bruising, and a fever of 10 days' duration. The patient had lost about 10 lb over a 6-month period and noted early satiety. On physical examination he was pale, underweight, and had a fever of 103°F. Massive splenomegaly, moderate hepatomegaly and pulmonary congestion were noted. Purpuric lesions were present on the upper extremities.

Initial laboratory studies disclosed the following values: WBC, 30.5×10^9/L; RBC, 2.9×10^{12}/L; Hgb, 8.3 g/dL; Hct, 25.8%; MCV, 89 fL; MCH, 28.6 pg; MCHC, 32.2%;

platelets, 650×10^9/L. The differential count revealed 45% segmented neutrophils, 6% band neutrophils, 20% lymphocytes, 9% monocytes, 3% eosinophils, 3% basophils, 4% metamyelocytes, 3% myelocytes, 2% promyelocytes, 5% "dwarf" megakaryocytes, and 15 nucleated red blood cells (NRBCs) per 100 WBCs. Erythrocyte morphology demonstrated anisocytosis and poikilocytosis, with prominent teardrop red cells, polychromasia, and basophilic stippling. Platelet number was increased and platelet morphology was abnormal, as evidenced by the presence of giant platelets and hyper- and hypogranulated platelets, and megakaryocytic fragments. Other laboratory tests included reticulocyte count, 3.6%; LAP score, 132 (normal is 22 to 124); LDH, 3054 μ/L; uric acid, 13.2 mg/dL; stool occult blood, negative; Ph' chromosome, negative; and direct antiglobulin test (DAT), negative. A bone marrow aspirate was attempted several times but was unsuccessful because of a dry tap. The bone marrow biopsy revealed trilineage hyperplasia with many clumps of dysplastic atypical megakaryocytes. Extensive fibrosis was also noted. Bacterial and fungal bone marrow cell cultures were performed, and all results were negative.

Comment

The diagnosis of idiopathic myelofibrosis with myeloid metaplasia (IMF/MM) was made based on the classic findings of leukoerythroblastic anemia, marked splenomegaly, thrombocytosis with circulating megakaryocyte precursors, teardrop erythrocytes, and increased fibrosis of the bone marrow. Chronic myelogenous leukemia was excluded, because the majority of these patients have the Philadelphia chromosome, a low LAP, a higher proportion of myelocytes and myeloblasts, and a bone marrow showing predominantly granulocytic hyperplasia. Additionally the red cell morphological changes—in particular teardrop red cells—are more prominent in myelofibrosis.

Of patients with known polycythemia vera (PV), 15% to 20% undergo a transition to IMF; however, because there is no prior history of PV, this disease can be ruled out. Granulomatous disorders and acute leukemia can be excluded by careful scrutiny of the bone marrow and the negative microbiologic cultures. An increased platelet count and marked proliferation of bizarre megakaryocytes would be highly unusual in acute leukemia.

Another disorder considered in differential diagnosis is essential thrombocythemia (ET). Again, these patients rarely show the red cell abnormalities associated with fibrosis in the marrow and splenic hematopoiesis, and the bone marrow is easily aspirated. The platelet count in ET is almost always greatly elevated, generally greater than 1000×10^9/L, and immature granulocytes are rarely prominent.

Bulsulfan therapy was administered to this patient and continued over the course of 1 year. Blood transfusions were required every 3 to 4 weeks to counteract the impending anemia. Androgen therapy (danazol) was also initiated. The patient's condition gradually worsened, and it was evident that the chemotherapy was only mildly effective in decreasing splenic size. Splenectomy was per-

continued

formed in an attempt to ameliorate his anemia and relieve the constitutional symptoms of splenomegaly.

Four years after initial presentation, this patient developed acute myelogenous leukemia and underwent a rapidly progressive fatal course. This case illustrates a typical course of myelofibrosis. The median survival is approximately 5 years, and treatment often has little effect in prolonging the survival.

Questions

1. Referring to the WBC differential, is a "left shift" evident in this case? Why or why not?
2. What is the corrected WBC count, given the number of NRBCs?
3. Give reasons why the bone marrow aspirate resulted in a "dry tap" in this case.
4. What is the significance of the teardrop red cells?

Answers

1. Yes. Evidence of a "left shift" in the WBC differential is indicated by the presence of 4% metamyelocytes, 3% myelocytes, and 2% promyelocytes.
2. The corrected WBC is $26.5 \times 10^9/L$. The following calculation is used to derive the corrected WBC.

$$\text{Corrected WBCs/L} = \frac{\text{WBC/L} \times 100}{100 + \text{no. NRBCs/100 WBCs}}$$

$$26{,}522/L \text{ or } 26.5 \times 10^9/L = \frac{30{,}500 \times 100}{115}$$

(p. in 3rd ed. 608)

3. A "dry tap" occurred during the bone marrow aspiration procedure done on this patient because of the extensive fibrosis that is a hallmark feature of myelofibrosis. The reticulin and collagin fibers that cause fibrosis form a tight network, locking in the marrow contents. As a result, the bone marrow sinusoid blood is unaspiratable.
4. The teardrop cells are significant because they correlate with bone marrow fibrosis. The teardrop shape of the red cell occurs as the cell passes through the narrow, fibrotic sinusoids of the bone marrow and spleen.

► CASE STUDY 2

A 58-year-old white man was admitted to the hospital with pain and swelling of the left arm suggestive of thrombophlebitis. He had presented to his physician 2 days earlier with complaints of pounding headaches, blurred vision, tinnitus, and generalized pruritus, especially after bathing. The patient had been treated for gout for the past 2 months. Family history is unremarkable for any hematologic disorders. The patient is a nonsmoker.

On physical examination, the patient's face appeared flushed, and the retinal veins were engorged. Several ecchymoses were apparent on the legs. The spleen tip was palpable three fingerbreadths below the costal margin (indicating moderate splenomegaly). No hepatomegaly or lymphadenopathy was observed.

A complete blood count revealed the following values: WBC, $20.3 \times 10^9/L$; RBC, $7.53 \times 10^{12}/L$; Hgb, 18.2 g/dL; Hct, 58.0%; MCV, 77 fL; MCH, 24.2 pg; MCHC, 31.4%; platelets, $710 \times 10^9/L$. The differential count demonstrated 80% segmented neutrophils, 8% band neutrophils, 9% lymphocytes, and 3% monocytes. Red cell morphology was consistent with a microcytic, hypochromic classification.

Subsequent investigations were undertaken as part of the diagnostic workup of the erythrocytosis. Determination of the red cell mass (utilizing the ^{51}Cr dilution method) was performed and found to be 41 mL/kg (normal male is 36 mL/kg or less). The plasma volume was 40 mL/kg. Arterial oxygen saturation was 94%. The serum iron was 30 μg/dL (normal is 50 to 150) and total iron-binding capacity (TIBC), 460 μg/dL (normal is 250 to 450). Serum vitamin B_{12} was 925 pg/mL (normal is 205 to 876), and vitamin B_{12}–binding capacity was 2600 pg/mL (normal is 1000 to 1022). The LAP score was 198, and the uric acid determination was 10.3 mg/dL. A bone marrow examination revealed 95% cellularity, with pan-hyperplasia and many large megakaryocytes. Iron stores were absent, and the reticulin content was slightly increased.

Comment

Several findings in the history and physical examination suggest a presumptive diagnosis of PV. The nonspecific symptoms of headache and blurred vision are a result of cerebral circulatory disturbances caused by hyperviscosity. Thrombotic episodes, such as the phlebitis recorded in this patient, are vascular manifestations resulting from the thrombocytosis in conjunction with the hyperviscosity and increased blood volume. The facial plethora and engorged retinal veins are findings associated with conjunctival and mucosal blood vessel congestion. Generalized pruritus occurs in 30% of patients with PV and is related to hyperhistaminemia. The lack of cardiac or respiratory abnormalities, and the presence of normal arterial saturation is helpful in ruling out secondary erythrocytosis. The splenomegaly noted is a frequent finding in myeloproliferative disorders.

The most important clinical findings supportive of PV are the elevation of the Hgb and Hct, increased red cell mass, and normal plasma volume. Furthermore, evidence of trilineage involvement, leukocytosis, and thrombocytosis, in addition to erythrocytosis and bone marrow pan-hyperplasia, strongly suggests a diagnosis of PV. Abnormal elevation of the vitamin B_{12} and B_{12}-binding proteins, uric acid, and LAP are consistent with a myeloproliferative process and are helpful in establishing a diagnosis of PV. The low serum iron and absence of iron stores indicate concomitant iron deficiency. In most patients this is attributed to occult gastrointestinal blood loss and defective platelet function.

This patient fulfills all the diagnostic criteria for PV set forth by the PVSG. Because this 58-year-old patient has an elevated Hct and platelet count and is symptomatic (thrombophlebitis), both phlebotomy and myelosuppressive therapy were initiated. Colchicine and allopurinol were used to control the gout experienced by this patient. Pruritus was a persistent complaint despite the management of erythrocytosis by phlebotomy and hydroxyurea. Cyproheptadine was prescribed and found to be successful in controlling the pruritus.

Questions

1. What laboratory parameters listed in this case indicate a microcytic, hypochromic process?
2. How do the results of the iron studies in this case differ from those for a patient diagnosed with iron-deficiency anemia?
3. If an erythropoietin level were ordered on this patient, would the expected result be normal, increased, or decreased?
4. What is the reason for the splenomegaly in this patient?

Answers

1. The following red cell parameters indicate a microcytic, hypochromic process in this patient: MCV, 77 fL; MHC, 24.2 pg; MCHC 31.4%. Iron deficiency causes this process and results from the tremendous increase of iron required for the excessive erythropoiesis seen in PV.
2. Although the serum iron is decreased in both iron deficiency anemia (IDA) and in this case of PV, the transferrin levels, reflected in total serum iron-binding capacities (TIBC) is only mildly increased here, whereas in IDA the TIBC would be moderate or markedly increased. Another more obvious difference between the two disorders is that IDA is a microcytic, hypochromic anemic process, and PV is a microcytic, hypochromic—but **not** anemic process. (3rd ed. p 104)
3. The expected erythropoietin level in this patient would be decreased, indicating autonomous production of red cells by the bone marrow. This is a particularly cost-effective diagnostic tool for differentiating PV from other secondary and relative causes of erythrocytosis.
4. The characteristic mild to moderate splenomegaly seen in individuals with PV is attributed to extramedullary hematopoiesis. Splenic enlargement is seen in about 75% of patients and is an important finding.

➤ CASE STUDY 3

This 35-year-old white woman initially presented with the thrombocytosis (platelet count, 1200×10^9/L) discovered upon routine physical examination. Her WBC and Hgb values were normal. The history was unremarkable except for occasional epistaxis and minor bruising. She was advised to have a routine follow-up examination and CBC every 3 months and, despite a continually elevated platelet count, remained asymptomatic for 3 years. At that time she was seen by her physi-

cian with complaints of dizziness, visual disturbances, and erythromelalgia. She had also had recent dental surgery and experienced a major perioperative bleeding episode. Mild splenomegaly was noted. Her platelet count was 2500×10^9/L, and the platelet distribution width (PDW) was increased. Other laboratory values were as follows: WBC, 18.5×10^6/L; Hct, 28.5%; prolonged bleeding time; reduced platelet adhesion; and defective platelet aggregation with epinephrine. Bone marrow biopsy demonstrated megakaryocytic hyperplasia with massive platelet clumping. Erythroid and myeloid hyperplasia, as well as a mild increase in reticulin content, were also observed.

Plateletpheresis was performed to rapidly reduce the marked thrombocytosis. The patient was treated with the myelosuppressive agent hydroxyurea in dosages varying from 1 g/day to 500 mg five times per week, depending on the platelet counts. The bleeding and vaso-occlusive symptoms were resolved, and coagulation abnormalities were corrected. Close follow-up is necessary for this patient to ensure a continued beneficial clinical and laboratory response.

Comment

This case highlights the common findings in essential thrombocythemia (ET); namely, marked increased platelet counts, thrombohemorrhagic events, splenomegaly, and bone marrow megakaryocytic hyperplasia. Although this is primarily a disease of upper-middle-age (50 to 70 years) a second population of younger, predominantly female patients exists. Two-thirds of patients are asymptomatic, as was this patient initially. With the advent of automated cell counters that routinely generate platelet counts, asymptomatic patients are being discovered more frequently.

The erythromelalgia noted in this patient represents one of the most characteristic vaso-occlusive manifestations. Prolonged bleeding after trauma or surgery is a common finding related to platelet dysfunction.

In an asymptomatic young patient, it is advisable to withhold myelosuppressive therapy, because these patients do well for many years untreated. When a patient requiring surgery presents with markedly increased platelet count and hemorrhagic complications, plateletpheresis will lower the platelet count dramatically. Additionally myelosuppression is necessary to control the hyperproliferative process.

Causes of reactive thrombocytosis, such as iron-deficiency anemia, malignancy, inflammatory disorders, splenectomy, and so on, are generally easy to exclude based on the clinical and hematologic features of the individual patient. In order to reliably exclude the other chronic MPDs, the PVSG guidelines should be followed. To distinguish a patient with ET from an iron-deficient PV patient, a 1-month trial of oral iron should be instituted. The Hgb should not rise by more than 1 gm/dL to support a diagnosis of ET. In patients with anemia, splenomegaly, and thrombocytosis, the presence of the Ph[1] chromosome conclusively rules out the diagnosis of ET.

The outlook for long-term survival in ET is encouraging as long as appropriate measures are taken to min-

continued

imize thrombohemorrhagic complications. Many patients can tolerate markedly increased platelet counts for years without any complications. The introduction of plateletpheresis has allowed dramatic response in life-threatening or urgent surgical situations. Furthermore, hydroxyurea has proved to be an effective chemotherapeutic agent.

Questions

1. Why did this patient experience a major perioperative bleeding episode when her platelet count was 2500×10^9/L?
2. Erythromelalgia can progress into what clinical manifestation?
3. What is the reason for the megakaryocytic hyperplasia seen in the bone marrow biopsy?

Answers

1. Although the platelet number is elevated in ET, the platelets function abnormally. Besides abnormal platelet function, hemorrhage in individuals with ET has been attributed to: thrombosis with infarction, ulceration of the infaction, and subsequent bleeding; consumption of coagulation factors; and, excessive production of prostacyclin by endothelial cells stimulated by the increased numbers of platelets, resulting in suppression of platelet granule release and aggregation.
2. The erythromelalgia of the toes, feet, and fingers seen in ET patients can progress to cyanosis and/or necrosis of the extremities. This toxic effect is caused by the metabolites of platelet arachidonic acid.
3. The megakaryocytic hyperplasia of ET results from a neoplastic clonal disorder of multipotential stem cells, which gives rise to excessive numbers of circulating platelets. This disease can be contrasted with the various disorders that can be associated with a reactive, or non-neoplastic thrombocytosis.

QUESTIONS

1. What is the origin of MPDs?
   a. Fibroid infiltration of major organs
   b. Neoplastic transformation of multipotential stem cells
   c. Widespread deterioration of cellular function
   d. Splenic sequestration of normal blood cells

2. Which of the following is *not* a characteristic of a chronic MPD?
   a. Extramedullary hematopoiesis
   b. Possible termination in acute leukemia
   c. Cytogenetic abnormalities
   d. Hypoplasia of bone marrow

3. What is the predominant abnormal erythrocyte morphology associated with idiopathic myelofibrosis?
   a. Schistocytes
   b. Ovalocytes
   c. Teardrop cells
   d. Target cells

4. Which features of chronic myelogenous leukemia are the most important characteristics that distinguish it from myelofibrosis?
   a. Presence of increased platelets and fibroblasts
   b. Decreased erythrocytes with abnormal morphology
   c. Increased leukocytes with hypercellular bone marrow
   d. Low LAP score and presence of Ph' chromosome

5. Which of the following factors does *not* cause fibroblast proliferation?
   a. CSF
   b. TGF-β
   c. bFGF
   d. PDGF

6. What are the laboratory findings in polycythemia vera?
   a. Decreased hematocrit; increased RBCs and granulocytes; decreased platelets
   b. Increased hematocrit; increased RBCs, granulocytes, and platelets
   c. Normal hematocrit; normal RBCs; increased granulocytes and platelets
   d. Increased hematocrit; increased RBCs; decreased granulocytes and platelets

7. What is the expected erythropoietin value in polycythemia vera?
   a. Normal
   b. Increased
   c. Decreased

8. When is myelosuppression advocated in patients with polycythemia vera?
   a. If the patient is less than 20 years old
   b. When thrombosis-associated risk factors are present
   c. If the patient shows signs of glossitis
   d. If the patient has failed iron therapy

9. Which features help to distinguish secondary erythrocytosis and relative erythrocytosis from polycythemia vera?
   a. Absence of splenomegaly; normal leukocyte, platelet, and LAP levels
   b. Presence of splenomegaly; increased leukocyte, platelet, and LAP levels
   c. Presence of hepatomegaly; decreased leukocyte, platelet, and LAP levels
   d. Presence of both splenomegaly and hepatomegaly; increased leukocytes and platelets; decreased LAP score

10. What is the safest and least expensive treatment for patients with polycythemia vera?
    a. High altitude
    b. Decrease of iron levels
    c. Therapeutic phlebotomy
    d. Decrease of erythropoietin levels

11. Which condition will *not* cause an absolute erythrocytosis?
    a. High altitude
    b. Chronic pulmonary disease
    c. Polycythemia vera
    d. Dehydration

12. What condition is defined by a platelet count greater than 600×10^9/L, megakaryocytic hyperplasia, absence of Ph' chromosome, and hemoglobin of 13 g/dL or more (or normal red cell mass)?
    a. Essential thrombocythemia
    b. May-Hegglin anomaly
    c. Acute myelogenous leukemia
    d. Polycythemia vera

13. The thrombosis seen in patients with essential thrombocythemia is a result of which of the following?
    a. Protein C deficiency
    b. Marked fibroblast proliferation
    c. Intravascular clumping of sludged, hyperaggregable platelets
    d. Splenic sequestration of platelets

14. What condition is not characteristically associated with reactive thrombocytosis?
    a. Acute hemorrhage
    b. Aplastic anemia
    c. Chronic inflammatory disorders
    d. Iron-deficiency anemia

15. Which of the following chronic MPDs is associated with the best prognosis?
    a. CML
    b. IMF
    c. PV
    d. ET

> Giant, bizarre platelets and micromegakaryocytes (dwarf megakaryocytes) may be seen in the peripheral blood in IMF.
> Elevation of the hematocrit (above 58% in males and above 52% in females) is the most important hallmark of polycythemia vera (PV).
> Elevated red cell mass, splenomegaly, decreased erythropoietin, normal arterial oxygen saturation, and increased leukocyte alkaline phosphatase (LAP) are other important features of PV.
> Treatment of PV involves phlebotomy or use of cytotoxic myelosuppressive agents, or a combination of both.
> Increased secretion of erythropoietin has been implicated as the responsible stimulus for all cases of secondary erythrocytosis.
> The arterial oxygen saturation is usually decreased in patients with secondary erythrocytosis.
> Relative erythrocytosis occurs when there is depletion in circulating plasma volume (causing increased hematocrit but normal red cell mass), and it is often seen in patients with dehydration.
> The platelet count is markedly elevated in essential thrombocythemia (ET), often to more than 1000×10^9 per liter.
> Hemorrhage and thrombosis caused by dysfunctional platelets, splenomegaly, erythromelalgia, and neurologic manifestations are clinical features of ET.
> ET must be differentiated from the many causes of reactive thrombocytosis.

REFERENCES

1. Dameshek, W: Some speculations on the myeloproliferative syndrome. Blood 6:372, 1951.
2. Lewis, SM: Myelofibrosis, Pathology and Clinical Management, Hematology, vol 4. Marcel Dekker, New York, 1985.
3. Hueck, G: Zwei Falle von Leukamia mit eigenthum lichem blut-resp Knoch en Markesbefund. Virchow Arch, Pathol Anat 78:475, 1879.
4. Lee, GR, et al: Wintrobe's Clinical Hematology, ed 9. Lea and Febiger, Philadelphia, 1993.
5. Hoffbrand, AV, and Lewis, SM: Postgraduate Hematology, ed. 3. Heineman Professional Publishing, Oxford, 1989.
6. Williams, WJ: Hematology, ed 5. McGraw-Hill, New York, 1995.
7. Hippocrates: Dehumoribus. Chapter 1.
8. Vasquez, H: Sur une forme speciale de cuanose d'accompanant d'hypergloblie excessive et persistante. C R Soc Biol (Paris): 4:384, 1892 and suppl nute Buil Mem Soc Med Hop Paris, 12:60, 1895.
9. Osler, W: Chronic cyanosis with polycythemia and enlarged spleen; a new clinical entity. Am J Med Sci. 126:187, 1903.
10. Turk, W: Beitrage zur Kenntnis des Symptomenbildes Polyzythamie mit Milz-tumor und Zyanose. Wien Klin Wochenschr, 17:153, 1904.
11. Hirsch, R: Generalized osteosclerosis with chronic polycythemia vera. Arch Pathol 19:91, 1935.
12. Rosenthal, N, and Sessen, FA: Course of polycythemia. Arch Intern Med 62:903, 1938.
13. Berk, PD, et al: Therapeutic recommendations in polycythemia vera based on Polycythemia Vera Study Group Protocols. Semin Hematol 23:132, 1986.
14. Wasserman, LR: Polycythemia Vera Study Group: A historical perspective. Semin Hematol 23:183, 1986.
15. Weinfeld, A, et al: Acute leukaemia after hydroxyurea therapy in poly-cythemia vera and allied disorders: Prospective study of efficacy and leukae-mogenicity with therapeutic implications. Eur J Haematol 52:134, 1994.
16. Gaisbock, F: Die Bedeutung des Blutdruckmessung fur die arztlichen Praxis. Dtsch Arch Klin Med 83:363, 1905.
17. Murphy, S, et al: Essential thrombocythemia: An interim report from the Poly-cythemia Vera Study Group. Semin Hematol 23:177, 1986.

See the bibliography for this chapter at the end of the book.

SUMMARY CHART

> Myeloproliferative disorders (MPDs) arise from a malignant transformation of a single multipotential stem cell that is committed to differentiation of granulocytes, monocytes, erythrocytes, and platelets.
> MPDs are grouped together because of shared characteristics, the most important being panhyperplasia of the bone marrow, extramedullary hematopoiesis, bone marrow fibrosis, and predilection for leukemic transformation.
> Important features of idiopathic myelofibrosis (IMF) are anemia with teardrop poikilocytosis, leukoerythroblastic blood picture, marked bone marrow fibrosis, splenomegaly, and variable but often elevated platelet counts.
> Megakaryocyte growth factors stimulate bone marrow fibroblastic proliferation in IMF.

19 Myelodysplastic Syndromes

Giovanni D'Angelo, FCMLS
Martin Gyger, MD, FRCP(C)
Douglas Fish, MD, FRCP(C)
Lambert Busque, MD, FRCP(C)

OBJECTIVES

At the end of this chapter, the learner should be able to:

1. Give an overview of the clonal nature and stem cell origin of myelodysplastic syndromes (MDS).

2. Recognize the characteristic laboratory features of each subgroup of MDS.

3. List differential diagnostic criteria that are characteristic for each MDS subgroup.

4. Illustrate the complexity of diagnosis in refractory anemia.

5. Distinguish RAEB and RAEB-t from acute myeloid leukemia.

6. Differentiate between primary and secondary MDS.

7. Characterize the diagnostic and prognostic values of cytogenetic studies.

8. Recognize the most important prognostic criteria for survival and leukemic transformation.

9. Summarize the most important clinical manifestations and causes of mortality.

10. Describe the therapeutic regimen that is most likely to achieve long-term survival.

Myelodysplastic syndromes (MDS) are clonal hematologic malignancies characterized by peripheral blood cytopenias, dysplastic blood cells, and a propensity to transform into acute leukemia. MDS are relatively frequent with an incidence several times greater than that of the acute leukemias. MDS are composed of a group of several different entities that have a variable outcome ranging from a relatively indolent disorder to a rapidly progressing disease associated with a dismal vital prognosis.

MDS were first described in the1930s as preleukemic anemia. In 1982, the French-American-British (FAB) Morphology Cooperative Group classified these syndromes into five distinct entities according to specific morphological criteria.[1] These are refractory anemia (RA), refractory anemia with ringed sideroblasts (RARS), refractory anemia with excess blasts (RAEB), refractory anemia with excess blasts in transformation (RAEB-t), and chronic myelomonocytic leukemia (CMML). The anemia of patients with MDS is qualified as refractory in view of the fact that it is not responsive to iron, folic acid, vitamin B_{12}, or to the administration of other hematinic therapies.

The fundamental characteristic of MDS is the discrepancy between the presence of peripheral blood cytopenias and bone marrow hypercellularity. This ineffective hematopoiesis is probably caused by increased intramedullary death of blood cell precursors (apoptosis).[2] Although MDS may show variable clinical severity, they are almost always fatal. There is no curative treatment for MDS other than allogeneic bone marrow transplantation, a therapeutic modality available to a minority of patients because of the age limitation of the transplantation procedure combined with the limited availability of compatible donors. New therapeutic venues such as immunotherapy or apoptosis inhibitors show some promise for patients not amenable to transplantation. This chapter summarizes the current knowledge of the pathogenesis, clinical features, and treatment of MDS, emphasizing the role of the laboratory investigation in the diagnosis of this important hematologic disorder.

➤ EPIDEMIOLOGY AND ETIOLOGY

MDS affect predominantly the elderly, with a median age of onset of 70 years old and an incidence close to 45 per 10^5 in that age group.[3] MDS occur at a lower frequency in younger adults and in children. Men are slightly more frequently affected with the exception of the 5q− syndrome, which affects more women than men.

Little is known about the cause of MDS. Several risk factors have been associated with the development of MDS, such as exposure to environmental and occupational products, including ammonia, petrochemicals, and low-dose irradiation.[4] For most of these, the relative risk following exposure is low, and, in some cases, the associations have not been clearly established. In fact, only exposure to benzene has been convincingly associated with the development of MDS. Benzene, which is processed in vivo to hydroquinone, induces damage to hematopoietic progenitor cells that may lead to MDS.[5] MDS can also occur as a late complication in patients treated with chemotherapy or radiation therapy; in this case, it is referred to as secondary MDS (see later discussion).

In most cases of MDS, it is not possible to document a causative agent, and so the majority of patients are said to have de novo MDS. This has led to the hypothesis that environmental toxic agents that cause MDS are ubiquitous. It has been suggested that dietary exposure to foods that have a high phenol content, such as some fruits, vegetables, and coffee, may lead to an accumulation of toxic metabolites such as hydroquinone in the bone marrow and predispose selected individuals to MDS.[6] Another hypothesis suggests a genetic component. Persons with genetic polymorphisms for genes coding for the enzymes involved in the detoxification of metabolites, when associated with reduced enzyme activity, may be subject to more significant damage from the environment. One example is the 609C→T polymorphism of the NQ01enzyme, which confers a lesser capacity to detoxify potential carcinogens such as benzene.[7] More studies are needed to identify the causative factors of de novo MDS.

➤ PATHOGENESIS

As previously stated, the exact mechanisms that lead to the development of the MDS are not completely delineated. It is generally accepted that the pathogenesis is complex and involves the accumulation of different genetic alterations in a hematopoietic progenitor cell. Recent advances in molecular biology have allowed the characterization of some of the fundamental defects present in MDS.

MDS Are Clonal Proliferative Disorders

Monoclonal (clonal) derivation of cells is the hallmark of cancer. A somatic mutation giving rise to a growth advantage of the mutated cell leads to a clinically significant disorder. The clonal nature of MDS has been firmly established by the documentation of clonal cytogenetic anomalies in a significant proportion of patients with MDS.[8] X-inactivation assays have also confirmed the monoclonal nature of the MDS.[9] These assays are based on the principle of X inactivation in females, whereby early in embryogenesis one of the two X chromosomes is randomly inactivated by methylation in each cell. Each subsequent daughter cell will inactivate the same X chromosome as its precursor. Thus, most females are balanced mosaics at the cellular level, with half their cells in any given tissue carrying the paternal X in the active state and the other half with the maternal X in the active state. The documentation that blood cells of female patients with MDS have a preponderance of the same X chromosome in the active state instead of the predicted random X-inactivation pattern confirms the clonal derivation of the disease. This suggests that a somatic mutation conferring a selective growth advantage has occurred in a progenitor cell with repopulating ability.[10]

Cell of Origin of the Neoplastic Clone

The precise cellular origin of the neoplastic clone is central to the understanding of the pathogenesis of MDS. In which hematopoietic progenitor cell did the genetic defect causing MDS occur? This question has given rise to controversy in the past several years. Although some authors argue that the cellular origin of MDS is an omnipotent stem cell with the ability to differentiate into all cell lineages, including lymphoid cells, others favor a pluripotent stem cell already committed to myeloid differentiation (Fig. 19–1).

This question can be addressed first by looking at the nature of the blast cell population in patients undergoing leukemic transformation during the course of their disease. In the vast majority of cases, blasts are myeloid or myelomonocytic in phenotype.[11] Extremely rarely can a lymphoid phenotype be demonstrated.[12] Cytogenetic analysis of marrow metaphases and fluorescence in situ hybridization (FISH) performed on interphase nuclei have consistently documented cytogenetic anomalies in myeloid cells, with none being found in lymphoid cells.[13,14] The controversy has been fueled by the documentation that a significant proportion (30% to 40%) of female MDS patients had results compatible with a clonal derivation of cells in all lineages, including T and B lymphocytes, by the X-inactivation assay.[15] This was interpreted as evidence that, in some cases, MDS originated from a stem cell with the ability to differentiate into all cell lineages. These data have been subjected to reanalysis in the light of recent documentation that close to 40% of normal women aged over 60 demonstrate an abnormal pattern of X inactivation of blood cells that mimics clonal derivation of cells, known as *acquired skewing*.[16] Because the populations analyzed with MDS are usually in this same age group (more than 60 years old), it is possible that the skewing found in T and B lymphocytes reflects the normal change in clonality patterns with age and may not be interpreted as proof positive of primitive hematopoietic stem cell involvement in these patients.

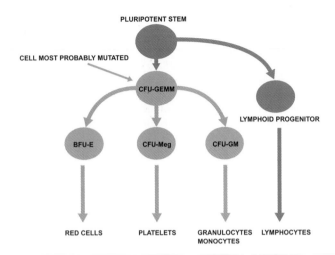

PLURIPOTENT STEM

CELL MOST PROBABLY MUTATED

CFU-GEMM

LYMPHOID PROGENITOR

BFU-E   CFU-Meg   CFU-GM

RED CELLS   PLATELETS   GRANULOCYTES   LYMPHOCYTES
                              MONOCYTES

➤ **FIGURE 19–1**   Schematic representation of marrow stem cell hierarchy showing the stem cell theoretically involved in the pathogenesis of myelodysplastic syndromes (MDS), according to cytogenetic and fluorescence in situ hybridization (FISH) analyses (see text). CFU-GEMM = colony-forming unit–granulocyte-erythrocyte-megakaryocyte-macrophage; BFU-E = burst-forming unit–erythroid; CFU-Meg = colony-forming unit–megakaryocyte; CFU-GM = colony-forming unit–granulocyte-macrophage.

In summary, most studies aimed at determining the cell of origin of MDS point to a defect arising in a repopulating stem cell already committed to myeloid differentiation. Whether molecular events not detectable by the present technology are present in the omnipotent stem cell remains to be shown.

Ineffective Hematopoiesis

The phenomenon by which each cell is able to trigger its own death is called *apoptosis* or *programmed cell death*. Apoptosis is essential to tissue homeostasis. An abnormal decrease in the rate of natural apoptosis will lead to cell accumulation, whereas an increase in the rate of apoptosis will lead to decreased cellular output.

Apoptosis is characterized by three sequential phases: (1) initiation, (2) commitment, and (3) execution.[17] A variety of factors can initiate apoptosis, such as chemotherapy, radiotherapy, corticosteroid administration, and growth factor deprivation; it may also occur as a direct effect of cytotoxic T-cell activity. Apoptosis can be initiated by inhibitory cytokines such as tumor necrosis factor-alpha (TNF-α), transforming growth factor-beta (TGF-β), and the action of *Fas*-ligand on its receptor FAS/CD95 (Fig. 19–2). The commitment phase is, in part, regulated by proteins belonging to the *Bcl-2* family. Some of these are proapoptotic (*Bax, Bak, Bad, Bcl-XS, Bik*), whereas others are antiapoptotic (*Bcl-2, Bcl-XL, Mcl-1*). If the balance of *Bcl-2* family protein activities favors apoptosis, a family of cysteine proteases called caspases will be activated, leading to cell death following a series of molecular cleavages affecting the cytoskeleton, cytosol, and nuclear proteins. This will lead to a pathognomonic phenotype characterized by chromatin condensation, oligodimerization of deoxyribonucleic acid (DNA), and nuclear disintegration.

Yoshida first proposed that the ineffective hematopoiesis seen in MDS was caused by an abnormally high rate of intramedullary apoptosis.[18] Several groups using different methods to assess this hypothesis by such methods as in situ end labeling (ISEL), nick-end labeling (TUNEL), and flow cytometry, have consistently shown an elevated rate of apoptosis in MDS patients compared with normal controls. Apoptosis seems to affect CD34+ progenitors as well as maturing cells. The degree of apoptosis is more important in early phase of the disease than in advanced or proliferative stage. Several lines of evidence suggest a major role for in-

hibitory cytokines in the initiation of apoptosis in MDS. TNF-α is elevated in the bone marrow of MDS patients, and correlates with the degree of apoptosis.[19] TGF-β has also been shown to be elevated in MDS, and may also play an important initiating role.[19] Growth-stimulatory cytokines such as granulocyte/macrophage-monocyte colony-stimulating factor (GM-CSF), which show some anti-apoptotic activity, are diminished in MDS. Therefore, the balance between growth-stimulatory and growth-inhibitory cytokines may favor apoptosis in MDS. As antigen and *Fas*-ligand are also abnormally elevated on the surface of MDS cells, the *Fas* pathway of apoptosis may also be important in the pathogenesis of MDS.

Although increased apoptosis is a key biologic manifestation of MDS, it is still not clear if it is central to the pathogenesis of this disease or merely an indication of ineffective hematopoiesis caused by other genetic anomalies of the involved clone. The investigation of the cause and mechanisms of apoptosis in MDS may shed new light on its pathogenesis and may lead to novel therapeutic approaches.

Genetic Anomalies in MDS

The most common genetic alteration associated with MDS is the loss of genetic material. The cytogenetic analysis of patients with MDS is characterized mainly by chromosomal deletions (see the later discussion of cytogenetics). These can involve part of or a whole chromosome. This is in sharp contrast to the acute leukemias, in which the finding of chromosomal translocations is dominant. The acute leukemias appear to follow the model of oncogene activation, resulting in the transformation of the cell of origin, whereas the deletional pattern found in MDS favors a tumor suppressor gene model. In this model, the lack of both copies (one from each parental chromosome) is necessary to lead to carcinogenesis. One allele may be mutated and the other deleted.[20] The best described examples of this model are found in retinoblastoma and the Li-Fraumeni syndrome (*p53*).[21] It is also possible that haploinsufficiency (the presence of only one active allele of a gene) alone may be sufficient to cause a malignant hematologic process in some cases. It has been recently shown that hereditary haploinsufficiency for *AML1* is associated with the development of acute leukemia in a family.[22] It is, therefore, possible to suggest that MDS patients are missing key genes

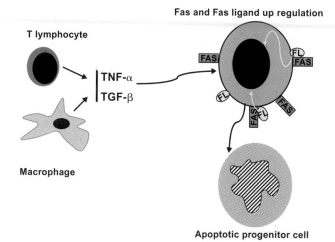

Fas and Fas ligand up regulation

T lymphocyte

TNF-α

TGF-β

Macrophage

Apoptotic progenitor cell

▶ **FIGURE 19–2** Apoptosis of progenitor cells in bone marrow of patient with MDS. There is an increased production of inhibitory cytokines such as TNF-α and TGF-β in MDS patients. This may contribute to upregulation of *Fas* and co-expression of *Fas*-ligand (FL). This is one of the several pathways that could activate programmed cell death. Cysteine proteases (caspases) will be activated and will execute the cell.

essential for maintaining normal hematopoiesis and that, with time, this leads to the accumulation of more severe and numerous genetic anomalies associated with disease progression and deterioration of the hematologic phenotype. No one gene that is commonly deleted in a significant proportion of MDS patients has been identified so far; however, the identification of such genes is the focus of intensive research by several groups.

Biologic Characteristics of Disease Progression in MDS

With progression toward leukemia, the MDS phenotype changes. The number of blast cells increases in the marrow, peripheral blood leukocytosis may replace leukopenia, and hepatosplenomegaly can occur. MDS then evolves into a proliferative peripheral blood disorder. A number of biologic phenomena have been observed on acceleration of MDS, such as a decrease in medullary apoptosis, a decrease in *Fas* expression, as well as mutations at the *p53* (tumor suppressor) and *RAS* (proto-oncogene) loci.[23] The *p15ink4b* gene, involved in the control of the cell cycle, becomes more heavily methylated and, therefore, less active to block abnormal cells in G phase, facilitating the proliferation of abnormal cells.[24] MDS is thus one of the best examples of the multistep pathogenesis of neoplasia for hematologic cancers. The accumulation of different genetic alterations changes the phenotype of the cell from normal to clonal and dysplastic, and further changes confer a full-blown malignant phenotype, leading to the development of acute leukemia.

▶ MORPHOLOGICAL ABNORMALITIES IN PERIPHERAL BLOOD AND BONE MARROW

Definitions of Specific Morphological Characteristics

At the laboratory level, the diagnosis of an MDS is made by the careful morphological study of blood and bone marrow smears using the Wright-Giemsa stain, and of the bone marrow biopsy specimen using hematoxylin-eosin (H & E) and reticulin stains (Table 19–1). The iron content of both marrow aspirate and biopsy specimens is revealed by the

use of Prussian blue (Perl's stain).[25] Other special stains, such as myeloperoxidase (MPO), Sudan black B (SBB), periodic acid–Schiff (PAS), and specific and nonspecific esterases may be used in the investigation of MDS. The review of these materials allows the distinction between MDS subtypes based on established criteria. MDS are most often suspected in patients presenting with anemia, which is usually normochromic, macrocytic, and refractory to all types of standard therapeutic approaches with or without accompanying cytopenias. A vast array of laboratory tools helps the physician to establish the diagnosis of each type of MDS.[26–28]

Blasts

Some types of myelodysplastic syndromes are diagnosed according to the number of blasts in the bone marrow at initial diagnosis. There are two types of blast, according to the FAB classification: type I refers to a myeloblast of variable size, without any azurophilic granules or Auer rods (Fig. 19–3); type II refers to a myeloblast that is slightly larger and contains few azurophilic granules (1 to 20) (Fig. 19–4); Goasguen and associates[29] have proposed a type III myeloblast, containing more than 20 azurophilic granules with a basophilic cytoplasm and absence of the Golgi zone similar to type I and II myeloblasts.

Sideroblasts

Type I refers to a normal sideroblast containing one to four cytoplasmic iron-containing granules, normally accounting for 15% to 50% of bone marrow erythroblasts. A type II sideroblast is considered abnormal, harboring 5 to 10 granules, scattered throughout the cytoplasm. Type III is synonymous with a ringed sideroblast, having more than 10 granules that cover at least one-third of the nuclear rim, sometimes forming a complete ring around the nucleus.[30]

Lineage Dysplasia

Dyserythropoiesis

Peripheral Blood

Anemia is present in at least 90% of cases and is most often macrocytic or normocytic with a decreased reticulocyte number (see Color Plate 213). Erythrocyte morphological

> **Table 19-1**
SUMMARY OF MORPHOLOGICAL HALLMARKS IN MDS

Erythrocytes	Leukocytes	Platelets
Peripheral Blood		
Macrocytosis	Hypogranulation	Giant forms
Dimorphism	Pelgeroid nuclei	Hypogranulation
Anisopoikilocytosis (fragmented cells)	Hyposegmented or hypersegmented	Megakaryocyte fragments
Acanthocytes (teardrop cells)	Ringed-shaped nuclei	
Stippling	Döhle bodies	
Polychromasia	Myeloblasts	
Nucleated red blood cells (NRBCs)	Immature granulocytes, monocytes	
Pappenheimer bodies		
Howell-Jolly bodies		
Bone Marrow Aspirate		
Erythropoiesis	Myelopoiesis	Thrombopoiesis
"Dyserythropoiesis"	"Dysmyelopoiesis"	"Dysmegakaryopoiesis"
Megaloblastic changes	Decreased primary granules	Micromegakaryocyte mononuclear
Multinuclearity	Giant primary granules	Decreased nuclear polyploidization
Ringed sideroblasts	Decreased secondary granules	Hypogranulation
Intranuclear bridging	Auer rods	Separated nuclei (botryoids, "pawn-ball" shape)
Nuclear fragments and budding	Pelgeroid forms	Mononuclear vacuolated basophilic cytoplasm
Vacuolization	Fragmented nuclei	
Maturation arrest	Maturation arrest	
Bone Marrow Biopsy		
Dysplasia		
Abnormal localization of immature myeloid precursors (ALIP)		
Fibrosis		

characteristics that may be encountered are macrocytosis, anisopoikilocytosis, basophilic stippling, a dual red blood cell population (normochromic, hypochromic), Pappenheimer bodies, dacryocytes (teardrop cells), fragmented cells, elliptocytes, Howell-Jolly bodies, and acanthocytes (see Color Plates 214 through 216).

Bone Marrow
Erythroblasts may harbor megaloblastoid changes with dense or fine chromatin with asynchronous cytoplasm maturation, internuclear bridging, and broad-based nuclear budding (Fig. 19–5; see also Color Plates 217 through 220). Cytoplasmic abnormalities may include intense basophilia, Howell-Jolly bodies, and ghost cells. With iron stains, abnormal sideroblasts of type II and type III may be found (Fig. 19–6; see also Color Plate 221).

Dysgranulocytopoiesis

Peripheral Blood
Neutropenia is found in almost 60% of patients, although neutrophilia may be encountered occasionally. Granulo-cytes show variable degrees of hyposegmentation with bilobulation (pseudo-Pelger-Huët anomaly) or monolobulation (pseudo-Stodtmeister anomaly),[31] abnormal chromatin, or, rarely, atypical hypersegmentation (Figs. 19–7 and 19–8; see also Color Plate 222). In the cytoplasm, one may find variable degrees of hypogranulation, persistent basophilic zones (pseudo-Döhle bodies), or, more rarely, hypergranulation with larger granules than usual (see Color Plate 223). Combined nuclear and cytoplasmic dysplasia is detected in over 90% of cases.

Bone Marrow
The nuclei of neutrophils often show variable degrees of hyposegmentation (pseudo-Pelger-Huët or Stodtmeister anomalies) (see Color Plates 224 and 225). Other nuclear abnormalities include hypersegmentation, ring formation, chromatin clumping, and formation of chromatin sticks. According to the specific type of MDS, there may be numerous immature myeloid cells presenting asynchronous nuclear-cytoplasmic maturation. The cytoplasm may be hypogranular or agranular, with persistent basophilia at the rim of the cell. One can also observe hybrid myelomonocytic cells with specific staining properties for granulocytes

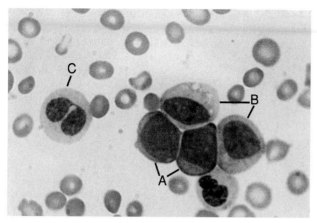

➤ **FIGURE 19–3** Refractory anemia with excess of blasts in transformation (RAEB-t) (bone marrow, magnification ×1000). *A.* Two blast cells. *B.* Two immature granulocytes with some degree of hypogranularity and vacuolization. *C.* Pelgeroid hypogranular neutrophil.

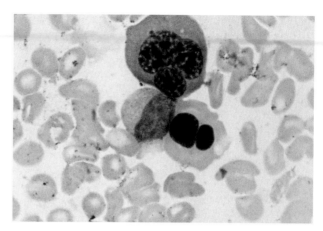

➤ **FIGURE 19–5** Wright-Giemsa stain, bone marrow (magnification ×1000). Dysplastic multinucleated erythroblasts with asynchronous maturation (RAEB-t).

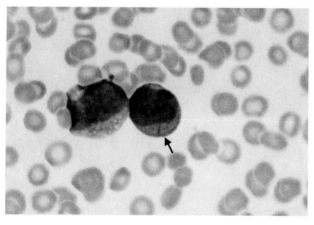

➤ **FIGURE 19–4** Two blasts with azurophilic rods, blast with an Auer rod *(arrow)* (bone marrow, magnification ×1000).

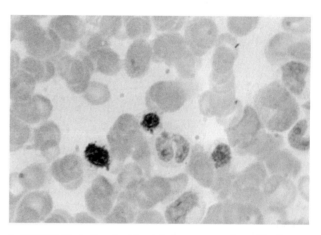

➤ **FIGURE 19–6** Prussian blue stain, bone marrow (magnification ×1000). Three-ringed sideroblasts (sideroblasts type III).

(chloroesterase) and monocytes (alpha-naphthol acetate or butyrate esterase). Vacuolated monocytes or myeloid precursors, or both, have been encountered in a few cases.

Dysmegakaryocytopoiesis

Peripheral Blood

Thrombocytopenia is present in almost 60% of patients, occasionally being severe (less than 20×10^9/L). Thrombocytosis is of rare occurrence and is usually associated with the 5q− syndrome. One may find variable morphological abnormalities such as platelet gigantism, ballooning, and more or less severe hypogranulation[32] (see Color Plates 213 and 215).

Bone Marrow

There are two characteristic morphological abnormalities of megakaryocytes in the bone marrow: the presence of micromegakaryocytes (dwarf or mononuclear megakaryocytes), and megakaryocytes with multiple small nuclei detached from one another or separated by a thin strand of nuclear material and cytoplasmic hypogranularity (botryoids, "pawn-ball" shape) (Figs. 19–9 and 19–10; and Color Plates 226 through 229). In rare cases, megakaryocytes may show large cytoplasmic vacuoles (see Color Plate 230).

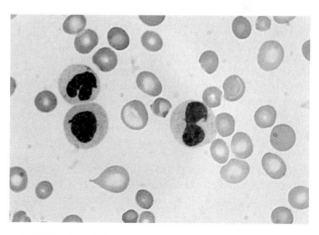

➤ **FIGURE 19–7** Refractory anemia with excess of blasts (RAEB) (peripheral blood, magnification ×1000). Pseudo-Pelger-Huët anomaly, mononuclear Stodtmeister type.

➤ FAB CLASSIFICATION OF MYELODYSPLASTIC SYNDROMES[1,33]

As discussed earlier, MDS are classified into five distinct subgroups: RA, RARS, RAEB, RAEB-t, and CMML. The distinction between each subgroup of MDS relies essen-

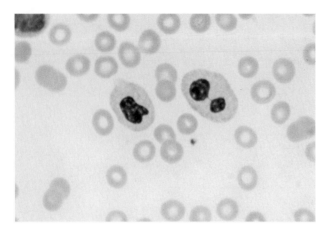

➤ **FIGURE 19–8**   Bilobulated and monolobulated neutrophil (peripheral blood, magnification ×1000).

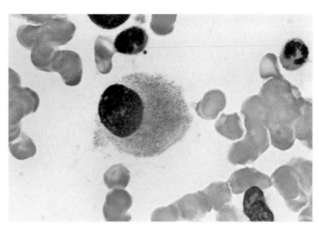

➤ **FIGURE 19–9**   RAEB (bone marrow, magnification ×1000). Monolobular (dwarf) megakaryocyte.

tially on the study of bone marrow aspirate stained with Wright-Giemsa and Prussian blue. The laboratory and hematologic distinctive features of each MDS subgroup are summarized in Table 19–2.

Refractory Anemia (RA)

This type of myelodysplastic syndrome is the most difficult to recognize and diagnose. Indeed, the diagnosis rests mainly on the subjective identification of qualitative abnormalities according to the FAB classification, involving one or more bone marrow hematopoietic cell lineages, in a patient suspected of having refractory anemia. Anemia is present in more than 90% of patients. It is usually normochromic and macrocytic, but in some cases, erythrocytes may be normocytic, with a variable degree of morphological abnormalities, usually more subtle than those found in other subgroups. Cytopenias are common, with a white blood cell count less than 3.9×10^9/L and a platelet count below 130×10^9/L. Morphological abnormalities such as dysgranulopoiesis or dysmegakaryopoiesis are more subtle than in other types of MDS. The bone marrow is usually normocellular or hypercellular. Infrequently, it may be slightly hypocellular or may present a variable degree of fibrosis. Blast cells, type I and type II, represent less than 5% of all nucleated cells. Erythroid hyperplasia is relatively common, with mild dyserythropoiesis and occasional ringed sideroblasts (less than 15% of nucleated red blood cells). Cytogenetic studies are crucial in the diagnosis of this particular subtype of MDS in view of the absence of quantitative criteria for its diagnosis. Indeed, the finding of a clonal chromosomal abnormality in such a setting confirms the diagnosis. Approximately 50% of patients are found to have such abnormalities. The diagnosis may also be supported by abnormal bone marrow culture results or an X-inactivation clonality assay showing a clonal pattern in myeloid cells in the presence of a normal somatic tissue control. In the absence of a clonal chromosomal abnormality, the establishment of this diagnosis based solely on single lineage dysplasia should be made with great caution. Isolated dyserythropoiesis on blood or bone marrow smears may be a feature shared by a variety of hematologic disorders, including relatively benign diseases with no potential to progress to acute leukemia and bearing no relationship to the MDS. A combination of two cell lineage dysplasias should be present to consider the diagnosis of RA.

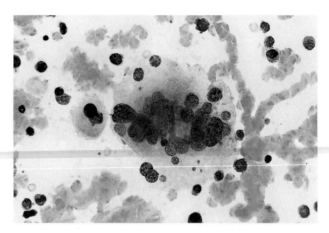

➤ **FIGURE 19–10**   RAEB (bone marrow, magnification ×1000). Large megakaryocyte with multilobulated nuclei, some of them distinctly detached and small in size (botryoid, "pawn-ball" shape).

Refractory Anemia with Ringed Sideroblasts (RARS)

RARS shares almost all the morphological features of RA, although generally to a lesser extent. Fortunately, the diagnosis rests on quantitative criteria: the presence of at least 15% ringed sideroblasts in the bone marrow (varying from 15% to 90% among nucleated red blood cells) (see Color Plate 221). Ringed sideroblasts are pathologic sideroblasts in which the usual migration of mitochondria from the nucleus toward the cytoplasm does not occur. As a result, they remain frozen around the nucleus, where insoluble iron conglomerates and further contributes to cell destruction. This feature, combined with lineage dysplasia as mentioned earlier, is satisfactory to establish the diagnosis. Red blood cells are usually macrocytic or normocytic with dimorphic features (dual population of hypochromic and normochromic red blood cells). Leukopenia and thrombocytopenia are relatively infrequent (10% to 15% of cases).

Refractory Anemia with Excess Blasts (RAEB)

In this type of MDS, the degree of lineage dysplasia is more significant. The anemia is macrocytic and normochromic, with important morphological abnormalities such as ovalocytosis and the presence of dacryocytes related to bone

> **Table 19-2**
LABORATORY FEATURES OF MDS

| | MORPHOLOGY* | | |
Type	**Peripheral Blood**	**Bone Marrow Aspirate**	**Dysplasia**
RA	Blasts < 1% Cytopenia	Blasts < 5% Ringed sideroblasts < 15%	+/++ 1–3 cell lineages
RARS	Blasts < 1% Cytopenia	Blasts < 5% Ringed sideroblasts > 15%	+ 1–3 cell lineages
RAEB	Blasts < 5% Cytopenia	Blasts 5%–20%, no Auer rods Ringed sideroblasts, variable	+++ 2–3 cell lineages
RAEB-t	Blasts > 5% Cytopenia	Blasts 20%–30%, or blasts 5%–20% with Auer rods	++++ 3 cell lineages
CMML	Blasts < 5% Monocytosis > 1 × 10^9/L WBC < 13 or > 13 × 10^9/L	Blasts 1%–20% Monocytes, promonocytes ≥ 20% Ringed sideroblasts, variable	++/+++ 2–3 cell lineages

Cytogenetic

Standard karyotyping: Single and complex abnormalities

Molecular cytogenetic: FISH and SKY technologies, PCR

Progenitor Cell Culture

Progenitor colonies are reduced or absent; *exception:* CMML

Immunology

Apoptosis greatly increased

CD34 increased in number

CD55, CD59 may be decreased in RBC, neutrophils, and possible other cells (PNH features)

Molecular Biology

Gene mutation, oncogenes changes (*p53, RAS*)

Abbreviations: FISH = fluorescence in situ hybridization; SKY = spectral karyotyping; PCR = polymerase chain reaction
*See text for details and specifics, in particular, the characteristic morphological abnormalities.

marrow dyserythropoiesis. On rare occasions, one can find a peripheral blood sample with an increased number of immature granulocytes. Although occasional blasts may be seen in the peripheral smear, the count is always below 5% (see Color Plate 231). Dysgranulopoiesis with nuclear hyposegmentation and hypogranulation is frequent. Thrombocytopenia is a common feature, with giant size and hypogranular platelets. Bone marrow cellularity is normal or increased, with myeloblasts of type I and type II ranging between 5% and 20% (see Color Plates 232 and 233). Dysmegakaryocytopoiesis and dyserythropoiesis with ringed sideroblasts, variable in number, can be significant (Color Plate 234).

Refractory Anemia with Excess Blasts in Transformation (RAEB-t)

This type of MDS is closely related to refractory anemia with excess blasts. The major difference lies in the number of blasts found in the bone marrow at initial diagnosis. In RAEB-t, the number of blasts ranges from 20% to 30%. In the peripheral blood, blasts frequently comprise more than 5%. Auer rods may be found. Their presence is diagnostic of RAEB-t, even if the number of blasts in the bone marrow is less than 20%. Acute myeloblastic leukemia, type M2, can mimic RAEB-t when the blast count is between

25% and 30%. The degree of dysplasia in the bone marrow and the presence of a t(8;21), typical for a small proportion of AML type M2, helps in differentiating between these two entities.[34]

Chronic Myelomonocytic Leukemia (CMML)

This type of MDS is controversial in regard to its classification as a myelodysplastic syndrome. In the blood and bone marrow, the same morphological abnormalities as those found in the other types of MDS may occur. On clinical grounds, this type of MDS is more closely related to the chronic myeloproliferative disorders, particularly when the white blood cell (WBC) count is higher than 13 × 10^9/L. Patients often present with splenomegaly or hepatomegaly. Peripheral WBC counts may be as high as 75 × 10^9/L, a picture resembling chronic myelogenous leukemia (CML) (see Color Plate 235). The bone marrow is usually hypercellular, with monocytosis and a blast cell count between 1% and 20% (see Color Plate 236). In some cases, cytogenetics may be the only means of distinguishing CMML from CML. Indeed, CML has a specific clonal marker, the Philadelphia chromosome t(9;22)(q34q11.2).[35] There are no specific chromosomal abnormalities in CMML. The diagnosis rests mainly on the presence of more than

1×10^9/L monocytes in the peripheral blood and the findings of lineage dysplasia in the peripheral blood or bone marrow, or both, as in other MDS.

➤ LABORATORY INVESTIGATION

Cytochemistry

Decreased enzymatic activity of myeloperoxidase, chloroesterase, and alkaline phosphatase; abnormal positivity in myeloid precursors; PAS positivity in erythroblasts; dual esterase in myeloid and monocytoid cells; and decreased SBB staining are often found in MDS (see Color Plates 237 through 239). An increase in the number of erythrocytes with HbF (positive Kleihauer-Betke acid elution test) is a common observation (see Color Plate 240). Cytochemistry is of less diagnostic value in MDS with major qualitative and quantitative abnormalities such as RARS, RAEB, RAEB-t, and CMML than in RA, where cytochemical studies of blood and bone marrow cells can lend credence to the diagnosis.

Following is a summary of the frequency of cytochemical anomalies in RA patients, based on our observations and those of others. For leukocytes, in 60% to 78% of cases, neutrophil peroxidase shows reduced activity in most of the neutrophils (polymorphonuclear neutrophils [PMNs]) or an absence of activity in a small percentage of cells; chloroesterase and leukocyte alkaline phosphatase (LAP) staining show decreased activity in mature neutrophils, but LAP activity may be increased in neutrophil precursors. In the erythrocyte lineage, 18% to 25% of erythroblasts stain positive for PAS, with basophilic erythroblasts and proerythroblasts showing granular and droplet reactions whereas more mature erythroblasts (polychromatophilic and orthochromatic) have diffuse cytoplasmic reactivity. Occasionally, some erythrocytes stain positive, with a more homogenous or diffuse pattern. Although no single cytoenzyme anomaly can be considered a specific early marker for leukemic transformation, a progressive deterioration of cytochemical enzymatic activities associated with morphological abnormalities can become indicators of an impending leukemic phase. These changes in enzymatic activity must, however, be interpreted with caution because infections, toxic bone marrow damage, and some congenital defects of hematopoiesis may present similar cytochemical abnormalities.[36-38]

Bone Marrow Histology

In patients with MDS, discrepancies between the cellularity estimates from aspirate smears and biopsy specimens occur in up to 20% of cases. It is well accepted that the most accurate estimate of bone marrow cellularity is made from an adequate biopsy specimen. In addition to the cellularity evaluation, the bone marrow biopsy specimen may be of great help in revealing typical histologic changes such as the disruption of normal hematopoietic architecture, with displacement of granulopoiesis, erythropoiesis, and megakaryocytopoiesis from their usual sites. Abnormal localization of immature precursors (ALIP),[39] clusters or aggregates of myeloblasts and promyelocytes of usually three or more cells distant from the bone marrow trabeculae, is also a feature of some MDS. This finding has been considered by some authors as an indicator of early leukemic transformation. Bone marrow biopsy is especially relevant in the rare cases of MDS with severe myelofibrosis (10%)[40,41] (Fig. 19–11) or associated

with bone marrow hypoplasia.[42,43] Although dyserythropoiesis and dysgranulopoiesis are difficult to assess on bone marrow biopsy specimens, dysmegakaryocytopoiesis can be fairly estimated.

Cytogenetics

A full description of the terminology and abbreviations used in describing chromosomes and their abnormalities is beyond the scope of this chapter. For detailed guidelines, the reader is referred to a specialty textbook.[44] A brief review adapted for the comprehension of this section is presented in Table 19–3.

Since the introduction of the FAB classification for MDS in 1982, cytogenetics has become one of the most informative laboratory tools in their investigation and management. The nature and complexity of clonal chromosomal abnormalities have proved to be essential in the diagnosis and establishment of the prognosis. Specific chromosomal abnormalities, when documented, contribute independent prognostic factors and, thus, provide the opportunity to individualize therapy.

Clonal cytogenetic abnormalities are detected in 30% to 60% of patients with MDS.[45] The incidence rises to close to 90% in secondary MDS.[46] Structural and numerical anomalies are found, but, as noted earlier, deletions are by far the most frequent and characteristic cytogenetic events observed. The most frequent anomalies are the deletion of the long arm of chromosome 5 (5q−), monosomy 7 (7−), and trisomy 8 (8+). Deletions of parts of chromosomes 11, 12, and 20 are also frequently reported (Fig. 19–12). The cytogenetic anomalies reported in secondary MDS are related to the type of therapy that patients have previously received. More than 90% of patients treated with an alkylating agent show anomalies of chromosome 5 or 7, or both.[46] Patients treated with agents of the epipodophyllotoxins class demonstrate anomalies (mainly translocations) involving chromosome 11q23, where the gene MLL resides.[47] No chromosome abnormalities are specifically associated with any FAB subgroup; however, the 5q− anomaly is documented more frequently in RA,[48] as is del(20q). Monosomy 7 is rarely seen in RA.[49] Complex karyotypes are more often found in RAEB and RAEB-t. A chromosome rearrangement involving 12p occurs in rare cases of CMML. Certain cytogenetic anomalies are associated with morphological or

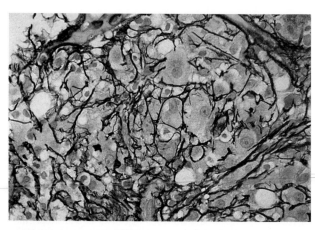

➤ **FIGURE 19–11**   RAEB (bone marrow, reticulin stain, magnification ×400). Severe fibrosis.

clinical particularities. Monosomy 7, especially in children, is associated with a greater risk of bacterial infection independent of the neutrophil count.[50] Anomalies involving the short arm of chromosome 17 (17p) where the *p53* gene resides, are associated with hypolobulated granulocytes with small cytoplasmic vacuoles.[51] Involvement of the 3q26 band (EVI-1) is associated with thrombocytosis and dysplastic megakaryocytes.[52] Stereotypic translocations, such as t(8;21), t(15;17), t(9;22), and others found in specific types of chronic and acute myeloid leukemia are, as a general rule, not found in de novo MDS.

Cytogenetic anomalies carry important prognostic significance. The risk of transformation to leukemia or severity of blood cytopenias may be predicted by specific cytogenetic changes. Patients with complex karyotypes (three or more chromosomal abnormalities within the same cell) have a shortened survival, as do patients with monosomy 7. On the other hand, patients with −Y, del(20q), or del(5q) as a sole anomaly have a more favorable clinical outcome, with a tendency for a long, leukemia-free survival. The remaining patients have an intermediate prognosis.[53]

The 5q− Syndrome

In the mid-1970s, van den Berghe[54] described patients with an acquired interstitial deletion of the long arm of chromosome 5 (Fig. 19–13). These patients had specific clinical features that included a macrocytic anemia, normal or elevated platelet count, mild leukopenia, and, in the bone marrow, monolobular or dwarf megakaryocytes and erythroid hypoplasia. Patients are usually classified as having RA according to the FAB classification and are, in contrast to other MDS patients, predominantly females. The 5q− syndrome is associated with a good prognosis with a median survival time of approximately 8 years. The deleted DNA segment lies between bands 5q13 and 5q33 (Fig. 19–14). Although there may be variable breakpoints within this region, band 5q31 seems to be consistently deleted.[55] Interestingly, several genes related to hematopoiesis are located in the involved region, including those coding for GM-CSF, interleukin-3 (IL-3), IL-4, IL-5, CD14, macrophage colony-stimulating factor (CSF-1), colony-stimulating factor 1 receptor (CSF1R), and platelet-derived growth factor (PDGF).[56] No one of these has been shown to be consistently deleted and, therefore, causative of the syndrome. Intense research is under way to try to identify the causative gene or genes involved. It is important to note that a 5q anomaly found in conjunction with other cytogenetic anomalies, or in a patient with a history of treatment with an alkylating agent, is not associated with this clinical syndrome and is not associated with a good prognosis.

The Future of Cytogenetics

One limitation of traditional cytogenetic analysis is the necessity to obtain cell metaphases through marrow culture, which is at times unsuccessful or leads to suboptimal chromosome identification. The use of gene- or chromosome-specific probes in the FISH technique allows the analysis of the interphase nuclei. FISH is particularly useful for numerical anomalies (e.g., 8+) and for some deletions (e.g, del[5]) (see Color Plate 241). Newer technologies such as spectral karyotyping (SKY) will allow the identification of hidden translocations by distinctly coloring each individual chromosome. This powerful new technique will reinforce the already predominant role of cytogenetics in the investigation of MDS.

> **Table 19-3**
> ### ABBREVIATIONS AND TERMINOLOGY USED IN DESCRIBING CHROMOSOMES AND THEIR ABNORMALITIES

Abbreviation	Significance
p	Short arm of a chromosome
q	Long arm of a chromosome
p−, q−	Loss of chromosomal material to the short arm and long arm, respectively
p+, q+	Addition of chromosomal material to the short and long arm, respectively
del	Deletion of chromosomal material
t	Translocation of chromosomal material (DNA exchange between 2 chromosomes)
mar	Marker chromosome that is not fully characterized
+	Addition of a chromosome
−	Loss of a chromosome
Hypodiploid	Cells having fewer than 46 chromosomes
Hyperdiploid	Cells having more than 46 chromosomes
Complex karyotype	The presence of more than 2 chromosomal abnormalities in the same cell

Example: 47.XX.del(7)(q22).+8. The description in order of chromosome abnormalities in a karyotype is the following: sec aberrations are specified first, followed by abnormalities of the autosomes, listed in numerical order, irrespective of aberration type. In this example, a breakpoint in the long arm of chromosome 7, at region (band) 22(q22) has resulted in the loss (del) of chromosomal material →del(7)(q22); there is also a gain of 1 chromosome 8 → +8.

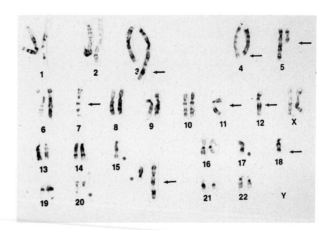

> **FIGURE 19–12** Karyotype GTG banding, resolution 450 bands, showing complex clonal abnormalities involving at least 8 chromosomes within the same cell, including del(5)(q13q33), −7, del(20)(q11.2).

Immunology

Cell surface antigens of peripheral blood cells, bone marrow, biopsy specimens can be studied by flow cytometry or immunocytochemistry using alkaline phosphatase antialkaline phosphatase methodology (APAAP) and other techniques. An increase in the percentage of CD34+ cells (stem cell progenitors) in the bone marrow is of prognostic significance and usually correlates with impending leukemic transformation.[57] Blasts from patients evolving toward acceleration or transformation in any type of MDS may carry antigens characteristic of other cell lineages, mostly myeloid, monocytic, and lymphoid. In the rare cases in which a lymphoblastic proliferation is found, the immunophenotypic pattern is consis-

tently of the early B type (CD19+, CD10−, TdT+). RAEB and RAEB-t show a higher frequency of myeloblastic and megakaryoblastic immunologic markers, whereas in RA, RARS, and CMML, a granulomonocytic phenotype predominates. Hybrid lymphoid-myeloid cells or the coexpression of granulomegakaryocytic antigens are also frequently observed. At the molecular level, rearrangements of the immunoglobulin H (IgH) and the T-cell antigen receptor-gamma (TCR-γ) and -delta (TCR-δ) genes can be found.

Patients with type I and II blasts expressing the H blood group antigen[58] have a poor prognosis as opposed to those expressing a purely myeloid phenotype. Expression of surface antigens from monocytes and granulocytes may vary considerably, with either loss or gain of specific or nonspecific antigens. Lymphopenia is frequently observed, with a decrease in the number of CD4+ cells and a slight increase of CD8+ cells.[59] It has been reported that an increased number of CD8+ cells at initial diagnosis in RA and RARS is associated with a decreased incidence of ANLL transformation. Although natural killer lymphocytes are decreased, antibody-dependent cellular cytotoxicity is observed.

Fewer B-lymphocyte abnormalities have been reported. B-cell Epstein-Barr virus (EBV) receptors are decreased in number.[60] Immunoglobulin synthesis may be abnormally regulated. Polyclonal hypergammaglobulinemia is observed in approximately 30% of patients with MDS; 12% have a monoclonal gammopathy, whereas 13% are hypogamma-globulinemic. In patients with CMML, polyclonal hyper-gammaglobulinemia may be observed in more than 60% of cases.[61] Autoantibodies, in general, have been reported in 22% of all patients with MDS, but in patients with CMML, they are a more frequent occurrence (present in more than 50% of patients). Platelet antibodies are present in 55% of the cases studied, and erythrocyte autoantibodies in 46%. The direct antiglobulin test was positive in 8% of the cases where IgG1 and C3d were detected on the RBCs.[62]

Evaluation of Progenitor Cell Growth in Semisolid Media

Several investigators have studied in vitro growth patterns from MDS patients. There is a specific pattern of colony clusters that grow in culture from normal progenitor cells. Marrow cells pass through all stages of maturation to become morphologically recognizable mature cells. In vitro cultures of bone marrow cells from individuals with MDS have provided information about the nature of the pathophysiologic defect. In general, the ability of hematopoietic progenitor cells to form colonies is found to be either reduced or absent.[63] Aberrant growth patterns are mostly observed in the more severe subgroups of MDS, such as RAEB and RAEB-t. CMML is a notable exception and is distinguished by increased colony growth.[64] Investigators have tried to correlate these growth patterns with the propensity to evolve to acute leukemia, dividing them into leukemic and nonleukemic types. Given the lack of standardization and results that are often conflicting, no firm conclusions can be made about growth patterns with respect to either prognosis or leukemic potential in individual patients with MDS at this time. In vitro bone marrow culture from patients with MDS is a valuable complementary tool to be considered together with cytogenetics and other laboratory studies.

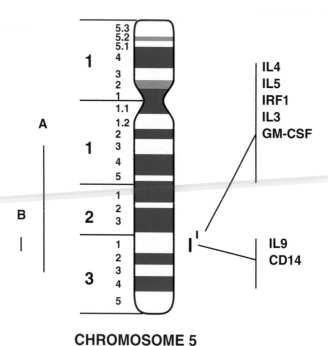

CHROMOSOME 5

➤ FIGURE 19–13   The 5q− syndrome. Several genes related to hematopoiesis are localized on 5q. *A.* The interstitial deletion may comprise any region located between band 5q13 and 5q33. *B.* The band 5q31 is consistently deleted in most patients.

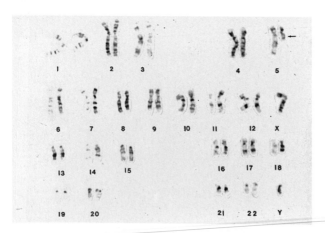

➤ FIGURE 19–14   Karyotype with GTG banding, 450 bands resolution, showing the interstitial deletion of chromosome 5 → 46XY, del(5)(q13q33) characteristically found in the 5q− syndrome.

X-Inactivation Clonality Studies

The documentation of clonal derivation of cell populations may support the diagnosis of MDS in the appropriate clinical setting. Unfortunately this type of investigation is limited to female patients, because it is based on the principle of random X inactivation that occurs in the female embryo. The X inactivation clonality assay requires the differentiation of the paternal and maternal X chromosomes as well as the active from the inactive one. Highly polymorphic markers such as the multiallelic CAG tandem repeat of the first exon of the human androgen receptor gene *(HUMARA)*, coupled with the study of the different methylation sites between the active X and the inactive X chromosomes, allows these distinctions to be made in 90% of cases.[65]

The applicability of the X-inactivation clonality assay is limited by the skewing phenomenon, which mimics a clonal derivation of cells and is found in a significant proportion of aging women.[16] This phenomenon can be ruled out by analyzing a somatic tissue not involved in the disease process. Clonality results are interpretable if the somatic tissue shows a balanced pattern of X inactivation (both alleles active). The somatic tissue used as a control should be embryologically related to the sample to be analyzed and should not be involved in the disease process, because tissue-specific variation of X-inactivation patterns occurs. T lymphocytes are thus a good control for MDS patients. Because the *HUMARA* clonality assay is polymerase chain reaction (PCR)–based, small numbers of cells obtained by flow cytometry or colonies grown in semisolid media suffice for analysis. The X-inactivation assay is particularly useful for the female patient with a normal karyotype and a low or normal blast count, because it may be the only proof of a clonal hematologic disorder. It is of note that close to 25% of patients with MDS have preserved polyclonal hematopoiesis and that a polyclonal result does not exclude the diagnosis.

Cellular Dysfunction

Genetic mutations or other abnormalities such as chromosomal deletions, translocations, or gene amplification are responsible for a vast array of functional abnormalities within specific cell lineages.

Red Blood Cells (RBCs)

Several metabolic abnormalities may be encountered, the most frequent being acquired pyruvate kinase deficiency and an increased level of fetal hemoglobin. Acquired hemoglobin H, increased expression of the i antigen, loss of ABO blood group antigens, demasking of the Tn antigen, and increased sensitivity to complement (positive serum acid or sugar water test) have also been reported.[66–69] At times, loss of erythrocyte membrane proteins such as decay-accelerating factor (DAF) CD55, and glycosyl phosphatidyl inositol (GPI)–linked antigen CD59. Concomitantly, such loss may be observed on neutrophils and other cells overlapping with paroxysmal nocturnal hemoglobinuria.

White Blood Cells (WBCs)

Abnormal granulocyte function is frequently observed with decreased cytoplasmic granules and myeloperoxidase deficiency. Alkaline phosphatase and alpha-naphthol acetate esterase isoenzyme activities may also be decreased in granulocytes. Chemotaxis, adhesion, phagocytosis, and microbicidal capacity may be impaired.[70,71] These functional abnormalities are not necessarily related to cellular hypogranulation. Abnormal phagocytosis, chemotaxis, or bactericidal activities in neutrophils have been closely associated with chromosome 7 anomalies (monosomy 7 and del[7q]). These specific dysfunctions are associated with a high frequency of bacterial infections. In these situations, the GP130 molecule, produced by a gene located on chromosome 7, is secreted in inadequate amounts, and is responsible for the major defect in chemotaxis and phagocytosis.[72]

Platelets (PLTs)

Platelet aggregation, adhesion, and other platelet functions are also frequently impaired in MDS.[73]

Other laboratory findings may be abnormal in MDS, including vitamin B_{12} and folate levels; serum ferritin and transferrin saturation (both increased); and muramidase, which is increased both in serum and urine in CMML.

➤ SECONDARY MYELODYSPLASTIC SYNDROMES (sMDS)

MDS are said to be secondary when they occur after significant exposure to chemotherapy, radiotherapy, or other toxic agents.[74–76] The term *secondary myelodysplastic syndromes* seems more appropriate than the often-seen "therapy-related MDS," because exposure to toxic agents is also responsible for sMDS. The laboratory findings, clinical manifestations, and evolution resemble those of de novo MDS, although sMDS show a higher frequency of clonal chromosomal abnormalities and a greater tendency to early leukemic transformation, particularly if a complex karyotype is present. The prognosis is generally worse in sMDS than in de novo MDS.

There has been an increase in the number of patients presenting with sMDS at hematology and oncology centers in recent years. From 5% to 10% of patients undergoing autologous bone marrow transplantation with chemotherapy with or without combined radiotherapy as preparative regimens will develop sMDS.[77–79] Most cases are causally related to previous therapy with alkylating agents, almost all of which have been shown to be leukemogenic. This undesirable potential seems to be enhanced by the use of radiotherapy. The period of latency between exposure and the development of sMDS is usually 6 to 8 years, and patients have a poor response to therapy with the exception of allogeneic bone marrow transplantation. Recently, the use of the epipodophyllotoxins etoposide and tenoposide has been shown to be leukemogenic if administered in combination with cisplatinum, doxorubicin, or alkylating agents.[80] In patients with MDS and a history of previous exposure to alkylating agents, cytogenetic studies usually show unbalanced cytogenetic aberrations, primarily −7, −5, 5q−, and 7q−. Recently, an increasing number of patients with sMDS have been observed with balanced chromosomal translocations. Studies have revealed that the majority of these patients have been previously exposed to epipodophyllotoxins and antracyclines, which target DNA topoisomerase II, often in combination with other drugs including alkylating agents. DNA topoisomerases are a class of enzymes important in various DNA transactions such as replication, transcription, and recombination.[81] Most of the balanced translocations involve 11q23 and different partners such as chromosomes 4, 6, 9, or 19. Usually the gene *MLL1* at band q23 of chromosome 11 is rearranged. Balanced translocations involving the gene *AML1* at 21q21 are also reported in this setting. Patients with these translocations usually have a short latency between exposure and development of sMDS, and tend to present with acute leukemia with monocytic features. Response to therapy is better than with classical sMDS resulting from exposure to alkylating agents.

MDS in Children

MDS occurs rarely in children. RAEB and RAEB-t are the most frequent FAB subtypes in that age group. Children are most often symptomatic with fever, pallor, and asthenia.[82] In contrast to adults, children more commonly have normocytic, normochromic anemia than macrocytosis. Several syndromes such as Fanconi's anemia, Down's syndrome, Kostmann's agranulocytosis, and Shwachman's syndrome are associated with an increased risk of development of acute myeloblastic leukemia in children and should be investigated.[83,84] Monosomy 7 syndrome and juvenile chronic myeloid leukemia usually present with leukocytosis and hepatosplenomegaly and are considered myeloproliferative disorders rather than MDS.[85]

➤ CLINICAL MANIFESTATIONS

Most commonly, the presenting symptoms are those attributable to progressive bone marrow failure. Clinical manifestations develop in relationship to the degree of anemia, neutropenia, or thrombocytopenia. Symptoms related to infection, hemorrhage, or anemia with cardiac failure, such as severe dyspnea on exertion, may be encountered in patients with MDS and severe bone marrow failure. Fatigue and weakness may also be noted. In patients with RAEB and RAEB-t, these may appear relatively early in the course of the disease. Those patients not having excess numbers of blasts in the bone marrow may be asymptomatic for a long period of time. Rarely, patients may present systemic symptoms such as infection, arthralgias, weight loss, fever, and cutaneous vasculitis.

Abnormal physical findings are neither prominent nor specific. The spleen may be palpable in 20% of patients, and the liver may be enlarged in approximately 10%. Enlarged lymph nodes are not usually present. As opposed to the other types of MDS, in CMML, splenomegaly, hepatomegaly, lymphadenopathy, and nodular cutaneous leukemic infiltrates are more common.[86,87] The overall clinical picture of CMML is more closely related to the myeloproliferative disorders such as CML, polycythemia vera, essential thrombocytosis, and primary myelofibrosis.

➤ EVOLUTION AND PROGNOSIS

Although the overall survival is less than 2 years, the MDS are a heterogeneous group of bone marrow disorders with survival that can vary from weeks to several decades after the initial diagnosis. The causes of mortality are also not uniform. One-third of patients will die of leukemic transformation whereas close to 40% will suffer complications related to bone marrow failure, such as infection or bleeding. Almost one-third will die of conditions unrelated to MDS.[88,89]

There is a need for a classification system that allows the prospective categorization of patients at diagnosis into different prognostic groups in order to select appropriate therapy for an individual patient. The FAB classification has been useful in this regard, although it requires further refinements. It incorporates the single most important prognostic factor: the blast count. The survival and leukemic transformation rates according to FAB subtype are shown in Figure 19–15.

Several other prognostic risk factors have been identified, including (1) the nature and number of chromosome abnormalities,[90] (2) the severity of pancytopenia at diagnosis,[91] (3) the age of the patient, and (4) the presence of ALIP.[39] Different systems have been proposed to quantify the overall prognostic score of individual patients using a combination of these factors. These include the Bournemouth,[88] Dusseldorf,[92] Sanz,[93] and Goasguen[94] scoring systems (Table 19–4). Although they all contribute to a better evaluation of the prognosis of MDS patients, they have been recently supplanted by the International Prognostic Scoring System (IPSS)[95] (Table 19–5). The latter has been thoroughly validated and offers a more precise estimate of overall survival than the previously published systems. The IPSS score is based on the number of peripheral blood cytopenias, the bone marrow blast cell count, and cytogenetic results.

➤ DIAGNOSTIC PROBLEMS IN MDS

Some MDS patients carry features shared with other hematologic disorders (Fig. 19–16). These clinical situations may lead to confusion concerning the appropriate diagnosis for the patient. The most common of these difficult diagnostic quandaries are presented next.

MDS with Hypoplastic Marrow

Between 8% and 22% of MDS patients have a marrow cellularity inferior to 25%.[96] It may be difficult to differentiate such cases from aplastic anemia, which also presents with peripheral blood cytopenias and a hypocellular marrow. The single most important test that may allow the differentiation between these two entities is the demonstration of a clonal cytogenetic anomaly that will confirm the diagnosis of MDS. If the karyotype is normal, careful analysis of the bone marrow smear for dysplastic changes may provide some clues to the correct diagnostic category. In some cases, it may not be possible to differentiate between the two.

MDS with Severe Myelofibrosis

Close to 15% of MDS patients show significant bone marrow fibrosis on biopsy.[97] This is more frequently seen in the setting of sMDS. Patients may have a dry tap on bone marrow aspirate. They often have trilineage dysplasia, profound cytopenias, and no organomegaly. The differential diagnosis includes acute myelofibrosis (AML, M7) and a myeloproliferative disorder such as myeloid metaplasia. The absence of organomegaly and the presence of a characteristic cytogenetic anomaly may support the diagnosis of MDS.

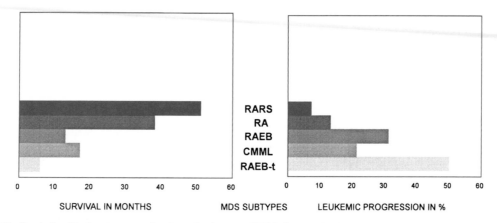

> FIGURE 19–15 Survival and leukemic progression for each subgroup of MDS. Data pooled from several series with a total of 3554 patients.

MDS with Thrombocytosis

This presentation is associated with either the 5q− syndrome or a translocation or other anomaly involving chromosome 3q. Essential thrombocytosis should be considered. Cytogenetic analysis is mandatory to establish the diagnosis.

MDS with Features of Chronic Myelogenous Leukemia

Because CMML may present with a very high WBC count and a significant number of immature myeloid cells in the peripheral blood, this disease entity may mimic CML. Cytogenetic studies are of major importance in order to distinguish between these two entities. The finding of t(9;22) is diagnostic of CML and resolves the problem. Because 5% to 10% of patients with CML may not exhibit the t(9;22) chromosome abnormality by standard cytogenetics, molecular studies by FISH or PCR techniques may be necessary. MDS with the t(5;12) fuses the *TEL* oncogene with the gene for PDGF and gives rise to a clinical picture almost identical to CML.[98]

MDS with Close to 30% Myeloblasts

The boundary between RAEB-t and acute myeloid leukemia (AML) is a mathematical one. RAEB-t, as stated earlier, is defined by a blast count ranging between 20% and 30%. Acute myeloblastic leukemia of FAB M2 type may present with a blast count below or close to 30%. Thus, it can be difficult for the clinician to distinguish between RAEB-t and M2 acute myeloid leukemia. This distinction is of major importance in view of the different therapeutic strategies available for each of these diseases. The degree of dysplasia and cytogenetic findings such as t(8;21), typical for M2 AML, or monosomy 7, 7q−, monosomy 5, or 5q−, more consistently found in MDS, may help to resolve the question.

MDS versus Erythroleukemia (FAB M6)

MDS are often difficult to differentiate from erythroleukemia (FAB M6) when the total population of marrow erythroblasts exceeds 50% of all nucleated cells. In that situation, the number of blasts may not exceed the minimal requirement of 30% of all nucleated cells. FAB has suggested

> ## Table 19-4
> ## DIFFERENT SCORING SYSTEMS IN MDS

Parameter	FAB	Bournemouth	Düsseldorf	Sanz	Goasguen	Bournemouth Modified	Pediatric	IPSS
Hemoglobin	−	+	+	−	+	+	−	*+
Neutrophils	+	+	−	−	−	+	−	*+
Platelets	+	+	+	+	+	+	+	*+
BM Blasts	−	+	+	+	+	+	−	+
ALIP	−	−	−	−	−	+	−	−
Cytogenetics	−	−	−	−	−	+	+	+
Dysplasia	+	−	−	−	−	−	−	−
LDH	−	−	+	−	−	−	−	−
Age	−	−	−	+	−	−	−	−
HbF	−	−	−	−	−	−	+	−
Megakaryocytes	+	−	−	−	−	−	−	−

Abbreviations: BM = bone marrow; ALIP = abnormal localization of immature precursors; LDH = lactate dehydrogenase; HbF = fetal hemoglobin; IPSS = International Prognostic Scoring System; *score 0–2 of cytopenia (see Table 19–5 for more detail)

> **Table 19-5**

INTERNATIONAL PROGNOSTIC SCORING SYSTEM (IPSS) FOR MDS

	SCORE BASED ON THREE PARAMETERS				
BM Blasts %	<5	5–10	•*	11–20	21–30
Score value	0	0.5	1.0	1.5	2.0
Karyotype	Good		Intermediate		Poor
	Normal or −Y del(5q) only del(20q) only		Other abnormalities		Complex (≥3 abnormalities) or chromosome 7 anomalies
Score value	0		0.5		1.0
Cytopenias†		None or one cytopenia		Two or three types of cytopenias	
Score value		0 or 1.0		2.0 or 3.0	

PROGNOSTIC SUBGROUPS	
Overall Sum Score	**Median Survival**
Low Risk = score 0	5–7 yr
Intermediate risk 1 = score 0.5 or 1.0	3–5 yr
Intermediate risk 2 = score 1.5 or 2.0	1–2 yr
High risk = score ≥ 2.5	0.4 yr

Abbreviation: BM = Bone marrow

*Score value 1.0 per number BM blasts was not attributed.

†Hemoblogin   Absolute neutrophils   Platelets
<10 g/dL   <1.5 × 10⁹/L   <100 × 10⁹/L

Note: Using these features: (1) number of BM blast cells, (2) cytogenetic abnormalities, (3) cytopenias. The international MDS risk analysis workshop generated an IPSS with four prognostic subgroups of patients who showed significant clinical outcomes.

Sources: From Greenberg, P, et al: International scoring system for evaluating prognosis in myelodysplastic syndromes. Blood 89:2079, 1997; and Heany, ML, and Golde, DW: Myelodysplasia (review article). N Eng J Med 340: 1649, 1999.

that to establish the correct diagnosis, the number of blasts should be calculated as a percentage of nonerythroid cells (NEC). If the percentage exceeds 30% of NEC, the diagnosis is AML of the FAB subtype M6 rather than MDS (Fig. 19–17).

➤ TREATMENT

MDS are associated with major therapeutic dilemmas. The disease is not curable, except in patients eligible for an allogeneic bone marrow transplantation from a matched related or unrelated donor. Unfortunately, this procedure is associated with treatment-related mortality (within 6 months of transplantation) that varies from 10% to 25%, depending on age of recipient, degree of compatibility, and relatedness of donor. The risk associated with bone marrow transplantation may be inappropriately high for a patient with a good initial prognosis, whereas supportive care alone may be as inappropriate for patients with an impending leukemic transformation. Bone marrow transplantation is usually limited to patients younger than 60 years of age if a matched sibling donor is being considered, and to persons younger than 50 years of age if the donor is matched but unrelated to the recipient. Overall survival is between 55% and 60% for patients with low-risk MDS, 40% for intermediate-risk patients, and only 20% for high-risk patients.[99] The chance of relapse post–bone marrow transplantation is less than 10% for low- and intermediate-risk patients, and 30% if high risk. Bone marrow transplantation may become more widely applicable in the future with prophylactic and therapeutic improvements in the areas of graft-versus-host disease and infection, and perhaps with the introduction of nonmyeloablative preparative regimens (mini-transplantation), associated with fewer toxic side effects than standard regimen transplantation.

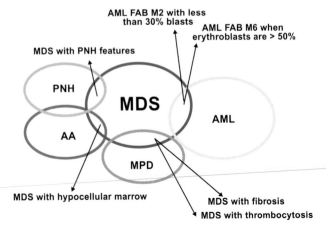

➤ FIGURE 19–16   Overlap between MDS and other hematologic disorders. AA = aplastic anemia; MPD = myeloproliferative disorder; PNH = paroxysmal nocturnal hemoglobinuria; AML = acute myeloid leukemia.

Because this disease group affects mostly elderly people not admissible to transplantation, the mainstay of treatment is restricted to supportive measures such as blood component therapy and antibiotics. The transfusion of red cell concentrates may alleviate symptoms related to anemia. Chelation therapy with desferrioxamine may be indicated for patients who have an otherwise-favorable prognosis and important transfusion requirements in order to prevent secondary hemochromatosis. Platelets can also be transfused for bleeding patients when necessary.

Hematinics such as vitamin B$_{12}$, folic acid, and pyridoxine are notoriously ineffective in the absence of a documented deficiency. Steroid or androgen therapy has been associated with no satisfactory response.

Immunosuppressive therapy using antithymocyte globulin (ATG) has recently been associated with clinically interesting results in patients with a normocellular or hypocellular marrow, no ringed sideroblasts, and a normal karyotype. Close to 60% of such patients may become transfusion-independent for several years.[100] Treatment with cyclosporine A has also been associated with hematologic im-

provement in patients with hypoplastic marrows.[101] Other immune response modifiers such as interferon have not shown adequate clinical response.

Differentiating agents such as retinoids have also failed to show any significant effect. Low-dose cytarabine therapy has led to a positive outcome in 10% to 25% of patients so treated, but no survival advantage could be demonstrated over supportive therapy.[102] Treatment with 5-azacitidine, which demethylates DNA, has resulted in hematologic improvement in close to 50% of patients in small trials.[103] Larger, randomized clinical trials are under way to evaluate its therapeutic benefit.

The use of growth factors has been widely studied in MDS. Erythropoietin (Epo) significantly increases the hemoglobin level in a minority of patients.[104] Good responders are not transfusion-dependent, have an inappropriately low endogenous level of basal Epo, and a diagnosis of RA. G-CSF therapy restores neutrophil counts in most neutropenic patients as long as therapy is maintained.[105] It is generally used for short-term treatment during episodes of severe infection, because long-term therapy is associated

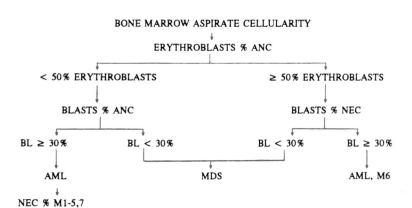

When the erythroblasts (erythroid precursors) are ≥ 50% of ANC, the percentage of myeloblasts (type I, type II) from bone marrow smears is then calculated by excluding erythroblasts (% of NEC). If the result is < 30%, a diagnosis of MDS can be made. If BL ≥ 30%, the diagnosis is then AML, M6.

On the other hand, if the erythroblasts are < 50% of ANC, then the percentage of myeloblasts from bone marrow smears is calculated by including ANC. If BL < 30%, we are facing a MDS diagnosis. If BL ≥ 30%, then diagnoses of AML M1-M5 and M7 can be ascertained by excluding NEC.

Example: Erythroblasts 53%;   blasts 10%;   others 37%.
            10 of 47 is 21% total blasts excluding erythroblasts.
            We are thus dealing with a MDS.

Other Examples:	**Myeloblasts**	**Erythroblasts**	**Diagnosis**
	5 - 20%	< 50%	RAEB
	20 - 30%	< 50%	RAEB-t
	> 30%	< 50%	AML
	> 30%	> 50%	AML-M6

➤ FIGURE 19–17   Algorithm according to FAB criteria proposed to distinguish MDS from different types of acute myeloid leukemia (AML).

with a prohibitively high cost. Other cytokines, such as IL-3, or combinations of cytokines have also been evaluated with only modest benefit.

High-dose chemotherapy with regimens similar to those used to induce remission in acute leukemia has met with disappointing results. A hematologic response is achieved in 20% to 50% of patients; however, these responses are short-lived, with fewer than 20% of patients still in remission 2 years after such therapy.[106] Younger age of patients, the presence of Auer rods, and normal cytogenetic results tend to be associated with a better response rate. Consolidation with autologous transplantation in patients achieving a complete response is being investigated in some centers. Other agents such as topotecan, a topoisomerase I inhibitor, are under evaluation. Thalidomide, which may interfere with angiogenesis, may also have some value in the future.

Therapeutic options for MDS outside of the allogeneic bone marrow transplantation setting are disappointing. It is expected that a better understanding of the fundamental biology of this disorder at the cellular and subcellular levels through research may allow the development of novel and more effective therapeutic approaches in the future.

> **CASE STUDY**
___

A 72 year-old man was admitted to hospital with complaints of increasing weakness. Physical examination revealed pallor but no organomegaly. His previous medical history was unremarkable.

The laboratory results were as follows:

CBC:

WBC	2.9×10^9/L
RBC	2.43×10^{12}/L
Hgb	91 g/L
Hct	0.27 g/L
MCV	111 fL
MCH	37.4 pg
MCHC	337 g/L
RDW	19.0%
PLT	90×10^9/L
PDW	17.4%

Blood Smear Differential and Morphology:

Blasts	2%
Polymyelocytes	0%
Myelocytes	1%
Metamyelocytes	0%
Band	3%
Segmented neutrophils	69%
Eosinophils	1%
Basophils	1%
Lymphocytes	20%
Monocytes	3%

Occasional pseudo-Pelger-Huët neutrophils with hypogranulation, and occasional giant platelets.
Aniso-macrocytosis and occasional basophilic stippling were noted.

Bone Marrow Smear:
Hypercellular.
Blast cells (type I and type II), 23%; a few blasts with Auer rods.
Myeloid dysplasia with immature cells with asynchronous nuclear-cytoplasmic maturation.
Pelgeroid cells with hypogranulation.
Erythroblasts (35%) with megaloblastoid changes.
Micromegakaryocytes (mononuclear).
Prussian blue stain showed 10% ringed sideroblasts (type III).
Cytogenetics: complex karyotype, including monosomy 7.
Diagnosis: RAEB-t.
Treatment: Supportive therapy (transfusion).

QUESTIONS

1. Which type of anemia is most common in MDS?
   a. Microcytic, hypochromic
   b. Normocytic, hypochromic
   c. Macrocytic, normochromic
   d. Dimorphic

2. Which of the following morphological abnormalities are helpful in the diagnosis of MDS?
   a. Pseudo-Pelger-Huët and hypogranulation
   b. Ringed sideroblasts
   c. Micromegakaryocytes, monolobular megakaryocytes
   d. All of the above

3. Which of the following criteria will differentiate RAEB-t from AML of the M2 type?
   a. Thrombocytopenia
   b. Anemia
   c. The finding of t(8;21)
   d. Blasts less than 5%

4. Which of these cell surface antigens is of prognostic significance in MDS?
   a. CD19
   b. CD HLA-DR
   c. CD34
   d. CD33

5. Which one of these MDS subgroups has the most favorable prognosis?
   a. RAEB
   b. CMML
   c. RA
   d. RARS

6. Which type of treatment may offer a cure in patients with MDS?
   a. Chemoradiotherapy
   b. Allogeneic bone marrow transplantation
   c. Autologous bone marrow transplantation
   d. Growth factors such as GM-CSF

7. Which of following agents may lead to secondary MDS (sMDS)?
   a. Hydrocortisone
   b. Alkylating agents
   c. Irradiated blood components
   d. Folic acid

8. Which of the following is most likely to affect prognosis in MDS?
   a. Leukopenia
   b. Increased bone marrow myeloblasts
   c. Erythroid hyperplasia
   d. Thrombocytosis

9. In female patients with RA and elevated platelet counts, which chromosome abnormality is most often found?
   a. (5q–)
   b. t(8;21)
   c. (7q–)
   d. t(15;17)

10. Which of the following biologic or genetic anomalies are important in the pathogenesis of MDS?
    a. Chromosomal translocations
    b. Chromosomal deletions
    c. Hemolysis
    d. Increased intramedullary apoptosis

11. Which of the MDS subtypes is more closely related to the chronic myeloproliferative disorders?
    a. RAEB
    b. CMML with WBC > 13 × 10⁹/L
    c. CMML with WBC < 13 × 10⁹/L
    d. RARS

12. Which MDS scoring system is most often used today?
    a. FAB
    b. IPSS
    c. Sanz
    d. Bournemouth

SUMMARY CHART

➤ Myelodysplastic syndromes (MDS) are clonal hematologic malignancies characterized by peripheral blood cytopenias, dysplastic blood cells in the peripheral blood and in the bone marrow, and a propensity to transform into acute leukemia.

➤ Diagnosis of MDS is based on the morphological study of the blood and bone marrow smears.

➤ Morphological abnormalities are present in all cell lines and are characterized by dyserythropoiesis (abnormal red cells), dysgranulopoiesis (abnormal granulocytes), and dysmegakaryocytopoiesis (abnormal megakaryocytes and platelets).

➤ Anemia is present in 90% of cases and is often macrocytic or normocytic with decreased reticulocyte count.

➤ The abnormal red cell morphologies noted on the peripheral smear are macrocytosis, a dual red cell population, red cell fragments, teardrop-shaped cells, ovalocytes, and acanthocytes; inclusions may include Pappenheimer bodies, Howell-Jolly bodies, and basophilic stippling.

➤ Neutropenia is found in 60% of patients with MDS. Nuclear and cytoplasmic dysplasias are detected in over 90% of cases.

➤ Granulocytes show variable degrees of hyposegmentation and hypogranulation. Hypersegmentation and hypergranulation are rare findings.

➤ Thrombocytopenia is present in almost 60% of patients. The platelet morphology includes gigantism and hypogranulation.

➤ The bone marrow picture indicates erythroid hyperplasia with megaloblastic changes such as asynchronous cytoplasmic maturation, internuclear bridging, nuclear budding, and Howell-Jolly bodies. With iron stain, abnormal sideroblasts may be found. Megakaryocyte abnormalities are micromegakaryocytes, mononuclear megakaryocytes, or megakaryocytes with multiple small nuclei detached from one another by a thin strand of nuclear materials.

➤ Myelodysplastic syndromes are classified into five distinct subgroups: refractory anemia (RA), refractory anemia with ringed sideroblasts (RARS), refractory anemia with excess of blasts (RAEB), refractory anemia with excess of blasts in transformation (RAEB-t), and chronic myelomonocytic leukemia (CMML). The distinction between each subgroup relies on the study of bone marrow aspirate stained with Wright-Giemsa stain.

➤ RA is characterized by macrocytic or normocytic anemia with variable degrees of morphological abnormalities. Leukopenia and thrombocytopenia are common findings. Dysgranulopoiesis and dysmegakaryopoiesis are less common. The bone marrow is usually normocellular or hypocellular with erythroid hyperplasia and a mild dyserythropoiesis. There are less than 5% blasts and occasional (less than 15%) ringed sideroblasts in the bone marrow.

➤ RARS shares all the morphological feature of RA, with the exception of more than 15% ringed sideroblasts in the bone marrow. Cytopenia is relatively infrequent.

➤ RAEB is associated with a significant dysplasia. Immature granulocytes and occasional blasts (5%) may be seen in the peripheral blood. Hyposegmented and hypogranulated granulocytes are frequent. Thrombocytopenia with giant and hypogranular platelets is a common finding. The number of bone marrow blasts increases to between 5% and 20%. Dysmegakaryocytopoiesis and dyserythropoiesis with ringed sideroblasts are variable.

➤ RAEB-t is closely related to RAEB. The number of blasts increases to between 20% and 30% in the

➤ bone marrow and more than 5% blasts in the peripheral blood.

➤ Chronic myelomonocytic leukemia contains all the same morphological abnormalities as those found in the other types of MDS. Patients often present with hepatosplenomegaly. White blood cell counts are high, with an increase in monocytes. The bone marrow is usually hypercellular, with monocytosis and a blast cell count of 1% to 20%.

➤ Cytochemical abnormalities in MDS include decreased or abnormal positivity of enzymatic activities of myeloperoxidase, chloroesterase, alkaline phosphatase, Sudan black B, and dual esterase in myeloid and monocytic cells.

➤ Bone marrow biopsy is helpful to estimate cellularity, histologic changes, and abnormal localization of immature precursors.

➤ Clonal cytogenetic abnormalities are detected in 30% to 60% of patients with MDS. The most frequent abnormalities are deletion of long arm of chromosome 5 (5q−), monosomy (7−), trisomy 8 (8+), and deletion of part of chromosomes 11, 12, and 20. No chromosomal abnormalities are specifically associated with any subgroup; however, the 5q− anomaly is documented with more frequently in RA.

➤ The 5q− syndrome has specific clinical features that include macrocytic anemia, normal or elevated platelet count, mild leukopenia, and in the bone marrow, monolobular or dwarf megakaryocytes and erythroid hypoplasia. Patients usually are classified as RA according to FAB classification and are predominantly female.

➤ Cell surface antigens of peripheral blood cells, bone marrow, or biopsy specimens can be studied by flow cytometry or immunocytochemistry using alkaline phosphatase antialkaline phosphatase (APAAP) and other techniques.

➤ Generally, the ability of hematopoietic progenitor cells to form colonies in vitro is decreased or absent. Aberrant growth patterns are mostly observed in RAEB and RAEB-t. In CMML, increased colony growth is noted.

➤ Functional abnormalities of red blood cells, white blood cells, and platelets are frequently associated with MDS.

➤ Secondary myelodysplastic syndrome (sMDS) occurs after significant exposure to chemotherapy, radiotherapy, or other toxic agents. The laboratory findings, clinical manifestations, and evolution resemble those of de novo MDS, with a higher frequency of chromosomal abnormalities and a greater tendency to early leukemic transformation.

➤ MDS occurs rarely in children. RAEB and RAEB-t are the most frequent FAB subtype.

➤ Clinical manifestations in patients with MDS are related to the degree of anemia, neutropenia, or thrombocytopenia.

➤ Progenitor cell growth in semisolid media is dramatically decreased in MDS, with the exception of CMML.

➤ Several factors influence the prognosis in MDS. The most significant are cytogenetic abnormalities, severity of pancytopenia, age of patient, and percentage of blasts.

➤ The International Prognosis Scoring System (IPSS) facilitates effective evaluation of the prognosis for individual patient.

➤ Allergenic bone marrow transplantation is a curative treatment for MDS.

References

1. Bennett, JM, et al: Proposals for the classification of the myelodysplastic syndromes. Br J Haematol 51:189, 1982; Clin Haematol 15:909, 1986; Br J Haematol 87:749, 1994.
2. Greenberg, PL: Apoptosis and its role in the myelodysplastic syndromes: Implication for disease natural history and treatment. Leuk Res 22:1123, 1998.
3. Aul, C, et al: Age-related incidence and other epidemiological aspects of myelodysplastic syndrome. Br J Haematol 82:385, 1992.
4. Rigolin, GM, et al: Exposure to myelocytic agents and myelodysplasia: Case-control study and correlation with clinicobiological findings. Br J Haematol 103:189, 1998.
5. Aksoy, M, and Erden, S: Following study on the mortality and development of leukemia in 44 pancytopenic patients with chronic exposure to benzene. Blood 52:285, 1978.
6. De Caprio, AP: The toxicity of hydroquinone-relevance to occupational and environmental exposure. Crit Rev Toxico 29:283,1999.
7. Rothman, N, et al: Benzene poisoning, a risk factor for hematological malignancy, is associated with NQO1 609C→ T mutation and rapid fractional excretion of chlorzoxazone. Cancer Res 57:2839, 1997.
8. Mecucci, C, and van den Berghe, H: Cytogenetics. Hematol Oncol Clin North Am 6:522, 1992.
9. Janssen, JWG, et al: Clonal analysis of myelodysplastic syndromes: Evidence of multipotent stem cell origin. Blood 73:248, 1989.
10. Busque, L, and Gilliland, DG: Clonal evolution in acute leukemia. Blood 82:337,1993.
11. Tricot, G: The myelodysplastic syndromes: Different evolution patterns based on sequential morphological and cytogenetic investigations. Br J Haematol 59:659, 1985.
12. Berneman, ZN: A myelodysplastic syndrome preceding acute lymphoblastic leukemia. Br J Haematol 60:353, 1985.
13. Kere, J, et al: Monosomy 7 in granulocytes and monocytes in myelodysplastic syndrome. N Engl J Med 316:499, 1987.
14. Gerritsen, WR, et al: Clonal analysis of myelodysplastic syndrome: Monosomy 7 is expressed in the myeloid lineage, but not in the lymphoid lineage as detected by fluorescent in situ hybridization. Blood 80:217, 1992.
15. Tsukamoto, N, et al: Clonality in MDS: Demonstration of pluripotent stem cell origin using X-linked restriction fragment length polymorphisms. Br J Haematol 83:589, 1993.
16. Busque L, et al: Nonrandom X-Inactivation patterns in normal females: Lyonization ratios vary with age. Blood 88:59, 1996.
17. Mufti, GJ: Ineffective haemopoiesis and apoptosis in myelodysplastic syndromes. Br J Haematol 101:220, 1998.
18. Yoshida, Y: Hypothesis: Apoptosis may be the mechanism responsible for the premature intramedullary cell death in the myelodysplastic syndrome. Leukemia 7:144, 1993.
19. Shetty, V, et al: Measurement of apoptosis, proliferation and three cytokines in 46 patients with myelodysplastic syndromes. Leuk Res 20:891, 1996.
20. Knudson, AG: Mutation and cancer: Statistical study and retinoblastoma. Proc Natl Acad Sci USA 68:820, 1971.
21. Santibanez-Koref, MF, et al: P53 germline mutations in Li-Fraumeni syndrome. Lancet 338:1490, 1991.
22. Song, WJ, et al: Haploinsufficiency of CBFA2 causes familial thrombocytopenia with propensity to develop acute myelogenous leukaemia. Nat Genet 23:166, 1999.
23. Carter, G, et al: Genetic lesions in preleukemia. Crit Rev Oncogenet 3:339, 1992.
24. Quesnel, B, et al: Methylation of the p15^{INK4b} gene in myelodysplastic syndromes is frequent and acquired during disease progression. Blood 91(8):2985, 1998.
25. Dacie, JV, and Lewis, SM: Practical Haematology, ed 6. Churchill Livingstone, Edinburgh,1984, p 107.
26. Kouides, PA, and Bennett, JM: Morphology and classification of myelodysplastic syndromes. Hematol Oncol Clin North Am 6:485, 1992.
27. Hamblin, TJ, and Oscier, DG: The myelodysplastic syndrome—A practical guide. Hematol Oncol 5:19, 1987.
28. Hast, R, et al: Diagnostic significance of dysplastic features of peripheral blood polymorphs in myelodysplastic syndromes. Leuk Res 13:173, 1989.
29. Goasguen, JE, et al: Prognostic implication and characterization of the blast cell population in the myelodysplastic syndrome. Leuk Res 15:1159, 1991.
30. Hast, R: Sideroblasts in myelodysplasia: Their nature and clinical significance. Scand J Haematol 36 (suppl 45):53, 1986.
31. Lindriz, EA: Pelger-Huet anomaly, the Stodtmeister type. Atlas of Haematol-

ogy, ed 2. Sandoz, Medyczne Wydawnictwo Multimedialne, Gdansk, Poland, 2001, p 82, Plate 143-B.

32. Jakobsen, P: Ballooning platelets in the myelodysplastic syndromes. Eur J Haematol 53:175, 1994.
33. Bennett, JM, et al: Proposed revised criteria for the classification of acute myeloid leukemia. Ann Intern Med 103:626, 1985.
34. Swirsky, DM, et al: 8;21 translocation in acute granulocytic leukemia: Cytogenetical, cytochemical and clinical features. Br J Haematol 56:199, 1984.
35. Gale, RP, and Cannani, E: Review. The molecular biology of chronic myelogenous leukaemia. Br J Haematol 60:395, 1985.
36. Schmalzl, F: The value of cytochemical investigations in the diagnosis of the myelodysplastic syndromes. In Schmalzl, F, and Mufti, GJ (eds): Myelodysplastic Syndromes. Springer-Verlag, NY, 1992, p 44.
37. De Pasquale, A, and Quaglino, D: Enzyme cytochemical studies in myelodysplastic syndromes. In Schmalzl, F. and Mufti, GJ (eds): Myelodysplastic Syndromes. Springer-Verlag, NY, 1992, p 51.
38. Seo, IS, et al: Myelodysplastic syndrome: diagnostic. Implications of cytochemical and immunocytochemical studies. Mayo Clin Proc 68:47, 1993.
39. Tricot, G, et al: Prognostic factors in the myelodysplastic syndromes: Importance of initial data on peripheral blood counts, bone marrow cytology, trephine biopsy and chromosomal analysis. Br J Haematol 60:10, 1984.
40. Delacretaz, F, et al: Histopathology of myelodysplastic syndromes: The FAB classification (proposals) applied to bone marrow biopsy. Am J Clin Pathol 87:180, 1987.
41. Rios, A, et al: Bone marrow biopsy in myelodysplastic syndromes: Morphological characteristics and contribution to the study of prognostic factors. Br J Haematol 75:26, 1990.
42. Tricot, G, et al: Bone marrow histology in myelodysplastic syndromes. I. Histological findings in myelodysplastic syndromes and comparison with bone marrow smears. Br J Haematol 57:423, 1984.
43. Yoshida, Y, et al: Refractory myelodysplastic anaemias with hypocellular bone marrow. J Clin Pathol 41:763, 1988.
44. Gersen, L, and Keagle, MB: The Principles of Clinical Cytogenetics. Humana Press, NJ, 1999.
45. Heim, S, and Mitelman, F: Chromosome abnormalities in the myelodysplastic syndromes. Clin Haematol 15:1003, 1986.
46. Le Beau, MM, et al: Clinical and cytogenetic correlations in 63 patients with therapy-related myelodysplastic syndromes and acute nonlymphocytic leukemia: Further evidence for characteristic abnormalities of chromosomes no. 5 and 7. J Clin Oncol 4:325, 1986.
47. Pedersen-Bjergaard, J, and Philip, P: Balanced translocations involving chromosome bands 11q23 and 21q22 are highly characteristic of myelodysplasia and leukemia following therapy with cytostatic agents targeting at DNA topoisomerase II. Blood 78:1147, 1991.
48. Van den Berghe, H, et al: The 5q− anomaly. Cancer Genet Cytogenet 17:189, 1985.
49. Johnson, E, and Cotter, FE: Monosomy 7 and 7q− associated with myeloid malignancy. Blood Rev 11:46, 1997.
50. Hasle, H, et al: Myelodysplastic syndrome, juvenile myelomonocytic leukemia, and acute myeloid leukemia associated with complete or partial monosomy 7. Leukemia 13:376, 1999.
51. Lai, JL, et al: Myelodysplastic syndromes and acute myeloid leukemia with 17p deletion. An entity characterized by specific dysgranulopoiesis and a high incidence of P53 mutations. Leukemia 9:370, 1995.
52. Testoni, N, et al: 3q21 and 3q26 cytogenetic abnormalities in acute myeloblastic leukemia: Biological and clinical features. Haematologica 84:690, 1999.
53. Greenberg, PL: Risk factors and their relationship to prognosis in myelodysplastic syndromes. Leuk Res 22:S3, 1998.
54. Van den Berghe, H, et al: Distinct haematological disorder with deletion of long arm of no. 5 chromosome. Nature 251:437, 1974.
55. Le Beau, MM, et al: Cytogenetic and molecular delineation of the smallest commonly deleted region of chromosome 5 in malignant myeloid diseases. Proc Natl Acad Sci USA 90:5484, 1993.
56. Le Beau, MM, et al: Molecular and cytogenetic analysis of chromosome 5 abnormalities in myeloid disorders: Chromosomal localization and physical mapping of IL-4 and IL-5. Cancer Cells 7:53, 1989.
57. Sullivan, SA, et al: Circulating CD34+ cells: An adverse prognostic factor in the myelodysplastic syndromes. Am J Hematol 39:96, 1992.
58. Koeller, U, et al: Immunological phenotyping of blood and bone marrow cells from patients with myelodysplastic syndromes. In Schmalzl, F, and Mufti, GJ (eds): Myelodysplastic Syndromes. Springer-Verlag, NY, 1992, p 60.
59. Knox, SJ, et al: Studies of T-lymphocytes in preleukemic disorders and acute nonlymphocytic leukemia: In vitro radiosensitivity, mitogenic responsiveness, colony formation, and enumeration of lymphocytic subpopulations. Blood 61:449, 1983.
60. Anderson, RW, et al: Lymphocyte abnormalities in preleukemia. I. Decreased NK activity, anomalous immunoregulatory cell subsets and deficient EBV receptors. Leuk Res 7:389, 1983.
61. Mufti, GJ, et al: Immunological abnormalities in myelodysplastic syndromes. I. Serum immunoglobulins and autoantibodies. Br J Haematol 63:143, 1986.
62. Sokol, RJ, et al: Erythrocyte autoantibodies, autoimmune haemolysis, and myelo-dysplastic syndromes. J Clin Pathol 42:1088, 1989.
63. Richert-Boe, KE, and Bagby, GC: In vitro hematopoiesis in myelodysplasia: Liquid and soft-gel culture studies. Hematol Oncol Clin North Am 6:543, 1992.
64. Geissler, K, et al: Colony growth factors for chronic myelomonocytic leukemia cells. Blood 74:1472, 1989.
65. Allen RC, et al: Methylation of HpaII and HhaI sites near the polymorphic

66. Kahn, A: Abnormalities of erythrocyte enzymes in dyserythropoiesis and malignancies. Clin Haematol 10:123, 1976.
67. Newman, DR, et al: Studies on the diagnostic significance of hemoglobin F levels. Mayo Clin Proc 48:199, 1973.
68. Salmon, C: Blood group changes in preleukemic states. Blood Cells 2:211, 1976.
69. Hauptman, GM, et al: False positive acidified serum test in a preleukemic dyserythropoiesis. Acta Haematol 59:73, 1978.
70. Martin, S, et al: Defective neutrophil function and microbicidal mechanisms in the myelodysplastic disorders. J Clin Pathol 36:1120, 1983.
71. Boogaerts, MA, et al: Blood neutrophil function in primary myelodysplastic syndromes. Br J Haematol 55:411, 1983.
72. Gyger, M, et al: Childhood monosomy 7 syndrome. Am J Hemat 13:329, 1982.
73. Lintula, R, et al: Platelet function in preleukaemia. Scand J Haematol 26:65, 1981.
74. Iurlo, A, et al: Cytogenetic and clinical investigations in 76 cases with therapy-related leukemia and myelodysplastic syndrome. Cancer Genet Cytogenet 43:227, 1989.
75. Pedersen-Bjergaard, J, et al: Therapy-related myelodysplasia and acute myeloid leukemia. Cytogenetic characteristics of 115 consecutive cases and risk in seven cohorts of patients treated intensively for malignant diseases in the Copenhagen series. Leukemia 7:1975, 1993.
76. LeBeau, MM, et al: Clinical and cytogenetic correlations in 63 patients with therapy-related myelodysplastic syndromes and acute nonlymphocytic leukemia: Further evidence of characteristic abnormalities of chromosomes no. 5 and 7. J Clin Oncol 4:325, 1986.
77. Stone, RM, et al: Myelodysplastic syndrome as a late complication following autologous bone marrow transplantation for non-Hodgkin's lymphoma. J Clin Oncol 12:2535, 1994.
78. Miller, JS, et al: Myelodysplastic syndrome after autologous bone marrow transplantation: An additional late complication of curative cancer therapy. Blood 83:3780, 1994.
79. Darrington, DL, et al: Incidence and characterization of secondary myelodysplastic syndrome and acute myelogenous leukemia following high-dose chemoradiotherapy and autologous stem-cell transplantation for lymphoid malignancies. J Clin Oncol 12:2527, 1974.
80. Pedersen-Bjergaard, J, and Philip, P: Two different classes of therapy-related and de novo acute myeloid leukemia. Cancer Genet Cytogenet 55:119, 1991.
81. Liu, LF: DNA topoisomerase poisons as antitumor drugs. Annu Rev Biochem 58:351, 1989.
82. Blank, J, and Lange, B: Preleukemia in children. J Pediatr 98:565, 1981.
83. Linman, JW, and Bagby, GC: The preleukemic syndrome (hemopoietic dysplasia). Cancer 42:854, 1978.
84. Kleihauer, E: The preleukemic syndromes (hematopoietic dysplasia) in childhood. Eur J Pediatr 133:5, 1980.
85. Sieff, CA, et al: Monosomy 7 in childhood: A myeloproliferative disorder. Am J Hematol 49:235, 1981.
86. Copplestone, JA, et al: Monocytic skin infiltration in chronic myelomonocytic leukaemia. Clin Lab Haematol 8:115, 1986.
87. Da Silva, MAP, et al: Extramedullary disease in myelodysplastic syndromes. Am J Med 85:589, 1988.
88. Mufti, GJ, et al: Myelodysplastic syndromes: A scoring system with prognostic significance. Br J Haematol 59:425, 1985.
89. Kerkhofs, H, et al: Utility of the FAB classification for myelodysplastic syndromes: Investigation of prognostic factors in 237 cases. Br J Haematol 65:73, 1987.
90. Yunis, JJ, et al: Refined chromosome analysis as an independent prognostic indicator in de novo myelodysplastic syndromes. Blood 67:1721, 1986.
91. Tricot, G, et al: Prognostic factors in the myelodysplastic syndromes: Importance of initial data on peripheral blood counts, bone marrow cytology, trephine biopsy and chromosomal analysis. Br J Haematol 60:19, 1985.
92. Aul, C: Primary myelodysplastic syndromes: Analysis of prognostic factors in 235 patients and proposals for an improved scoring system. Leukemia 6:52, 1992.
93. Sanz, GF: Two regression models and a scoring system for predicting survival and planning treatment in myelodysplastic syndromes: A multivariate analysis of prognostic factors in 370 patients. Blood 74:395, 1989.
94. Goasguen, JE: Prognostic factors in myelodysplastic syndromes—A simplified 3-D scoring system. Leuk Res 14:255, 1990.
95. Greenberg, P, et al: International scoring system for evaluating prognosis in myelodysplastic syndromes. Blood 89:2079, 1997.
96. Yoshida, Y, et al: Refractory myelodysplastic anaemias with hypocellular bone marrow. J Clin Pathol 41:763, 1988.
97. Pagliuca, A, et al: Myelofibrosis in primary myelodysplastic syndromes: A clinico-morphological study of 10 cases. Br J Haematol 71:499, 1989.
98. Golub, TR, et al: Fusion of PDGF receptor beta to a novel ets-like gene, tel, in chronic myelomonocytic leukemia with t(5;12) chromosomal translocation. Cell 77(2):307, 1994.
99. Applebaum, FR, and Anderson, J: Bone marrow transplantation for myelodysplasia in adults and children: When and who? Leuk Res 22:S35, 1998.
100. Molldrem, JJ, et al: Antithymocyte globulin for patients with myelodysplastic syndrome. Br J Haematol 99:699, 1997.

101. Biesma, DH, et al: Immunosuppressive therapy for hypoplastic myelodysplastic syndrome. Cancer 79:1548, 1997.
102. Baccarani, M, et al: Low dose arabinosyl cytosine for treatment of
myelodysplastic syndromes and subacute myeloid leukemia. Leuk Res
7:539, 1983.
103. Wijermans, PW, et al: Continuous infusion of low-dose 5-Aza-2'-deoxycyti-
dine in elderly patients with high-risk myelodysplastic syndrome. Leukemia
11:S19, 1997.
104. Bessho, M, et al: Improvement of anemia by recombinant erythropoietin in
patients with myelodysplastic syndromes and aplastic anemia. Int J Cell
Cloning 8:445, 1990.
105. Negrin, RS, et al: Maintenance treatment of patients with myelodysplastic
syndromes using recombinant human granulocyte colony stimulating factor.
Blood 78:36, 1992.
106. Fenaux, P, et al: Aggressive chemotherapy in adult primary myelodysplastic
syndromes: A report on 29 cases. Blut 57:297, 1988.

See the bibliography for this chapter at the end of the book.

20 Multiple Myeloma and Related Plasma Cell Disorders

JAMES M. LONG, MD, LTCOL (SEL) USAF

MULTIPLE MYELOMA

Overview
Plasma Cell Development and Abnormal Clones
Etiology and Epidemiology
Pathophysiology of Multiple Myeloma
Cytogenetics in Multiple Myeloma
Laboratory and Radiologic Evaluation of Plasma Cell Disorders
Diagnosis and Differential Diagnosis of Multiple Myeloma
Treatment of Multiple Myeloma and Its Variants

MONOCLONAL GAMMOPATHY OF UNDETERMINED SIGNIFICANCE

WALDENSTRÖM'S MACROGLOBULINEMIA

HEAVY-CHAIN DISEASE

CASE STUDY 1 Multiple Myeloma

CASE STUDY 2 MGUS

CASE STUDY 3 Waldenström's Macroglobulinemia

OBJECTIVES

At the end of this chapter, the learner should be able to:

1. List laboratory tests that are useful for the evaluation of immunoglobulin disorders.

2. Describe the significance of an M-spike and its evaluation by immunoelectrophoresis.

3. State what Bence-Jones proteins are, how they are detected, and why they are important.

4. List the diagnostic criteria for multiple myeloma.

5. List tests useful for staging and prognosis of patients with multiple myeloma.

6. List diagnostic criteria for monoclonal gammopathy of undetermined significance.

7. List diagnostic criteria for Waldenström's macroglobulinemia.

8. Describe heavy-chain disease.

➤ MULTIPLE MYELOMA

Overview

Multiple myeloma is a disorder characterized by the overproduction of abnormal plasma cells. This single cellular excess has far-reaching effects, as listed in Table 20–1. Patients with multiple myeloma may have markedly different symptoms at the time of diagnosis because of the variety of body functions affected by the disease. Multiple myeloma may cause bone destruction, high serum calcium levels, kidney failure, infections, nerve compression with paralysis, and changes in mental status ranging from mild confusion to coma. This disease is diagnosed in some patients with no symptoms after a screening blood test reveals abnormally high serum protein levels or x-rays reveal excess calcium loss from the bones. In some rare cases, patients are diagnosed only after they have developed marked changes in their mental status with extensive bone destruction, high calcium levels, and kidney failure. Most patients found to have multiple myeloma fall somewhere between these two extremes.

The causes of multiple myeloma and the population it affects are discussed in this chapter. The wide-ranging effects

of myeloma on the body follow in a "cause-and-effect" format. The use of the clinical laboratory in evaluating plasma cell disorders is discussed, followed by an introduction to the various radiologic procedures used in the evaluation of these diseases. The evolving field of molecular biology and its relevance to the study of multiple myeloma are briefly introduced.

Following this technical information, the clinical usefulness of this testing is presented. Specifically, it is shown how physicians are able to use this information to determine whether a patient has multiple myeloma or one of the other related plasma cell disorders listed in Table 20–2. These other disorders are briefly introduced. Because the prognosis of the patient and treatment decisions depend on the extent and aggressiveness of the disease, various "staging" systems have been developed. These systems, which attempt to group together patients with similar disease conditions and expected outcomes, are briefly presented.

Principles of the treatment of multiple myeloma are summarized, but extensive discussion of the details of treatment is beyond the scope of this text. References are supplied for those seeking further information.

> ## Table 20-1
> ### SIGNS AND SYMPTOMS OF PLASMA CELL DISORDERS

Signs	Symptoms
Anemia	Tiredness Fatigue Shortness of breath
Hypercalcemia	Mental status changes Bone pain Kidney stones Constipation and abdominal pain
Renal failure	None (until late)
Bone lesions on radiograph	Bone pain Mass Pathologic fractures
Elevated serum globulins	Possible hyperviscosity syndrome
Serum hyperviscosity	Confusion Increased bleeding tendency Raynaud's phenomenon Visual complaints

> ## Table 20-2
> ### PLASMA CELL DISORDERS

Solitary plasmacytoma

Multiple myeloma

   Smoldering myeloma

   Classic multiple myeloma

   Advanced myeloma

   Nonsecretory myeloma

Monoclonal gammopathy of undetermined significance (MGUS)

Waldenström's macroglobulinemia

Heavy-chain disease (HCD)

   Gamma HCD

   Mu HCD

   Alpha HCD

Plasma Cell Development and Abnormal Clones

The plasma cell is the final stage in the development of B lymphocytes (refer to Chap. 1 and Fig. 20–1). It is characterized by the production and release of specific immunoglobulin molecules (see Fig. 20–1).

During cellular replication and differentiation, a genetic mistake may occur. Evolving evidence supports the theory that mutations in multiple myeloma occur during the period when mature B lymphocytes are becoming plasmablasts. A mutated plasmablast is then relocated via the blood to the bone marrow, where it produces a colony of identical mutated plasma cells referred to as a *clone*. A single tumor mass composed of a clone of abnormal plasma cells is called a *plasmacytoma*. Some of these abnormal cells travel by the blood to other locations in the bone marrow where new colonies are established.[1] These multiple plasmacytomas lead to the name multiple myeloma.

There is clear evidence that one of the primary changes that occur as a result of these mutated plasma cells is the production of interleukin-6 (IL-6). IL-6 is one of a broad class of molecules referred to as *cytokines*. Cytokines provide "communication" among cells leading to stimulation or suppression of cellular reproduction, production of cell products, or secretion of other cytokines (see Chap. 1). Abnormal plasma cells in multiple myeloma proliferate when exposed to IL-6 and other growth factors. Blocking IL-6 stops the growth of myeloma cells in the laboratory. Although it is not the only cytokine involved, it appears to be one of the most important.[2] IL-6 has been shown to inhibit apoptosis in multiple myeloma in conjunction with adhesion molecules, tumor suppressor genes, and oncogenes. As these mutated plasma cells induce the production of the IL-6 and other cytokines that cause further replication, the malignancy known as multiple myeloma develops.

Etiology and Epidemiology

The overall incidence of myeloma is 5 cases per 100,000 persons each year. Men have approximately 50% greater risk than women. The rates of occurrence in black individuals (8 per 100,000) are double the rates in white individuals (4 per 100,000). Hawaiians, Alaskans, female Hispanics, and female Native Americans also have higher rates than whites, whereas persons of Japanese and Chinese descent experience less. There is a steady increase in the incidence of multiple myeloma with age, the disease being distinctly rare under the age of 40 and the highest risk (70 cases per 100,000 population) being in black men over the age of 80 (Fig. 20–2).[3]

Environmental factors play a clear role in causing multiple myeloma. Atomic bomb survivors and individuals exposed to radiation in the workplace (such as radium watch dial painters and radiologists) have an increased risk of multiple myeloma.[4] Studies of workers at nuclear power plants also suggest that chronic exposure to low levels of radiation may lead to increased risk of myeloma. Chronic stimulation of the immune system has been a suspected cause of myeloma. Increased risk of myeloma in the agricultural industry has implicated grain dust, molds, engine exhaust, viruses, insecticides, fertilizers, herbicides, and other agricultural chemicals. Workers in the metal, rubber, wood, leather, and textile industries may be at increased risk, as are those who work with benzene and other organic solvents.[5] The debate still rages about the significant evidence linking the use of hair dyes to increased risk of myeloma in women and men. In a study conducted by Johns Hopkins University from 1966 to 1996, evaluations suggested associations with the use of permanent hair dyes with particular attention to duration, frequency, age at first use, and dark colors; however, associations were not consistent within and between studies.[6] No relationship to tobacco or alcohol use has been shown. Certain medical conditions, such as rheumatoid arthritis, chronic allergic

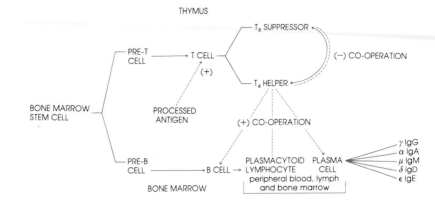

> ➤ **FIGURE 20–1** Development of T and B lymphocytes showing interaction. T_4 and T_8 are equivalent to CD4 and CD8, respectively.

conditions, and chronic infections, may also increase the risk for myeloma.[7]

Pathophysiology of Multiple Myeloma

Overview

There are three primary disease processes that lead to the complex disruption of various organ systems. The understanding of multiple myeloma can be simplified by examining these processes. Each has multiple effects and is discussed in turn. First, the effects of the expanding plasma cell mass are presented, followed in turn by discussions of the overproduction of monoclonal immunoglobulins, and the production of osteoclast activating factor (OAF) and other cytokines.

Expanding Plasma Cell Mass

Mutated plasmablasts in the bone marrow undergo continued clonal replication under the influence of IL-6 and other growth factor cytokines.[2] As this relentless growth proceeds, individual actively dividing cells again circulate in the blood to find rest at other locations in the bone marrow. Each new colony establishes an independent local production of growth factor, and the process continues.

Normal bone marrow is gradually replaced by the steadily growing individual malignant plasma cell colonies. As the replacement progresses, normal circulating blood cells decrease in number, a condition referred to as *pancytopenia*. These cellular deficiencies commonly appear in sequence. First, a decrease in the number of red blood cells (anemia) is observed. Later, decreases in the numbers of platelets occur (thrombocytopenia), and in advanced myeloma, neutrophils also decrease (neutropenia). Anemia results in fatigue, shortness of breath, and rapid heart rate. Thrombocytopenia results in delayed hemostasis, with resultant prolonged bleeding and injuries. Neutropenia causes a dramatically increased susceptibility to bacterial infections.

The expanding cell masses originating in the bone marrow frequently cause destruction of the surface "cortex" of the bone. Stretching of the overlying nerve-rich periosteum leads to pain. Pain is present at diagnosis in more than two-thirds of patients.[8,9] The expanding plasmacytoma may extend beyond the boundaries of the bone to compress adjacent neurologic structures. This occurs most frequently in the vertebrae, where the nerve roots exiting from the spine and even the spinal cord itself may be compressed. This causes pain and may lead to paralysis and loss of sensation. Less commonly, plasmacytomas may occur in areas other than the bone and bone marrow (Fig. 20–3). These "extramedullary plasmacytomas" may occur in the nasopharynx, paranasal sinuses, liver, spleen, skin, kidneys, and gastrointestinal tract. Symptoms result from the growing tumor and vary according to the site involved.

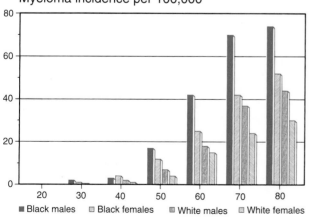

Myeloma incidence per 100,000

Decade of age (years)

■ Black males ▨ Black females ▨ White males ▨ White females

> ➤ **FIGURE 20–2** Average annual age-specific incidence of multiple myeloma in the United States, 1973 to 1988. Age is plotted as the average of two 5-year age groups. Rates are per 100,000 persons per decade of age in years. (From Ries, LAG, et al: Cancer Statistics Review 1973–1988. US Government Printing Office, Washington, DC, 1991 [DHHS publication (NIH) No. 92789].)

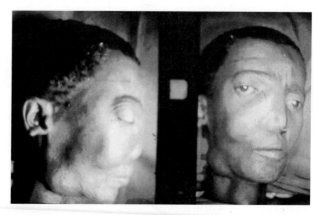

> ➤ **FIGURE 20–3** Plasmacytomas of the face and jaw in a patient with multiple myeloma.

Production of Immunoglobulin: "Monoclonal Gammopathy"

Normal Immunoglobulin Structure

Most malignant plasma cells actively produce immunoglobulin (Ig). Immunoglobulin units are composed of two identical heavy chains (50,000 daltons) and two identical light chains (25,000 daltons) (Fig. 20–4). These chains are held together by varying numbers of disulfide bonds. The antibody produced by each plasma cell has only one type of light chain and one type of heavy chain. There are two types of light chains named kappa (κ) and lambda (λ). There are five types of heavy chains named gamma (γ), alpha (α), mu (μ), delta (δ), and epsilon (ε). They correspond to the five classes of antibodies named IgG, IgA, IgM, IgD, and IgE. The heavy-chain subunit identifies the immunoglobulin class.

Each immunoglobulin class has a specific function. IgG is the primary antibody class involved in fighting infection and is produced in measurable amounts long after the antigen stimulus is removed. IgA is characteristically a secretory antibody providing protection of body surfaces in the gastrointestinal tract and the airways. IgM is produced as the earliest, but temporary, response to infections and becomes unmeasurable within weeks after it first appears. The IgE class is involved in allergic or hypersensitivity reactions. The role of IgD remains unclear. IgA and IgG have varying numbers and location of the disulfide bonds linking the heavy chains together and the heavy chains to the light chains. These differing "isotypes" are named IgG1, IgG2, IgG3, IgG4, IgA1, and IgA2. The functions and properties vary slightly as a result of these differences.

Most antibodies are composed of two identical heavy chains and two identical light chains making a single immunoglobulin unit. IgM, however, exists primarily as a "pentameric" molecule composed of five such units. IgA and IgG2 tend to exist in pairs of units as "dimers" or may polymerize to larger molecules. An antibody is named by its heavy-chain class as well as the type of light chain (e.g., IgG-κ or IgA-λ).

Monoclonal and Incomplete Immunoglobulins

In multiple myeloma, the normally controlled and purposeful production of antibodies is replaced by the inappropriate production of even larger amounts of useless immunoglobulin molecules. The normally equal production of light chains and heavy chains may be imbalanced. The result is the release of excess free light chains or free heavy chains. The immunoglobulins produced by a clone of myeloma cells are identical. Any abnormal production of identical antibodies is referred to by the general name of *monoclonal gammopathy*. Rarely (in less than 1% of cases), myelomas may produce no antibodies; 6% produce only light chains. Two antibody classes are produced in 3.5% of cases and probably represent the coexistence of two different malignant clones (Fig. 20–5). The overproduction of immunoglobulin is one of the hallmarks of multiple myeloma. IgG is the immunoglobulin produced in more than 50% of cases, followed by IgA (20%), and, rarely, IgD and IgE (less than 2%).[1]

Hyperviscosity Syndrome

The presence of excess immunoglobulin can lead to alteration in the physical characteristic of blood known as viscosity. Overly viscous blood has higher resistance to flow. The result is decreased flow through the smallest blood vessels of the brain, heart, and other organs as well as an increased workload on the heart. Patients suffering from hyperviscosity syndrome may complain of confusion, blurred vision, headache, chest tightness or angina, or numbness or tingling of the fingertips. The increased oncotic pressure caused by these proteins leads to expansion of blood volume. The heart may be unable to tolerate these changes, leading to congestive heart failure. Such patients experience fluid weight gain, swelling of the ankles, and difficulty in breathing.

Any class of immunoglobulins can cause hyperviscosity syndrome if the blood levels are sufficiently high. IgM, a large molecule composed of five immunoglobulin units, causes a much higher increase in viscosity than would five individual units (of IgG, for example). For this reason, most cases of clinical hyperviscosity syndrome are seen as a result of excess IgM, IgA, and IgG3; these may exist as dimers or polymers and are somewhat more likely to cause

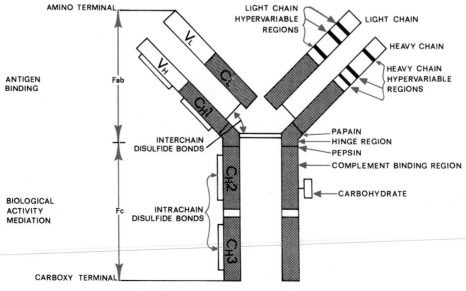

➤ FIGURE 20–4 Structure of the basic immunoglobulin unit.

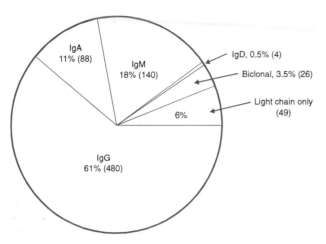

➤ **FIGURE 20–5** Monoclonal serum protein in 787 Mayo Clinic patients.

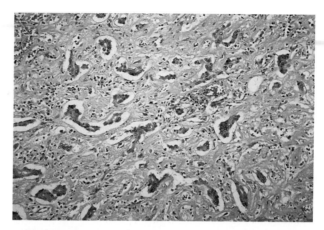

➤ **FIGURE 20–6** Amorphous amyloid deposits replacing normal liver architecture.

hyperviscosity syndrome than IgG monomers.[10]

Decreased Production of Normal Immunoglobulins

Patients with multiple myeloma often have decreased levels of the normal circulating antibody classes. The low levels are probably caused by suppressed function of normal B lymphocytes and plasma cells as a response to the presence of the abnormal immunoglobulins. The lower level of immunoglobulins leads to increased susceptibility to infections such as sinusitis, bronchitis, and pneumonia. Infection remains the leading cause of death of patients with multiple myeloma.

Bence-Jones Protein and Kidney Damage

Imbalanced immunoglobulin production most frequently yields an excess of light chains. These light chains are rapidly metabolized in the blood and are small enough to be filtered into the urine. The excess is thus most frequently detected by finding light chains in the urine and is often not detected in the blood. Light chains have the unique property of precipitating out of solution when urine is heated to approximately 56°C, and then dissolving again as the temperature rises. As the urine is allowed to cool to 56°C, a precipitate will again form, followed by dissolution on further cooling. These urinary light chains are named Bence-Jones proteins after the physician who first noted this unusual property. Light chains are toxic to the kidneys and can lead to leakage of protein into the urine (proteinuria) and kidney failure.

Amyloidosis

Immunoglobulin κ or λ light chains may settle or deposit in many organs such as the heart, kidneys, nerves, liver, spleen, gastrointestinal tract, and skin. This nonstructural protein which accumulates in these organs is called *amyloid* (Fig. 20–6; and Color Plate 242). Amyloidosis causes progressive loss of function of the involved organs and may lead to death caused by heart or kidney failure.[10]

Autoimmune Phenomena

Rarely, the antibodies produced by myeloma plasma cells are specifically targeted on the patient's own cells. If the targeted cells are red cells, this may lead to the red cell destruction known as *autoimmune hemolytic anemia*. If the antibodies are directed against one of the clotting factor proteins, the patient may develop a bleeding disorder. Although rare, many different manifestations of this type of autoimmune phenomena have been reported.

Bleeding Disorders and Cryoglobulins

Increased levels of immunoglobulins in the blood may interfere with the function of the clotting factor proteins of the coagulation cascade. This is usually not clinically significant, but may result in prolongation of tests of blood coagulation such as the prothrombin time (PT) and activated partial thromboplastin time (APTT). In advanced stages, bruising and abnormal gum or nose bleeding may occur.

Cryoglobulins are immunoglobulins that precipitate on exposure to cold.[11] Cryoglobulinemia may rarely occur in patients with multiple myeloma. Patients with this syndrome often complain of pain in the extremities on exposure to cold. This usually affects the fingers, nose, and ears. Cryoglobulins can cause more serious complications such as vasculitis and kidney damage after cold exposure. Recently, amorphous deposits of cryoglobulins have been described in neutrophils and monocytes as cytoplasmic inclusions consistent with phagocytosed immunoglobulins.[12]

Production of Osteoclast-Activating Factor and Cytokines

Osteoclasts and Bone Destruction

Normal bone is a dynamic structure with ongoing remodeling as a result of a balance between bone resorption and new bone formation. Osteoclasts are bone cells active in locally reabsorbing bone and releasing calcium into the blood. Nearby osteoblasts are equally active in utilizing calcium in the blood to form new bone.

Multiple myeloma interrupts this balance by the secretion of at least two substances. These are IL-6 and OAF, mentioned earlier. Osteoclast-activating factor, as its name implies, stimulates osteoclasts to increase bone resorption and release of calcium. Because osteoblasts are not stimulated, the net result is progressive destruction of the bone, with corresponding loss of calcium and weakening of the bone structure. In x-rays, bone appears dense because of the calcium in the cortex. Because the individual plasmacytomas growing in the marrow each stimulate local destruction of the cortical bone and loss of calcium, radiographs demonstrate clear or lucent areas referred to as *lytic lesions* (Fig. 20–7). These weakened areas may break under everyday stresses such as standing up, lifting objects, or even bending over (Fig. 20–8). Such breaks caused by weakening of the bone from malignancy are called pathologic fractures.

IL-6 as well as other factors have been found to have a critical role in stimulating osteoclast activity as well as inhibit-

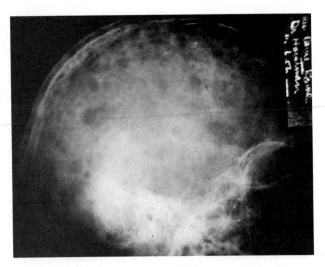

> **FIGURE 20–7**   Extensive lytic skull lesions in a patient with multiple myeloma.

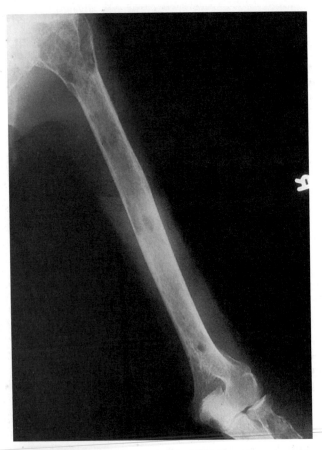

> **FIGURE 20–8**   Radiologic film of the left humerus of a patient with multiple myeloma. Areas with severe cortical bone destruction may be fractured by everyday activities such as lifting or walking (pathologic fractures).

ing osteoblasts and new bone formation. It is likely that the inhibition of osteoblastic activity is as important as the stimulation of osteoclasts in the formation of lytic bone lesions. IL-6 has a local effect on bone destruction, as does OAF, but also is found in measurable levels in the blood. Occasionally, myeloma patients have a generalized loss of calcium from the bones known as osteoporosis that may appear earlier than the lytic lesions. It is possible that circulating IL-6 or other cytokines may be partly responsible for this finding.[13,14]

Hypercalcemia

Balance of calcium in the body is critical because of its role in many cellular processes. As calcium is released from the bones, the result is excess free calcium in the blood. This may cause several symptoms. One of the earliest is constipation and cramping from altered motility of the intestine. Muscle weakness may occur. Varying degrees of change in mental status may develop, such as confusion, psychosis, and even coma. The extent of mental status change is dependent on both the level of calcium and the rate of rise. Bone pain is common with high calcium levels. Increased calcium in the urine can lead to formation of kidney stones and kidney failure. Figure 20–9 outlines the disorders associated with multiple myeloma.

Cytogenetics in Multiple Myeloma

Chromosomal studies in multiple myeloma and the plasma cell dyscrasias have been somewhat staggered in the last decade owing to variability of marrow infiltration by malignant plasma cells and low proliferative states. The chromosomal aberrations that have been reported are depicted in Table 20–3. Chromosomal abnormalities have been found in 20% to 60% of patients, with monosomy 13, and trisomy or tetrasomy in chromosome 9, being the most common in multiple myeloma.[15,16]

In a recent study conducted by the Mayo Clinic, 24 cases of multiple myeloma exhibited the t(11;14)(q13;q32) abnormality, with plasma cells comprising 60% of bone marrow cells. A positive correlation was found with the presence of this translocation and overexpression of the cyclin D1 nuclear protein. The cyclin D1 nuclear protein has valuable diagnostic significance in predicting survival in patients with multiple myeloma.[17,18]

Laboratory and Radiologic Evaluation of Plasma Cell Disorders

Laboratory Studies

Protein Electrophoresis

Protein in the serum consists primarily of albumin, immunoglobulins, and smaller amounts of other proteins. Serum proteins are measured as total protein on routine automated chemistry panels. Measurement of albumin allows approximate quantitation of the immunoglobulin-containing fraction by subtraction (i.e., Total protein − Albumin = Immunoglobulin fraction). Thus, one can detect a substantial increase in immunoglobulins by an automated chemistry panel alone. It is important to differentiate between increased immunoglobulins formed as a result of normal processes and the monoclonal antibodies seen in disorders of plasma cell function such as multiple myeloma. This can best be performed by protein elec-

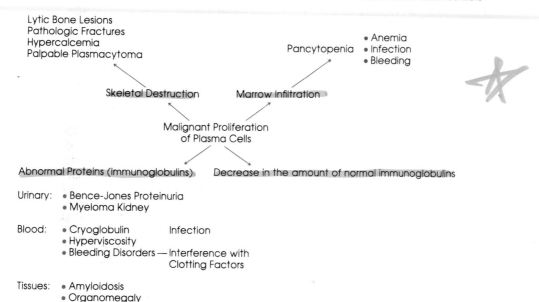

➤ FIGURE 20–9 Mechanisms of disease in multiple myeloma. Skeletal destruction, abnormal immunoglobulin production, marrow failure, and decreased production of normal immunoglobulin all play a role.

➤ Table 20-3
CYTOGENETIC ABNORMALITIES IN MULTIPLE MYELOMA

Abnormality	Chromosome Number
Trisomy/Tetrasomy	3
	5
	7
	9
	11
	15
	18
	19
	21
Monosomy/Nullosomy	8
	13
	14
	X*
	Y
Translocations	t(11;14)(q13;q32)
	t(8;14)(q24;q32)
	t(14;18)(q32;q21)
	t(6;14)(p21;q32)
	t(1;16)(p11;p11)
	t(1;16)(q10;p10)

*Females.

Source: Zandecki M, et al: Multiple myeloma: Almost all patients are cytogenetically abnormal. Br J Haematol 94:217, 1996, with permission.

trophoresis. Figure 20–10 illustrates and compares different patterns of protein electrophoresis for the various plasma cell disorders.

The spike on protein electrophoresis caused by monoclonal immunoglobulins is called a *monoclonal spike* or an *M-spike* (see Fig. 20–10). Thus, a primary reason for performing a protein electrophoresis is to determine whether an M-spike is present or not. The same procedure is used for analyzing urine samples for M-spikes. It is performed on an aliquot of a 24-hour urine collection. Further identification of the proteins causing the M-spike is carried out by a technique called immunoelectrophoresis, which is critical in the diagnostic evaluation of multiple myeloma.

Immunoelectrophoresis

In immunoelectrophoresis, the proteins are separated by electrical charge and antibodies to IgG, IgM, IgA, κ light chains, and λ light chains are then diffused into the gel. Precipitation occurs when the antibody from the reagent meets the corresponding light-chain or heavy-chain molecule. An M-spike may be identified because it will form a line of precipitation only with the antibody targeted to its specific heavy-chain class and with the antibody targeted toward its specific light chain.

Quantitative Immunoglobulins

Immunoglobulin classes IgG, IgA, and IgM and both κ and λ light chains are quantitated by either radial immunodiffusion or rate nephelometry. The latter is the most accurate technique (less than 5% variation in results) and is based on light scatter caused by antigen-antibody complexes formed by mixing a serum sample with an appropriate specific antibody reagent.[19] Decreased levels of normal immunoglobulins are characteristic of multiple myeloma.

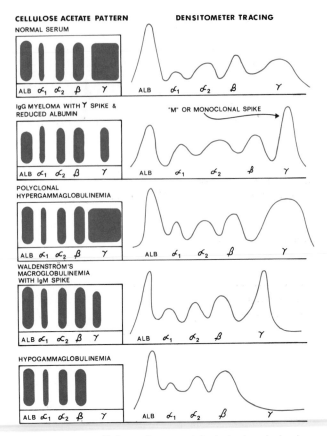

CELLULOSE ACETATE PATTERN   DENSITOMETER TRACING
NORMAL SERUM

IgG MYELOMA WITH γ SPIKE &   "M" OR MONOCLONAL SPIKE
REDUCED ALBUMIN

POLYCLONAL
HYPERGAMMAGLOBULINEMIA

WALDENSTRÖM'S
MACROGLOBULINEMIA
WITH IgM SPIKE

HYPOGAMMAGLOBULINEMIA

➤ **FIGURE 20–10**   Patterns of serum protein electrophoresis showing characteristic patterns of normal serum, monoclonal M-spike, polyclonal antibody production, IgM M-spike, and the absence of antibody production seen in hypogammaglobulinemia.

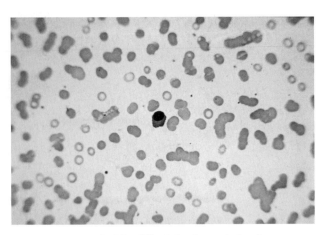

➤ **FIGURE 20–11**   Peripheral blood showing marked rouleaux formation. Note the "stacked-coin" appearance of the red cells.

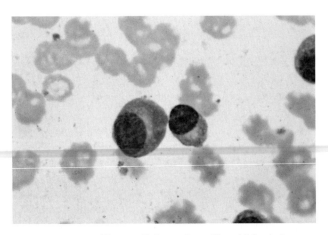

➤ **FIGURE 20–12**   Plasma cells in a patient with multiple myeloma peripheral blood.

Complete Blood Count and Peripheral Blood Smear

The automated complete blood count (CBC) is the most readily available assessment of bone marrow function. The most common finding in multiple myeloma is a decrease in the number of red blood cells with no change in size (normocytic anemia). In more advanced disease, the platelet count and even the white blood cell count may also decrease.

The peripheral smear allows microscopic examination of the blood cells. The most characteristic finding in multiple myeloma is rouleaux formation of the red cells. Rouleaux is the stacking of red cells together like coins (Fig. 20–11 and Color Plate 243). It is caused by increased amounts of immunoglobulins in the blood causing red blood cells to adhere to each other. The same phenomenon results in the increased erythrocyte sedimentation rate described next. With progressive replacement of bone marrow by myeloma, plasma cells may be identified in the peripheral blood (Fig. 20–12 and Color Plate 244). Replacement of bone marrow may also cause teardrop-shaped red cells and earlier forms of white blood cells such as metamyelocytes and myelocytes to appear in the blood. Gross examination of the stained glass slide may reveal a bluish background tint because of the staining of immunoglobulin in the plasma.

Erythrocyte Sedimentation Rate

The erythrocyte sedimentation rate (ESR) is often performed, but adds little to the evaluation of or treatment de-

cisions in myeloma. An increased ratio of serum protein to number of red cells results in adherence of the red cells to each other. Stacked red cells have an increased weight compared to their surface area, resulting in a faster rate of settling out of solution because of gravity. The ESR is measured in millimeters settled per hour and is often elevated in myeloma.

Bone Marrow Biopsy

In evaluations for possible multiple myeloma, the bone marrow biopsy is performed to evaluate the numbers of plasma cells present and to examine the appearance of the cells. Because myeloma may be a patchy process, biopsies are usually taken at two different sites. Characteristic findings on marrow biopsy in patients with myeloma include increased numbers of plasma cells, often forming "sheets," with immature, binucleate, and large forms commonly seen (Fig. 20–13 and Color Plate 245). A differential count of marrow cells, usually from 300 to 1000 cells counted, is performed to establish percentages of various cell types present. Patients with myeloma have more than 10% plasma cells, often more than 30%, and in some cases much higher percentages (Fig. 20–14 and Color Plate 246). Flame cells (Fig. 20–15 and Color Plate 247) are large, intensely staining plasma cells sometimes found in the bone marrow of patients with IgA myeloma.

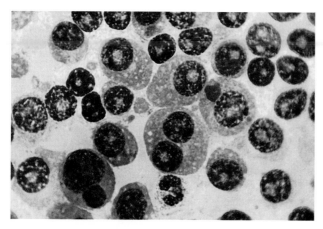

> FIGURE 20–13 Bone marrow aspirate showing atypical and binucleated plasma cells and Russell bodies (*arrow*).

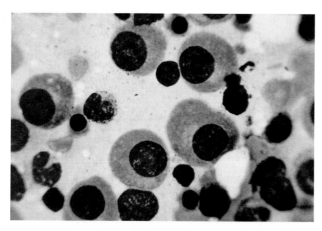

> FIGURE 20–14 Bone marrow biopsy sample showing replacement of marrow by plasma cells.

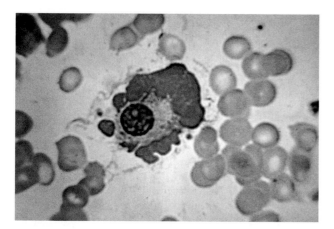

> FIGURE 20–15 Flame cell, sometimes associated with IgA myeloma.

Chemistry Studies

Routine chemistry panels yield useful information in myeloma. Serum blood urea nitrogen (BUN) and creatinine are measures of kidney function that directly correlate with survival of myeloma patients. Serum lactate dehydrogenase (LDH) is another nonspecific marker of disease activity with shorter survival correlating with high levels of LDH. Calcium levels are elevated in the great majority of patients at

some time in the course of the disease. Calcium is primarily bound to albumin. It is the unbound or free calcium that is of concern, and calcium levels must always be interpreted with the albumin level in mind. For each 1 g/dL of albumin below normal, the serum calcium should be considered increased by 0.8 mg/dL. High serum uric acid levels may be seen and can cause kidney damage. This level should be evaluated initially and when increased disease activity is suspected.

Beta₂ Microglobulin and C-Reactive Protein

Beta$_2$ microglobulin (β_2m) is the light chain of the histocompatibility locus antigen (HLA). It is a nonspecific but useful predictor of disease activity and prognosis in multiple myeloma. A level of 6 μg/mL or greater is associated with decreased survival. β_2m takes on even greater significance when considered along with serum albumin, as discussed later.

C-reactive protein (CRP) is another marker of disease activity, reflecting activity of IL-6, the importance of which has been previously discussed. It also has prognostic value and will probably play an increasingly prominent role in the management of patients with multiple myeloma.

Radiologic Studies

Plain Film Radiography

Plain film radiography is what is usually known as x-rays. Definition of soft tissues is poor because of small differences in density to x-rays. Bones are visualized quite well in most areas of the body because of the calcium in the cortex of the bones. Multiple myeloma decreases the calcium in bones, producing both discrete lytic or "punched-out" lesions (Fig. 20–16) and the general decrease in bone density known as osteoporosis (Fig. 20–17). A full skeletal survey is usually performed to evaluate patients with possible myeloma. Special attention is given to the weight-bearing bones such as the femurs, spine, and humerus. Extensive destruction in these areas may lead to pathologic fractures. Multiple lytic lesions are very suggestive of multiple myeloma and are present in 76% of patients at diagnosis.

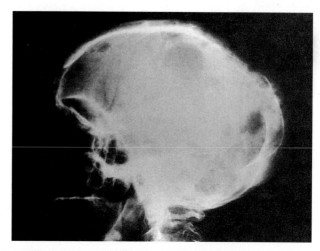

> FIGURE 20–16 Skull radiograph showing discrete punched-out lesions characteristic of multiple myeloma, caused by production of osteoclast-activating factor by clusters of malignant plasma cells.

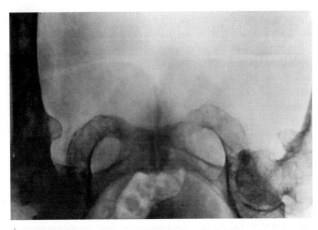

> **FIGURE 20–17**   Pelvic radiograph of a patient with multiple myeloma showing the diffuse loss of bone seen in this disease.

Nuclear Medicine Studies

In multiple myeloma, the usefulness of nuclear medicine studies is very limited. This is because technetium radioisotope used in bone scans is actively taken up by osteoblasts. Because there is little osteoblastic activity in myeloma, most myeloma lesions are not detected.

Magnetic Resonance Imaging

Magnetic resonance imaging (MRI) produces computer-generated images based on tissue absorption of radiofrequency energy while in a powerful magnetic field. It excels at imaging neurologic tissues and the spine because of its ability to detect differences between normal and abnormal soft tissues and its ability to image the spine longitudinally. MRI can clearly demonstrate the presence of plasmacytomas in the spine and evaluate for nerve compression. Myeloma involving the bone marrow in vertebrae can be seen even with no destruction of the cortical bone visible on spinal radiographs.

Diagnosis and Differential Diagnosis of Multiple Myeloma

Diagnostic Criteria for Multiple Myeloma

The currently agreed-on diagnostic criteria are listed in Table 20–4. Multiple myeloma is considered present if (1) two major criteria, (2) one major criterion and one unrelated minor criterion, or (3) three minor criteria are present. Thus, an M-spike of 5 g/dL or IgG-κ light chains with multiple lytic lesions would fulfill the criteria for diagnosis. Forty percent plasma cells in the bone marrow with an IgG-κ M-spike of 1.8 g/dL without bone lesions would fulfill the criteria. Plasma cells comprising 15% of the bone marrow with an M-spike measuring 1.2 g/dL with an IgA level of 20 mg/dL and an IgM level of 30 mg/dL would also fulfill the criteria.

Only six tests are required to make or exclude the diagnosis of multiple myeloma. These include bone marrow biopsy, serum protein electrophoresis, urine protein electrophoresis, immunoelectrophoresis, serum quantitative immunoglobulins, and a radiologic bone survey. If a mass is present, a biopsy should be performed to evaluate for plasmacytoma. Other tests are important in the staging and prognosis of myeloma.

> **Table 20–4**
> ### DIAGNOSTIC CRITERIA FOR MULTIPLE MYELOMA

I.   Biopsy-proven plasmacytoma

II. > 30% plasma cells in bone marrow

III. Monoclonal protein (M-spike)

   > 3.5 g/dL of serum IgG or

   > 2.0 g/dL of serum IgA or

   > 1.0 g/24 hr of lambda or kappa urinary light chains (in absence of amyloidosis)

Minor Criteria

a. 10%–30% plasma cells in bone marrow

b. M-spike present but less than levels above

c. Multiple lytic bone lesions

d. Low-normal immunoglobulins

   IgM < 50 mg/dL

   IgA < 100 mg/dL

   IgG < 600 mg/dL

Rules of Combination

A. One major and one minor criterion

   1. I + b; I + c; I + d (not I + a)

   2. II + b; II + c; II + d (not II + a)

   3. III + a; III + c; III + d (not III + b)

B. Three minor criteria (must include a + b)

   1. a + b + c

   2. a + b + d

Source: Adapted from Durle, BGM, and Salmon, SE: Staging kinetics and flow cytometry of multiple myeloma. In Wiernik, P, et al (eds): Neoplastic Diseases of the Blood. Churchill Livingstone, New York, 1985, with permission.

Differential Diagnosis

Frequently a patient has a monoclonal gammopathy and fails to meet the criteria for diagnosis of multiple myeloma. A list of other disorders that may be responsible must then be considered. Such a list of alternative diagnoses is called a *differential diagnosis*. A review of 856 patients at Mayo Clinic who underwent evaluation for monoclonal gammopathy is shown in Figure 20–18.[20] Table 20–5 lists the standard battery of tests used for evaluating monoclonal gammopathies and plasma cell disorders. A complete physical examination (always done), computed tomographic (CT) scans of the chest and abdomen, with biopsies of suspicious enlarged lymph nodes, may also be required. "Monoclonal gammopathy of undetermined significance" is often diagnosed after multiple myeloma, B-cell lymphoma, and chronic lymphocytic leukemia are excluded. Much less commonly, Waldenström's macroglobulinemia, heavy-chain disease, or amyloidosis may be diagnosed. The spectrum of plasma cell disorders is listed in Table 20–2.

Staging

Once a diagnosis of multiple myeloma has been established, an estimate is made of the extent of disease to help

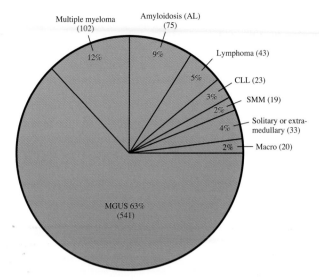

➤ **FIGURE 20–18** Monoclonal gammopathies in 856 Mayo Clinic patients (1990). CLL = chronic lymphocytic leukemia; SMM = smoldering multiple myeloma; Macro = macroglobulinemia; MGUS = monoclonal gammopathy of undetermined significance.

➤ **Table 20–5**
STANDARD EVALUATION OF PLASMA CELL DISORDERS

Determine whether monoclonal protein is present

  Serum protein electrophoresis (SPEP)

  24-hour urine protein and protein electrophoresis (UPEP)

Characterize monoclonal protein

  Immunoelectrophoresis (IEP) of urine and serum

  Immunofixation electrophoresis if results are questionable

Evaluate bones with skeletal survey

Evaluate renal function

  Serum BUN

  Serum creatinine

  24-hour urine for creatinine clearance

Screening serum chemistry panel

  Calcium

  Total protein

  Albumin

  Uric acid

Evaluate bone marrow function

  CBC with reticulocyte count and WBC differential

  Bone marrow aspirate and biopsy

Evaluate for suppression of normal immunoglobulins

  Quantitative immunoglobulins

Serum viscosity

Miscellaneous

  Erythrocyte sedimentation rate (ESR)

  C-reactive protein

  Biopsy of mass or bone lesion if bone marrow is normal

  β_2 microglobulin if multiple myeloma diagnosed

determine the appropriate treatment plan and the patient's prognosis. This procedure, called *staging,* is also useful for reporting treatment outcomes and providing a common means of communication between physicians.

Various staging systems have been proposed and are currently in use.[21,22] The older and probably most used staging system, described by Durie and Salmon in 1975,[23] is outlined in Table 20–6. This system uses hemoglobin, M-spike magnitude, serum calcium level, bone radiographs, and serum creatinine level (kidney function) to estimate the mass of myeloma cells in the body. It associates low myeloma mass (stage I) with a median survival of greater than 5 years. An intermediate myeloma mass (stage II) is associated with a survival of approximately 3.5 years, although a patient with a high myeloma mass (stage III) may survive less than 2 years.

Other systems have been proposed that make use of serum beta$_2$ microglobulin (β_2m) and albumin, or β_2m and C-reactive protein (CRP). The use of serum albumin and β_2m is illustrated in Table 20–7 and demonstrates identification of groups surviving 55 months, 29 months, and 4 months. A similar staging system may be used for β_2m and CRP levels to establish survival groups of 54, 27, and 6 months.[24] In practice, it is common to collect all this information to use in formulating a composite prognosis.

Treatment of Multiple Myeloma and Its Variants

General Principles of Treatment

Chemotherapy is the primary treatment of multiple myeloma. Radiation therapy may be used for treating localized painful areas, lytic lesions endangering the strength of a bone, or masses compressing nerve structures. It is highly effective for localized processes, but has limited usefulness for treating the full extent of the disease.

Although various combinations of chemotherapy have been used, the standard treatment remains the use of alkylators and glucocorticoids.

Standard chemotherapy does not cure myeloma. Of all patients, 50% to 60% have at least a 50% reduction in the size of the M-spike. There is a clear prolongation of survival in patients who receive chemotherapy compared with those who do not.

Patients under the age of 65 who are otherwise in good health may consider high-dose chemotherapy with autologous marrow or peripheral stem cell support. This treatment first removes bone marrow or peripheral blood stem cells (or both) and preserves them by freezing in liquid nitrogen. High doses of chemotherapy are given (often high-dose melphalan with or without other agents) followed by reinfusion of the thawed stem cells or bone marrow. In a recent study, investigators tested the efficacy of a 100 mg/m^2 dose of melphalan (MEL100). Patients were treated with two or three MEL100 courses followed by stem cell support. Complete remission was 47% with greater than a 56-month survival rate.[25]

Younger patients (under the age of 55) may be treated experimentally with allogeneic bone marrow transplantation using a treatment regimen similar to that just men-

➤ **Table 20-6**
MYELOMA STAGING SYSTEM

Criteria	Median Survival
Stage I (low myeloma mass) (*all* criteria *must* be met)	> 60 months
1. Hemoglobin > 10 g/dL	
2. Corrected serum calcium < 12 mg/dL	
3. Less than 2 lytic bone lesions	
4. Small M-spike	
IgG < 5 g/dL	
IgA < 3 g/dL	
Urine light chains < 4 g/24 hr	
Stage II (intermediate myeloma mass)	41 months
1. Does not meet *all* stage I criteria	
2. Does not meet *any* stage III criteria	
Stage III (high myeloma mass) (any of the following criteria)	23 months
1. Hemoglobin < 8.5 g/dL	
2. Corrected serum calcium > 12 mg/dL	
3. ≥ 2 lytic bone lesions	
4. Large M-spike	
IgG > 7 g/dL	
IgA > 5 g/dL	
Urine light chains > 12 g/24 hr	
Substaging	
A. Serum creatinine < 2.0 mg/dL	
B. Serum creatinine > 2.0 mg/dL	

Source: Adapted from Durie, BGM, and Salmon, SE: Staging kinetics and flow cytometry of multiple myelomas. In Wiernik, P, et al (eds): Neoplastic Diseases of the Blood. Churchill Livingstone, New York, 1985, with permission.

tioned, but infusing donor marrow, usually from an HLA-matched sibling. This has the benefits of not reintroducing myeloma cells with the bone marrow and possibly allowing the new bone marrow to reject the myeloma (graft-versus-disease effect). This procedure is associated with a 30% to 50% chance of death from infections or complica-tions from the donor-recipient mismatch known as graft-versus-host disease.

Interferon α, which has been proved to inhibit myeloma cell growth, has met with variable results in patients with multiple myeloma. Used as a single agent, interferon produced a response rate of 10% to 25%. In untreated patients the time to response was short, patients with the IgA myeloma type were more likely to benefit, and the median duration of response was analogous to the duration of response in patients receiving chemotherapy. The benefit of interferon may be as a maintenance therapy in patients who are responding to first-line chemotherapeutic agents.[26]

Smoldering Myeloma

If a patient meets the criteria for the diagnosis of stage I, low-mass multiple myeloma, and has normal kidney function, normal serum calcium, and no lytic bone lesions, then he or she falls into the category of smoldering myeloma. Because there is no curative treatment, and because these patients are not suffering ill effects from the myeloma, treatment may often be delayed with close monitoring for signs of disease progression. Treatment is usually required within 1 to 3 years, when progression to stage II or III occurs.

Multiple Myeloma

When a patient has stage II or III (intermediate or high-mass) multiple myeloma, treatment is initiated with chemotherapy at the time the diagnosis is made. Supportive care is given to resolve high calcium levels with intravenous saline and medications that inhibit osteoclasts such as glucocorticoids, bisphosphonates, and calcitonin. If needed, radiation treatments for plasmacytomas or large lytic bone lesions may be given. Vaccines for the encapsulated bacteria (*Streptococcus pneumoniae, Haemophilus influenzae,* and *Neisseria meningitidis*) should be given early. In patients with recurrent bronchitis or sinusitis, intravenous pooled immunoglobulins given at monthly intervals may be of significant benefit. Chemotherapy continues until maximum reduction in M-spike is achieved. Interferon injections have been shown to prolong the remission achieved by chemotherapy. When the disease progresses, chemotherapy is reinstituted.

Nonsecretory Myeloma

Less than 1% of multiple myelomas may be found to have no abnormal immunoglobulins in the blood or urine. The numbers of plasma cells in the bone marrow, elevation of serum calcium, and formation of plasmacytomas with bone pain all still occur. The immunoglobulin levels are usually normal. Treatment is the same as for multiple myeloma. Because of a normal immune response, infectious complications are fewer. Absence of light-chain excretion via the

➤ **Table 20-7**
MYELOMA STAGING BASED ON β₂ MICROGLOBULIN AND SERUM ALBUMIN

Stage	β_2 Microglobulin	Serum Albumin	Median Survival
I. Low risk	< 6 μg/mL	> 3.0 g/dL	55 months
II. Intermediate risk	> 6 μg/mL	> 3.0 g/dL	29 months
III. High risk	> 6 μg/mL	< 3.0 g/dL	4 months

Source: Adapted from Bataille, R, et al: C-reactive protein and beta 2 microglobulin produce a simple and powerful staging system. Blood 80:733, 1992, with permission.

kidneys preserves renal function, and survival is often improved. Evaluation of response to therapy is impaired because of the lack of M-spike. Treatment decisions are commonly based on changes in β_2m or CRP levels.

Solitary Plasmacytoma

Of patients with plasmacytomas, 5% are found to have a single tumor. The usual presentation is pain at the site of the growing tumor. The tumor may secrete immunoglobulin, resulting in a small serum M-spike, but no other signs of myeloma are present, including lytic bone lesions. The bone marrow has less than 10% plasma cells. Solitary plasmacytomas occur more often in men, and with an average age 7 years younger than the average age of multiple myeloma patients. The standard treatment for solitary plasmacytomas is radiation therapy given over 4 to 6 weeks. It is estimated that only 15% of patients treated for solitary plasmacytoma remain disease-free. On relapse, the myeloma tends to have a comparatively mild course, with an average survival of 10 years or more. Treatment decisions on relapse are the same as for multiple myeloma.[27]

Solitary plasmacytomas of nonbone structures also occur. These extramedullary plasmacytomas can be found in the sinuses, gastrointestinal tract, skin, and other locations (see Fig. 20–3). Principles of treatment are the same as for skeletal plasmacytomas, but the risk of conversion to multiple myeloma is lower.[28,29]

Plasma Cell Leukemia

The presence of significant numbers of plasma cells in the peripheral blood constitutes plasma cell leukemia (Fig. 20–19 and Color Plate 248). Half of these rare cases are found in advanced multiple myeloma, late in the course of the illness, in the final weeks of the disease. Near-complete replacement of the bone marrow by malignant plasma cells results in increased numbers of circulating cells.

Half of cases are caused by a variation of multiple myeloma referred to as primary plasma cell leukemia. This variant has circulating plasma cells at the time of diagnosis. It is complicated by more frequent high-calcium levels and more kidney failure, and much more anemia and thrombocytopenia. Enlargement of the liver, spleen, and lymph nodes is common. Treatment is the same as for multiple myeloma, often using one of the more aggressive regimens. Prognosis is poor, with expected survival of only several months.[30]

➤ MONOCLONAL GAMMOPATHY OF UNDETERMINED SIGNIFICANCE

Monoclonal gammopathy of undetermined significance (MGUS) was previously named benign monoclonal gammopathy. The only critical finding is a small M-spike on serum protein electrophoresis and no other findings of multiple myeloma. This is found in approximately 1% of individuals over the age of 50 and up to 3% of those over the age of 70.[31] Considering that the incidence of multiple myeloma in the same age group is 70 per 100,000 or less, most patients with a small M-spike will not have multiple myeloma. By definition, MGUS is diagnosed when a patient has a small M-spike, urine light chains less than 1 g per 24 hours, no lytic bone lesions, and less than 10% plasma cells in the bone marrow as listed in Table 20–8. No treatment is indicated.

This condition is no longer referred to as benign monoclonal gammopathy because it is well recognized that as many as 11% of such patients eventually develop an overt malignant process such as lymphoma, chronic lymphocytic leukemia, or multiple myeloma over a 5-year period (Table 20–9). After completing the initial screening tests for mul-

> **Table 20–8**
DIAGNOSTIC CRITERIA FOR MONOCLONAL GAMMOPATHY OF UNDETERMINED SIGNIFICANCE

I. M-spike present

   IgG < 3.5 g/dL

   IgA < 2.0 g/dL

   Urinary light chains < 1.0 g/24 hr

II. < 10% plasma cells in bone marrow

III. No bone lesions

IV. No symptoms

   (*all* criteria must be met)

Source: Adapted from Durie, BGM, and Salmon, SE: Staging kinetics and flow cytometry of multiple myeloma. In Wiernik, P, et al (eds): Neoplastic Diseases of the Blood. Churchill Livingstone, New York, 1985, with permission.

> **Table 20–9**
MONOCLONAL GAMMOPATHY OF UNDETERMINED SIGNIFICANCE: 5-YEAR FOLLOW-UP

Course of Illness	Fraction of Patients
No significant progression of M-spike	57%
> 50% increase in M-spike	9%
Progression to malignant monoclonal gammopathy	11%
Death from unrelated cause	23%

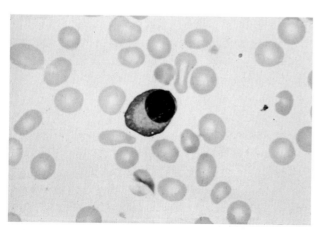

➤ **FIGURE 20–19**   Peripheral blood in plasma cell leukemia showing presence of circulating plasma cells. (From Dutcher, T: Hematology. In: Listen, Look, and Learn. Health and Education Resources, Inc, Bethesda, MD, with permission.)

tiple myeloma, a second M-spike measurement is taken approximately 3 months later. If it remains stable, the patient is followed at 6-month intervals for life. If significant changes occur, appropriate testing is repeated.

➤ WALDENSTRÖM'S MACROGLOBULINEMIA

Waldenström's macroglobulinemia (WM) is the overproduction of monoclonal IgM antibodies by cells called *plasmacytoid lymphocytes* or *prolymphs* (Fig. 20–20 and Color Plate 249). Prolymphs appear to be an intermediate stage of maturation between mature B lymphocytes and early plasma cells. It is diagnosed by finding a monoclonal M-spike and the presence of plasmacytoid lymphocytes infiltrating the bone marrow (Fig. 20–21 and Color Plate 250).

WM has an overall incidence of 2.5 million cases per year and a median age of diagnosis of 63 years.[32] It is found equally in both men and women. Patients with this disease come to physicians with early complaints of fatigue, weight loss, and generalized weakness. As the levels of IgM rise, the liver, spleen, and lymph nodes may become enlarged because of infiltration with abnormal lymphocytes. Prolymphocytes may also infiltrate nerves, the meninges, and even the brain, resulting in a variety of neurologic manifestations.

When levels of IgM rise sufficiently, symptoms of "hyperviscosity syndrome" may arise. Clinical features of hyperviscosity syndrome are listed in Table 20–10. Blurred vision, headache, and confusion are common neurologic changes. Worsening can lead to somnolence and even coma. Examination of the eyes may reveal characteristic "sausage-link" veins in 50% of patients with WM caused by hyperviscosity (Fig. 20–22). Congestive heart failure may occur because of the high protein levels resulting in expansion of fluid volume within the blood vessels.

Patients with WM often have extensive bruising called *cryoglobulinemic purpura* (Fig. 20–23) and may have bleeding from the gums and nose. More severe bleeding may be seen. This is caused by interference with platelets and blood clotting factor proteins by the abnormal IgM. Bleeding time is often prolonged, as are the clotting factor assays, PT and APTT (see Chap. 32).

Cryoglobulins are proteins (often IgM) that precipitate on exposure to cold. Some patients with WM develop symptoms of cryoglobulinemia. Patients with cryoglobulinemia may develop pain and color changes in cold exposed areas (Raynaud's phenomenon), clotting or thrombosis of small blood vessels, and kidney damage.

WM is not curable at this time. Chemotherapy is the primary treatment, using alkylators such as chlorambucil, cy-

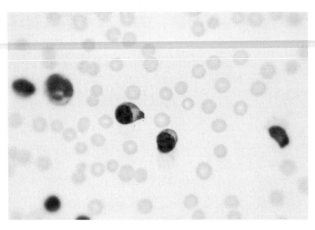

➤ FIGURE 20–20   Plasmacytoid lymphocytes; note the red-staining accumulation of immunoglobulin in the cytoplasm.

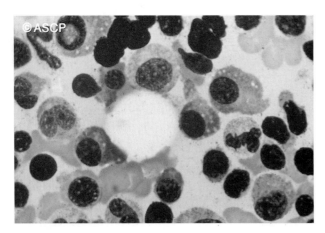

➤ FIGURE 20–21   Plasmacytoid lymphocytes in marrow aspirate from a patient with Waldenström's macroglobulinemia. (From Hyun, BH: Morphology of Blood and Bone Marrow. American Society of Clinical Pathologists, Workshop 5121, Philadelphia, September 7, 1983, with permission.)

➤ **Table 20-10**
CLINICAL FEATURES OF HYPERVISCOSITY SYNDROME

Sign or Symptom	Fraction of Patients
Neurologic changes	20%
Retinopathy	35%
Hypervolemia/congestive heart failure	20%
Abnormal bleeding	20%
Enlarged liver and spleen	35%
Enlarged lymph nodes	45%

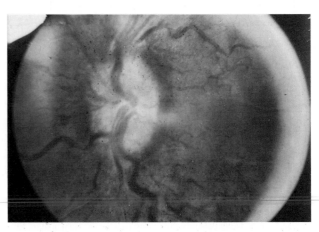

➤ FIGURE 20–22   Tortuous veins with sausage-link appearance in the fundus of the eye.

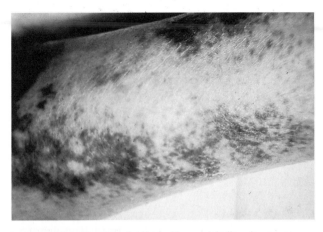

> **FIGURE 20–23** Arm of patient with cryoglobulinemic purpura. Note the skin manifestations.

clophosphamide, and L-phenylalanine mustard. If severe symptoms are present at diagnosis, IgM may be quickly removed by plasmapheresis, resulting in rapid improvement in symptoms.[10] Table 20–11 compares WM with multiple myeloma.

Survival is estimated based on the percentage of prolymphs in the bone marrow. Less than 20% replacement of bone marrow by prolymphs results in survival approaching 5 years, whereas 50% replacement or more results in survival of less than 1 year.

> ## Table 20-11
> **COMPARISON OF MULTIPLE MYELOMA AND WALDENSTRÖM'S MACROGLOBULINEMIA**

	Macroglobulinemia	Myeloma
Organomegaly	+++	+
Hyperviscosity	+++	+
Lytic bone lesions	+	+++
Renal failure	+	+++
Length of survival	++	+

► HEAVY-CHAIN DISEASE

Heavy-chain disease (HCD) is the excessive production of the heavy-chain portion of the antibody unit. It appears to be a disorder in which the plasma cells have lost the ability to synthesize the light-chain component. An HCD has been identified for each of the major immunoglobulin classes: IgG, IgA, and IgM.[33–36] These diseases are very rare. Table 20–12 summarizes the characteristics of heavy-chain diseases.

> ## ► CASE STUDY 1: Multiple Myeloma
>
> A 71-year-old man went to his physician with complaints of a constant aching in his back that had progressively worsened over a 6-month period. His wife noted that he was frequently confused, slept much of the day, and made occasional nonsensical statements.
>
> On examination, the patient appeared normal. However, he was unable to state the correct date and could not name the current president of the United States. His spine was tender to examination. Lymph nodes, liver, and spleen were not enlarged, and his examination was otherwise normal.
>
> Radiographs of the spine were ordered and revealed osteoporosis with compression fractures of the third and fourth lumbar vertebrae. Blood tests revealed a mild normocytic anemia with a hemoglobin (Hgb) level of 10 g/dL and a mean corpuscular volume (MCV) of 91 fL. Platelets and white blood cells were normal. The laboratory reported that rouleaux were noted on his blood smear. His chemistry panel revealed a calcium level of 10.6 mg/dL (normal range is 8.8 to 10.5) with a low albumin level of 2.6 g/dL. Total protein was 8.2 g/dL. The physician subtracted the albumin from the total protein and realized that the antibody-containing protein level was elevated at 5.6 g/dL. The serum calcium was then corrected because of the low albumin levels, and found that the equivalent calcium level was 11.7 g/dL. The patient's kidney function was normal.
>
> *continued*

> ## Table 20-12
> **HEAVY-CHAIN DISEASES (HCDs)**

Disease	Antibody Heavy Chain (M-spike)	Organ Involvement	Other Characteristics	Survival Rate
Gamma (γ) HCD	γ chains (IgG)	Liver and spleen may be enlarged Enlarged lymph nodes	Disease of elderly people	Few weeks to a few years
Alpha (α) HCD	α chain (IgA)	GI tract (abdominal mass)	Commonly called Mediterranean lymphoma because it is frequently reported in younger individuals in the Mediterranean area	Few months
Mu (μ) HCD	μ chains (IgM)	Enlargement of liver and spleen	May be a variation of CLL because of high number of lymphs in blood BM: vacuolated plasma cells	Not available

Abbreviations: BM = bone marrow findings; CLL = chronic lymphocytic leukemia

The patient was hospitalized. Hydration with normal saline rapidly lowered the calcium levels, and the patient's mental status quickly improved over the following 3 days. Because of continued back pain, an MRI scan of his spine was obtained that revealed destruction of the bone structure at several levels, with bone marrow signal alteration consistent with malignancy, but no compression of the spinal cord. Serum protein electrophoresis revealed an M-spike measuring 4.7 g/dL. Immunoelectrophoresis revealed that the M-spike was composed of an IgG-κ antibody. His serum IgM level was 63 mg/dL, and IgA level was 120 mg/dL. A 24-hour urine collection demonstrated no protein. Bone marrow biopsies were obtained and revealed 32% plasma cells, forming sheets, with binucleated forms present. A radiologic skeletal survey revealed classic lytic lesions in the skull, pelvis, both arms, and both femurs, with diffuse osteoporosis.

Questions

1. What major and minor criteria for multiple myeloma are met in this patient?
2. What stage myeloma does he have?
3. What other tests could be ordered to help estimate this patient's survival prognosis?
4. Should he be considered for bone marrow transplantation? Why?

Answers

1. Major criteria met were (a) more than 30% plasma cells in the bone marrow; (b) IgG-κ M-spike greater than 3.5 g/dL. Minor criteria met were (a) lytic bone lesions; (b) low-normal immunoglobulins (see Table 20–4).
2. The patient has stage III disease based on the presence of multiple lytic bone lesions. Any single stage III criterion is sufficient (see Table 20–6).
3. Low albumin is an adverse prognostic factor. Beta$_2$ microglobulin and C-reactive protein are also useful in determining prognosis (see Table 20–7).
4. The patient is not a candidate for bone marrow transplantation. The patient's age makes it likely that the danger of the procedure would outweigh the potential benefit.

► CASE STUDY 2: MGUS

A 55-year-old man was seen by a physician at the primary care clinic for prolonged back pain after lifting some heavy boxes several months before. Examination of the patient's back revealed some tenderness in the muscles with no bone tenderness. X-rays of the back were read as normal. As part of his evaluation, a serum protein electrophoresis was ordered; it revealed an M-spike measured at 1.1 g/dL. Immunoelectrophoresis identified the M-spike as IgG-λ. He was referred to a hematologist to rule out multiple myeloma.

The hematologist performed a thorough physical examination and found no significant abnormalities, including normal lymph nodes, liver, and spleen. A full skeletal survey and 24-hour urine collection for protein evaluation, serum calcium, and serum quantitative immunoglobulins were ordered, and bilateral iliac crest bone marrow biopsies were performed. The x-rays were normal. No protein was detected in the urine. Calcium, IgM, and IgA levels were normal. The bone marrow revealed 6.4% normal-appearing plasma cells. To be thorough, the hematologist also ordered CT scans of the chest and abdomen, which revealed no enlarged lymph nodes suspicious for lymphoma, and confirmed a normal size spleen. The hematologist felt satisfied that this patient had MGUS.

Questions

1. Which explanation should be given to the patient?
   a. You have an incurable disease, probably a cancer that has not yet been found. I want to see you back every 3 months for tests.
   b. Nothing of concern was found. There is nothing to worry about. Have a nice day.
   c. Your body is producing some abnormal antibodies. It is a common disorder that will probably never cause you any problems. A small percentage of patients may develop a more serious problem later, so I need to see you back in 3 months, and then periodically to see if there has been any change.
2. Besides multiple myeloma, what other malignancies can be associated with monoclonal gammopathies?
   (1) Lung cancer
   (2) Chronic lymphocytic leukemia
   (3) Acute myeloid leukemia
   (4) Non-Hodgkin's lymphoma
      a. 1, 2, and 3
      b. 1 and 3
      c. 2 and 4
      d. All of the above
3. What follow-up schedule would be appropriate?
   a. Monthly serum protein electrophoresis.
   b. Bone marrow biopsy repeated every 6 months for 2 years. If there is no evidence of myeloma at that time, the patient does not have to return anymore.
   c. Repeat the complete evaluation every 6 months.
   d. Repeat the serum protein electrophoresis in 3 months, then every 6 months thereafter if there has been no change.

Answers

1. c. Although a few patients develop multiple myeloma, non-Hodgkin's lymphoma, or chronic lymphocytic leukemia, most patients with MGUS are not adversely affected by this disorder (see Table 20–9).
2. c. Choices (2) and (4) are correct. Lymphoid malignancies may produce measurable amounts of immunoglobulin. Nonlymphoid malignancies such as lung cancer and acute myeloid leukemia do not (see Fig. 20–18).
3. d. Once the initial evaluation is complete, no further testing needs to be done unless there is a change in the production of the M-spike im-

munoglobulin. Three months is considered a reasonable interval because of the known growth rate of these disorders. If the patient's condition is stable after that time interval, the period of time may safely be increased to 6-month follow-ups for life.

➤ CASE STUDY 3: Waldenström's Macroglobulinemia

A 59-year-old woman was seen by her physician for a 35-lb unintentional weight loss from her usual 165 lb over the past 18 months. She had been having trouble concentrating at work, had decreased energy, and had two frightening episodes during which she could not make sense of the words she was reading in a novel. She was otherwise in excellent health.

On physical examination, she was noted to be a tall, thin woman with no enlarged lymph nodes. Her spleen was enlarged, and easily felt approximately 7 cm below her left ribs. Her neurologic examination was normal. Blood tests revealed Hgb of 9.7 g/dL, hematocrit (Hct) of 29.2%, and MCV of 89 fL. Platelets, white cells, and white cell differential were normal. Chemistry panel was normal with the exception of a total protein level of 8.7 g/dL and a low albumin of 2.7 g/dL. Calcium level was 8.3 mg/dL. A serum protein electrophoresis was ordered and revealed a 5.7 g/dL M-spike.

Immunoelectrophoresis identified the protein as an IgM-κ. A bone marrow biopsy revealed that 23% of the marrow consisted of abnormal plasmacytoid lymphocytes consistent with Waldenström's macroglobulinemia. Blood viscosity was measured and found to be moderately increased.

Questions

1. Which of the following is a possible cause of the patient's problems in concentrating and reading?
   a. The calcium level is actually high when the low albumin level is considered. High calcium is well known to cause mental status changes.
   b. The increased viscosity of the blood is causing poor circulation through the blood vessels in the brain, resulting in these symptoms.
   c. On exposure to cold, cryoglobulins in the patient's head precipitate and block blood vessels.
   d. Osteolytic lesions in the spine.
2. Which statement is most correct about the patient's diagnosis?
   a. This is a terminal disease that may end her life within a year.
   b. This is a chronic disorder that often requires treatment, but she will probably live a relatively normal life.
   c. This disease is rapidly fatal and does not respond to treatment.
   d. This is a terminal disease, but the numbers of abnormal cells in the bone marrow suggest that, with treatment, she may live another 4 or 5 years.

3. If the patient developed more severe neurologic problems, what could be done to rapidly lower the IgM in the blood?

Answers

1. b. Hyperviscosity syndrome is common with Waldenström's macroglobulinemia, and these are classic symptoms. The plasmacytoid lymphocytes may infiltrate nerves, meninges, and the brain and may be a less common cause of mental status changes and neurologic changes. Hypercalcemia is uncommon with WM, and correcting the albumin to 4 g/dL (1.3 g/dL increase) would result in a correction of serum calcium level of $0.8 \times 1.3 = 1.04$ mg/dL, totaling 9.34 mg/dL. This is within the normal range. Chilling of the scalp would not result in precipitation of cryoglobulins in the brain, but might affect the tips of the ears and nose.
2. d. The prognosis of patients with WM is associated with extent of plasmacytoid lymphocytes in the bone marrow. This patient may live for 3 to 4 years after diagnosis.
3. Plasmapheresis is useful in removing IgM-rich plasma from the patient within 1 to 2 hours and may result in dramatic resolution of symptoms.

QUESTIONS

1. Which laboratory test(s) for whole blood is/are used in the evaluation of plasma cell disorders?
   a. CBC
   b. Peripheral blood smear
   c. ESR
   d. All of the above

2. What laboratory serum tests are used for evaluation of plasma cell disorders, and how are they used?
   a. First, serum protein electrophoresis (SPEP); then, if an M-spike is seen, immunoelectrophoresis (IEP) or immunofixation to determine the specific antibody class
   b. IEP, used to determine the antibody group and immunofixation or SPEP, used to determine if light or heavy chains are increased
   c. First, SPEP; then, if no abnormalities are seen, IEP or immunofixation, used as a more sensitive indicator of increased antibody class(es)
   d. First, either SPEP or IEP; then, if an M-spike is seen, immunofixation to determine the specific antibody class

3. Which of the following tests can directly detect urinary light chains and is used to distinguish between κ and λ light chains?
   a. Heat precipitation test
   b. Urine immunoelectrophoresis
   c. Sulfosalicylic acid (SSA) test
   d. Both b and c

4. Which list would contain diagnostic criteria for multiple myeloma?
   a. Biopsy-proven plasmacytoma and 10% to 30% plasma cells
   b. More than 30% plasma cells in bone marrow
   c. Biopsy-proven plasmacytoma and M-spike present
   d. Monoclonal protein and M-spike present

5. Which of the following would be diagnostic criteria for Waldenström's macroglobulinemia?
   a. IgM M-spike and hyperviscosity
   b. Lytic bone lesions and rouleaux
   c. Renal failure and more than 30% plasma cells
   d. M-spike of IgM, IgG, or IgA; low-normal levels of other immunoglobulins; inability to make light chains

6. What are the characteristics of heavy-chain disease? (*Use the answer choices for question 5.*)

7. Which of the following might be found on the peripheral blood smear in a patient with multiple myeloma?
   a. Bite cells
   b. Target cells
   c. Rouleaux
   d. Howell-Jolly bodies

8. What does staging refer to?
   a. Bone marrow compatibility
   b. Estimate of disease severity
   c. Chemotherapy regimen
   d. Determination of specific immunoglobulin in heavy-chain disease

9. Which heavy-chain disease primarily involves the gastrointestinal tract and is associated with poor survival?
   a. Gamma
   b. Mu
   c. Alpha
   d. Delta

10. Which values for $\beta_2 m$ and albumin are associated with the best prognosis in multiple myeloma?
    a. $\beta_2 m$ less than 6 μg/mL; albumin greater than 3 g/dL
    b. $\beta_2 m$ greater than 6 μg/mL; albumin greater than 3 g/dL
    c. $\beta_2 m$ greater than 6 μg/mL; albumin less than 3 g/dL
    d. $\beta_2 m$ greater than 10 μg/mL; albumin greater than 3 g/dL

SUMMARY CHART

➤ Multiple myeloma is a disorder characterized by the overproduction of abnormal plasma cells. Bone destruction, hypercalcemia, kidney failure, hyperviscosity, and paralysis are common manifestations.

➤ A single tumor mass composed of a clone of abnormal plasma cells is called a *plasmacytoma*.

➤ Multiple myeloma is evident when mutated plasma cells induce the proliferation of interleukin-6 (IL-6) and other cytokines, causing further replication of this malignancy.

➤ Multiple myeloma is associated with pancytopenia, causing anemia, bleeding diathesis, and increased susceptibility to infection.

➤ Any abnormal production of identical antibodies is referred to as *monoclonal gammopathy;* excess production of IgG is the most common in patients with multiple myeloma.

➤ Bence-Jones proteins are common in multiple myeloma; they are characterized as excess light chains found in the urine which precipitates at 56°C.

➤ Amyloidosis occurs in multiple myeloma when immunoglobulin kappa (κ) or lambda (λ) light chains settle or deposit in organs such as the heart, kidneys, nerves, liver, spleen, and gastrointestinal tract.

➤ IL-6 and osteoclast-activating factor (OAF) play major roles in the production of the lytic bone lesions associated with multiple myeloma by stimulating the development of osteoclasts and subsequent release of calcium from bone, thereby weakening the bone structure.

➤ An M spike is a spike caused by increased levels of monoclonal immunoglobulins on protein electrophoresis.

➤ Laboratory evaluation in multiple myeloma includes immunoelectrophoresis, quantitative immunoglobulin assay, complete blood count (CBC), peripheral blood smear, erythrocyte sedimentation rate (ESR), bone marrow biopsy examination, chemistry panel, beta$_2$ microglobulin ($\beta_2 m$), and C-reactive protein (CRP). Diagnostic procedures include radiography and magnetic resonance imaging (MRI).

➤ Patients with multiple myeloma have more than 10% plasma cells, which often form "sheets" with immature and binucleate forms on bone marrow biopsy examination.

➤ The most characteristic finding in multiple myeloma is rouleaux formation of the red cells, which occurs when increased amounts of immunoglobulins in the blood cause red blood cells to adhere to each other.

➤ Staging in multiple myeloma provides an estimated extent of disease to help determine the appropriate treatment plan and patient prognosis.

➤ Chemotherapy is the primary treatment in multiple myeloma.

➤ The presence of significant numbers of plasma cells in the peripheral blood constitutes plasma cell leukemia.

➤ Monoclonal gammopathy of undetermined significance (MGUS) is evident when a patient has a small M spike, urine light chains of less than 1 g per 24 hours, no lytic bone lesions, and less than 10% plasma cells in the bone marrow.

➤ Waldenström's macroglobulinemia is the overproduction of monoclonal IgM antibodies by cells called *plasmacytoid lymphocytes* or *prolymphs*.

➤ Manifestations associated with Waldenström's macroglobulinemia include hyperviscosity syndrome, increased levels of IgM, fatigue, cryoglobulinemic purpura, and bleeding diathesis.

➤ Standard treatment in Waldenström's macroglobulinemia includes chemotherapy and plasmapheresis to remove increased levels of IgM.

➤ Heavy-chain disease refers to the excessive production of the heavy-chain portion of the antibody unit; immunoglobulins IgG, IgA, and IgM are implicated.

References

1. Foerster, J, and Paraskevas, F: Multiple myeloma. In Lee, RG, et al (eds): Wintrobe's Clinical Hematology, ed 10. Williams & Wilkins, Baltimore, 1999, p 2638.
2. Gado, K, et al: Role of interleukin-6 in the pathogenesis of multiple myeloma. Cell Biol Int 24:195, 2000.
3. Ries, LAG, et al: Cancer Statistics Review 1973–1988. US Government Printing Office, Washington, DC, 1991.
4. Lundberg, I, and Milatou-Smith, R: Mortality and cancer incidence among Swedish pain industry workers with long-term exposure to organic solvents. Scand J Work Environ Health 24:270, 1998.
5. Bergsagel, DE, et al: Benzene and multiple myeloma: Appraisal of the scientific evidence. Blood 94:1174, 1999.
6. Correa, A, et al: Use of hair dyes, hematopoietic neoplasms, and lymphomas: A literature review. II. Lymphomas and multiple myeloma. Cancer Invest 18:467, 2000.
7. Riedel, DA, and Pottern, LM: The epidemiology of multiple myeloma. Hematol Oncol Clin North Am 6:225, 1992.
8. Umeno, Y, et al: A case of multiple myeloma which developed into multiply extramedullary involvement in the terminal stage. Fukuoka Igaku Zasshi 91:55, 2000.
9. Shaheen, H, et al: Clinicopathological features and management of Pakistani patients with multiple myeloma. JPMA J Pak Med Assoc 49:233, 1999.
10. Siami, GA, and Siami, FS: Plasmapheresis and paraproteinemia: Cryoprotein-induced diseases, monoclonal gammopathy, Waldenström's macroglobulinemia, hyperviscosity syndrome, multiple myeloma, light chain disease, and amyloidosis. Ther Apher 3:8, 1999.
11. Kallemuchikkal, U, and Gorevic, PD: Evaluation of cryoglobulins. Arch Pathol Lab Med 123: 119, 1999.
12. Maitra, A, et al: Cytoplasmic inclusions in leukocytes. An unusual manifestation of cryoglobulinemia. Am J Clin Pathol 113:107, 2000.
13. Manolagas, SC: The role of IL-6 type cytokines and their receptors in bone. Ann NY Acad Sci 840:194, 1998.
14. Ershler, WB, and Keller, ET: Age-associated interleukin-6 gene expression, late-life diseases, and frailty. Annu Rev Med 51:245, 2000.
15. Zandecki, M, Lai, JL, Facon, T: Multiple myeloma: Almost all patients are cytogenetically abnormal. Br J Haematol 94:217–227, 1996.
16. Moscinski, LC, and Ballester, OF: Recent progress in multiple myeloma. Hematol Oncol 12:111, 1994.
17. Lai, JL, et al: Improved cytogenetics in multiple myeloma: a study of 151 patients including 117 patients at diagnosis. Blood 85:2490, 1995.
18. Hoyer, JD, et al: The (11;14)(q13;q32) translocation in multiple myeloma. A morphologic and immunohistochemical study. Am J Clin Pathol 113:831, June 2000.
19. Hoechtlen-Vollmar, W, et al: Amplification of cyclin D1 gene in multiple myeloma: Clinical and prognostic relevance. Br J Haematol 109:30, 2000.
20. Kyle, RA: Sequence of testing for monoclonal gammopathies. Arch Pathol Lab Med 123:114, 1999.
21. Kyle, RA: Diagnostic criteria of multiple myeloma. Hematol Oncol Clin North Am 6:347, 1992.
22. Greipp, PR: Advances in the diagnosis and management of myeloma. Semin Hematol 29:24, 1992.
23. Lymphoma Tumor Group: Plasma cell disorders. In: Cancer Treatment Policies. British Columbia Cancer Agency, 1994, pp 4–6. (www.bccancer.bc.ca)
24. Durie, BGM, and Salmon, SE: A clinical staging system for multiple myeloma: Correlation of measured myeloma cell mass with presenting clinical features, response to treatment and survival. Cancer 36:842, 1975.
25. Bataille, R, et al: C-reactive protein and beta 2 microglobulin produce a simple and powerful myeloma staging system. Blood 80:733, 1992.
26. Palumbo, A, et al: Dose-intensive melphalan with stem cell support (MEL100) is superior to standard treatment in elderly myeloma patients. Blood 94:1248, 1999.
27. Blade, J, and Esteve, J: Viewpoint on the impact of interferon in the treatment of multiple myeloma: Benefit for a small proportion of patients? Med Oncol 17:77, 2000.
28. Dimopoulos, MA, et al: Solitary plasmacytomas of bone and asymptomatic multiple myeloma. Hematol Oncol Clin North Am 6:359, 1992.
29. Matsumura, S, et al: Radiographic findings for solitary plasmacytoma of the bone in the anterior wall of the maxillary sinus: A case report. Oral Surg Oral Med Oral Pathol Oral Radiol Endod 89:651, 2000.
30. Hidaka, H, et al: A case of extramedullary plasmacytoma arising from the nasal septum. J Laryngol Otol 114:53, 2000.
31. Blade, J, and Kyle, RA: Nonsecretory myeloma, immunoglobulin D myeloma, and plasma cell leukemia. Hematol Oncol Clin North Am 13:1259, 1999.
32. Kyle, RA, and Rajkumar, SV: Monoclonal gammopathies of undetermined significance. Hematol Oncol Clin North Am 13:1181, 1999.
33. Gertz, MA, et al: Waldenström's macroglobulinemia. Oncologist 5:63, 2000.
34. Kambham, N, et al: Heavy chain deposition disease: The disease spectrum. Am J Kidney Dis 33:954, 1999.
35. Fine, KD, and Stone, MJ: Alpha-heavy chain disease, Mediterranean lymphoma, and immunoproliferative small intestinal disease: A review of clinicopathological features pathogenesis, and differential diagnosis. Am J Gastroenterol 94:1139, 1999.
36. Liapis, H, et al: Nodular glomerulosclerosis secondary to mu heavy chain deposits. Hum Pathol 31:122, 2000.

21 The Lymphomas

Dan M. Hyder, MD

OBJECTIVES

At the end of this chapter, the learner should be able to:

1. List distinguishing features for lymphocyte-predominant, mixed cellularity, lymphocyte-rich, lymphocyte depletion, and nodular sclerosing Hodgkin's lymphoma.

2. Describe the morphological and immunophenotypic features of Reed-Sternberg cells.

3. List distinguishing features for the four stages of Hodgkin's lymphoma.

4. Describe the classification criteria for non-Hodgkin's lymphomas by the Working Formulation and REAL classification.

5. Describe tests that may be needed to provide a differential diagnosis for lymphomas.

6. Describe the prognosis and treatment options for Hodgkin's lymphoma and the more common categories of non-Hodgkin's lymphomas.

The malignant lymphomas are a heterogeneous group of diseases that arise from cells of the lymphoid tissue (lymphocytes, histiocytes, and reticulum cells). They are broadly divided into the two major categories of Hodgkin's disease (Hodgkin's lymphoma) and the lymphocytic lymphomas. Although the vast majority of lymphomas within the second category are of lymphocytic origin, occasional cases do appear to arise from nonlymphoid cells. Consequently, the lymphocytic lymphomas are also frequently referred to as the non-Hodgkin's lymphomas (NHL). This subdivision of the malignant lymphomas into two general categories has both biologic and therapeutic implications.

It is important for the student and clinician alike to be aware of the diagnostic difficulties often faced by the pathologist in evaluating lymphoid proliferations. Perhaps no area in pathology has produced so many subcategories of a basic disease process as the area of lymphoma diagnosis. The distinction between benign and malignant lymphoid proliferations, Hodgkin's lymphoma versus non-Hodgkin's lymphoma, and the subcategorization of these two major types of lymphoma is frequently difficult and may require additional studies beyond light microscopy. In some circumstances, a definitive diagnosis may not be possible.

➤ HODGKIN'S LYMPHOMA

Hodgkin's disease was the first of the lymphomas to be recognized. In 1832 Thomas Hodgkin described what he believed to be a primary yet benign disease of the lymphoid tissue.[1] Samuel Wilks in 1865 suggested that the disorder described by Hodgkin was a malignant process and was the first to apply the term *Hodgkin's disease* in honor of Hodgkin's original description of the process.[2] It was not until 1898 that Sternberg[3] and later in 1902 that Reed[4] described the distinctive histologic features of Hodgkin's disease, including the peculiar cell that is the morphological hallmark of Hodgkin's disease and that now bears their names; that is, the Sternberg-Reed (or Reed-Sternberg) cell (Figs. 21–1 and 21–2*A;* and Color Plate 251).

Etiology and Pathogenesis

The continued use of the term *Hodgkin's disease* rather than *Hodgkin's lymphoma* attests to the fact that the etiology and even the very nature (i.e., inflammatory/reactive versus malignant) of Hodgkin's disease remains uncertain. There has been considerable intrigue focusing on a possible viral etiology of Hodgkin's lymphoma, with particular attention to certain ribonucleic acid (RNA) tumor viruses

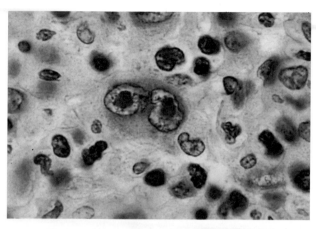

> ► **FIGURE 21–1** Classic Reed-Sternberg cell (*center*), characterized by large size, multilobed nucleus, and inclusion-like nucleoli.

and Epstein-Barr virus (EBV). Conclusive experimental evidence, however, is lacking. Certain epidemiologic data, such as the occasional occurrence of several cases of Hodgkin's lymphoma within a small locale and brief space of time (time-space clustering), would also suggest an infectious etiology. Other epidemiologic studies, however, have failed to support an infectious mode of transmission.

Although an infectious mode of transmission is unlikely, an infectious cofactor would appear to be operational in the pathogenesis of Hodgkin's lymphoma. The probable infectious agent is EBV, although cytomegalovirus and herpes virus 6 have also been implicated. EBV nucleic acids can be demonstrated in the lesions of approximately 80% of cases of Hodgkin's lymphoma, and EBV antigens such as latent membrane protein can be detected in approximately 50% of the cases. The mechanism by which a virus such as EBV promotes the development of Hodgkin's lymphoma is unclear; however, it is postulated that a preceding state of immunosuppression permits an abnormal immune response to an EBV infection. The resulting genetic errors in the immunoregulatory cells (T and B lymphocytes) are hypothesized to lead to the development of Hodgkin's lymphoma.

The current view of Hodgkin's lymphoma is that it is truly a malignant proliferation and, therefore, more properly referred to as *Hodgkin's lymphoma* rather than Hodgkin's disease. The malignant cells are the Reed-Sternberg cell and its variants, which usually represent only a small percentage of the total cells in a Hodgkin's lymphoma lesion (see Fig. 21–2A through E). Despite the prevailing view that the Reed-Sternberg cell is the malignant cell of Hodgkin's lymphoma, the origin of this cell remains an enigma. Kinship to almost every cell of the mononuclear phagocytic and lymphoreticular system has been proposed for the Reed-Sternberg cell. Functional, enzymatic, immunophenotypic, and genotypic data are conflicting, but the weight of the data strongly favors a B-lymphocyte origin of the Reed-Sternberg cell.[5]

Pathology

The cytologic hallmark of Hodgkin's lymphoma is the presence of an unusual giant cell, the Reed-Sternberg cell. The features of this cell include large size (up to 45 μm in diameter), abundant acidophilic cytoplasm, multinucleated or poly-

lobated nucleus, and gigantic (more than 5 μm in diameter), inclusion-like nucleoli (see Figs. 21–1 and 21–2A). There is often clearing of the chromatin around the macronucleoli, resulting in a distinct halo effect. Formerly, it was necessary to identify at least one of these "diagnostic" Reed-Sternberg cells before a primary diagnosis of Hodgkin's lymphoma could be made; however, with current immunophenotyping techniques, this is no longer a requirement. The identification of Reed-Sternberg (or Reed-Sternberg–like) cells, however, is not a sufficient condition for the diagnosis of Hodgkin's lymphoma. Reed-Sternberg–like cells are commonly seen in a variety of benign and malignant conditions other than Hodgkin's lymphoma (Table 21–1). The diagnosis of Hodgkin's lymphoma should be based on finding Reed-Sternberg cells (morphologically or immunophenotypically) in the proper cellular, stromal, and clinical setting. Many nondiagnostic variants of Reed-Sternberg cells have been described (see Fig. 21–2A through E). Observation of these cells is helpful in suggesting the possibility of Hodgkin's lymphoma and in the subclassification of Hodgkin's lymphoma.

Several classification schemes for Hodgkin's lymphoma are in use; however, they all share the fact that they are primarily based on growth pattern and cellular composition. Clinicians commonly utilize the Rye classification (Table 21–2), which is a simplification of the Lukes and Butler classification.[6,7] Recent advances in understanding the biology of Hodgkin's lymphoma indicates that there are two pathologically distinct forms of Hodgkin's lymphoma, lymphocyte-predominant Hodgkin's lymphoma and "classic" Hodgkin's lymphoma.[8] The classic group may be further subdivided based on cellular composition. The recently proposed World Health Organization (WHO) classification of Hodgkin's lymphoma (Table 21–3) incorporates this new information.[9]

Lymphocyte-predominant Hodgkin's Lymphoma

Lymphocyte-predominant (LP) Hodgkin's lymphoma is a relatively uncommon (5% of cases) but pathologically and clinically distinct variety of Hodgkin's lymphoma.

The growth pattern is generally characterized by a vague nodularity although in some cases it may be well developed. It is questionable whether a purely diffuse form of LP Hodgkin's lymphoma exists.[10] The cellular milieu is composed of a mixture of small, normal-appearing lymphocytes, benign histiocytes, rare or absent Reed-Sternberg cells, and variable numbers of a characteristic, though nondiagnostic, Reed-Sternberg variant referred to as an *L & H* or *popcorn cell* (see Fig. 21–2C). This cell has a variable amount of pale staining cytoplasm, a convoluted nucleus prosaically referred to as popcorn-shaped, and an indistinct nucleolus. Phenotypic studies suggest that L & H cells are closely related to proliferating germinal center cells (centroblasts).[11] Plasma cells, eosinophils, fibrosis, and necrosis are usually absent. The histologic features of LP Hodgkin's lymphoma must be distinguished from various reactive conditions such as infectious mononucleosis as well as other subcategories of Hodgkin's and non-Hodgkin's lymphoma. Such differentiation may require special phenotypic and genotypic studies.

Classic Hodgkin's Lymphoma

Classic Hodgkin's lymphoma is morphologically defined by the observation of classic Reed-Sternberg cells in the appro-

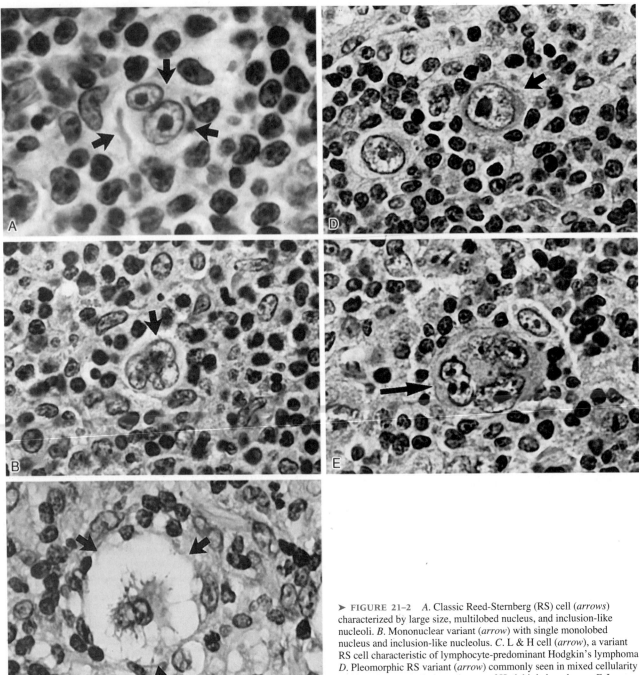

► FIGURE 21–2   *A.* Classic Reed-Sternberg (RS) cell (*arrows*) characterized by large size, multilobed nucleus, and inclusion-like nucleoli. *B.* Mononuclear variant (*arrow*) with single monolobed nucleus and inclusion-like nucleolus. *C.* L & H cell (*arrow*), a variant RS cell characteristic of lymphocyte-predominant Hodgkin's lymphoma. *D.* Pleomorphic RS variant (*arrow*) commonly seen in mixed cellularity and lymphocyte depletion subtypes of Hodgkin's lymphoma. *E.* Lacunar cell (*arrows*), a variant RS cell characteristic of nodular sclerosing Hodgkin's lymphoma.

priate cellular and stromal background. It is the background that determines the subcategory of classic Hodgkin's lymphoma to which the lesion belongs.

Nodular Sclerosing Hodgkin's Lymphoma

Nodular sclerosing (NS) Hodgkin's lymphoma is the most common subtype of Hodgkin's lymphoma, representing 60% to 80% of cases. The cardinal histologic features of NS Hodgkin's lymphoma are the presence of birefringent collagenous sclerosis, classic Reed-Sternberg cells, and a distinctive Reed-Sternberg variant called a *lacunar cell.* The sclerosis observed in NS Hodgkin's lymphoma is different from that seen in the other subtypes of Hodgkin's lymphoma. It is found in the form of well-organized bands of collagen

that subdivide the tissue into distinct nodules (Fig. 21–3). Within the nodules is a variable mixture of lymphocytes, classic Reed-Sternberg cells, lacunar cells, plasma cells, eosinophils, and neutrophils. The lacunar cells often form distinct collections within the central region of the nodule ("grouped lacunars"), and these collections may be associated with focal necrosis (Fig. 21–4). The lacunar cell is best identified in formalin-fixed tissue sections in which the artifact of formalin fixation produces a distinctive appearance of this Reed-Sternberg variant. The lacunar cell is separated from the surrounding cells by a large clear or pale-staining space (lacuna) (see Fig. 21–2E). Wisps of cytoplasm may be seen in this space. The nucleus is large and often polylobated, and the nucleoli are small to intermediate in size.

> ➤ **Table 21-1**
> ## DISEASES OR DISORDERS IN WHICH REED-STERNBERG–LIKE CELLS HAVE BEEN REPORTED

Viral infection, e.g., infectious mononucleosis

Anticonvulsant-induced lymphadenopathy

Epithelial and stromal malignancies

Melanoma

Various lymphomas and leukemias

Myeloproliferative disorders

> ➤ **Table 21-2**
> ## RYE CLASSIFICATION OF HODGKIN'S LYMPHOMA

Nodular sclerosis

Lymphocyte predominance

Mixed cellularity

Lymphocyte depletion

Unclassified

Source: From Lukes, RJ, et al: Report of the Nomenclature Committee. Cancer Res 26:1311, 1966, with permission.

> ➤ **Table 21-3**
> ## WHO CLASSIFICATION OF HODGKIN'S LYMPHOMA

	Frequency
Nodular lymphocyte-predominant	5%
Classic Hodgkin's lymphoma	
Nodular sclerosis, grades I and II	60%–80%
Lymphocyte-rich	5%
Mixed cellularity	15%–30%
Lymphocyte depletion	< 1%

Source: From Harris, NL: Hodgkin's disease: Classification and differential diagnosis. Mod Pathol 12:159, 1999, with permission.

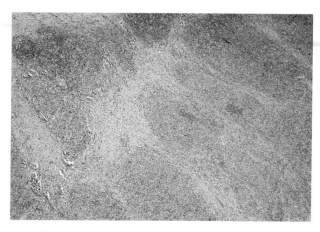

➤ **FIGURE 21–3** Nodular sclerosing Hodgkin's lymphoma characterized by orderly bands of collagen that subdivide the tissue into cellular nodules containing a mixture of cell types, including large numbers of lacunar cells.

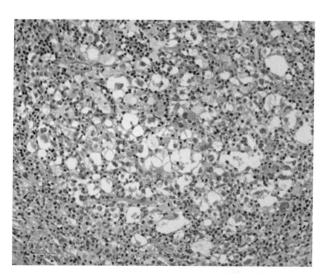

➤ **FIGURE 21–4** Grouped lacunar cells in nodular sclerosing Hodgkin's lymphoma. A cluster of lacunar cells and other Reed-Sternberg variant cells forms a distinctive nodule referred to as "grouped lacunar cells." Necrosis is often present in the center of these nodules.

Mixed Cellularity Hodgkin's Lymphoma

As its name implies, mixed cellularity (MC) Hodgkin's lymphoma is characterized by a heterogeneous mixture of cells, including lymphocytes, histiocytes, plasma cells, eosinophils, Reed-Sternberg cells, and Reed-Sternberg variants (Fig. 21–5). Classic Reed-Sternberg cells and mononuclear variants are usually readily apparent. MC Hodgkin's lymphoma represents 15% to 30% of cases of Hodgkin's lymphoma.

In addition to the cellular milieu, there is usually an increase in the background stroma in the form of a disorderly, noncollagenous fibrosis distinct from that seen in NS Hodgkin's lymphoma. Small areas of necrosis are commonly present. In some cases, clusters of epithelioid histiocytes may be numerous, making distinction from Lennert's lymphoma (a T-cell lymphoma with high content of epithelioid histiocytes) difficult. The lymphocytes of Lennert's lymphoma are cytologically atypical as opposed to the small, uniform features of the lymphocytes in all forms of Hodgkin's lymphoma, including MC Hodgkin's lymphoma. There is often only partial involvement of nodes involved by MC Hodgkin's lym-

In some cases of Hodgkin's lymphoma, the characteristic cellular milieu of NS Hodgkin's lymphoma may be seen, including the presence of large numbers of lacunar cells; however, the sclerotic bands are absent. These cases have been assigned by some authorities to a subcategory of NS Hodgkin's lymphoma referred to as the *cellular phase* of NS Hodgkin's lymphoma. Others have assigned cases with this pattern to mixed cellularity Hodgkin's lymphoma.

Sclerosis may be seen in many other lymphoid and nonlymphoid malignancies. For example, agnogenic myeloid metaplasia (see Chap. 18) may produce a histologic pattern of fibrosis and cellular atypia virtually indistinguishable from NS Hodgkin's lymphoma. Sclerosis alone, even when present as orderly bands of collagen, is not sufficient for a diagnosis of NS Hodgkin's lymphoma.

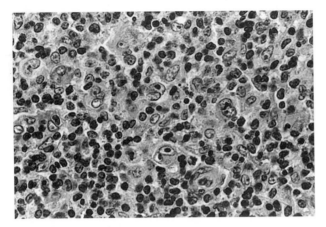

➤ **FIGURE 21–5** Mixed cellularity Hodgkin's lymphoma characterized by a polymorphous cellular milieu including small lymphocytes, eosinophils, plasma cells, and frequent Reed-Sternberg (RS) cells and RS variants characterize this subtype of Hodgkin's lymphoma.

phoma. This is usually an interfollicular pattern, which may be missed on casual examination or confused with a reactive process.

Lymphocyte-Rich Hodgkin's Lymphoma

Approximately 5% of Hodgkin's lymphoma cases may exhibit small numbers of classic Reed-Sternberg cells in a background rich in lymphocytes. The Reed-Sternberg cells exhibit the immunophenotype of classic Reed-Sternberg cells rather than the immunophenotype of L & H cells seen in LP Hodgkin's lymphoma. These cases have recently been assigned to a new category of Hodgkin's lymphoma referred to as lymphocyte-rich (LR) classic Hodgkin's lymphoma. LR Hodgkin's lymphoma shares pathologic and clinical features more akin to MC Hodgkin's lymphoma than to LP Hodgkin's lymphoma.[10]

Lymphocyte Depletion Hodgkin's Lymphoma

Lymphocyte depletion (LD) Hodgkin's lymphoma is the rarest form of Hodgkin's lymphoma, with less than 1% of cases so classified. Lymphocytes are sparse in this disorder whereas Reed-Sternberg cells and Reed-Sternberg variants are numerous. Other types of cells such as plasma cells, histiocytes, and eosinophils are infrequently found. In addition, irregular sclerosis is a major histologic component of LD Hodgkin's lymphoma. Several histologic variants of LD Hodgkin's lymphoma have been described. Their recognition primarily serves to aid the pathologist in differentiating LD Hodgkin's lymphoma from other malignancies with which it is easily confused.

There has been a marked decrease in the diagnosis of LD Hodgkin's lymphoma during the past two decades. This is not due to a decreased incidence of this form of Hodgkin's lymphoma but to the recognition that many cases previously diagnosed as LD Hodgkin's lymphoma are actually misdiagnosed cases of non-Hodgkin's lymphoma, particularly polymorphous T-cell lymphomas.[12] It may, in fact, be impossible in some cases, even after detailed phenotypic and genotypic studies, to resolve the differential diagnosis between a pleomorphic non-Hodgkin's and LD Hodgkin's lymphoma.

Unclassified Hodgkin's Lymphoma

A small percentage of cases exhibit sufficient histologic features for a diagnosis of Hodgkin's lymphoma but insufficient features to be assigned to one of the preceding subcategories. These cases are assigned to the unclassified subcategory.

Histologic Progression

The concurrent evaluation of multiple sites of involvement with Hodgkin's lymphoma usually demonstrates similar histology at each site. On the other hand, with the passage of time, reevaluation often reveals histologic progression in the sequence: LR Hodgkin's lymphoma to MC Hodgkin's lymphoma to LD Hodgkin's lymphoma. Although it is often stated that NS Hodgkin's lymphoma does not undergo such progression but remains NS Hodgkin's lymphoma, there may be progression over time within the histologic spectrum of NS Hodgkin's lymphoma. That is, cases of NS Hodgkin's lymphoma initially rich in lymphocytes may undergo a progressive decrease in the number of lymphocytes, with concomitant increase in the number of Reed-Sternberg cells and Reed-Sternberg variants equivalent to that seen in the non-NS types. This progression, however, maintains the overall nodular sclerosing pattern of NS Hodgkin's lymphoma. Eventually a stage of extreme cellular depletion may be reached, referred to as *obliterative total sclerosis,* in which few cellular elements, including Reed-Sternberg cells, are found.

Clinical Features

In the United States, Hodgkin's lymphoma accounts for approximately one-third of newly diagnosed cases of lymphoma. The incidence of Hodgkin's lymphoma exhibits a bimodal distribution, with peaks between the ages of 15 and 35 and in the over-50 age group.

Most patients with Hodgkin's lymphoma present with a complaint of nonpainful lymph node swelling. Each subtype of Hodgkin's lymphoma is associated with rather characteristic, but not totally specific, clinical features. LP Hodgkin's lymphoma demonstrates a male predominance and is generally a disease of younger patients. The disease is usually localized at presentation to one peripheral node or node group. Patients with LP Hodgkin's lymphoma experience an increased frequency of late relapses compared with classic Hodgkin's lymphoma. NS Hodgkin's lymphoma shows a female predominance and is usually associated with cervical, scalene, or supraclavicular adenopathy. An anterior mediastinal mass is often detected by chest x-ray. Most patients with NS Hodgkin's lymphoma are asymptomatic on presentation. MC and LD Hodgkin's lymphoma are most often seen in symptomatic patients with widely disseminated disease. Extranodal involvement is common in these two subcategories of Hodgkin's lymphoma.

Diagnostic Evaluation and Staging

The diagnosis of Hodgkin's lymphoma requires tissue biopsy and microscopic evaluation. Because of the complexities involved in accurate diagnosis and subclassification, adequate tissue should be obtained at the time of initial biopsy for routine light microscopic studies as well as for ancillary studies such as immunophenotypic and genotypic analysis if these are found to be necessary.

Following a tissue diagnosis of Hodgkin's lymphoma, the patient should be appropriately staged to determine the extent of disease and permit selection of appropriate therapy. The staging evaluation of Hodgkin's lymphoma has become standardized and can be divided into clinical and pathologic staging. Clinical staging should be performed on all newly diagnosed patients with Hodgkin's lymphoma. The elements of clinical staging are listed in Table 21–4. Pathologic staging requires exploratory laparotomy with multiple node samplings and splenectomy. Except at certain institutions, routine pathologic staging is not performed and is reserved for those cases in which the results of pathologic staging would alter the therapy. The results of the staging evaluation are used to assign the patient to staging groups. The most widely utilized staging scheme is the Ann Arbor classification (Table 21–5), which was proposed in 1971.[13] A modification of the Ann Arbor staging classification was proposed in 1984 and is referred to as the Cotswolds scheme.[14] The principal modification was the subdivision of the Ann Arbor stage III category into two substages, III1 and III2. These staging schemes may be used with the data obtained from either clinical or pathologic staging, or both. In addition to the anatomic extent of the disease implicit in the staging categories, the disease is further classified based on the presence or absence of specific symptoms (Table 21–6). The letter "A" (asymptomatic) or "B" (symptomatic) is then appended to the appropriate stage number.

The clinical utility of the Ann Arbor and Cotswolds staging schemes stems from the predictable behavior of Hodgkin's lymphoma. Hodgkin's lymphoma is a lymph node–based disease and rarely, if ever, starts in extranodal sites. It spreads by the lymphatic route in an orderly and predictable pattern to contiguous lymph nodes. Only late in the disease course when hematogenous spread may occur is a more disorderly pattern seen.

Treatment and Prognosis

Current modalities for the therapy of Hodgkin's lymphoma are radiation, chemotherapy, or a combination of the two. The selection of therapy is directed by the results of the staging evaluation rather than the specific histologic subtype. With appropriate therapy, the 10-year survival for stages I and II Hodgkin's lymphoma now exceeds 80%. Ten-year survival for stages III and IV Hodgkin's lymphoma has been improved with aggressive chemotherapy and now approaches 70%.[15]

> **Table 21-4**
> **STAGING WORKUP FOR HODGKIN'S LYMPHOMA**

1. Initial tissue biopsy demonstrating Hodgkin's lymphoma
2. Careful history
3. Detailed physical examination
4. Laboratory studies (CBC, sedimentation rate, chemistry panel to include liver, kidney, and bone profiles)
5. Chest x-ray (anterior and lateral)
6. CT scan of thorax, abdomen, and pelvis
7. Bipedal lymphangiography (unless chemotherapy intended)
8. Bone marrow biopsy if "B" symptoms* or cytopenias are present

*See Table 21–6.
Abbreviations: CBC = complete blood count; CT = computed tomography

> **Table 21-5**
> **ANN ARBOR STAGING**

Stage I	Involvement of single lymph node region or localized involvement of a single extralymphatic organ or site (I$_E$)
Stage II	Involvement of 2 or more lymph node regions on the same side of the diaphragm or localized involvement of a single associated extralymphatic organ or site and its regional lymph node(s) with or without involvement of other lymph node regions on the same side of the diaphragm (II$_E$)
Stage III	Involvement of lymph node regions on both sides of the diaphragm, which may also be accompanied by localized involvement of an associated extralymphatic organ site (III$_E$)
Stage IV	Disseminated (multifocal) involvement of 1 or more extralymphatic organs, with or without associated lymph node involvement, or isolated extralymphatic organ involvement with distant (nonregional) nodal involvement

Source: From Carbone, PP, et al: Report of the Committee on Hodgkin's Staging Classification. Cancer Res 31:1860, 1971, with permission.

▶ NON-HODGKIN'S LYMPHOMA

Virchow (1858)[16] and Billroth (1871)[17] were the first to employ the terms *lymphoma* and *malignant lymphoma*. The distinction between the two major categories of malignant lymphoma (i.e., the lymphocytic lymphomas and Hodgkin's lymphoma) was suggested in 1893 by Dreschfield[18] and Kundrat.[19]

Etiology and Pathogenesis

It seems certain that a prerequisite for the development of lymphoma is damage to the regions of the genetic code that regulate the growth and reproduction of cells of the immune system. The inciting agents for this damage remain unknown; however, it is felt that mutagenic factors such as chemicals, ionizing radiation, and certain viruses may play a role in initiating and promoting the damage. Although viruses such as EBV do not appear to be directly mutagenic, they may function via persistent antigenic stimulation as polyclonal mitogens that somehow favor the eventual selection of a single clone of non–growth-regulated (malignant) cells. Support for this hypothesis comes from the increased incidence of lymphomas in individuals with conditions associated with primary or acquired immunodeficiency (Table 21–7).

The genetic damage associated with the development of a lymphoma is often associated with numerical or structural

> **Table 21-6**
> **"B" SYMPTOMS OF HODGKIN'S LYMPHOMA**

1. Unexplained loss of more than 10% of body weight in the 6 months before admission
2. Unexplained fever with temperature above 38°C
3. Drenching night sweats

> **Table 21-7**
CONDITIONS ASSOCIATED WITH INCREASED RISK OF DEVELOPING NON-HODGKIN'S LYMPHOMA (NHL)

Sjögren's syndrome

Sarcoidosis

Systemic lupus erythematosus

Rheumatoid arthritis

Celiac disease

Dermatitis herpetiformis

Acquired immunodeficiency syndrome (AIDS)

Organ transplant recipients

Congenital immunodeficiency disorders

alterations of chromosomes, or both.[20] With high-resolution karyotyping techniques, nonrandom chromosomal abnormalities can be demonstrated in approximately 60% of cases of lymphoma. Certain types of lymphoma are highly correlated with specific chromosomal abnormalities, particularly translocations involving chromosomes 2, 8, 14, and 22 (Table 21–8).

The pathogenic significance of these chromosomal translocations relates to the function of the genetic material located at or near the site of these translocations. One of the breakpoints commonly involved in B-cell lymphomas is at the site of the transcriptionally active immunoglobulin heavy- or light-chain (kappa [κ] and lambda [λ]) genes located on chromosomes 14, 2, and 22, respectively. For many T-cell lymphomas, a common breakpoint is in the region of one of the T-cell receptor genes. The other breakpoint is in the vicinity of a gene important in the regulation of cell growth and division. This growth-regulating gene, referred to as a proto-oncogene when it is normally located in the genome, is translocated to the region of one of the immunoglobulin genes (B-cell lymphomas) or T-cell receptor genes (T-cell lymphomas). In this new location, the growth-regulating gene functions abnormally and is now referred to as an oncogene.

One of the best-studied examples of this process occurs in Burkitt's lymphoma, a B-cell lymphoma, in which the c-myc proto-oncogene located at region q24 on chromosome 8 is translocated to the immunoglobulin heavy-chain locus at 14q32 (Fig. 21–6). This occurs in about 90% of Burkitt's lymphoma cases. It also is found in about 40% of high-grade large-cell lymphomas and, therefore, is not specific for Burkitt's lymphoma. The c-myc proto-oncogene normally functions in the nuclear signaling that switches cell proliferation on and off. The translocation of c-myc to the heavy-chain locus deregulates the function of the c-myc gene, resulting in uncontrolled cell proliferation.

Chromosomal translocations are only one mechanism for oncogene activation. Other mechanisms include deletions, base pair mutations, and gene amplification. Oncogene activation-deregulation is believed to play a role in the development of most, if not all, lymphomas.

Pathology

Since the original suggestion by Dreschfield[18] that the lymphocytic lymphomas represent distinct histologic entities, a number of lymphoma classification schemes have been proposed. At least nine major classification schemes have been extensively utilized since the mid-1960s. Most of these schemes are based on the growth pattern, for example, nodular or diffuse (Fig. 21–7A and B), and the cytologic features of the malignant cells. At present, the most widely utilized scheme in use by pathologists and clinicians in the United States is the Working Formulation for Clinical Usage (Table 21–9). The Working Formulation was developed by a multi-institutional study group in response to a need for a clinically useful standardized grouping of the lymphomas based on prognosis.[21] Despite the success of

> **Table 21-8**
COMMON CHROMOSOMAL ABNORMALITIES ASSOCIATED WITH MALIGNANT LYMPHOMAS

Abnormality	Genetic Loci Involved	Associated Lymphoma
Trisomy 12	?	B-CLL/SLL
t(9;14)	PAX5/IgH	Lymphoplasmacytoid cell lymphoma
t(11;14)	bcl-1/IgH (Prad 1)	Mantle cell lymphoma
t(14;18)	IgH/bcl-2	Follicle center lymphoma
t(11;18)	?	Marginal zone lymphoma (extranodal)
Trisomy 3	?	Marginal zone lymphoma (extranodal)
t(8;14)	c-myc/IgH	Burkitt's lymphoma
t(2;8)	kappa/c-myc	Burkitt's lymphoma
t(8;22)	c-myc/lambda	Burkitt's lymphoma
t(3;14)	bcl-6/IgH	Diffuse large B-cell lymphoma
inv 14 (q11;q32)	?	T-CLL/PLL
t(2;5)	ALK-NPM	Systemic anaplastic large cell

Abbreviations: B-CLL = B-cell chronic lymphocytic leukemia; SLL = small cell lymphocytic lymphoma; *ALK* = kinase gene; NPM = nucleolar protein gene; T-CLL = T-cell lymphocytic leukemia; PLL = prolymphocytic leukemia

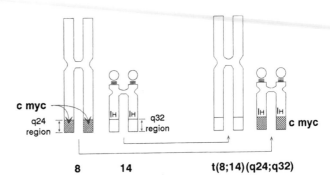

> ► FIGURE 21–6 Reciprocal translocation t(8;14) (q24;q32) is seen in majority of cases of Burkitt's lymphoma as well as some non–Burkitt's high-grade lymphomas. A reciprocal translocation of genetic material occurs between chromosomes 8 and 14. A distal portion of the long arm of chromosome 8, containing the c-myc oncogene, is translocated to a site adjacent to the immunoglobulin heavy-chain locus on chromosome 14.

the Working Formulation, it fails to recognize several clinically distinct types of lymphomas that have been described since publication of the Working Formulation. It is now generally accepted that accurate lymphoma classification cannot be based strictly on morphological features but requires immunophenotypic and genotypic information.

In 1994 the International Lymphoma Study Group published the Revised European-American Classification of Lymphoid Neoplasms (REAL) (Table 21–10), which utilized clinical, morphological, immunophenotypic, and genotypic features to subclassify the lymphomas.[22] The utility of this more "biologically correct" classification scheme has been subsequently verified.[23]

A conceptual understanding of the common classification schemes requires knowledge of the morphological ontogeny

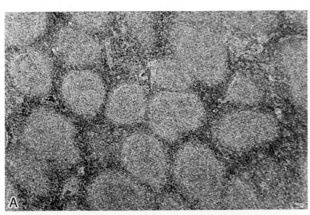

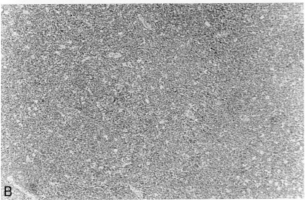

> ► FIGURE 21–7 Growth patterns of the non-Hodgkin's lymphomas. A. Nodular (follicular) pattern resulting from closely packed neoplastic follicles without mantle zones. B. Diffuse pattern in which neoplastic cells are distributed as sheets of cells without follicular organization.

of normal lymphocytes. Although it is customary to discuss the lymphomas with reference to one of the classification schemes, taking a more conceptual approach will facilitate understanding the relationship between the various lymphomas as well as the various classification schemes. The lymphocytic lymphomas may be conceptualized as a malignant population of lymphocytes arrested at a particular stage (morphological, genotypic, phenotypic, or functional) of lymphocyte maturation (see Chap. 18). Thus, we would expect to see lymphomas that express the attributes of normal lymphoid cells found in each of the various normal lymphoid compartments; that is, the precursor (bone marrow), intrafollicular, mantle zone, marginal zone, and interfollicular compartments. As illustrated in Figures 21–8 and 21–9A and B, each of the lymph node compartments is occupied by morphologically characteristic cells. These cells are also immunophenotypically and genotypically distinct.

Lymphomas Related to Intrafollicular (Follicular Center) Lymphocytes

Two principal morphologically distinct lymphocyte cell types are found in the normal follicle (see Fig. 21–9); namely, the small cleaved (centrocyte) and large noncleaved (centroblast) lymphocytes. The follicular center lymphomas are composed of various mixtures of these two cell types.

Follicular center lymphomas composed predominantly of small cleaved lymphocytes (centrocytes) are referred to as poorly differentiated lymphocytic (Rappaport); centroblastic-centrocytic, small-cell type (Kiel); follicular, predominantly small cleaved-cell (Working Formulation); and follicular, grade I (REAL) lymphomas. The predominant malignant cell in this lymphoma is the counterpart of the small cleaved follicular center cell (centrocyte), although a few large lymphocytes (centroblasts) are always present.

The small cleaved cell is relatively small (6 to 12 μm in diameter) with scant cytoplasm, slightly to distinctly irregular nucleus (angulated, clefted), and indistinct nucleoli (Fig. 21–10). A predominantly follicular or mixed follicular and diffuse growth pattern is most commonly found. Pure diffuse lymphomas of this type are rare and most cases classified as such are usually some other type of lymphoma, most commonly mantle cell lymphoma.

Follicular center lymphomas composed predominantly of large lymphocytes are referred to as histiocytic (Rappaport); centroblastic-centrocytic, large-cell (Kiel); follicular large-cell (Working Formulation); and follicular grade III (REAL) lymphomas. These lymphomas are composed predominantly (more than 50%) of large cleaved (large centrocytes) and large noncleaved (centroblasts) cells.

➤ Table 21–9
WORKING FORMULATION FOR CLINICAL USAGE

Low Grade

Malignant lymphoma, small lymphocytic

    Consistent with CLL

    Plasmacytoid

Malignant lymphoma, follicular, predominantly small cleaved cell

    Diffuse areas

    Sclerosis

Malignant lymphoma, follicular, mixed small cleaved and large cell

    Diffuse areas

    Sclerosis

Intermediate Grade

Malignant lymphoma, follicular, predominantly large cell

    Diffuse areas

    Sclerosis

Malignant lymphoma, diffuse, small cleaved cell

    Sclerosis

Malignant lymphoma, diffuse, mixed, small and large cell

    Sclerosis

    Epithelioid cell component

Malignant lymphoma, diffuse, large cell

    Cleaved cell

    Noncleaved cell

    Sclerosis

High Grade

Malignant lymphoma, large cell, immunoblastic

    Plasmacytoid

    Clear cell

    Polymorphous

    Epithelioid cell component

Malignant lymphoma, lymphoblastic

    Convoluted cell

    Nonconvoluted cell

Malignant lymphoma, small noncleaved cell

    Burkitt's

    Follicular areas

Source: Heim S, and Mitelman, F: Cancer Cytogenetics. Alan R. Liss, NY, 1995.

➤ Table 21–10
REVISED EUROPEAN-AMERICAN LYMPHOMA CLASSIFICATION

B-Cell Neoplasms

I. Precursor B-cell neoplasm

  1. Precursor B-lymphoblastic leukemia/lymphoma

II. Peripheral B-cell neoplasms

  1. B-cell chronic lymphocytic leukemia/ prolymphocytic leukemia/small lymphocytic lymphoma

  2. Lymphoplasmacytoid lymphoma (immunocytoma)

  3. Mantle cell lymphoma

  4. Follicle center lymphoma, follicular (Provisional cytologic grades I, II, III) (Provisional subtype: follicle center lymphoma, diffuse, predominantly small cell)

  5. Marginal zone B-cell lymphoma

    a. Extranodal (low grade B-cell lymphoma of mucosa-associated lymphoid tissue type)

    b. Nodal (± monocytoid B-cells) (Provisional entity)

  6. Splenic marginal zone B-cell lymphoma (± circulating villous lymphocytes) (Provisional entity)

  7. Hairy-cell leukemia

  8. Plasmacytoma/myeloma

  9. Diffuse large B-cell lymphoma (Subtype: Primary mediastinal large B-cell lymphoma)

  10. Burkitt's lymphoma

  11. High-grade B-cell lymphoma, Burkitt-like (Provisional entity)

T-Cell and Postulated Natural Killer (NK) Cell Neoplasms

I. Precursor T-cell neoplasm

  1. Precursor T-lymphoblastic lymphoma/leukemia

II. Peripheral T-cell and postulated NK cell neoplasms

  1. T-cell chronic lymphocytic leukemia/prolymphocytic leukemia

  2. Large granular lymphocyte leukemia

    a. T-cell type

    b. Natural killer cell type

  3. Mycosis fungoides/Sézary syndrome

  4. Peripheral T-cell lymphomas; unspecified (Provisional cytologic categories: medium-sized cell; mixed medium and large cell; large cell) (Subtypes: subcutaneous panniculitic T-cell lymphoma; hepatosplenic gamma/delta T-cell lymphoma)

  5. Angioimmunoblastic T-cell lymphoma

  6. Angiocentric lymphoma

  7. Intestinal T-cell lymphoma (± enteropathy)

  8. Adult T-cell lymphoma/leukemia, HTLV1+

  9. Anaplastic large cell lymphoma (T- and null-cell types)

  10. Anaplastic large cell lymphoma, Hodgkin's-like (Provisional entity)

Source: Harris, NL, et al: A revised European-American classification of lymphoid neoplasms: A proposal from the International Lymphoma Study Group. Blood 84:1361, 1994, with permission.

    Large cleaved (Fig. 21–11) cells are from 15 to 20 μm in diameter and have modest amounts of cytoplasm, irregular vesicular nuclei, and indistinct nucleoli. Large noncleaved cells (centroblasts) (see Fig. 21–11) are 20 to 40 μm in diameter, have a modest amount of pyranophilic (RNA-rich)

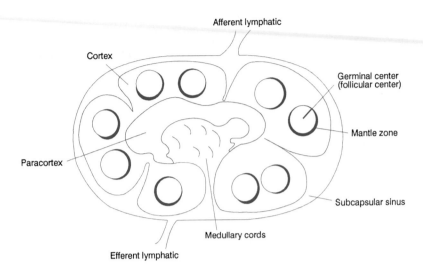

➤ FIGURE 21–8   Anatomic compartments of the lymph nodes.

cytoplasm, round to oval vesicular nuclei, and small but distinct nucleoli. All three growth patterns (follicular, diffuse, or mixed follicular and diffuse) may be observed.

All follicular center lymphomas are a mixture of small cleaved and large cells (Table 21–11). When neither cell type dominates, a mixed pattern is recognized by some classification schemes. However the significance of subcategorizing follicular lymphomas based on the frequency of small cleaved and large cells has been called into question.[24]

Lymphomas derived from follicular center cells are, by definition, B-cell lymphomas. The expected immunophenotype of a follicular center lymphoma is as follows: surface immunoglobulin–positive (sIg+), B cell–associated antigen–positive (e.g., CD19+, CD20+), CD10 usually positive (more than 50%), CD5-negative, CD23 usually negative, CD43-negative, and CD11c-negative (Table 21–12). Follicular lymphomas are distinguished at the genetic level by a unique chromosomal translocation, t(14;18), involving the *bcl-2* proto-oncogene on chromosome 18 and the

immunoglobulin heavy-chain gene on chromosome 14 (see Table 21–8). This translocation is detectable in 70% to 95% of cases of follicular lymphoma.

Follicular center lymphomas accounts for approximately 40% of adult non-Hodgkin's lymphomas in the United States. The disease most commonly affects adults and is usually widespread at diagnosis (Table 21–13). Although the disease course is usually indolent, it is not often curable with current therapy (median survival is 6 to 8 years). Progression with time from a follicular pattern to a more aggressive, diffuse large-cell pattern occurs in approximately 40% of cases (Table 21–14); however, spontaneous remissions have also been described.

Lymphomas Related to Mantle Zone Lymphocytes (Mantle Cell Lymphoma)

Lymphomas composed of lymphocytes with the morphological and immunophenotypic features of mantle cells have only recently been accepted as a distinctive subcategory of

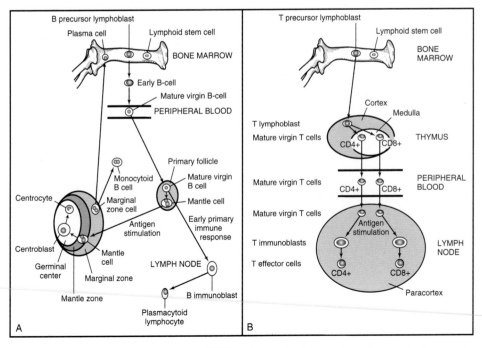

➤ FIGURE 21–9   Maturation (ontogeny) of *A.* B lymphocytes and *B.* T lymphocytes in relation to the pertinent anatomic compartments.

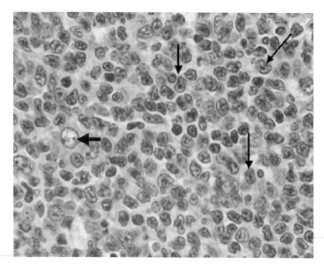

➤ **FIGURE 21-10**   Follicular small cleaved-cell lymphoma. Center of malignant follicle is composed predominantly (more than 75%) of small cleaved cells (centrocytes) (*small arrows*). Large transformed lymphocytes (centroblasts) (*large arrow*) are always present but do not exceed 25% of the cells within the follicle.

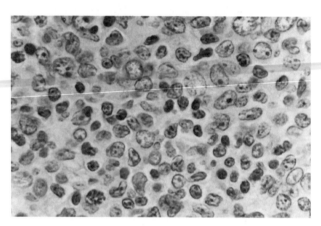

➤ **FIGURE 21-11**   Malignant lymphoma, follicular large cell. Center of malignant nodule is composed predominantly (more than 50%) of a mixture of large cleaved and large noncleaved cells (centroblasts).

non-Hodgkin's lymphoma.[25] The cytologic features of mantle cell lymphoma are somewhat variable, creating difficulty in differentiating on histologic grounds mantle cell lymphoma from other low-grade non-Hodgkin's lymphomas. The cells of mantle cell lymphoma are most commonly small- to medium-sized lymphocytes with scant pale cytoplasm, irregular nuclei, and inconspicuous nucleoli (Fig.

21–12). Most often, mantle cell lymphoma has a diffuse or vaguely nodular pattern; however, occasionally a distinct mantle zone pattern is observed. In this form the malignant cells are distributed as an expanded mantle zone surrounding benign (polyclonal) germinal centers. This pattern of mantle cell lymphoma must be distinguished from mantle zone hyperplasia.

The immunophenotype of mantle cell lymphomas aids in differentiating this subcategory of lymphoma from other morphologically similar lymphomas. Characteristically, the malignant cells express monoclonal sIg, B cell–associated antigens, CD5, and CD43, but are negative for CD23, CD11c, and usually CD10 (see Table 21–12). This immunophenotype corresponds to the normal CD5-positivie, CD23-negative B cell of the inner follicle mantle.[26] Most cases of mantle cell lymphoma demonstrate a unique chromosomal translocation, t(11;14), involving the *bcl-1* proto-oncogene on chromosome 11 and the immunoglobulin heavy-chain gene on chromosome 14 (see Table 21–8). This translocation results in the overexpression of the cell cycle protein cyclin D1, which may be detected in the nuclei of mantle cell lymphoma by immunocytochemical techniques.

Mantle cell lymphoma is a disease of older adults with high male-to-female ratio (see Table 21–13). The disease is usually widespread at diagnosis and, despite its moderately aggressive course (3- to 5-year median survival), behaves similarly to other low-grade lymphomas in that it is generally not curable with current therapies.[27] A peculiar extranodal presentation of the disease in the intestine is referred to as lymphomatous polyposis (Fig. 21–13). Several histologic variants of mantle cell lymphoma (pleomorphic, large cell, and blastoid) have been described and are associated with a more aggressive clinical course.[28]

Lymphomas Related to Marginal Zone Lymphocytes

The marginal zone of lymph nodes is a poorly defined anatomic compartment.[29] However, in other lymphoid tissues (i.e., spleen and Peyer's patches), the marginal zone is better defined.[30] The typical marginal zone cell is a centrocyte-like cell (small cleaved cell) with more abundant pale-staining cytoplasm than a true centrocyte. Under antigenic stimulation, these marginal zone B cells are believed, by some investigators, capable of differentiation into monocytoid (parafollicular) B cells and plasma cells (see Fig. 21–9A and B). Monocytoid B cells are medium-sized lymphocytes morphologically resembling monocytes that are found predominantly in the lymphoid sinuses and paracortex of some reactive lymph nodes but not in normal lymph nodes. They are par-

➤ **Table 21-11**
INDOLENT B-CELL LYMPHOMAS: MORPHOLOGICAL FEATURES

Lymphoma Subtype	Small Cells	Large Cells
B-cell CLL/SLL	Round (rarely cleaved)	Paraimmunoblasts/prolymphocytes
Mantle cell	Cleaved (rarely round)	Usually absent
Follicular center cell (CB/CC)	Cleaved (centrocytes)	Centroblasts
Immunocytoma	Round	Immunoblasts
Marginal cell	Round, cleaved, and/or monocytoid	Centroblasts/Immunoblasts

Abbreviations: CLL = chronic lymphocytic leukemia; SLL = small cell lymphocytic lymphoma; CB/CC = centroblastic/centrocytic

> **Table 21-12**
LOW-GRADE B-CELL LYMPHOMAS: IMMUNOPHENOTYPIC PROFILE

Lymphoma Subtype	CD5	CD10	CD23	CD43	Cyclin D1
B-cell CLL/SLL	+	−	+	+	−
Mantle cell	+	−/+	−	+	+
Follicular center cell (CB/CC)	−	+/−	−	−	−
Immunocytoma	−/+	−	−	−/+	
Marginal cell					
Extranodal	−	−	−	−/+	−
Nodal	−	−	−	+/−	−

Abbreviations: −/+ = less than 50% of cases positive; +/− = more than 50% of cases positive; CLL = chronic lymphocytic leukemia; SLL = small lymphocytic lymphoma; CB/CC = centroblastic/centrocytic

ticularly common in the reactive lymphadenopathies associated with human immunodeficiency virus (HIV) infection and toxoplasmosis.

Lymphomas related to marginal zone cells are a group of recently described and controversially related entities.[31] A common form of presentation of marginal zone lymphoma is at extranodal sites, particularly stomach, salivary gland, lung, thyroid, and orbit, where they have been referred to as lymphomas of mucosal-associated lymphoid tissue (MALT lymphomas).[32] Collections of lymphoid tissue normally occur in extranodal mucosal sites such as the small bowel (Peyer's patches). Mucosal-associated lymphoid tissue, however, does not normally occur in the most common sites for MALT lymphomas. Under conditions of chronic antigenic stimulation (e.g., infection or autoimmune disease), such lymphoid tissue may develop in these sites. Examples of such conditions are *Helicobacter pylori* gastritis, Sjögren's syndrome, and Hashimoto's thyroiditis. Lymphomas that develop in the setting of chronic antigenic stimulation may remain dependent on the presence of benign antigen-driven T cells, a fact that has important therapeutic and prognostic implications. For example, in the case of the MALT-type marginal cell lymphoma of the stomach, eradication of the offending antigen (*H. pylori*) with antimicrobial therapy has been demonstrated to be effective in treating this specific lymphoma.[33]

The histologic features of extranodal marginal zone lymphoma (MALT) are highly characteristic. Reactive follicles or their remnants are uniformly present (Fig. 21–14). Subjacent to the mucosal lining or glandular epithelium of involved organs and surrounding the reactive follicles are collections of small- to medium-sized lymphocytes with a moderate amount of pale-staining cytoplasm and irregular nuclei (centrocyte-like cells) (Figs. 21–15 and 21–16). In addition to centrocyte-like cells, neoplastic cells with features similar to small lymphocytes or monocytoid B cells, or both, are present. Plasma cell differentiation in a portion of the cells is also a common finding. A constant feature of these lymphomas is infiltration of the associated epithelium by neoplastic lymphocytes, resulting in the formation of lymphoepithelial lesions (Fig. 21–17). The neoplastic cells may also infiltrate the reactive follicles, giving the impression of a follicular center cell lymphoma, a process referred to as *follicular colonization.*

A second pattern of marginal zone lymphoma is lymph node–based and is often referred to as monocytoid B cell lymphoma by hematopathologists in the United States.[34] Node-based marginal zone lymphoma is frequently observed in patients with autoimmune disorders such as Sjögren's syndrome or coexistent extranodal (MALT) type of marginal zone lymphoma, suggesting a close relationship between extranodal (MALT) and node-based (monocytoid B cell) lymphomas.

> **Table 21-13**
LOW-GRADE B-CELL LYMPHOMAS: CLINICAL FEATURES

Lymphoma Subtype	Male: Female	Stage 1 (%)	Extranodal (%)	BM (%)	PB (%)	NED at 5 years (%)	Survival Rate at 5 years (%)
B-cell CLL/SLL	2:1	0	Rare	100	> 90	< 10	90
Mantle cell	3:1	< 10	> 50	> 50	25	0	< 40
Follicular center cell (CB/CC)	1:1	< 10	< 50	> 50	< 15	< 25	> 60
Immunocytoma	1.3:1	Rare	Rare	100	< 30	0	> 70
Marginal cell							
Extranodal	1:2	> 80	100	< 15	Rare	> 80	100
Nodal	1.2	50?	?*	50?	Rare	50?	50

*Pure nodal marginal cell lymphomas are uncommon.
Abbreviations: BM = bone marrow involvement; PB = peripheral blood involvement; NED = no evidence of disease

Histologically, node-based marginal zone lymphoma is characterized by infiltration of the paracortex and sinuses with a monoclonal population of monocytoid B cells. These cells have oval, reniform, or sometimes quite irregular nuclei; bland chromatin pattern; and relatively abundant pale-staining cytoplasms with distinct cytoplasmic borders. Benign secondary follicles with hyperplastic germinal centers are present, which serve to accent the pale-staining infiltrate of monocytoid B cells.

The characteristic immunophenotype of the marginal zone

> ## Table 21-14
> ## LOW-GRADE B-CELL LYMPHOMAS: LARGE-CELL TRANSFORMATION

Lymphoma	Secondary Large-Cell Type	Incidence of Transformation
Chronic lymphocytic leukemia/ small lymphocytic lymphoma	Richter's transformation (diffuse large cell)	5%
	Paraimmunoblastic/prolymphocytoid transformation	15%
Mantle cell lymphoma	Blastic variant (lymphoblastoid)	?%
	Centrocytoid/centroblastic (centroblastoid variant)	?%
Follicular center cell lymphoma	Secondary centroblastic (diffuse large cell)	40%
Immunocytoma	Secondary immunoblastic	5%
Marginal zone cell lymphoma	Secondary high-grade lymphoma	?%

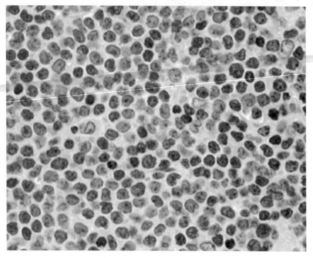

> FIGURE 21-12   Mantle cell lymphoma. The cytologic features are "intermediate" between those of small lymphocytic lymphoma and small cleaved-cell lymphoma.

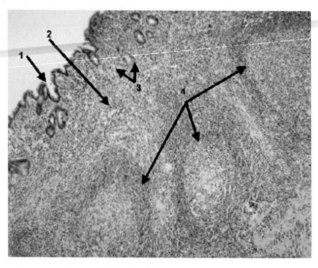

> FIGURE 21-14   Mucosal-associated lymphoid tissue (MALT) lymphoma of the stomach: (1) gastric epithelium; (2) malignant lymphoid infiltrate; (3) lymphoepithelial lesions; (4) reactive follicles.

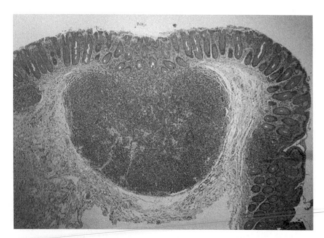

> FIGURE 21-13   Lymphomatous polyposis, a form of mantle cell lymphoma, is characterized by the presence of multiple malignant lymphoid polyps of the gastrointestinal tract. The malignant cells have the cytologic and phenotypic features of mantle cells.

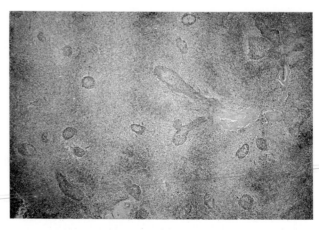

> FIGURE 21-15   MALT lymphoma of the parotid gland. Pale zones of malignant cells surround and infiltrate remnants of parotid gland epithelium. Collections of dark-staining cells are benign (reactive) lymphocytes.

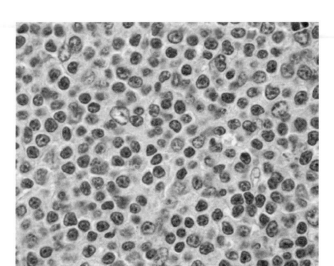

➤ **FIGURE 21-16** MALT lymphoma of the parotid gland, a type of lymphoma thought to be related to marginal zone lymphocytes, is composed of a mixture of cells with features of lymphoplasmacytoid cells, centrocyte-like cells, and monocytoid B cells. One of the morphological types often predominates.

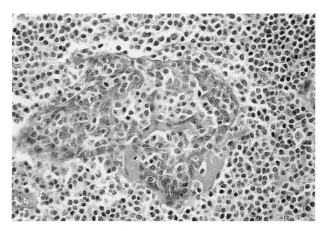

➤ **FIGURE 21-17** Lymphoepithelial lesion. Detailed view of a lymphoepithelial lesion (MALT lymphoma of parotid gland) composed of metaplastic parotid gland epithelium infiltrated by the atypical lymphoid cells of MALT lymphoma.

lymphomas is as follows: sIg+, cytoplasmic Ig+ (40%), B-cell antigen+, CD5−, CD10−, CD23−, CD43−/+, and CD11c+/− (see Table 21–12). The extranodal form (MALT lymphoma) is associated with the chromosomal abnormalities trisomy 3 and t(11;18) (see Table 21–8).

The clinical features of marginal zone lymphoma correspond to the two modes of presentation discussed earlier (see Table 21–13). The extranodal (MALT) form is a disease of adults with a slight female predominance and is highly associated with autoimmune disease or infection (*Helicobacter* gastritis). The disease is usually localized (stage I or II) at presentation and the prognosis is excellent following therapy for localized disease. Dissemination occurs, however, in approximately 30% of cases. Although the disease course is usually indolent following dissemination, disseminated disease appears to be incurable with current therapy. Transformation to a large-cell lymphoma occasionally occurs (see Table 21–14).

Node-based marginal zone lymphoma (monocytoid B-

cell lymphoma) in most cases probably represents dissemination of extranodal (MALT) lymphoma. However, pure nodal presentations, usually in the cervical region, have been observed. The majority of patients present with advanced disease (stage III or IV).

Adding to the complexity and controversy of the category of marginal zone lymphomas is the entity splenic marginal zone lymphoma with or without villous lymphocytes.[35] Its relationship to nodal and extranodal marginal zone lymphoma is not well understood; however, most investigators consider it a distinct entity separate from marginal zone lymphoma of the nodal and MALT types.[36] Patients characteristically have massive splenomegaly with minimal adenopathy. Bone marrow and peripheral blood involvement are common. The spleen exhibits nodular expansion of the white pulp by intermediate-sized lymphocytes resembling splenic marginal zone cells surrounding a central core of small lymphocytes. The phenotype of the cells of splenic marginal zone lymphoma is similar to those of marginal zone lymphomas. The clinical course is indolent and incurable; however, splenectomy may result in long remissions.

Lymphomas Related to Interfollicular Lymphocytes

The normal interfollicular zone of lymphoid tissue is a complex mixture of cell types. Although it is often referred to as the *T-cell zone,* because of the predominance of T cells, several other cell types are found in this region, notably recirculating B cells, histiocytes, and reticulum cells. Despite the prevalence of T cells in the interfollicular zone, the majority of lymphomas whose normal counterpart is an interfollicular cell are B-cell lymphomas.

Small Lymphocytic Lymphoma

This low-grade lymphoma is also commonly referred to as *well-differentiated lymphocytic lymphoma* (Rappaport classification). The growth pattern is diffuse, although a pseudofollicular pattern may be observed (Fig. 21–18A). These pseudofollicles, also called *growth centers,* do not have the cytologic or histologic features of true neoplastic follicles.[37] In the early phase of nodal involvement, the neoplastic cells may be confined to the interfollicular areas with sparing of the normal follicles. Later, there is total effacement of lymph node architecture. The majority of the neoplastic cells are small, uniform lymphocytes with scant cytoplasm, round nucleus, clumped chromatin, and absent to small nucleoli; that is, they appear cytologically similar to normal small lymphocytes (Fig. 21–18B). Admixed with these small lymphocytes are variable numbers of intermediate to large lymphocytes referred to as *prolymphocytes* and *paraimmunoblasts.* These cells are most commonly found in increased numbers within the pseudofollicles (growth centers). In approximately 40% of the cases of small lymphocytic lymphoma, a leukemic phase identical to chronic lymphocytic leukemia develops. Small lymphocytic lymphoma and chronic lymphocytic leukemia are now considered to represent different clinical expression of the same basic disease process.

Small lymphocytic lymphomas may show evidence of plasmacytoid differentiation, including the presence of cytoplasmic immunoglobulin and a small amount of circulating monoclonal immunoglobulin in the peripheral blood. These cases are phenotypically and clinically similar to

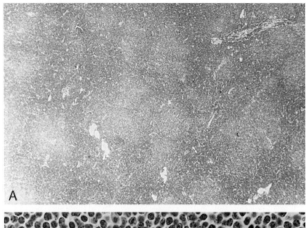

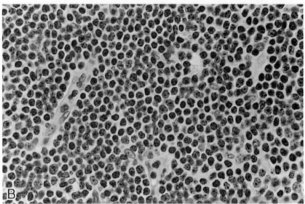

➤ FIGURE 21-18 Malignant lymphoma, small lymphocytic. *A.*
Pseudofollicular pattern is evident because of presence of numerous
growth centers. *B.* Outside the growth centers, this subtype of lymphoma
is composed predominantly of sheets of small, uniform lymphocytes.

small lymphocytic lymphoma and as such should be distinguished from true immunocytoma (see later discussion). Diagnostic difficulty may also occur when there is overgrowth
of the lymphoma by the larger cells of the growth centers
(paraimmunoblastic and prolymphocytoid transformation).
Transformation to a large-cell lymphoma (Richter's transformation) can occur and portends a more aggressive clinical course (see Table 21–14).

The normal counterpart cell to the malignant cell of small
lymphocytic lymphoma is believed to be a recirculating B or
T lymphocyte. The vast majority of small lymphocytic lymphomas express a B-cell phenotype (98% in western countries). In addition to the expression of B cell–associated antigens (CD19, CD20, and CD22), with sensitive techniques,
low-density monoclonal sIg is detectable. The B-cell small
lymphocytic lymphomas are also positive for CD5, CD23,
and CD43 but lack CD10 (see Table 21–12). A small number
of cases are weakly positive for CD11c. Two percent of small
lymphocytic lymphomas express a mature T-cell phenotype,
usually of the "helper" type (CD2+/CD3+/CD4+/CD5+/
CD7+/CD8−). Approximately 20% of T-cell cases coex-
press CD4 and CD8, and only very rare cases are CD8-
positive, CD4-negative.

Trisomy 12 has been reported in one-third of cases of
B-cell small lymphocytic lymphoma, whereas T-cell small
lymphocytic lymphoma is characterized cytogenetically in
75% of the cases by inv 14 (q11;q32) (see Table 21–8).

Small lymphocytic lymphoma/chronic lymphocytic leukemia is a disease of older adults and is usually widespread

at diagnosis. The disease, although indolent in behavior, is
considered incurable with standard therapy. Aggressive
treatment, including bone marrow transplantation, in the
hope of achieving durable remissions or even cure is under
investigation.

Lymphoplasmacytoid Cell Lymphoma/ Immunocytoma

A phenotypically and clinically distinct form of lymphoma
of small lymphoid cells exists in which the cells exhibit maturation to plasma cells and a phenotype distinct from typical small lymphocytic lymphoma.[38] Specifically, they express surface and cytoplasmic immunoglobulin, usually of
the IgM class; are positive for B–cell associated antigens
(CD19, CD20, CD22, and CD79a); but lack CD5 and CD10
(see Table 21–12). Less than 50% of cases are positive for
CD43. The normal counterpart of this lymphoma is believed
to be a recirculating CD5-negative cell, which has been
stimulated to differentiate to plasma cells. Approximately
50% of uses of lymphoplasmacytoid cell lymphoma will
demonstrate t(9;14), involving the IgH and *PAX5* genes (see
Table 21–8). Clinically, these lymphomas usually correspond to the syndrome of Waldenström's macroglobulinemia. A monoclonal gammopathy of the IgM type is often
present and is associated with hyperviscosity symptoms.
Similar to other low-grade lymphomas, this disease is indolent but incurable, and large-cell lymphoma transformation
may occur (see Table 21–14).

Diffuse Large-Cell Lymphoma

During the initial phase of the normal primary immune
process, antigenic stimulation effects the transformation of
"virgin" T and B cells to T and B immunoblasts (see Fig.
21–9). B immunoblasts are also produced via the germinal
center pathway during the latter phases of the primary immune process and during the secondary immune response
(see Fig. 21–9). Normal T and B immunoblasts are found
in the interfollicular compartment (paracortex) of reactive
lymph nodes.

Lymphomas corresponding to the immunoblast stage of
differentiation and morphologically resembling immunoblasts are referred to as *immunoblastic lymphomas.* This
category of lymphoma falls within the broad category of
diffuse large-cell lymphoma. Diffuse large-cell lymphomas
are conceptualized in the Working Formulation as composed of two subcategories: diffuse large-cell lymphomas
of follicular origin (centroblastic), and diffuse large-cell
lymphomas of interfollicular origin (immunoblastic). Controversy exists as to whether these two subcategories can be
reliably distinguished on morphological grounds alone and
whether there is any clinical justification for separating
these two subcategories of large-cell lymphoma.[39]

Diffuse large-cell lymphomas exhibit a spectrum of morphological features. In general, the nuclei of these neoplastic cells are larger than those of the admixed benign macrophages. The most common histologic picture is a mixture
of large cells resembling centroblasts (large noncleaved
cells) and immunoblasts (Fig. 21–19).

Diffuse large-cell lymphomas most commonly exhibit a
B-cell phenotype; however, T-cell types may also be observed. The histologic features are helpful but not infallible
in predicting the immunophenotype. The B-cell diffuse
large-cell lymphomas are usually CD5- and CD10-negative

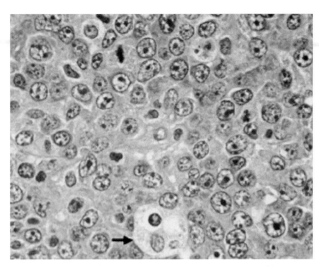

➤ **FIGURE 21–19** Diffuse large-cell lymphoma is characterized by malignant cells whose nuclei are larger than the nucleus of a benign macrophage (*arrow*). Usually a mixture of cell types is present, including large noncleaved cells (centroblasts), large cleaved cells, and immunoblasts.

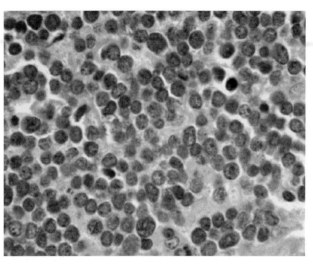

➤ **FIGURE 21–20** Lymphoblastic lymphoma, a form of high-grade lymphoma, is cytologically characterized by cells with scant cytoplasm, finely dispersed chromatin ("blastic"), and brisk mitotic rate.

and, at the molecular level, do not show rearrangement of the *bcl-2* gene or the t(14;18) characteristic of follicular lymphomas. The 20% of B-cell diffuse large-cell lymphomas that are *bcl-2* rearranged may represent transformation of a preexisting follicular lymphoma. The T-cell subtype is further discussed under Peripheral T-cell Lymphoma, Unspecified, later in this chapter.

Diffuse large-cell lymphoma is mainly a disease of adults, with the median age of onset in the sixth decade. At presentation, the disease is often confined to one side of the diaphragm, and bone marrow involvement occurs in only 10% of affected patients. Involvement of extranodal sites, including privileged sites such as the testis or central nervous system, frequently occurs. Diffuse large-cell lymphoma is aggressive but potentially curable with multiagent chemotherapy. Relapse is more common and survival shorter with the T-cell type than with B-cell diffuse large-cell lymphoma.[40]

Lymphomas Related to Precursor Lymphocytes (Lymphoblastic Lymphomas)

The cells of lymphoblastic lymphoma are cytologically identical to the lymphoblasts of acute lymphoblastic leukemia (Fig 21–20). They have scant cytoplasm and nuclei, with finely dispersed chromatin and absent or indistinct nucleoli. The nuclear contour may be either convoluted or nonconvoluted, and mitotic activity is high. The cells are slightly larger than normal lymphocytes, and the cytologic and histologic features of this lymphoma may be confused with those of small, noncleaved cell lymphoma. Attention to nuclear features as well as immunophenotypic and cytogenetic data can resolve the distinction between these two lymphoma types.

Approximately 70% of lymphoblastic lymphomas are of the T-cell type. Their phenotype is complex; however, most are terminal deoxynucleotidyl transferase (TdT)–positive (see Chap. 18), which serves to distinguish them from other categories of lymphoma. In addition to TdT, most T-cell lymphoblastic lymphomas are CD7- and CD3-positive, whereas cases of T-cell acute lymphoblastic leukemia usually express a more immature phenotype (CD7+, CD3−).

The B-cell type of lymphoblastic lymphoma also shows a high frequency of expression of TdT. It is usually CD19+, CD79a+, CD22+, CD20−/+, CD10+/−, HLA-DR+, and CD34+/−. Surface immunoglobulin is rarely present. Both the B- and T-cell types of lymphoblastic lymphomas are believed to be derived from committed precursor B- and T-cells, respectively.

Lymphoblastic lymphoma most commonly affects male adolescents and young adults. The disease is very aggressive, with rapidly enlarging mediastinal mass or peripheral lymph nodes, or both. Central nervous system involvement is frequent, and a leukemic phase is a common terminal event. Despite the aggressive course that is rapidly fatal if untreated, lymphoblastic lymphoma is potentially curable with multiagent chemotherapy.

Common Lymphomas Whose Normal Counterpart Cell Is Poorly Defined

The normal counterpart cell of many of the rare lymphomas has not been defined; however, this is also true for some relatively common lymphomas, for example, Burkitt's lymphoma.

Burkitt's lymphoma, first described in 1958 by Dennis Burkitt,[41] is endemic to Africa but also accounts for approximately one-third of non-African pediatric lymphomas and a high percentage of lymphomas in immunocompromised patients, particularly patients with acquired immunodeficiency syndrome (AIDS).

The monotonously uniform cells of Burkitt's lymphoma are described as small noncleaved cells in the Working Formulation. They are medium-sized cells with uniformly round nuclei, multiple small nucleoli, and a modest amount of intensely basophilic cytoplasm (Fig. 21–21). Lipid vacuoles are readily evident in the cytoplasm on smears or imprints of the tissue. The mitotic rate of Burkitt's lymphoma is very high, and the estimated volume doubling time of this lymphoma is the highest of any tumor (approximately 1 day). Programmed tumor cell death (apoptosis) is also very high, and a starry sky pattern of tingible-body macrophages is usually evident owing to phagocytosis of the apoptotic debris (Fig. 21–22). The normal counterpart to the Burkitt

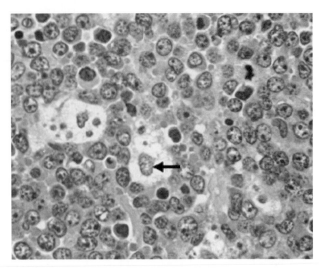

> ➤ **FIGURE 21–21**   Malignant lymphoma, small noncleaved cell (Burkitt's) is characterized by uniform cells (15 μm in diameter) with moderate amounts of pyranophilic cytoplasm. The nuclei are round, with multiple small nucleoli, and are smaller in diameter than the nuclei of the associated macrophages (*arrow*).

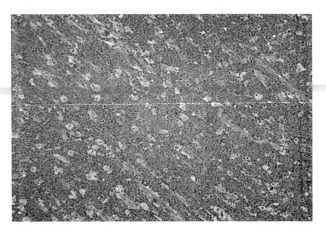

> ➤ **FIGURE 21–22**   Malignant lymphoma, small noncleaved cell type: "Starry sky" pattern is produced by the clear cytoplasm of numerous tingible-body macrophages, which are admixed with the neoplastic small noncleaved cells.

lymphoma cell is believed to be a proliferating B cell of unknown stage.

As previously discussed, Burkitt's lymphoma is cytogenetically characterized by a t(8;14) in the majority of cases or less often by t(2;8) or t(8;22). In the endemic (African) form of this disease, the breakpoint on chromosome 14 involves the heavy-chain joining region, suggesting an early B-cell origin of the Burkitt cell. However, in the nonendemic form, the breakpoint is in the heavy-chain switch region, consistent with origin at a latter stage (possibly follicular center cell) of B-cell development. The endemic and immunodeficiency-related cases are also associated with a high frequency of tumor cell incorporated EBV genomes. The immunophenotype of Burkitt's lymphoma is surface IgM-positive, B-cell antigen–positive, CD10-positive, CD5- negative, CD23-negative, and TdT-negative.

The male-to-female ratio for Burkitt's lymphoma is approximately 2.5 to 1. The facial bones, particularly the jaw, are the most common sites of involvement for the African (endemic) variety (Fig. 21–23). In the nonendemic variety,

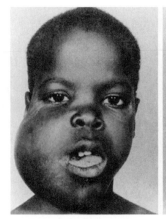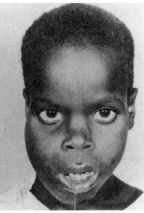

> ➤ **FIGURE 21–23**   Burkitt's lymphoma before (*left*) and after treatment (*right*).

an abdominal mass is the most common presenting pattern. The distal ileum, cecum, and mesentery are the most frequent sites of involvement. Other less common sites of involvement include the kidneys, ovaries, and breasts. Burkitt's lymphoma is a highly aggressive and rapidly fatal disease if untreated; however, this disease is potentially curable and prognosis correlates with tumor bulk (see staging).

Miscellaneous Lymphomas

A plethora of uncommon, unusual, and sometimes difficult to classify lymphomas have been described (Table 21–15). Most of these fall within the general category of peripheral T-cell lymphomas, also referred to as *post-thymic T-cell lymphomas*.[42] Peripheral T-cell lymphomas are defined immunologically as TdT/CD1-negative, CD3-positive T-cell lymphomas; that is, they correspond to normal T cells at the post-thymic stage of T-cell ontogeny. Some peripheral T-cell lymphomas behave as distinct clincopathologic entities and are named accordingly. The remainder are placed in the general category of peripheral T-cell lymphoma, unspecified.

Peripheral T-Cell Lymphoma, Unspecified

The REAL and WHO classifications incorporate a wastebasket category for the large number of peripheral T-cell lymphomas that do not fall into a defined clinicopathologic category. Morphologically, this is a heterogeneous category with individual cases usually composed of a polymorphous mixture of atypical small-, medium-, and large-sized cells. Occasionally, one cell size may predominate, giving a more monomorphic picture. Benign eosinophils, plasma cells, and epithelial histiocytes are often admixed with the neoplastic cells, and high endothelial venules may be prominent. Both nodal and extranodal (skin, subcutaneous tissue, spleen, viscera) sites are often involved. Involved lymph nodes demonstrate either a diffuse effacement of nodal architecture or an interfollicular growth pattern of the neoplastic cells with preservation of benign follicles. Immunophenotypically, this group of lymphomas usually exhibits a mature (post-thymic) T helper cell phenotype (TdT−, CD3+, CD4+, CD8−) although other phenotypes (CD4−, CD8+ or CD4+, CD8+) may occasionally be observed. Clinically, peripheral T-cell lymphoma, unspecified, is a disease of adults that usually behaves in an aggressive fashion. Overall 5-year survival is 25%.[43] Multiagent chemotherapy, however, offers the potential for cure for some patients.

> **Table 21–15**
MISCELLANEOUS LYMPHOMAS

Type of Lymphoma	Characteristics
Cutaneous T-cell lymphomas	
Mycosis fungoides	Epidermotropic T-cell lymphoma infiltrate of skin progressing from patches to plaques to tumor nodules; affects adults; usually indolent but progressive
Sézary syndrome	Epidermotropic T-cell lymphoma producing erythroderma, generalized lymphadenopathy, and peripheral blood involvement; affects adults; unfavorable prognosis.
Primary cutaneous anaplastic large-cell lymphoma, T-cell/null-cell type	Large, CD30+ lymphoid cells infiltrate the skin; usually solitary lesion, may regress, rarely becomes systemic; highly favorable prognosis
Subcutaneous pannicultic T-cell lymphoma	Subcutaneous T-cell lymphoma producing nodules, often in the extremities; may be associated with fatal hemophagocytic syndrome
Angioimmunoblastic T-cell lymphoma	Mixture of atypical T cells, eosinophils, plasma cells, extrafollicular dendritic cells, and arborizing venules; systemic symptoms including skin rash, hypergammaglobulinemia, and hemolytic anemia; aggressive course; patients often die of infection
Adult T-cell leukemia/lymphoma	HTLV-1–associated, rapidly fatal disease; endemic to Japan, Caribbean, and Brazil; highly variable histology; widely disseminated disease at presentation
Systemic anaplastic large-cell lymphoma, T-cell/null-cell type	Aggressive lymphoma with bimodal age distribution; often shows good response to chemotherapy; nodal and extranodal infiltration by CD30+, ALK-NPM+ (t(2;5)) lymphoma with variable cytology and tendency for sinusoidal involvement
Hepatosplenic T-cell lymphoma	Aggressive lymphoma affecting young adults; marked hepatosplenomegaly without lymphadenopathy; sinus infiltration by CD3+, TCR-gamma/delta+, medium-sized lymphoma cells
Intestinal T-cell lymphoma (with or without enteropathy)	Gastrointestinal T-cell lymphoma associated with adult onset celiac disease; ulcerative lesions of jejunum often lead to intestinal perforation; poor prognosis
Angiocentric lymphoma	Rare lymphoma affecting extranodal sites (lung, nose, skin, central nervous system) composed of polymorphic infiltrate, including atypical lymphoid cells, which is angiocentric/angiodestructive; indolent to aggressive course, T-cell natural killer cell phenotype

Primary Cutaneous T-Cell Lymphoma

Primary involvement of the skin by lymphoma is usually of the T-cell type. B-cell lymphomas may occasionally secondarily involve the skin; however, this is seldom an isolated or presenting finding in B-cell lymphoma. Hodgkin's lymphoma rarely involves the skin in the form of direct extension from adjacent involved lymph nodes.

The category of cutaneous T-cell lymphoma includes a broad group of dysplastic and frankly malignant T-cell proliferations with a predilection for infiltration of the skin.[44] Disorders within the umbrella of this category include mycosis fungoides, Sézary syndrome, lymphomatoid papulosis, and primary cutaneous anaplastic large-cell lymphoma.

Mycosis fungoides and Sézary syndrome, two related disorders, are characterized by infiltration of the dermis and epidermis by malignant T cells with a peculiar cerebriform nucleus. Thin sections of well-fixed paraffin-embedded material or plastic-embedded sections are required to appreciate this nuclear detail. In 90% of cases, these cells exhibit a mature "helper" phenotype (pan-T+, CD4+, CD8−) and in 10%, a mature suppressor phenotype (pan-T+, CD4−, CD8+). In many cases, mycosis fungoides progresses through three clinical phases. In the premycotic (erythroderma) phase, lasting from 6 months to 50 years, the T-cell infiltrate produces a nonspecific eczematous dermatosis that is difficult to differentiate from a benign inflammatory infiltrate. As the disease progresses, the infiltrate thickens to form distinct plaques (plaque stage) and finally tumor nodules (tumor stage) (Fig.

21–24). Systemic dissemination with lymph node, peripheral blood, and visceral organ involvement is more likely to develop in the later stages. Transformation to a large-cell lymphoma similar to anaplastic large-cell lymphoma may occur and is most frequently seen as a terminal event. The prognosis for mycosis fungoides confined to the skin is relatively good, with median survival of greater than 10 years. Extracutaneous spread, however, is associated with a median survival of less than 1 year.

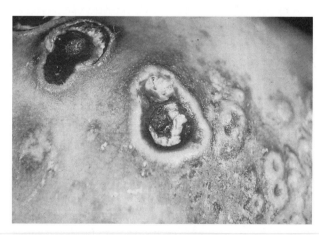

> **FIGURE 21–24** Mycosis fungoides, tumor stage. Tumor nodules are produced by massive local infiltrates of the skin by the characteristic cerebriform cells of mycosis fungoides.

In the related Sézary syndrome, the early erythroderma stage is associated with leukemia of the characteristic cerebriform T cells (Sézary cells) (Fig. 21–25 and Color Plate 252). Progression to the tumor stage is unusual in Sézary syndrome.

Primary cutaneous anaplastic large-cell lymphoma and lymphomatoid papulosis are related, cutaneous T-cell proliferations that are extremely difficult to differentiate by histologic features alone.[45] These morphologically similar disorders are both cytologically malignant; however, lymphomatoid papulosis generally pursues a clinically benign course whereas cutaneous anaplastic large-cell lymphoma, by definition, behaves in a malignant fashion. With the passage of time, 10% to 20% of patients with lymphomatoid papulosis develop overt lymphoma with dissemination beyond the skin. It is, therefore, probable that these two disorders represent a continuum. In addition to their morphological similarity, they are immunophenotypically indistinguishable, and both appear to be clonal proliferations of T cells.

Cutaneous anaplastic large-cell lymphoma is probably a different disease than systemic anaplastic large-cell lymphoma, discussed later. The atypical cells of the cutaneous disease, although CD30-positive, similar to the systemic disorder, are epithelial membrane antigen (EMA)–negative, and the t(2;5) chromosomal translocation associated with the systemic disease is absent in the cutaneous disease (see Table 21–8). Furthermore, cutaneous anaplastic large-cell lymphoma is an indolent, incurable disorder compared with the more aggressive but potentially curable systemic lymphoma.

Angioimmunoblastic Lymphadenopathy with Dysproteinemia (AILD)–like T-Cell Lymphoma

In 1979, Shimoyama and colleagues described a lymphoma with clinical and morphological features similar to that of immunoblastic lymphadenopathy (IBL) and angioimmunoblastic lymphadenopathy with dysproteinemia (AILD).[46] These disorders are associated with evidence of hyperimmunity (fever, skin rash, hypergammaglobulinemia) and often develop following exposure to certain drugs and infectious agents. There is a high frequency of evolution of these disorders to frank lymphoma. It is now generally recognized that within this category, there is a spectrum of clinicopathologic entities that run the gamut from benign (possibly premalignant) disorders to aggressive, rapidly fatal lymphomas. The affected lymph nodes of AILD-like lymphoma exhibit a mixture of atypical lymphoid cells, follicular dendritic cells, and thick-walled high endothelial venules.

Angiocentric T-Cell Lymphomas

Angiocentric T-cell lymphoma[47] is the malignant member of a family of diseases that encompasses a variety of angiocentric and angiodestructive disorders (lymphocytic vasculitis, lymphomatoid granulomatosis, polymorphic reticulosis, lethal midline granuloma, and angiocentric T-cell lymphoma). The lymphoma is characterized by tissue nodules of atypical lymphoreticular cells centered about blood vessels, often resulting in their destruction. The lung is the most common site of involvement; however, involvement of other extranodal sites (e.g., nose, palate, and skin) is frequent. The disease course, ranging from indolent to aggressive, appears to be dependent on the number of large cells present.

HTLV-1–Associated T-Cell Lymphoma/ Leukemia

This aggressive lymphoma is associated with infection by the type C retrovirus, HTLV-1, and is most common in the endemic areas of southwestern Japan, the Caribbean basin, and the tropical islands of the Pacific and Indian Oceans.[48] A low frequency of infection is observed in the United States, mainly among blacks of the southeastern region. This type of lymphoma is, therefore, rare in the United States. It is often widely disseminated at presentation and clinically is characterized by lymphadenopathy, hepatosplenomegaly, and involvement of the peripheral blood, skin, and cerebrospinal fluid. Hypercalcemia is usually present. Skin involvement is common and mimics mycosis fungoides. In involved fluids such as peripheral blood or cerebrospinal fluid, the distinctive bizarre polypoid malignant cells are readily identified. These cells express a mature "helper" phenotype and also are positive for the T-cell growth factor receptor (IL-2 receptor). The expression of IL-2 and clinical presentation, including positive HTLV-1 serology, serve to distinguish this disease from mycosis fungoides. In its classic form this disease is rapidly fatal despite aggressive therapy (less than 1 year survival). Chronic or smoldering subtypes of this lymphoma are recognized, with disease mainly limited to the skin. Survival with these indolent subtypes usually exceeds 2 years.

Anaplastic Large-Cell Lymphoma

A peculiar form of node-based lymphoma in which the large, atypical malignant cells preferentially infiltrate the lymph node sinuses is referred to as *anaplastic large-cell lymphoma*.[49] This disease appears clinically distinct from the primary cutaneous large-cell lymphoma previously discussed. Because of the cytologic features and sinus pattern of node involvement, this disease is easily mistaken for metastatic carcinoma, germ cell tumor, melanoma, or malignant histiocytosis. The phenotype of anaplastic large-cell lymphoma is variable, which can contribute to the confusion. Although these lymphomas are uniformly CD30-positive (Fig. 21–26), there is variable expression of CD45, CD15, and various T-cell antigens from case to case. The frequent expression of epithelial membrane antigen by the malignant cells further adds to the ease of misdiagnosing this disorder.

This disease may present at any age but preferentially occurs in children. It is commonly associated with a unique

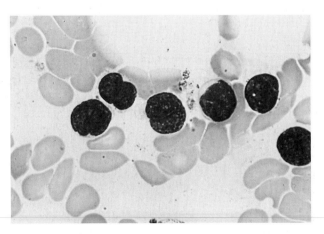

► FIGURE 21–25   Sézary cells observed in the peripheral blood from a patient with Sézary syndrome. (From the American Society of Clinical Pathologists, with permission.)

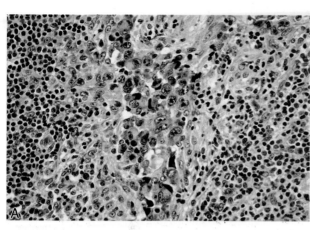
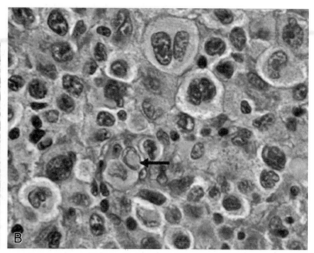

➤ FIGURE 21–26 *A*. Anaplastic large-cell lymphoma (ALCL). Large pleomorphic cells of ALCL infiltrate in a sinus pattern that may be easily misinterpreted as metastatic carcinoma or melanoma. *B*. ALCL nuclei are often lobulated, resulting in pseudonuclear inclusions (*arrow*).

chromosomal translocation, t(2;5) (p23;q35), which results in overexpression of the *ALK-NPM* protein that can be detected by immunocytochemical techniques. Aggressive chemotherapy often leads to complete remissions.

Lymphomas Derived from Nonlymphoid Cells

The vast majority of lymphomas are derived from the various types of lymphocytes. Rare cases present clinically as lymphomas, and the malignant cells are morphologically indistinguishable from the lymphocytic lymphomas; however, at the immunologic and genetic level they are nonlymphoid. These rare cases most often exhibit either a histiocyte or reticulum cell phenotype.

Diagnostic Evaluation

Tissue biopsy is required for the diagnosis and subcategorization of non-Hodgkin's lymphoma. The mainstay of diagnosis is the histologic evaluation of well-stained tissue sections by an experienced pathologist. Ancillary studies, however, are often required. These include immunophenotypic studies, nucleic acid (DNA and RNA) content analysis, cytogenetics, gene rearrangement, and functional studies (Table 21–16). The diagnostic difficulties fall into a relatively small number of categories; namely, differentiating (1) benign versus malignant lymphoproliferations, (2) lymphoma versus nonlymphoma, (3) T-cell versus B-cell lymphoma, and (4) Hodgkin's lymphoma versus non-Hodgkin's lymphoma. One or more of the ancillary tests may be required to resolve the differential diagnostic dilemma, and rarely, the dilemma may be irresolvable.

Benign versus Malignant

If light microscopic evaluation fails to distinguish a benign from a malignant lymphoproliferation, the demonstration of immunophenotypic or genotypic monoclonality would favor a malignant diagnosis. For B cells, immunophenotypic monoclonality is defined as restriction of immunoglobulin light-chain production by a population of cells to a single light-chain class, either κ or λ.[50–53] Operationally, light-chain monoclonality is present if the percentage of κ-positive cells to λ-positive cells (κ-to-λ ratio) falls outside of the expected ("normal") range or if "clonal excess" can be demonstrated by statistical comparison (Kolmogorov-

Smirnov test)[54] of the κ and λ fluorescence intensity distributions (see Chap. 29). An example of immunophenotypic monoclonality demonstrated by two-color flow cytometry is illustrated in Figure 21–27.

Unfortunately, at the present time, no practical method exists to define immunophenotypic T-cell clonality. Evidence for T-cell malignancy, however, may be suggested by immunophenotypically demonstrating an aberrant T-cell phenotype. Benign T-cell proliferations generally express a "normal" T-cell phenotype in which all pan–T-cell antigens (CD2, CD3, CD5, CD7) are expressed by the individual T cells. On the other hand, T-cell malignancies that might be confused with a benign T-cell proliferation often express an aberrant T-cell phenotype in which one or more of the pan–T-cell antigens are not expressed. Approximately 60% of peripheral T-cell lymphomas will express such an aberrant phenotype, with CD5 and CD7 being the most frequently absent antigens.[55]

A genotypic definition of both B- and T-cell clonality is possible. Clonal rearrangements of the T-cell receptor or immunoglobulin genes are detectable by several methods, including Southern blot analysis and the polymerase chain reaction (PCR) (see Chap. 33). Figure 21–28 illustrates the

---

➤ Table 21-16
ROUTINE AND ANCILLARY TESTS USEFUL IN THE EVALUATION OF LYMPH NODE BIOPSIES

Fresh Tissue

- Bacterial/viral studies
- Cell suspension for surface marker, cytogenetic studies, and genotypic studies
- Frozen material for rapid diagnosis, histochemical and immunohistochemical stains

Fixed Tissue

- Paraffin embedded for light microscopy and limited histochemical, immunohistochemical, and genotypic studies
- Resin (plastic) embedded for electron microscopy and thin-section light microscopy

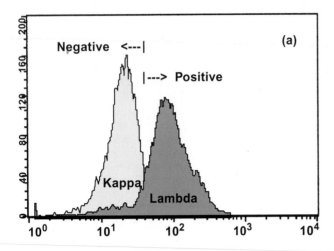

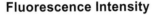

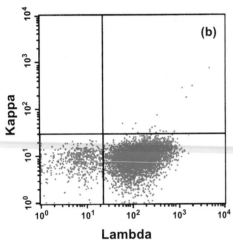

> ➤ FIGURE 21-27   B-cell monoclonality detected by flow
> cytometry. *A.* Overlay of two single-color (one-parameter)
> histograms demonstrating a monoclonal lambda population. *B.*
> Two-color (dual-parameter) histogram with simultaneous analysis
> for kappa (y-axis) and lambda (x-axis) light chains. The dense
> cluster of events in the lower right quadrant indicates a monoclonal
> lambda population.

results of Southern blot analysis in which a clonal population
of T cells is indicated by the presence of nongermline bands
in the Southern blot analysis. The identification of a clonal
rearrangement is presumptive evidence of a malignant proliferation.[56-58] Although biphenotypic rearrangements (both
T-cell receptor and immunoglobulin genes rearranged) may
rarely occur, the specific type of rearrangement is generally
useful in assigning lineage to the lymphoma; that is, a B-cell
lymphoma if immunoglobulin gene rearrangement is found,
and a T-cell lymphoma if T-cell receptor gene rearrangement
is found.

Although karyotypic analysis in a search for nonrandom
chromosome abnormalities might be useful in distinguishing benign from malignant lymphoproliferations or subcategorizing the non-Hodgkin's lymphomas, the technical difficulties in performing this type of analysis have made
cytogenetic studies an uncommon ancillary test in lymphoproliferation evaluation. The development of DNA probes
for specific chromosomal alterations may obviate the necessity of performing karyograms in the cytogenetic evaluation of lymphoproliferations. Southern blot analysis, PCR,
and fluorescence in situ hybridization (FISH) are commonly used techniques for demonstrating diagnostically
important chromosomal translocation (see Table 21–8)
without the need for complete karyotype analysis.

Lymphoma versus Nonlymphoma

The differential diagnoses of large-cell lymphoma and nonlymphoid malignancies, such as amelanotic melanoma,
poorly differentiated carcinoma, germ cell neoplasms, and
round cell sarcomas, is a frequently occurring problem in
surgical pathology. Differential diagnosis is facilitated by
determining the antigenic phenotype of the tumor cells.
This is most commonly done by staining of the cells with
an immunoenzyme technique using a panel of antibodies
directed against normal cellular differentiation antigens.[59]
Although no single antibody is either 100% specific or sensitive for identifying the "cell of origin" of a tumor, with the
aid of a panel of antibodies it is generally possible to define
a phenotypic profile that permits identification of the type
of tumor. From a therapeutic perspective it is most important to resolve the differential—carcinoma versus lymphoma versus sarcoma versus melanoma—which can usually be accomplished by a relatively small antibody panel
(Table 21–17). Additional refinement of the diagnosis may
be possible with larger panels.

T-cell versus B-cell Lymphoma

Although morphological features may suggest a B-cell or
T-cell phenotype, ancillary tests are required for specific
distinction between B-cell and T-cell lymphoma. The im-

Hodgkin's Lymphoma versus Non-Hodgkin's Lymphoma

On morphological grounds alone, it is sometimes difficult, if not impossible, to distinguish Hodgkin's lymphoma from non-Hodgkin's lymphoma.[60] For this reason, as well as important therapeutic implications, there has been considerable interest in the utility of ancillary techniques to resolve this differential diagnosis. The literature is replete with contradictory studies concerning the significance of various tests in distinguishing Hodgkin's lymphoma from non-Hodgkin's lymphoma.[61] This state of affairs reflects defects in our understanding of the basic biologic differences between these disorders as well as the nonspecificity of the tests. At present the only specific immunophenotypic distinction between these disorders is the presence of light-chain monoclonality in B-cell non-Hodgkin's lymphomas and its absence in Hodgkin's lymphoma. Clonal rearrangement of the immunoglobulin heavy-chain and T-cell receptor genes has been described in some cases of Hodgkin's lymphoma and, therefore, limits the utility of such tests in the differential diagnosis of Hodgkin's from non-Hodgkin's lymphomas.[62]

Although the immunophenotypic differences between Hodgkin's and non-Hodgkin's lymphoma are not sufficient alone to distinguish these entities when viewed in the context of histologic and clinical data, immunophenotypic analysis may be a useful adjunct. The differential diagnosis of Hodgkin's lymphoma, excluding lymphocyte-predominant Hodgkin's lymphoma, generally includes peripheral T-cell lymphoma and anaplastic large-cell lymphoma. The Reed-Sternberg cells and Hodgkin's cells of Hodgkin's lymphoma are characteristically CD45-negative, CD15-positive, and CD30-positive (Table 21–18), whereas peripheral T-cell lymphomas are usually CD45-positive, CD15-negative, and CD30-negative. Unfortunately the Reed-Sternberg–like cells of peripheral T-cell lymphoma are occasionally CD15- or CD30-positive, or both,[63] and careful attention to histologic features and the presence of CD45 positivity on the Reed-Sternberg–like cells are required to prevent misdiagnosis in these cases. Similarly, anaplastic large-cell lymphomas are by definition CD30-positive, yet the usual absence of CD15 and presence of CD45 on the large atypical cells aids in distinguishing anaplastic large-cell lymphoma from Hodgkin's lymphoma.

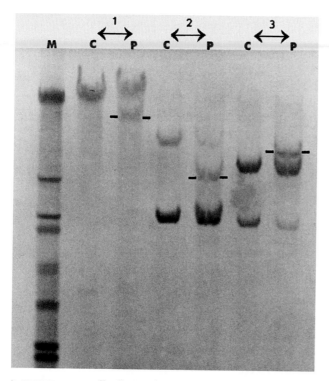

► FIGURE 21–28 T-cell monoclonality demonstrated by Southern blot analysis: Abnormal bands designated by small bars indicate clonal rearrangement of the T-cell receptor gene. M = molecular weight markers; C = control DNA to locate position of germ-line (nonrearranged) bands; P = patient DNA; 1 = Bam HI digest; 2 = Eco RI digest; 3 = Hind III digest (for details, see Chap. 33).

munophenotypic demonstration of light-chain monoclonality and the expression of B-lineage antigens (CD19–22), or of an aberrant B-cell phenotype by the cells of a malignant lymphoma, are indicative of a B-cell lymphoma.[52] Similarly, the expression of a normal or abnormal T-cell phenotype by the malignant cells is associated with T-cell malignancy.[52] Gene rearrangement studies appear to be more sensitive than immunophenotypic studies in distinguishing T-cell versus B-cell lymphoma; however, relatively few lymphomas require this technically more demanding procedure to make this distinction.

► Table 21-17
ANTIBODY PANEL FOR DISTINGUISING AMONG THE FOUR MAJOR CATEGORIES OF CANCER

Cancer Type	ANTIBODY			
	Cytokeratin*	Vimentin†	LCA‡ (CD45)	S100¶
Carcinoma	+	−	−	−
Sarcoma	−	+	−	−
Lymphoma	−	±	+	−
Melanoma	−	±	−	+

*Antibody directed against the cytokeratin group of intermediate filament proteins found in epithelial cells.
†Antibody directed against the 58-kd intermediate filament protein found in mesenchymal cells.
‡Antibody directed against the 200-kd leukocyte common antigen found in various hematopoietic and lymphoreticular cells.
¶Antibody directed against the 25-kd protein found in selected cells of the nervous system, melanocytes, interdigitating reticulum cells, etc. The antibody HMB-45 is more specifically restricted to melanocytes than anti-S100.

> ## Table 21-18
> ## IMMUNOPHENOTYPE OF HODGKIN'S LYMPHOMA

Antibody	RS Cells and Variants*	L & H Cells
CD45	−	+/−
CD15	+	−/+
CD30	+	−/+
CD20	−/+	+/−
CD74	+	+
CD75	−/+	+
EMA	−	+/−

*Excludes L & H cells.
Abbreviations: +/− = usually positive; −/+ = usually negative;
EMA = Epithelial membrane antigen

> ## Table 21-19
> ## STAGING CLASSIFICATION OF BURKITT'S LYMPHOMA

Stage A	Single extra-abdominal site
Stage B	Multiple extra-abdominal sites
Stage C	Intra-abdominal tumor
Stage D	Intra-abdominal tumor with multiple extra-abdominal sites
Stage AR	Stage C disease with > 90% of tumor surgically removed

Expression of the *ALK-NPM* protein also serves to distinguish systemic anaplastic large-cell lymphoma from Hodgkin's lymphoma. Nodular lymphocyte-predominant Hodgkin's lymphoma must be distinguished from low-grade non-Hodgkin's lymphomas, particularly follicular center lymphomas and reactive conditions such as progressive transformation of follicle centers. The expression of monoclonal surface immunoglobulin by the low-grade lymphomas definitively distinguishes them from nodular lymphocyte-predominant Hodgkin's lymphoma.

Staging

The staging evaluation of the non-Hodgkin's lymphomas is similar to that for Hodgkin's lymphoma. The same staging scheme, the Ann Arbor classification (see Table 21–5), which was designed for Hodgkin's lymphoma, is also used for the staging of non-Hodgkin's lymphomas. Because the natural history of Hodgkin's lymphoma is different from that of non-Hodgkin's lymphoma, there are certain problems with using the Ann Arbor classification in staging the non-Hodgkin's lymphomas. Despite these drawbacks, the Ann Arbor scheme remains the staging scheme of choice. One major exception to this statement is Burkitt's lymphoma. In this lymphoma the bulk of tumor, rather than sites of involvement, is a primary determinant of prognosis. Consequently, a different staging scheme is in use for Burkitt's lymphoma (Table 21–19).

Treatment and Prognosis

For the purposes of prognostic assessment and therapeutic selection, the non-Hodgkin's lymphomas can be grouped into two broad categories: the indolent lymphomas and the diffuse aggressive lymphomas. The indolent lymphomas are composed of the low-grade lymphomas of the Working Formulation and the more recently described group of mantle cell and marginal zone lymphomas (see Table 21–11). They are so designated because the median survival without therapy for this group of lymphomas is relatively long (7 to 9 years). The diffuse aggressive lymphomas encompass the intermediate- and high-grade lymphomas of the Working Formulation. Without treatment, these lymphomas are rapidly fatal (median survival is 6 to 12 months).

Therapy for the indolent lymphomas is controversial. As a group, relatively few present with localized disease (stages I and II). Strictly localized indolent lymphoma (stage I/IE) can be effectively treated with radiotherapy, resulting in durable complete remission. Approximately 90% of these lymphomas are stage III or IV at presentation, and although they are sensitive to both radiation and chemotherapy, the disease is essentially incurable with standard or aggressive multiagent chemotherapy. Furthermore, because existing therapies were ineffective in prolonging survival in the low-grade lymphomas, a "watch and wait" approach was adopted by many oncologists during the 1970s and 1980s.[64] When symptoms warranted, or the lymphoma progressed to a higher grade, therapy was instituted. More recently, aggressive multiagent chemotherapy has been shown to be effective at prolonging survival; however, this does not equate to cure.

Prior to the development of modern chemotherapeutic modalities, the indolent lymphomas were considered "favorable" lymphomas and the diffuse aggressive lymphomas were considered the "unfavorable" category. The situation is now reversed. The indolent lymphomas are recognized as clinically indolent but incurable with current therapies. On the other hand, the diffuse aggressive lymphomas are rapidly fatal if untreated but are potentially curable with aggressive chemotherapeutic strategies. The 10-year survival for the diffuse aggressive lymphomas treated aggressively with multiagent chemotherapy is now greater than that for the indolent lymphomas. Long-term survival depends on achieving an initial complete remission. Utilizing intensive multiagent chemotherapy, complete remission rates of 60% to 85% have been achieved in the advanced stage, diffuse aggressive lymphoma category. Relapse-free survival at 2 years is between 40% and 70%. Therapy following relapse is usually ineffective. Patients who survive for 2 years without evidence of recurrence are considered "cured," because relapses seldom occur after a 2-year disease-free interval. As survival is increased with aggressive therapy, the risk of secondary (chemotherapy-induced) acute nonlymphocytic leukemia is also increasing. Approximately 8% of patients develop acute nonlymphocytic leukemia within 10 years of chemotherapy for non-Hodgkin's lymphoma, and these leukemias are usually resistant to therapy.

The therapeutic response of lymphoblastic lymphoma to aggressive chemotherapy has not been as impressive as with the other aggressive lymphomas. Adults older than 45 years tend to have longer survival than younger patients; however, median survival is still short.[65]

► CASE STUDY

A 68-year-old male auto mechanic presents to his primary care physician with a chief complaint of bilateral, painless masses in the neck region of at least 6 months' duration. He has a 120 pack-year smoking history, and his family history includes a father and brother with thyroid cancer. His past medical history is positive for rheumatoid arthritis. On physical examination, the patient is found to have bilateral supraclavicular and cervical lymphadenopathy consisting of matted groups of lymph nodes that were painless to palpation. The patient was afebrile and had experienced an unintentional decrease in weight from 195 pounds to 180 pounds over a 6-month interval.

Questions

1. What pathologic processes must be considered in the evaluation of lymphadenopathy?
2. What are some of the important diagnostic tests that should be performed?

All parameters of the initial complete blood count (CBC) were normal, and the peripheral smear was without morphological abnormality. A chest x-ray demonstrated hilar adenopathy without any recognizable parenchymal lung lesions. Excisional biopsy of a group of nodes was performed. On microscopic examination there was diffuse effacement of lymph node architecture by a population of relatively uniform cells, averaging 20 to 40 μm in diameter, with round to slightly irregular nuclei and occasional prominent nucleoli. Immunophenotypically, the cells were characterized by the expression of CD45, CD19, CD20, and κ light chains. No T-cell antigens were detected on the abnormal cells.

Questions

3. What is the most likely diagnosis based on the available data?
4. What additional studies should be performed before therapy is instituted?

Bilateral bone marrow biopsy specimens demonstrate several aggregates of abnormal cells, similar to those observed in the lymph nodes, randomly distributed within the marrow. A computed tomographic (CT) scan of the abdomen and pelvis reveals para-aortic adenopathy and modest enlargement of the spleen.

Questions

5. What stage is this lymphoma?
6. What therapy would be appropriate?
7. What is the probability of "cure"?

Answers

1. The causes of lymphadenopathy are myriad and include various benign and malignant etiologies. Benign disorders producing localized or generalized adenopathy are most commonly infectious or inflammatory in nature (e.g., viral illness, cat scratch fever), but may be secondary to autoimmune disorders (e.g., lupus, rheumatoid arthritis). Metastatic malignancies (carcinoma, melanoma, or sarcoma) produce lymphadenopathy, but on physical examination are usually more localized. Lymphoma must always be considered in the differential diagnosis of lymphadenopathy, regardless of the patient's age.

2. The formed elements (white cells, red cells, and platelets) of the peripheral blood often exhibit changes that are helpful in accessing the cause of lymphadenopathy; therefore, a CBC with peripheral smear evaluation is indicated. A chest x-ray should be performed in a search for intrathoracic disease, particularly lung lesions. The definitive test to distinguish benign from malignant processes is microscopic examination of an enlarged lymph node. This may be achieved by fine needle aspiration or excisional biopsy. Excisional biopsy is preferred if lymphoma is high on the differential diagnostic list.

3. Malignant lymphoma, diffuse large B-cell (REAL classification).

4. For staging purposes, bilateral bone marrow biopsies and CT scanning of the abdomen and pelvis should be performed.

5. Stage IV.

6. Multiagent chemotherapy.

7. The probability of 2-year relapse-free survival is 40% to 70% for advanced, aggressive-grade non-Hodgkin's lymphomas. If relapse does not occur within 2 years after achieving complete remission, the patient is considered cured. Therefore, the probability of cure in this case is 40% to 70%.

QUESTIONS

1. What infectious agent is most commonly associated with the pathogenesis of Hodgkin's lymphoma?
   a. Echovirus
   b. Herpesvirus
   c. *Helicobacter pylori*
   d. Epstein-Barr virus

2. The cell characteristic of all types of classic Hodgkin's lymphoma is the:
   a. Lacunar cell
   b. L & H cell
   c. Reed-Sternberg cell
   d. Sézary cell

3. An asymptomatic mediastinal mass affecting a young woman is a common form of presentation for which type of Hodgkin's lymphoma?
   a. Nodular sclerosing
   b. Lymphocyte-predominant
   c. Mixed cellularity
   d. Lymphocyte depletion

4. All follicular center lymphomas are composed of a mixture of:
   a. Small cleaved and small noncleaved cells
   b. Centrocytes (small cleaved) and centroblasts (large noncleaved) cells

   c. Large cleaved cells and immunoblasts
   d. Prolymphocytes and paraimmunoblasts

5. Small lymphocytic lymphoma is characterized by all of the following except:
   a. Indolent but incurable
   b. Usually CD19+, CD5+, CD23+, CD10−
   c. Growth centers
   d. t(14;18)

6. Translocations involving the bcl-1 and IgH genes are commonly associated with which low-grade B-cell lymphoma?
   a. Small lymphocytic
   b. Immunocytoma
   c. Mantle cell
   d. Marginal cell

7. Lymphomatous polyposis is a type of:
   a. Small lymphocytic lymphoma
   b. Large-cell lymphoma
   c. Mantle cell lymphoma
   d. MALT lymphoma

8. MALT lymphomas are characterized by all of the following except:
   a. Extranodal involvement
   b. Associated follicular hyperplasia
   c. CD19+, CD5+, CD10+ phenotype
   d. t(11;18)

9. A lymphoma expressing a monoclonal B-cell phenotype with coexpression of CD10 and rearrangement of the bcl-2 gene is most likely derived from:
   a. Follicular center cells
   b. Mantle cells
   c. Marginal zone cells
   d. Interfollicular cells

10. Burkitt's lymphoma is histologically characterized by which of the following?
    a. Uniform nuclei
    b. High mitotic rate
    c. "Starry sky" pattern
    d. All of the above

11. Lymphoblastic lymphomas are associated with all the following except:
    a. High frequency of developing acute lymphoblastic leukemia
    b. Mediastinal mass
    c. Usually express B-cell phenotype
    d. Potentially curable in young patients

12. All of the following are T-cell disorders except:
    a. Mycosis fungoides
    b. Sézary syndrome
    c. Hepatosplenic gamma/delta lymphoma
    d. Burkitt's lymphoma

13. A lymphoma associated with infection by a type C retrovirus is:
    a. Endemic to Japan
    b. Associated with hypercalcemia
    c. Usually rapidly fatal
    d. All of the above

14. The immunophenotypic definition of B-cell monoclonality is:
    a. Clonal rearrangement of the IgH gene
    b. Loss of B-cell antigens by the malignant cells
    c. Expression of a single light-chain class
    d. Expression of a single heavy-chain class

15. Alternatives to karyotypic analysis for the demonstration of chromosomal translocations include:
    a. Southern blot analysis
    b. PCR
    c. FISH
    d. All of the above

16. Reed-Sternberg cells usually express the following immunophenotype:
    a. CD45+, CD30+, CD15+
    b. CD45−, CD30+, CD15+
    c. CD45+, CD30+, CD15−
    d. CD45−, CD30−, CD15+

17. All of the following are true regarding the low-grade non-Hodgkin's lymphomas except:
    a. Survival without treatment averages more than 5 years
    b. Disease is usually advanced at diagnosis
    c. Multiagent chemotherapy can prolong survival
    d. Cure is possible in more than 50% of cases

18. The diffuse aggressive lymphomas are:
    a. Seldom curable
    b. Rapidly fatal if untreated
    c. Best treated with a combination of surgery and radiotherapy
    d. Single-agent chemotherapy is the treatment of choice

19. The staging system for Hodgkin's lymphoma and the non-Hodgkin's lymphomas is:
    a. Working Formulation
    b. Duke's staging system
    c. Rye staging system
    d. Ann Arbor staging system

20. A patient with Hodgkin's lymphoma that is localized to lymph nodes above and below the diaphragm and is associated with drenching night sweats would be classified as:
    a. Stage IIIE
    b. Stage IIB
    c. Stage IIIB
    d. Stage IIIA

SUMMARY CHART

➤ The malignant lymphomas are a heterogeneous group of diseases that arise from cells of the lymphoid tissue (lymphocytes, histiocytes, reticulum cells).

➤ The Reed-Sternberg cell is the hallmark of Hodgkin's disease; the morphological features of the Reed-Sternberg cell include large size (up to 45 μm in diameter), multinucleated, and inclusion-like nucleoli.

➤ The probable infectious agent of Hodgkin's lymphoma is Epstein-Barr virus.

➤ Lymphocyte-predominant Hodgkin's lymphoma consists of a mixture of small, normal-appearing lymphocytes; benign histiocytes; rare, classic Reed-Sternberg cells; and many variant Reed-Sternberg cells (L & H cells).

➤ The most common type of Hodgkin's lymphoma is nodular sclerosing Hodgkin's lymphoma, which is characterized by birefringent collagenous sclerosis, classic Reed-Sternberg cells, and lacunar cells.

➤ Mixed cellularity Hodgkin's lymphoma is characterized by a heterogeneous mixture of cells, including lymphocytes, histiocytes, plasma cells, eosinophils, Reed-Sternberg cells, and Reed-Sternberg variants.

➤ Lymphocyte-rich Hodgkin's lymphoma is characterized by small numbers of Reed-Sternberg cells in a background of lymphocytes.

➤ Lymphocyte depletion Hodgkin's lymphoma is the rarest form of Hodgkin's disease. It is characterized by numerous Reed-Sternberg cells and variants, and rare lymphocytes, plasma cells, histiocytes, and eosinophils; irregular sclerosis is also present.

➤ The usual histologic progression in Hodgkin's disease is lymphocyte-rich to mixed cellularity to lymphocyte depletion lymphoma.

➤ Most patients with Hodgkin's lymphoma present with nonpainful lymph node swelling.

➤ The most widely used staging scheme in Hodgkin's disease is the Ann Arbor classification.

➤ The Revised European-American Classification of Lymphoid Neoplasms (REAL) utilizes clinical, morphological, immunophenotypic, and genotypic features to classify the lymphomas.

➤ The follicular center lymphomas (non-Hodgkin's lymphoma) are composed of various mixtures of centrocytes (small cleaved) and centroblasts (large noncleaved) cells and represent the B-cell phenotype (CD19+, CD20+, CD5−); t(14;18) is associated with this disorder.

➤ Mantle cell lymphoma is characterized by small- to medium-sized lymphocytes with scant pale-staining cytoplasm, irregular nucleus, and inconspicuous nucleoli; cells express surface immunoglobulin, CD5, and CD43; t(11;14) is also found.

➤ The MALT lymphomas are related to marginal zone cells and usually present in extranodal sites (stomach, salivary gland, lung, thyroid, and orbit); hence, the name mucosal-associated lymphoid tissue (MALT).

➤ The immunophenotype of Burkitt's lymphoma is surface IgM–positive, CD10-positive, CD5-negative, CD23-negative, and TdT-negative.

➤ Lymphomas that involve the skin are typically of the T-cell type.

➤ Characteristics of the systemic form of anaplastic large-cell lymphoma include overexpression of the *ALK-NPM* protein, t(2;5), CD30-positive, and infiltration of the lymph node sinuses by large atypical malignant cells.

References

1. Hodgkin, T: On some morbid appearances of the absorbent glands and spleen. Med-Chir Trans 17:68, 1832.
2. Wilks, Sir S: Cases of enlargement of the lymphatic glands and spleen (or, Hodgkin's disease), with remarks. Guy's Hosp Rep 11:56, 1865.
3. Sternberg, C: Uber eine eigenartige unter dem Bilde der Pseudoleukamie verlaufende Tuberculose des lymphatischen Apparates. Ztschr Heilk 19:21, 1898.
4. Reed, DM: On the pathological changes in Hodgkin's disease, with special reference to its relation to tuberculosis. Johns Hopkins Hosp Rep 10:133, 1902.
5. Kuppers, R, et al: Hodgkin's disease: Hodgkin and Reed-Sternberg cells picked from histological sections show clonal immunoglobulin gene rearrangement and appear to be derived from B cells at various stages of development. Proc Natl Acad Sci USA, 91:1092, 1994.
6. Lukes, RJ, et al: Report of the Nomenclature Committee. Cancer Res 26:1311, 1966.
7. Lukes, RJ, and Butler, JJ: The pathology and nomenclature of Hodgkin's disease. Cancer Res 26:1063, 1966.
8. Harris, NL: Hodgkin's disease: Classification and differential diagnosis. Mod Pathol 12:159, 1999.
9. Jaffe, ES, et al: World Health Organization classification of neoplastic diseases of the hematopoietic and lymphoid tissues: A progress report. Am J Clin Path, 110(Suppl 1):58, 1998.
10. von Wasielewski, R, et al: Lymphocyte-predominant Hodgkin's disease: An immunohistochemical analysis of 208 reviewed Hodgkin's disease cases from the German Hodgkin's Study Group. Am J Pathol 150:793, 1997.
11. Marafioti, T, et al: Origin of nodular lymphocyte-predominant Hodgkin's disease from a clonal expansion of highly mutated germinal center B cells. N Eng J Med 337:453, 1997.
12. Kant, JA, et al: A critical reappraisal of the pathologic and clinical heterogeneity of "lymphocyte depleted Hodgkin's disease." J Clin Oncol 4:284, 1986.
13. Carbone, PP, et al: Report of the Committee on Hodgkin's Staging Classification. Cancer Res 31:1860, 1971.
14. Lister, TA, et al: Report of a committee convened to discuss the evaluation and staging of patients with Hodgkin's disease: Cotswolds meeting. J Clin Oncol 7(11):1630, 1989.
15. DeVita, VT, et al: Curability of advanced Hodgkin's disease with chemotherapy. Ann Intern Med 92:587, 1980.
16. Virchow, RLK: Die cellulare Pathologie in ihrer Begruendung auf physiologische und pathologische Gewebelehre. Hirschwald, Berlin, 1858.
17. Billroth, T: Multiple Lymphome: Erfolgreiche Behandlung mit Arsenik. Wien Med Wochenschr 21:1066, 1871.
18. Dreschfield, J: Ein Beitrag Zur Lehre von den Lymphosarkomen. Dtsch Med Wochenschr 17:1175, 1893.
19. Kundrat, H: Uber Lympho-sarkomatosis. Wien Klin Wochnschr 6:211, 234, 1893.
20. Heim, S, and Mitelman, F: Cancer Cytogenetics. Alan R Liss, New York, 1995.
21. Rosenberg, SA, et al: National Cancer Institute sponsored study of classification on non-Hodgkin's lymphomas: Summary and description of a working formulation for clinical usage. Cancer 49:2112, 1982.
22. Harris, NL, et al: A Revised European-American Classification of Lymphoid Neoplasms: A Proposal from the International Lymphoma Study Group. Blood 84:1361, 1994.
23. Grogan, TM, et al: A Southwest Oncology Group Perspective on the revised European-American Lymphoma Classification. Hematol Oncol Clin North Am 11(5):819, 1997.
24. Miller, TP, et al: Follicular lymphomas: Do histologic subtypes predict outcome? Hematol Oncol Clin North Am Oct 11(5):893, 1997.
25. Banks, PM, et al: Mantle cell lymphoma. A proposal for unification of morphologic, immunologic, and molecular data. Am J Surg Pathol 16:637, 1992.
26. Inghirami, G, et al: Autoantibody-associated cross-reactive idiotype-bearing human B lymphocytes: Distribution and characterization, including IgVH gene and CD5 antigen expression. Blood 78:1503, 1991.
27. Argatoff, L, et al: Mantle cell lymphoma: A clinicopathologic study of 80 cases. Blood 89:2067, 1997.

28. Majilis, A, et al: Mantle cell lymphoma: Correlation of clinical outcome and biologic features with three histologic variants. J Clin Oncol 15:1664, 1997.

29. Van den Oord, J, et al: The marginal zone in the human reactive lymph node. Am J Clin Pathol 86:475, 1986.

30. VanKrieken, JHJM, et al: Splenic marginal zone lymphocytes and related cells in the lymph: A morphologic and immunohistochemical study. Hum Pathol 20:320, 1989.

31. Harris, NL: Low-grade B-cell lymphoma of mucosa-associated lymphoid tissue and monocytoid B-cell lymphoma: Related entities that are distinct from other low-grade B-cell lymphomas. Arch Path Lab Med 117:771, 1993.

32. Isaacson, P, et al: Malignant lymphoma of mucosa-associated lymphoid tissue. Histopathology 11(5) 445, 1987.

33. Witherspoon, A, et al: Regression of primary low-grade B-cell gastric lymphoma of mucosa-associated lymphoid tissue after eradication of *Helicobacter pylori*. Lancet 342:575, 1993.

34. Ngan, B-Y, et al: Monocytoid B-cell lymphoma: A study of 36 cases. Hum Pathol 22:409, 1991.

35. Schmid, C, et al: Splenic marginal zone cell lymphoma. Am J Surg Pathol 16:455, 1992.

36. Hammer, RD, et al: Splenic marginal zone lymphoma: A distinct B-cell neoplasm. Am J Surg Pathol 10:613, 1996.

37. Nathwani, BN: Classifying non-Hodgkin's lymphomas. In Berard, CW, et al (eds): Malignant Lymphoma (IAP Monographs in Pathology; no. 29). Williams & Wilkins, Baltimore, 1987.

38. Swerdlow, SH: Small B-cell lymphomas of the lymph nodes and spleen: Practical insights to diagnosis and pathogenesis. Mod Pathol 12:125, 1998.

39. Salar, A, et al: Diffuse large B-cell lymphoma: Is morphologic subdivision useful in clinical management? Eur J Haemotol 60:202, 1998.

40. Gascoyne, R: Prognostic factors in diffuse aggressive non-Hodgkin's lymphoma. Hematol Oncol Clin North Am 11:847, 1997.

41. Burkitt, D: A sarcoma involving the jaws in African children. Br J Surg 46:218, 1958.

42. Chen, JKC: Peripheral T-cell and NK-cell neoplasms: An integrated approach to diagnosis. Mod Pathol 12:177, 1999.

43. The Non-Hodgkin's Lymphoma Classification Project: A clinical evaluation of the International Lymphoma Classification of non-Hodgkin's lymphomas. Blood 89:3909, 1997.

44. Edelson, RL: Cutaneous T cell lymphoma. J Dermatol Surg Oncol 6:358, 1980.

45. Willemze, R, et al: Spectrum of primary cutaneous CD30 (Ki-1)-positive lymphoproliferative disorders. J Am Acad Dermatol 28:973, 1993.

46. Shimoyama, J, et al: Immunoblastic lymphadenopathy (IBL)-like T cell lymphoma. Jpn J Clin Oncol 9(Suppl):347, 1979.

47. Jaffe, ES: Post thymic lymphoid neoplasia. In Jaffe, ES, and Bennington, JL (eds): Surgical Pathology of the Lymph Nodes and Related Organs. WB Sanders, Philadelphia, 1985.

48. Gallo, RC: Human T cell leukemia/lymphoma virus and T cell malignancies in adults. Cancer Surv 3:113, 1984.

49. Lennert, K, et al: Large cell anaplastic lymphoma of T-cell type (Ki-1+). In Lennert, K, and Feller, AC (eds.) Histopathology of Non-Hodgkin's Lymphomas, ed 2. Springer-Verlag, New York, 1992, pp 229–244.

50. Picker, LJ, et al: Immunophenotypic criteria for the diagnosis of non Hodgkin's lymphoma. Am J Pathol 128:181, 1987.

51. Tubbs, R, et al: Tissue immunomicroscopic evaluation of monoclonality of B cell lymphomas. Am J Clin Pathol 76:24, 1986.

52. Hsu, SM: The use of monoclonal antibodies and immunohistochemical techniques in lymphoma: Review and overlook. Hematol Pathol 2:183, 1988.

53. Little, JV, et al: Flow cytometric analysis of lymphomas and lymphoma-like disorders. Semin Diag Pathol 6:37, 1989.

54. Ault, KA: Detection of small numbers of monoclonal B lymphocytes in blood of patients with lymphoma. N Engl J Med 300:1401, 1979.

55. Weiss, LM, et al: Morphologic and immunologic characterization of 50 peripheral T cell lymphomas. Am J Pathol 118:316, 1985.

56. Korsmeyer, SJ, and Walkman, TA: Immunoglobulin genes: Rearrangement and translocation in human lymphoid malignancy. J Clin Immunol 4:1, 1984.

57. Bertness, VO, et al: T cell receptor gene rearrangements as clinical markers of human T cell lymphomas. J Engl J Med 313:534, 1985.

58. Cossman, J, et al: Molecular genetics and the diagnosis of lymphoma. Arch Pathol Lab Med 112:117, 1988.

59. Battifora, H: Recent progress in the immunohistochemistry of solid tumors. Semin Diagn Pathol 1:251, 1984.

60. Braziel, RM, et al: Mistaken diagnoses of Hodgkin's disease. Hematol Oncol Clin North Am 11:863, 1997.

61. Grogan, T: Hodgkin's Disease in Surgical Pathology of the Lymph Nodes and Related Organs, ed 2. WB Saunders, Philadelphia, 1995.

62. Griessler, H, et al: Clonal rearrangements of T-cell receptor and immunoglobulin genes and immunophenotypic antigen expression in different subclasses of Hodgkin's disease. Int J Cancer 40:157, 1987.

63. Chittal, SM, et al: Monoclonal antibodies in the diagnosis of Hodgkin's disease. Am J Surg Pathol 12:9, 1988.

64. Horning, SJ, and Rosenberg, SA: The natural history of untreated low grade non Hodgkin's lymphomas. J Engl J Med 311:1471, 1984.

65. Weinstein, JH, et al: Long term results of the APO protocol for treatment of mediastinal lymphoblastic lymphoma. J Clin Oncol 1:537, 1983.

22 Lipid (Lysosomal) Storage Diseases and Histiocytosis

DENISE M. HARMENING, PhD, MT(ASCP), CLS(NCA)
CATHERINE M. SPIER, MD

LIPID (LYSOSOMAL) STORAGE DISEASES
  Gaucher's Disease
  Niemann-Pick Disease
  Tay-Sachs Disease
  Mucopolysaccharidoses
HISTIOCYTOSIS
  Sea-Blue Histiocyte Syndrome
  Other Histiocytic Disorders (Eosinophilic Granuloma, Hand-Schüller-Christian Disease, Letterer-Siwe Disease)
CASE STUDY

OBJECTIVES

At the end of this chapter, the learner should be able to:

1. Name the enzyme deficiency seen in Gaucher's disease.
2. List characteristics for type I, type II, and type III Gaucher's disease.
3. Describe the appearance of Gaucher's cells.
4. Name the enzyme deficiency seen in Niemann-Pick disease.
5. List clinical features of Niemann-Pick disease.
6. Name the enzyme deficiency seen in Tay-Sachs disease.
7. List clinical features of Tay-Sachs disease.
8. Describe clinical features of Hurler's syndrome, Hunter's syndrome, and other mucopolysaccharidoses.
9. List laboratory findings in mucopolysaccharidosis disorders.
10. Describe the characteristic cell of sea-blue histiocyte syndrome.

➤ LIPID (LYSOSOMAL) STORAGE DISEASES

The lipid storage diseases are rare, autosomally inherited disorders. They are known as *lysosomal storage diseases* because there is subcellular accumulation of unmetabolized material in the lysosomes of various cells. Lipid or lysosomal storage diseases are caused by various enzyme defects (inborn errors) in lipid metabolism linked to an enzyme deficiency (Fig. 22–1). Although many different types of lipid storage disorders have been documented, the most widely known and well established include Gaucher's, Niemann-Pick, and Tay-Sachs diseases and mucopolysaccharidoses (Table 22–1). Although all ethnic groups are known to be affected by lipid storage diseases, there is an increased incidence of selected disorders such as Gaucher's and Tay-Sachs diseases in certain ethnic groups, most notably Ashkenazi Jews (Jews who trace their origin to the Baltic Sea region).

Lipid storage diseases have a wide clinical expression, ranging from essentially asymptomatic to severe and incapacitating with early death. The aim of control in these disorders has been directed at prenatal detection. The only currently effective practical therapy is enzyme replacement, which has initiated a new age of treatment for genetic disorders and has improved the lives of many patients. The greatest controversy regarding enzyme replacement therapy, however, is the optimum amount and frequency of treatment.[1] In addition, allogeneic bone marrow transplantation has been used to treat some patients and can be considered curative.[2] However, bone marrow transplantation is an extremely aggressive, expensive, and high-risk therapy considering that these conditions now have an effective and practical treatment in enzyme replacement therapy. Table 22–2 summarizes the general characteristics of lipid storage diseases.

Gaucher's Disease

Historical Perspectives

This disorder was first described in 1882 by Philippe C. Gaucher in a 32-year-old woman with an enlarged spleen. Gaucher believed that the abnormal cells found in her spleen at autopsy were part of a primary splenic tumor. This abnormal cell, later named *Gaucher's cell*, is the result of the defi-

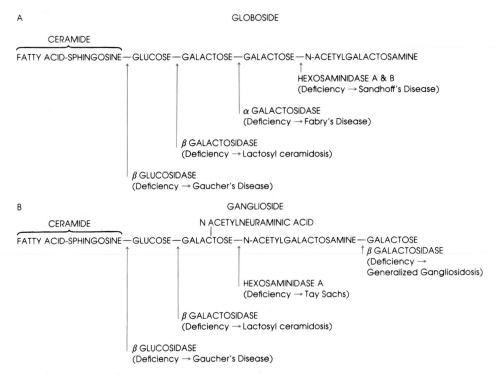

➤ FIGURE 22–1   Schematic structure of globoside and ganglioside to show site of action of the several catabolic enzymes, which, when defective, result in one of the storage diseases. (From Wintrobe, MM, et al: Clinical Hematology, ed 8. Lea & Febiger, Philadelphia, 1981, p 1341, with permission.)

ciency of the enzyme beta (β)-glucocerebrosidase, which leads to an accumulation of unmetabolized substrate glucocerebroside in cells, predominantly the monocyte-macrophage system (the reticuloendothelial system) (Fig. 22–2 and Color Plate 253). Gaucher's observations were studied further, and the entity known as Gaucher's disease was defined and characterized as a familial disorder at the turn of the century.[3] In 1920, another variation or type of Gaucher's disease that is characterized by neurologic involvement was first described. It was after this date that Gaucher's disease was classified as a lysosomal storage disorder resulting from an enzyme deficiency with an autosomal-recessive inheritance pattern. Although Gaucher's disease is the most frequent lysosomal storage disease, it was not until 1965 that the actual enzyme deficiency was identified as glucocerebrosidase. In 1984 the gene for glucocerebrosidase was cloned, and in 1991 an important breakthrough occurred with the initiation of clinical trials for enzyme replacement therapy at the National Institutes of Health (NIH).[2] Gaucher's disease became the first enzyme-deficiency disorder to be successfully treated with infusion of replacement enzyme.[4–7] Table 22–3 summarizes the chronology of Gaucher's disease.

Classification and Clinical Features

Gaucher's disease has three clinically recognizable types: the adult or nonneuronopathic form (type I); the infantile, acute, or malignant neuronopathic form (type II); and the juvenile or subacute neuronopathic form (type III). Gaucher's types I, II, and III all have in common the triad of hepatosplenomegaly, Gaucher's cells in the bone marrow, and an increase in serum acid phosphatase (Table 22–4).[8] The severity of the disease and the patient's age when the disease is first manifested are related to the magnitude of the enzyme deficiency. Table 22–5 briefly summarizes the characteristics of each type of Gaucher's disease.

The accumulation of glucocerebrosides, the result of the

➤ **Table 22–1**
LIPID STORAGE DISEASES

Gaucher's disease

Niemann-Pick disease

Tay-Sachs disease

Mucopolysaccharidoses

➤ **Table 22–2**
GENERAL CHARACTERISTICS OF LIPID STORAGE DISEASES

• Rare, inherited autosomal-recessive disorders

• Also known as lysosomal storage diseases because of accumulation of unmetabolized material in lysosomes

• Caused by enzyme deficiencies in lipid metabolism

• Increased incidence of some lipid storage diseases in certain ethnic groups (i.e., Gaucher's disease in Ashkenazi Jews)

• Great variation in clinical expression (i.e., asymptomatic to severe with early death)

• Effective therapy: enzyme replacement

• Most well-known and characterized: Gaucher's disease, Niemann-Pick disease, Tay-Sachs disease, and mucopolysaccharidoses

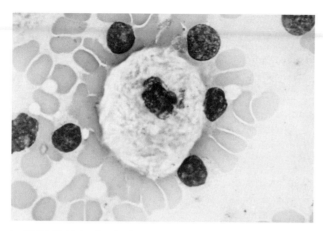

> ➤ FIGURE 22-2   Gaucher's cell, bone marrow aspirate.

enzyme deficiency of β-glucocerebrosidase, produces the distinctive Gaucher's cells (see Fig. 22–2). These cells are histiocytes that are 20 to 100 μm in diameter with a displaced nucleus. One or more round to oval nuclei are present in each cell. The cytoplasm is faintly blue with white stain and has a "crumpled tissue paper" or finely folded appearance, possibly a result of glycolipid deposition. The presence of Gaucher's cells alone is not pathognomonic for Gaucher's disease, because these cells are also found in other lymphoproliferative disorders. Gaucher's cells can be deposited in any bone in the body, which leads to a predisposition for fractures, loss of bone, and avascular necrosis (particularly in the femoral head).[2]

Bone involvement in Gaucher's disease may be presented as chronic bone pain or severe crises similar to those described in patients with sickle cell anemia.[9] The accuracy and severity of such episodes of bone involvement are unpredictable. Skeletal involvement in Gaucher's disease includes a spectrum of findings radiographically ranging from minimal bone loss and osteopenia to severe evidence of bone destruction, including osteolytic and sclerotic lesions.[2] Table 22–6 summarizes the radiologic classification of bone pathology.[9] Figure 22–3 demonstrates the osteolytic lesions seen in the x–ray of the knee of a patient with Gaucher's disease.

The underlying mechanisms of the bone complications of Gaucher's disease are not well defined. It is assumed that

> ➤ **Table 22-3**
> ## GAUCHER'S DISEASE: CHRONOLOGY

- 1882: First described by Philippe Gaucher
- Abnormal cell named Gaucher's cell
- 1900: Gaucher's disease defined as a familial disorder
- 1920: Another type of Gaucher's disease described, characterized by neurologic involvement
- Gaucher's disease classified as a lysosomal storage disorder inherited as autosomal-recessive
- 1965: Enzyme deficiency identified as glucocerebrosidase
- 1984: Gene for glucocerebrosidase cloned
- 1991: Enzyme replacement therapy in clinical trials

Gaucher's cells infiltrate the medullary space and eventually replace trabecular bone and initiate a series of events that lead to osteopenia, osteolytic lesions, and osteonecrosis. Gaucher's disease is clearly a multisystemic disorder characterized not only by skeletal disease but also by organomegaly, hematologic complications, and occasionally pulmonary involvement.[8]

Type I: Adult Gaucher's Disease (Chronic Non-neuronopathic)

Type I nonneuronopathic Gaucher's disease is the most common type of this disorder and the most common of the lipidoses. It is the most frequently inherited disorder in the Ashkenazi Jewish population. There is a remarkable degree of variability in the clinical signs and symptoms. Some patients with type I Gaucher's disease may display anemia, thrombocytopenia, massively enlarged livers and spleens, and extensive skeletal disease. In contrast, other type I Gaucher's disease patients have no symptoms at all, and the disorder is identified in their adult years only during the screening or evaluation for other diseases. The average age of onset is between 30 and 40 years. In most cases of a severe disorder, the diagnosis is made in childhood or early adulthood. Approximately two-thirds of the patients with type I Gaucher's disease are of Ashkenazi Jewish descent.[2] The remaining one-third of patients with type I disease have a panethnic distribution.

Three clinical presentations occur in the type I nonneuronopathic form of Gaucher's disease: (1) the mild presentation, which represents from 10% to 25% of patients who are essentially asymptomatic and live without the need for any treatment or intervention; (2) the moderate clinical presentation, in which the patient has hepatosplenomegaly, near-normal blood counts, and a normal physical appearance; and (3) the most severe form, in which patients present with massive hepatosplenomegaly, significant thrombocytopenia, anemia, and skeletal complications.[10] A few patients with the severe forms of the disease may develop central nervous system damage, delayed sexual maturation, severe wasting, and eventually death. It should be noted that clinical presentations can be misleading because some of these patients may still develop underlying skeletal complications (Table 22–7). It is important, therefore, to perform a baseline skeletal evaluation even in patients with a mild case of the disease. The femoral head is the most common initial bone site to be affected by the disease, and this area should be evaluated by magnetic resonance imaging (MRI) to assess for avascular necrosis.[2]

The definitive diagnosis of Gaucher's disease is made with an assay for the enzyme acid β-glucocerebrosidase activity of the leukocytes. Bone marrow examination alone is insufficient for confirming the diagnosis because Gaucher's cells may be present in other disorders.

> **Table 22-5**
GAUCHER'S DISEASE: CLINICAL SUBTYPES

Clinical Features	Type I: Nonneuronopathic (Adult Form)	Type II: Acute Neuronopathic (Infant Form)	Type III: Subacute Neuronopathic (Juvenile Form)
Clinical onset	Childhood/adulthood	Infancy	Childhood/juvenile
Estimated frequency	1/450–1/1,000	1/100,000	1/100,000
Hepatosplenomegaly	+	+	+
Hematologic complications secondary to hypersplenism	+	+	+
Skeletal deterioration (bone crises/fractures)	+	–	+
Neurodegenerative course	–	+++	++
Life expectancy	6–80+ yr	2 yr	20–40 yr
Ethnic predilection	Ashkenazi Jew	Panethnic	Swedish (Norrbottnian)

The gene for the enzyme glucocerebrosidase is located on chromosome 1q21–31. Since the characterization, cloning, and sequencing of the glucocerebrosidase gene in 1984, more than 40 genetic mutations have been described.[1] The mutations include both single insertional and point mutations as well as crossover mutations. All of the mutations that cause Gaucher's disease have complex effects on the properties of this enzyme.[11] The normal enzyme, glucocerebrosidase (acid β-glucosidase), is a lysosomal enzyme responsible for the degradation of the glucosylceramide molecule, preventing its buildup in tissue cells.[12] Protein synthesis of the normal enzyme occurs in the endoplasmic reticulum, with transport to the Golgi apparatus for glycosylation and delivery to the lysosomes of the cell. Mutations at the genetic level that code for the production of this enzyme have direct effects on the catalytic activity, with decreases from 5- to 100-fold.[13] In addition, enzyme stability and half-life activity (normal is 60 hours) are also decreased for acid β-glucosidase as a result of these mutations.[14]

Type II: Infantile Gaucher's Disease (Acute or Malignant Neuronopathic)

Type II Gaucher's disease is a much rarer form that occurs in infancy, and patients rarely survive past the age of 2 years. Type II acute neuronopathic Gaucher's disease is seen in all ethnic groups, although it is uncommon in the Jewish population.[2] The frequency of type II disease is estimated at approximately 1 in 100,000.[2] The hallmark of type II Gaucher's disease is neurologic involvement, including multiple signs such as difficulty swallowing, opisthotonos (extreme arching of the spine), and other manifestations of brain stem involvement that are noted early in infancy.[15] The infant has difficulty in feeding and fails to grow. Death usually occurs before the age of 2 years. Familial intermarriage is frequently found in the infant's family history.

The clinical presentation of this type II disease is much more uniform than that observed in type I Gaucher's disease and is very severe. The disease exhibits a progressive pattern of clinical symptoms, with hepatosplenomegaly evident within the first 6 months of life, and is often discovered by 3 months of age. The principle cause of death in infants with type II Gaucher's disease is brain stem damage.

Type III: Juvenile Gaucher's Disease (Subacute Neuronopathic)

Type III Gaucher's disease may be present from early childhood to the teenage years and is characterized by clinical and physical findings and survivals ranging between those of type I and type II.[2] Type III has been noted, especially, in a group of children from northern Sweden, the off-

> **Table 22-6**
RADIOLOGIC CLASSIFICATION OF GAUCHER BONE PATHOLOGY

Stage	Description
1. Osteopenia	Coarse trabecular pattern of decreased bone density, which may be localized or diffuse
2. Medullary expansion	Loss of normal concavity above femoral condyles
3. Localized destruction (osteolysis)	Small erosions, well-defined or moth-eaten, cortex rarefied and endosteally notched, ground-glass veiling
4. Ischemic necrosis of long bone, sclerosis, osteitis	Patchy densities and erosions serpiginous sclerotic streaks, layered periostitis, sequestra
5. Diffuse destruction, epiphyseal collapse, osteoarthrosis	Flattening or irregular destruction of femoral heads with mixed lytic and sclerotic foci, larger "soap bubble" pattern

Source: Wenstrup, RJ (ed): Antiresorptive bone therapy in Gaucher disease. Gaucher Clin Persp 6:12,1998.

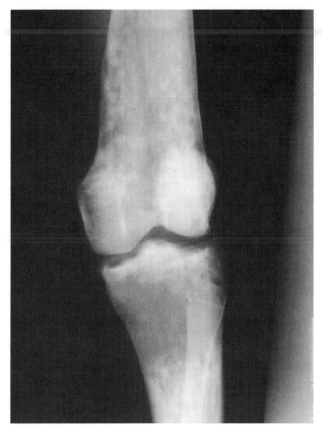

➤ **FIGURE 22–3** Anteroposterior radiograph of the knee shows diffuse mottled increased density of the distal femur and proximal tibia, characteristic of widespread bone infarction in Gaucher's disease. The metaphyseal regions are broader than normal, resembling an Erlenmeyer flask deformity. (Courtesy of Charles S. Resnik, MD, Department of Diagnostic Radiology, University of Maryland Medical Center, Baltimore, Maryland.)

vival. Table 22–8 compares the clinical characteristics of type IIIa and type IIIb Gaucher's disease.

Laboratory Diagnosis

Peripheral blood, bone marrow, and spleen are the sites most frequently examined in patients with Gaucher's disease. The peripheral blood nearly always demonstrates a moderate normocytic, normochromic anemia with thrombocytopenia because of the replacement of normal hematopoietic cells with Gaucher's cells in the bone marrow. There is pooling of blood in the enlarged spleen and some degree of ineffective erythropoiesis, with decreased incorporation of iron in erythroid precursors in the bone marrow. As a result, active signs of a compensated anemia such as polychromasia and nucleated red blood cells are usually absent on the peripheral smear.[18] Leukocytes are commonly decreased in number. Platelets are also usually decreased in number as a result of splenic sequestration. These patients may have a bleeding tendency, with nosebleeds especially common. Gaucher's cells are noted only rarely in the peripheral blood. Bone marrow aspirates are often the first tissue in which Gaucher's cells are detected; these cells are required for diagnosis (see Fig. 22–2). They are histiocytes, 20 to 100 μm in diameter, found in moderate numbers and as clumps of cells in the thickest areas of the smear. One or more round to oval nuclei are present in each cell. The cytoplasm is faintly blue with Wright's stain and has a "crumbled tissue paper" or finely folded appearance, possibly as a result of glycolipid deposition. Electron microscopy has demonstrated that this appearance is the result of lamellar bodies stacked inside secondary phagolysosomes. These cells stain positive with periodic acid–Schiff (PAS), acid phosphatase, Giemsa, iron, Sudan black B, and oil red O stains because of the accumulation of the unmetabolized glucocerebroside. It is important to note that the presence of Gaucher's cells is not pathognomonic for Gaucher's disease, because these cells are also found in other lymphoproliferative disorders.

The spleen is variably enlarged, owing to the accumulation of masses of Gaucher's cells. The enlargement is commonly up to 10 times normal splenic weight and can cause considerable discomfort to the patient. Other organs and systems commonly affected include the liver and, in type II, the nervous system, pituitary gland, kidneys, lung, and ovaries. These organs contain massive deposits of Gaucher's cells.

The serum acid phosphatase level is increased, and isozyme measurement of this enzyme has shown that the tartrate-resistant fraction is what is increased in patients with Gaucher's disease. Table 22–9 summarizes the laboratory findings in Gaucher's disease.

Although the Gaucher's cell is associated with the disease, so-called pseudo-Gaucher's cells have also been described. They are seen in disease states with increased cellular turn-

spring of several related intermarriages. The frequency of type III Gaucher's disease among some Swedes is approximately 1 in 100,000.[2] Neurologic involvement is also characteristic of type III Gaucher's disease; however, the clinical manifestations are much more heterogeneous than those observed in type II.

Two distinct subtypes of type III Gaucher's disease have been described.[16] The classic form, type IIIa, usually presents itself clinically between early childhood and mid-adult life. Type IIIb Gaucher's disease is characterized by a clinically aggressive systemic disease with neurologic involvement of isolated horizontal supranuclear gaze palsy as the major sign.[17] Ocular motor disorder is the distinctive neurologic feature of type IIIb Gaucher's disease. Generally, in type III Gaucher's disease regardless of the subtype, the more severe the neurologic disease, the shorter the sur-

➤ **Table 22–7**
CLINICAL PRESENTATIONS OF TYPE I GAUCHER'S DISEASE

Mild	Moderate	Severe
10%–25% of patients	Hepatosplenomegaly	Massive hepatosplenomegaly
Asymptomatic	Near-normal blood counts	Significant thrombocytopenia
No need for treatment	Normal physical appearance	Anemia, skeletal complications

> **Table 22-8**
COMPARISON OF TYPE IIIa AND IIIb GAUCHER'S DISEASE

	Type IIIa	Type IIIb
Clinical onset	Early childhood to mid-adult	Infancy to early childhood
Clinical course	Mild to moderately severe	Aggressive systemic disease
Neurologic involvement	At onset; multifocal rapid jerky movements, ataxia, spasticity, dementia, and seizures	Ocular motor disorder, horizontal supranuclear gaze palsy; mild cognitive impairment

over, especially chronic myelogenous leukemia, in which the phenomenon was first described. In theory, the increased cell turnover presents so much glycosylceramide to the reticuloendothelial system that its enzyme system is overwhelmed and cannot adequately metabolize all of the material. The excess is therefore stored in histiocytes, with their end morphological expression identical to that of true Gaucher's cells. This phenomenon is also seen in a variety of other disorders, including acute myelocytic leukemia, chronic lymphocytic leukemia, plasma cell myeloma, aplastic anemia, idiopathic thrombocytopenic purpura, thalassemia major, and rheumatoid arthritis[19] (Table 22–10). The presence of Gaucher-like cells in patients with these diseases has no known prognostic significance. It should be emphasized that in each of these diseases there is no deficiency of the β-glucocerebrosidase, as there is in Gaucher's disease, but rather an overtaxation of a normal system.

Prognosis
As previously stated, the length of survival in patients with Gaucher's disease is variable and depends on the type. The adult form (type I) has the longest survival, with patients surviving commonly into adulthood. In the infantile form (type II), survival beyond 2 years of age is rare. Like the clinical features, survival in the juvenile form (type III) is intermediate between the first two, and patients usually live into adolescence. A relatively increased risk of cancer in patients with Gaucher's disease has been reported,[20] primarily because of an increased incidence of hematologic malignancy. Patients with Gaucher's disease are 15 times more likely to develop a hematologic malignancy than a healthy individual. Table 22–11 lists the most frequently reported hematologic malignancies. This increased risk of malignancy may be associated with immunologic abnormalities found in patients

with Gaucher's disease. These abnormalities include increased helper-to-suppressor (T_4:T_8) cell ratio, decreased natural killer (null) cells, polyclonal B-cell lymphocytosis, and plasmacytosis.[20] Table 22–12 lists the immunologic abnormalities described in Gaucher's disease.

Treatment
Before the advent of the newer treatment modality of enzyme replacement therapy, Gaucher's disease was traditionally managed by supportive therapy. Total or partial splenectomy was frequently performed. In addition, transfusions, orthopedic procedures, and occasionally bone marrow transplantation were used in some patients. Although potentially curative, allogeneic bone marrow transplantation is an extremely aggressive and high-risk therapy. In 1991, a major advancement occurred in the treatment of Gaucher's disease type I. The U.S. Food and Drug Administration approved the use of enzyme replacement therapy for this disorder. Gaucher's disease is the first lysosomal storage disorder for which enzyme replacement therapy is available. Enzyme replacement therapy has successfully reversed many of the clinical complications of this disorder, including correcting blood counts and reducing the organomegaly that occurs in these patients.[21–25]

> **Table 22-9**
GAUCHER'S DISEASE: LABORATORY FINDINGS

Normocytic, normochromic or normocytic, hypochromic anemia

Leukopenia

Thrombocytopenia

Gaucher's cells in bone marrow (BM) aspirate

Increased serum acid phosphatase

Positive staining of Gaucher's cells in BM with PAS, acid phosphatase, Giemsa, iron, Sudan black B, and oil red O stains

Abbreviation: PAS = para-aminosalicylic acid

> **Table 22-10**
DISORDERS IN WHICH "PSEUDO-GAUCHER'S" CELLS HAVE BEEN DESCRIBED

Acute myelocytic leukemia (AML)

Chronic lymphocytic leukemia (CLL)

Plasma cell myeloma

Aplastic anemia

Idiopathic thrombocytopenic purpura (ITP)

Thalassemia major

Rheumatoid arthritis

> **Table 22-11**
MOST FREQUENTLY REPORTED HEMATOLOGIC MALIGNANCIES IN GAUCHER'S DISEASE

Multiple myeloma

Chronic lymphocytic leukemia (CLL)

Hodgkin's disease and non-Hodgkin's lymphoma

Acute leukemia

> **Table 22-12**
> ## IMMUNOLOGIC ABNORMALITIES DESCRIBED IN GAUCHER'S DISEASE

Increased helper-to-suppressor (T_4:T_8) cell ratio

Decreased natural killer (null) cells

Polyclonal B-cell lymphocytosis

Plasmacytosis

> **Table 22-14**
> ## CLINICAL MANIFESTATIONS OF NIEMANN-PICK DISEASE

Growth retardation

Hepatosplenomegaly

Lymphadenopathy

Pigmentation

Neurologic impairment

The first enzyme replacement therapy utilized was a purified enzyme from human placenta. This enzyme, which is an alglucerase injection, is manufactured by Genzyme Corporation as Ceredase and has demonstrated effectiveness by the reversal of signs and symptoms of Gaucher type I, nonneuronopathic disease.[4] Another form of the enzyme, the recombinant form, which is also produced by Genzyme Corporation as Cerezyme, is genetically engineered and has the advantage of being unlimited in supply. In addition, the recombinant Cerezyme has the advantage of a very low risk of transmitting any infectious agent and also has a lower rate of patients developing IgG antibodies to the glucocerebrosidase enzyme.[26]

Niemann-Pick Disease

This inherited form of lipid storage disease was first described in 1914 by Niemann and subsequently by Pick in 1933.[27]

Niemann-Pick disease is caused by a deficiency of the enzyme sphingomyelinase, with a secondary accumulation of the unmetabolized lipid sphingomyelin as well as cholesterol. Sphingomyelin is a sphingophospholipid that is a common constituent of cell membranes as well as cellular organelles. As a result, a deficiency of sphingomyelinase is a serious disorder. Table 22–13 summarizes the general characteristics of Niemann-Pick disease.

A wide variety of clinical manifestations of variable severity have been reported in patients with Niemann-Pick disease. These include growth retardation, hepatosplenomegaly, lymphadenopathy, pigmentation, and impaired neurologic functions (Table 22–14).[28] A large number of lipid-laden giant foam cells known as *Niemann-Pick cells* can be found in affected tissues and organs (Fig. 22–4 and Color Plate 254). The detection of Niemann-Pick cells in patients with this disorder is essential for the diagnosis of this disease. There is an increased incidence of Niemann-Pick disease in the Jewish population, especially in consanguineous groups. Because of

the very different clinical manifestations of the disease, five types, A through E, have been described.[29] Only types A, B, and C are discussed here. Type E, which is very rare, has been found only in adults and is characterized by a mild chronic course and a lack of neurologic manifestations. Table 22–15 compares types A, B, and C of Niemann-Pick disease.

Classification and Clinical Features

Type A
This form is also known as *infantile* or *classic Niemann-Pick disease.* It is the most common form, accounting for up to 85% of all cases of Niemann-Pick disease. The onset is early in infancy and is associated with failure to thrive, difficulty feeding, and retarded physical and mental development. The skin has a waxy consistency. There is often jaundice at birth and, usually, hepatosplenomegaly with a distended abdomen. The lymph nodes are enlarged as well. A cherry-red spot in the macula of the eye is found in approximately 50% of the affected infants. The neurologic symptoms are more pronounced in this type of Niemann-Pick disease than in any of the other types. Deterioration is rapid, and survival past the age of 1 or 2 years is rare.

Type B
Also called the *chronic* or *adult form,* type B Niemann-Pick disease is much more rare than type A, with approximately 20 reported cases in the literature. Clinical onset consisting of hepatosplenomegaly usually occurs in infancy, but the central nervous system is not involved. Individuals with this type of disease may live longer than those with type A, but they do not survive beyond childhood or early adolescence.

> **Table 22-13**
> ## GENERAL CHARACTERISTICS OF NIEMANN-PICK DISEASE

Inherited lipid storage disease

Caused by a deficiency of the enzyme sphingomyelinase

Niemann-Pick cells (lipid-laden giant foam cells) found in bone marrow aspirate, tissues, and organs

Increased incidence in the Jewish population

Five types, A to E, have been described

Wide variety of clinical manifestations

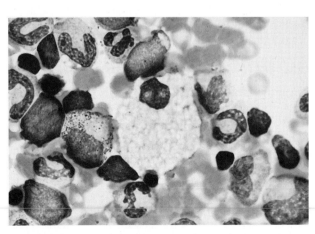

> **FIGURE 22-4** Niemann-Pick cell, bone marrow aspirate.

> **Table 22-15**
COMPARISON OF TYPES A, B, AND C NIEMANN-PICK DISEASE

Classification	Type A, Infantile or Classic	Type B, Chronic or Adult	Type C, Two Forms: Infantile or Juvenile Form and Adolescent or Adult Form
Incidence	Accounts for 85% of all cases	Rare	Rare
Clinical manifestations	Jaundice at birth, hepatospleno-megaly, enlarged lymph nodes, cherry-red spot in macula of the eye, neurologic symptoms, retarded physical and mental development	Hepatosplenomegaly	Hepatosplenomegaly in infantile form, splenomegaly in the adult form, neurologic abnormalities, neuro-ophthalmologic findings, seizures
Survival	1–2 yr	Childhood or early adolescence	Juvenile or adulthood

Type C

Type C Niemann-Pick disease has been described in two forms, an infantile or juvenile form with a prolonged life span, and an adolescent or adulthood form, which is generally slower in evolution and progression.[30] The primary defect in type C Niemann-Pick disease is still unknown. However, this type is characterized by a milder defect in sphingomyelinase activity and an abnormality in cholesterol transport reflected in an alteration in cholesterol esterification from exogenous cholesterol.

Type C Niemann-Pick disease is an autosomal-recessive disease characterized by a gradual and ill-defined onset of neurologic abnormalities, which include unsteady gait, poor motor coordination, slurred speech, dysphagia, and ophthalmoplegia.[29] When neurologic symptoms appear, psychotic manifestations may also be predominant. Neuro-ophthalmologic findings in which the oculomotor system is often affected are also characteristic. In addition, seizures often appear with neurologic involvement, with grand mal seizures most frequently observed. Frequent seizures may contribute to the mental deterioration observed in patients with type C Niemann-Pick disease. Hepatosplenomegaly is a constant finding in the infantile or juvenile form, whereas hepatomegaly is often absent in the adult form. Splenomegaly, however, is present in the adult form, with thrombocytopenia being a sign of hypersplenism. The characteristic foam cell, Niemann-Pick cell, or sea-blue histiocytes, or a combination, are a consistent finding in the bone marrow of patients with type C Niemann-Pick disease. Diagnosis of type C Niemann-Pick disease is made with the finding of the characteristic abnormality in cholesterol transport and esterification from exogenous cholesterol.

Laboratory Diagnosis

There is a distinct pattern to the histiocytes in Niemann-Pick disease. These cells are most commonly seen in bone marrow and spleen, although they accumulate throughout the body and in the nervous system in patients with type A disease. They are large cells, 20 to 90 μm in diameter, with an inconspicuous nucleus. The cytoplasm is filled with and distended by round, uniformly sized droplets of accumulated lipid, turning the cell a very pale or light blue when Wright-stained (see Fig. 22–4). Stains producing a positive reaction with Niemann-Pick cells are the lipid stains oil red O, Sudan black, and luxol fast blue; and acid phosphatase and nonspecific esterase. The PAS staining is weak, and the myeloperoxidase stain is negative.

The bone marrow of some adult patients with certain varieties of Niemann-Pick disease contains a mixture of Niemann-Pick cells and sea-blue histiocytes (histiocytes distended with blue-staining ceroid on Wright's stain). It is believed that the sphingomyelin is gradually metabolized to ceroid, thus generating the sea-blue histiocytes. A marrow specimen with these findings would then need to be distinguished from the entity of sea-blue histiocytosis (see the section at the end of this chapter).

Other disorders that may cause Niemann-Pick–like cells in the bone marrow are GM_1 gangliosidosis, lactosyl ceramidosis, and Fabry's disease.

The peripheral blood is most remarkable for the vacuoles that may be found in lymphocytes and monocytes of a routine peripheral blood smear (Fig. 22–5 and Color Plate 255). These vacuoles are round, and from 2 to 20 may be found within one cell. Anemia and leukopenia may be present but do not usually present any threat to the patient. Serum lipids are not usually increased. An assay of the enzyme sphingomyelinase activity in leukocytes and fibroblasts can also be performed.

Prognosis and Treatment

There may be a slightly longer survival in patients with the other types of Niemann-Pick disease, but those with type A

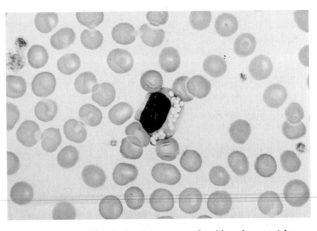

> **FIGURE 22–5**   Tay-Sachs disease, vacuolated lymphocytes (also characteristic of Niemann-Pick disease).

have a very short life expectancy. Survival past the age of 2 years is uncommon. Currently there is no treatment for Niemann-Pick disease. However, successful allogeneic bone marrow transplants have been reported for type B.[18] In addition, research studies have focused on finding a source of enzyme replacement for sphingomyelinase[31] and gene therapy using retroviruses.[32]

Tay-Sachs Disease

Also known as GM$_2$ gangliosidosis, Tay-Sachs disease was first described in 1881 by the British ophthalmologist Warren Tay. In 1886, the New York neurologist Bernard Sachs used the term *familial amaurotic infantile idiocy* to describe this disorder. Its incidence in the Ashkenazi Jewish population is 100 times greater than that in the non-Jewish population.[33] It is estimated that this high-risk group has a 1 in 30 carrier rate. This autosomal-recessive sphingolipidosis is the result of a deficiency of the enzyme hexosaminidase A, with an increase of the other isoenzyme, hexosaminidase B. The gene for hexosaminidase A is located on chromosome 15.[33] Inheritance of two abnormal alleles (one from each parent) accounts for almost all infantile Tay-Sachs cases in the Ashkenazi Jewish population. The severity of the disease correlates with the level of residual enzyme activity. The unmetabolized GM$_2$ ganglioside accumulates in almost all tissues and has its most devastating effects within the central nervous system and eye.[34] Table 22–16 summarizes the general characteristics of Tay-Sachs disease.[35]

Clinical Features

Although affected infants appear normal at birth, by 6 months of age both physical and mental deterioration are notable. They have an exaggerated physical response to noise (the startle reflex) beginning at age 3 to 5 months. There is a progressive loss of motor function with weakness, decreased attentiveness to surroundings, hypotonia (diminished tone of skeletal muscles), and poor head control between the ages of 6 and 10 months.[35] In addition, a cherry-red spot in the macula of each eye is found; this is the most characteristic feature of Tay-Sachs disease. The central nervous system steadily degenerates after 1 year of age. Along with the continual deterioration, there is enlargement of the head (macrocephaly), seizures, and paralysis. Spasticity with hyperactive reflexes, deafness, and

> **Table 22-16**
> **GENERAL CHARACTERISTICS OF TAY-SACHS DISEASE**

Known as GM$_2$ gangliosidosis

Autosomal-recessive inheritance

Caused by deficiency of hexosaminidase A

Higher incidence in Ashkenazi Jewish population

Central nervous system degeneration

Physical and mental deterioration

Cherry-red spot in the macula of each eye

Macrocephaly (enlargement of head)

Seizures and paralysis

Death by 4 years old

blindness follow. The neurons are greatly enlarged by accumulation of the unmetabolized ganglioside in vacuoles in the cytoplasm. In contrast to many other lipid storage diseases, the spleen, liver, and lymph nodes are not enlarged. Feeding is poor, and death occurs by 4 years of age. It should be noted that cherry-red spots are not pathognomonic for Tay-Sachs disease; however, this clinical finding in a Jewish infant with the absence of organomegaly is strongly suggestive of Tay-Sachs disease.[36]

Laboratory Diagnosis

A deficiency of hexosaminidase A is the basic cause of this disease. Hexosaminidase A is the enzyme responsible for hydrolyzing GM$_2$ ganglioside, the glycolipid that accumulates in neurons. This deficiency can be demonstrated in the serum, plasma, leukocytes, and cultured fibroblasts of infants with Tay-Sachs disease.

The major site of pathology is in the central nervous system, and examination of other tissues is less informative. The peripheral blood contains vacuolated lymphocytes (see Fig. 22–5). The number and size of the vacuoles are related to the duration of the disease. It is postulated, but not definitely proven, that they contain the unmetabolized lipid GM$_2$ ganglioside. Vacuolated lymphocytes, however, are not pathognomonic for Tay-Sachs disease, because they are also seen in Niemann-Pick disease and in certain types of leukemias. Foam cells, or vacuolated histiocytes, are found in the bone marrow. The presence of these cells is helpful but not diagnostic for the disease.

Because of the high frequency of this disease in certain populations, prenatal detection has taken on greater importance. Culture of fetal fibroblasts from the amniotic fluid can be undertaken to detect hexosaminidase A levels in the fetus. Mass screening programs of adults at possible risk for transmitting the disease have been undertaken, with variable success.

Prognosis and Treatment

The infantile form of Tay-Sachs disease is uniformly fatal before age 4. Enzyme replacement is now being attempted, and the final results of the potential therapy are not yet known. Patients with the juvenile and adult forms of Tay-Sachs disease have longer survival than those with the infantile form, although it is quite variable. Supportive treatment remains the mainstay of this disorder, which includes management of hydration, recurrent infections, and seizures with conventional fluids, antibiotics, and drugs, respectively. Prenatal diagnosis can be performed by measuring hexosaminidase A in amniotic fluid, cultured amniocytes, or chorionic villus samples.

Mucopolysaccharidoses

The mucopolysaccharidoses (MPSs) are rare disorders that constitute a group of lysosomal storage diseases caused by a deficiency in one of the enzymes involved in the breakdown of mucopolysaccharides.[34]

Similar to the previously described disorders, the MPSs show accumulations of unmetabolized material within lysosomes (Fig. 22–6 and Color Plate 256); however, it is mucopolysaccharides, not sphingolipids, that accumulate. Products are found in the reticuloendothelial system (spleen, bone marrow, liver), lymph nodes, blood vessels, brain, heart, connective tissue, and urine. The clinical severity of these disor-

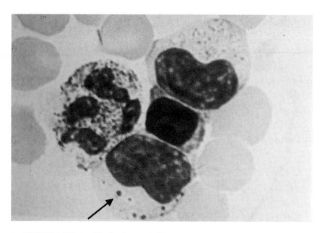

➤ **FIGURE 22–6** Hurler's anomaly.

ders varies widely, with mild, intermediate, and severe forms. Multiple clinical presentations exist, including skeletal abnormalities, organomegaly, facial dysmorphism, and corneal opacities.

The original description of children affected with different forms of the MPSs was published within a relatively short time span at the turn of the century. In London in 1900, Dr. John Thompson first described three young brothers with the characteristics of MPS. Gertrud Hurler elaborated on his description, describing two unrelated boys in Munich in 1919 with very similar characteristics, now known as Hurler's syndrome. In 1917, Hunter described two brothers with a constellation of abnormalities now recognized as Hunter's syndrome. Table 22–17 summarizes the general characteristics of MPSs.

Classification

The MPSs have been arranged into seven categories, but there are only four possible unmetabolized products that build up in tissues: keratan sulfate, dermatan sulfate, heparan sulfate, and chondroitin sulfate. Table 22–18 gives an abbreviated classification scheme for MPSs.[34] With the exception of Hunter's syndrome, which is X-linked recessive, these disorders have an autosomal-recessive mode of inheritance. There does not appear to be a significant increase of affected individuals within any one ethnic group.

In terms of the biochemical classification of MPS, very different clinical phenotypes can result from different mutations at the same locus. Characterization of these mutations showed deletions for MPS I, II, and III, and point mutation for MPS IV.[37]

> ## Table 22–17
> ## GENERAL CHARACTERISTICS OF MUCOPOLYSACCHARIDOSES
>
> Rare lyosomal storage disease
>
> Autosomal-recessive inheritance
>
> Deficiency of one of the enzymes involved in the breakdown of mucopolysaccharides
>
> Panethnicity
>
> Different clinical phenotypes resulting from different mutations at the same locus

For example, in MPS I H (Hurler's disease) and in MPS I S (Scheie's syndrome), mutations at the same locus of the enzyme alpha (α)-iduronidase occur for both disorders, producing quite different clinical phenotypes.[38] In Hurler's disease, there is a progressive mental and physical deterioration, with death occurring usually in the first decade of life. This is in contrast to the course in Scheie's disease, in which the condition is milder, intellect is normal into adult life, and life expectancy is normal. The presence of many different mutations at the α-iduronidase enzyme locus that may be inherited in either the homozygous or heterozygous state accounts for the wide variation in clinical phenotypes. The use of molecular probes to characterize these mutations will eventually allow correlations to be made between mutations and phenotypes.

Clinical Features

Many clinical abnormalities are found within each type of MPS, which are outlined in Table 22–18. The findings in Hurler's syndrome are given in the most detail, because it is considered the prototype of the MPSs.

In patients with Hurler's syndrome (MPS I), there may be a short period of apparently normal development, but this is only temporary. These individuals are abnormally short and have coarse facial features, with a broad, flat nose, widely spaced eyes, and thickened tongue and lips.[39] Some authors have described their appearance as similar to that of a gargoyle (the carved heads sometimes found on older European churches). The amount of body hair is increased, dark, and especially prominent on the forehead. The skin is thickened. Patients are mentally retarded. Clouding of the corneas of the eyes is present. These individuals may have hearing loss or be completely deaf. The heart is damaged, owing to the accumulation of mucopolysaccharides in the valves and blood vessels. There is a hump on the back and a prominent abdomen, with enlarged liver and spleen. The arms and legs are abnormal, with contractures of many joints. In addition, the hands are very wide and the fingers shortened.

In Hunter's syndrome (MPS II), the changes are similar, although not as severe. Corneal clouding is much less common. Patients affected with Sanfilippo's syndrome (MPS III) have a more normal stature but unfortunately many more severe neurologic problems and decreased survival. Compared with patients with Hurler's syndrome, those with Scheie's syndrome (MPS I S) have more prominent corneal clouding but less abnormality in stature, facial appearance, and mental development. Patients with Maroteaux-Lamy syndrome (MPS VI) have growth and skeletal abnormalities but no mental retardation. In Morquio's syndrome (MPS IV), patients have numerous skeletal changes, giving a markedly abnormal physical appearance; however, there is no mental retardation.[34]

Laboratory Diagnosis

An accurate enzymatic diagnosis should be established for all suspected cases of MPS, as clinical diagnosis alone is often impossible because of overlapping phenotypes. The diagnosis of MPS can be made by performing simple enzyme assays using leukocytes, serum, or fibroblasts.[40] The identification of heterozygotes, however, is still a difficult process because of the overlays of normal and heterozygous levels of enzyme activity. Molecular studies such as

> **Table 22-18**
MUCOPOLYSACCHARIDOSES (MPSs)

Category	Mode of Inheritance	Accumulated Product	Enzyme Deficiency	Clinical Features	Life Expectancy
MPS I H (Hurler's)	Autosomal recessive	Heparan sulfate Dermatan sulfate	α-L-iduronidase	Onset 6–8 months, severe mental retardation, dwarfism, large long head, flat broad nose with upturned nostrils (coarse facies), corneal clouding, hepatosplenomegaly, valvular lesions, coronary artery lesions, skeletal deformities, joint stiffness	6–10 yr
MPS I S (Scheie's)	Autosomal recessive	Heparan sulfate Dermatan sulfate	α-L-iduronidase	Onset after 5 yr, normal intelligence, stiff joints (especially of the hands), near-normal height, corneal clouding, valvular lesions, coronary artery lesions	Normal
MPS I H-S (Hurler-Scheie)	Autosomal recessive	Heparan sulfate Dermatan sulfate	α-L-iduronidase	Onset infancy, mild retardation (may be normal), dwarfism, facial and bony lesions of Hurler's syndrome, cardiac lesions	3rd decade
MPS II (Hunter's) (wide range of severity)	X-linked recessive	Heparan sulfate Dermatan sulfate	Iduronate α-sulfatase	Mild retardation to normal intelligence, similar to Hurler's syndrome, but not corneal clouding, retinal degeneration, deafness, nodular skin infiltrates	2nd decade to normal
MPS III (Sanfilippo's A) (Sanfilippo's B) (Sanfilippo's C) (Sanfilippo's D) (wide range of severity)	Autosomal recessive	Heparan sulfate	Heparan N-sulfatase, α-N-Acetyl-glucosaminidase, α-Glucosaminide transferase N-Acetylglucosamine-6-sulfatase	Onset after 3 yr, mild to severe mental retardation, normal growth, Hurler's facies, no corneal clouding, no heart disease, no hepatosplenomegaly, mild skeletal changes	2nd–3rd decade
MPS IV A (Morquio's) (wide range of severity)	Autosomal recessive	Keratan sulfate Chondroitin sulfate	N-Acetylgalactosamine, 6-sulfate sulfatase	Normal intelligence, severe skeletal deformities, dwarfism, thoracolumbar gibbus	3rd–6th decade
MPS IV B (Morquio's)			β-Galactosidase	Kyphoscoliosis, facies similar to Hurler's syndrome, corneal clouding, valvular and coronary artery lesions, joint hypermobility, genu valgum	

continued

➤ **Table 22-18**
MUCOPOLYSACCHARIDOSES (MPSs) (Continued)

Category	Mode of Inheritance	Accumulated Product	Enzyme Deficiency	Clinical Features	Life Expectancy
MPS VI (Maroteaux-Lamy)	Autosomal recessive	Dermatan sulfate	N-Acetylgalac-tosamine 4-sulfatase, (arylsulfa-tase B)	Similar to Hurler's syndrome, but normal intelligence, longer survival	2nd decade
MPS VII (Glucuronidase deficiency disease)	Autosomal recessive	Dermatan sulfate Heparan sulfate Chondroitin sulfate	β-Glucuroni-dase	Variable from severe mental retardation with dysostosis multiplex and hep-atosplenomegaly to a milder form; also severe neonatal form with hydrops fetalis	Variable, 1–40 yr

Source: Modified from Fensom, AH, and Benson PF: Recent advances in the prenatal diagnosis of the mucopolysaccharidoses. Prenatal Diagn 14:1, 1994.

the cloning of complementary deoxyribonucleic acids (cDNAs) can complement accurate enzyme assays.[40] Several specialized substrates used for the diagnosis of MPS are now available commercially.

In contrast to findings in the other lysosomal storage diseases, nonmetabolized products may be detected in the urine of patients with MPS.[39] Using the toluidine blue spot test or the turbidity test to detect acid mucopolysaccharides is the initial screening test. The spot test may be unreliable, however, with up to 32% false-negative test results in patients with Hurler's syndrome reported. Also of note is that the urine of normal healthy newborn infants may give false-positive results, a phenomenon that disappears by 2 weeks of age. Any positive screening test result should be confirmed by lysosomal enzyme assays.

An interesting but somewhat inconsistent finding in the peripheral blood of patients with MPS is the presence of large granules in leukocytes, especially lymphocytes. These are known as *Alder-Reilly bodies* (see Fig. 22–6). In polymorphonuclear leukocytes this needs to be distinguished from toxic granulation, but the large size of the granules in MPS usually leaves little doubt. A metachromatic stain, such as toluidine blue, aids in confirmation. These granules are found with much greater regularity, however, in histiocytes and lymphocytes in the bone marrow.

Prognosis

The prognosis of the MPSs varies somewhat with the type. Patients with Hurler's syndrome may live only one decade, whereas those affected with Hunter's syndrome may live into their twenties.[39] The theoretical aid of enzyme replacement therapy has yet to be translated into practical results.

Treatment

Bone marrow transplantation has been used successfully in treating some patients with MPS.[41] More studies are needed, however, to prove that bone marrow transplanta-

tion can be a practical treatment leading to a complete cure. Prenatal diagnosis is still important, including first-trimester diagnosis by chorionic villus sampling, early amniocentesis for more sensitive lysosomal enzyme assays, use of DNA analysis for detecting mutations, and the possibility of preimplantation diagnosis of early embryos after in vitro fertilization.

➤ HISTIOCYTOSIS

Sea-Blue Histiocyte Syndrome

Although initially described in isolated case reports of young adults with an enlarged spleen, the syndrome of the sea-blue histiocyte is a genetic disorder with a benign course. The striking blue color of the histiocytes after staining with Wright's or May-Grünwald-Giemsa stain gives the syndrome its name.

The mode of transmission has not been clearly established, but autosomal-recessive inheritance, with a variable degree of expression, appears most likely. Most patients receive the diagnosis before they reach 40 years of age. The earlier in life the disease is found, the more severe it is likely to be. Major findings on physical examination are splenomegaly and usually hepatomegaly. Also described, but occurring less consistently, are abnormalities of the eyes, skin, and nervous system. Involvement of the lung may be noted on radiographic examination. Involvement of the lymph nodes is not seen.

Significant laboratory findings are usually confined to the blood. In the peripheral blood, thrombocytopenia is found with great frequency. Consequently, clinical manifestations such as epistaxis, gastrointestinal tract bleeding, and purpura may be expected. However, there is no correlation of the degree of thrombocytopenia with the size of the spleen. Blood lipid levels are normal. Abnormal liver function study results are only rarely seen.

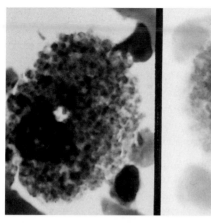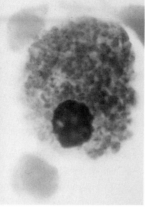

➤ **FIGURE 22–7** Sea-blue histiocytes. Note the abnormally coarse azurophilic granules present in neutrophils, lymphocytes, and monocytes. (From Hyun, BH, et al: Bone marrow. In: Practical Hematology. A Laboratory Guide with Accompanying Filmstrip. WB Saunders, Philadelphia, 1975, with permission.)

The bone marrow aspirate is usually the site of diagnosis. Histiocytes of variable size (20 to 60 μm) are present in greatly increased numbers. They contain the blue-to-green staining granules that vary in size, shape, and ability to take up the stain (Fig. 22–7 and Color Plate 257). Thus, not all cells will have the same staining intensity. It is not currently known why the granules stain blue with these stains. The cells also react with the PAS, Sudan black B, and acid-fast stains, but not with toluidine blue or iron stains.[42]

Most patients with this syndrome do well and have normal life spans. Splenectomy is not always required; many patients never have the spleen removed. As previously mentioned, manifestations of the disease at an early age may imply more severe symptoms. Table 22–19 summarizes the general characteristics of sea-blue histiocytosis.

Other Histiocytic Disorders (Eosinophilic Granuloma, Hand-Schüller-Christian Disease, Letterer-Siwe Disease)

This group of "histiocytic" disorders represents an abnormal proliferation and accumulation of mature histiocytes, or Langerhans' cells. Langerhans' cells are large but inconspicuous cells in the skin whose function is to process and present antigen to other cells in the area, including lymphocytes.[29] These cells, as well as histiocytes, are normally found in small numbers in the skin and reticuloendothelial system. Most patients with these disorders are either children or young adults. A favorable outcome may be expected in most cases, with the exception of Letterer-Siwe disease, which may be fatal. These disorders may actually represent a continuum, from the unifocal and benign eosinophilic granuloma to the generalized and sometimes fatal Letterer-Siwe disease.[29] The term *histiocytosis X* is generally used to describe these disorders. Table 22–20 summarizes the major characteristics of histiocytic disorders.

➤ **Table 22–19**
GENERAL CHARACTERISTICS OF SEA-BLUE HISTIOCYTOSIS

Autosomal-recessive, benign genetic disorder

Striking blue histiocytes with Wright's stain

Splenomegaly and hepatomegaly

Thrombocytopenia

➤ **Table 22–20**
CHARACTERISTICS OF HISTIOCYTIC DISORDER

Disease	Age at Onset	Main Site(s) of Involvement	Disease
Eosinophilic granuloma	Children and young adults, especially males, often no symptoms until bone fracture	Unifocal—skull, rib, femur most common	Rare spontaneous healing; most require surgical removal; occasional patients develop recurrence later
Hand-Schüller-Christian disease	Usually < 5 years old	Multifocal—bones, skin, lymphoid tissue; triad of pituitary, eye, and skull involvement is characteristic but uncommon	50%: spontaneous recovery 50%: recovery with chemotherapy
Letterer-Siwe disease	Usually < 3 years old	Generalized—skin, lymphoid tissue, bones, +/− bone marrow; more severe and extensive than Hand-Schüller-Christian disease	Chemotherapy has improved prognosis, which was previously considered poor

➤ CASE STUDY

A 32-year-old man visited his physician complaining of pain in his forearms and fatigue. Physical examination revealed an enlarged spleen (2 cm) and multiple bruises down the patient's forearms. His physician ordered the following laboratory workup:

RBC count	3.1×10^{12}/L
WBC count	4.9×10^{9}/L
Hemoglobin	11.0 g/dL
Hematocrit	32%
MCV	92 fL
MCHC	31%
Reticulocytes	0.4%

Differential:

Segmented neutrophils	52%
Lymphocytes	41%
Monocytes	4%
Bands	3%

A bone marrow aspiration was performed at the left posterior iliac crest and revealed a histiocytic-appearing cell (see Fig. 22–2). These cells stained positive with PAS, Sudan black B, and Prussian blue.

Questions

1. This case history is representative of what lipid storage disease?
2. What further testing must be done to confirm the diagnosis?
3. Is "effective erythropoiesis" apparent in this case? Why or why not?
4. Classify the anemia according to the red blood cell (RBC) indices.
5. What treatment is available to this patient?

QUESTIONS

1. What defect is found in lipid storage diseases?
   a. Subcellular accumulation of unmetabolized material in lysosomes
   b. Cellular accumulation of metabolites in cytoplasm
   c. Protein accumulation in cellular mitochondria
   d. Abnormal sequestration of minerals and trace elements in cellular nuclear organelles

2. What is the enzyme deficiency seen in Gaucher's disease?
   a. Sphingomyelinase
   b. Hexosaminidase A
   c. β-Glucocerebrosidase
   d. α-Galactosidase

3. Which description best characterizes type I Gaucher's disease?
   a. Found in any ethnic group; multiple neurologic signs, including difficulty in swallowing and

manifestations involving brain stem; enlargement of liver and spleen
   b. Found primarily in Ashkenazi Jews; enlargement of liver and spleen; anemia thrombocytopenia
   c. Found in northern Sweden; neurologic disorders, bone disorders, skin pigment changes
   d. Found in Mediterranean populations; hypermetabolic manifestations; fever, lethargy, poor musculature, bone deformities

4. What are the characteristics of Gaucher's cells?
   a. Atypical lymphocytes with foamy cytoplasm
   b. Hypersegmented neutrophils with Auer's rods
   c. Large, multilobed monocytes with prominent red granules
   d. Histiocytes with blue, folded cytoplasm

5. What is the enzyme deficiency seen in Niemann-Pick disease?
   a. Sphingomyelinase
   b. Hexosaminidase A
   c. β-Glucocerebrosidase
   d. α-Galactosidase

6. What are the characteristics of Niemann-Pick cells?
   a. Atypical lymphocytes with large vacuoles
   b. Cytoplasm filled with lipid droplets, inconspicuous nucleus
   c. Vacuolated histiocytes or foam cells
   d. Lymphocytes with Alder-Reilly bodies

7. What is the enzyme deficiency seen in Tay-Sachs disease?
   a. Sphingomyelinase
   b. Hexosaminidase A
   c. β-Glucocerebrosidase
   d. α-Galactosidase

8. What are the clinical features of Tay-Sachs disease?
   a. Waxy, jaundiced skin; retarded physical and mental development; cherry-red spot in macula of eye
   b. Startle reflex; blindness; macrocephaly; no enlargement of liver, spleen, or lymph nodes
   c. Abnormal facial features; deafness; increased body hair, mental retardation; heart damage; structural deformities
   d. Splenomegaly; hepatomegaly; eye, skin, nervous system, and lung abnormalities

9. Which cell is found in Tay-Sachs disease, but is not considered diagnostic?
   a. Atypical lymphocytes with large vacuoles
   b. Cytoplasm filled with lipid droplets; inconspicuous nucleus
   c. Vacuolated histiocytes or foam cells
   d. Lymphocytes with Alder-Reilly bodies

10. Which cell may be found in MPS disorders?
   a. Large, foamy histiocytes with blue or green granules
   b. Neutrophils with toxic granulation
   c. Neutrophils with Döhle bodies
   d. Lymphocytes with Alder-Reilly bodies

SUMMARY CHART

➤ Lipid storage diseases range from essentially asymptomatic to severe and incapacitating, resulting in death.

➤ Gaucher's disease results from a deficiency of the enzyme β-glucocerebrosidase, which leads to an accumulation of unmetabolized substrate glucocerebroside in cells, predominantly the monocyte-macrophage system. This accumulation of glucocerebrosides produces the distinctive Gaucher's cells.

➤ Gaucher's disease has three clinically recognizable types: the adult or nonneuronopathic form (type I); the infantile, acute, or malignant neuronopathic form (type II); and the juvenile or subacute neuronopathic form (type III).

➤ Type I (chronic nonneuronopathic) adult Gaucher's disease is the most common type of Gaucher's disease. It occurs frequently as an inherited disorder in the Ashkenazi Jewish population. Clinical features include anemia, thrombocytopenia, massively enlarged liver and spleen, and extensive skeletal disease.

➤ Type II (acute or malignant neuronopathic) infantile Gaucher's disease occurs in infancy. Patients rarely survive past the age of 2 years. It is found in all ethnic groups, although it is uncommon in the Jewish population. The clinical presentation of type II disease is much more uniform than that of type I, and is very severe. Features include difficulty swallowing, opisthotonos, and other manifestations of brain stem involvement, which are noted in early infancy.

➤ Type III (subacute neuronopathic) juvenile Gaucher's disease may be present from early childhood to the teenage years. Two distinct subtypes of type III have been described. Type IIIa usually presents clinically between early childhood and mid-adult life. Type IIIb is a clinically aggressive systemic disease, with neurologic involvement characterized by isolated horizontal supranuclear gaze palsy.

➤ Gaucher's disease is the first lysosomal storage disorder for which enzyme replacement therapy is available.

➤ Niemann-Pick disease is caused by a deficiency of the enzyme sphingomyelinase, with a secondary accumulation of the unmetabolized lipid sphingomyelin as well as cholesterol. Type A is also known as infantile or classic Niemann-Pick disease. Type B is also called the chronic or adult form. Type C has been described in two forms: infantile and juvenile.

➤ Tay-Sachs disease, also known as GM_2 gangliosidosis, is an autosomal-recessive sphingolipidosis that occurs as a result of deficiency of the enzyme hexosaminidase A, with an increase in hexosaminidase B.

➤ Mucopolysaccharidoses are rare disorders that constitute a group of lysosomal storage diseases caused by a deficiency in one of the enzymes involved in the breakdown of mucopolysaccharides.

➤ Sea-blue histiocyte syndrome is a genetic disorder with a benign course. The striking blue color of the histiocytes after staining with Wright's or May-Grünwald-Giemsa stain gives the syndrome its name.

➤ Histiocytic disorders represent an abnormal proliferation and accumulation of mature histiocytes, or Langerhans' cells.

References

1. Barranger, JA, and Rice, EO (eds): Gaucher disease: Diagnosis, monitoring, and management. Gaucher Clin Persp 5:6, 1997.
2. Neudorf, SML (ed): Bone marrow transplantation for the correction of Gaucher disease. Gaucher Clin Persp 5:9, 1997.
3. Desnick, RJ: Gaucher disease (1882–1982): Centennial perspectives on the most prevalent Jewish genetic disease. Mt Sinai J Med 49:443, 1982.
4. Grabowski, GA (ed): A comparison of imiglucerase and alglucerase therapy for type 1 Gaucher disease. Gaucher Clin Persp 6:6, 1998.
5. Cox, TM, and Mistry, PK (eds): Therapeutic targeting of human mannose-terminated glucocerebrosidase. Gaucher Clin Persp 5:9, 1997.
6. Erikson, A, et al: Enzyme replacement therapy of infantile Gaucher disease. Neuropediatrics 24:237, 1993.
7. Schiffmann, R (ed): Enzyme replacement therapy for type 3 Gaucher disease. Gaucher Clin Persp 5:12, 1997.
8. Clarke, JTR (ed): Gaucher disease: Differential diagnosis. Gaucher Clin Persp 5:6, 1997.
9. Wenstrup, RJ (ed): Antiresorptive bone therapy in Gaucher disease. Gaucher Clin Persp 6:12, 1998.
10. Hammert, LC, and Ball, ED (eds): Hematologic complications associated with Gaucher disease. Gaucher Clin Persp 5:9, 1997.
11. Grace, ME, et al: Analysis of human acid beta-glucosidase by site-directed mutagenesis and heterologous expression. J Biol Chem 269:2283, 1994.
12. Berg-Fusman A, et al: Human acid beta-glucosidase. N-glycosylation site occupancy and the effect of glycosylation on enzymatic activity. J Biol Chem 268:14861, 1993.
13. Miao, S, et al: Identification of Glu340 as the active-site nucleophile in human glucocerebrosidase by use of electrospray tandem mass spectrometry. J Biol Chem 269:10975, 1991.
14. Sibille, A, et al: Phenotype/genotype correlations in Gaucher disease type I: Clinical and therapeutic implications. Am J Hum Genet 52:1094, 1993.
15. Brady, RO, et al: The role of neurogenetics in Gaucher disease. Arch Neurol 50:1212, 1993.
16. Kaye, EM (ed): Type 3 Gaucher disease. Gaucher Clin Persp 5:12, 1997.
17. Patterson, MC, et al: Isolated horizontal supranuclear gaze palsy as a marker of severe systemic involvement in Gaucher's disease. Neurology 43:1993, 1993.
18. McGovern, MM, and Desnick, R: Abnormalities of the monocyte macrophage system. In Lee, GR, et al (eds): Wintrobe's Clinical Hematology, ed 10. Lippincott, Williams & Wilkins, Philadelphia, 1999.
19. Savage, RA: Specific and not-so-specific histiocytes in bone marrow. Lab Med 15:467, 1984.
20. Shiran, A, et al: Increased risk of cancer in patients with Gaucher disease. Cancer 72:219, 1993.
21. Grabowski, GA, and Pastores, GM: Enzyme replacement therapy in type 1 Gaucher disease. Gaucher Clin Persp 1:8, 1993.
22. Aggio, MC, and Fernandez, V (eds): Enzyme replacement treatment of Gaucher disease in Argentina. Gaucher Clin Persp 6:12, 1998.
23. Machado de Paula, MT, et al (eds): Gaucher patients treated at HEMORIO. Gaucher Clin Persp 6:12, 1998.
24. Richards, SM, et al: Antibody response in patients with Gaucher disease after repeated infusion with macrophage-targeted glucocerebrosidase. Blood 82:1402, 1993.
25. Gaucher Disease Conference, National Institutes of Health, Bethesda, MD, Feb 27–Mar 1, 1995.
26. Pastores, GM (ed): Recombinant enzyme therapy for Gaucher disease: Long-term clinical experience and therapeutic outcomes with cross-over from alglucerase. Gaucher Clin Persp 6:6, 1998.
27. Pick, L: Niemann-Pick's disease and other forms of so called xanthomatosis. Am J Med Sci 185:601, 1933.
28. Das, S, et al: Niemann-Pick disease. J Indian Med Assoc 92(3):87, 1994.
29. Cotran, RS, et al: Pathologic Basis of Disease. WB Saunders, Philadelphia, January 1994.
30. Turpin, JC, et al: Clinical aspects of Niemann-Pick, type C disease in the adult. Dev Neurosci 13:304, 1991.
31. Bembi, B, et al: Treatment of sphingomyelinase deficiency by repeated implantations of amniotic epithelial cells. Am J Med Genet 44:427, 1992.
32. Dinur, T, et al: Toward gene therapy for Niemann-Pick disease (NPD): Separation of retrovirally corrected and noncorrected NPD fibroblasts using a novel fluorescent sphingomyelin. Hum Gene Ther 3:633, 1992.

33. Triggs-Raine, BL, et al: Screening for carriers of Tay-Sachs disease among Ashkenazi Jews. N Engl J Med 323:6, 1990.

34. Robb, RM: Ocular abnormalities in childhood metabolic disease and leukemia. In Nelson, LB, et al (ed): Pediatric Ophthalmology, ed 3. WB Saunders, Philadelphia, 1991, p 468.

35. Sandhoff, K, et al: The GM$_2$ gangliosidoses. In Scriver, CR, et al (eds): The Metabolic Basis of Inherited Disease, ed 6. McGraw-Hill, New York, 1989, pp 1807–1839.

36. Di Natale, P, et al: Biochemical diagnosis of mucopolysaccharidoses: Experience of 297 diagnoses in a 15-year period (1977–1991). J Inher Metab Dis 16:473, 1993.

37. Wicker, G, et al: Mucopolysaccharidosis VI (Maroteaux-Lamy syndrome). An intermediate clinical phenotype caused by substitution of valine for glycine at position 137 of arylsulfatase B. J Biol Chem 266:21386, 1991.

38. Roubicek, M, et al: The clinical spectrum of α-L-iduronidase deficiency. Am J Hum Genet 20:471, 1985.

39. Hopwood, JJ, and Morris, C: The mucopolysaccharidoses. Diagnosis, molecular genetics and treatment. Mol Biol Med 7:381, 1990.

40. Fensom, AH and Benson, PF: Recent advances in the prenatal diagnosis of the mucopolysaccharidoses. Prenatal Diagn 14:1, 1994.

41. Hoogerbrugge, PM, and Vossen, JMJJ: Bone marrow transplantation in the treatment of lysosomal storage disease. In Fernandes, J, et al (eds): Inborn Metabolic Diseases. Diagnosis and Treatment. Springer-Verlag, Berlin, 1990, pp 659–670.

42. Henry, JB: Clinical Diagnosis and Management by Laboratory Methods. WB Saunders, Philadelphia, 1990, p 454.

Hemostasis and Introduction to Thrombosis

Part IV

23 Introduction to Hemostasis

CLAUDIA E. ESCOBAR, MT(ASCP)SH
DENISE M. HARMENING, PHD, MT(ASCP), CLS(NCA)
DIANE M. JOINER MAIER, MLT(ASCP)
VICKIE L. SIMMONS, MT(ASCP)SH
KELLY M. SMITH-MOORE, MT(ASCP)SH
JANIS WYRICK-GLATZEL, MS, MT(ASCP)

OBJECTIVES

At the end of this chapter, the learner should be able to:

1. Define the terms *coagulation, fibrinolysis, petechiae, ecchymosis,* and *hemorrhage.*
2. List the major and minor systems involved in maintaining hemostasis.
3. Describe the events that take place in primary hemostasis.
4. Name the three structural zones of platelets.
5. Describe the composition and functions of the peripheral zone, sol-gel zone, and organelle zone.
6. List steps in platelet plug formation and describe the process of platelet adhesion and aggregation.
7. Describe the events that take place in secondary hemostasis.
8. Name the product responsible for stabilization of the hemostatic plug.
9. List characteristics for the contact coagulation

proteins, prothrombin proteins, and fibrinogen group.

10. Define the extrinsic system, intrinsic system, and common pathway.

11. Describe the events that take place in fibrinolysis.

12. Describe the use of the prothrombin time test in monitoring hemostasis.

13. Describe the use of the activated partial thromboplastin time test in monitoring hemostasis.

14. Describe the thrombin-mediated reactions in hemostasis.

➤ PLATELETS AND HEMOSTATIC MECHANISMS

Overview

Hemostasis is the complex process by which the body spontaneously stops bleeding and maintains blood in the fluid state within the vascular compartment. The major role of the hemostatic system is to maintain a complete balance of the body's tendency toward clotting and bleeding (Fig. 23–1). Normal hemostasis is both rapid and localized. Hemostasis is achieved by the highly integrated and regulated interaction of (1) blood vessels, (2) platelets, (3) coagulation proteins, and (4) fibrinolysis (Table 23–1). Minor ancillary systems involved are also listed in Table 23–1. Through a complex series of molecular interactions involving cells and biochemicals, a balance between procoagulant and fibrinolytic activity is achieved. A fine line separates clot formation in circulating blood from bleeding. It has long been recognized that an imbalance, either acquired or inherited, in any one of the many factors that contribute to hemostasis often leads to hemorrhage or thrombosis. Significant changes in blood flow have a profound effect on cellular function, notably endothelial cell function. Mechanical or pathologic disruption of intact endothelium within the vessel wall initiates localized hemostatic and thrombotic responses. If the vascular injury exceeds the capacity of the platelets mediated by thrombin to form a hemostatic platelet plug, then the clinical signs and symptoms of hemorrhage occur. Stagnation of blood flow as a result of arterial disease or mechanical impedance disturbs the endothelial cell anticoagulant effect, thus leading to the formation of a thrombus clot and hypercoagulable states.[1]

Protective mechanisms exist that prevent thrombin formation in normal healthy vessels. Intact endothelial cells within a vessel wall are nonreactive or thromboresistant through the interaction of receptors and proteoglycans. Coagulation proteins circulate in blood as inactive enzymes or zymogens held in balance by anticoagulant and fibrinolytic pathways, and platelet procoagulant membrane lipids are internalized within the cell. These combined mechanisms serve to keep hemostasis in balance.

Hemostasis can be divided into two stages: primary and secondary hemostasis. Simply stated, *primary hemostasis* is defined by platelet adhesion to exposed collagen within the endothelium of the vessel wall. Platelet adhesion is mediated by platelet membrane glycoprotein Ib (GPIb) and von Willebrand's factor (vWF).[2] The interaction of platelets and vascular endothelium is the first step in a series of reactions that lead to thrombus formation and serve to halt bleeding after vascular injury. However, the primary response alone is ineffective for any duration of time.

Secondary hemostasis involves the enzymatic activation of the coagulation proteins to produce fibrin from fibrinogen, thereby stabilizing the fragile clot formed during primary hemostasis. The cascade of coagulation reactions is a result of complexes that form between enzymes, substrates, phospholipid surfaces, and cofactors.

Gradually, the stable clot is dissolved through a process known as *fibrinolysis*. Fibrinolysis involves the proteolytic digestion of fibrinogen and fibrin by the enzyme plasmin. Through the release of platelet-derived growth factor (PDGF), vascular healing and repair is promoted, completing the process of hemostasis.[3]

In general, the relative importance of the hemostatic mechanisms varies with vessel size (Table 23–2). Basically, the larger the area of bleeding, the larger the vessel involved. Ecchymoses, epistaxis, petechiae, gastrointestinal, and genitourinary bleeding represent mucocutaneous hemorrhage highly suggestive of qualitative or quantitative platelet disorders. Bleeding into joint cavities and into the retroperitoneum is characteristic of factor deficiencies or

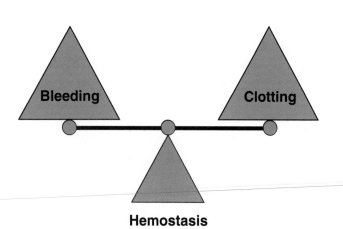

➤ FIGURE 23–1   Hemostasis: A system in balance.

➤ **Table 23-1** **SYSTEMS INVOLVED IN MAINTAINING HEMOSTASIS**	
Major Systems	**Minor Systems**
Vascular system	Kinin system
Platelets	Serine protease inhibitors
Coagulation system	Complement system
Fibrinolytic system	

> ### ► Table 23-2
> ### VESSELS AND GENERAL BREACH-SEALING REQUIREMENTS

Vessel	Relative Sizes	General Breach-Sealing Requirements*
Capillary	Smallest	Generally direct sealing
Venule		Mostly fused platelets
Arteriole		Mostly fused platelets
Vein		Vascular contraction, fused platelets, perivascular and intravascular hemostatic factor activation
Artery	Largest	Great vascular contraction, more fused platelets, greater perivascular and intravascular hemostatic factor activation

*In general, the larger the vessel, the more hemostatic system involvement is required to seal the breach.

> ### ► Table 23-4
> ### VESSEL LAYER COMPOSITION AND FUNCTION

Vessel Layer	Composition and Function
Tunica adventitia	Connective tissue cell support
Tunica media	Elastic tissue and smooth muscle, controlling vasoconstriction and sometimes vasodilation
Tunica intima	Broad flat endothelial cells with an underlying basement membrane supported by a few connective tissue cells, providing a smooth nonwettable surface but facilitating migration of cells through the spaces as needed

warfarin (Coumadin) toxicity. The hemorrhagic condition characteristically seen in disseminated intravascular coagulation (DIC) presents with both mucocutaneous and joint bleeding, evidence of both platelet and coagulation protein deficiencies.[4] Some sources and types of bleeding are listed in Table 23–3.

The focus of this chapter is to provide a comprehensive review of present-day knowledge of the biochemistry, function, interaction, and regulation of each of the major components that participate in hemostasis. Subsequent chapters further define the genetic and molecular mechanism, laboratory diagnosis, and current treatment of the various thrombotic and hemorrhagic disorders of hemostasis.

Vascular System

Advanced Concepts

The blood vessel, with its smooth and continuous endothelial lining and fibrous coat, is designed to facilitate blood flow as well as participate in the process of hemostasis. Table 23–4 outlines the structure of the vessel wall, which includes the outermost layer (adventitia), the middle layer (media), and the inner layer (intima). The endothelial surface of the blood vessel is usually inert to platelets and coagulation factors. It is termed a *nonwettable* surface because the physical and biochemical characteristics of the

endothelium render the cell surface thromboresistant. This is achieved through (1) synthesis and secretion of a vasodilator, prostacyclin (PGI_2); (2) secretion of tissue plasminogen activator (t-PA); (3) inactivation and clearance of thrombin; (4) activity of the cofactor thrombomodulin in the thrombin-dependent activation of protein C; and (5) the degradation of proaggregating substances such as adenosine diphosphate (ADP) and vasoactive amines.[5]

However, when the endothelial lining is disrupted, the vascular system acts to prevent bleeding by promoting rapid vasoconstriction of the injured vessel as well as adjacent vessels. This process diverts blood flow around the damaged vessel and enhances contact activation of platelets and coagulation factors (Table 23–5). Platelet adhesion occurs almost immediately to the exposed collagen fibers of the subendothelium. The principal mechanism of platelet adhesion involves (1) vWF, (2) collagen fibers, and (3) platelet membrane glycoprotein Ib (GPIb; the receptor for vWF).[6] The adherent platelet undergoes activation events, including shape change, platelet aggregation, and secretion of ADP from the platelet-dense body. Secretion of platelet ADP acts in the recruitment of additional platelets to form the primary hemostatic plug. Activated platelets provide an important phospholipid surface that enhances activation of the coagulation proteins in both the intrinsic and extrinsic system. In addition, platelet secretion of thromboxane A_2 (TXA_2), a prostaglandin, and serotonin further promotes vasoconstriction. Endothelial release of tissue factor (formerly known as tissue thromboplastin) during vascular injury represents one of the body's major procoagulant abil-

> ### ► Table 23-3
> ### SOME SOURCES AND TYPES OF BLEEDING

Source	Type
Arteriole, venule	Pinpoint petechial hemorrhage (diapedesis or leakage of blood out of small vessels)
Veins	Ecchymosis (large, ill-defined soft tissue bleeding)
Artery	Rapidly expanding "blowout" hemorrhage

> ### ► Table 23-5
> ### ACTIONS OF THE VASCULAR SYSTEM TO PREVENT BLEEDING

1. Contraction of vessels (vasoconstriction) and reflex stimulation of adjacent vessels
2. Diversion of blood flow around damaged vasculature
3. Initiation of contact activation of platelets with subsequent adhesion, release reaction, and aggregation
4. Contact activation of the coagulation system (both extrinsic and intrinsic) leading to fibrin formation

ities. The initiation of the extrinsic pathway of coagulation requires tissue factor, factor VII/VIIa, calcium, and a negatively charged phospholipid membrane. The factor VIIa—tissue factor complex is now known to initiate the activation of both factor X and factor IX. Release of t-PA by the damaged endothelial cell provides the mechanism for clot dissolution, necessary to reestablish vascular patency.[7] PDGF, secreted by platelets, assists in proliferation and repair of damaged endothelium. The vascular response involved in the hemostatic mechanisms usually lasts less than 1 minute. Table 23–6 lists some of the major substances contained within the endothelium or subendothelium, or both, that play primary roles in hemostasis. Other substances known to bind to endothelial cells that promote coagulation are listed in Table 23–7.

➤ PRIMARY HEMOSTASIS

Platelet Structure (Basic Information)

Platelets are anucleated cytoplasmic fragments measuring 2 to 4 μm in diameter and originate from bone marrow megakaryocytes. On Wright's stain, platelets appear as pale blue cells with fine azurophilic granules (Fig. 23–2). During megakaryopoiesis, the interval from megakaryoblast to production of platelets is approximately 1 week. In the peripheral blood, about 70% of the platelets are circulating, whereas 30% are sequestered in the microvasculature of the spleen and serve as functional reserves after their release from the bone marrow. Platelets survive for 7 to 10 days in circulation and are active in hemostasis.

The normal platelet count ranges from 150,000 to 350,000 per microliter (μL), depending on the methodology employed. Normal platelet function in vivo and in vitro requires more than 100,000 platelets per microliter.[8] It is unusual for a patient with a platelet count greater than 20,000/μL to have major hemorrhages. Assuming normal platelet function, a platelet count greater than 50,000/μL will minimize the chance of hemorrhage during surgery.

Platelets must be adequate in both number and function

➤ Table 23-7
OTHER SUBSTANCES THAT BIND TO ENDOTHELIAL CELLS AND THEIR ROLE IN COAGULATION

High-molecular-weight kininogen (HMWK)	Cofactor required for efficient activation of the contact phase
Factors X and Xa	On endothelial cells mediates prothrombin activation
Factor IX/IXa	Cell-bound factor IXa functions in factor VIII–dependent activation of factor X
Prothrombinase complex	Complex (Xa, Va, Ca++, and phospholipid) assembled on endothelial cells further propagates coagulation and triggers intracellular signaling events
Fibrinogen and fibrin	Present in healing blood vessel subendothelium (fibrinogen); binds to endothelial cells; reinforces platelet plug
Fibronectin	Functions as an adhesive protein for platelets, promoting spreading

➤ Table 23-6
MAJOR HEMOSTASIS-RELATED SUBSTANCES PRESENT IN THE ENDOTHELIUM AND/OR SUBENDOTHELIUM AND THEIR FUNCTION IN HEMOSTASIS

Substance(s)	Some Function(s) in Hemostasis
Collagen	Binds to platelet membrane GPIb/IIa; activates plasma coagulation factors via intrinsic pathway
Heparin sulfate	A glycosaminoglycan that has anticoagulant activity and contributes to the activation of antithrombin III
von Willebrand's factor (vWF)	Protein synthesized in endothelial cells and megakaryocytes; primarily binds to platelet membrane receptor GPIb to promote adhesion; also functions as a carrier for factor VIII, providing factor stability in circulation; may also bind to platelet GPIIb/IIIa in conditions of high shear stress to promote adhesion
PGI$_2$	A prostacyclin synthesized by endothelial cells that physiologically inhibits platelet aggregation and limits thrombus formation beyond the damaged vessel
Tissue factor (TF)	A lipoprotein released following vascular trauma that initiates coagulation by activating factor VII with ionized calcium (extrinsic pathway) and contributes to the activation of factors X and IX (intrinsic pathway)
Tissue factor pathway inhibitors (TFPIs)	A glycoprotein found on endothelial surfaces that serves as an anticoagulant by inhibiting factors VIIa/TF and Xa
Thrombomodulin	A large protein found on the endothelial surfaces that serves as a cofactor in protein C activation when bound to thrombin
Tissue plasminogen activator (t-PA)	Serine proteinase secreted by endothelial cells that regulate fibrinolysis; when bound to fibrin, t-PA inactivates plasminogen
Plasminogen activator inhibitors (PAIs)	Proteins found in endothelial cells that regulate fibrinolysis by neutralizing the activity of plasmin, plasminogen, and t-PA; associated with risk of thrombosis

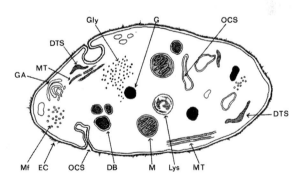

> ➤ FIGURE 23-2 Normal platelets: Wright-stained blood smear (peripheral blood).

to participate optimally in hemostasis. Platelets participate in hemostasis by (1) providing a negatively charged phospholipid surface for factor X and prothrombin activation; (2) releasing substances that mediate vasoconstriction, platelet aggregation, coagulation (thrombin generation), and vascular repair; and (3) providing surface membrane glycoproteins such as GPIIb and IIIa to attach to other platelets via fibrinogen, and GPIb to bind to collagen and subendothelium via vWF. Platelets achieve these tasks, by functioning in shape change, adhesion, aggregation, and secretion (release). A basic understanding of the platelet's ultrastructure and its organelles (Fig. 23–3) is crucial to understanding how the platelet performs each of its vital functions. Each of these individual functions can be assessed by clinical testing; however, all functions are required during the formation of the hemostatic platelet plug known as primary hemostasis.

Platelet Structure (Advanced)

The platelet structure is quite distinct, leading to subdivision into three defined zones, each possessing unique functional capabilities. These zones are prominently delineated by the circumferential band of microtubules found in the platelet, as seen in Figure 23–4. Table 23–8 summarizes the three described zones and their contents. Impaired cellular function of the platelet membrane, cytoskeleton, granular constituents, and secreted proteins often leads to platelet dysfunction and abnormal hemostasis.

Peripheral Zone

Basic Concepts
The peripheral zone is a complex region of the platelet consisting of the glycocalyx (an amorphous exterior coat), platelet membrane, numerous deeply penetrating surface-connecting channels known as the *open canalicular system (OCS),* and a submembranous area of specialized microfilaments (see Fig. 23–3).

A number of glycoproteins anchored in the platelet membrane are present in the glycocalyx and mediate the critical events of platelet adhesion and aggregation. Specific binding of platelet membrane receptors to adhesive macromolecules such as fibronectin, collagen, and vitronectin in plasma or vascular subendothelium further facilitates the spreading of platelets on the damaged vessel wall and leads to platelet activation and the formation of large platelet aggregates. Platelet membrane glycoproteins serve as receptors and facilitate transduction of activation signals across the platelet membrane in response to various external stimuli.

Adhesion of platelets to exposed collagen within the subendothelium involves the interaction of platelet membrane receptor, GPIb and vWF, a plasma component. Platelet adhesion typically occurs 1 to 2 seconds following vascular injury. Following adhesion, release of adenosine diphosphate (ADP)

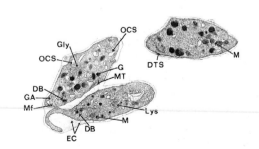

> ➤ FIGURE 23-3 Discoid platelets; *(top)* summary diagram of the platelet organelles; *(bottom)* transmission electron micrograph (TEM) of cross-sectioned platelets illustrating basic ultrastructure.

MT —— Microtubules
G —— Other Granules
DB —— Dense Bodies
DTS —— Dense Tubular System
M —— Mitochondria
Gly —— Glycogen Lakes (particles)
Lys —— Lysosomes
OCS —— Open Canalicular System
Mf —— Microfilaments
EC —— Exterior Coat (Glycocalyx)
GA —— Golgi Apparatus

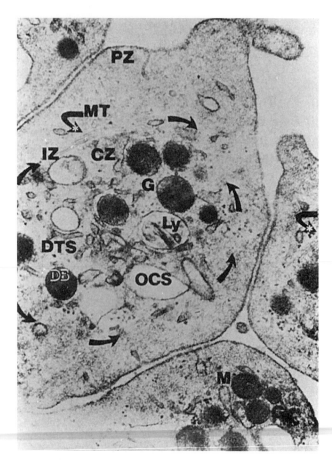

> **FIGURE 23–4**   Internal anatomy of a stimulated platelet. Circumferential band of microtubules (MT) leads to reorganization of the internal structure of the platelet into three zones. The peripheral zone (PZ) is the region external to a circumferential band of microtubules (MT with * on curved arrows). The intermediate zone (IZ) *(encircling arrows)* includes the microtubules and the closely adjacent cytoplasmic material. The central zone (CZ) is internal to the microtubule band and contains many organelles such as granules (G), dense bodies (DB), dense tubular system (DTS), lysosomes (Ly), mitochondria (M), and many profiles of the open canalicular system (OCS). Magnification ×49,700. (From Barnhart, MI: Platelet responses in health and disease. Mol Cell Biochem 22:115, 1978, with permission.)

> ### Table 23–8
> ## PLATELET ULTRASTRUCTURAL ZONES

> I. Peripheral zone (stimulus receptor/transmitter region)
>   a. Glycocalyx
>   b. Platelet membrane
>   c. Open canalicular system (OCS)
>   d. Submembranous region
> II. Sol-gel zone (cytoskeletal/contractile region)
>   a. Circumferential microtubules
>   b. Microfilaments
> III. Organelle zone (Metabolic/organellar region)
>   a. Granules
>   1. α Granules
>   2. Dense granules
>   3. Lysosomes
>   4. Glycogen granules
>   b. Mitochondria
>   c. Dense tubular system
>   d. Peroxisomes

platelets causes the activation of additional platelets, thus augmenting the primary hemostatic response.

The platelet membrane, similar to other plasma membranes, contains a phospholipid component. Activated platelets undergo shape change, develop stickiness, and expose platelet membrane phospholipids. Platelet factor 3 (PF3) is known to move to the outer surface of the platelet membrane, thus allowing for the assembly of the vitamin K–dependent coagulation factors.[9] PF3 serves as a cofactor in the complex. Coagulation factors V and VIII are also present on the surface of the platelet membrane, as are various platelet factors (PFs) that participate in the formation of fibrin. At least seven PFs have been identified; they are listed in Table 23–9. PF3 and PF4 seem to be the most important platelet factors.[9]

Advanced Concepts
A number of glycoproteins present in the glycocalyx are responsible for blood group specificity (ABO), tissue com-

and adenosine triphosphate (ATP) from intracellular platelet granules cause platelet shape change in adjacent platelets. Platelet aggregation requires a conformational change in platelet membrane receptor GPIIb/IIIa (and GPV), thus allowing the binding of fibrinogen. The binding of the two symmetric ends of fibrinogen to different platelets promotes platelet-to-platelet interaction, thus leading to the formation of a large platelet aggregate. Calcium or magnesium, or both, in the form of divalent cations are also required for fibrinogen binding. Platelet aggregation begins approximately 10 to 20 seconds following vascular injury.

The platelet membrane also includes receptors for substances such as ADP, thrombin, epinephrine, collagen, TXA$_2$, and serotonin, which play a role in platelet aggregation.[9] ADP and TXA$_2$ are potent platelet aggregators when bound to their specific platelet membrane receptors. These two platelet-derived aggregators are released during platelet activation in response to thrombin and amplify intracellular events, leading to platelet secretion and platelet aggregation. The secretion of such substances by activated

> ### Table 23–9
> ## PLATELET FACTORS (PFs) 1 TO 7

> | | |
> |---|---|
> | PF1 | Coagulation factor V |
> | PF2 | Thromboplastin-like material |
> | PF3 | Platelet thromboplastin* |
> | PF4 | Antiheparin factor* |
> | PF5 | Fibrinogen coagulant factor |
> | PF6 | Antifibrinolytic factor* |
> | PF7 | Platelet cothromboplastin |

*Most important.
   Source: Adapted from Bick, RL, and Murano, G: Physiology of hemostasis. In Bick, RL (ed): Hematology: Clinical and Laboratory Practice. CV Mosby, St. Louis, 1992, pp 1285–1309.

patibility (human leukocyte antigen [HLA]), and platelet antigenicity.

Although the primary receptor for vWF seems to be GPIb, in rapidly flowing blood with a high shear stress, vWF is more likely to bind to GPIIb/IIIa.

The membranous surface-connecting system referred to as the open canalicular system (OCS) consists of tubular invaginations of the plasma membrane that articulate throughout the platelet even though it is part of the peripheral zone. Chemical substances stored in the dense and alpha (α) granules of the platelet are released to the exterior through the OCS. The OCS also facilitates the collection of plasma procoagulants that aid in fibrin formation by providing increased surface absorptive area. This membrane system appears to be the calcium-regulating mechanism of the platelet.

Sol-Gel Zone

Basic Concepts

The term *cytoskeleton* is often used to describe this zone. Within the matrix of the platelet are microtubules, microfilaments, and submembranous filaments.

Microtubules encase the entire platelet, maintaining its discoid shape. Microtubules are composed of protein subunits called *tubulin*. In the stimulated platelet (see Fig. 23–4), contraction of the circumferential band of microtubules toward the center of the platelet appears to be responsible for both the movement of organelles toward the center and their reorganization, which facilitates the secretory process.[4]

Microfilaments are randomly interwoven throughout the cytoplasm of the platelet and are composed of two contractile proteins, actin and myosin. Also present is thrombosthenin, a contractile protein similar to actomyosin.[8] Actomyosin is complexed actin and myosin. Microfilaments can convert from an unorganized gelatinous state to organized parallel filaments capable of contraction within seconds as the platelet's shape changes.

Advanced Concepts

Microtubules disappear from the center of the platelet after secretion and reappear in other peripheral areas such as pseudopods. Microtubules appear to monitor the internal contraction of platelets, preventing platelet secretion in response to only minimal stimulation and thereby regulating the degree of platelet response to external stimuli.

Organelle Zone

Basic Concepts

The organelle region is responsible for the metabolic activities of the platelet. Like many other cells, platelets possess mitochondria and various cytoplasmic granules. Unlike many cells, platelets are anucleated and do not possess either a Golgi body or rough endoplasmic reticulum (RER).

Generally, the most numerous organelles are the platelet granules, which are heterogeneous in size, electron density, and chemical content. Platelets contain three morphologically distinct types of storage granules: dense granules, α granules, and lysosomes. The α granules are most numerous (20 to 200 per platelet) and store a number of different substances that are listed in Table 23–10, along with their major function in hemostasis.[4]

Dense granules or bodies, are smaller and fewer in number (2 to 10 per platelet) and appear as dense opaque granules in transmission electron microscope (TEM) preparations. Dense granules contain storage ADP, ATP, ionic calcium, serotonin, and phosphates.

Lysosomes appear similar to the azurophilic granules

> **Table 23–10**
> ## CHEMICAL CONTENTS OF PLATELET GRANULES AND THEIR MAJOR FUNCTION IN HEMOSTASIS

Alpha Granules	Function
Platelet-Specific Proteins	
Beta-thromboglobulin (β-TG)	Inhibits heparin; chemotactic; promotes smooth muscle growth for vessel repair
Platelet factor 4 (PF4)	Inhibits heparin
Platelet-derived growth factor (PDGF)	Promotes smooth muscle growth; involved in atherosclerosis and lipid metabolism
Thrombospondin	Promotes platelet-to-platelet interaction; mediates cell-to-cell interaction
Plasma Proteins	
Fibrinogen	Fibrin formation
von Willebrand factor (vWF)	Promotes platelet adhesion
Factor V	Cofactor in fibrin formation
Factor VIII	Cofactor in fibrin formation
Fibronectin	Cellular adhesion molecule; promotes platelet spreading
Albumin	Uncertain
High-molecular-weight kininogen (HMWK)	Activation of the intrinsic pathway via contact
α$_2$-Antiplasmin	Inhibits plasmin
Plasminogen	Precursor to plasmin; functions in fibrinolysis
Dense Granules	
ADP (nonmetabolic)	Promotes platelet aggregation
ATP (nonmetabolic)	Uncertain
Calcium	Primary and secondary messenger regulates platelet activation/aggregation
Serotonin	Promotes vasoconstriction
Lysosomes	
Neutral proteases*	Uncertain
Acid hydrolase*	Uncertain
Bacteriocidal enzymes*	Uncertain

*The specific function of these proteins is uncertain; they may serve to decrease platelet activation in response to thrombin.

found in granulocytes and contain microbicidal enzymes, neutral proteases, and acid hydrolases. Proteases may contribute to disruption of the subendothelial structure following vascular injury. Glycogen granules are also found within the organelle zone and function in platelet metabolism.

The contents of both α and dense granules are released during secretion into the OCS. Secretion promotes the recruitment of additional platelets to the platelet aggregate at the site of vascular injury. Platelet secretion is an energy-dependent reaction that relies on the metabolic function of mitochondria. The estimated 10 to 60 mitochondria present per platelet require glycogen as their source of energy for metabolism.[4] In the resting platelet, ATP (energy) production is generated by glycolysis and the oxidative Krebs cycle. In the activated state, about half the ATP production in platelets occurs through the glycolytic pathway. Table 23–10 summarizes the important platelet-secreted proteins and their known role in hemostasis.

The dense tubular system (DTS) is another important structure present in the cytoplasm of the organelle zone of platelets. Similar to the sarcotubules in skeletal muscle, the DTS is derived from the smooth endoplasmic reticulum (ER) of immature megakaryocytes. The DTS is the site of prostaglandin and thromboxane synthesis and sequestration of calcium. It is primarily the release of calcium from the DTS that triggers platelet contraction and subsequent internal activation of platelets.

> ## ► Table 23-11
> ### EVENTS THAT OCCUR IN PLATELETS AFTER VESSEL INJURY

Vasoconstriction	Regulates blood flow in damaged vessel; increases concentration of biochemicals to promote platelet activation events
Platelet shape change	Signals intracellular activation, leading to platelet plug formation
Platelet aggregation	A platelet-to-platelet interaction mediated by fibrinogen, Ca++, and platelet membrane activated glycoprotein IIb/IIIa complex
Platelet plug	Adhesion and aggregation of platelets to the site of injury
Platelet secretion	Release of chemical constituents contained in various granules; amplifies platelet response
Stabilization	Platelet plug stabilized by formation of fibrin mesh over the platelet aggregates

► PLATELET FUNCTION

Overview

Numerous stimuli can trigger platelet activation, which may be transient, reversible, or irreversible. Activation refers to several separate responses of platelet function that include adhesion, shape change, secretion, stickiness, and aggregation. Platelets respond in a graded fashion, depending on the strength and duration of the stimuli as well as the physiologic or pathologic state of the platelet.

In the initial stage of activation, platelets form pseudopods as they begin to contract. As activation progresses, contraction and pseudopod formation progress, organelles including the α granules and dense bodies are reorganized to the center of the platelet, and further contraction causes the granules to spill their contents into the OCS, which shunts the contents to the outside of the platelet.[10] Adjacent platelets are activated through receptor contact with the granular contents, amplifying the activation process. Therefore, it may be said that platelet activation spans shape change, platelet adhesion, granular secretion, cytoskeletal reassembly, and platelet aggregation.

Before proceeding further, the reader should review the structure of the platelet in order to visualize and understand subsequent events that occur in the platelet at the ultrastructural level during hemostasis (see Fig. 23–3). Table 23–11 outlines the basic events that occur in primary hemostasis after injury to a vessel.

Maintenance of Vascular Integrity

Basic Concepts

Platelets are involved in the nurturing of endothelial cells lining the vascular system. Maintaining the integrity of the vessel wall is a function of the endothelial cells, the connective tissue of the subendothelium, and platelets. A primary feature of intact endothelium is its thromboresistance to platelets, leukocytes, and coagulation proteins. Platelet and endothelial cell interaction is modulated by the prostaglandin PGI_2. PGI_2 is synthesized by endothelial cells from arachidonic acid (a membrane phospholipid) and has an antagonistic effect on platelet adhesion and platelet aggregation, thus serving to locally limit the hemostatic response. Routinely, circulating platelets survey the vessel wall for denuded endothelium. Once the vessel wall integrity is disrupted, platelets are incorporated into the vessel wall, releasing a substance called platelet-derived growth factor (PDGF) that nurtures the endothelial cells, maintaining normal vascular integrity and thromboresistant properties.[11] Figure 23–5 shows a scanning electron micrograph (SEM) demonstrating platelet adherence at the site of endothelial loss compared with the normal smooth contour of the endothelial cell.

Advanced Concepts

PDGF is a mitogen stored in and secreted from the α granule of the platelet. Specific receptors for PDGF have been isolated on cultured fibroblasts and smooth muscle cells.[11] When vessel injury occurs and platelets are activated, PDGF is secreted, stimulating endothelial cell migration and proliferation of smooth muscle growth, thereby mediating wound healing and vascular repair. PDGF is an important growth factor and is thought to be linked to the pathologic development of atherosclerosis through its influence on lipid metabolism. PDGF also demonstrates chemotactic properties for neutrophils and monocytes, as well as fibroblasts and smooth muscle cells. The characteristics of PDGF help to limit the hemostatic response; thus, the platelet plug remains local to the site of vascular injury.

In the absence of platelets, a large number of red cells migrate through the vessel wall, enter the lymphatic drainage,

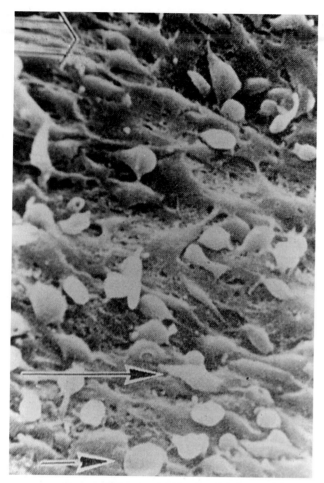

> FIGURE 23–5   SEM of platelet adherence at the site of endothelial loss. Short arrow points to a discoid intact platelet with a single pseudopod; long arrow points to an elongated adherent platelet; double arrow marks densely adherent platelets appearing as elongated humps fused to the subendothelial layer. (From Cotran, E: Robbins Pathologic Basis of Disease, ed 1. WB Saunders, Philadelphia, 1979, p 120, with permission.)

and appear as petechiae or purpura in the skin or mucous membranes. The process of maintenance of normal vascular integrity, involving nourishment of the endothelium by the platelet or actual incorporation of platelets into the vessel wall, utilizes a small minority of the platelets in circulation but is nevertheless an important function.

Platelet Plug Formation

Adhesion and aggregation of platelets to the site of vascular damage occurs in concert with cellular activation. These cellular events are mediated through specific receptors on the platelet membrane. The membrane is key to the interaction of extracellular agonists with intracellular biochemicals. A series of complex intracellular events occurs which lead to further biochemical and morphological change of the platelet. The culmination of these processes permits the platelet to perform its vital role in hemostasis, given normal platelet number and function.

Adhesion

Damage to the endothelial monolayer exposes flowing blood to the subendothelial connective tissue matrix, which is composed of adhesive molecules (i.e., collagen, vWF, fibronectin, and thrombospondin). The specific binding of platelet receptors to these adhesive molecules in plasma or vascular subendothelium mediates adhesion. Adhesion is a reversible process. The principal mechanism of adhesion involves three critical components: (1) vWF, a plasma protein that links the platelet to subendothelial binding sites; (2) a platelet membrane receptor, GPIb; and (3) collagen fibers. The adhesion of platelets to collagen facilitates platelet spreading on the subendothelial surface, which promotes release of dense granules' contents, leading to platelet aggregation. Activation of additional platelets, through the interaction with either collagen or other mediators (such as thrombin, ADP, or TXA_2), amplifies the response and provides a positive feedback mechanism that recruits platelets into the site.[2]

Evidence indicates that vWF is synthesized by endothelial cells and megakaryocytes. Once made, vWF is released into the plasma where it is absorbed onto the surface of the platelet bound to its receptor, GPIb (Fig. 23–6), or incorporated into the subendothelium. Platelets thus adhere to the area of injury at the endothelial lining, acting to arrest the initial episode of bleeding. In Figure 23–7, a TEM demonstrates platelet adhesion to subendothelial connective tissue at the focus of endothelial loss. A decrease in platelet number as well as platelet dysfunction results in increased bleeding.

Shape Change

The interaction of circulating platelets with external stimuli or agonists results in a series of complex reactions known col-

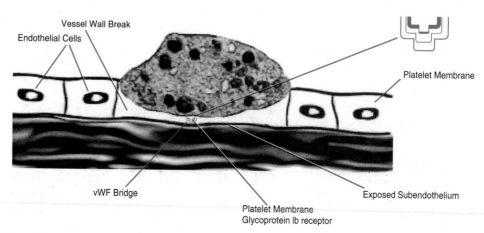

Vessel Wall Break
Endothelial Cells
Platelet Membrane
vWF Bridge
Platelet Membrane Glycoprotein Ib receptor
Exposed Subendothelium

> FIGURE 23–6   Pictorial representation of platelet adhesion to subendothelium through von Willebrand's factor (vWF) bridge.

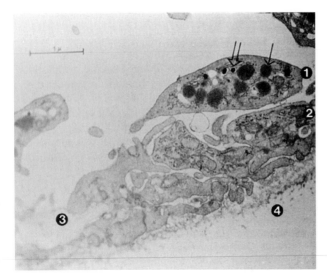

➤ FIGURE 23–7   TEM of platelet adherence to subendothelial connective tissue at the focus of endothelial loss. *(1)* Intact platelet with pseudopod (thin arrow indicates α granule; thick arrow indicates dense body), *(2)* partially degranulated platelet, *(3)* degranulated platelet "ghost," (4) internal elastic lamina. (From Cotran, E: Robbins Pathologic Basis of Disease, ed 1. WB Saunders, Philadelphia, 1979, p 116, with permission.)

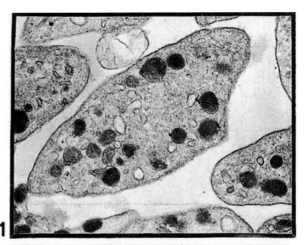

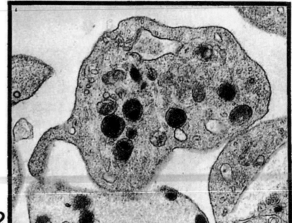

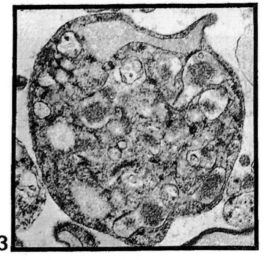

➤ FIGURE 23–8   TEM showing disk-to-sphere transformation of an activated platelet. Note progression from *(1)* disk shape to *(2)* pseudopod formation to *(3)* degranulated ballooned sphere.

lectively as *platelet activation* that precede the ultimate activation event of platelet aggregation and platelet secretion. Platelet activation occurs when an external agonist interacts with its specific membrane receptor on the platelet. Signal transduction occurs, transmitting the signal from outside the cell to inside the cell. Activation of second messenger pathways within the platelet lead to further intracellular biochemical changes, culminating in platelet activation events such as shape change, secretion, cytoskeletal reassembly, and platelet aggregation. Following vessel injury and exposure to external stimuli, platelets change shape from circulating discs to spheres with pseudopods, indicating platelet activation (Fig. 23–8).

Many agonists such as collagen, ADP, thrombin, and TXA_2 alter the internal levels of cytosolic calcium, thus promoting shape change. The normal discoid shape of the platelet is defined by the circumferential microtubules. Increases in cytosolic calcium cause dissolution of the circumferential microtubules, thereby altering platelet shape. Shape change is thought to represent the most sensitive parameter of platelet activation. TXA_2 and ADP are potent platelet agonists when bound to their specific membrane receptors. During platelet activation in response to thrombin, these two platelet-derived agonists (ADP and TXA_2) are released, serving to amplify intracellular events that result in platelet secretion and platelet aggregation.[12] When platelets become activated, shape change and exposure of platelet membrane phospholipids such as PF3 occurs. Exposure of PF3 promotes the assembly of vitamin K–dependent factors on the platelet membrane surface. Activated platelets adhere to exposed collagen, mediated by GPIb and vWF. Dependent on the strength of the agonist, shape change and signaling platelet activation may be followed by platelet aggregation.

Aggregation

Platelet-to-platelet interaction is known as *aggregation* and usually begins 10 to 20 seconds following vascular injury and platelet adhesion. Platelet aggregation is an energy-dependent process that requires ATP, which is primarily derived from glycolysis. Ionized calcium (Ca^{2+}), fibrinogen receptors GPIIb and IIIa, and fibrinogen are necessary for platelet aggregation. Fibrinogen must bind to the activated platelet membrane GPIIb/IIIa complex.[13] Once fibrinogen binds to this membrane complex, extracellular Ca^{2+}-dependent fibrinogen bridges form between adjacent platelets, thereby promoting platelet aggregation. ADP induces the exposure of fibrinogen receptor sites on the platelet membrane. It should be noted that normal plasma fibrinogen levels support platelet aggregation. In the absence of plasma fibrinogen, platelet fibrinogen, stored in the α granules, is released, promoting platelet aggregation. Platelets deficient in GPIIb/IIIa (Glanzmann's thrombasthenia) do not aggregate in response to platelet-aggregating agents.[13] Thus, platelets will not aggregate in the absence of membrane glycoproteins, fibrinogen, or divalent calcium.

In vitro platelet aggregation can be initiated by a variety of agents (Table 23–12). In vitro aggregation can be visualized as a two-phase process that may be reversible or irreversible, depending on the strength of the stimulus. Primary aggregation of platelets is caused by the release of small amounts of ADP from electron-dense granules of adherent platelets in an initial release wave. This initial *aggregation wave is* referred to as *primary* or *reversible aggregation*.[10] At this point in platelet aggregation, small platelet aggregates are formed with low ambient concentrations of aggregating agents. ADP in this concentration is a weak platelet agonist and, thus, platelet aggregates dissociate into individual platelets. Primary aggregation involves contraction of the circumferential microtubules and reorganization and centralization of platelet organelles.

The secondary wave of aggregation is dependent on the activation stimulus being strong enough to evoke the secretion of platelet granules, particularly nonmetabolic ADP from the electron-dense granule, as a consequence of a stronger more complete contraction of the circumferential microtubules. The beginning of secondary aggregation actually defines the activation event of secretion. Ultrastructural analysis shows the internal reorganization of organelles is more severe, and degranulation is evident by the lack of density of the granules with TEM (Fig. 23–9). Biochemical studies have confirmed the release of substances such as ADP, serotonin, and epinephrine. Secondary aggregation is often considered to be irreversible.

Various laboratory methods are employed to evaluate platelet aggregation. The standard aggregometer is a spectrophotometer to which platelet-rich plasma and exogenous aggregating agents are added. As platelets aggregate, decreased optical density results in increased light transmittance. The change in density (percent transmittance) is recorded, creating typical aggregation "patterns" for each

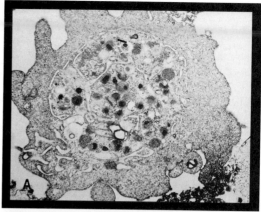
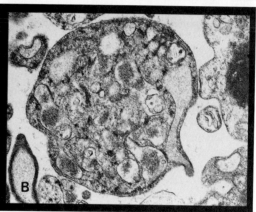

➤ **FIGURE 23–9** TEM of an activated and a degranulated platelet. *A.* Early aggregation of activated platelet (the primary wave of aggregation, a reversible process). *B.* Degranulated platelet (the secondary wave of aggregation, an irreversible process). (From Barnhart, MI: Platelet responses in health and disease. Mol Cell Biochem 22:117, 1978, with permission.)

aggregating agent. The pattern produced is analyzed for reaction time, shape change, primary aggregation, release reaction, and secondary aggregation. The lumi-aggregometer employs both photometric and fluorometric methods in measuring platelet aggregation and simultaneous release of ATP. Figure 23–10 depicts a typical biphasic response of in vitro platelet aggregation to ADP, as recorded by an aggre-

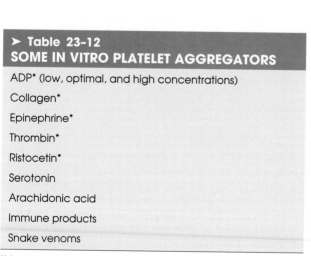

➤ **Table 23–12**
SOME IN VITRO PLATELET AGGREGATORS

ADP* (low, optimal, and high concentrations)

Collagen*

Epinephrine*

Thrombin*

Ristocetin*

Serotonin

Arachidonic acid

Immune products

Snake venoms

*More commonly used.
Abbreviation: ADP = adenosine diphosphate

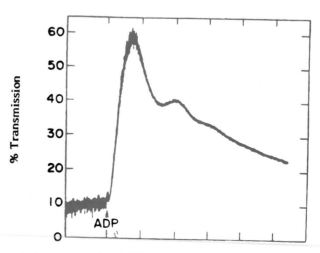

➤ **FIGURE 23–10** A typical biphasic response of in vitro platelet aggregation to ADP, as recorded by an aggregometer.

gometer. It should be noted that aggregation is an energy-dependent process that requires and exhausts the ATP resources of the platelet. (see Chap. 32 for discussion of the principles, instrument methods, and interpretation of platelet aggregation).

Secretion (The Release Reaction)

Platelet secretion (release) and secondary aggregation are intimately related and occur almost simultaneously; therefore, the discussion of the two topics is difficult to separate. As stated previously, the beginning of secondary aggregation actually defines the activation event of secretion. For secondary aggregation to occur, there must be secretion, particularly ADP, from the electron-dense granules. A sufficiently strong stimulus is necessary for the secretion or release reaction to occur. The release reaction from dense granules involves the secretion of ADP, serotonin, and calcium. During the various stages of aggregation, platelet-secreted proteins are released from cellular organelles, thus serving as markers of platelet activation. ADP is responsible for both primary and secondary aggregation (depending on the amount secreted) and serves to amplify the process. Amplification of the initial aggregation of platelets (a reversible phenomenon) results in secondary aggregation and the recruitment of many other platelets into a large platelet mass. The transformation of irreversibly aggregated platelets into a mass of degenerative platelet material without membranes is termed *viscous metamorphosis* (Fig. 23–11). The biochemical contents of the platelet lysosome are also released during secretion. It is thought that these enzymes function in *viscous metamorphosis* and *dissolution of the platelet plug* at the site of vascular injury.

Specific platelet-secreted proteins are released from α and dense granules as well as from platelet lysosomes following appropriate stimulation. Four platelet-specific proteins secreted from the α granule have been well characterized to date and are currently used as "markers of platelet activation." These include beta-thromboglobulin (β-TG), platelet factor 4 (PF4), thrombospondin, and PDGF, which confirm the degranulation of platelet α granules.[1] Because β-TG, PF4, thrombospondin, and PDGF are proteins virtually absent from normal plasma and found in small concentrations within platelet α granules, these proteins specifically mark platelet activation.[1] A number of clinical conditions such as arteriosclerosis, cerebrovascular disease, cardiopulmonary by-

pass, shock, venous thrombosis, and DIC are associated with increased plasma levels of these markers, thus signifying platelet activation.

Stabilization of the Hemostatic Plug

The last stage involved in arresting bleeding after vessel damage is the formation of a stable platelet plug. This stabilization is achieved through the activation of the coagulation cascade and formation and deposition of fibrin (the end product of coagulation) on the platelet aggregates. Exposure of collagen within the subendothelium of the damaged vessel (via the intrinsic pathway) and the release of tissue factor (via the extrinsic pathway) directly initiate fibrin formation. Thus, fibrin interweaves through and over the initial platelet aggregate or platelet plug, compressing the plug into place at the site of the vessel injury. What originally starts as a small gelatinous mass or clot gradually increases in size. In pathologic conditions, thrombus formation may often occlude the lumen of a vessel, producing ischemia to the affected organ or tissue.[14] During thrombus formation, thrombin, plasminogen, t-PA, and antiplasmin are all incorporated into the clot.[14] As thrombin is incorporated into the clot, it is protected from degradation by its inhibitors, antithrombin (AT-III) and heparin cofactor II. Thrombin now trapped within the meshwork of the clot activates factor XIII, resulting in the cross-linking of fibrin strands and, thus, clot stabilization.

Fibrinolysis, the complex series of enzymatic reactions that promote clot dissolution, is simultaneously activated during the process of clot formation. As previously mentioned, plasminogen, the precursor of the proteolytic enzyme plasmin, is incorporated into the fibrin clot. Endothelial cells of the damaged vessel wall secrete t-PA, which catalyzes the conversion of plasminogen to plasmin.[14] Release of both endothelial cell t-PA and its inhibitor, plasminogen activator inhibitor (PAI), is mediated by thrombin. Any excess plasmin is controlled by its inhibitor, antiplasmin. Thus, fibrinolysis is initiated in the final phase of thrombus formation. It is important to mention that thrombin also stimulates the secretion of endothelial cell substances as well as the secretion of platelet proteins that promote tissue repair and play a major role in wound healing. Clot dissolution, therefore, provides a critical means by which formed thrombi are removed from the vascular system, blood vessels are repaired, and blood flow returns to normal. Protective mechanisms prevent thrombin formation in healthy intact blood vessels.

Figure 23–12 provides a review of the sequence of events involved in platelet plug formation and the approximate time involved in each stage.

Advanced Concepts

PLATELET ACTIVATION

Binding of ADP to the platelet membrane activates phospholipase, an enzyme that cleaves the phospholipids present in the platelet membrane, freeing fatty acids such as arachidonic acid. Arachidonic acid is converted in the cytoplasm of the platelet into the (prostaglandin) endoperoxides by prostaglandin synthetase, commonly known as cyclooxygenase. These endoperoxides are converted to TXA_2, a potent platelet aggregator, a mediator of platelet release reaction, and a promoter of vasoconstriction (Fig. 23–13).

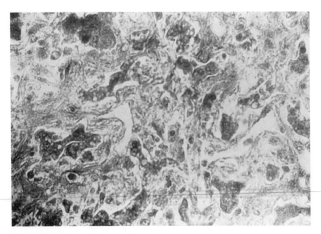

➤ **FIGURE 23–11**   TEM of viscous metamorphosis.

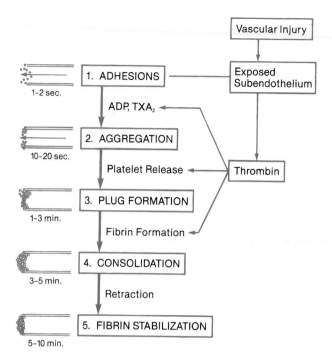

> ➤ **FIGURE 23–12** Sequence of events in hemostatic plug formation. *(1)* Platelet adhesion to exposed subendothelial connective tissue structures. *(2)* Platelet aggregation by ADP, thromboxane A_2, and thrombin recruitment through transformation of discoid platelets into reactive spiny spheres that interact with one another through calcium-dependent fibrinogen bridges. *(3)* Contribution of platelet coagulant activity to the coagulation process, which stabilizes the plug with a fibrin mesh. *(4)* Consolidation of the platelet mass to provide a dense thrombus. *(5)* Fibrin polymerization and fibrin stabilization by factor XIII. (From Thompson, AR, and Harker, LA: Manual of Hemostasis and Thrombosis, ed 3. FA Davis, Philadelphia, 1983, with permission.)

With its in vivo half-life of 3 seconds, TXA_2 activity is limited in time because it hydrolyzes spontaneously within the platelet to an inactive form thromboxane B_2 (TXB_2). As TXA_2 is generated with subsequent aggregating effects on platelets, calcium, sequestered in the dense tubular system of the platelet, is extruded in the sol-gel zone. Thrombin, also a potent platelet aggregator, can induce secretion of all platelet granules. Serotonin, secreted by the dense bodies of the platelet, is a weak aggregating agent as the sole stimulus, but amplifies the aggregating effect of other agonists such as ADP. Serotonin serves as an important vasoconstrictor, and a potent stimulator of smooth muscle PGI_2 production.

EFFECT OF ASPIRIN ON PLATELET PLUG FORMATION
Aspirin is a widely used antithrombotic agent for the clinical treatment of arterial thrombi. Aspirin exerts a permanent yet limited effect on platelet aggregation by inhibiting the action of the cyclo-oxygenase enzyme and production of TXA_2.[15] Platelets are anucleated cells; thus, they lack the ability to synthesize new mRNA or protein. Exposure of platelets in the portal circulation to a relatively small dose of aspirin (60 to 325 mg) results in the irreversible inactivation (acetylation) of the platelet enzyme cyclo-oxygenase, and inhibition of TXA_2 synthesis for the life span of the circulating platelet.[15] It is this quality that gives aspirin its tremendous therapeutic effect on platelet activation. Megakaryocytes, however, are capable of synthesizing cyclo-oxygenase, and newly formed platelets show normal enzyme activity. Aspirin also inhibits endothelial cell cyclo-oxygenase consistent with the fact that they are genetically identical cellular products. However, endothelial cells possess the organelles necessary to synthesize cyclo-oxygenase, thereby regenerating enzyme activity as the level of circulating aspirin decreases.

Aspirin's effect on platelet cyclo-oxygenase is highly sensitive yet quite limited. Platelets activate and aggregate in response to stimuli such as thrombin and collagen. There are several other intracellular signaling pathways that mediate platelet activation and aggregation, but only one, TXA_2 synthetase, is inhibited by aspirin.[15] Thus, aspirin has a modest effect on platelet function in vivo, causing moderate prolongation of the bleeding time and moderate inhibition of platelet aggregation. Despite its limited effect on platelet function, aspirin provides a clinically significant antithrombotic effect.

➤ SECONDARY HEMOSTASIS: FIBRIN-FORMING (COAGULATION) SYSTEM
The fibrin-forming (coagulation) system is that system through which coagulation factors interact to eventually form a fibrin clot. The purpose of fibrin clot formation (secondary hemostasis) is to reinforce the platelet plug (primary hemostasis).

This system is mediated by many coagulation proteins (coagulation factors), normally present in the blood in an inactive state (coagulation factors). Table 23–13 lists the coagulation factors and their most commonly used designations. *Secondary hemostasis* is the phrase used to encompass the coagulation factors' role in the hemostatic mechanism.

Most of the coagulation factors are designated by Roman numerals. The numerical system adopted assigns the number to the factors according to the sequence of discovery and not to the point of interaction in the cascade. Some factors are routinely referred to by their common names, such as fibrinogen and prothrombin, whereas others are more commonly referred to by Roman numeral (such as factor XI, plasma thromboplastin antecedent factor).

Activation of a factor is designated by addition of a small "a" next to the Roman numeral in the coagulation cascade (e.g., XII → XIIa) unless convention dictates otherwise. For example, most references incorporate "thrombin" into the coagulation cascade rather than its alternate designation, IIa. Some of the common names are derived from the original patients who exhibited symptoms leading to elucidation of that factor deficiency and an understanding of the role of that factor in the cascade (e.g., Christmas factor, Hageman factor). Other common names describe the action of the factor in the coagulation system (e.g., fibrin-stabilizing factor).

All the coagulation proteins are produced in the liver. The von Willebrand portion of factor VIII is produced in other body sites as well; namely, endothelial cells and megakaryocytes.

Classification of Coagulation Factors by Hemostatic Function
In terms of general hemostatic function, the coagulation factors can be divided into three categories: substrate, cofactors, and enzymes (Table 23–14).

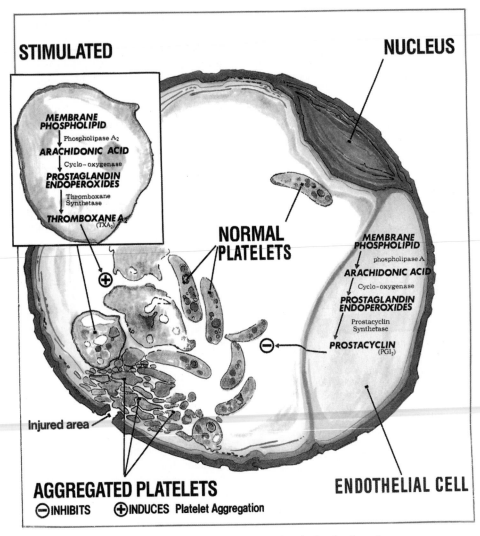

➤ FIGURE 23–13   Synthesis of prostaglandins in platelets and endothelial cells during platelet plug formation.

Factor I, fibrinogen, is regarded as the main substrate of the blood coagulation system, because the formation of a fibrin clot from fibrinogen is the ultimate goal. Cofactors are proteins that accelerate the enzymatic reactions involved in the coagulation process. Some examples of blood coagulation cofactors are V (labile factor) and VIII:C (antihemophilic factor, or AHF).

The last general category of blood coagulation factors is the enzyme category. Enzymes involved in coagulation can be subdivided into two groups: serine proteases and transaminases. Except for factor XIII (fibrin-stabilizing factor), all the enzymes are serine proteases when they are in their activated form. These proteases have serine as a portion of their active enzymatic site and function to cleave peptide bonds.

Factor XIII (fibrin-stabilizing factor) is the only member of the transaminase subgroup. It functions to create cross-linkages between the fibrin monomers formed during the coagulation process to produce a stable fibrin clot.

Classification of Coagulation Factors by Physical Properties

On the basis of their physical properties, the coagulation proteins may also be divided into three other groups: (1) the contact proteins, (2) the prothrombin proteins, and (3) the

fibrinogen- or thrombin-sensitive proteins. Refer to Table 23–15 for details on each group.

The contact group includes factor XII (Hageman factor), factor XI (plasma thromboplastin antecedent), prekallikrein (Fletcher factor), and high-molecular-weight kininogen (HMWK; Fitzgerald factor). These proteins are involved in the initial phase of intrinsic system activation. Although deficiencies of these coagulation proteins are associated with markedly abnormal laboratory tests, an isolated factor XI deficiency is associated with a mild bleeding disorder. Interestingly, problems with thrombosis have been reported in patients with factor XII (Hageman factor) and prekallikrein (Fletcher factor) deficiencies.

The prothrombin group (see Table 23–15) generally consists of low-molecular-weight proteins that include factors II (prothrombin), VII (stable factor), IX (Christmas factor), and X (Stuart-Prower factor). This group is also known as the vitamin K–dependent coagulation proteins. Each member of this group contains a unique amino acid—gamma carboxyglutamic acid—that is necessary for both calcium binding and attraction of these coagulation factors to the surface of activated platelets, where the formation of a fibrin clot occurs.

Drugs that act as antagonists to vitamin K (such as war-

Table 23-13
NOMENCLATURE OF COAGULATION FACTORS

Factor I	Fibrinogen
Factor II	Prothrombin
Factor III	Tissue thromboplastin (tissue factor)
Factor IV	Ionized calcium (Ca++)
Factor V	Labile factor (proaccelerin)
Factor VI	Not assigned*
Factor VII	Stable factor (serum prothrombin conversion accelerator (SPCA) proconvertin)
Factor VIII	Antihemophilic factor (AHF), factor VIII:C (coagulant portion)
Factor IX	Christmas factor (plasma thromboplastin component (PTC), antihemophilic factor B)
Factor X	Stuart-Prower factor
Factor XI	Plasma thromboplastin antecedent (PTA)
Factor XII	Hageman factor (contact factor)
Factor XIII	Fibrin-stabilizing factor (FSF)
Fitzgerald factor	High-molecular-weight kininogen (HMWK)
Fletcher factor	Prekallikrein

*The factor VI designation was dropped because a substance originally thought to be factor VI was found to be a precursor to factor V, and to avoid confusion, factor VI has not been reassigned.

farin, which is commonly used for oral anticoagulant therapy, and indanediones, which are used in therapy for individuals who exhibit warfarin sensitivity[10]) inhibit this vitamin K–dependent reaction, which is required for functionally active coagulation factors of the prothrombin group. Factors II (prothrombin), VII (stable factor), IX (Christmas factor), and X (Stuart-Prower factor), and proteins C and S, are still synthesized by the liver but are not complete because they lack spe-

Table 23-14
CLASSIFICATIONS OF COAGULATION FACTORS BY HEMOSTATIC FUNCTION

Substrate

Fibrinogen (factor I)

Cofactors

Labile factor (factor V)

Factor VIII:C (antihemophilic factor, coagulant portion)

Enzymes

Serine Proteases

  IIa, VIIa, IXa, Xa, XIa, XIIa, prekallikrein

Transaminase

  Factor XIIIa

cific binding receptors for calcium.[10] These proteins may be present physically but are impaired functionally as they cannot enter into the formation of an enzyme-substrate complex.[10] Therefore, patients who are vitamin K–deficient exhibit decreased production of functional prothrombin proteins (normal amounts of the proteins may be present, but the proteins themselves are dysfunctional). These dysfunctional factors are called proteins induced by vitamin K absence or antagonists (PIVKAs).

Acquired deficiencies of the vitamin K–dependent coagulation factors are relatively common because the body does not contain appreciable stores of vitamin K. Characteristic prototypes for developing a vitamin K deficiency include patients who have just had surgery and are receiving parenteral feeding, patients who are receiving high doses of intravenous antibiotics, and patients suffering from liver disease.

The fibrinogen group (see Table 23–15) consists generally of high-molecular-weight proteins that include factors I (fibrinogen), V (labile factor), VIII:C (antihemophilic factor), and XIII (fibrin-stabilizing factor). During coagulation, generated thrombin acts on all the factors in the fibrinogen group. Thrombin enhances the activity of factors V (labile factor) and VIII:C (antihemophilic factor) by converting these proteins to active cofactors, which are involved in the assembly of macromolecular complexes on the surface of activated platelets. Thrombin also activates factor XIII (fibrin-stabilizing factor) and converts fibrinogen to fibrin.

Factors V (labile factor) and VIII:C (antihemophilic factor) are the least stable factors, because their activity is relatively labile to degradation and denaturation. Therefore, testing for factor V (labile factor) and VIII:C (antihemophilic factor) should be rapid, or else appropriate storage measures should be taken. In addition to the presence of the fibrinogen group in plasma, these factors are also found within platelets. Some of the fibrinogen group of coagulation factors have been reported to increase with inflammation, pregnancy, and with the use of oral contraceptives. Table 23–16 summarizes other physical properties of the coagulation factors.

Blood Coagulation: The "Cascade" Theory

The process of blood coagulation involves a series of biochemical reactions that transforms circulating substances into an insoluble gel through conversion of soluble fibrinogen to fibrin. This process requires plasma proteins (coagulation factors) as well as phospholipids and calcium.

Blood coagulation leading to fibrin formation can be separated into two pathways, extrinsic (Fig. 23–14) and intrinsic (Fig. 23–15), both of which share specific coagulation factors with the common pathway[16] (Fig. 23–16). Both extrinsic and intrinsic pathways require initiation, which leads to subsequent activation of various coagulation factors in a cascading, waterfall, or domino effect. Useful demonstrations can be derived from the waterfall or domino concept. According to the cascade theory, each coagulation factor is converted to its active form by the preceding factor in a series of biochemical chain reactions. Ca^{2+} participates in some of the reactions as a cofactor. Each reaction is promoted by the preceding reaction, and if there is a deficiency of any one of the factors, the consequences listed in Table 23–17 result.

Eventually, both the extrinsic and intrinsic systems lead to the common pathway with generation of the enzyme

➤ **Table 23-15**
CLASSIFICATION OF COAGULATION PROTEINS BY PHYSICAL PROPERTIES

	Contact Group	Prothrombin Group	Fibrinogen Group
Factors	XII, XI, PK, HMWK	II, VII, IX, X	I, V, VIII, XIII
Consumed during coagulation	No	No (except II)	Yes
Present in serum	Yes	Yes (except II)	No
Present in stored plasma	Yes	Yes	No*
Absorbed by BaSO₄	No	Yes	No
Present in adsorbed plasma	Yes	No	Yes
Vitamin K–dependent	No	Yes	No

*Factors V and VIII are not present in stored plasma because of their labile nature, but factors I and XIII are present.
Abbreviations: PK = prekallikrein; HMWK = high-molecular-weight kininogen

thrombin, which converts fibrinogen to fibrin (Figs. 23–17 and 23–18). The term *extrinsic* is used because this pathway is initiated when tissue factor, a substance not found in blood, enters the vascular system (see Fig. 23–14). The tissue factor includes a phospholipid component that is the source of required phospholipid in the extrinsic system (Fig. 23–19). Phospholipid provides a surface for interaction of various factors. The phospholipids required in the intrinsic pathway are provided by the platelet membrane. In the intrinsic pathway, all the factors necessary for clot

➤ **Table 23-16**
PHYSICAL PROPERTIES OF THE COAGULATION FACTORS

Factor	Clotting Pathway	Molecular Weight	Half-Life in Vivo (hr)	Plasma Concentration (mg/dL)	Storage Stability	Other Characteristics*
I	Intrinsic, extrinsic, common pathway	340,000	90–150	200–400	Stable	Activity destroyed during coagulation process, present in absorbed plasma
II	Intrinsic, extrinsic, common pathway	70,000	50–100	10–15	Stable	Consumed during coagulation process
III	Extrinsic system only	45,000	—	0	Stable	Found in tissues
V	Intrinsic, extrinsic, common pathway	330,000	12–36	0.5–1.2	Labile	Activity destroyed during coagulation process, present in absorbed plasma
VII	Extrinsic system only	48,000	4–6	0.05–2.0	Stable	Present in serum
VIII/vWF	Intrinsic system only	350,000	8–12	0.01–0.1	Labile	Activity destroyed during coagulation process, present in absorbed plasma
IX	Intrinsic only	60,000	20–24	0.3–0.4	Stable	Present in serum
X	Intrinsic, extrinsic common pathway	59,000	24–65	0.5–1.0	Stable	Present in serum
XI	Intrinsic only	160,000	40–80	0.5–12	Stable	Present in serum and absorbed plasma
XII	Intrinsic only	80,000	50–70	3.0–4.0	Stable	Present in serum and absorbed plasma
XIII	Intrinsic, extrinsic, common pathway	320,000	72–150	1.0–2.5	Stable	Activity destroyed during coagulation process, present in absorbed plasma
PK	Intrinsic only	85,000	35	3.0–5.0	? Stable	Present in serum and absorbed plasma
HMWK	Intrinsic only	150,000	150–160	6.0–9.0	? Stable	Present in serum and absorbed plasma

*All factors are present in normal fresh plasma.
Abbreviations: PK = prekallikrein; HMWK = High-molecular-weight kininogen

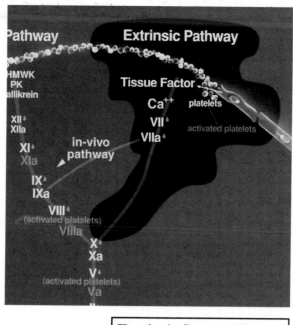

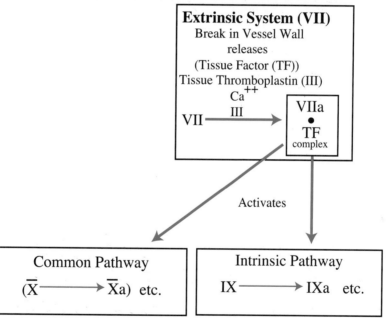

> ➤ FIGURE 23–14   The extrinsic pathway and the role of factor VIIa in activation of factor X and IX. (From American Bioproducts Company, modified with permission).

formation are intrinsic to the vascular compartment because they are all found within the circulating blood (see Fig. 23–15).

Extrinsic Pathway (Factors VII)

In the extrinsic pathway, factor VII is activated to factor VIIa in the presence of Ca^{2+} (factor IV) and the tissue factor (factor III), which is released from the injured vessel wall (see Fig. 23–14). Only factor VIIa, Ca^{2+}, and factor III (tissue factor) are needed to activate factor X to Xa.

Figures 23–17 and 23–18 show that the extrinsic pathway provides a means for very quickly producing small amounts of thrombin, leading to fibrin formation. In addition, the VIIa tissue factor complex can activate factor IX to IXa in the intrinsic pathway. In the laboratory, the prothrombin time (PT) test is used to monitor the extrinsic pathway (for a review of the procedure, see Chap. 32).

Intrinsic Pathway (Factors XII, XI, IX, and VIII)

Basic Concepts

Following exposure to negatively charged foreign substances such as collagen, subendothelium, or phospholipids, activation of factor XII involving "contact factors" and factor XI initiates clotting through the intrinsic pathway (see Fig. 23–15).

Once generated, factor XIIa in the presence of Fitzgerald factor (HMWK) and Fletcher factor (prekallikrein) converts factor XI to XIa. Factor XIIa is capable of activating factor XI without HMWK, but the activation takes place much more slowly.[8]

The next reaction in the intrinsic pathway is the activation of factor IX to factor IXa by factor XIa, in the presence of Ca^{2+}. Activated factor IX (IXa) participates, along with

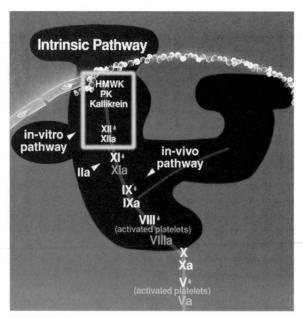

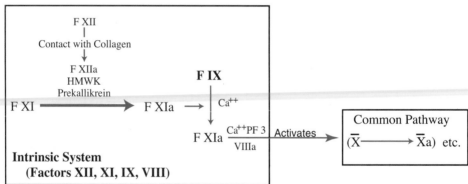

➤ **FIGURE 23–15**   The intrinsic pathway and its role in activation of factor X. HMWK = high-molecular-weight kininogen; PF3 = platelet factor 3. (From American Bioproducts Company, modified with permission).

the essential cofactor VIII:C, in the presence of ionized calcium and PF3, a source of phospholipid, to activate factor X, which leads to the generation of thrombin and formation of fibrin. The complex consisting of factor IXa–factor VIIIa–phospholipid–Ca^{2+} has been called *tenase complex* because it activates factor X[10] (Fig. 23–20).

The macromolecular complex of factors IXa, VIIIa, X, PF3, and Ca^{2+} assembles on the surface of the activated platelet (providing the phospholipid) during the intrinsic pathway of blood coagulation. This surface provides a protective environment that facilitates the enzymatic reactions of the coagulation cascade without interference from the physiologic anticoagulants normally present in plasma.

In regard to the intrinsic pathway, it is also important to be familiar with the properties of the factor VIII complex (Table 23–18). Factor VIII complex consists of two main portions, factor VIII:C (the procoagulant portion) and vWF (the carrier protein).

It should be noted that factor VIII requires enhancement by the generated enzyme thrombin to amplify its activity. In the laboratory, the activated partial thromboplastin time (APTT) test is used to evaluate the intrinsic pathway. During laboratory testing, the intrinsic pathway is initiated in vitro by activation on negatively charged surfaces such as glass or kaolin (for a review of this procedure, see Chap. 32).

Factor VIII complex, which consists of several components, comprises the largest protein involved in the coagulation cascade. The major portion of this protein complex is considered to be the carrier protein called *von Willebrand's factor (vWF)*, although this is not the portion active in the coagulation cascade. There seems to be a movement to use the designation "vWF" rather than factor VIII:vWF when referring to the vWF portion of the factor VIII complex.[10]

A smaller subunit or protein that is associated with factor VIII is responsible for the clotting or procoagulant activity of factor VIII (VIII:C). The C in the expression VIII:C stands for "coagulant." It is factor VIII:C that is functionally active in the coagulation cascade.

The vWF portion of the complex carries the VIII:C procoagulant portion. The vWF portion may exhibit a stabilizing effect over factor VIII:C by protecting it from proteolytic activity.[10] Because of vWF's extremely large size and its ability to bind to the platelet membrane GPIb and IIb/IIIa receptors, it appears to have a role in anchoring the platelet plug to the vessel breach.

Common Pathway (Factors X, V, II, and I)

The common pathway begins with the activation of factor X by the intrinsic system, the extrinsic system, or both (see

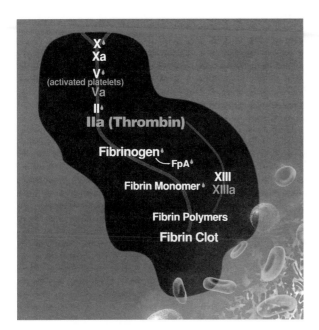

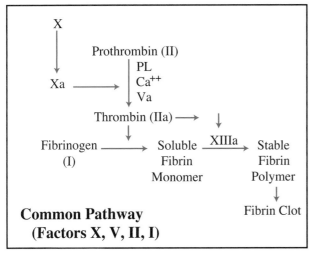

**Common Pathway
(Factors X, V, II, I)**

➤ FIGURE 23-16   The common pathway and formation of fibrin clot. PL = phospholipid source. (From American Bioproducts Company, modified with permission).

Figs. 23–16 and 23–17). Factor Xa, in the presence of factor V, Ca^{2+}, and phospholipid (PF3), converts prothrombin to its active form, thrombin. Thrombin then takes the following actions: it feeds back to activate factors VIII and V, converts fibrinogen to soluble fibrin monomer, and helps to stabilize the fibrin monomer by converting factor XIII to XIIIa, which cross-links the fibrin monomers to form stable

➤ **Table 23-17**
CONSEQUENCES OF FACTOR DEFICIENCY

- Coagulation cannot proceed at a normal rate
- Initiation of the next subsequent reaction is delayed
- The time required for the clot to form is prolonged
- Bleeding from the injured vessel continues for a longer time (or there may be a physiologic tendency toward thrombosis present if the patient is deficient in factor XII)

ble fibrin polymer. Thrombin also has other actions (see later discussion of Thrombin-Mediated Reactions in Hemostasis [Advanced Concepts]). Because the common pathway contains the factors X, V, II, and I, these factors may be monitored by both the PT and the APTT.

From the extrinsic system, factor VIIa in the presence of tissue factor and ionized calcium converts factor X to Xa. From the intrinsic system, the tenase complex (factor IXa in the presence of factor VIII:C, phospholipid [PF3], and Ca^{2+}) converts factor X to Xa (see Figs. 23–17 and 23–18).

After the formation of factor Xa, this activated factor, along with cofactor V, in the presence of Ca^{2+} and phospholipid (PF3), converts factor II, prothrombin, to the active enzyme thrombin. The phospholipid is present to provide surfaces so that prothrombin and factor X can be bound by bridges of ionized calcium.[10] The association of factor Xa, factor V, phospholipid, and Ca^{2+} is called the *prothrombinase complex* (or the prothrombin activator) because it enzymatically converts the substrate prothrombin to the enzymatically active thrombin[10] (Fig. 23–21). This additional macromolecular complex of factors Xa, V, IV (Ca^{2+}), PF3 (the platelet membrane phospholipid), and prothrombin also assembles on the surface of activated platelets.

Activation of thrombin is slow, but once generated, it further amplifies coagulation (Table 23–19). Thrombin acts on fibrinogen to form fibrin monomers. Fibrinogen is composed of three pairs of polypeptide chains (two alpha [α] chains, two beta [β] chains, and two gamma [γ] chains). Thrombin cleaves a portion of each of the α and β polypeptides to form fibrinopeptides A and B. Most of the α and β chains are still left on the fibrinogen molecule. After this cleavage of fibrinopeptides A and B, the remainder of the fibrinogen molecule is called *fibrin monomer* (Fig. 23–22).

By using the PT and APTT test results in the laboratory, one can identify defects or deficiencies as occurring in the intrinsic, extrinsic, or common pathways of blood coagulation with the exception of factor XIII functional deficiency. Using Table 23–20, the reader can practice interpretation of these tests in identifying possible factor deficiencies. However, the most common cause of a prolonged PT or APTT is anticoagulant therapy.

➤ **THROMBIN-MEDIATED REACTIONS IN HEMOSTASIS (ADVANCED CONCEPTS)**

Each of the four major components of coagulation, and the various substances produced by each component, help to regulate the basal state of hemostasis by which blood remains fluid and cell surfaces remain nonthrombogenic. Vascular damage initiates physical, cellular, and molecular changes to platelets, endothelium, and circulating coagulation proteins. When the inert proenzymes of coagulation become activated, inhibitors irreversibly bind to these activated factors, thus controlling the hemostatic response. Numerous pathways exist that ultimately lead to the generation of *thrombin,* and consequently *fibrin* formation, following vascular injury. Thus, thrombin has a central role in the bioregulation of hemostasis in both normal and pathologic conditions. The following discussion provides an overview of thrombin-mediated mechanisms in hemostasis. Refer to Table 23–21 to summarize the various roles of thrombin in hemostasis.

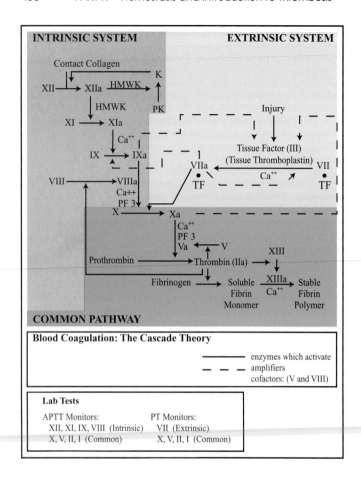

INTRINSIC SYSTEM   EXTRINSIC SYSTEM

Contact Collagen   K

XII ──► XIIa ──HMWK──►
              HMWK   PK
XI ──► XIa
        Ca⁺⁺   Injury
IX ──► IXa   Tissue Factor (III)
VIII ──►VIIIa   (Tissue Thromboplastin)
        Ca++   VIIa   ──Ca⁺⁺──   VII
        PF 3   ●TF   ●TF
X ──────► Xa
          Ca⁺⁺
          PF 3
          Va ◄── V   XIII
Prothrombin ──────► Thrombin (IIa) ───►
Fibrinogen ──────► Soluble ──XIIIa──► Stable
                    Fibrin   Ca⁺⁺   Fibrin
                    Monomer   Polymer

COMMON PATHWAY

Blood Coagulation: The Cascade Theory

────── enzymes which activate
– – – – amplifiers
          cofactors: (V and VIII)

Lab Tests

APTT Monitors: PT Monitors:
  XII, XI, IX, VIII (Intrinsic)   VII (Extrinsic)
  X, V, II, I (Common)   X, V, II, I (Common)

➤ **FIGURE 23–17** Blood coagulation: The "cascade" theory of coagulation. The extrinsic system, the intrinsic system, and the common pathway and the appropriate laboratory tests for evaluation of each. HMWK = high-molecular-weight kininogen; PF3 = platelet factor 3; PK = prekallikrein; PT = prothrombin time; APTT = activated partial thromboplastin time.

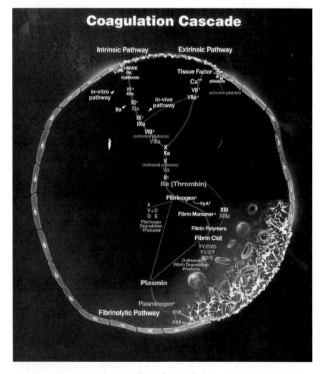

Coagulation Cascade

➤ **FIGURE 23–18** An overview of coagulation cascade, the intrinsic and extrinsic pathways, and the interaction between the two. The fibrinolytic pathway and its action on fibrinogen and fibrin. HMWK = high-molecular-weight kininogen; PK = prekallikrein; FpA = fibrinopeptide A. (From American Bioproducts Company, with permission.)

Thrombin-Mediated Platelet Aggregation

Thrombin is considered to be a potent platelet-aggregating agent. The binding of thrombin to specific platelet membrane receptors initiates cellular events leading to platelet secretion and aggregation. Thrombin promotes secretion of serotonin, a vasoconstrictor, and TXA_2, a platelet-aggregating agent. As a result of thrombin-induced secretion, vessels constrict, limiting blood flow, and platelets aggregate. The hemostatic plug grows in size, eventually being enmeshed within fibrin. Activated platelets provide surface phospholipids for the assembly of coagulation factors and further thrombin generation.

Thrombin Formation: Role of Extrinsic Pathway

Formation of thrombin occurs by way of the extrinsic pathway and tissue factor. Tissue factor, a membrane glycoprotein, is released from cells and tissues and binds to factor VII in circulation, thus activating factor VII to factor VIIa. The TF-VIIa complex then activates either factor IX or X. The prominent pathway is thought to be activation of factor IX to promote coagulation and fibrin formation.

Thrombin Formation: Role of Common Pathway

Factors X, II (prothrombin), I (fibrinogen), and cofactor V are critical to the formation of a thrombus in circulation. Activated factor IXa (via factor VIIa) factor X, Ca^{2+}, and thrombin-activated VIIIa assemble on membrane platelet phospholipid and catalyze the activation of factor X. Newly generated factor Xa, membrane-bound thrombin-activated

Phospholipid, Ca^{++}-Dependent Reactions of Extrinsic and Common Pathway.

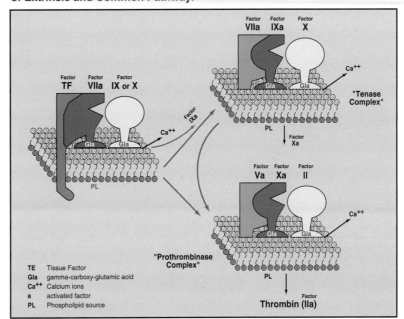

➤ **FIGURE 23–19** Platelet membrane phospholipid provides a surface for the interaction of coagulation factors and the formation of "tenase complex" and "prothrombinase complex."

factor Va, Ca^{2+}, and factor II (prothrombin) assemble on the platelet membrane, forming the prothrombinase complex. This complex catalyzes the conversion of prothrombin to thrombin. Thus, this thrombin-modulated pathway provides a positive feedback mechanism to amplify the generation of thrombin from prothrombin at a faster rate. Increased thrombin concentrations serve to amplify the activation of cofactors V and VIII, which, in turn, leads to enhanced thrombin formation from its precursor prothrombin.

Thrombin-Mediated Anticoagulant Activity

Antithrombin III (AT-III) is the main physiologic inhibitor of thrombin, factors Xa, IXa, XIa, and XIIa, activated protein C, and kallikrein (Fig. 23–23). In the presence of heparin, the inactivation of thrombin and factor Xa by AT-III is significantly increased. AT-III is consumed in the inhibition of thrombin.

The role of protein C (a vitamin K–dependent factor) as an anticoagulant is related to the presence of thrombin, thrombomodulin, and protein S.[17] Protein C is activated by thrombin and endothelial cell thrombomodulin. The formation of thrombin-thrombomodulin complex accelerates the activation of protein C. Activated protein C exerts an anticoagulant effect by inactivating cofactors Va and VIIIa, thus slowing the rate of thrombin formation. It is important to note that activated protein C does not inhibit the other regulatory roles of thrombin in hemostasis. The inhibition of cofactors Va and VIIIa by protein C is enhanced by the presence of protein S, another vitamin K–dependent factor. Activated protein C is also inhibited by other plasma proteins. The role of activated protein C is to turn off the amplification pathway of thrombin generation. It is interesting to note that the reactions that lead to thrombin formation from its precursor prothrombin are regulated in part by thrombin-mediated mechanisms (see Chap. 27 for a detailed discussion of anticoagulant therapy).

Fibrinogen Conversion and Fibrin Stabilization via Thrombin

Thrombin proteolytically cleaves first fibrinopeptide A, then fibrinopeptide B from the α and β chains of fibrinogen, respectively, forming a soluble fibrin monomer. Fibrin monomers polymerize in an end-to-end and side-to-side manner held together by weak hydrogen bonds. Factor XIII is activated to factor XIIIa by thrombin (in the presence of Ca^{2+}) and catalyzes the cross-linking of glutamine and lysine, thus polymerizing soluble fibrin monomers to an insoluble fibrin meshwork.

Thrombin-Mediated Tissue Repair

Thrombin has numerous effects on the cells that play a role in tissue repair and wound healing. Shortly after thrombin generation, there is increased vascular permeability and increased adhesion of leukocytes to endothelial cells mediated by various adhesion molecules secreted by platelets and endothelial cells. Neutrophils and monocytes undergo chemotaxis in response to thrombin. Thrombin mediates the release of a potent smooth muscle mitogen (PDGF, or platelet-derived growth factor) as well as stimulates the proliferation of fibroblasts, smooth muscle cells, and endothelial cells, thus aiding in vascular repair.

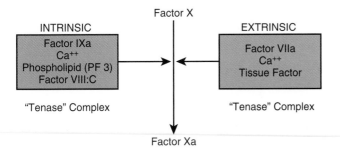

➤ **FIGURE 23–20** Activation of factor X at the beginning of the common pathway and the "tenase" complex.

> ## Table 23-18
> ## FACTOR VIII COMPLEX

I. Smaller protein subunit

  1. Nomenclature

     VIII (referring to the procoagulant portion)

     VIII:C (for coagulant)

     VIII:AHF (the antihemophilic factor)

  2. Components

     a. VIII:CAg—antigen determinant of VIII, measured by immunoassays with human antibodies to VIII

     b. VIII:C—procoagulant property of normal plasma measured in the APTT test as procoagulant activity

  3. Characteristics

     a. Inherited as sex-linked recessive

     b. Acts as a cofactor in a complex with factor IXa, Ca++, and PF3 to activate factor X to Xa

II. Major protein portion

  1. Nomenclature

     a. vWF (von Willebrand factor)

     b. VIII:vWF

     c. VIII:R (factor VIII–related protein)

  2. Components

     a. vWF:Ag—antigen determinant on vWF that is detected by using the heterologous antibodies to vWF

     b. Ristocetin cofactor (VIIIR:Rco)—the property of normal plasma VIIIR that supports ristocetin-induced agglutination of washed normal platelets

  3. Characteristics

     a. Usually inherited as autosomal dominant

     b. Responsible for platelet adhesion

     c. Responsible for ristocetin-induced aggregation of platelets

     d. Stabilizes VIII:C when bound to vWF during circulation, and functions in prevention or protection of VIII:C from proteolytic inactivation or removal from the circulation

Abbreviation: APTT = activated partial thromboplastin time

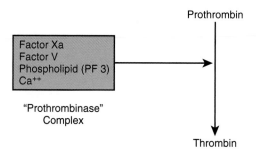

> **FIGURE 23–21**   Conversion of prothrombin to thrombin by prothrombinase complex.

The fibrinolytic system is mediated mainly by the enzyme plasmin, which acts primarily on fibrin to produce lysis of the clot. Plasmin is generated from the inactive zymogen called *plasminogen*. Plasminogen is activated to plasmin by t-PA and other substances (see Chap. 26).

A number of plasmin inhibitors exist to keep fibrinolysis from getting out of control. In addition to plasmin, plas-

> ## Table 23-19
> ## ACTIONS OF THROMBIN

- Converts fribrinogen to fibrin
- Activates factor XIII
- Enhances activity of factors V and VIII
- Induces platelet aggregation

► FIBRIN-LYSING (FIBRINOLYTIC) SYSTEM

The fibrin-forming and fibrin-lysing systems are intimately related. Activation of coagulation also activates fibrin lysis. Fibrinolysis, the physiologic process of removing unwanted fibrin deposits, represents a gradual progressive enzymatic cleavage of fibrin to soluble fragments. These fragments are then removed from the circulation by the fixed macrophages of the reticuloendothelial system (RES). This action of the fibrinolytic system reestablishes blood flow in vessels occluded by a thrombus and facilitates the healing process following injury. For a detailed description of the fibrinolytic system refer to Chapter 26.

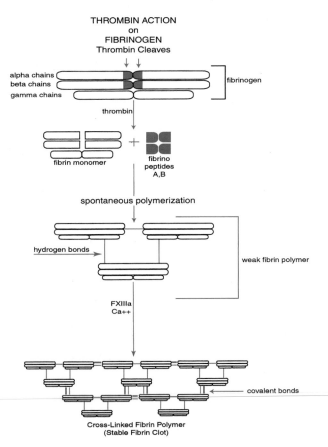

> **FIGURE 23–22**   Thrombin activity on fibrinogen.

➤ **Table 23-20**
INTERPRETATION OF COAGULATION TEST RESULTS

Test Battery	Results	Possible Cause
APTT	Abnormal	1. Vitamin K defect
PT	Abnormal	2. Liver disease
TT	Normal	3. Inhibitor present
		4. Factor deficiency in common pathway (X, V, II)
APTT	Abnormal	1. Factor deficiency in the intrinsic pathway
PT	Normal	2. Lupus anticoagulant
		3. Specific factor inhibitor (VIII inhibitor)
APTT	Normal	1. Factor deficiency in the extrinsic pathway
PT	Abnormal	2. Specific factor inhibitor
APTT	Abnormal	1. Factor deficiency (I)
PT	Abnormal	2. Severe liver disease
TT	Abnormal	3. DIC
		4. Potent inhibitor
		5. Hypofibrinogenogenemia or dysfibrinogenemia

Abbreviations: PT = prothrombin time; APTT = activated partial thromboplastin time; TT = thrombin time; DIC = disseminated intravascular coagulation

minogen, and plasminogen activators, inhibitors of plasmin are a part of the fibrinolytic system.[18] Table 23–22 lists some inhibitors of plasmin.

It is important to realize that some of the same substances that initiate or enhance clot formation also initiate clot degradation. For example, in tissue, both tissue thromboplastin (initiator of extrinsic pathway of fibrin formation)

➤ **Table 23-21**
THROMBIN-MEDIATED REACTIONS IN HEMOSTASIS

Procoagulant

- Induces platelet activation and aggregation
- Activates cofactor VIII to VIIIa
- Converts fibrinogen to fibrin
- Activates factor XIII to XIIIa
- Via autocatalysis converts prothrombin to thrombin

Coagulation Inhibitor

- Binds with antithrombin III to inhibit serine proteases (XIIa, XIa, Xa, IXa, and kallikrein)
- Promotes endothelial cell release of t-PA
- Binds to thrombomodulin to activate protein C (inhibits Va and VIIIa)

Tissue Repair

- Induces cellular chemotaxis
- Stimulates proliferation of smooth muscle and endothelial cells

and t-PA (which activates plasminogen) are released with endothelial damage. t-PA is produced by vascular endothelial cells and selectively binds to fibrin as it activates fibrin-bound plasminogen. Because circulating plasminogen is not activated by t-PA, this biologic substance is efficient in dissolving a clot without causing systemic fibrinolysis and serves as an ideal therapeutic fibrinolytic agent.

Biologic t-PA has been successfully produced by recombinant deoxyribonucleic acid (DNA) technology and is currently available. Inhibitors of t-PA also exist and contribute to controlling its actions.[18] It is also important to note that thrombin generates both fibrin and plasmin formation.

Action of Plasmin

Plasmin is a broad-spectrum endopeptidase (proteolytic enzyme) that acts nonspecifically, with a strong affinity for fibrin.[16] Plasmin, however, cannot distinguish between the protein fibrin and fibrinogen. The action of plasmin begins by splitting off pieces of each of the α and β polypeptides (a larger portion than that cleaved by thrombin) and a smaller piece of each of the two γ polypeptides from fibrinogen. The remaining molecule is called the *X monomer* (which is still thrombin-clottable).

As plasmin continues its action, it further splits the X monomer into a Y fragment (not clottable by thrombin) and a smaller D fragment. Further action of plasmin cleaves the Y fragment into D and E fragments.[10] Therefore, the final fibrin-split products are two D fragments and one E fragment generated from one molecule of fibrinogen (Fig. 23–24). These products are collectively known as either fibrin(ogen) degradation products (FDPs) or fibrin(ogen)-split products (FSPs).[10]

The term *fibrin(ogen)* means that the FDPs can come from either fibrinogen or fibrin. Early FDPs include X

Antithrombin III and Protein C Pathways

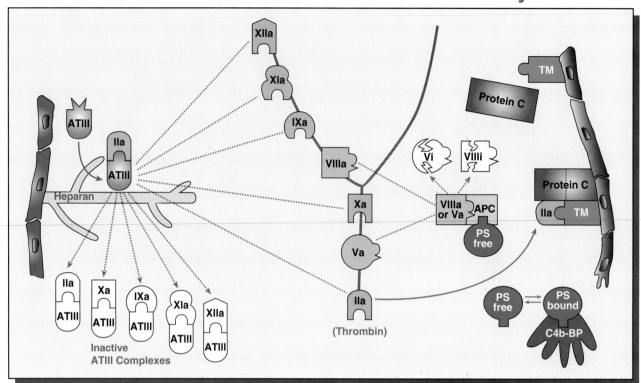

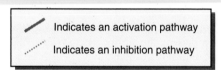

> Indicates an activation pathway
>
> Indicates an inhibition pathway

➤ **FIGURE 23–23**   The inhibitor pathway of coagulation. AT-III = antithrombin III; PC = protein C; APC = activated protein C; PS = protein S; C4b-BP = C4b-bound protein; TM = thrombomodulin.

monomer and Y fragments; late FDPs include D and E fragments. These fragments are important clinically because they can increase vascular permeability and interfere with thrombin-induced fibrin formation. In patients with certain disease conditions, when plasmin is activated, FDPs are measured (see Chaps. 26 and 27 for further information).

In addition to its action on fibrin and fibrinogen, plasmin also destroys factors V, VIII, and other coagulation factors. The actions of plasmin are summarized in Table 23–23.

➤ KININ SYSTEM

The kinin system, important in inflammation, vascular permeability, and chemotaxis, is activated by both the coagulation and fibrinolytic systems (see Chap. 26).

Fletcher factor (prekallikrein) and Fitzgerald factor (HMWK) are additionally needed to enhance or amplify the contact factors involved in the intrinsic system (Fig. 23–25).

> ## ➤ Table 23-22
> ## SOME INHIBITORS OF PLASMIN
>
> • α₂-Antiplasmin (a rapid inhibitor of plasmin)
>
> • α₂-Macroglobulin (a slower inhibitor of plasmin)
>
> • Others (see later discussion of protease inhibitors)

Specifically, factor XIIa in the presence of HMWK converts prekallikrein to kallikrein. Kallikrein feeds back to accelerate the conversion of factor XII to XIIa, speeding up intrinsic system processes.

The activation of factor XII acts as the common link between many aspects of the hemostatic mechanism, including the fibrinolytic system, the kinin system, and the complement system (see Fig. 23–25 and Chap. 26).

➤ PROTEASE INHIBITORS

Because the fibrinolytic system is activated when coagulation is activated, extra fibrin is degraded and eliminated along with some of the coagulation factors. However, enzymes such as plasmin and kallikrein still circulate until they are eliminated by (1) liver hepatocytes (which have an affinity for activated enzymes), (2) RES cells (which pick up particulate matter), or (3) serine protease inhibitors present in plasma.[19]

Serine protease inhibitors attach to various enzymes and inactivate them. Some important serine protease inhibitors are listed in Table 23–24.

➤ COMPLEMENT SYSTEM

The complement system is composed of approximately 22 serum proteins that, working together with antibodies and

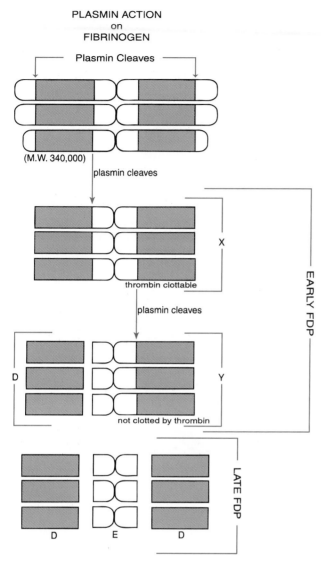

PLASMIN ACTION
on
FIBRINOGEN

Plasmin Cleaves

(M.W. 340,000)

plasmin cleaves

X

thrombin clottable

plasmin cleaves

D

Y

not clotted by thrombin

EARLY FDP

D   E   D

LATE FDP

➤ **FIGURE 23–24** Plasmin activity on fibrinogen. FDP = fibrin degradation product.

clotting factors, play an important role as mediators of both immune and allergic reactions. The reactions in which complement participates take place in the blood or in other body fluids. The most important biologic role of comple-

---

➤ **Table 23–23**
THE ACTIONS OF PLASMIN

- Destroys fibrinogen and fibrin
- Produces FDPs, which increase vascular permeability and interfere with thrombin-induced fibrin formation
- Produces D-dimer, a degradation product specifically derived from cross-linked stabilized fibrin polymer
- Destroys factors V, VIII, IX, XI, and other plasma proteins
- Indirectly enhances or amplifies conversion of factor XII to XIIa
- Enhances or amplifies conversion of prekallikrein to kallikrein, liberating kinins from kininogen
- Cleaves C3 into fragments (see later discussion of complement system)

---

ment is the production of cell membrane lysis of antibody-coated target cells. Two independent pathways of activation of the complement cascade may occur along with a common cytolytic pathway. These are designated the classic and alternate pathways of complement activation (see Chap. 13 for a review of the complement system).

Plasmin activates complement by cleaving C3 into C3a and C3b. C1 esterase inhibitor inactivates complement and also has a role in hemostasis, as described earlier.

Both the coagulation system and the fibrinolytic system are interrelated with the complement system.[20] The interrelationship of the coagulation, complement, and fibrinolytic systems is discussed in Chapter 26.

➤ LABORATORY EVALUATION OF HEMOSTASIS

The diagnosis of any hemostatic disorder is made by the systematic evaluation of information obtained in the history and physical examination, along with the appropriate laboratory testing. Diagnostically, the most valuable data from a patient's history include:

1. Documentation of the physical appearance, site, severity, and frequency of bleeding episodes
2. A reliable patient and family history of bleeding disorders
3. An accurate drug history
4. Other contributing or underlying illnesses

Bleeding disorders present themselves differently, depending on the causative problem. Two general rules apply: firstly, patients with platelet disorders usually exhibit petechiae and mucous membrane bleeding. In general, this is because a defect of primary hemostasis is present, resulting in the formation of a defective platelet plug. Secondly, patients with coagulation defects may develop deep spreading hematomas and bleeding into the joints with evident hematuria. In general, this is because a defect of secondary hemostasis is present, resulting in the inadequate fibrin reinforcement of a functionally normal platelet plug.

Alteration of any aspect of the hemostatic mechanism may cause abnormal bleeding in a wide variety of familial and acquired clinical disorders. These defects may be classified into three broad categories that can be diagnostically approached by a systematic laboratory evaluation. These include vascular and platelet disorders, coagulation factor deficiencies or specific inhibitors, and fibrinolytic disorders.

Although many laboratories differ in their approach to a bleeding disorder, a general profile of laboratory tests is usually established. This profile can often be used as a means of differentiating various hemostatic problems. Laboratory screening tests routinely ordered to assess hemostatic dysfunction are listed in Table 23–25 (see Chap. 32).

The PT and APTT are both variations of plasma recalcification times accelerated by the addition of a thromboplastic substance. The PT reagent contains thromboplastin and calcium that, when added to patient plasma, initiates rapid formation of a fibrin clot. The APTT reagent contains phospholipid substitute, activator, and calcium chloride to initiate fibrin clot formation.

As mentioned previously, the PT test measures the factors of the extrinsic and common pathways of coagulation (factors VII, X, V, II, and I). Factor VII is the only factor

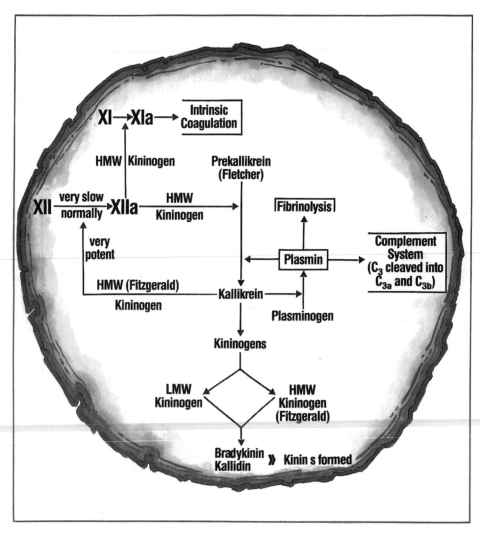

➤ **FIGURE 23–25**   Interrelationship of coagulation, fibrinolytic, kinin, and complement systems. HMW = high molecular weight; LMW = low molecular weight.

listed that is restricted to the extrinsic system, as factors X, V, II, and I are part of the common pathway (see Figs. 23–17 and 23–18). The PT test is ideally used to detect early vitamin K deficiencies, because factor VII has the shortest half-life of the coagulation factors and is vitamin K–dependent. The PT test is also used to monitor oral anticoagulant therapy. Any abnormalities of these factors, a vitamin K defect, liver disease, or the presence of inhibitors will result in an abnormally prolonged PT.

The APTT test measures factors of the intrinsic and common pathways of blood coagulation (XII, Fletcher, Fitzgerald, XI, IX, VIII, X, V, II, and I). It should be noted that factors XII, XI, IX, VIII, Fletcher, and Fitzgerald are limited to the intrinsic system. Deficiencies or inhibitors of any of these factors will result in an abnormally prolonged APTT. Both the PT and APTT tests will show prolonged results with an abnormality of the shared factors of the common pathway (X, V, II, and I). A factor abnormality refers to a

➤ **Table 23-24**
SOME IMPORTANT SERINE PROTEASE INHIBITORS

- Antithrombin III
- α_2-Macroglobulin
- α_2-Antiplasmin
- α_2-Antitrypsin
- C1 esterase inhibitor
- Protein C inhibitor
- Protein S inhibitor

➤ **Table 23-25**
SOME COMMON LABORATORY SCREENING TESTS FOR HEMOSTATIC DISORDERS

- Platelet count
- Peripheral blood smear examination
- Template bleeding time (TBT)
- Prothrombin time (PT)
- Activated partial thromboplastin time (APTT)
- Thrombin time (TT)*

*Included less often.

deficiency of that factor in plasma for any one of the following reasons:

1. Decreased synthesis
2. Synthesis of a dysfunctional factor molecule
3. Excessive destruction of factors through acquired disorders
4. Inactivation of factors through circulating inhibitors

Table 23–20 summarizes the interpretation of the PT and APTT test results.

As the reader will note, neither the PT nor the APTT screens adequately for factor XIII activity. The PT and APTT test for the initial conversion of fibrinogen to fibrin. Cross-linked stabilized fibrin, which develops later through mediation of factor XIIIa, does not have an impact on the PT or APTT. Special testing to assess factor XIII activity must be done (see Chap. 32).

PT and APTT can be reported in a variety of ways, such as patient seconds and control seconds, percent activity, and ratio. Recent changes have occurred in PT reporting that bear mention. The International Normalized Ratio (INR) now seems to be the mode of choice for PT reporting[21] because it adjusts for source-related thromboplastin sensitivity differences through use of a mathematical exponent, the International Sensitivity Index (ISI). The ISI is unique to each batch of thromboplastin and is furnished by the manufacturer.

Numerous articles state the method for reporting INR values. INR standardizes PT reporting worldwide by adjusting all reported values to a World Health Organization international reference thromboplastin standard (so that all PT results reported by INR methodology are theoretically comparable), and facilitates optimal oral anticoagulant therapy in patients at risk for thrombosis, especially those on warfarin who travel extensively and require frequent monitoring. Thromboplastins with a low ISI (less than 1.2) seem to correlate better to human brain thromboplastin,[21] which is the most sensitive of reagents with an ISI of 1.

The thrombin time is a measure of the ability of thrombin to convert fibrinogen to fibrin and is particularly useful in the evaluation of circulating anticoagulants (pathologic inhibitors). The thrombin time is prolonged in the following conditions:

1. Hypofibrinogenemia and dysfibrinogenemia
2. Treatment with heparin
3. Circulating FDPs
4. Pathologic circulating inhibitors

Table 23–26 can be used as a general guide toward categorizing bleeding disorders into the groups previously listed, using the suggested screening tests. Additional laboratory testing is designed to narrow down the abnormality to one of these specific areas. As a result, laboratory testing can be divided into the following categories:

1. Screening tests for vascular or platelet dysfunction (such as bleeding time, platelet adhesion, platelet aggregation, and PF3 assay)
2. Tests for coagulation (such as factor assays)
3. Special tests (e.g., for fibrinolytic disorders such as tests for determination of FDPs and D-dimers, and protamine sulfate and ethanol gel tests for detection of fibrin monomers)

The reader may refer to subsequent chapters for a detailed discussion of vascular and platelet-related disorders, plasma clotting factor defects, hemostatic system interaction, thrombosis and anticoagulant therapy, and laboratory methods.

➤ CASE STUDY

A 4-year-old boy was brought to the emergency department by his parents. The boy had fallen off of the monkey bars in a park and hit his thigh against one of the bars during the fall. His thigh became swollen and painful. There was a history of bleeding in the male family members. They had been labeled as "bleeders" in their family history. Coagulation studies were performed that showed a normal PT, prolonged APTT, and normal platelet count and bleeding time.

Because the PT was normal, all extrinsic and common pathway deficiencies were ruled out. The abnormal APTT led the laboratory technologist to believe the child had a problem with a factor deficiency in the intrinsic pathway (VIII, IX, XI, and XII). Factor XII deficiency was ruled out, because it does not present with bleeding and patients with this disorder are more likely to develop thromboses. Factor assays were performed for VIII, IX, and XI, to rule out any deficiencies. Results of the factor IX and XI assays were normal. However, factor VIII assays revealed abnormal results. vWF antigenic assays were also performed to rule out von Willebrand's disease.

The results of all the assays confirmed a diagnosis of hemophilia A resulting from deficiency of factor VIII.

continued

➤ Table 23–26
CLASSIFICATION OF BLEEDING DISORDERS BY SCREENING TESTS

Test	Vascular Disorder	Quantitative Platelet Disorder	Qualitative Platelet Disorder	Factor Deficiency
Platelet count	N	AbN	N	N
PT	N	N	N	AbN*
APTT	N	N	N	AbN*
TBT	AbN	AbN	AbN	N

*Dependent on the factor deficiency; see Table 23–20 for specific information.
Abbreviations: N = normal; AbN = abnormal; PT = Prothrombin time; APTT = activated partial thromboplastin time; TBT = template bleeding time

Hemophilia A is an X-linked, recessive disorder passed from the mother, who is the carrier, to her male children. Because of inheritance patterns, male children have a 25% chance of being affected, depending on what X gene is inherited. Female children will be carriers if they inherit the affected gene. More information on hemophilia A and other factor deficiencies can be found in Chapter 27.

QUESTIONS

1. Which of the following is true concerning the organelle zone?
   a. Responsible for metabolic activities of the platelet
   b. Contains dense granules, α granules, and glycocalyx
   c. Contains the dense tubular system which is the site of prostaglandin synthesis, calcium release, and platelet relaxation
   d. Contains the OCS to deliver stored products to the platelet surface

2. What events are involved in the normal formation of a platelet plug?
   a. Adhesion, activation, fibrinolysis, secondary hemostasis
   b. Aggregation, coagulation, release reaction, lupus anticoagulant
   c. Release action, adhesion, lupus anticoagulant, secondary hemostasis
   d. Activation, adhesion, aggregation, release reaction

3. What product is responsible for stabilization of the hemostatic plug?
   a. TXA_2
   b. PF3
   c. Fibrin
   d. GPIIb

4. Which of the following are classified as contact group proteins?
   a. Factors II, VII, IX, X
   b. Factors XII, XI, PK, HMWK
   c. Factors I, V, VIII, XIII
   d. Factors I, II, V, X

5. Which of the following are classified as prothrombin group proteins?
   a. Factors II, VII, IX, X
   b. Factors XII, XI, PK, HMWK
   c. Factors I, V, VIII, XIII
   d. Factors I, II, V, X

6. Which of the following are classified as fibrinogen group proteins?
   a. Factors II, VII, IX, X
   b. Factors XII, XI, PK, HMWK
   c. Factors I, V, VIII, XIII
   d. Factors I, II, V, X

7. Which of the following factors are dependent on vitamin K for synthesis?
   a. Factors II, VII, IX, X
   b. Factors XII, XI, PK, HMWK
   c. Factors I, V, VIII, XIII
   d. Factors I, II, V, X

8. Which of the following factors are unique to the extrinsic system?
   a. Factors XII, XI, X, IV, VIII, V, II, I
   b. Factors III, VII
   c. Factors VII, X, V, II, I
   d. Factors XII, XI, IV, PF3, VIII

9. What events take place in the extrinsic system?
   a. Activation of factor X to Va
   b. Acceleration of intrinsic pathway by enhancement of the activity of factors XII and XI
   c. Activation of factor XII to XIIa to initiate clotting
   d. Activation of factor VII to VIIa in the presence of Ca^{2+} and factor III

10. Which of the following factors are unique to the intrinsic system?
    a. Factors XII, XI, IX, VIII, X, V, II, I, Fletcher, Fitzgerald
    b. Factors XII, XI, IX, VIII, Fletcher, Fitzgerald
    c. Factors VII, X, V, II, I
    d. Factors III, VII, X, V, II, I

11. What factor is not found in the common pathway?
    a. Factor X
    b. Factor V
    c. PF3
    d. Factor XII

12. Which of the following is a function of thrombin?
    a. Conversion of fibrinogen to fibrin
    b. Activation of factor XIII to stabilize fibrinolysis
    c. Conversion of factor VII to XIIa
    d. Enhancement of factor V, VIII, and XI activity

13. Which of the following is a function of plasmin?
    a. Cleavage of T-PA
    b. Destruction of fibrin
    c. Conversion of XII to XIa
    d. Inhibition of XIa

14. What is the purpose of the PT test in monitoring hemostasis?
    a. Measures factors of the extrinsic pathway
    b. Detects platelet decrease or dysfunction
    c. Detects presence of aspirin
    d. Monitors heparin therapy

15. What is the purpose of the APTT test in monitoring hemostasis?
    a. Measures factors of the intrinsic pathway
    b. Detects deficiency of factors for both intrinsic and extrinsic pathways
    c. Measures circulating FDPs
    d. Detects platelet dysfunction

SUMMARY CHART

➤ Hemostasis is the complex process by which the body spontaneously stops bleeding and maintains blood in the fluid state within the vascular compartment.

➤ Hemostasis can be divided into two stages: primary and secondary. Primary hemostasis is defined by platelet adhesion to exposed collagen within the endothelium of the vessel wall. Secondary hemostasis involves the enzymatic activation of the coagulation proteins to produce fibrin from fibrinogen, thereby stabilizing the fragile clot formed during primary hemostasis.

➤ Biochemical characteristics of the endothelium render the cell surface thromboresistant by (1) synthesis and secretion of a vasodilator prostacyclin (PGI_2); (2) secretion of tissue plasminogen activator (t-PA); (3) inactivation and clearance of thrombin; (4) activity of the cofactor thrombomodulin in the thrombin-dependent activation of protein C; and (5) the degradation of proaggregating substances such as adenosine diphosphate (ADP) and vasoactive amines.

➤ The principal mechanism of platelet adhesion involves (1) plasma, (2) collagen fibers, and (3) platelet membrane glycoprotein GPIb (the receptor for von Willebrand's factor [vWF]).

➤ Platelets measure roughly 2 to 4 μm in diameter. Normal platelet count ranges from 150,000 to 350,000 cells/μL. Platelets participate in hemostasis by (1) providing a negatively charged phospholipid surface for factor X and prothrombin activation; (2) release of substances that mediate vasoconstriction, platelet aggregation, coagulation (thrombin generation), and vascular repair; and (3) providing surface membrane glycoproteins such as GPIb and IIIa to attach to other platelets via fibrinogen.

➤ Within the matrix of the platelet are microtubules, microfilaments, and submembranous filaments.

➤ The initial stage of platelet activation is as follows: platelets form pseudopods, organelles including α granules and dense bodies are reorganized to the center, and contraction causes the granules to spill their contents into the open canalicular system (OCS).

➤ Platelet-derived growth factor (PDGF) is a mitogen stored in and secreted from the α granule of the platelet.

➤ Platelet adhesion involves three components: (1) vWF, (2) glycoprotein Ib (GPIb), and (3) collagen fibers.

➤ Activation of second messenger pathways within the platelet leads to intracellular biochemical changes, culminating in platelet activation events such as shape change, secretion, cytoskeletal reassembly, and platelet aggregation.

➤ Platelet aggregation (platelet-to-platelet interaction) is an energy-dependent process that requires adenosine triphosphate (ATP), primarily derived from glycolysis.

➤ Four platelet-specific proteins secreted from the α granules are currently used as "markers of platelet activation." These include β-thromboglobulin, platelet factor 4, thrombospondin, and PDGF.

➤ During thrombus formation, thrombin, plasminogen, tissue plasminogen activator, and antiplasmin are incorporated into the clot.

➤ Aspirin exerts a permanent yet limited effect on platelet aggregation by inhibiting the action of the cyclo-oxygenase enzyme and production of thromboxane A_2 (TXA_2).

➤ Coagulation factors are designated by Roman numerals. Activation of a particular factor is designated by a lower case "a."

➤ Coagulation factors may be divided into three categories: substrate, cofactors, and enzymes. On the basis of physical properties, coagulation proteins may be divided into three groups: contact proteins, prothrombin proteins, and fibrinogen or thrombin-sensitive proteins.

➤ Blood coagulation leading to fibrin formation can be separated into three pathways: extrinsic, intrinsic, and the common pathway.

➤ The role of protein C (a vitamin K–dependent factor) as an anticoagulant is related to the presence of thrombin, thrombomodulin, and protein S.

➤ Fibrinolysis is the physiologic process of removing unwanted fibrin deposits.

➤ The kinin system, important in inflammation, vascular permeability, and chemotaxis, is activated by both the coagulation and fibrinolytic systems.

➤ The complement system is composed of approximately 22 serum proteins that, working together with antibodies and clotting factors, play an important role as mediators of both immune and allergic reactions.

➤ A patient's history should include (1) physical appearance, site, severity, and frequency of bleeding episodes; (2) patient and family history; (3) drug history; and (4) contributing or underlying illnesses.

➤ Factor abnormality may occur as a result of decreased synthesis, dysfunctional factor molecule(s), excessive destruction of factors, or inactivation of factors.

➤ Thrombin time may be prolonged because of hypofibrinogenemia and dysfibrinogenemia, treatment with heparin, circulating fibrin degradation products (FDPs), and pathologic circulating inhibitors.

References

1. Colman, RW, et al: Hemostasis and Thrombosis: Basic Principles and Clinical Practice, ed 4, Lippincott-Raven, Philadelphia, November, 2000.
2. Li, JM, et al: Adhesion of activated platelets to venous endothelial cells is mediated via GPIIb/IIIa. J Surg Res 61:543, 1996.
3. Michelson, AD: Platelet function in the newborn. Semin Thromb Hemost 24:507, 1998.
4. Beutler, E, et al: William's Hematology, ed 6. McGraw-Hill, New York, 2000.
5. Hoffman, R, et al: Hematology: Basic Principles and Practice, ed 3. Churchill Livingstone, New York, 1999.
6. Claytor, B, et al: Laser scanning cytometry: a novel method for the detection of platelet-endothelial cell adhesion. Thromb Haemost 82:527, 1999.
7. Bick, RL, and Kaplan, H: Syndromes of thrombosis and hypercoagulability: Congenital and acquired causes of thrombosis. Med Clin North Am 82(3):409–58, 1998.

8. Richard, LG, et al: Wintrobe's Clinical Hematology, ed 10, vols I and II. Lea & Febiger, Philadelphia, 1999.
9. Barnard, MR, et al: Fresh liquid-preserved, and cryopreserved platelets: Adhesive surface receptors and membrane procoagulant activity. Transfusion, 39:880, 1999.
10. Bick, RL: Hematology: Clinical and Laboratory Practice. Mosby, St Louis, 1993.
11. Hart, MN, and Kent, TH: Introduction to Human Disease. Prentice-Hall, Englewood Cliffs, NJ, 1998.
12. Michelson, AD, and Furman, MI: Laboratory markers of platelet activation and their clinical significance. Curr Opin Hematol 6:342, 1999.
13. Wilcox, DA, et al: Megakaryocyte-targeted synthesis of the integrin β_3-subunit results in the phenotypic correction of Glanzman thrombasthenia. Blood 95(12):3645–3651, 2000.
14. Loscalzo, J, and Schafer, AI: Thrombosis and Hemorrhage, ed 2. Williams & Wilkins, Baltimore, 1998, pp 1027–1063.
15. Michelson, AD, et al: The effects of aspirin and hypothermia on platelet function in vivo. Br J Haematol 104:64, 1999.
16. Tapper, H, and Herwald, H: Modulation of hemostatic mechanisms in bacterial infectious diseases. Blood 96(7), 2329–2337, October 2000.
17. Hosaka, Y, et al: Thrombomodulin in human plasma contributes to inhibit fibrinolysis through acceleration of thrombin-dependent activation of plasma procarboxypeptidase. Thromb Haemost 79:371, 1998.
18. Vaughn, D: Update on plasminogen activator inhibitor-1. Can J Cardiol 14(Suppl D):14, 1998.
19. Norbis, F, et al: Diluted Russell's viper venom time and colloidal silica clotting time for the identification of the phospholipid-dependent inhibitors of coagulation. Thromb Res 85:427, 1997.
20. Bick, RL: Disseminated intravascular coagulation: Pathophysiological mechanisms and manifestations. Semin Thromb Hemost, 24:3, 1998.
21. Jensen, R: Oral Anticoagulation and the INR. Clin Hemost Rev 13(5), May 1999.

See the bibliography for this chapter at the back of the book.

24 Disorders of Primary Hemostasis

Quantitative and Qualitative Platelet Disorders and Vascular Disorders

DARLA K. LILES, MD
CHARLES L. KNUPP, MD

QUANTITATIVE PLATELET DISORDERS
Deficient Platelet Production
Ineffective Erythropoiesis
Congenital Disorders
Abnormal Distribution of Platelets
Increased Destruction of Platelets

QUALITATIVE PLATELET DISORDERS
Congenital Disorders of Platelet Function
von Willebrand's Disease
Acquired Qualitative Platelet Disorders

VASCULAR DISORDERS
Primary Purpura
Secondary Purpura
Vascular and Connective Tissue Disorders

CONGENITAL CONNECTIVE TISSUE DISORDERS

CASE STUDY 1

CASE STUDY 2

CASE STUDY 3

CASE STUDY 4

OBJECTIVES

At the end of this chapter the learner should be able to:

1. Describe the laboratory tests that may be utilized in the evaluation of quantitative and qualitative platelet disorders.

2. Understand the pathophysiologic processes that cause thrombocytopenia. List the thrombocytopenic disorders caused by each process.

3. Describe how the diagnosis of idiopathic thrombocytopenic purpura (ITP) is made.

4. Compare ITP and thrombotic thrombocytopenic purpura (TTP).

5. Understand the characteristics of the inherited platelet membrane defects and compare Bernard-Soulier syndrome to Glanzmann's thrombasthenia.

6. Describe the types of von Willebrand's disease and how they differ in the management of bleeding.

7. Differentiate von Willebrand's disease from Bernard-Soulier syndrome and hemophilia A.

8. Understand the pathophysiology responsible for storage pool and platelet release defects and how it relates to laboratory studies used for diagnosis of these disorders.

9. Differentiate between reactive and primary thrombocytosis and describe the hemostatic problems expected.

10. Differentiate among the vascular disorders associated with purpura.

Disorders of primary hemostasis include abnormalities that clinically result in bleeding. These include quantitative and qualitative platelet disorders, and defects of the blood vessel wall. Despite the number of disorders that one encounters in primary hemostasis, the clinical manifestations are typically limited to skin and mucosal bleeding (Table 24–1). Spontaneous hemarthrosis and hematomas of deep structures are typical features of coagulation protein deficiency states and not platelet or vascular defects. This chapter reviews the etiology, pathophysiology, clinical manifestations, and laboratory tests used to identify the various quantitative and qualitative platelet disorders as well as the numerous vascular disorders.

Table 24–2 lists laboratory tests that aid in the evaluation of disorders of primary hemostasis.

The automated platelet count is one of the most important

> ## Table 24-1
> ### CLINICAL MANIFESTATIONS OF PLATELET AND VASCULAR DISORDERS (PRIMARY HEMOSTASIS)

Ecchymosis

Petechiae

Purpura

Mucosal bleeding

Epistaxis

Gingival bleeding

Gastrointestinal bleeding

Menorrhagia

Hematuria

initial tests to evaluate a bleeding tendency, because acquired quantitative platelet disorders are the most common disorders of primary hemostasis. Visual inspection of the peripheral smear can be used to confirm the automated platelet count and reveal platelet morphology. The peripheral smear should be carefully inspected for evidence of large or dysplastic platelets. Direct inspection should also assess for platelet satellitism or platelet clumping, which may cause a falsely low automated platelet count termed *pseudothrombocytopenia*. When pseudothrombocytopenia is suspected, a "true" automated count can often be obtained by performing a platelet count in alternative anticoagulants such as citrate or heparin. This phenomenon does not result in clinical bleeding. It is usually a result of ethylene diaminetetraacetic acid (EDTA)–dependent cold agglutinins.[1,2]

The bleeding time has been utilized as a screening test to

> ## Table 24-2
> ### LABORATORY TESTS TO ASSESS DISORDERS OF PRIMARY HEMOSTASIS

Platelet count

Peripheral blood smear

Template bleeding time

Von Willebrand studies

FVIII:C

vWF antigen

vWF activity

Platelet antibody testing

Flow cytometry

Platelet glycoprotein analysis

Platelet-associated IgG

Platelet aggregation studies

Lumiaggregometry

^{51}Cr release

Bone marrow aspiration and biopsy

Abbreviations: FVIII:C = factor VIII:C; vWF = von Willebrand factor

evaluate platelet and vascular disorders. There are several standard methods for performing bleeding times as described in Chapter 32; however, the Ivy bleeding time is the most commonly utilized method for performing this test. Templates are utilized to allow uniformity of the incision to improve the reproducibility of this test. Bleeding times may be abnormal with qualitative or quantitative platelet disorders, certain vascular defects, and von Willebrand's disease. The bleeding time must be interpreted with caution in the context of a carefully obtained history and other platelet tests, especially an automated platelet count. A medication history is essential, because ingestion of aspirin and nonsteroidal analgesics may cause a prolonged bleeding time.[3] The bleeding time has been utilized as a screening tool to determine the risk of bleeding in many clinical settings; however, there is now a large body of literature that has shown no correlation with risk of bleeding in these instances.[4,5]

Because von Willebrand's disease mimics the bleeding diathesis of platelet disorders, assays to exclude this diagnosis are an integral part of the evaluation. To determine the presence or absence of von Willebrand's disease, factor VIII coagulant activity, von Willebrand's antigen (vWF:Ag), von Willebrand's activity by ristocetin-induced platelet aggregation, and von Willebrand's multimers must be assayed together. Further discussion of these tests can be found later in this chapter in the section on von Willebrand's disease.

Platelet antibody testing determines the amount of immunoglobulin G (IgG) bound on the platelet surface by various methodologies. Increased amounts of platelet-associated IgG are often found in immune-mediated thrombocytopenias, but this finding is not specific enough to establish a diagnosis of an immune origin. Flow cytometry can be used to measure surface glycoproteins and platelet-bound IgG.

Platelet aggregation assesses platelet function by measuring the response of the platelet to various stimuli such as epinephrine, adenosine diphosphate (ADP), collagen, and ristocetin. The procedure for performing platelet aggregation is described in Chapter 32. Abnormalities of the platelet surface and release defects can be identified with this test. Drugs and disorders such as liver or renal disease can interfere with platelet function and make interpretation of this test difficult. Lumi-aggregation or ^{51}Cr release assays may be useful to specifically measure platelet release.

Bone marrow aspiration and biopsy are useful in determining the etiology of quantitative platelet disorders. The bone marrow specimen can be used to assess adequacy of megakaryocytes and overall cellularity, myelodysplasia, and infiltrative processes such as malignancy or fibrosis.

▶ QUANTITATIVE PLATELET DISORDERS

Platelets must be present in adequate numbers to maintain normal hemostasis. The average platelet count ranges from 150 to 400 $\times$ 10^9/L of whole blood. *Thrombocytopenia* is defined as a platelet count below the lower limit of normal, although clinical signs and symptoms of thrombocytopenia typically are not manifested until the platelet count falls below 100 $\times$ 10^9/L and usually not until the platelet count falls below 50 $\times$ 10^9/L. Overt spontaneous hemorrhage is not usually seen until the platelet count falls to less than 20 $\times$ 10^9/L. Quantitative platelet disorders are the most commonly encountered group of platelet abnormalities discussed in this chapter and result from three distinct mecha-

► Table 24-3
CLASSIFICATION OF DISORDERS CAUSING THROMBOCYTOPENIA

Deficient Platelet Production

Myelophthisic (marrow infiltrative processes)

    Leukemia

    Lymphoma

    Multiple myeloma

    Metastatic carcinoma

    Myelofibrosis

Aplasia

    Aplastic anemia (Fanconi's anemia)

    Amegakaryocytic thrombocytopenia

    Drug effect (chemotherapy)

    Radiation therapy

Ineffective erythropoiesis

    Pernicious anemia (vitamin B_{12} deficiency)

    Folic acid deficiency

    Alcohol ingestion

    Myelodysplasia

    Paroxysmal nocturnal hemoglobinuria

Congenital disorders

    May-Hegglin syndrome

    Thrombocytopenia with absent radii (TAR) syndrome

    Bernard-Soulier syndrome

Abnormal Platelet Distribution

    Hypersplenism (splenomegaly)

    Hemangiomas (Kasabach-Merritt syndrome)

Increased Platelet Destruction

Immune (primary)

    Idiopathic thrombocytopenic purpura (ITP)

    Posttransfusion purpura

    Neonatal isoimmune purpura

    Drug-induced thrombocytopenia

    Heparin-induced thrombocytopenia and thrombosis

Immune (secondary)

    Lymphoproliferative disorders

    Systemic lupus erythematosis/Collagen vascular disorders

    Viral infection (mononucleosis, measles, HIV)

Microangiopathic thrombocytopenia

    Thrombotic thrombocytopenic purpura (TTP)

    Hemolytic uremic syndrome (HUS)

    Disseminated intravascular coagulation (DIC)

Pregnancy-associated thrombocytopenia

    Gestational thrombocytopenia

    Preeclampsia-eclampsia and HELLP syndrome

Abbreviations: HIV = human immunodeficiency virus; HELLP = hemolysis elevated liver enzymes, and low platelet count

---

nisms: deficient platelet production, splenic sequestration, or peripheral destruction (Table 24–3). Qualitative platelet defects may coexist with quantitative platelet defects to increase bleeding risk.

Deficient Platelet Production

Impaired platelet production resulting in thrombocytopenia may be caused by many disorders. These disorders produce megakaryocytic hypoplasia often with erythroid and granulocytic hypoplasia, resulting in pancytopenia. These platelet disorders may occur spontaneously (aplastic anemia) or as a result of injury to the bone marrow (radiation or chemotherapy). Replacement of marrow hematopoietic tissue as a result of infiltrative processes such as myelofibrosis, leukemia, Hodgkin's and non-Hodgkin's lymphoma, and metastatic cancer results in pancytopenia (anemia, thrombocytopenia, and leukopenia) and a blood smear characterized by nucleated red blood cells, teardrop-shaped cells (dacryocytes), and immature granulocytes These characteristic findings on the peripheral smear are often referred to as a *myelophthisic picture* and should make one highly suspicious of an infiltrative process within the bone marrow. Bone marrow aspiration and biopsy are indicated to confirm a diagnosis of marrow aplasia or infiltration when these findings are present.

Ineffective Erythropoiesis

Ineffective erythropoiesis is associated with normal to increased marrow cellularity but peripheral blood cytopenias.

Megaloblastic anemia associated with vitamin B_{12} or folic acid deficiency is commonly associated with thrombocytopenia as a result of impaired deoxyribonucleic acid (DNA) synthesis. Serum lactate dehydrogenase (LDH) levels are high as a result of intramedullary death of hematopoietic progenitors. Thrombocytopenia is generally mild. Platelet life span has been reported as being normal to only slightly decreased. Myelodysplasia may simulate vitamin deficiencies but does not respond to vitamin replacement. Chromosomal abnormalities may be present. Paroxysmal nocturnal hemoglobinuria, a rare disorder with increased cellular sensitivity to complement, also is associated with cytopenias resulting from intramedullary cellular destruction. These disorders are discussed in detail in Part II of this book.

Alcohol has a direct toxic effect on the marrow, thereby producing thrombocytopenia in the absence of a folic acid or vitamin B_{12} deficiency. Mild thrombocytopenia and acquired platelet function defects appear to improve after stopping the use of alcohol.

Congenital Disorders

A number of congenital disorders produce thrombocytopenia; however, all are rare. Bernard-Soulier syndrome and May-Hegglin anomaly do not have associated skin or skeletal defects. Patients with TAR syndrome have absent radii in addition to the thrombocytopenia. Some of these disorders also exhibit a qualitative abnormality in platelet function. A list of congenital disorders and their associated abnormalities is found in Table 24–4.

Abnormal Distribution of Platelets

Normally the spleen pools approximately one-third of the platelets produced by the marrow. When the spleen enlarges, more platelets can be sequestered in the spleen, leading to thrombocytopenia. Many conditions, including liver cirrho-

> ## ➤ Table 24-4
> ## CONGENITAL DISORDERS ASSOCIATED WITH DECREASED PLATELET PRODUCTION

Disorder	Associated Abnormalities
Alport's syndrome	Giant platelets
	Thrombocytopenia
	Deafness
	Nephritis
Chédiak-Higashi syndrome	Partial oculocutaneous albinism
	Increased susceptibility to pyogenic infections
	Storage pool defect of dense granules
Hermansky-Pudlak syndrome	Platelet deficiency of nonmetabolic ADP
	Oculocutaneous albinism
May-Hegglin anomaly	Thrombocytopenia
	Giant platelets
	Döhle bodies
TAR syndrome	Multiple skeletal and cardiac abnormalities
	Storage pool defect
Wiskott-Aldrich syndrome	Disorders of dense granules
	Recurrent pyogenic infections
	Eczema
	Thrombocytopenia

sis, hematologic malignancies, and portal vein thrombosis, can cause hypersplenism. Typically, the platelet count remains greater than 50×10^9/L in patients with hypersplenism. Kasabach-Merritt syndrome, a rare disorder, results in platelet sequestration in giant hemangiomas.

Increased Destruction of Platelets

Immunologic Thrombocytopenias
This group of thrombocytopenias all have an immune-mediated mechanism by which there is increased platelet destruction.

Idiopathic Thrombocytopenic Purpura
Idiopathic thrombocytopenic purpura (ITP) is one of the most common disorders causing severe isolated thrombocytopenia. There is not a specific test that readily confirms the diagnosis of ITP, so it is typically a diagnosis of exclusion. ITP can present in children and adults; however, there are important differences between the two groups in terms of the long-term prognosis.[6]

Young children may present with an immune thrombocytopenia that typically develops within 1 to 3 weeks following an acute viral illness. The onset of symptoms is usually abrupt, with initial platelet counts of less than 20×10^9/L. This disorder is usually self-limiting and sponta-

neous remissions, with or without therapy, occur in the majority of these patients.

In adults, ITP commonly presents in the 20- to 50-year-old group, with a greater predilection for women. There is usually not a recent history of drug exposure or infectious illness that can be related to the onset of thrombocytopenia. Platelet counts are typically less than 30×10^9/L in patients who present with bleeding manifestations. Clinically, patients present with mucosal bleeding typical of a primary hemostatic defect, such as menorrhagia, epistaxis, easy bruisability, or petechiae (Figs. 24–1 and 24–2 and Color Plates 258 and 259). Some patients are diagnosed while still asymptomatic based on a low platelet count on a routine complete blood count obtained for other reasons. These patients usually have a platelet count greater than 50×10^9/L. ITP in the adult age group is typically a chronic problem and does not usually remit spontaneously.

The bone marrow is characterized by increased or normal numbers of megakaryocytes (Fig. 24–3 and Color Plate

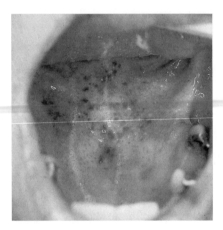

➤ FIGURE 24–1   Oral cavity of a patient with idiopathic thrombocytopenic purpura (ITP).

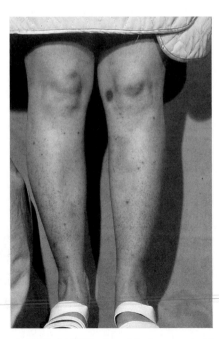

➤ FIGURE 24–2   Petechial bleeding of the lower extremities in a patient with ITP.

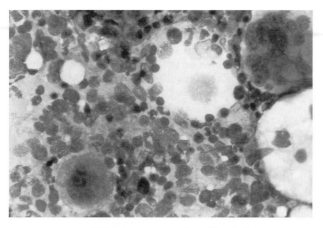

➤ **FIGURE 24–3** ITP, bone marrow aspirate. Note the increased number of megakaryocytes with normal cellularity (M/E 3:1).

260). Platelet life span is shortened and circulating platelets are morphologically large on the smear, reflecting the early release from the marrow in response to the peripheral destruction. There are also changes in the splenic microcirculation which cause a reduction of platelet transit time in the spleen and increased destruction of the antibody-coated platelets.[7] The bleeding time in ITP may not be as prolonged as the bleeding time in other disorders associated with the same degree of thrombocytopenia, suggesting that the younger platelets in ITP may be more effective at maintaining hemostasis.

Because ITP is a diagnosis of exclusion, other causes of thrombocytopenia must be considered and eliminated first. Drugs that may cause thrombocytopenia must be stopped, and consideration given to a bone marrow aspirate and biopsy to exclude a primary bone marrow disorder. Antiplatelet antibody tests have been utilized by some to help confirm the diagnosis of ITP; however, these tests are not specific.

Splenectomy and corticosteroids are the conventional therapies used to treat patients with ITP.[8] Patients with ITP are initially treated with corticosteroids to rapidly increase the platelet count and improve hemostasis. Corticosteroids are thought to reduce autoantibody production and to suppress splenic sequestration of moderately sensitized platelets, thereby increasing the platelet life span and ameliorating the thrombocytopenia. The aim of therapy is to give high-dose daily prednisone sufficient to obtain a satisfactory increase in the platelet count initially, and then to reduce the dosage to a level that maintains the platelet count at hemostatic levels. Approximately 70% to 90% of patients treated respond favorably to steroids. Most patients also usually respond to intravenous gamma globulin. Recently published guidelines for the treatment of ITP recommend the use of corticosteroids initially unless there is active bleeding for which the addition of gamma globulin is recommended.[9] There does not appear to be a more rapid increase of the platelet count with both of these agents compared to either alone. Anti-D globulin (Win Rho SDF) can be used in some individuals with ITP who are Rh-positive. Its mechanism of action is probably similar to gamma globulin but has the benefits of being a short infusion over 5 minutes and not requiring the volume necessary to administer gamma globulin. There is often an associated mild hemolysis of red cells associated with the administration of Win Rho SDF; there-

fore, the dosage should be adjusted according to the hemoglobin level at time of treatment. The response to Win Rho SDF is highest prior to splenectomy, with only rare responses reported in patients who have failed to respond to splenectomy. The time to response with any of these initial treatments varies with each individual, although most responses are seen within a week or two of initiation of therapy. Thrombocytopenia usually recurs when these treatments are stopped.

Splenectomy is the long-term treatment of choice for ITP after an initial response to steroid therapy or gamma globulin. Significant improvement following splenectomy is obtained in 70% to 90% of patients. The benefit of splenectomy results from the removal of the organ responsible for the autoantibody production and the sequestration of moderately sensitized platelets.

In patients who do not respond to splenectomy or who relapse after splenectomy, many other agents have been utilized.[10] Unfortunately, the studies of efficacy of these treatments have involved relatively small numbers of patients. Some of the agents that have been attempted include danazol, dapsone, colchicine, vitamin C, chemotherapeutic agents such as vincristine and cytoxan, intravenous gamma globulin (IVIgG), and plasma exchange with or without extracorporeal immunoadsorption of plasma by staphylococcal protein A columns. The next most effective agent when there is failure of response to splenectomy has not been clearly defined, and the decision about which treatment modality to utilize varies according to the treating physician.[11]

In patients who are actively bleeding, antifibrinolytic agents such as epsilon (ϵ)-aminocaproic acid (EACA) can be used to help control bleeding until the platelet count can be corrected. These agents are safe to use either prior to or after splenectomy and are most effective at sites of high fibrinolytic activity (i.e., urinary tract, nose, and mouth). Platelet transfusions are usually not effective because transfused platelets are usually rapidly destroyed; however, in some patients a platelet response may occur and bleeding may improve.[12]

Posttransfusion Purpura

In this disorder, sudden onset of thrombocytopenia occurs approximately one week after transfusion of blood or blood products containing platelets (Fig. 24–4 and Color Plate 261). It is believed that posttransfusion purpura (PTP) results from an anamnestic immune response. The majority of cases are a

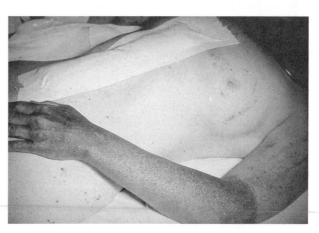

➤ **FIGURE 24–4** Posttransfusion purpura (PTP).

result of an alloantibody directed against the platelet antigen Pl^{A1}, also referred to as HPA-1a.[13] Rare reports of cases of PTP have occurred in association with other platelet antigens, including Pl^{A2}, Bak^a, Bak^b, Pen^a, and Br^a.[14] The Pl^{A1} antigen is found in approximately 97% of the normal population; the 3% of people who lack the Pl^{A1} (HPA-1a) antigen on their platelets are considered at risk for developing PTP. Most reported cases have been in middle-aged women who have had children. It is believed that primary immunization occurs in pregnancy, when Pl^{A1}-positive fetal platelets sensitize a Pl^{A1}-negative mother (see the following discussion of isoimmune neonatal thrombocytopenia.) Other mechanisms for the development of PTP have been suggested.[13]

Complement fixation, release of ^{51}Cr, or ^{14}C-serotonin have been some of the reliable laboratory tests used to detect and measure anti-Pl^{A1} (HPA-1a) antibodies in PTP. Currently, direct and indirect laboratory tests have been developed to increase specificity and sensitivity in the detection of platelet antibodies. These tests employ some of the following techniques: enzyme-linked immunosorbent assay (ELISA), western blot followed by ELISA or radioimmunoassay (RIA), platelet suspension immunofluorescence, and immunoprecipitation of radiolabeled glycoprotein IIIa (GPIIIa). To confirm the presence of a platelet-specific antibody, a panel with Pl^{A1}-positive cells should be run. The patient's platelets should also be phenotyped. In some cases of PTP, isosensitization to HLA antigens found on platelets occurs, as well as the appearance of platelet-specific antigens other than Pl^{A1}, making serologic typing difficult.

Plasmapheresis without exchange and gamma globulin have been effective means of treating the hemorrhagic complications associated with PTP. In a number of cases, patients have had repeated episodes of PTP following reexposure to Pl^{A1}-positive blood. Pl^{A1}-negative blood is indicated for all subsequent transfusions when possible because patients are considered at risk for recurrence of PTP.

Isoimmune Neonatal Thrombocytopenia

Similar to the pathogenesis of erythroblastosis fetalis, isoimmune neonatal thrombocytopenia results from immunization of the mother by fetal platelet antigens and placental transfer of maternal antibody.[15] Isoimmune neonatal thrombocytopenia is most often caused by maternal antibodies to the Pl^{A1} (HPA-1a) antigen; however, as in posttransfusion purpura, isoimmune neonatal thrombocytopenia has been reported rarely with other platelet antigens such as Pl^{A2}, Bak^a, Bak^b, Br^a, and Br^b. It is an uncommon disorder, generally affecting the firstborn child. Based on gene frequency of the Pl^{A1} (HPA-1a) antigen in fathers, there is a high probability that a Pl^{A1}-negative mother will have a Pl^{A1}-positive child. Once isoimmune neonatal thrombocytopenia has developed, there appears to be an increased risk of the next child being affected, because most fathers are homozygous for Pl^{A1}.

A large percentage of Pl^{A1}-negative mothers who give birth to an affected child are phenotype-positive for the HLA-B8 antigen. It has been suggested that the HLA-B8 antigen serves to protect from immunization, which accounts for the relatively low incidence of isoimmune neonatal thrombocytopenia, despite the frequency of the Pl^{A1} antigen and the chance for maternal sensitization. The relationship of ABO incompatibility to symptomatic isoimmune neonatal thrombocytopenia is unclear.

Infants who develop isoimmune neonatal thrombocytopenia appear normal at birth but within hours develop scattered petechiae and purpuric hemorrhages, with platelet counts below $30 \times 10^9/L$. Intracranial hemorrhage is the primary cause of mortality in these infants. Characteristically, in this disorder the platelet count begins to decrease shortly after birth with low levels reached several hours later.

Therapy is aimed at preventing intracranial hemorrhage and keeping platelet counts at hemostatically safe levels. Cesarean delivery is recommended to prevent birth trauma when this disorder is suspected prior to delivery, thereby eliminating the potential for intracranial bleeding. Corticosteroids and gamma globulin have been used as a means of antenatal treatment. Postnatal treatment is not necessary as long as the infant remains asymptomatic and the platelet count remains above $30 \times 10^9/L$. When the infant manifests clinical signs of bleeding and the platelet count falls below $10 \times 10^9/L$, compatible platelet transfusion utilizing maternal platelets or Pl^{A1}-negative donor platelets is indicated.

Drug-Induced Immune Thrombocytopenia

Drugs may cause thrombocytopenia that can recur if the drug is administered again to the patient. Quinine has been recognized as a frequent cause of thrombocytopenia since the first report in 1928.[16] The drug appears to act as a hapten, eliciting an antibody response when complexed with a larger carrier molecule. The antibody-drug-platelet complex leads to thrombocytopenia. Antibody binding with drug appears to be the initial step in the formation of the complex. Cellular binding or adsorption of the antibody-drug complex to the platelet membrane results in platelet injury and splenic sequestration.

The list of drugs that can cause immune drug purpura is rather extensive. The drugs most frequently implicated are quinine, quinidine, salicylates, thiazides, and sulfa drugs.[17] When possible, any suspect drug should be stopped in a thrombocytopenic patient.

Drug-induced immune purpura appears to occur more frequently in the elderly population as a result of the increased usage of medication; however, cases have been reported in children and young adults. Purpura occurs approximately 7 days after initial use of the drug but may occur within 3 to 5 days owing to an anamnestic response on reexposure to the drug. It is estimated that 1 in 100,000 individuals using prescription medication per year will require hospitalization as a result of a drug-induced blood disorder. The frequency for users of quinine and quinidine is approximately 1 in 1000. The disorder is generally self-limiting because the platelet count returns to normal once the drug has been removed from circulation. Readministration of a drug known to cause purpura should be avoided.

Heparin Therapy

Heparin therapy is associated with the development of two distinct types of thrombocytopenia. One type develops early in treatment and is benign. The platelet count rarely falls below $100 \times 10^9/L$, and there is no resultant bleeding or thrombotic complications. The second type is associated with severe thrombocytopenia and paradoxically thrombotic instead of hemorrhagic complications. Initially, it may be difficult to distinguish between these two types of thrombocytopenia based on laboratory values alone.

In the second type of thrombocytopenia, platelet counts as

low as 20×10^9/L or below occur in association with arterial and venous thrombosis; this type has been termed *heparin-induced thrombocytopenia and thrombosis syndrome (HITTS)*. The actual incidence of this syndrome is not well defined, but it probably occurs in fewer than 1% of patients receiving heparin.[18] It is reported more often with bovine heparin administration than porcine heparin. HITTS typically develops 4 to 7 days after initial exposure to heparin; however, in individuals who have been previously exposed to heparin it can develop within 1 to 3 days after reexposure. Patients with myocardial infarction and cardiogenic shock or those who have undergone major vascular surgery may be particularly susceptible. Venous or arterial thrombosis results in an incidence of morbidity and mortality of 20% of the patients who develop HITTS.

Pathologically, this syndrome develops secondary to antibody produced to platelet factor 4–heparin complex with immune complex Fc receptor–induced activation of platelets.[19,20]

Laboratory confirmation of HITTS is difficult. The most readily available test to confirm HITTS is a platelet aggregation test utilizing donor platelets mixed with patient serum after the patient has been off heparin for 8 or more hours.[21] Heparin is added to the patient samples at low and high concentrations, and platelet aggregation is observed in the heparin sample compared to a control sample without heparin. In patients with HITTS the aggregation test should show aggregation of platelets at the low concentration of heparin but not at the high concentration of heparin or the sample without heparin. This test is approximately 40% sensitive but 90% specific for confirming the diagnosis of HITTS. Platelet release assays increase the sensitivity of detection. Newer tests utilizing flow cytometry or ELISA are even more sensitive for the diagnosis of HITTS and can be performed in the presence of heparin. However, these tests may detect the presence of antibody that has not caused the syndrome in patients with thrombocytopenia resulting from other causes.

In patients with HITTS, heparin must be discontinued. This may be sufficient if thrombosis is not present. The platelet count will return to normal within 4 to 6 days. If the patient has a thrombotic complication, alternative anticoagulation must be utilized. In some instances patients can be administered warfarin without need for intravenous anticoagulation; however, recent reports have suggested warfarin may increase the risk for skin necrosis and venous limb gangrene in this syndrome.[22] In patients who have life- or limb-threatening thrombosis, there are a limited number of choices for intravenous anticoagulation that all have potential hemorrhagic risk.[23] Dextran has been administered; however, there is no laboratory measure other than clinical observation to measure its efficacy. Dextran coats circulating red blood cells, complicating type and crossmatch for red cell transfusion products. Newer agents that have been used in this setting include low-molecular-weight heparins, heparinoids, hirudin, and hirudin analogs.[24] Low-molecular-weight heparins may cross-react with heparin promoting the clinical syndrome. Hirudin is a leech-derived peptide with antithrombin activity that is effective as an anticoagulant but has been associated with a high risk of bleeding. Lepthirudin, a recombinant form of hirudin, is clinically available for this indication. The antithrombin defect induced by hirudin cannot be easily corrected. Fibrinolytics may play a role, especially in individuals who develop neurovascular compromise related to their thrombosis.

Secondary Immune Thrombocytopenia

Lymphoproliferative Disorders/Collagen Vascular Disorders

Lymphoproliferative disorders such as Hodgkin's disease and non-Hodgkin's lymphoma, as well as other hematologic malignancies such as chronic lymphocytic leukemia, have been reported with an ITP-like thrombocytopenia associated with decreased platelet survival. In systemic lupus erythematosus (SLE), roughly 14% of the patients develop thrombocytopenia resembling ITP during the course of the disease. The hematologic manifestations of SLE, which include ITP and thrombocytopenia secondary to bone marrow suppression, may precede the other clinical manifestations of the disease. Thrombocytopenia resulting from either etiology in SLE responds well to corticosteroid therapy.

Viral Infections

Viral infections may also transiently impair megakaryopoiesis without a reduction in marrow cellularity. Chronic viral infections such as human immunodeficiency virus (HIV) or hepatitis may lead to marrow hypocellularity and, subsequently, to thrombocytopenia in affected individuals.

Thrombocytopenia as a result of acute viral, bacterial, or parasitic infections has been well documented. An immunologic mechanism appears likely in the development of thrombocytopenia as a result of infection.[25,26] Viral infections such as mononucleosis, mumps, and rubeola may be complicated by severe thrombocytopenia. In bacterial sepsis, thrombocytopenia may be present with or without disseminated intravascular coagulation (DIC). Malaria is frequently associated with thrombocytopenia as a result of increased destruction and splenic sequestration.

HIV-Related Immune Thrombocytopenic Purpura

An array of hemostatic complications have been described in association HIV. The most common hemostatic abnormality in these patients is immune thrombocytopenic purpura. The incidence of immune thrombocytopenic purpura appears to vary according to the stage of the disease. Significant hemorrhagic complications may occur but are difficult to predict based solely on the platelet count.

The pathogenesis of HIV-related immune thrombocytopenic purpura appears to be heterogeneous and, at present, is still speculative. The pattern of IgG subclasses found in HIV-infected patients, as well as the level of anti-IgG immune complexes on platelet surfaces in HIV disease, are significantly different from patients with "classic ITP." Immunohistochemical markers show increased CD8+ T cells in the spleens of patients with HIV-related immune thrombocytopenic purpura. Viral infection of hematopoietic cells, altered platelet production, and dysfunction of the reticuloendothelial system may all play a prominent role in HIV-mediated thrombocytopenia.

To date, the optimal treatment modality for HIV-related immune thrombocytopenic purpura appears to be IVIgG. Splenectomy and antiretroviral therapy may also be effective. Corticosteroids may be effective but have the potential to increase the risk of infection in these individuals.

Microangiopathic Thrombocytopenia

Thrombotic Thrombocytopenic Purpura

Thrombotic thrombocytopenic purpura (TTP) is a rare and often fatal syndrome associated with thrombocytopenia and microangiopathic hemolytic anemia (Fig. 24–5). Despite being recognized since 1924, the pathogenesis of this syndrome remains poorly understood. Both familial and sporadic nonfamilial forms of the syndrome occur. This disorder was first described as a pentad of signs and symptoms that included thrombocytopenia, microangiopathic hemolytic anemia, fever, neurologic abnormalities, and renal dysfunction.[27] As TTP is recognized more readily, it has become clear that thrombocytopenia and microangiopathic hemolytic anemia characterize this disorder, and the fluctuating neurologic abnormalities, fever, and renal dysfunction occur less frequently. The diagnosis should be suspected in any individual who presents acutely with thrombocytopenia, and consideration should be given to initiation of appropriate treatment even in the absence of other signs or symptoms. Hyaline microthrombi are the characteristic pathologic feature and are found in multiple organs. When the diagnosis of TTP is in question, a biopsy of superficial arterioles and capillaries from the skin or gingiva is often helpful to confirm the diagnosis. However, the microthrombi are not solely diagnostic for TTP, as they occur in other microangiopathic processes such as DIC (Fig. 24–6). The coagulation screening tests are normal in TTP in contrast to DIC, where they abnormal.

The exact pathogenic mechanisms responsible for this disorder remain uncertain. Endothelial cell damage, possibly secondary to drugs or infectious agents, appears to be critical in the development of vascular injury. Once endothelial cell damage occurs, inhibition of fibrinolysis and deficiency of prostacyclin (PGI$_2$) synthesis may then lead to platelet aggregation and thrombosis. The presence of platelet microparticles may increase the thrombotic tendency. A genetic predisposition or an underlying disorder may be necessary for expression of the disease. In the familial variant of TTP, there is now evidence that the protease in vascular endothelial cells that is responsible for cleaving von Willebrand's multimers may be defective or absent.[28] In nonfamilial cases, autoantibody against von Willebrand–cleaving protease is present.[29] The large von Willebrand's multimers that are secreted by endothelial cells may then persist in circulation and appear to promote development of microvascular thrombosis.

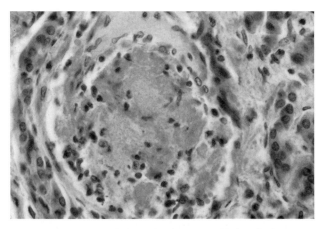

➤ FIGURE 24–6 Renal biopsy from a patient with thrombotic thrombocytopenic purpura (TTP) showing glomerular deposits of platelet-fibrin microvascular occlusion.

The incidence of TTP is thought to be approximately one per million, however, increased awareness of the diagnosis may change these statistics.[30] Women appear to be affected more often than men, with a female-to-male ratio of 3:2. The peak incidence occurs between the third and fourth decade of life. Patients who are pregnant, have viral infections, ingest certain drugs such as ticlopidine, or have autoimmune disorders appear to be predisposed to development of TTP.

Patients with TTP initially present with nonspecific symptoms of malaise, weakness, fatigue, fever, or abdominal pain.[31] Neurologic dysfunction and renal abnormalities are part of the classic pentad but need not be present to make the diagnosis. The degree of severity of these signs and symptoms can be quite variable; fever is typically less than 38.3°C, and the renal abnormalities may be as mild as proteinuria or microscopic hematuria. Overt renal failure requiring dialysis is uncommon in TTP, in contrast to hemolytic uremic syndrome (HUS). Neurologic manifestations can be as mild as headaches or as severe as coma, seizures, or obtundation. Abdominal pain, pancreatitis, and gastrointestinal bleeding may also be associated findings. Any organ system may become involved in TTP; however, symptomatic pulmonary and cardiac involvement are unusual. Pericarditis is rare in TTP, but diffuse cardiac ischemia mimicking pericarditis with diffuse ST segment elevation on electrocardiogram (ECG) can be seen and is typically fatal despite appropriate treatment.

Laboratory features of TTP are those of a severe microangiopathic hemolytic anemia with schistocytes, reticulocytosis, and nucleated red blood cells on the peripheral blood smear. Signs of hemolysis are reflected by increases in LDH and indirect bilirubin, and decreased haptoglobin levels. There is severe thrombocytopenia and evidence of decreased peripheral platelet survival despite megakaryocytic hyperplasia in the bone marrow. However, early in the course of TTP, schistocytes and nucleated red blood cells may not be prominent, and severe thrombocytopenia may be the predominant finding. Prothrombin time (PT), activated partial thromboplastin time (APTT), and fibrinogen level are generally normal in patients with TTP, with slight elevations in the fibrinogen degradation products (FDPs).

Before the development of newer treatment modalities such as plasma exchange, the mortality in TTP exceeded 90%. With the development of plasma exchange, there has

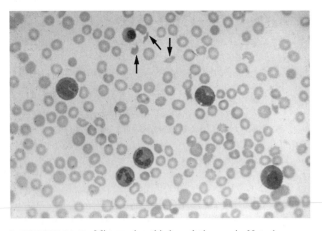

➤ FIGURE 24–5 Microangiopathic hemolytic anemia. Note the presence of schistocytes (*arrows*) and nucleated red cell (*top border*).

been a significant improvement in the survival of patients with TTP; however, the mortality in patients diagnosed with this syndrome remains high at approximately 20% to 40%.[32] Plasma exchange is presently the only treatment modality with proven efficacy in this disorder and should be instituted as soon as the diagnosis is made.[33] The frequency, volume of plasma utilized, and type of plasma for exchange has not been standardized, although most experts support daily exchanges of at least one complete plasma volume utilizing fresh frozen plasma or cryoprecipitate-poor plasma. The length of time plasma exchange should be continued is also not clearly defined, although most clinicians support continuation of the plasma exchange until the platelet count and LDH level have both normalized. Corticosteroid therapy when used as the sole therapeutic agent is ineffective. However, corticosteroids in addition to plasma exchange may offer some benefit, although the amount of corticosteroids needed and the length of therapy have not been clearly defined. Patients should be monitored closely following discontinuation of plasma exchange for evidence of relapse, because relapse is common. Platelet transfusions should be avoided unless the patient is overtly bleeding, because platelet transfusions may accelerate the microangiopathy and have been temporally related to deterioration and death.

In patients who do not respond to plasma exchange or who relapse on plasma exchange, there is no standard treatment intervention. The literature has case reports of many interventions effective in small numbers of patients. Splenectomy is often considered the next best therapeutic intervention once patients fail plasma exchange or for those patients prone to relapses of the disorder. The majority of patients undergoing splenectomy have also received corticosteroids and blood products, which may also increase the response rate. Antiplatelet drugs such as aspirin, dipyridamole, sulfinpyrazone, and dextran have been used. Often these antiplatelet drugs are used in variable combinations, making their efficacy difficult to evaluate. Because patients initially present with thrombocytopenia, antiplatelet agents may increase the risk of hemorrhage and usually are not administered until the platelet count is rising after initiation of plasma exchange. Immunosuppressive drugs, such as vincristine, and intravenous synthetic prostacyclin have been reported to induce remission. Heparin therapy has been used in the past but has shown no benefit.

Hemolytic Uremic Syndrome

HUS is characterized clinically by microangiopathic hemolytic anemia, thrombocytopenia, and renal failure (see Color Plate 126). Renal vascular damage may initiate intravascular hemolysis with subsequent red cell ADP and platelet membrane phospholipid release. Renal damage may also promote coagulant activity, resulting in fibrin deposition and endothelial damage but no consumption of coagulation factors.

HUS resembles TTP pathologically but unlike TTP, which typically affects adults, HUS is more commonly seen in the pediatric population. Following viral and bacterial infections, HUS usually takes a mild course. The prognosis of adult-onset HUS is worse than that of childhood-onset HUS, with both a higher mortality rate and higher incidence of long-term morbidity from permanent renal damage.[34] The pathologic thrombi in HUS are almost always limited to the glomerular capillaries and afferent arterioles of the kidney. Fever, hypertension, and renal failure are common findings, whereas neurologic manifestations are usually less common and less severe. Severe neurologic problems or evidence of systemic thrombi are more likely to suggest the diagnosis of TTP. The hereditary form of HUS, which is more common in adults, is associated with an unfavorable prognosis.

Therapeutic management of HUS is usually conservative. Supportive therapy may include hemodialysis, antihypertensive therapy, anticoagulants, blood transfusions, antiplatelet drugs, corticosteroids, and antifibrinolytic agents. Unlike TTP, plasma exchange is not always necessary in HUS and is usually reserved for adults with the familial form of the disorder.

Disseminated Intravascular Coagulation

Acute DIC is caused by many illnesses, sepsis, obstetric emergencies, and severe trauma, and may cause bleeding. Chronic DIC may be seen with cancer and may result in thrombosis rather than bleeding. Thrombocytopenia is usually seen in acute DIC; however, the platelet count may be normal or elevated in chronic DIC. In all instances, there appears to be accelerated platelet destruction in combination with coagulation factor consumption. DIC must be differentiated from other causes of microangiopathy causing thrombocytopenia, because the treatments differ. Pathogenesis and treatment of DIC is discussed in Chapter 26.

Pregnancy-Associated Thrombocytopenia

Thrombocytopenia may occur in pregnancy owing to coincidental development of disorders discussed earlier in this chapter, or it may occur as a consequence of the pregnancy.[35] Disorders resulting from pregnancy include gestational thrombocytopenia and thrombotic microangiopathies such as preeclampsia-eclampsia and HELLP syndrome (*h*emolysis, *e*levated *l*iver enzymes, *l*ow *p*latelets).

Gestational Thrombocytopenia

Mild thrombocytopenia with platelets counts of 50 to 80 $\times$ 10^9/L may occur in about 8% of normal pregnant women. This most commonly develops in the third trimester of pregnancy and does not cause bleeding in the mother or baby. No treatment is necessary for this disorder. The platelet count returns to normal after delivery. This gestational thrombocytopenia must be differentiated from other thrombocytopenic disorders of pregnancy such as eclampsia, HELLP syndrome, ITP, or TTP, because these disorders may cause harm to the mother or the fetus and require treatment to prevent maternal or fetal morbidity and mortality.

Preeclampsia-Eclampsia and HELLP Syndrome

Preeclampsia is a relatively common disorder of pregnancy that causes hypertension, elevation of uric acid, and thrombocytopenia. Eclampsia is a more severe form of the disorder and may result in seizures and renal dysfunction; it also has a greater association with thrombocytopenia. A variant of eclampsia termed *HELLP syndrome* is also described.[36] These disorders are thrombotic microangiopathies with clinical manifestations resulting from platelet activation and consumption. The more severe forms of these syndromes must be differentiated from TTP or HUS. Preeclampsia and eclampsia typically occur with the first pregnancy and usually occur in the last trimester, whereas TTP and HUS may occur at any time in pregnancy. Delivery of the fetus usually is effective in reversing these disorders. Aspirin appears to be useful in treating preeclampsia. However, when these disorders are severe or serious complications have developed, plasma exchange therapy is used.

Thrombocytosis

Thrombocytosis, defined as platelet count above the normal range, may be either a reactive process or due to a primary myeloproliferative disorder (MPD). Reactive thrombocytosis, unlike thrombocytosis from a primary MPD, is rarely associated with bleeding and thrombotic complications, and the platelet count usually does not exceed 1×10^{10}/L . The morphology of platelets in a reactive process is usually normal in contrast to those in a myeloproliferative disorder, where the platelets are often large and dysplastic. Tests of platelet function are also typically normal in reactive thrombocytosis. Bone marrow examination may demonstrate increased numbers of megakaryocytes; however, in contrast to MPDs, the megakaryocytes are neither clustered nor dysplastic.

Primary Thrombocytosis

Because all of the myeloproliferative syndromes are characterized by an autonomous proliferation of a pluripotent stem cell, they can all be associated with thrombocytosis. Bleeding, thrombosis, and platelet function defects can also be seen with any of the MPDs. (The MPDs as they relate to specific platelet defects are discussed later in the section on acquired qualitative platelet disorders.) Patients with essential thrombocythemia typically have the highest platelet counts of all of the MPDs, often exceeding 1×10^{10}/L. Idiopathic myelofibrosis and chronic myelogenous leukemia (CML) are also associated with milder degrees of thrombocytosis. Based on observations of patients with reactive thrombocytosis and normal platelet function, in which bleeding and thrombotic complications are uncommon, thrombocytosis alone is not the sole factor in the development of bleeding and thrombosis in the myeloproliferative syndromes. These complications are suggested to result from qualitative platelet defects.

Reactive Thrombocytosis

Reactive thrombocytosis may be attributed to many causes and may be either a transient or chronic process. Thrombocytosis is a common finding associated with acute hemorrhage. The platelet count is generally elevated within a day or so after hemorrhage as a result of increased marrow stimulation. Similar responses may be seen following therapeutic phlebotomy for polycythemia vera and hemochromatosis.

Iron-deficiency anemia has classically been associated with mild thrombocytosis that does not usually exceed 750 $\times 10^9$/L. This associated thrombocytosis may help to differentiate iron deficiency from other causes of red blood cell microcytosis that are not typically associated with thrombocytosis. Repletion of iron stores corrects the platelet count to normal.

Thrombocytosis is also associated with underlying malignancy, and with chronic inflammatory or infectious processes.

Thrombocytosis can be seen postoperatively after almost any surgical procedure but is most common and pronounced after splenectomy. Within the first 2 weeks, platelet counts rise and then decline to a higher normal or slightly above normal level over a period of months after splenectomy. Platelet counts may initially increase to as much as two to

six times preoperative levels. Platelet survival has been documented to be normal. It has been suggested that the thrombocytosis seen after splenectomy is caused by increased platelet production, because elimination of the splenic pool can account for no more than a 50% rise in the platelet count. Regulation of thrombopoiesis is thought to be a moderated by a humoral factor produced by the spleen.

Certain drugs may also induce thrombocytosis. Administration of epinephrine will cause a rapid but transient increase in platelet count secondary to platelet release from the spleen. Recovery of marrow suppression from alcohol or chemotherapeutic agents will elevate the platelet count. Growth factors such as interleukin-11 (IL-11), IL-6, and thrombopoietin stimulate platelet production and are generally administered to aid in platelet recovery after chemotherapy.

➤ QUALITATIVE PLATELET DISORDERS

Congenital Disorders of Platelet Function

Congenital disorders of platelet function are rare and can be classified based on the platelet function or response that is abnormal. This classification currently includes (1) platelet surface membrane defects, (2) platelet release or secretion defects, and (3) defects associated with abnormal platelet-coagulant protein interactions shown in Table 24–5. Some disorders also exhibit thrombocytopenia in addition to platelet dysfunction. Other cutaneous, skeletal, and other congenital abnormalities may also be present. Tables 24–4 and 24–5 list the various congenital disorders as they relate to abnormal platelet function.

Platelet Membrane Defects

As noted in Chapter 23, the platelet surface includes a glycocalyx containing various glycoproteins that function as receptors to bind molecules or proteins and transmit signals to the interior of the platelet to effect platelet reactions. Glanzmann's thrombasthenia and Bernard-Soulier syndrome are congenital disorders with surface glycoprotein deficiencies that result in platelet dysfunction. The laboratory abnormalities in these syndromes are noted in Table 24–6.

Glanzmann's Thrombasthenia

Glanzmann's thrombasthenia is a rare autosomal-recessive disorder of platelet function caused by an absence or deficiency of the membrane GPIIb/IIIa complex. GPIIb/IIIa

> ### ➤ Table 24-5
> ### CONGENITAL DISORDERS OF PLATELET FUNCTION

Platelet membrane defects

   Glanzmann's thrombasthenia

   Bernard-Soulier syndrome

Platelet release (secretion defects)

   Storage pool deficiency (granule defects)

   Primary secretion defects (enzymatic pathway defects)

von Willebrand disease

> **Table 24-6**
COMPARISON OF GLANZMANN'S THROMBASTHENIA AND BERNARD-SOULIER SYNDROME

	Glanzmann's Thrombasthenia	Bernard-Soulier Syndrome
Platelet count	Normal	Decreased
Platelet morphology	Normal	Giant platelets
Bleeding time	Prolonged	Prolonged
Platelet aggregation		
ADP	Abnormal	Normal
Thrombin	Abnormal	Abnormal
Collagen	Abnormal	Normal
Epinephrine	Abnormal	Normal
Ristocetin	Normal	Abnormal
Clot retraction	Abnormal	Normal
Platelet glycoprotein defect	GPIIb/IIIa	GPIb/IX

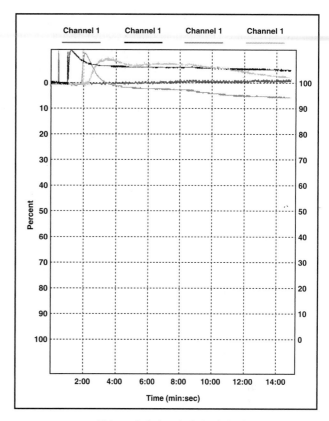

> **FIGURE 24-7** This graph depicts the lack of platelet aggregation to epinephrine, 10 μm (blue); ADP, 5 μm (black); collagen, 2 μg/mL (red); and arachidonic acid, 0.5 μg/mL (green)—typical of a patient with Glanzmann's thrombasthenia.

mediates the binding of fibrinogen, von Willebrand's factor (vWF), and fibronectin to activated platelets. GPIIb/IIIa also serves to connect adhesive proteins to contractile proteins of the platelet following activation, thereby facilitating clot retraction. These two proteins exist within the platelet membrane as heterodimers. Calcium is required for stabilization of the complex. GPIIb/IIIa must exist as a complex in order to function as a ligand to bind fibrinogen. Both megakaryocytes and platelets express the GPIIb/GPIIIa complex.

The gene that codes for GPIIb and GPIIIa is located on chromosome 17. Gene deletion and gene rearrangement of GPIIIa may account for the phenotypic defects seen in Glanzmann's thrombasthenia.

Clinical manifestations of Glanzmann's thrombasthenia are quite variable, ranging from minor bruising to severe and potentially fatal hemorrhages, with the severity of bleeding consistent within single families.[37] Although uncommon, Glanzmann's thrombasthenia occurs with greater frequency than Bernard-Soulier syndrome, another surface glycoprotein abnormality. Glanzmann's thrombasthenia appears to cluster in ethnic populations where consanguinity is prevalent. Bleeding is most commonly from mucosal surfaces and includes easy bruisability, epistaxis, spontaneous gingival bleeding, prolonged bleeding from minor cuts, and menorrhagia. Gastrointestinal hemorrhages are less common. The formation of deep hematomas and recurrent hemarthroses that are typical features in hemophilia are not present in Glanzmann's thrombasthenia.

Criteria for diagnosing Glanzmann's thrombasthenia include (1) an autosomal-recessive trait with clinical manifestations expressed in homozygotes only; (2) normal platelet count and normal platelet morphology, (3) prolonged bleeding time, (4) absent platelet aggregation to ADP, thrombin, collagen, and epinephrine, with normal platelet agglutination to ristocetin (Fig. 24–7); (5) flow cytometric assessment of GPIIb/IIIa surface protein, revealing deficiency or absence; (6) normal lumi-aggregation and ^{51}Cr release; and (7) abnormal clot retraction.

Patients with Glanzmann's thrombasthenia who present with severe bleeding episodes require platelet transfusions to replace dysfunctional platelets. Supportive therapy should be used judiciously, because patients may develop alloantibodies to GPIIb and GPIIIa on the transfused platelets or anti-HLA antibodies and become refractory to platelet transfusions. Antifibrinolytic agents such as EACA may help in controlling hemorrhage, especially from the nose and mouth where fibrinolytic activity is prominent. Topical measures such as thrombin or pressure packing may be effective. DDAVP has been used but has not been helpful. Estrogen therapy in the form of birth control pills is especially useful in controlling menorrhagia.

Bernard-Soulier Syndrome

Bernard-Soulier syndrome is a rare autosomal-recessive bleeding disorder caused by a deficiency of the platelet GPIb/IX complex. GPV, which is associated with the GPIb/IX complex on the platelet surface and is a thrombin substrate, has also been documented to be deficient in Bernard-Soulier platelets. As discussed in Chapter 22 GPIb/IX plays a major role in various hemostatic events. GPIb/IX is the platelet receptor involved in the vWF-dependent contact adhesion of unactivated platelets to exposed subendothelium at high shear rates and for the binding of platelets to fibrin. It also serves as a high-affinity thrombin-binding site and regulates platelet shape and reactivity. Because the platelet membrane is attached to the cytoskeleton via GPIb, the loss of normal membrane-cytoskeletal function may account for the abnormal platelet morphology seen in Bernard-Soulier platelets.[38]

Patients with Bernard-Soulier syndrome present with the typical symptoms of a primary hemostatic disorder with varying severity. Gingival bleeding, epistaxis, purpura, menorrhagia, and gastrointestinal bleeding are the typical hemorrhagic manifestations. Symptoms occur early in life and have a tendency to decrease with age.

Laboratory abnormalities in patients with Bernard-Soulier syndrome include normal or moderately reduced platelet counts with large irregularly shaped platelets noted on the peripheral smear, and a prolonged bleeding time. The platelets may be large enough to resemble lymphocytes. Normal numbers of megakaryocytes are found on bone marrow examination. Platelet aggregation is normal with ADP, epinephrine, and collagen, and is reduced with thrombin. Ristocetin-induced platelet aggregation is absent in Bernard-Soulier syndrome, similar to von Willebrand's disease. However, the deficient ristocetin-induced aggregation defect is corrected by the addition of normal plasma in von Willebrand's disease, but not in Bernard-Soulier syndrome, where the deficiency of GPIb/IX (which is the receptor for vWF) is the cause for the aggregation defect. Crossed immunoelectrophoresis or flow cytometry of platelet membrane glycoproteins should demonstrate a decrease in GPIb, GPIX, and GPV to confirm a diagnosis of Bernard-Soulier syndrome.

Heterogeneity among the glycoprotein abnormalities in Bernard-Soulier indicates that there are multiple genetic defects. Heterozygotes present with recognizable abnormalities such as occasional large platelets on the peripheral smear, with a history of bleeding yet few clinical problems. Homozygotes present with abnormal platelet function and morphology, thrombocytopenia, and hemorrhagic disease.

Rather specific criteria for the diagnosis of this bleeding syndrome have been established. These criteria are (1) an autosomal trait with clinical manifestations expressed in homozygotes (or double heterozygotes with combined genetic abnormalities of GPIb, GPV, and GPIX); (2) normal platelet count or moderate thrombocytopenia (despite a normal number of marrow megakaryocytes); (3) a significant number of giant or large platelets present on the peripheral blood smear and prolonged bleeding time in excess of the degree of thrombocytopenia; (4) absent platelet agglutination in response to human vWF and ristocetin; (5) normal platelet aggregation in response to ADP, collagen, and epinephrine, with reduced aggregation in response to thrombin; and (6) normal factor VIII coagulant activity (FVIII:C) and vWF antigen.

Affected individuals who present with active bleeding should be treated with red blood cell transfusions to replace blood loss and an antifibrinolytic agent such as EACA. Antifibrinolytic agents do not correct the defect but only allow the primary hemostatic plug to remain intact at the site of injury. DDAVP has been reported to shorten the bleeding time in some individuals[39] but not in others. Estrogen therapy may be helpful in controlling bleeding.[39,40] In instances in which bleeding is not controlled by these measures, platelet transfusions may be necessary; however, these should be used judiciously to avoid alloimmunization to GPIb.

Platelet Release (Secretion) Defects

As described in Chapter 23, platelet glycoprotein receptors transmit signals intracellularly to cause release of platelet granule substances and platelet shape change. Phospholipases (A and C) are liberated from the internal surface of the platelet membrane in response to platelet agonists and cause an increase in intracellular calcium levels. This produces centralization of granules and fusion of granule membrane with the open canalicular system to transport granule proteins to the environment to allow adhesion and aggregation. The disorders of platelet release primarily involve absence of platelet granules or defective enzymatic pathways.

Storage Pool Deficiencies (Granule Defects)

Storage pool deficiencies are classified according to an analysis of the granule proteins and the morphological appearance of the platelets. Most commonly, a decrease in platelet dense granules is present, with decreased amounts of secretable ADP, adenosine triphosphate (ATP), calcium, and serotonin (delta [δ] storage pool deficiency). In other patients, alpha (α) granules and dense granules are decreased, and decreases in amounts of α-granule proteins such as platelet factor 4, beta (β)-thromboglobulin, and platelet-derived growth factor as well as the dense granule proteins are noted ($\alpha\delta$ storage pool deficiency). Other patients have a decrease in α granules, only, with normal dense granules and normal amounts of dense granule constituents (α storage pool deficiency). Deficiency of the α granules leads to an agranular appearance of platelets on the Wright-stained peripheral blood smear and has been termed *gray platelet syndrome*. Platelet factor 3 (PF3) activity is reduced in these disorders and appears related to the defects in platelet aggregation.

The inheritance pattern of these disorders has not been well defined but in some instances appears to be an autosomal-dominant pattern. Patients with storage pool deficiency have a mild to moderate mucosal bleeding tendency. Easy bruising, epistaxis, menorrhagia, postpartum bleeding, and bleeding after dental extractions and tonsillectomy are often present. Gastrointestinal bleeding is uncommon, and hemarthrosis is not present. Storage pool deficiencies have been found in association with other congenital abnormalities (see Table 24–4). The Hermansky-Pudlak syndrome describes patients with oculocutaneous albinism and dense granule storage pool deficiency. Individuals with Chédiak-Higashi syndrome also have oculocutaneous abnormalities, including ocular albinism and characteristic silver-gray hair with dense granule storage pool deficiency. Other congenital abnormalities including Wiskott-Aldrich syndrome and the syndrome of thrombocytopenia with absent radii (TAR syndrome) have been described to have an associated platelet storage pool deficiency.

Laboratory features of storage pool deficiencies include a prolonged or normal template bleeding time. Aspirin ingestion may cause a marked prolongation of the bleeding time. Plasma coagulation screening tests and factor assays are normal in these disorders. Platelet aggregation testing is abnormal, with primary wave aggregation but absent or reduced secondary wave aggregation in response to ADP and epinephrine. Collagen-induced aggregation is reduced at lower but not high collagen concentrations. Platelet counts are normal, and the morphology of platelets is normal except in the gray platelet syndrome or Chédiak-Higashi syndrome.

Primary Secretion Defects (Enzymatic Pathway Defects)

These disorders resemble storage pool deficiencies but have no abnormalities of the platelet granules and have normal amounts of platelet granule contents. The causes of release defects are deficiencies of enzymes and other "second messengers" that transmit the signal from surface receptors to cause platelet release of granule contents. The bleeding tendency and laboratory findings in these disorders are similar to those found in the storage pool deficiencies.

Cyclo-oxygenase deficiency results in deficient conversion of membrane-associated arachidonic acid to thromboxane A_2. Thromboxane synthetase deficiency and other defects of thromboxane A_2 generation and calcium mobilization have been described.[41]

Treatment of storage pool deficiencies and primary secretion defects has primarily been with judicious use of platelet transfusions for prevention or treatment of bleeding. For procedures with low risk of bleeding or where bleeding is easily controlled by local measures, no additional treatment may be needed. Prednisone has been reported to improve the bleeding time but not platelet aggregation defects, presumably owing to an effect to promote vascular integrity. Cryoprecipitate and DDAVP have improved the bleeding time in patients with Hermansky-Pudlak syndrome. DDAVP has been used in patients with gray platelet syndrome to shorten the prolonged bleeding time. However, efficacy in treating bleeding has not been reported in those studies. Red blood cell transfusion may also improve the platelet adhesion defect, possibly by supplying ADP. Avoidance of nonsteroidal anti-inflammatory agents or other drugs that induce platelet dysfunction is important in the management of these disorders.

von Willebrand's Disease

von Willebrand's disease is an inherited deficiency of vWF that may be confused with a primary platelet defect because of the similarities in clinical presentations between von Willebrand's disease and platelet disorders. von Willebrand's disease was originally termed *parahemophilia,* because it is a congenital bleeding disorder; however, it has a different inheritance pattern and different bleeding pattern than hemophilia.

vWF is a large, multimeric glycoprotein coded for by a gene located on chromosome 12 (Fig. 24–8). vWF is synthesized by vascular endothelial cells and stored in Weibel-Palade bodies. A small amount of vWF is also synthesized in megakaryocytes and stored in the platelet α granules. Polymerization of vWF occurs in endothelial cells with the production of high-molecular-weight multimers. vWF-cleaving protease reduces the size of the multimers at the time vWF is secreted into the plasma. Circulating vWF forms a complex with factor VIII, the protein that is deficient or defective in hemophilia A. vWF acts as a carrier protein for factor VIII, serving to protect the factor VIII molecule from proteolytic degradation and increase its concentration at the site of tissue injury. In normal individuals, plasma levels of factor VIII closely correlate with plasma levels of vWF.

The role that vWF plays in hemostasis is quite important, as seen from the bleeding manifestations in patients with von Willebrand's disease. vWF is an important adhesive protein following vascular injury. It serves as a ligand between platelets, vascular endothelium, and other adhesive proteins such as fibronectin (Fig. 24–9). vWF has distinct domains for binding to platelet GPIb/IX, GPIIb/IIIa, and subendothelial components heparin and collagen. Platelet GPIb serves as the major receptor for vWF. Platelet adhesion is dependent on subendothelium, GPIb, and vWF. In von Willebrand's disease, the platelets that are intrinsically normal exhibit abnormal adhesion because of the absence or dysfunction of vWF. vWF promotes secondary hemostasis by functioning as a carrier for factor VIII. In von Willebrand's disease, absence or dysfunction of vWF results in decreases in factor VIII and abnormal secondary hemostasis.

vWF can be measured antigenically and functionally using the antibiotic ristocetin. Ristocetin was removed from use after clinical trials revealed it produced thrombocytopenia. Further evaluation revealed it produced agglutina-

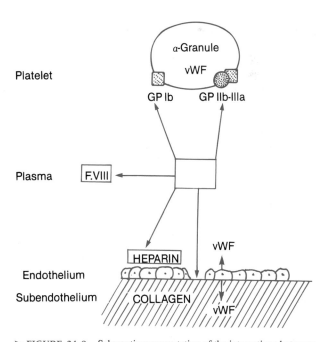

> **FIGURE 24–9** Schematic representation of the interactions between vWF, platelets, and collagen of the subendothelium. vWF synthesized by endothelial cells is released in plasma and is stored in the α granules of platelets, and can be released after stimulation. vWF mediates platelet adhesion through binding to collagen and to platelet glycoprotein Ib (GPIb) in the presence of ristocetin, as well as the platelet GPIIb/IIIa in the presence of physiologic agonists (thrombin, collagen, ADP). vWF also binds to factor VIII (FVIII) and heparin.

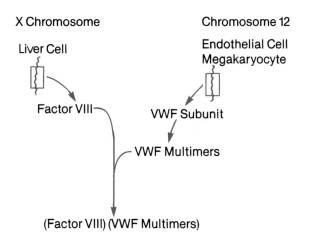

The Factor VIII/VWF Complex in Plasma

> **FIGURE 24–8** Factor VIII/von Willebrand factor (vWF) complex in plasma.

tion of platelets in the presence of vWF. This has led to its use as a diagnostic agent in the evaluation of von Willebrand's disease in vitro with the ristocetin-induced platelet aggregation (RIPA) test. Factor VIII is measured by a functional clotting assay. Measurements of factor VIII, vWF antigen, and vWF activity are important in differentiating von Willebrand's disease from hemophilia A and to define the types of von Willebrand's disease.

von Willebrand's disease comprises both quantitative and qualitative abnormalities of the large multimeric vWF glycoprotein. Affected individuals exhibit mucocutaneous bleeding typical of defects of primary hemostasis, in contrast to the joint and deep muscle bleeding typical for hemophilia. The disorder has an autosomal pattern of inheritance but has variable penetrance for expression in affected individuals.[42] Severe cases are characterized by recurrent, potentially life-threatening bleeding, whereas mild cases may go undetected. Diagnosis of von Willebrand's disease is often difficult because of the variability of abnormal laboratory results within affected individuals or family members. vWF and factor VIII are both acute phase reactant proteins, and plasma levels may be increased with stresses such as inflammation, surgery, and pregnancy or with estrogen therapy. Furthermore, the levels of vWF vary with ABO blood types, with the lowest levels being seen in individuals of O blood type.

von Willebrand's disease can be classified into three general categories: (1) type 1, an autosomal-dominant disorder accounting for 70% of all cases, which is characterized by a quantitative decrease in normal vWF and mild bleeding; (2) type 2, which has variable inheritance with numerous subtypes, accounts for most of the remaining cases, and is characterized by a qualitative abnormality in the structure of vWF; and (3) type 3, a rare autosomal-recessive disorder characterized by absent levels of vWF multimers and a severe bleeding diathesis very similar in presentation to hemophilia A.[43] von Willebrand Normandy is an unusual type 2 variant of von Willebrand's disease that is characterized by a defect in the vWF binding to factor VIII. This disorder is sometimes confused with mild hemophilia A, because the factor VIII coagulant level is reduced but the vWF antigen and activity levels are normal or elevated. Clinically, the bleeding diathesis associated with von Willebrand Normandy is similar to other patients with type 2 von Willebrand's disease.[44]

A platelet-type von Willebrand's disease has also been described. It is a platelet disorder characterized by increased binding of normal vWF to platelets caused by a point mutation in platelet glycoprotein Ibα (GPIbα).[45,46]

The routine laboratory evaluation of patients suspected of having von Willebrand's disease includes a bleeding time, platelet count, factor VIII coagulant activity, quantitative measurements of plasma vWF antigen (vWF:Ag) by crossed immunoelectrophoresis or agarose gel electrophoresis, and functional assays of plasma vWF by RIPA (vWF activity).[47] Subtypes of von Willebrand's disease can be distinguished according to the vWF:Ag, vWF activity, factor VIII coagulant activity, and multimeric pattern on gel electrophoresis.

For patients with type 1 von Willebrand's disease, DDAVP is considered the initial treatment of choice.[48] DDAVP stimulates the release of vWF from endothelial cell Weibel-Palade bodies. Baseline plasma vWF antigen and activity increase about three- to fourfold after DDAVP administration. vWF stores within the endothelial cells are depleted after about 3 to 4 days of DDAVP treatment. Patients requiring longer treatment or those who do not achieve an adequate response to DDAVP may require the use of intermediate purity factor VIII products such as Humate P, which contain intact vWF or cryoprecipitate. In type 1 patients who receive cryoprecipitate, there is evidence that the endothelial cells are also stimulated to increase de novo synthesis of vWF.

Patients with type 3 von Willebrand's disease do not make vWF and do not respond to DDAVP: therefore, they must be treated with intermediate purity factor VIII products or cryoprecipitate.

There are many subtypes of type 2 von Willebrand's disease, some of which respond to DDAVP and some of which do not. DDAVP has been reported to cause thrombocytopenia in the type 2b variant.[45] In many of the type 2 variants, response to therapy is difficult to quantitate and may require measurement of the bleeding time and determination of correction of a prolonged bleeding time after administration of appropriate therapy. Addition of DDAVP to cryoprecipitate has been utilized as an effective combination in certain patient populations.

Antifibrinolytic agents can be utilized as an adjunctive therapy in all patients with von Willebrand's disease. For dental procedures, local measures are used and replacement therapy may not be necessary.

Acquired Qualitative Platelet Disorders

Platelet dysfunction can also be caused by many systemic illnesses and medications (Table 24–7). In these diseases, the platelet dysfunction is a secondary manifestation and not typically one of the primary presenting features of these disorders. Acquired causes of platelet dysfunction are more commonly encountered than congenital platelet disorders; however, the results of platelet function tests can appear similar to those seen with congenital disorders. To differentiate between acquired and congenital causes of platelet dysfunction, a careful history and physical examination as well as family history must be obtained.

Renal Disease: Uremia

Bleeding has long been recognized as a common complication of uremia. Patients with acute and chronic renal failure generally exhibit bleeding from mucous membranes. Petechiae, purpura, epistaxis, ecchymosis, and gastroin-

> **Table 24–7**
> **ACQUIRED QUALITATIVE PLATELET DISORDERS**

Renal disease (uremia)

Liver disease

Paraproteinemias

Myeloproliferative disorders

Acquired von Willebrand disease

Cardiopulmonary bypass

Acquired storage pool deficiencies

Drug therapy

testinal bleeding are common. Severe hemorrhage within serous cavities and muscles may also occur.

A number of different laboratory findings and clinical symptoms suggest that platelet dysfunction with abnormal platelet–vessel wall interaction is the major cause of hemorrhage. Studies have shown an abnormality in the interaction of vWF and platelet GPIIb/IIIa complex in uremic patients; however, platelet membrane glycoproteins Ib, IIb, and IIIa are quantitatively normal. Other platelet abnormalities seen in uremia include abnormal prostaglandin synthesis, decreased membrane procoagulant activity, decreased platelet serotonin release, abnormal β-thromboglobulin levels, elevated intracellular calcium, and decreased thromboxane synthesis. Increased levels of "uremic toxins," such as guanidosuccinic acid and phenols, are rather consistent findings in patients with uremia. The acquired platelet defects associated with uremia are thought to be primarily mediated by these products. A correlation of the metabolic changes with the exact mechanism of the functional defect has not yet been firmly established.

Mild thrombocytopenia with platelet counts as low as 100 $\times 10^9$/L, decreased adhesion, abnormal aggregation, and increased bleeding times are abnormal laboratory findings often seen in patients with uremia. Platelet aggregation studies in uremic patients typically show no characteristic patterns.

The anemia of renal failure may contribute to the hemostatic defects observed in uremic patients. Hematocrit values of less than 25% may prolong bleeding times. Red cells may play a role in hemostasis by improving factor VIII coagulant function and by providing ADP, a platelet-aggregating agent. Erythropoietin (r-HuEPO) therapy has proved to be effective in improving hemostasis and decreasing the bleeding tendencies in uremic patients on dialysis. It has been theorized that r-HuEPO may also increase platelet number and aid aggregation.

Hemodialysis or peritoneal dialysis is the treatment of choice to correct the hemostatic defect in uremia. However, platelet function abnormalities may remain. Administration of cryoprecipitate to patients unresponsive to dialysis has been reported to shorten the prolonged bleeding time and decrease bleeding. The use of DDAVP in uremic patients has also prevented clinical bleeding in patients following surgical procedures and has shortened the prolonged bleeding time.[49]

Liver Disease

Chronic liver disease is often associated with a significant hemorrhagic diathesis as a result of multiple alterations in hemostasis, including platelet dysfunction. Mild to moderate thrombocytopenia is seen in approximately one-third of patients with chronic liver disease as a result of splenic sequestration secondary to congestive splenomegaly associated with portal hypertension. Abnormal platelet function tests found in patients with chronic liver disease include reduced platelet adhesion; abnormal platelet aggregation to ADP, epinephrine, and thrombin; and abnormal PF3 availability. An acquired storage pool deficiency has also been suggested. The exact mechanism responsible for the platelet defects seen in chronic liver disease is not known.

Treatment of bleeding in a patient with chronic liver disease may require several modalities simultaneously to correct the multiple abnormalities present. Transfusion with platelet concentrates may ameliorate the bleeding and thrombocytopenia associated with chronic liver disease; however,

the expected rise in platelet count following transfusion may be blunted if splenic sequestration or increased platelet consumption occurs. DDAVP may improve the qualitative platelet defect associated with this disorder. The numerous coagulation factor deficiencies common in chronic liver disease typically require the administration of fresh frozen plasma to correct the coagulation abnormalities. Use of conjugated estrogens may decrease the overall bleeding tendency after an acute episode.

Paraproteinemias

Patients with lymphoproliferative malignances may exhibit both hemorrhagic diatheses and hypercoagulability. These hemostatic alterations are complex and multifactorial. Clinically significant bleeding is a manifestation associated with multiple myeloma, Waldenström's macroglobulinemia, and other related malignant paraprotein disorders. The pathogenesis of hemorrhage and other recognized hemostatic abnormalities has been proposed to be caused by the interaction of the paraprotein with platelets and coagulation factors. Clinical bleeding and platelet dysfunction are seen in approximately 60% of patients with IgM myeloma or Waldenström's macroglobulinemia as compared to approximately 40% of the patients with IgA myeloma and 15% of patients with IgG myeloma.

The hemorrhagic diathesis of paraproteinemias is characterized by a prolonged bleeding time and platelet dysfunction. The occurrence of bleeding correlates with the impairment of platelet function. Thrombocytopenia and inhibition of coagulation factors may also contribute to the bleeding tendency. Patients may present clinically with spontaneous epistaxis and ecchymosis, or unexplained postoperative bleeding in the face of a normal platelet count and coagulation profile. Patients with malignant paraprotein disorders should not ingest aspirin or aspirin-containing drugs because this may exacerbate the platelet defect. Uremic platelet dysfunction associated with renal failure often seen in the malignant paraproteinemias may also contribute to the hemorrhagic episodes.

Platelet abnormalities include decreased aggregation in response to various aggregating agents, altered shape change, abnormal release reactions, and a prolonged bleeding time. Acquired von Willebrand's syndrome causing reduced levels of vWF/factor VIII complexes, other circulating anticoagulants, amyloid-associated coagulopathies, impaired fibrin formation and polymerization, hyperviscosity syndrome, nephrosis, and DIC represent additional abnormalities that predispose patients with paraproteinemia to bleeding.

Thrombocytopenia, unrelated to the paraprotein effect, may result from marrow replacement, chemotherapy, or hypersplenism and is a common finding contributing to the incidence of significant bleeding.

Therapy for patients with qualitative defects resulting from multiple myeloma and related disorders includes plasmapheresis to reduce the circulating paraprotein concentrations and chemotherapy to inhibit paraprotein production. Blood product support and other therapies may be required when additional hemostatic abnormalities are present.

Myeloproliferative Disorders

The MPDs include polycythemia vera (PV), idiopathic myelofibrosis, CML, and essential thrombocythemia (ET). This group of disorders has many clinical and hematologic features in common, but the hemostatic and thrombotic problems are variable. The hemorrhagic manifestations include ecchymosis, epistaxis, and mucocutaneous bleeding from the gastrointestinal and genitourinary tracts. Thrombosis occurs in both the arterial and venous circulation and includes deep vein thrombosis, pulmonary embolism, stroke, myocardial infarction, and thrombosis of the hepatic, portal, splenic and mesenteric veins. The precise mechanisms that cause the problems are unknown.[50] In many cases, thrombocytosis is a contributing factor, especially for thrombotic problems in patients with an MPD. Patients may present with bleeding and thrombosis simultaneously, or alternate with bleeding and thrombotic episodes as the disease progresses.

Aggregation patterns in these disorders are usually not characteristic. The most consistently noted laboratory abnormalities include abnormal release and aggregation in response to epinephrine, collagen, and ADP, but these findings vary from patient to patient with the same type of MPD. The bleeding time is prolonged in many cases but does not correlate with the risk for bleeding or thrombosis in these patients. Other reported abnormalities include acquired storage pool defects, abnormal prostaglandin and arachidonic acid metabolism, and platelet hyperactivity.

Thrombosis is a major complication of PV owing to an increased red cell mass and whole blood viscosity and thrombocytosis. Thrombocytosis is generally moderate, in the range of $500 \times 10^9/L$ to $1 \times 10^{10}/L$, and is seen in approximately 50% to 60% of cases. Platelet function defects are thought to be responsible for many of the hemostatic problems seen. Abnormal platelet aggregation in response to epinephrine, ADP, and collagen has been reported in PV. Platelet activation and intravascular coagulation with increased plasma levels of β-thromboglobulin, low platelet serotonin levels, and abnormal levels of fibrinogen and prothrombin have also been reported in cases of PV.

Patients with idiopathic myelofibrosis may experience bleeding, such as ecchymosis and urogenital hemorrhage. Thromboembolic complications, with the exception of hepatic and portal vein thrombosis, occur rather infrequently. It has been suggested that of all the MPDs, idiopathic myelofibrosis has the greatest degree of platelet function defects. Decreased platelet adhesion and prolonged bleeding times are relatively common findings in patients with idiopathic myelofibrosis. Storage pool deficiencies and impaired platelet aggregation have also been reported.

ET presents with thrombocytosis and is associated with both bleeding and thrombosis, although bleeding episodes occur more often. Evidence suggests that thrombocytosis alone does not account for the bleeding and thrombotic episodes seen in ET, but the combination of thrombocytosis and abnormal platelet function determine the hemostatic defects in ET. Decreased platelet aggregation in response to epinephrine as well as decreased platelet retention are noted in patients with ET. Impaired PF3 availability and platelet hyperactivity have been reported in patients with thrombosis in ET. Several platelet defects have been described in ET, but what predisposes patients to bleeding or thrombotic manifestations is still uncertain.

Bleeding and thrombosis occur least frequently in patients with CML. When present, bleeding includes mucocutaneous hemorrhages, retinal hemorrhages, and hematuria. It is thought that acquired platelet defects may be responsible for this bleeding as a result of dysplastic platelet production. Thrombocytopenia, as occurs with transformation

to blast crisis, also results in a bleeding tendency. Decreased or absent platelet aggregation in response to ADP, epinephrine, and collagen have been reported in cases of CML. A prolonged bleeding time is quite frequently seen in patients with CML in remission as well as in a blast crisis. A factor V deficiency has been reported in some cases of CML. Increases in platelet vWF have also been noted.

Management of patients with MPDs aims at reducing the risk of hemorrhage and thrombotic complications.[51] Cytoreductive chemotherapy is often used. In patients with marked thrombocytosis and cerebral ischemia, plateletpheresis in addition to chemotherapy may be helpful. The use of antiplatelet drugs such as aspirin is controversial. Antiplatelet therapy may be useful to prevent recurrences of thrombosis or to treat a specific complication of pain and erythema of the hands termed *erythromelalgia* but may worsen a preexisting bleeding tendency. Hemorrhage may require administration of platelets to replace endogenous dysfunctional platelets.

Acquired von Willebrand Disease

Acquired von Willebrand disease is a rare bleeding disorder that has been found in patients with myeloproliferative disorders, lymphoproliferative diseases, monoclonal gammopathies, and collagen vascular diseases, and after certain infectious processes.[52] Most patients are 40 years of age or older, with no previous history of bleeding. Bleeding presents with an insidious onset and manifests as mucocutaneous or posttraumatic hemorrhage.

Pathologically, this disorder is caused by production of an antibody that specifically interacts with vWF. Acquired von Willebrand disease is caused by a diverse group of disorders, and the associated antibodies are a heterogeneous group that interact differently with the vWF protein from patient to patient. Because these antibodies are so varied, the laboratory findings seen in acquired von Willebrand disease are also variable from patient to patient but may include a prolonged bleeding time, decreased plasma levels of factor VIII coagulant activity, vWF:Ag, and vWF activity, and abnormalities in vWF multimeric patterns. Platelet vWF is generally normal. The typical rise in factor VIII coagulant activity and vWF activity after infusion of cryoprecipitate seen in congenital von Willebrand disease is not seen in the acquired form because of neutralization of these activities by antibody.

Spontaneous remission or remission after therapy for the underlying disease is typical of this disorder. Therapeutic use of DDAVP has been observed to correct the bleeding time and increase the level of vWF. A response to the use of corticosteroid therapy has been documented. Plasmapheresis to remove antibody has been reported to be effective in a few patients who are bleeding and do not respond to other measures.

Cardiopulmonary Bypass

In the United States, more than 200,000 patients per year undergo cardiopulmonary bypass surgery. Alterations in hemostasis and life-threatening hemorrhage have been documented. Various hemostatic abnormalities are implicated in the development of the hemorrhagic manifestations of cardiopulmonary bypass surgery. These abnormalities include decreases in platelet number and function, factor deficiencies resulting from consumption and hemodilution, increased fibrinolytic activity, DIC, and inadequate or excess neutralization of heparin with protamine.[53] Postbypass diffuse microvascular bleeding occurs with greater frequency in patients undergoing repeat surgery or complicated cardiac procedures as compared with patients undergoing surgery for the first time. During cardiopulmonary bypass, a prolonged bleeding time can be seen even though the platelet count is only mildly low, in the range of 100×10^9/L. Platelet activation and platelet dysfunction account for the majority of bleeding complications seen during this procedure.[54] Proposed mechanisms include platelet activation with α granule release during exposure to the extracorporeal unit, and plasmin degradation of platelet membrane receptors.

Platelet concentrates are administered to stop bleeding. Fresh frozen plasma and cryoprecipitate should be given only to treat bleeding associated with coagulation factor deficiencies. DDAVP is often given prophylactically for high-risk patients or to stop bleeding after it occurs. Aprotinin is also used to decrease postoperative bleeding, particularly in those patients undergoing repeat or complicated procedures. It is thought that aprotinin maintains platelet function by inhibiting plasmin degradation of platelet membrane receptors.

Acquired Storage Pool Deficiencies

Acquired storage pool deficiencies have been reported in patients with SLE, ITP, TTP, DIC, HUS, MPDs, hairy-cell leukemia, acute nonlymphocytic leukemia, chronic lymphocytic leukemia, and in cardiopulmonary bypass. The acquired platelet defect in each disorder may be variable and can be caused by either production of dysfunctional platelets (i.e., MPDs) or depletion of storage pool constituents resulting from injury or activation (DIC).

Drug Therapy

A large variety of pharmacologic drugs may affect platelet function. Some drugs may induce thrombocytopenia. Other drugs alter platelet responses. Drug-induced alterations of hemostasis that cause activation of platelet function clinically manifest as thrombosis whereas drugs that inhibit platelet function clinically manifest as hemorrhage. Individual susceptibility to the effects of these drugs varies greatly. Most often, the acquired drug-induced hemostatic abnormalities observed are transitory and disappear when the drug is discontinued. However, other effects, such as those seen in heparin-induced thrombocytopenia and thrombosis, may be irreversible or disappear more slowly.

Drugs that inhibit platelet function do so by a variety of mechanisms that include altering prostaglandin synthesis, phosphodiesterase activity, platelet membrane or membrane receptors, and cyclic adenosine monophosphate (cAMP) levels. However, the mechanism of platelet inhibition for many drugs is still uncertain.

Aspirin has been well documented to inhibit platelet aggregation and platelet secretion in response to ADP, epinephrine, and low concentrations of collagen. Prolonged bleeding times may be associated with the use of aspirin. The effect of aspirin on the bleeding time is generally dose-dependent, but extremely prolonged bleeding times at lower dosages have been reported in susceptible individuals (syndrome of intermediate platelet dysfunction). Aspirin inhibits prostaglandin synthesis by irreversible acetylation and inactivation of cyclo-oxygenase (COX-1), thereby inhibiting endoperoxide and thromboxane A_2 synthesis, which are two important mediators of platelet release. The inhibitory effect of aspirin on thromboxane A_2 synthesis remains for the life span of the platelet. Aspirin also inhibits endothelial cell synthesis of prostacyclin; however, inhibitory action is predominantly against platelet cyclo-oxygenase. Low-dose aspirin treatment takes advantage of this differential effect on vascular and platelet cyclo-oxygenase. Patients with hemophilia, von Willebrand disease, or major underlying hemostatic defects may develop significant or spontaneous bleeding after aspirin ingestion and should avoid aspirin or aspirin-containing compounds. Salsalate and choline magnesium trisalicylate do not contain an acetyl group and do not inhibit cyclo-oxygenase. These drugs are preferable in patients with underlying hemostatic disorders.

Certain other nonsteroidal anti-inflammatory agents (NSAIDs), such as indomethacin, ibuprofen, phenylbutazone, and naproxen, can induce significant platelet dysfunction by inhibiting prostaglandin synthesis. These drugs inhibit cyclo-oxygenase, but the effect is reversible. Newer NSAIDs, such as COX-2 inhibitors, do not affect platelet function but have been reported to cause gastrointestinal bleeding. The cause for the bleeding remains uncertain.

Sulfinpyrazone is a competitive inhibitor of platelet cyclo-oxygenase. Bleeding times are not prolonged, and platelet aggregation is generally normal. Its complete mechanism of action is not well understood as an antiplatelet agent.

Other drugs suppress platelet function by inhibiting cAMP production. cAMP plays a major role in mediating platelet activity. Platelet response is inhibited when intracellular levels of cAMP are raised. Drugs such as dipyridamole inhibit phosphodiesterase, an enzyme capable of inactivating cAMP, resulting in increased cAMP levels in platelets. Dipyridamole has a mild effect on platelet function by itself and does not prolong the bleeding time; however, when administered with aspirin, it exerts a greater antiplatelet effect.

Ticlopidine is utilized in patients undergoing cardiac catheterization and coronary stent placement and in patients with transient ischemic attacks or completed strokes to inhibit platelet function. Ticlopidine's mechanism of action is inhibition of ADP-induced platelet-fibrinogen binding. The effect of ticlopidine is irreversible and lasts the life of the affected platelet. Ticlopidine is occasionally used in conjunction with aspirin therapy to induce two separate mechanisms of platelet inhibition. When drugs such as these with differing mechanisms are utilized together, the hemorrhagic complications may increase. Clopigridol has a similar mechanism of action.

Antimicrobial drugs such as penicillin, ampicillin, and carbenicillin may inhibit platelet function through interference with membrane or membrane receptors. When administered in high doses, bleeding may occur. Cephalosporin antibiotics may also inhibit platelet function. These drugs affect platelet aggregation, platelet secretion, and platelet adhesion.

Dextran is also known to prolong the bleeding time. Platelet function tests such as aggregation, PF3 availability, and platelet retention have all been shown to be abnormal with the use of dextran. It is believed that dextran interferes with the platelet surface membrane to cause platelet dysfunction.

Several GPIIb/IIIa receptor antagonists have been developed and approved for intravenous human use in acute coronary syndromes or for percutaneous coronary interventions, such as angioplasty or stent placement, to prevent reocclusion. Abciximab (Reopro) is a mouse-human chimeric Fab fragment that exhibits irreversible, noncompetitive binding to platelets. Recovery of platelet function is noted by 48 hours after administration, but platelet-bound antibody is still detectable for 14 days after administration. Eptifibatide (Integrelin) is a cyclic heptapeptide that contains a lysine-glycine–aspartic acid (KGD) sequence similar to that found on adhesive proteins such as fibrinogen or vWF. This peptide has reversible, competitive binding to platelets, with recovery of platelet function 2 to 4 hours after administration. Tirofiban (Aggrastat) is a nonpeptide GPIIb/IIIa inhibitor that also exhibits reversible, competitive binding to platelets with a similar recovery of platelet function in 2 to 4 hours.

Bleeding is a potential complication of all of these drug treatments and is usually noted when excessive doses of heparin are used concomitantly with these drugs. Heparin dosing based on body weight has reduced the risk of serious and fatal bleeding complications. Thrombocytopenia is a less frequent complication but may be severe (less than 10 $\times$ 10^9/L). Onset of thrombocytopenia is rapid, usually within 12 to 24 hours of treatment, and increases the hemorrhagic risk in patients treated with these agents. Thrombocytopenia caused by these agents is often mistaken for heparin-induced thrombocytopenia because patients typically are given both agents concomitantly. The precipitous onset of thrombocytopenia after initiation of therapy may be helpful in differentiating GPIIb/IIIa inhibitor-induced thrombocytopenia from heparin-induced thrombocytopenia. Thrombocytopenia appears to occur more frequently with abciximab than with eptifibatide or tirofiban. The mechanism responsible for thrombocytopenia is not known but may be a result of accelerated immune clearance of platelets from the circulation.

Numerous other conditions have been associated with an acquired platelet defect. These include paroxysmal nocturnal hemoglobinuria, infectious mononucleosis, severe B_{12} deficiency, diabetes, hyperbetalipoproteinemia, congenital heart defects, and hypothyroidism. The pathogenesis in these various disorders in uncertain.

► VASCULAR DISORDERS

Purpura can be caused by abnormalities of skin, connective tissue, or blood vessels, or may be a result of inflammatory processes that are not associated with quantitative or qualitative platelet disorders. These may be congenital or acquired vascular disorders and are listed in Table 24–8.

Primary Purpura

Primary purpura comprises disorders that result in bruising but are not associated with any specific disease. Simple purpura or "devil pinches" occur as a result of skin fragility. The bruising is usually mild and occurs with minimal trauma. Often, there may be a family history of easy bruising. Mechanical purpura occurs as a result of sudden increases in capillary pressure and usually manifests as petechiae. Sneezing, coughing, Valsalva maneuvers, or seizures may cause this problem. Senile purpura, which is seen in older individuals, is similar to that occurring in individuals who are receiving corticosteroid therapy. In these disorders, the purpuric lesions usually occur on the hands and arms and result from loss of subcutaneous tissue and support of blood vessels in affected skin. Factitious purpura is caused by self-induced trauma and usually is found on areas of the body that are easily accessible. The purpura may be caused by pinching, suction applied to the skin, or a blow to the skin. Factitious bleeding may also be produced to mimic oral, vaginal, or urinary tract hemorrhage by placing blood in various areas of the body or in bodily fluids. Some individuals ingest oral warfarin or inject heparin to induce a coagulopathy to pro-

► **Table 24-8**
VASCULAR PURPURAS

Primary Purpura

Simple purpura

Mechanical purpura

Senile purpura

Factitious purpura

Schamberg's purpura

Secondary Purpura

Infectious purpura

   Waterhouse-Friderichsen syndrome

   Purpura fulminans

   Septic emboli

Allergic purpura

   Schönlein-Henoch purpura

   Drug sensitivity

Metabolic purpura

   Scurvy

   Cushing's syndrome

   Diabetes mellitus

   Protein C deficiency

Psychogenic purpura

   Gardner-Diamond syndrome

   DNA hypersensitivity

Purpura secondary to dysproteinemia

   Waldenström's purpura

   Cryoglobulinemia

   Amyloidosis

   Hyperviscosity syndrome

Vascular and connective tissue disorders

   Hereditary hemorrhagic telangiectasia

   Angiodysplasia

   Giant hemangiomas (Kasabach-Merritt syndrome)

   Ehlers-Danlos syndrome

   Marfan syndrome

   Pseudoxanthoma elasticum

   Osteogenesis imperfecta

voke bleeding. This is most commonly seen in health-care professionals who have access to anticoagulants. Factitious purpura is usually an indication of a severe psychiatric disturbance. Various skin disorders such as Schamberg's purpura (progressive pigmentary dermatosis) and related conditions result in purpuric lesions. These lesions are usually seen bilaterally on both lower legs and appear as a result of a non-inflammatory disorder of capillaries of the skin. If the disorder is long-standing, hemosiderin pigmentation is noted in previously involved areas.

Secondary Purpura

Secondary purpura results from another disease process and is just one of the manifestations of the disease process. These disorders are acquired and have no associated family history.

Infectious Purpura

Purpura may result from various infectious diseases. Bacterial infections such as meningococcemia, streptococcal or staphylococcal bacteremia, or diphtheria; rickettsial infection with Rocky Mountain spotted fever; and parasitic infection by malaria may cause purpura. The purpura may be caused by direct damage to blood vessels by the particular organism (vasculitis) or result from the effects of endotoxin on blood vessels. Septic emboli to the skin (ecthyma gangrenosum) may be seen in endocarditis. In the Waterhouse-Friderichsen syndrome, meningococcemia results in adrenal hemorrhage with adrenal insufficiency and shock. Purpura fulminans is an acute purpuric syndrome that usually occurs during septic shock, with development of ischemia followed by thrombosis and necrosis of affected areas, often the fingers and toes.[55] Meningococcemia, streptococcal infections, and viral infections may provoke this life-threatening problem.[56] If the individual survives, necrosis of the fingers and toes may require amputation. DIC is often seen with Waterhouse-Friderichsen syndrome or purpura fulminans.

Allergic Purpura

Allergic purpura is the result of an allergic vasculitis. Schönlein-Henoch purpura is a vasculitis involving the skin, gastrointestinal tract, kidneys, heart, and central nervous system.[57] This syndrome is considered an immune complex disease, and is characterized by involvement of capillaries with a diffuse perivascular infiltration by neutrophils, lymphocytes, and macrophages. Some patients have IgA deposition in the kidney and elevated serum IgA levels. This syndrome may be related to IgA nephropathy whereby similar IgA deposition in the kidney is noted. In Schönlein-Henoch purpura, the onset is abrupt, with a macular rash (usually symmetric) involving the lower extremities that becomes purpuric. In some individuals, the joint and gastrointestinal symptoms predominate and the cutaneous expression is minimal. This disorder is seen most commonly in children. Renal dysfunction is common and typically reversible in children. Overt renal failure is most common in affected adults. Schönlein-Henoch purpura may last several weeks and then recur (Fig. 24–10 and Color Plate 262).

Drug hypersensitivity may also result in allergic purpura. This must be differentiated from drug-induced thrombocytopenias that result in purpura. The mechanism by which these drugs cause purpura is not understood. Aspirin, at-

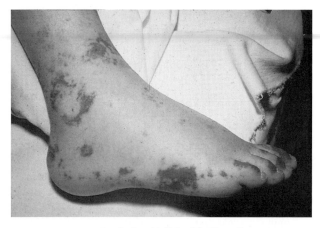

> FIGURE 24–10 Anaphylactoid (Schönlein-Henoch) purpura. Purpuric lesions of the foot.

ropine, iodides, penicillin, quinine, and sulfonamides have been described to cause allergic hypersensitivity purpura.

Metabolic Purpura

Metabolic purpura are caused by hormonal or biochemical abnormalities. Scurvy is caused by a deficiency of vitamin C. This was a common problem several centuries ago in sailors who did not have access to vitamin C on long voyages. In modern times, this disorder is found in refugees from war or famine, adults with inadequate or fad diets, and in alcoholics. Deficiency of vitamin C appears to cause a defect in the synthesis of collagen in the walls of small blood vessels. Vitamin C is a cofactor for hydroxylation of proline and lysine in the production of collagen and keratin. A platelet function defect may also be present, with a decrease in the platelet adhesion reaction. Scurvy may present with leg swelling, pain, or discoloration. Subperiosteal bone bleeding is characteristic of scurvy and may be noted radiologically. Gingival bleeding and hemarthrosis may also be present. Perifollicular hemorrhages with hyperkeratosis of the hair follicles and "corkscrew" hairs are characteristic of this problem. Vitamin C administration orally cures the disorder.

Cushing's syndrome caused by corticosteroid excess results in purpura (Fig. 24–11 and Color Plate 263). The pathogenesis is identical to that seen with steroid or senile purpura, including atrophy of the subcutaneous tissue and increased

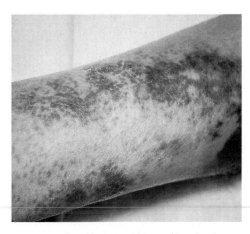

> FIGURE 24–11 Steroid purpura (skin manifestations).

blood vessel fragility. Other cutaneous stigmata of Cushing's syndrome include a "moon" face, pigmented abdominal striae, a "buffalo hump" on the lower neck and upper back, with wasting of the extremities and an obese abdomen.

Diabetes mellitus may be associated with retinal hemorrhages. This is a result of vascular proliferation caused by retinal hypoxia. These fragile vessels may leak fluid or hemorrhage because of their increased permeability. Laser photocoagulation and optimal control of hyperglycemia are treatments used for this problem. No endogenous platelet or coagulation disorder is present in this situation.

Protein C deficiency may occur on a congenital or acquired basis and is a risk factor for thrombosis. An unusual syndrome that resembles purpura fulminans can be present in neonates, resulting from inherited homozygous protein C deficiency.[58] This disorder presents hours after birth and is usually lethal. Protein C deficiency results from oral anticoagulant therapy, because protein C is a vitamin K–dependent protein. Rapid depletion of protein C by warfarin appears to cause a unique thrombotic disorder termed the *warfarin skin necrosis syndrome*. This unusual disorder presents as painful, erythematous areas on the buttocks, breasts, legs, or penis, which rapidly turn to hemorrhagic bullae and then become necrotic. Cessation of warfarin and administration of plasma that contains protein C are appropriate treatments. Vitamin K administration may be helpful but will usually not reverse the disorder soon enough to prevent necrosis.

Psychogenic Purpura

Psychogenic purpura comprises rare disorders that usually occur in individuals with emotional disorders. Patients with Gardner-Diamond syndrome present with spontaneous painful ecchymoses. Pain that may be described as stinging or burning occurs where the purpura subsequently develop. The lesions begin as erythema, become raised, and then turn ecchymotic. These lesions primarily occur on the extremities and appear episodically. In affected individuals, lesions can be reproduced by intradermal injection of blood, hemoglobin, or red cell stroma.[59] The disorder primarily affects middle-aged women. Often there is a history of physical abuse; there may be a history of extensive surgery or trauma. This disorder appears to be an entity different from factitious purpura.

DNA hypersensitivity syndrome is similar to Gardner-Diamond syndrome, involving development of painful purpura on the extremities. Injection of white blood cells or DNA from the individual can reproduce the lesions. Unlike Gardner-Diamond syndrome, in which most treatments other than psychiatric help are not beneficial, chloroquine often stops the purpura caused by DNA hypersensitivity.

Purpura Secondary to Dysproteinemia

Purpura caused by dysproteinemias encompasses several disorders. Benign hypergammaglobulinemic purpura (Waldenström's purpura) is a disorder of women that presents with recurrent purpura on the lower extremities and resultant hemosiderin staining of the skin similar to Schamberg's purpura.[60] Unlike Schamberg's purpura, polyclonal hypergammaglobulinemia and an elevated erythrocyte sedimentation rate are noted. Mild anemia may be present. Purpura are made worse by leg dependency or by wearing constrictive garments and improved with leg elevation and support stockings (Fig. 24–12 and Color Plate 264). Skin biopsy reveals necrotizing vasculitis. Patients may develop Sjögren's syndrome or ker-

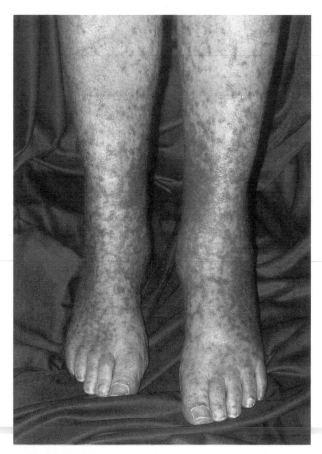

➤ **FIGURE 24–12**   Typical lower extremity vascular lesions seen in patients with paraproteinemia.

atoconjunctivitis sicca, suggesting this may be a vasculitis that results from a connective tissue disorder.

Cryoglobulinemia is caused by from production of cryoprecipitable serum proteins or protein complexes. This may result from primary plasma cell dyscrasias or from chronic viral infections such as hepatitis C. Exposure to cold may cause purpura on the skin of the extremities or face. The purpura may blister or ulcerate. The proposed pathogenesis for the purpura in the cryoglobulinemic disorders is vascular damage owing to precipitation of cryoglobulins.

Amyloidosis may cause purpura as a result of several mechanisms. Easy bruising is common in amyloidosis, with "pinch" purpura and ecchymosis from skin pressure during shaving. Postproctoscopic purpura occur when a patient with amyloidosis is placed in a head-down position for proctoscopic examination, with characteristic purpura around the eyelids (Fig. 24–13 and Color Plate 265). Bleeding is caused by deposition of amyloid protein around small blood vessels, resulting in vessel fragility. In addition, amyloid fibrils may bind factor X, and platelet function may be altered to enhance the bleeding tendency. Treatment for bleeding caused by amyloidosis involves treatment of the underlying disease with chemotherapy. Splenectomy has also been used. Administration of plasma and platelet transfusions are not usually effective.

Hyperviscosity syndrome results from hypergammaglobulinemia owing to an increase in plasma viscosity. Blood flow is restricted because of hyperviscosity involving development of ischemia and vascular injury, with resultant

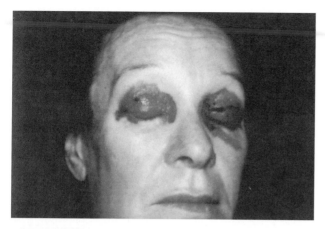

➤ FIGURE 24–13   Amyloid purpura. Note characteristic periorbital distribution.

hemorrhage. Purpura, gingival hemorrhages, and retinal hemorrhages are common. Central nervous system bleeding may be lethal. This disorder is usually seen in IgM syndromes such as Waldenström's macroglobulinemia, and IgA or IgG3 multiple myeloma. It is rarely seen in multiple myeloma with other IgG subtypes. Treatment is with plasmapheresis to remove excessive IgM or IgG, and chemotherapeutic treatment of the underlying plasma cell dyscrasia to reduce paraprotein production.

Vascular and Connective Tissue Disorders

These disorders result from abnormal blood vessel structure, with purpura and bleeding caused by increased permeability to blood. Most of these disorders are congenital.

Hereditary Hemorrhagic Telangiectasia

Hereditary hemorrhagic telangiectasia (Osler-Weber-Rendu syndrome) is caused by the development of telangiectases of mucous membranes and skin (Fig. 24–14 and Color Plate 266). This is an autosomal-dominant disorder that usually becomes obvious in adolescence or early adulthood. Lesions

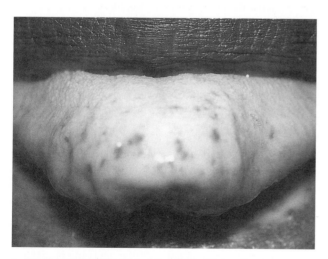

➤ FIGURE 24–14   The tongue of a patient with hereditary hemorrhagic telangiectasia. Note the multiple vascular telangiectases, which can occur in the nares, the oral mucous membranes, and throughout the gastrointestinal tract. Recurrent bleeding requiring transfusions is a common manifestation.

develop on the tongue, lips, palate, face, and hands. Similar lesions are present in nasal mucosa and throughout the gastrointestinal tract. The lesions blanch when pressure is applied, in contrast to petechiae, because these are vascular structures. Chronic epistaxis and gastrointestinal bleeding occur and usually worsen as the patient grows older. Iron-deficiency anemia is usual. The bleeding is difficult to control but may be treated with nasal packing, cauterization, or laser photocoagulation. Administration of parenteral iron or red blood cell transfusions is usually necessary. Estrogens and danazol have been reported to help in some patients.[61]

Angiodysplasia

Angiodysplasia is a disorder involving blood vessels of the gastrointestinal tract. The cutaneous lesions of hereditary hemorrhagic telangiectasia are not present. Vascular permeability leads to chronic gastrointestinal bleeding, anemia, and iron deficiency. This disorder has been associated with von Willebrand disease and may be caused by the effect of vWF on vascular structures. An acquired form of angiodysplasia has been reported in patients with aortic stenosis. In these patients, aortic valve surgery has improved the bleeding. Hemicolectomy has been used to treat the gastrointestinal bleeding.

Giant Hemangiomas (Kasabach-Merritt Syndrome)

Giant hemangiomas may occur congenitally soon after birth and affect the skin, liver, and spleen. Unless these lesions spontaneously regress, DIC may develop. These hemangiomas have numerous thin-walled blood vessels that produce thromboplastic substances to incite DIC. Treatment is usually surgical removal or radiation, if surgery is not possible. Interferon has been used in a single case report.

➤ CONGENITAL CONNECTIVE TISSUE DISORDERS

Several rare congenital disorders of connective tissue proteins have been described as producing purpura. Ehlers-Danlos syndrome is an autosomal-dominant disorder characterized by hyperelastic skin. Numerous subtypes of the disorder related to abnormal collagen synthesis have been described.[62] Bleeding is caused by abnormalities of the blood vessels or the supporting connective tissues. Some patients also have skeletal abnormalities. These patients may be mistaken for individuals with hemophilia because of the bleeding tendency and joint abnormalities. However, coagulation studies are normal in these individuals. Surgery and trauma should be avoided because of bleeding and poor wound healing.

Marfan syndrome is an autosomal-dominant disorder that results in bleeding and abnormalities of connective tissues. Individuals with this disorder are usually tall and have long limbs. Dislocation of the lens, aortic valvular regurgitation, and aortic dissection may occur. Easy bruising and bleeding at surgery are common. Studies of hemostasis are normal.

Pseudoxanthoma elasticum is an autosomal-recessive disorder affecting elastic fibers of the skin and arteries. Several types of the disorder have been described. Characteristic hyaline (angioid) streaks are noted in the retina. Easy bruising and gastrointestinal bleeding are common. Renal, uterine, or ocular hemorrhage may occur. Atherosclerosis as a result of calcification of medium-sized and large blood vessels usually occurs, and intermittent claudication is frequent. Tests of hemostasis are normal.

Osteogenesis imperfecta is another rare autosomal-dominant disorder that may result in easy bruising, epistaxis, hemoptysis, and, infrequently, intracranial bleeding. Affected individuals have blue-colored sclera.

➤ CASE STUDY 1

A 23-year-old African-American woman in the 14th week of her first pregnancy presents to the hospital with mild confusion, headaches, nausea, easy bruising, and petechiae. Physical examination reveals a temperature of 37.7°C, blood pressure of 150/100 mm Hg, pulse of 80 beats per minute, and respirations of 14 per minute. Mild confusion and decrease in light touch sensation of the right arm are noted. Scattered petechiae cover the inner thighs, and ecchymoses on the forearms are present. No other bleeding is observed. The uterus is enlarged, and a fetal heartbeat is detected. The spleen tip is not palpable.

Admission laboratory findings show a hematocrit of 21%, white blood count of 10×10^9/L, platelet count of 18.0×10^9/L, and reticulocyte count of 7%. PT, APTT, and fibrinogen are normal. FDP is positive, with a titer of 32, and D-dimer is positive at 0.5 to 1.0 μg/mL. The Direct Antiglobulin Test (DAT) is negative. The peripheral blood smear shows moderate poikilocytosis with schistocytes, nucleated red blood cells, and polychromasia. Serum creatinine is 2.5 mg/dL, blood urea nitrogen is 50 mg/dL, calcium is 7.6 mg/dL, and albumin is 2.4 mg/dL. Urinalysis is remarkable with 3+ proteinuria and numerous red blood cells. Bone marrow aspiration and biopsy reveal erythroid and megakaryocytic hyperplasia. Hyaline thrombi are seen in blood vessels of the biopsy. Electrocardiogram and chest radiograph are normal.

Questions

1. What is the most likely diagnosis? How should the patient be treated?
2. What other conditions should also be considered in the diagnosis? What additional testing could be performed to confirm or reject these diagnoses?

➤ CASE STUDY 2

An obese 36-year-old white female emergency medical technician complains of easy bruising of the arms and legs for several months. This bruising is episodic and seems unrelated to trauma during work. She reports no stinging or burning sensations prior to the appearance of bruises. No bleeding from the nose, mouth, or other mucous membranes is noted. No bleeding into joints or muscles has occurred. Family history is negative for bleeding or bruising. Physical examination reveals normal skin turgor with a few discrete fresh ecchymoses on the thighs and forearms but no other obvious bleeding. Platelet count is 380×10^9/L; bleeding time is 5 minutes, 30 seconds; APTT, PT, and fibrinogen studies are normal.

Questions

1. What additional information will be helpful in defining a cause for this bruising?
2. What conditions should be considered in the differential diagnosis? Why?
3. What additional testing can be performed to confirm a diagnosis?

➤ CASE STUDY 3

A 67-year-old white man with a history of cigarette smoking developed sudden onset of tingling and weakness of the left arm that lasted 10 minutes before resolving, consistent with a transient ischemic attack. He was examined soon afterward in the hospital emergency department and no residual neurologic abnormalities were found. The spleen was not palpable and no bleeding or bruising were present. Laboratory findings included a hematocrit of 43%, white blood count of 11.2×10^9/L, with a normal white blood cell differential, and platelet count of 760×10^9/L. Bone marrow aspirate and biopsy revealed megakaryocytic hyperplasia with clustering of megakaryocytes but no granulocytic or erythrocytic hyperplasia, no fibrosis, and normal storage iron. Bone marrow culture exhibited growth in the absence of added growth factors, consistent with a diagnosis of a myeloproliferative disorder. Smoking cessation and aspirin were advised to prevent recurrent thrombotic episodes. The patient refused hydroxyurea treatment.

Questions

1. What conditions are considered in the differential diagnosis of thrombocytosis in this patient?
2. Which characteristics present in this case differentiate myeloproliferative disorders from reactive causes of thrombocytosis?

➤ CASE STUDY 4

A 17-year-old Jewish woman complains of recurrent episodes of bleeding from the nose and mouth since birth and heavy menstrual bleeding since menarche. She has never had bleeding into joints or muscles. Her brother also has a history of nasal bleeding. Physical examination does not reveal any telangiectases of the nose or mouth. Skin and joints appear normal. Gynecologic examination is normal. Platelet count is 250×10^9/L. Bleeding time is prolonged at 18 minutes. Appearance of platelets on the peripheral blood smear is normal.

Questions
1. What conditions should be considered in the differential diagnosis for this bleeding? Why?
2. What additional testing can be performed to evaluate this bleeding tendency?
3. How would each of the possible conditions in the differential diagnosis be treated to minimize further bleeding episodes?

QUESTIONS

1. A patient presents with a platelet count of $212 \times 10^9/L$ and a bleeding time of 12 minutes. These results most probably suggest:
   a. Decreased platelet production
   b. Defective platelet function
   c. Increased platelet production
   d. Increased platelet destruction

2. Which of the following clinical manifestations is most characteristic of a platelet disorder:
   a. Mucosal bleeding
   b. Hemarthrosis
   c. Retroperitoneal hemorrhage
   d. Deep muscle hematomas

3. Which of the following is not characteristic of Bernard-Soulier syndrome?
   a. Prolonged bleeding time
   b. Absent platelet aggregation in response to bovine vWF or human vWF plus ristocetin
   c. Abnormal platelet aggregation in response to ADP, collagen, and epinephrine
   d. Abnormality in platelet membrane GPIb/IX

4. Which of the following is not characteristic of Glanzmann's thrombasthenia?
   a. Prolonged bleeding time
   b. Giant platelets with thrombocytopenia
   c. Absent platelet aggregation in response to ADP, thrombin, collagen, and epinephrine
   d. Normal platelet aggregation to ristocetin and bovine vWF

5. Which of the following statements is not true regarding acute idiopathic thrombocytopenia (ITP)?
   a. Thrombocytopenia occurs following a viral infection.
   b. Spontaneous remissions are common.
   c. It is found primarily in young children.
   d. Platelet counts are generally higher than in chronic ITP.

6. Thrombocytopenia, fever, renal disease, microangiopathic hemolytic anemia, and neurologic complications are hallmark characteristics of:
   a. Hemolytic uremic syndrome (HUS)
   b. Disseminated intravascular coagulation (DIC)
   c. Thrombotic thrombocytopenic purpura (TTP)
   d. Idiopathic thrombocytopenic purpura (ITP)

7. What disorders are classically associated with thrombocytosis?
   a. Myeloproliferative syndromes
   b. Autoimmune disorders
   c. Immunodeficiency syndrome (HIV)
   d. Renal disease

8. Which of the following is not an inherited vascular defect?
   a. Ehlers-Danlos syndrome
   b. Marfan syndrome
   c. Amyloidosis
   d. Giant hemangiomas

9. Which condition is classified as nonimmunologic thrombocytopenia?
   a. DIC
   b. ITP
   c. Storage pool defects
   d. Bernard-Soulier syndrome

10. Which condition is classified as immunologic thrombocytopenia?
    a. DIC
    b. ITP
    c. Storage pool defects
    d. Bernard-Soulier syndrome

SUMMARY CHART

➤ Quantitative and qualitative platelet disorders and vascular disorders are abnormalities of primary hemostasis that result in bleeding and purpura.
➤ Thrombocytopenia is the most common primary hemostatic disorder.
➤ The mechanisms responsible for thrombocytopenia include deficient marrow production of platelets, sequestration of platelets in the spleen or hemangiomas, or accelerated loss or destruction of platelets from the circulation.
➤ Thrombotic thrombocytopenic purpura (TTP) is a microangiopathic process that leads to thrombocytopenia with thrombosis and bleeding.
➤ Qualitative platelet disorders may be caused by abnormalities of the platelet surface glycoproteins (Bernard-Soulier syndrome and Glanzmann's thrombasthenia), deficiencies of platelet granules (storage pool defects), or abnormalities of the platelet release mechanism (release defects).
➤ von Willebrand disease is one of the most common congenital defects of primary hemostasis.
➤ von Willebrand factor results in a lack of binding of platelets at the site of injury, with bleeding characteristic of platelet defects.
➤ Vascular purpura is caused by abnormalities of blood vessels without associated platelet or plasma protein defects.

References

1. Pegels, J, et al: Pseudothrombocytopenia: An immunologic study on platelet antibodies dependent on ethylene diamine tetra-acetate. Blood 59:157, 1982.
2. Watkins, S, and Shulman, N: Platelet cold agglutinins. Blood 36:153, 1970.

3. Czapek, E, et al: Intermediate syndrome of platelet dysfunction. Blood 52:103, 1978.
4. Rodgers, RPC, and Levine, J: A critical appraisal of the bleeding time. Semin Thromb Hemast 16:1, 1990.
5. Gewirtz, A, et al: The preoperative bleeding time test: Assessing its clinical usefulness. Cleve Clin J Med 62:379, 1995.
6. George, J, et al: Chronic idiopathic thrombocytopenic purpura. N Engl J Med 331:1207, 1994.
7. Schmitz, E, et al: Changes in splenic microcirculatory pathways in chronic idiopathic thrombocytopenic purpura. Blood 78:1485, 1991.
8. Staso, R, et al: Long term observation of 208 adults with chronic idiopathic thrombocytopenic purpura. Am J Med 98:436, 1995.
9. George, J, et al: Idiopathic thrombocytopenic purpura: A practice guideline developed by explicit methods for the American Society of Hematology. Blood 89:1464, 1997.
10. McMillan, R: Therapy for adults with refractory chronic immune thrombocytopenic purpura. Ann Intern Med 126:307, 1997.
11. Picozzi, V, et al: Fate of therapy failures in adult idiopathic thrombocytopenic purpura. N Engl J Med 69:690, 1980.
12. Carr, JM, et al: Efficacy of platelet transfusions in immune thrombocytopenia. Am J Med 80:1051, 1986.
13. Kickler, T, et al: Studies on the pathophysiology of posttransfusion purpura. Blood 68:347, 1986.
14. Christie, D, et al: Posttransfusion purpura due to an alloantibody reactive with glycoprotein Ia/IIa (anti-HPA-5b). Blood 77:2785, 1991.
15. Bussell, J, et al: Fetal alloimmune thrombocytopenia. N Engl J Med 337:22, 1997.
16. Rosenthal, N: The blood picture in purpura. J Lab Clin Med 13:303, 1928.
17. Kaufman, D, et al: Acute thrombocytopenic purpura in relation to the use of drugs. Blood 82:2714, 1993.
18. Warkentin, T: Clinical presentation of heparin-induced thrombocytopenia. Semin Hematol 35(4 Suppl 5):9, 1998.
19. Suh, J, et al: Antibodies from patients with heparin-induced thrombocytopenia/thrombosis recognize different epitopes on heparin: Platelet factor 4. Blood 91:916, 1998.
20. Amiral, J: Antigens involved in heparin-induced thrombocytopenia. Semin Hematol 36(1 Suppl 1):7, 1999.
21. Walenga J, et al: Laboratory tests for heparin-induced thrombocytopenia: A multicenter study. Semin Hematol 36(1 Suppl 1):22, 1999.
22. Warkentin, T, et al: The pathogenesis of venous limb gangrene associated with heparin-induced thrombocytopenia. Ann Intern Med 127:804, 1997.
23. Warkentin, T: Limitations of conventional treatment options for heparin-induced thrombocytopenia. Semin Hematol 35(4 Suppl 5):17, 1998.
24. Ortel, T, and Chong, B: New treatment options for heparin-induced thrombocytopenia. Semin Hematol 35(4 suppl 5):26, 1998.
25. Kelton, J, et al: Elevated platelet-associated IgG in the thrombocytopenia of septicemia. N Engl J Med 300:760, 1979.
26. Francois, B, et al: Thrombocytopenia in the sepsis syndrome: Role of hemophagocytosis and macrophage colony-stimulating factor. Am J Med 103:114, 1997.
27. George, J, et al: Thrombotic thrombocytopenic purpura—hemolytic uremic syndrome: Diagnosis and management. J Clin Apheresis 13:120, 1998.
28. Furlan, M, et al: von Willebrand factor-cleaving protease in thrombotic thrombocytopenic purpura and the hemolytic-uremic syndrome. N Engl J Med 339:1578, 1998.
29. Tsai, H, and Lian, E: Antibodies to von Willebrand factor-cleaving protease in acute thrombotic thrombocytopenic purpura. N Engl J Med 339:1585, 1998.
30. Bukowski, R: Thrombotic thrombocytopenic purpura: A review. Prog Hemost Thromb 6: 287, 1982.
31. Thrompson, C, et al: Thrombotic microangiopathies in the 1980s: Clinical features, response to treatment, and the impact of the human immunodeficiency virus epidemic. Blood 80:1890, 1992.
32. Torok, TR, et al: Increasing mortality from thrombotic thrombocytopenic purpura in the United States—Analysis of national mortality data, 1968–1991. Am J Hematol 50:84, 1995.
33. Gillis, S: The thrombocytopenic purpuras: Recognition and management. Drugs 51:942, 1996.
34. Melnyk, A., et al: Adult hemolytic-uremic syndrome: A review of 37 cases. Arch Intern Med 155:2077, 1995.
35. McCrae, K, et al: Pregnancy-associated thrombocytopenia: Pathogenesis and management. Blood 80:2697, 1992.
36. Loos, W: HELLP syndrome: Clinical aspects and coagulation abnormalities. Biomed Progress 7:26, 1994.
37. George, J, et al: Glanzmann's thrombasthenia: The spectrum of clinical disease. Blood 75:1383, 1990.
38. Fox, J: Identification of a membrane skeleton in platelets. J Cell Biol 106:1525, 1988.
39. Cuthbert, R, et al: DDAVP shortens the bleeding time in Bernard-Soulier syndrome. Thromb Res 49:649, 1988.
40. Mant, M: DDAVP in Bernard-Soulier syndrome. Thromb Res 52:77, 1988.
41. Rao, K, et al: Impaired cytoplasmic calcium mobilization in inherited platelet secretion defects. Blood 74:664, 1989.
42. Ginsberg, D, and Bowie, E: Molecular genetics of von Willebrand disease. Blood 79:2507, 1992.
43. Sadler, J: A revised classification of von Willebrand disease for the subcommittee on von Willebrand factor of the scientific and standardization committee of the International Society on Thrombosis and Haemostasis. Thromb Haemost 71:520, 1994.
44. Elodee, S, et al: The mutation Arg53 → Trp causes von Willebrand disease Normandy by abolishing binding to factor VIII: Studies with recombinant von Willebrand factor. Blood 79:563, 1992.
45. Russell, S, and Roth, G: Pseudo-von Willebrand disease: A mutation in the platelet glycoprotein Ibα gene associated with a hyperactive surface receptor. Blood 81:1787, 1993.
46. Moriki, T, et al: Expression and functional characterization of an abnormal platelet membrane glycoprotein Ibα (Met 239 → Val) reported in patients with platelet-type von Willebrand disease. Blood 90:698, 1997.
47. Triplett, D: Laboratory diagnosis of von Willebrand disease. Mayo Clin Proc 66:832, 1991.
48. Mannucci, P: Desmopressin (DDAVP) in the treatment of bleeding disorders: The first 20 years. Blood 90:2515, 1997.
49. Eberst, M, and Berkowitz L: Hemostasis in renal disease: Pathophysiology and management. Am J Med 96:168, 1994.
50. Tefferi, A: Pathogenetic mechanisms in chronic myeloproliferative disorders: Polycythemia vera, essential thrombocythemia, agnogenic myeloid metaplasia, and chronic myelogenous leukemia. Semin Hematol 36(1 Suppl 2):3, 1999.
51. Barbui, T, and Finazzi, G: Clinical parameters for determining when and when not to treat essential thrombocythemia. Semin Hematol 36(1 Suppl 2):14, 1999.
52. Tefferi, A, and Nichols, W: Acquired von Willebrand disease: Concise review of occurrence, diagnosis, pathogenesis and treatment. Am J Med 103:536, 1997.
53. Woodman, R, and Harker, L: Bleeding complications associated with cardiopulmonary bypass. Blood 76:1680, 1990.
54. Kestin, A, et al: The platelet function defect of cardiopulmonary bypass. Blood 82:107, 1993.
55. Spicer, T, and Rau, J: Purpura fulminans. Am J Med 61:566, 1976.
56. Hautekeete, M, et al: Purpura fulminans in pneumococcal sepsis. Arch Intern Med 146:497, 1986.
57. Jennette, J, and Falk, R: Small vessel vasculitis. N Engl J Med 337:1512, 1997.
58. Marciniak, E, et al: Neonatal purpura fulminans: A genetic disorder related to the absence of protein C in blood. Blood 65:15, 1985.
59. Ratnoff, O: Psychogenic purpura (autoerythrocyte sensitization): An unsolved dilemma. Am J Med 87:16, 1989.
60. Ferreiro, J, et al: Benign hypergammaglobulinemic purpura of Waldenström associated with Sjögren's syndrome. Am J Med 81:734, 1986.
61. Vase, P: Estrogen treatment of hereditary hemorrhagic telangiectasias: A double blind controlled clinical trial. Acta Med Scand 209:393, 1981.
62. Hollister, DW: Heritable disorders of connective tissue: Ehlers-Danlos syndrome. Pediatr Clin North Am 25:57, 1978.

25 Disorders of Plasma Clotting Factors

SHARON L. SCHWARTZ, MT(ASCP)SH, CLS(NCA)
CAROL C. CARUANA, H(ASCP)SH

OBJECTIVES

At the end of this chapter, the learner should be able to:

1. List various defects that impair the coagulation system.
2. Name the vitamin K–dependent factors.
3. Describe the differences between hemophilia A and von Willebrand's disease.
4. Name the factor deficiency responsible for causing hemophilia A.
5. Name the factor deficiency responsible for causing hemophilia B.
6. Name the factor deficiency responsible for causing hemophilia C.
7. Describe laboratory methods used to identify factor deficiencies.
8. Describe circulating anticoagulants and inhibitors.
9. Describe laboratory methods used to identify anticoagulants and inhibitors.
10. Discuss various etiologies and treatment modalities for various factor deficiencies.
11. Describe the genetic mutations known to affect factor II and factor V and the consequences thereof.

This chapter covers disorders of plasma clotting factors and how these disorders directly affect hemostasis. Information is provided in detail on each of the coagulation factors, their deficiencies, and disorders (Table 25–1). Additionally, discussions include information on the lupus anticoagulant and specific factor inhibitors. The recommended blood component therapy for each specific plasma clotting defect is discussed. A summary of the materials presented and several case studies that illustrate the information are presented at the end of the chapter.

The transformation of liquid blood to a gel is a very complex process. The end result is the cessation of bleeding or hemostasis. Clotting factors circulate as inactive zymogens or precursors of serine proteases, which have serine as a portion of their active enzymatic site and function to cleave peptide bonds. Chapter 23 discusses the activation of the zymogens that participate in the coagulation pathways leading to the formation of an insoluble fibrin clot.

Plasma clotting factor defects can impair hemostasis. This can occur as a result of:

1. Decreased synthesis of the factors
2. Production of abnormal molecules that interfere with the coagulation pathways
3. Loss or consumption of the coagulation factors
4. Inactivation of these factors by inhibitors or antibodies[1]

Transmission of clotting factor disorders may be inherited as sex-linked or autosomal defects. They may also be acquired as a result of vitamin K deficiency, liver disease,

> **Table 25-1**
FACTOR DEFICIENCIES

Factor Deficiency		Minimum for Hemostasis	Half-life	Laboratory	Clinical
I	Afibrinogenemia (rare) Autosomal recessive– homozygous	50–100 mg%	120 hr	No clot formation Abnormal PT, APTT, TCT; no fibrinogen	Umbilical stump bleeding, easy bruising, ecchymosis, gingival oozing hematuria, poor wound healing
	Hypofibrinogenemia (rare) Autosomal recessive– heterozygous			Abnormal PT, APTT, TCT; low fibrinogen	Mild bleeding, thrombotic episodes
	Dysfibrinogenemia Variable inheritance Uncommon variants			Fibrinogen: qualitative— abnormal; quantitative— normal	Possible hemorrhage, possible thrombosis, possible asymptomatic
II	Hypoprothrombinemia (extremely rare) Autosomal recessive	30%–40%	100 hr	Abnormal PT, APTT	Postoperative bleeding, epistaxis, menorrhagia, easy bruising
V	Parahemophilia Autosomal recessive 1/1,000,000–homozygote	10%	25 hr	Abnormal PT, APTT, BT	Epistaxis, menorrhagia, easy bruising
VII	Hypoproconvertinemia Incomplete autosomal recessive–variable expression: 1/500,000	10%	5 hr	Abnormal PT, normal APTT	Epistaxis, menorrhagia, cerebral hemorrhage
VIII	Hemophilia A (classic hemophilia) Sex-linked recessive 1/10,000	30%	8–12 hr	Abnormal APTT; normal PT, BT	May be severe, moderate, mild—spontaneous hemor- rhage, hemarthroses, crippling, muscle hemorrhage, post- traumatic postoperative bleeding
	von Willebrand's syndrome Variable inheritance Variants: autosomal dominant– variable penetrance: 1/80,000	20%–40%	16–24 hr	Variable results Platelet studies, BT, APTT	Mucous membrane bleeding, superficial wound bleeding— variable depending on level of VIII:C levels
IX	Hemophilia B (Christmas disease) Sex-linked recessive: 1/100,000	30%–50%	20 hr	Abnormal APTT; normal PT	May be severe, moderate, mild—spontaneous hemorrhage, hemarthroses, crippling, muscle hemorrhage, posttraumatic postoperative bleeding, ecchymoses
X	Stuart-Prower defect Autosomal recessive: <1/500,000 Homozygous: 1/500 Heterozygous	10%	65 hr	Abnormal PT, APTT	Menorrhagia, ecchymoses, central nervous system bleeding, excessive bleeding after childbirth
XI	Hemophilia C–Incomplete Autosomal recessive pseudo- dominant: 1/100,000	20%–30%	65 hr	Abnormal APTT; normal PT	Mild bleeding, bruising, epistaxis retinal hemorrhage, menorrhagia
XII	Hageman trait (rare) Autosomal recessive	Unknown	60 hr	Abnormal APTT; normal PT	Asymptomatic—rarely bleed, thrombosis
XIII	Factor XIII deficiency Autosomal recessive	1%	150 hr	Normal PT, APTT; clot soluble in 5 M urea	Umbilical cord bleeding, delayed wound healing, minor injuries causing prolonged bleeding, fetal wastage, excessive fibrinolysis, male sterility, intracranial hemorrhage

Factor Deficiency		Minimum for Hemostasis	Half-life	Laboratory	Clinical
PK	Prekallikrein (Fletcher factor) Autosomal recessive	Unknown	35 hr	Abnormal APTT: shortening of time after prolonged incubation with activator	Asymptomatic
HMWK	Fitzgerald deficiency (rare) Autosomal recessive	Unknown	156 hr	Abnormal APTT	Asymptomatic

Abbreviations: PT = prothrombin time; APTT = activated partial thromboplastin time; BT = bleeding time; HMWK = high-molecular-weight kininogen; TCT = thrombin clotting time

   Source: From Pittiglio, DH, et al: Treating hemostatic disorders. A problem oriented approach. In Pittiglio, DH: Hemostasis Overview. American Association of Blood Banks, Arlington, VA, 1984, p 28, with permission.

hemorrhage, or a consumptive coagulopathy such as disseminated intravascular coagulation (DIC); induction of anticoagulant therapy; inflammatory disorders; and treatment with various drugs.

➤ DISORDERS OF PLASMA CLOTTING FACTORS AND LABORATORY EVALUATION

Factor I (Fibrinogen)

Fibrinogen is a large glycoprotein produced in the liver, with a molecular weight (M_r) of 340,000 daltons; it participates in the final stages of coagulation. The fibrinogen molecule consists of two sets of three different polypeptide chains—A-alpha (α), B-beta (β), and gamma (γ)—and has a half-life of about 3 days.[2] The interaction of these chains, combined with the activity of the enzyme thrombin, yields a network of insoluble strands called *fibrin*.[3] Fibrin monomers are produced by the cleavage of the fibrinopeptides A and B from the terminal ends of the α and β chains of the fibrinogen molecule. In the final stages, these soluble monomers then polymerize to form soluble fibrin strands. In order to stabilize the soluble fibrin strands, factor XIII, which is also activated by thrombin, acts as the stabilizing factor, cross-linking the fibrin monomers to produce insoluble fibrin. This process produces a stable fibrin clot. The normal plasma concentration of fibrinogen in the circulation is approximately 200 to 400 mg/dL.

Fibrinogen is also an acute-phase reactant. Physiologic stresses such as trauma, pregnancy, and tissue inflammation can cause fibrinogen concentrations to increase, resulting in an elevated erythrocyte sedimentation rate (ESR). High fibrinogen concentrations may also be seen in acute hepatitis and may be associated with atherosclerosis, arterial thrombosis, or both.[4]

Afibrinogenemia

Afibrinogenemia, the total absence of measurable fibrinogen in plasma, is a rare congenital disorder inherited as an autosomal-recessive trait. It can cause profuse bleeding after slight trauma and delay in wound healing. Initial symptoms include bleeding from the umbilical cord stump. Other symptoms can include intracranial bleeding, epistaxis, gastrointestinal bleeding, and menorrhagia. Hemarthrosis is

uncommon for this disorder. Mild to moderate thrombocytopenia can occur, but platelet counts are rarely less than 100,000/μL.[5,6] Platelet aggregation was found to be abnormal in two studies in which fibrinogen was absent in platelets of patients with this disorder.[7] Fibrinogen is required for normal platelet aggregation; it binds to stimulated platelets at the glycoprotein IIb/IIIa (GPIIb/IIIa) receptor, forming a "molecular bridge" with adjacent platelets, thus reinforcing the platelet plug at the site of vascular injury.[8] Afibrinogenemia would, therefore, produce a prolonged bleeding time.

The laboratory evaluation for this disorder should include: prothrombin time (PT), activated partial thromboplastin time (APTT), fibrinogen (activity and antigen), reptilase time (RT), and thrombin time (TT) (Table 25–2). The results of these tests will show marked abnormalities: prolongation of the PT, APTT, RT, and TT, and the absence of measurable fibrinogen. Mixture of the patient's plasma with adsorbed plasma or pooled normal plasma will correct these defects.

Treatment for this disorder can include cryoprecipitate, fresh frozen plasma, and whole blood transfusions if profuse bleeding has occurred.

Hypofibrinogenemia

Hypofibrinogenemia, below-normal levels of fibrinogen in plasma, may be inherited as an autosomal-recessive disorder. The level of fibrinogen is found to be in the range of 20 to 100 mg/dL. Umbilical stump bleeding is a common manifestation, as are other hemorrhagic symptoms noted with afibrinogenemia. Unlike afibrinogenemia, hemorrhage after trauma is an infrequent finding. It may also be acquired as a result of either liver disease or DIC.

In hypofibrinogenemia, the degree of laboratory test abnormalities is dependent on the level of fibrinogen present in the plasma.

Treatment for this condition may include cryoprecipitate or fresh frozen plasma.

Dysfibrinogenemia

Alteration of the structure of the fibrinogen molecule, either in amino acid sequence or in carbohydrate composition, leads to the formation of an abnormal protein. The normal interactions of fibrinogen with its enzymes and cofactors is disrupted, thereby causing defective fibrin formation.

Dysfibrinogenemia is a qualitative defect that can be either inherited, mostly as an autosomal-dominant trait, or ac-

> **Table 25-2**
DIFFERENTIAL DIAGNOSIS OF FIBRINOGEN DISORDERS AND HEPARIN

Test	Afibrinogenemia	Hypofibrinogenemia	Dysfibrinogenemia	Heparin
Bleeding time	P	N	N	N
Prothrombin time	P	P	P/N	P/N
APTT	P	P	P/N	P
Thrombin time	P	P	P	P
Reptilase time	P	P	P	N
Thrombin coagulase	P	P	N	N
Fibrinogen level (clotting assay)	ABN (undetectable)	ABN	N/ABN	N/ABN
Fibrinogen (immunologic assay)	Absent	ABN	N	N
Platelet aggregation	Abnormal	N	N	N(ABN)
Fibrinolytic test	N	N	N	N

Abbreviations: N = normal; P = prolonged; ABN = abnormal; APTT = activated partial thromboplastin time
   Source: From Girolami, A, et al: Rare and quantitative and qualitative: Abnormalities of coagulation. Changes Hematol 14:388, 1985, with permission.

quired as a result of some underlying disease, most often liver disease.

Polymerization of fibrin monomers, prepared by treating the abnormal molecules with a high concentration of thrombin (as in the clottable fibrinogen assay), has been found to be normal in several cases.[9] However, with lower thrombin concentrations, as in the diluted thrombin time (DTT) test, polymerization is delayed because of the lower cleavage rate of the abnormal peptide.[10] A common laboratory finding is a normal quantitative value of functional (clottable) fibrinogen with a mild to markedly prolonged DTT. The level obtained by immunochemical (antigenic) assay of fibrinogen is very often higher than the level determined by functional assay. The anticoagulants heparin, hirudin, and the antithrombins can also prolong the DTT. To evaluate the cause of an abnormal DTT, a reptilase time should be performed.[11,12] Reptilase, a thrombin-like enzyme extracted from the snake venom of *Bothrops atrox,* can be used to evaluate for the presence of these anticoagulants or for confirmation of dysfibrinogenemia.[13] Reptilase is unaffected by heparin, hirudin, and antithrombins, and remains normal in their presence (see Table 25–2).

Dysfibrinogenemia is usually asymptomatic, although occasionally associated with bleeding resulting from ineffective polymerization. However, recent reports indicate an association with thrombosis.[14] This may be a result of abnormalities in the interaction of fibrinolytic enzymes (tissue plasminogen activator, plasminogen, or plasmin) with the abnormal fibrinogen.

Treatment for dysfibrinogenemia and accompanying thrombosis consists of anticoagulant therapy.

Factor II (Prothrombin)

Prothrombin (M_r 71,600 daltons) is synthesized in the liver. It is the most abundant and has the longest half-life of the vitamin K–dependent clotting proteins, and circulates as a zymogen to a serine protease.[15] Prothrombin is converted to thrombin by the reactions of factor Xa in the presence of factor Va, acting as a "cofactor" of phospholipid and calcium ions. Deficiencies of prothrombin delay the generation of thrombin, thus contributing to hemorrhagic symptoms.

Hypoprothrombinemia

It has been suggested that the mode of inheritance of hypoprothrombinemia is autosomal recessive.[16] Patients who are either doubly heterozygous or homozygous with this rare condition may have hemorrhagic symptoms with prothrombin levels from 2% to 25% of normal activity. Deficiency may also be acquired via vitamin K deficiency or oral anticoagulant (warfarin) therapy. However, the type and severity of symptoms may vary with the level of functional prothrombin available. Epistaxis, menorrhagia, postpartum hemorrhage, and hemorrhage following surgery or trauma and broad spectrum antibiotic use are exhibited with prothrombin levels ranging from less than 2% to less than 50%. Ingestion of aspirin has exacerbated bleeding tendencies. Prothrombin levels approaching 50% of normal activity generally do not cause bleeding problems. Variable prolongation of both the PT and APTT and a normal thrombin time are obtained in individuals with this deficiency. These screening assays are not specific for this deficiency. Diagnosis is dependent on specific assays for functional activity or antigenic concentration of prothrombin, or both. In hypoprothrombinemia, both functional activity and antigenic concentration of prothrombin are decreased. Mixing studies with either aged serum or adsorbed plasma show no correction of the PT or APTT. Full correction will occur with pooled normal plasma.

Treatment of this deficiency may include fresh frozen plasma, prothrombin-complex concentrates, and concentrates of factors II, VII, IX, and X. Vitamin K supplementation will restore low factor levels associated with dietary deficiency or oral anticoagulation.

Dysprothrombinemia

The mode of inheritance of dysprothrombinemia is the same as in hypoprothrombinemia.[17] A structural defect causes impaired functional activity, although the antigenic concentration is normal. Bleeding manifestations may occur that are similar to those described for hypoprothrombinemia. Vitamin K deficiency, induction and therapeutic warfarin therapy, liver disease, and the presence of antibodies to prothrombin must be distinguished from dysprothrombinemia and hypoprothrombinemia to determine the proper course of therapy.

Treatment may include administration of fresh frozen plasma, prothrombin-complex concentrates, or concentrates containing factors II, VII, IX, and X.

Prothrombin Mutation (G20210A)

A single point mutation in the prothrombin gene, located on chromosome 11, was discovered in 1996 that was associated with elevated prothrombin concentration and an increased risk of venous thrombosis.[18] The mutation, prothrombin G20210A, consists of a single base pair substitution resulting from a G (guanine) to A (adenine) transition at nucleotide 20210 of the prothrombin gene.[19] It is the second most common cause of inherited thrombophilia (predisposition to thrombosis). Patients who are heterozygous for this mutation carry a two- to fivefold increased risk of venous thromboembolism as compared with normal individuals. This genetic defect is not commonly found in patients with arterial thromboembolic disease, but it has been identified as a risk factor for myocardial infarction in young women[20] and cerebrovascular ischemic disease in young patients.[21] This genetic variant is predominantly (although not exclusively) restricted to the Caucasian population. In the presence of other acquired risk factors, such as pregnancy, oral contraceptives, malignancy, antiphospholipid antibody (lupus anticoagulant), recent surgery, or trauma, the incidence of thrombosis is increased.[22,23]

The elevation of prothrombin (factor II) activity may still be within normal limits. Therefore, the mutation must be detected via direct deoxyribonucleic acid (DNA) analysis by polymerase chain reaction (PCR) technology.

Factor V (Proaccelerin)

Rapid enzymatic reactions that include protein cofactors have a vital role in normal blood coagulation. Factor V and factor VIII (antihemophilic factor) enhance these reactions. The absence of either of these factors leads to bleeding. Owren[24,25] discovered factor V deficiency in a 21-year-old woman with a lifelong bleeding history. The discovery showed that this clotting factor was not vitamin K–dependent. Congenital factor V deficiency, also known as *parahemophilia,* is inherited as an autosomal-recessive trait.[26] This extremely rare condition has a probability of occurrence of 1 person per 1 million population.[27] This factor is synthesized by the liver and is present in the α granules of platelets.[28] Factor V (M_r 350,000 daltons) has a short half-life, and is heat-labile. It functions as a cofactor in the conversion of prothrombin to thrombin. It is converted to its active cofactor, factor Va, by the action of thrombin or factor Xa, in the presence of calcium ions and phospholipids. The enzymes of Russell's viper venom can also activate factor V.

Ecchymoses, epistaxis, menorrhagia, and gingival, gastrointestinal tract, umbilical, and central nervous system bleeding are associated with deficiencies of factor V. Hemorrhagic manifestations are usually noted in individuals with less than 10% activity. Hemarthrosis seldom occurs even in severely deficient patients. Combined deficiencies of factors V and VIII have been reported in several families.

Acquired factor V deficiency can be the result of the appearance of specific antibodies or associated with a variety of diseases, such as liver disease, carcinoma, tuberculosis, DIC, and other causes.[29]

In the laboratory evaluation, the PT and APTT are prolonged, and both are corrected upon mixing with pooled normal or adsorbed plasma. However, mixing studies with aged serum do not correct the prolongation of either the PT or the APTT. The thrombin time is normal. Prior to analysis, the centrifuged plasma must be platelet-poor (platelet count less than $10,000/\mu L$) to avoid contamination of the plasma factor V level, because platelets contain endogenous factor V. Functional factor activity is decreased or absent. Correction with the addition of pooled normal plasma will not occur in the presence of an inhibitor.

Factor V–deficient patients are often treated with fresh or fresh frozen plasma. Cryoprecipitate does not contain adequate amounts of factor V to be used in therapy.

Factor V Mutation (Factor V Leiden)

Under normal conditions, activated factor V (and, as will be discussed, activated factor VIII) must be inactivated to prevent ongoing thrombin generation. This is accomplished via the naturally occurring anticoagulant protein C, and its cofactor, protein S. Protein C is activated by thrombin (which is bound to thrombomodulin on the endothelial cell surface; see Chap. 23). Activated protein C (APC) is responsible for this inactivation.

In 1993, a new and very common inherited thrombophilic syndrome was described: activated protein C resistance (APCR). It was found to be present in 3% to 7% of the Caucasian population of northern European decent.[30] The first molecular defect (mutation) was identified involving the transition of a G (guanine) to A (adenine) in position 1691 of the factor V gene. The resulting amino acid substitution replaces arginine with glutamine at amino acid 506; it is in this location where APC must bind to the factor V molecule.[31] This mutation, named *factor V Leiden* (R506Q), leads to impaired degradation of factor V by APC and results in continued thrombin generation, producing thrombosis (Fig. 25–1). This mutation is present in more than 90% of cases of APCR and in approximately 20% to 60% of patients with venous thrombosis.[32] The clottable activity of factor V is unaffected by this mutation. Therefore, detection of this defect must be by PCR technology.

Factor VII (Proconvertin)

The division of the coagulation system into the intrinsic and extrinsic systems was created as a useful tool for laboratory diagnoses. It has recently been recognized that this division does not occur in vivo as tissue factor–factor VIIa complex is responsible for the activation of factor IX as well as factor X.

The initiation of the coagulation pathways in vivo begins with the extrinsic system, involving components of the vascular and blood elements. A major component is tissue factor, which functions as a cofactor. Tissue factor is synthesized by macrophages and endothelial cells and is composed of a single polypeptide chain. The predominant plasma protein of the extrinsic system is factor VII (M_r 50,000 daltons), a vitamin K–dependent protein. It is produced in the liver, its activity is increased by factor XIIa or IXa, and it requires tissue factor, thrombin, and calcium ions to become factor VIIa.

Congenital factor VII deficiency is a rare, inherited autosomal-recessive trait.[33,34] Clinically, factor VII–deficient patients have deep muscle hematomas, joint hemorrhage, epistaxis, and menorrhagia. The PT is prolonged, with a normal APTT (factor VII is not measured in the APTT test

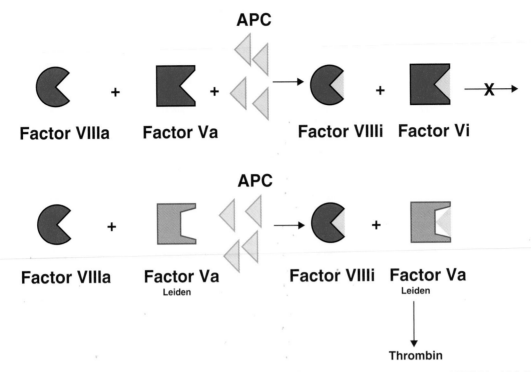

> FIGURE 25-1   Activated protein C (APC) resistance of factor V Leiden. (*Top*) Normal inactivation of factors V and VIII:C by APC. (*Bottom*) The binding site for APC on the factor V Leiden molecule is altered, thereby permitting activated factor V (factor Va Leiden) to continue thrombin generation and subsequent fibrin formation.

system). The PT can be fully corrected with Russell's viper venom (as it directly activates factor X), and mixing with aged serum (Table 25–3). Documentation of factor VII deficiency requires the one-stage factor assay. Patients who have less than 1% clottable activity can have severe hemorrhagic manifestations.

Factor VII deficiency can be acquired with liver disease, warfarin therapy, or dietary vitamin K deficiency. Treatment includes fresh frozen plasma, prothrombin-complex concentrates, and vitamin K supplementation.

Factor VIII

Factor VIII (FVIII), a large glycoprotein (M_r 330,000 daltons), is essential in the middle phase of coagulation.[35] It is not completely known where FVIII is synthesized, although studies have tended to support the liver as the source.[36,37] However, severe hepatic failure does not cause FVIII deficiency. Some evidence suggests that a cell type present in several organs may be the major source, such as fibroblasts, lymphocytes, monophages or macrophages, and vascular endothelial cells.[38]

Factor VIII is secreted into the plasma, where it circulates as a complex with von Willebrand's factor (FVIII:vWF) (Table 25–4).[39] Von Willebrand's factor, also a glycoprotein, is synthesized by megakaryocytes and endothelial cells. Only 1% to 2% of the complex functions as the procoagulant (FVIII:C), measurable by clotting assays, and the remaining portion is FVIII:vWF, which mediates platelet adhesion. When injury occurs, FVIII:vWF serves as a carrier to concentrate the FVIII:C at the site of injury. FVIII:C, whose half-life is approximately 8 to 12 hours, functions as a cofactor, accelerating the conversion of factor X to factor Xa in the presence of factor IXa, calcium ions, and phospholipids (see Chap. 23). Table 25–5 summarizes selected properties of FVIII:C and von Willebrand's factor. It must be activated (FVIIIa) by thrombin or other serine protease in order to possess cofactor activity. Inactivation of FVIIIa by APC is required to prevent ongoing thrombin generation and thromboembolic complications. FVIII:C is thermolabile and can rapidly lose activity unless the plasma is stored at or below −70°C.

Factor VIII is an acute-phase reactant; inflammation, stress, pregnancy, and infection can cause elevated levels. Recent studies have found a link between elevated levels of FVIII:C and a hypercoagulable state.[40] During some acute or chronic inflammatory processes, the elevated factor level, in combination with other vascular and stimulated platelet-derived substances, promotes the formation of thrombi. Oral contraceptives can elevate FVIII levels. If there are predisposing factors such as surgery, trauma, systemic infection, immobilization or an unrecognized abnormality of the anticoagulant–fibrinolytic mechanism, the

> ## Table 25-3
> ### LABORATORY FINDINGS FOR FACTOR VII DEFICIENCY

Test	Results	Normal Values
PT	> 20 sec	10.0–14.0 sec
APTT	< 36 sec	23.0–36.0 sec
Factor VII assay	< 0.01 U/mL	1.00 U/mL
Russell's viper venom	18.0 sec	< 25.0 sec
Other factor activity	1.00 U/mL	1.00 U/mL

Abbreviations: PT = prothrombin time; APTT = activated partial thromboplastin time

➤ **Table 25-4**
PROPOSED ABBREVIATIONS FOR FACTOR VIII AND VON WILLEBRAND'S FACTOR*

	ABBREVIATION	
Attribute	**Proposed**	**Outmoded**
Factor VIII		
Protein	VIII	VIII:C
Antigen	VIII:Ag	VIIIC:Ag
Function	VIII:C	—
von Willebrand's factor		
Protein	vWF	VIIIR:Ag, VIII/vWF, AHF-like protein
Antigen	vWF:Ag	VIIIR:Ag, AHF-like antigens
Function	—	VIIIR:RCo, VIIIR:vWF†

*The two proteins form a bimolecular complex that can be abbreviated as VIII/vWF.

†These abbreviations have been used to indicate the ristocetin cofactor activity of von Willebrand's factor. Because neither this test nor any other in vitro test completely reflects vWF activity, no abbreviation is recommended as representative of its function.

Source: From Marder, VJ, et al: Standard nomenclature for factor VIII and von Willebrand factor: A recommendation by the International Committee on Thrombosis and Haemostasis. Thromb Haemost 54:871, 1985, with permission.

risk of pulmonary embolism, deep vein thrombosis, or stroke increases dramatically.

Hemophilia A

Hemophilia A (classic hemophilia) is the most common hereditary coagulation disorder. It is a sex-linked bleeding disorder that has been documented for centuries. The fifth-century Talmud described a bleeding episode that occurred after circumcision. Modern rabbinic command forbids the circumcision of any child in whom the diagnosis of hemophilia has been made.[41] The disorder was found in the Royal House of Stuart in Europe and Russia. Queen Victoria, a carrier, was the source of hemophilia in four subsequent generations.[42,43]

The defect in hemophilia A is not an absence of the factor VIII complex but rather a molecular defect or absence of its procoagulant portion (FVIII:C).[44] The von Willebrand's factor antigenic component (vWF:Ag) of the FVIII complex is found to be normal in patients with hemophilia A. The gene for FVIII:C resides on the X chromosome, thereby producing sons with the disease and daughters who will be obligatory carriers of the trait. The female carrier does not usually exhibit clinical bleeding; she has two X chromosomes, only one of which produces functional FVIII:C. The ratio of antigenic FVIII to procoagulant FVIII (vWF:Ag/FVIII:C) should be approximately 2:1 in the carrier.[45] In approximately one-third of newly diagnosed cases of hemophilia A, there may be no previous family history of bleeding. This suggests that a mutation may be evident, or there could be several generations of "silent carriers" of the sex-linked recessive trait.[46,47]

Patients with FVIII:C levels of less than 1% (less than 0.01 U/mL) have severe hemorrhagic disease that requires constant transfusion therapy. These patients are classified as severe hemophiliacs. Patients with levels greater than 5% (greater than 0.05 U/mL) are considered mild hemophiliacs and have a less severe hemorrhagic disease. The moderately severe hemophiliac has levels that fall between the two ranges. Hemarthrosis is a primary symptom involving knees, elbows, ankles, shoulders, hips, and wrists. Other symptoms include hematuria, intracranial bleeding, hematomas, and unexplained spontaneous hemorrhage.

Approximately 10% to 15% percent of patients with hemophilia A develop antibodies or inhibitors to FVIII:C.[48] The inhibitors are usually temperature-dependent in vitro and are immunoglobulin (IgG) in nature. These inhibitors are capable of neutralizing FVIII:C at 37°C.[49] Administration of antihemophilic factor (AHF) may lead to a rise in antibody titers in patients who have developed antibodies (an anamnestic response) to AHF.[48]

➤ **Table 25-5**
SELECTED PROPERTIES OF FACTOR VIII:C AND VON WILLEBRAND'S FACTOR*

	Factor VIII:C	**von Willebrand's Factor**
Cellular site of biosynthesis	Hepatic	Endothelial cells and megakaryocytes
Plasma concentration	0.50–1.50 U/mL	50%–150%
Molecular weight	330,000 daltons	600,000–2 million daltons
Principal biologic activity	Procoagulant factor	Platelet adhesion to vessel wall
Functional assay	APTT factor Xa formation	Bleeding time, platelet adhesion, platelet agglutination (e.g., ristocetin-induced)
Immunologic assay	IRMA, ELISA, immunoblot: inhibitor neutralization	Quantitative: IRMA, ELISA, electroimmunoassay (Laurell)
Inheritance	X-linked recessive	Autosomal
Clinical disorder caused by deficiency	Hemophilia A	von Willebrand's disease

*In plasma, the two proteins are present as a bimolecular complex called the factor VIII–von Willebrand factor (FVIII:vWF) complex.
Abbreviations: IRMA = immunoradiometric assay; ELISA = enzyme-linked immunosorbant assay
Source: From Marder VJ, et al: Standard nomenclature for factor VIII and von Willebrand factor: A recommendation by the International Committee on Thrombosis and Hemostasis. Thromb Haemost 54:871, 1985 with permission.

Many forms of treatment are available for hemophilia A. Concentrates of human plasma such as AHF are widely used. Many hemophiliacs are treated with highly purified, heat-treated, lyophilized preparations of FVIII concentrate. Although cryoprecipitate is a rich source of FVIII, it is not the product of choice because of the high incidence of parenterally transmitted human immunodeficiency virus (HIV), hepatitis C, and other serious viral illnesses. New technologies that produce synthetic recombinant-DNA FVIII significantly lower the incidence of viral transmission. Patients who have developed antibodies to human FVIII concentrates often respond to treatment with porcine FVIII. Factor IX concentrates or prothrombin-complex concentrates (containing factors II, VII, IX, and X) have been used in severe cases. Thirty percent of normal activity is the ideal therapeutic level for maintaining hemostasis.

The laboratory findings for patients with hemophilia A are a prolonged APTT, normal PT, and a normal bleeding time (Table 25–6). Mixing studies with pooled normal or adsorbed plasma corrects the prolongation of the APTT. Aged serum does not correct the prolongation. The deficiency is further characterized by low to absent levels of FVIII:C, normal levels of vWF:Ag, and normal platelet function assays. Figure 25–2 shows how vWF:Ag is measured quantitatively using immunoelectrophoresis. The presence of an inhibitor can be established when mixing studies with pooled normal plasma do not correct the prolonged APTT. The functional activity is measured using a modified one-stage factor assay using the APTT test and quantitating the inhibitor in Bethesda units (see Specific Factor Inhibitors, later).[50]

von Willebrand's Disease

In 1926, a 5-year-old girl from the Åland Islands off the coast of Finland was evaluated by Dr. Erich von Willebrand

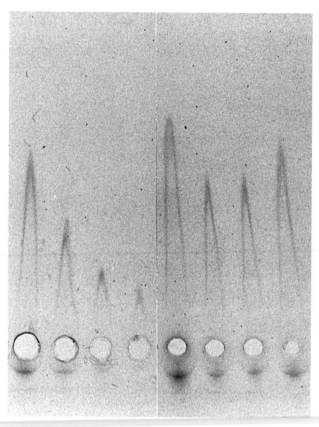

➤ **FIGURE 25–2** Quantitative immunoelectrophoresis of vWF:Ag; Laurell rockets in agarose gel. The first four peaks are the standard curve dilutions, followed by various vWF:Ag levels. Peak height is proportional to concentration.

➤ **Table 25-6**
COMPARISON OF HEMOPHILIA A AND CLASSIC VON WILLEBRAND'S DISEASE

	Hemophilia A	von Willebrand's Disease (Type 1)
Deficiency	FVIII:C; VIII:AHF	VIII:vWF
Inheritance	Recessive, X-linked	Dominant, autosomal
Clinical bleeding presentation	Hemarthroses, muscle, soft tissue, visceral	Gingival, gastrointestinal, mucous membrane
Bleeding tendency	Moderate to severe	Mild to moderate
Laboratory tests		
Bleeding time	N	A/N
Clot retraction	N	N
Glass bead adhesion	N	A
Platelet count	N	N
Ristocetin aggregation	N	A
PT	N	N
APTT	A	A/N
FVIII:C activity	A	A/N
vWFR:Co	N	A
vWF:Ag	N	A

Abbreviations: N = normal; A = abnormal; FVIII:C = factor VIII coagulant activity; AHF = antihemolytic factor; PT = prothrombin time; APTT = activated partial thromboplastin time; vWF:Ag = von Willebrand's factor antigen

for a severe bleeding disorder. After thoroughly investigating the family members and patient, Dr. von Willebrand concluded that this was a previously undescribed bleeding disorder. Von Willebrand's disease (vWD) differs from classical hemophilia A in three cardinal manifestations: autosomal inheritance rather than sex-linked; consistently prolonged bleeding times; and mucocutaneous bleeding rather than hemarthroses and deep muscle hemorrhage. It was not until the 1970s that von Willebrand's factor (vWF) and factor VIII (FVIII:C) were found to be different proteins produced by different cells under different genetic control.[51]

vWF is composed of a series of high-molecular-weight multimers with M_r ranging from 600,000 to 20 million daltons.[52] It circulates in the plasma as a heterogeneous mixture, produced by megakaryocytes and endothelial cells. vWF is stored and secreted from granules in endothelial cells called Weibel-Palade bodies, and α granules in platelets.[53] It binds to the subendothelium because of interaction with collagen.[54] After injury, vWF interacts with the glycoprotein Ib (GPIb) receptor on platelets, resulting in their activation and adhesion to the subendothelium. This action can be initiated in vitro using platelet-rich plasma and the antibiotic ristocetin, or the snake venom extract botrocetin. Ristocetin, an antibiotic similar in structure to vancomycin, was removed from clinical use when it was discovered that it caused thrombocytopenia. Shortly thereafter, ristocetin was shown to aggregate normal platelets but to cause little or no aggregation in patients with vWD.[55] Normal or hemophiliac plasma can correct this defect because of the presence of vWF. This platelet aggregation assay may not be sensitive to mild reductions of vWF and is not quantitative. A quantitative assay, using normal, formalin-fixed washed platelets, allows for a more sensitive measurement. This is known as the ristocetin cofactor activity (vWFR:Co) assay. In this method, the fixed platelets are not metabolically active and the response to ristocetin is termed ristocetin-induced platelet agglutination. When metabolically active platelet-rich plasma is exposed to ristocetin, the response is termed *aggregation*, because once vWF binds to its receptor, GPIb, it will induce subsequent GPIIb/IIIa receptor-dependent aggregation (ristocetin-induced platelet aggregation)[56] (Fig. 25–3). GPIIb/IIIa is normally the physiologic binding site for fibrinogen during in vitro aggregation, but in the absence of fibrinogen or when vWF is at high concentrations, such as at the site of vascular injury, vWF may also induce this receptor-mediated aggregation process.[57]

As stated previously, vWF circulates as a complex with FVIII:C. Patients with von Willebrand's disease who may have reduced or absent levels of vWF may also have reduced levels of FVIII:C. However, levels of FVIII:C are usually slightly greater than the level of vWF:Ag, presumably because there is a normal gene present for FVIII:C and the potential binding sites are saturated when levels of vWF:Ag are reduced.[58] The effects of ABO blood grouping have a significant effect on the amount of vWF:Ag produced. Individuals who are type A, B, and AB have much greater mean plasma vWF:Ag concentrations than blood type O individuals.[59]

Patients with von Willebrand's disease present with mucocutaneous bleeding as well as frequent instances of epistaxis, ecchymosis, easy bruisability, gastrointestinal bleeding, menorrhagia, and hemorrhage following surgery. These

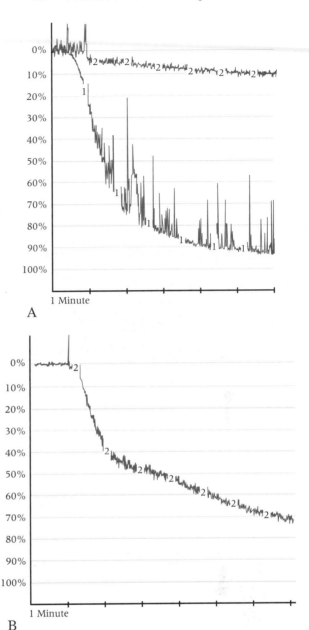

> **FIGURE 25–3** Ristocetin-induced platelet aggregation. *A.* (*1*) Normal response to ristocetin 1.2 U/mL. (*2*) Normal response to ristocetin 0.6 U/mL (low-dose). *B.* Abnormal response to ristocetin 0.6 U/mL characteristic of type 2B von Willebrand's disease. Each mark on the x axis represents 1-minute intervals.

manifestations are caused by the inability of platelets to adhere to the subendothelial surface following injury to the blood vessel.[60,61] vWF is an acute-phase reactant that increases during stress or pregnancy, or after surgery. This makes diagnosis or evaluation difficult in patients suspected of having von Willebrand's disease. Therefore, it may be necessary to study these patients on multiple occasions to rule out von Willebrand's disease as the cause of mild bleeding symptoms.[62,63]

Because of the variant forms of von Willebrand's disease that have been described, the clinical presentation may vary. vWF is the carrier protein for factor VIII:C, and thus it is not unusual for patients with von Willebrand's disease to have reduced concentrations. Patients who have severe forms of von Willebrand's disease generally present with a normal PT, prolonged APTT that corrects on mixing with pooled normal plasma, normal platelet counts, and an abnormal bleeding time test (see Table 25–6). The bleeding time (BT) is used to assess the function of platelets in hemostasis. Although the bleeding time is not a good screening test because of problems with standardization and interpretation, it is virtually always prolonged in patients with von Willebrand's disease. In milder forms of von Willebrand's disease, the bleeding time may be normal.[64] The most commonly used bleeding time test is known as the Ivy template bleeding time. This procedure uses a spring-loaded device that makes an incision of standard length and depth.

The laboratory assessment should include assays for FVIII:C activity, vWF:Ag concentration, vWFR:Co activity, platelet aggregation studies, and vWF multimeric analysis. Multimeric analysis will further confirm the specific variant form. Identification is essential for proper treatment. The von Willebrand variants include type 1, 2A, 2B, 2C, 3, and platelet-type (Table 25–7).

Type 1 von Willebrand's disease, inherited as an autosomal-dominant trait, is a partial quantitative deficiency and the most common type. Patients have a reduced level of normally functioning vWF activity; FVIII:C activity can be normal or decreased, and there is usually a parallel decrease of vWF:Ag concentration and vWFR:Co activity. With type 1 there is a normal distribution of multimers.

Type 2A, also inherited as an autosomal-dominant trait, is

▶ Table 25-7
LABORATORY DIAGNOSIS OF CLASSIC VON WILLEBRAND'S DISEASE (TYPE 1) AND VARIANTS*

	AUTOSOMAL DOMINANT				AUTOSOMAL RECESSIVE	
	Type 1	Type 2A	Type 2B	Platelet-type	Type 2C	Type 3
Bleeding time	Increased or normal	Increased	Increased	Increased	Increased	Increased
Platelet count	Normal	Normal	Normal or decreased	Low normal or decreased	Normal	Normal
Factor VIII:C	Normal or decreased	Normal or decreased	Normal or decreased	Normal or decreased	Normal	Markedly decreased
vWF:Ag	Decreased	Decreased or normal	Decreased or normal	Normal or decreased	Decreased or normal	Markedly decreased
Ristocetin cofactor	Decreased	Markedly decreased	Decreased or normal	Decreased or normal	Decreased	Markedly decreased
Crossed immunoelectro-phoresis of plasma vWF	Normal	Abnormal	Abnormal	Abnormal	Abnormal	Variable
Multimeric structure of vWF						
Plasma	Normal	Absence of largest and intermediate multimers	Absence of largest multimers	Absence of largest multimers	Absence of largest multimers and abnormal band structure	Variable
Platelets	Normal	Absence of largest and intermediate multimers	Normal	Normal	Absence of largest multimers and abnormal band structure	Variable
Ristocetin-induced platelet-aggregation in patient PRP	Decreased or normal	Markedly decreased	Increased	Increased	Decreased	Markedly decreased
Ristocetin-induced binding of vWF to platelets						
Patient plasma + normal platelets		Decreased	Increased	Normal or decreased		
Normal plasma + patient platelets		Normal	Normal	Increased		
vWF-induced aggregation of unstimulated patient platelets in PRP			Absent	Present		

Abbreviations: Factor VIII:C = VIII coagulant activity; vWF:Ag = von Willebrand's factor antigen; PRP = platelet-rich plasma
Source: From Miller JL: Blood coagulation and fibrinolysis. In Henry JB(ed): Clinical Diagnosis and Management, ed 17. WB Saunders, Philadelphia, 1984, p 777, with permission.

a qualitative defect of vWF. The absence of intermediate and high-molecular-weight multimers decreases the platelet-dependent functions. The vWFR:Co activity is disproportionately lower than the vWF:Ag concentration, which may indicate a dysfunctional molecule.

Type 2B, autosomal-dominant inheritance, is also a qualitative defect of vWF; the plasma shows a lack of only the high-molecular-weight multimers, whereas the platelet-associated vWF multimers are normal. A very important distinguishing feature of this variant is that patients have enhanced aggregation studies using low concentrations of ristocetin; this is because of the production of an abnormal vWF protein that spontaneously binds to normal platelets and increases their clearance from the circulation, causing mild thrombocytopenia in some patients. There is an increased affinity for the GPIb receptor, which is not an intrinsic abnormality of the platelets.

Type 2C von Willebrand's disease shares similar clinical and laboratory characteristics as type 2A, although the mode of inheritance is autosomal recessive, and multimeric analysis reveals an abnormal band structure in addition to the loss of the high-molecular-weight multimers.[65]

Type 3, inherited as an autosomal-recessive trait, is a complete quantitative deficiency of vWF. vWF:Ag concentration, vWFR:Co activity, and multimers are virtually undetectable. FVIII:C activity is usually 2% to 5% of normal because of the lack of its carrier protein. Development of anti-vWF antibodies is possible if patients are infused with plasma products, which may further complicate their therapy.

Platelet-type von Willebrand's disease, also known as pseudo-von Willebrand's disease, is an abnormality intrinsic to the platelet, although its laboratory findings are identical to those of type 2B von Willebrand's disease. It is inherited as an autosomal-recessive trait. A molecular abnormality in GPIb, the platelet receptor for vWF, causes increased binding of the high-molecular-weight multimers, clearing them from the plasma and, therefore, causes increased platelet turnover. A mild thrombocytopenia develops and larger-than-normal platelets are present on a peripheral smear. The presence of a response to low concentrations of ristocetin on platelet aggregation, as in type 2B, makes differential diagnosis difficult. Different treatments are required for these two disorders; therefore, it is imperative that they by identified. This can be accomplished by testing the response of the patient's plasma vWF, tagged with a monoclonal antibody to vWF, against normal formalin-fixed platelets at various concentrations of ristocetin. A patient with platelet-type von Willebrand's disease would, therefore, produce a normal result, whereas a patient with type 2B would show increased binding at lowered concentrations of ristocetin.[66]

Concentrates of FVIII, cryoprecipitate, and vWF have been used to treat von Willebrand's disease. However, commercial FVIII concentrates are not useful because they lack the high-molecular-weight multimers of vWF (Fig. 25–4). Desmopressin (DDAVP), a synthetic analog of vasopressin used to treat patients with diabetes insipidus, can be useful in treating patients with von Willebrand's disease. This medication causes both the vWF and FVIII:C activities to increase temporarily. Patients with type 1 von Willebrand's disease can be treated with DDAVP before dental work or surgery and after bleeding episodes, thereby avoiding exposure to blood products. The use of DDAVP as a treatment for type 2B can cause the increased release of ab-

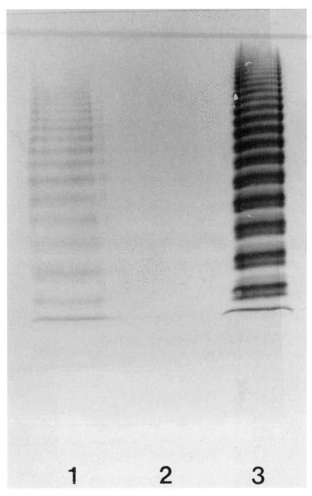

➤ FIGURE 25–4 vWF multimers. Samples of (*1*) normal plasma, (*2*) von Willebrand's plasma, and (*3*) cryoprecipitate, underwent electrophoresis in sodium dodecyl sulfate (SDS)-agarose gel. A western blotting technique was performed. The gel on nitrocellulose paper was incubated first with a rabbit anti–human vWF:Ag antibody and then with goat anti–rabbit IgG; then it was stained.

normal vWF molecules, increasing the binding to normal platelets, and thus causing accelerated clearance of normal platelets, resulting in thrombocytopenia. Because of this increased response, treatment with DDAVP is contraindicated in type 2B. Platelet concentrates are used to treat patients with platelet-type von Willebrand's disease.

Factor IX (Christmas Factor)

Factor IX is a single-chain glycoprotein (M_r approximately 60,000 daltons) that is synthesized in the liver, and is vitamin K–dependent. In the coagulation sequence, factor IX participates in the intrinsic pathway, where it is activated by factor XIa in the presence of calcium ions to become a serine protease, factor IXa_β.[67] A second mechanism of activation, which bypasses contact activation, occurs via tissue factor and factor VIIa.[68] Additionally, factor IX can be activated by a protease from Russell's viper venom[69,70] which leads to the formation of factor IXa_α. This activated factor, in the presence of FVIIIa, calcium ions, and phospholipid, activates factor X.[71] Although factor IXa alone is capable of slowly activating factor X in the presence of phospholipid and calcium ions, neither FVIII alone nor FVIII plus thrombin activates factor X in the absence of factor IXa.[72]

Hemophilia B

Factor IX deficiency, also known as *hemophilia B,* is a sex-linked recessive bleeding disorder. Females with the deficiency are quite rare, but carrier states and spontaneous mutations do occur. Although the clinical symptoms are quite similar, it was observed that mixing plasmas from two unrelated hemophilic patients would normalize the clotting time in the mixed plasma.[73,74] Hemophilia B became known as "Christmas disease" by Biggs and colleagues,[75] named after the first patient they had seen with the disease. Since then factor IX has also been known as Christmas factor, and plasma thromboplastin component (PTC).

The incidence of inherited factor IX deficiency in the normal population is approximately 1 per 100,000.[76] The level of factor IX activity determines the severity of the disorder, with the most severe deficiencies having less than 1% activity, and the milder deficiencies having 5% to 25% activity. In severe hemophilia B, there is a total absence of factor IX, demonstrated by the absence of clottable activity as well as antigen. Some hemophilia B patients synthesize a nonfunctional variant of the factor IX molecule, whereas others do not have identifiable factor IX antigen in the plasma and, therefore, have a true absence of synthesis of the molecule.[77] Measurement of factor IX antigen and clottable activity levels greatly increases the accuracy of determining carrier status.[78] Acquired deficiency states can be seen in patients with liver disease or vitamin K deficiency and in patients on oral anticoagulant therapy.

Treatment of patients with severe to moderate factor IX deficiency consists of regular infusions of fresh frozen plasma, prothrombin-complex concentrates, or factor IX concentrates. Patients with mild deficiencies usually receive treatment in association with minor as well as major surgery. The most serious complication in patients with hemophilia B is the formation of antibodies to factor IX. These are extremely difficult to handle, especially in life-threatening situations, and occur in approximately 10% of patients with this deficiency.[79,80]

The laboratory findings in factor IX deficiency include normal values for PT, thrombin time, and bleeding time. There is prolongation of the APTT, which corrects upon mixing with pooled normal plasma or aged serum. One-stage factor assays of factor IX activity produce decreased to absent levels.

Factor X (Stuart-Prower Factor)

Factor X (M_r 58,800 daltons) is a vitamin K–dependent glycoprotein. It is composed of a light chain and a heavy chain held together by a single disulfide bond.[81,82] The heavy chain contains the catalytic domain of the protein.[83] It is synthesized in the liver and released into the plasma as a precursor to a serine protease. The conversion of factor X to its proteolytic form, factor Xa, involves the cleavage of a peptide bond in the heavy chain. This reaction, in the intrinsic system, is catalyzed by factor IXa in the presence of factor VIIIa, calcium ions, and phospholipid. This same bond is cleaved by factor VIIa in the presence of tissue factor in the extrinsic system.[84]

Inherited factor X deficiency is extremely rare. Its transmission is autosomal recessive, with an occurrence of less than 1 per 500,000; however, the heterozygous state can occur in approximately 1 per 500.

Deficiency of factor X may occur at any age, but the most severe hemorrhagic symptoms occur in the very young. Bleeding sites vary according to the severity of the deficiency. Clinical symptoms range from easy bruising, epistaxis, gastrointestinal bleeding, or menorrhagia in mildly affected patients to hemarthrosis, central nervous system hemorrhage, and severe postoperative hemorrhage in the most severely affected patients.

Usually, the diagnosis of inherited factor X deficiency can be made by an appropriate family history and laboratory data. However, differentiating between inherited and acquired deficiencies should include the consideration of liver disease and vitamin K deficiency. Acquired factor X deficiencies usually coincide with other vitamin K–dependent factor disorders. Factor X deficiencies have been reported in patients with amyloidosis.[85]

Variant forms of factor X deficiency exist because of amino acid substitutions or deletions. As a result of these genetic changes, the function of the molecule is altered. This manifests itself in vitro as variable results with standard coagulation studies[86] (Table 25–8).

The laboratory results seen in this deficiency include a prolonged PT and APTT, which corrects upon mixing with pooled normal plasma or aged serum. Adsorbed plasma does not correct the prolongation of the PT or APTT. Thrombin times and bleeding times are normal. The "Stypven" time or Russell's viper venom time are prolonged because this assay is dependent on factors II, V, and X in the presence of phospholipid. Factor activity, typically using PT methodology, is decreased or absent, resulting in prolonged times (see Table 25–8). It is interesting to note, however, that factor assays based on either the PT or APTT may be used to determine factor activity, but in variant forms of factor X deficiency, discrepancies can occur in the values obtained, depending on which methodology is used.

Treatment consists of transfusions with fresh frozen plasma or prothrombin-complex concentrates. However, the need for such measures should be guided by the severity of the hemorrhagic episode. Levels of 10% are considered adequate for hemostasis. Unless the deficiency is acquired by poor diet or oral anticoagulant therapy, the disorder does not usually respond to vitamin K therapy.

Factor XI (Plasma Thromboplastin Antecedent)

Factor XI (M_r 143,000 daltons) is a plasma glycoprotein that participates in the intrinsic coagulation pathway.[87] It is one of the contact factor proteins involved in early coagulation. It is synthesized by the liver and secreted into the plasma as

> ## Table 25–8
> ## LABORATORY FINDINGS FOR FACTOR X DEFICIENCY

Test	Results	Normal Values
PT	> 30.0 sec	10.0–14.0 sec
APTT	> 70.0 sec	23.0–36.0 sec
Factor X assay	< 0.01 U/mL	1.00 U/mL
Russell's viper venom	55.0 sec	< 25.0 sec
Other factor activity	1.00 U/mL	1.00 U/mL

a zymogen to a serine protease that circulates as a complex with high-molecular-weight kininogen (HMWK).[88] Structurally, it is composed of two identical polypeptide chains linked by a single disulfide bond.[89,90] After contact with a negatively charged surface, factor XI is activated by factor XIIa. The resulting serine protease is composed of two light chains containing the active sites and two heavy chains bridged by disulfide bonds.[91,92] The heavy chains of factor XIa are necessary for binding to HMWK and its substrate, factor IX.[93]

Hemophilia C

Factor XI deficiency, also once known as Rosenthal syndrome or hemophilia C, is seen predominately in the Ashkenazi Jewish population. It is inherited as an autosomal-recessive trait. The incidence in the general population is approximately 1 in 100,000.[94] The heterozygous frequency within the Ashkenazi Jewish population is nearly 1 in 8.[95]

Factor XI is the only factor of the contact system (which also consists of factor XII, HMWK, and prekallikrein), in which a deficiency may lead to a bleeding diathesis. However, plasma levels do not always predict the occurrence of postoperative or posttraumatic bleeding. Symptoms can be mild, ranging from bruising, epistaxis, menorrhagia, hematuria, prolonged or delayed postpartum bleeding, and bleeding following dental extractions, to severe hemorrhage requiring massive replacement therapy. Levels of factor XI may fluctuate with time, and bleeding episodes vary in response to a variety of surgical procedures.[96] There is, however, some degree of correlation between the severity of hemostatic challenge and severe bleeding.[97] Levels of less than 15% factor activity are considered severely deficient and result in postoperative bleeding.

Replacement therapy is not needed in patients with factor XI deficiency unless they are scheduled for surgery. Preoperative infusion of fresh or fresh frozen plasma, or the supernatant plasma after the removal of cryoprecipitate, may be required to avoid severe hemorrhage. Increase in factor activity levels to 20% to 30% of normal is adequate for hemostasis.[98] Circulating alloantibodies (inhibitors) can arise in patients with severe factor XI deficiency after exposure to plasma products. Further plasma infusions will not control bleeding, but it may respond to activated prothrombin-complex concentrates, such as those used to treat patients with factor VIII or IX inhibitors.[99]

The laboratory features associated with a factor XI deficiency include a normal PT, and a prolonged APTT, which corrects upon mixing with pooled normal plasma, adsorbed plasma, and aged serum. The bleeding time and thrombin time are both normal. Specific factor XI activity assay produces decreased or absent levels. Freezing and thawing the plasma can cause activation of the contact system and significantly shorten the APTT in factor XI–deficient patients. Therefore, it is advisable to perform the factor activity assay on fresh plasma drawn in plastic syringes and placed into anticoagulated siliconized or nonwettable test tubes.[100] Normal factor XI activity is considered to be 70% to 130% (0.70 to 1.30 U/mL). Heterozygous individuals have levels ranging between 20% and 70% (0.20 to 0.70 U/mL), whereas patients homozygous for factor XI deficiency have levels of less than 15% (less than 0.15 U/mL). Because of the variability of factor activity in some individuals, repeat testing is warranted in questionable cases.

Chapter 23 discussed the "cascade" theory of blood coagulation, which included the intrinsic, extrinsic, and common pathways of hemostasis. Activation of the surface-mediated pathway (contact system) can be achieved with factor XII, prekallikrein, factor XI, and HMWK. With the exception of factor XI, which is associated with hemorrhagic tendencies, the remaining proteins participate in the inflammatory response, complement activation, fibrinolysis, and kinin formation.[101]

Recent studies have found that a high level of factor XI activity (greater than 120%; and more than 1.2 U/mL) was a risk factor for venous thrombosis.[102] Factor XI participates in the intrinsic coagulation pathway leading to the formation of thrombin; however, factor XI can also be activated by thrombin, both in the presence and in the absence of negatively charged surfaces.[103] This feedback mechanism leads to further thrombin generation, necessary for the formation of fibrin, and for protection against fibrinolysis.[104] Thrombin mediates this protective mechanism by activating thrombin-activatable fibrinolysis inhibitor (TAFI),[105] which removes the sites necessary for binding and activating plasminogen. Therefore, the risk of thrombosis associated with high levels of factor XI may be explained by the role of factor XI in the inhibition of fibrinolysis.

Factor XII (Hageman Factor)

Factor XII (FXII) (M_r 76,000 daltons) is a single-chain β-globulin.[106] It is one of the members of the contact factor system, is believed to be synthesized by the liver, and circulates as an inactive zymogen. Contact with negatively charged surfaces in vitro, such as glass, celite, kaolin, or ellagic acid (solid-phase activation), causes autoactivation of FXII and its conversion to a serine protease.[107] This process initiates the intrinsic pathway of coagulation. In-vivo (fluid-phase) activation occurs by contact with the contents of cell membranes and components of leukocytes. In this process, FXII undergoes a conformational change exposing its active site, which then converts prekallikrein to kallikrein and activates factor XI.[108] Factor XIIa is formed by enzymatic cleavage by enzymes such as trypsin, plasmin, or kallikrein, forming a two-chain molecule composed of a heavy chain and a light chain held by a disulfide bond.[109] The presence of small amounts of FXIIa leads to activation of its substrates: prekallikrein, factor XI, and HMWK.

Deficiency of FXII, known as Hageman trait, is inherited in an autosomal-recessive fashion. This disorder is not associated with clinical bleeding or hemorrhage. There may, however, be an increased incidence of thrombotic diseases, such as myocardial infarction or thromboembolism. Patients are asymptomatic and pose no hemorrhagic surgical risk. The deficiency is usually coincidentally discovered during presurgical screening. Laboratory analysis indicates a normal PT and prolonged APTT, which corrects upon mixing with pooled normal plasma, adsorbed plasma, or aged serum. Specific factor analysis yields decreased or absent levels of functional FXII, which is required for definitive diagnosis. Care should be exercised to prevent contact activation during specimen collection by drawing into plastic syringes and placing the blood into siliconized anticoagulated test tubes. Freezing and thawing should be avoided by testing the plasma when freshly drawn. Normal FXII activity levels fall in the range of 70% to 140% (0.70 to 1.40 U/mL), with heterozygotes having 40% to 60% activity.

Factor XIII (Fibrin-Stabilizing Factor)

In the final stages of the coagulation process, there is generation of thrombin, polymerization of fibrin, and activation of factor XIII (FXIII), which is responsible for the formation of a stable fibrin clot. FXIII is a proenzyme for plasma transglutaminase, and in the presence of fibrin, thrombin converts FXIII to an enzyme called *factor XIIIa*.[110,111] It is the only enzyme in the coagulation system that is not a serine protease. Factor XIIIa functions as a catalyst, forming bonds between various protein substrates such as fibrin monomers, α_2-plasmin inhibitor, fibronectin, and collagen.[112] The action of this cross-linking of various plasma and extracellular matrix proteins contributes to hemostasis, wound healing, and the maintenance of pregnancy.

FXIII (M_r 320,000 daltons) circulates with fibrinogen. Extracellular or plasma FXIII has two subunits, α_2 and β_2 chains. The α_2 chains exist in various tissues and cells such as the placenta, platelets, macrophages, and prostate, and contain the active catalytic site for transglutaminase activity. The β subunit is synthesized in the liver and circulates as a free dimer or as a complex with the subunit. It is postulated that the β subunit contributes to the stabilization of the α subunit; however, the function of the β subunit remains unknown.

Congenital FXIII deficiency is inherited as an autosomal-recessive trait, with a high frequency of consanguinity in families with this disorder.[113] Clinically, the homozygous deficiency has moderate to severe hemorrhagic diatheses. This is characterized by the initial stoppage of bleeding followed by recurrence of bleeding 36 hours or more after the initial traumatic event. This results from the dissolution of the fibrin clot that initially formed and was not stabilized by FXIII. These soluble fibrin clots are highly susceptible to degradation by plasmin. This disorder can be diagnosed at birth because the most common clinical symptom is bleeding from the umbilical stump. Acquired partial deficiency has been reported with several diseases, including leukemias, DIC, and severe liver disease. Treatment includes transfusion with fresh frozen plasma or cryoprecipitate.

All routine laboratory screening tests for hemostasis will indicate normal results; PT, APTT, fibrinogen, bleeding time, and platelet count. The screening test for FXIII deficiency is based on the solubility of a recalcified plasma clot in a 5-molar urea solution. If the plasma is deficient in FXIII, the clot will dissolve within 24 hours. This is a qualitative test only and does not reflect the level of FXIII present, although activity of approximately 1% of normal is sufficient to prevent both an abnormal test result and symptoms in vivo.[114]

Prekallikrein (Fletcher Factor)

Prekallikrein (PK) (M_r of approximately 100,000 daltons), is a single-chain protein synthesized in the liver.[115] Prekallikrein is the substrate for factor XII to form kallikrein and factor XIa. Approximately 75% circulates bound to HMWK,[116] and 25% circulates as free PK.

There appears to be no ethnic or racial predilection for this disorder. However, both functional and antigenic PK lacking in Fletcher trait plasma have been most often reported in black Americans.[117] It has been reported to be inherited as both an autosomal-dominant and recessive trait with no apparent associated clinical bleeding disorders.[118] Patients with this deficiency have experienced thrombotic events (i.e., myocardial infarction, thromboembolism, and

multiple cerebral thromboses),[119–121] and vascular permeability is also defective.[122]

A marked prolongation of the APTT is characteristic of this disorder. Mixtures of patient plasma with pooled normal plasma, adsorbed plasma, or aged serum will correct the APTT. Additionally, this particular deficiency can be demonstrated by extending the contact activation time of the patient's plasma with kaolin-like APTT reagents. Interval incubations (e.g., 5 minutes, 10 minutes, and 15 minutes) will progressively shorten the APTT.

High-Molecular-Weight Kininogen (Fitzgerald Factor)

High-molecular-weight kininogen (HMWK) (M_r 200,000 daltons) is a single-chain glycoprotein. The deficiency has been described as an autosomal-recessive trait, and like PK shows no predilection to race. HMWK is known as the contact activation cofactor as it is required for contact activation.[123] Studies indicate that plasma HMWK exists as a procofactor that can be activated by cleavage with kallikrein.[124] Its binding to endothelial cells is necessary for the binding of factor XI and its activation to factor XIa as well as for the activation of factor IX to IXa by factor XIa.[125] This deficiency presents with a markedly prolonged APTT that corrects upon mixing with pooled normal plasma, adsorbed plasma, or aged serum. Although there is no apparent associated clinical bleeding disorder, patients have been observed with deep vein thrombosis and pulmonary embolus.[126]

Because there is no bleeding associated with factor XII, PK, or HMWK deficiencies, replacement therapy is not needed. Patients who require major surgery have had no incidence of bleeding.

➤ CIRCULATING ANTICOAGULANTS— INHIBITORS

Circulating anticoagulants are acquired inhibitors of the coagulation mechanism. These are endogenously produced and interfere with various in vitro coagulation tests. When detected, it is important to differentiate their specificity because some are clinically significant, whereas others are inconsequential. These defects are composed of immunoglobulins (autoantibodies or alloantibodies) directed against either specific clotting factors or components of the assay system.

Specific Factor Inhibitors

The specific inhibitors are characterized as antibodies. They either directly inhibit (neutralize) clotting factor activity or cause increased clearance by binding to a nonactive site. They may occur secondary to transfusion, clotting factor replacement therapy, or both. They can also arise spontaneously in patients with no known coagulopathy.

Factor VIII:C inhibitors, the most frequently encountered, can develop in patients with hemophilia A as a result of transfusion. These would be classified as alloantibodies. The inhibitor has also been found as an autoantibody in patients with rheumatoid arthritis, systemic lupus erythematosus, drug reaction, postpartum, different forms of malignancy, and in elderly patients with no apparent underlying disease. The mortality rate is approximately 20%. Spontaneous remission has been reported in approximately 38% of cases.[127]

Factor VIII:C inhibitors are predominantly IgG antibodies and do not interfere with the function of vWF. Additionally, the antibodies do not interfere with the bleeding time. The inhibitor should be suspected in patients with hemophilia when transfused factor VIII product has a short half-life, hemostasis is difficult to achieve, or both. Also, a spontaneous inhibitor should be suspected in anyone with no prior history who presents with massive bruising or hematoma.[128] A normal PT and a prolongation of the APTT with little to no correction when mixed with pooled normal plasma is a laboratory finding. Preincubation for 1 to 2 hours may sometimes be required to further demonstrate the time and temperature dependency of the antibody. The inhibitor titer can be quantitated by incubating pooled normal plasma with various dilutions of the patient's plasma for 2 hours at 37°C and measuring the residual FVIII:C activity. This is known as the Bethesda assay. A test specimen having 50% residual FVIII:C activity is considered to contain 1 Bethesda unit of inhibitor. The inhibitor titer then becomes the reciprocal of the dilution, which neutralizes 50% of the FVIII:C activity.

Treatment of patients with specific inhibitors can include factor VIII concentrates; steroids, alone or in combination; immunosuppressive therapy; cytotoxic agents; porcine factor VIII; prothrombin-complex concentrates; or plasmapheresis for patients with very high inhibitor levels.

Spontaneously acquired inhibitors to factors II, VII, and X are very rare. Factor II inhibitors are described in association with the lupus anticoagulant (see Nonspecific Inhibitors, following). There have been several reports of factors XI and XII inhibitors. Several cases were reported as factor XI deficiency with acquired inhibitors posttransfusion and other cases occurring in patients with systemic lupus erythematosus.[129,130] Acquired factor V inhibitor is also rare; it has occurred in only one reported case of factor V deficiency. The remaining cases occurred in elderly patients who previously had normal levels.[131] Patients who exhibit this inhibitor vary in clinical bleeding. The laboratory findings include prolongation of both the PT and the APTT, and mixing with pooled normal plasma does not correct the prolongations.

Nonspecific Inhibitors—Lupus Anticoagulants

Nonspecific inhibitors, as their name implies, are not directed against specific clotting factors. These are usually not associated with a bleeding risk and are usually not temperature-dependent, as in the case of anti-VIII:C or anti-V.[132–134] However, these inhibitors have been associated with thrombosis, fetal loss, and thrombocytopenia, with or without autoimmune disorder.

The nonspecific inhibitors belong to a family of disorders known as the antiphospholipid antibody syndrome (APS). The APS refers to the association of autoantibodies against phospholipid with clinically evident arterial and venous thrombosis. It is one of the most common causes of acquired coagulation defects associated with both venous and arterial thrombosis.[135] The APS is comprised of two related but clinically distinct syndromes involving members of the antiphospholipid family, anticardiolipin antibody (ACA) and the lupus anticoagulants (LAs). Thrombosis associated with ACA is markedly more common than thrombosis associated with LAs.[136]

LAs were first recognized in patients with systemic lupus erythematosus (SLE).[137] This designation is a misnomer, however, because these inhibitors often occur in patients without SLE and who are otherwise healthy and have no underlying medical condition. Therefore, it is more appropriate that they be termed lupus-like anticoagulants. LAs are immunoglobulins that interfere with one or more phospholipid-dependent tests of coagulation. They are usually polyclonal IgG or IgM, also IgA or in combination. They occur spontaneously (primary), or secondary, associated with autoimmune diseases, SLE, acquired immune deficiency syndrome (AIDS), infectious diseases (bacterial, viral, protozoal), antibiotic and other drug exposure, inflammation, malignancies, and lymphoproliferative disorders.[118]

The ability to detect LAs is dependent on the sensitivity of the reagent and the preparation of the plasma prior to analysis. Depletion of platelets, which are rich in phospholipids, is essential to avoid neutralization of the inhibitor, especially if the sample is to be frozen. Patients possessing lupus-like anticoagulants present in the laboratory with a prolonged APTT and a normal PT (usually because PT reagents have much higher phospholipid content). In some cases, both the PT and APTT are prolonged. These results give the impression that the patient may have a bleeding tendency. It should be noted that some patients with lupus-like anticoagulants have had clinically significant bleeding. The bleeding can be attributed to a depression of prothrombin activity. In these cases, the factor II activity has been found to be approximately 20%, resulting in severe and even fatal bleeding.[138,139] However, thrombosis is the major problem in patients with LAs. A mixing study with pooled normal plasma usually shows no correction of the prolonged APTT. What is occurring in vitro is a direct reaction against ionic phospholipids, which are present in the reagents used for coagulation screening assays (PT and APTT). This will also affect any factor assays based on these methodologies; however, LAs do not inactivate the clotting factors in vitro: they inhibit the formation of the prothrombinase complex (factors Xa, Va, calcium ions, factor II, and phospholipid surfaces), causing a prolongation of the clotting time.[129,130,140–142] There is also evidence that plasma immunoglobulins are affected by nonprocoagulant phospholipid cardiolipin. There is a high incidence of thrombotic disease in patients with elevated anticardiolipin antibody.[143] This was first noted with a high prevalence of falsely positive tests for syphilis (VDRL), the reagent component of which is the antigen cardiolipin. Patients who have lupus-like anticoagulants have been found to have elevated levels of anticardiolipin antibodies in their plasma.[144] LA is much more frequently associated with venous than arterial thrombosis. Conversely, clinical signs of ACA include deep vein thrombosis (DVT) and pulmonary embolism (PE) in addition to premature cerebrovascular disease and coronary artery disease.[126]

Testing for confirmation of the LA should include the use of test systems that have high phospholipid content that neutralizes or bypasses the inhibitor. These tests include the platelet neutralization procedure (PNP) and the high phospholipid APTT. PNP phospholipid is derived from washed, buffered, frozen platelets. This increase in phospholipid will correct the abnormal APTT. Methodologies using altered phospholipid structures (i.e., hexagonal phospholipids) have also been used as confirmatory techniques (Table 25–9). False-positive tests may occur in heparinized patients. Prolonged APTT results in patients with clotting factor deficiencies are not corrected with the PNP. An additional method using a low concentration of phospholipid is known as the diluted Russell's viper venom time (dRVVT) (Table 25–10).

Table 25-9
CONFIRMATORY TEST FOR LUPUS ANTICOAGULANTS: INCREASED PHOSPHOLIPID*

Test	Nature of Phospholipid	Other Features	Sensitivity	Heparin	Oral Anticoagulant	Factor Deficiency	Specific Inhibitors	Comments
Platelet neutralization procedure (PNP)	Outdated washed platelets freeze-thawed	Use with sensitive APTT system	Sensitive in most cases with APTT >2 sec above upper limit of normal	False positive	False positive	—	Weak factor V inhibitor may be positive	Stored aliquots of platelets Stable 3 mo. at −20°C
High phospholipid APTT	Cephalin 1:200, 1:50, 1:25 (4–8× normal concentration)	Kaolin activator	—	—	—	—	—	In original study, time-dependent pattern noted
Rabbit brain neutralization procedure (RBNP)	Cephalin high concentration (use 4× more lipid)	Kaolin, tilt tube	Original study 30/31 patients had + test; only 18/30 had + TTI	False positive	No effect	No effect	Slight shortening with factor VIII and XI inhibitors	—
PS-liposome APTT	PS vehicle final PS concentration (24 × 10⁶ moles/L)	Kaolin Manchester APTT reagent	—	False positive	No effect	No effect	No effect with factor VIII and IX inhibitor	Other lipids (PA, PE, PG, and PS) no effect
"Inside-out membrane absorption test"	Washed fresh human RBCs, lysed with phosphate buffer	Use APTT in mixture	—	No effect, since ECTEOLA is used to absorb heparin	—	No effect	No effect with factor VIII inhibitor	—

*The confirmatory test for lupus anticoagulants may be divided into two categories. First is the use of test systems that seek to accentuate the effect of the anticoagulant by decreasing the amount of phospholipid in the test. Thus, the available phospholipid surfaces necessary for the prothrombinase complex are limited and the presence of a low titer antiphospholipid antibody will prolong the coagulation time. The TTI (tissue thromboplastin inhibitor) and the dRVVT (dilute Russell's viper venom time) are examples of this system. The second group of tests rely on increased amounts of phospholipid to either neutralize or bypass the phopholipid antibodies and shorten the prolonged coagulation time (PNP).

Abbreviations: PA = phosphatidic acid; PE = phosphatidyl ethanol; PG = phosphatidyl glycerol; PS = phosphatidylserine

Source: From Triplet, DA, and Brandt, JT: Confirmatory test for lupus anticoagulant. Hematol Pathol 2:121, 1988, with permission.

CONFIRMATORY TESTS FOR LUPUS ANTICOAGULANTS: DECREASED PHOSPHOLIPID

Test	Nature of Phospholipid	Other Features	Sensitivity	Heparin	Oral Anticoagulant	Factor Deficiency	Specific Inhibitors	Comment
Tissue thrombo-plastin inhibition (TTI)	Thromboplastin diluted with saline 1:50 and 1:500	—	Sensitive but not specific; positive in 30% normal subjects	False positive 0.2–0.8 U/mL of heparin	False positive	False positive with factor VII, X, V, VIII, IX deficiency	False positive with factors VIII, IX, or V inhibitors	May be negative with IgM drug-induced LA
Dilute Russell viper venom test (dRVVT)	Cephalin PTT diluted 1:8 TBS Correction: 0.1 mL ionophore treated platelets	RVV diluted 1:200 in TBS	Sensitive when compared with APTT and TTI	False positive	False positive corrected by mixing studies	False positive with factor V or X deficiency	False positive with factor V inhibitor	Correction studies may use ionophore* treated platelets or PNP
KCT	No added phospholipid; KCT very sensitive to residual platelets	May use mixture of normal and patient plasma	Presence of platelets will significantly shorten KCT in presence of LA	—	—	—	—	Use of filtered plasma will increase sensitivity
Dilute phospholipid APTT (PL-APTT)	Cephalin PTT diluted 1:5, 1:10; 1:20; 1:40	Mixing patient and normal plasma 1:1 and 0.5 silica	—	No effect if protamine is added	No effect	No effect	Strong inhibitor (> 10 Bethesda units) may give false positive	

Abbreviations: KCT = kaolin clotting time; TBS = Tris-buffered saline

*Ionophore treated platelets = platelets treated to allow transmission of ions across its all membrane.

Source: From Triplett, DA and Brandt, JT: Confirmatory test for lupus anticoagulants. Hematol Pathol 2:121, 1988, with permission.

> **Table 25-11**
FACTOR DEFICIENCIES AND TEST RESULTS

Factor	BT	PT	APTT	Adsorbed Plasma	Aged Serum	TT	Fibrinogen	Urea Solubility	Platelet Count	D-Dimer	FDP
I	N	A	A	C	NC	A	A	N	N	—	—
II	N	A	A	NC	NC	N	N	N	N	—	—
V	A	A	A	C	NC	N	N	N	N	—	—
VII	N	A	N	NC	C	N	N	N	N	—	—
VIII:C	N	N	A	C	NC	N	N	N	N	—	—
VIII:vWF	A	N	A	C	C	N	N	N	N	—	—
IX	N	N	A	NC	C	N	N	N	N	—	—
X	N	A	A	NC	C	N	N	N	N	—	—
XI	N	N	A	C	C	N	N	N	N	—	—
XII	N	N	A	C	C	N	N	N	N	—	—
XIII	N	N	N	—	—	N	N	A	N	—	—
Prekallikrein	N	N	A*	C	C	N	N	N	N	—	—
HMWK	N	N	A	C	C	N	N	N	N	—	—
Plasminogen	N	N	N	—	—	N	N	N	N	—	—
DIC	—	A	A	—	—	A	A	N	A	A	A
Antithrombin III	N	N	N	—	—	N	N	N	N	—	—

*The APTT will shorten after prolonged activation of the contact system.
Abbreviations: N = normal; C = correction; NC = no correction; BT = bleeding time; PT = prothrombin time; APTT = activated partial thromboplastin time; DD = D-dimer; FDP = fibrin degradation products
   Source: From Pittiglio, DH, et al: Treating hemostatic disorders. A problem-oriented approach. In Pittiglio, DH: Hemostasis Overview. American Association of Blood Banks, Arlington, VA, 1984, p 31, with permission.

This reagent, which is an extract from the venom of *Vipera russellii,* directly activates factor X. By diluting the venom, whereby there is enough to activate factor X, and providing a dilute, buffered phospholipid as the cofactor for prothrombinase production, the sensitivity to inhibitors directed at phospholipid is increased and a prolonged clotting time is achieved. One-stage factor assays show artificially decreased factor activity caused by impaired reactivity of the phospholipid reagent used in the test system. The dRVVT is also affected by the presence of heparin[145] (unless the heparin is neutralized prior to assay) and warfarin.

The continuing association between antiphospholipid antibodies and thrombotic episodes has supported advances in the diagnosis of this syndrome. No one assay is specific for LA. The most recent guidelines for LA testing were developed by the Scientific and Standardization Committee (SSC) Subcommittee for the Standardization of Lupus Anticoagulants. In its 1995 report, the SSC states its criteria for the laboratory diagnosis of LA as follows:

1. Prolongation of at least one phospholipid-dependent clotting test
2. Evidence of inhibitor activity shown by the effect of patient plasma on pooled normal plasma
3. Evidence that the inhibitor activity is dependent on phospholipid
4. LA must be distinguished carefully from other coagulopathies that may give similar results or occur concurrently with LA.[146]

A complete personal and family history is of utmost importance in beginning a workup for a hemostatic defect. This should also include a list of any prescription or over-the-counter medications. Table 25–11 summarizes the test results for the factor deficiencies presented in this chapter.

> **CASE STUDY 1**

A 12-year-old boy underwent tooth extraction in preparation for orthodontia. Persistent bleeding followed. The history was remarkable for bruising and frequent epistaxis. The patient's mother also experienced easy bruising and menorrhagia.

Physical examination revealed several medium-sized ecchymotic lesions on the lower extremities. Laboratory findings were as follows (reference ranges in parentheses):

PT	12.0 sec	(10–14 sec)
APTT	39.5 sec	(23–36 sec)
BT	> 15min	(2–9 min)
Platelet count	$300 \times 10^9/L$	(150–$450 \times 10^9/L$)
FVIII:C	0.30 U/mL	(0.50–1.50 U/mL)
vWF:Ag	45 %	(50%–150 %)
vWFR:Co	41%	(50%–150%)
RIPA*	Depressed response	(Normal response)
Multimers	Normal	(Normal)

*Ristocetin-induced platelet aggregation

The history of bruising, epistaxis, and dental bleeding with a prolonged APTT, BT, and reduced FVIII:C, vWF:Ag, vWFR:Co, and RIPA are indicative of classic von Willebrand's disease (type 1).

Questions

1. What blood product can correct the RIPA value in this case?
2. What laboratory values reflect a type 1 von Willebrand's disease?
3. What form of therapy would be indicated here?

Answers

1. Concentrates of factor VIII, cryoprecipitate, and von Willebrand factor can correct the RIPA response in this case.
2. Reduced levels of factor VIII:C (0.30 U/mL), vWf:Ag (45%), and vWfR:Co (41%) along with the prolonged bleeding time and depressed RIPA are classically seen with Type 1 von Willebrand's disease.
3. DDAVP would be advantageous as a prophylactic treatment prior to any future dental extractions or minor surgical procedure. This avoids exposure to any blood products by causing a transient increase in factor VIII:C and vWf.

► CASE STUDY 2

A full-term male infant was born by normal vaginal delivery. Thirty hours postpartum, there was new onset of oozing of blood at the umbilical stump. Laboratory analysis included:

CBC and platelet count	Normal	(10–14 sec)
PT	14.0 sec	
APTT	36 sec	(23–36 sec)
Fibrinogen	400 mg/dL	(160–450 mg/dL)

Clinical presentation did not indicate a hemorrhagic tendency. Late onset of umbilical stump bleeding prompted the evaluation of factor XIII. A recalcified plasma clot exposed to a 5-molar urea solution dissolved within 4 hours. This is conclusive for factor XIII deficiency.

Questions

1. Is the 5-molar urea dissolution test a qualitative or quantitative determination?
2. What treatment is indicated for this patient?

Answers

1. 5M Urea dissolution for factor XIII deficiency is a qualitative determination, however, the test is positive when activity is less than 1%.
2. Treatment would consist of fresh frozen plasma or cryoprecipitate infusion.

► CASE STUDY 3

A 5-year-old boy presented in the emergency department with a hemarthrosis of the right knee after falling off a playground swing. Physical examination revealed a well-nourished child with no fractures or other ecchymoses. He was afebrile. Laboratory findings were as follows:

CBC and platelet count	Normal	
PT	13 sec	(10–14 sec)
APTT	87 sec	(23–36 sec)
Fibrinogen	325 mg/dL	(160–450 mg/dL)
BT	6 min	(2–9 min)

Further studies included:

APTT 1:1 mix	32 sec	(23–36 sec)
FVIII:C	0.10 U/mL	(0.50–1.50 U/mL)
vWF:Ag	90%	(50%–150%)

This patient was known to have hemophilia A.

Questions

1. What material did the laboratory professional use when performing this mixing study?
2. What treatment is indicated for this patient?
3. Which factors are present in adsorbed plasma? In aged serum?

Answers

1. The mixing study in this case would have been performed with pooled normal plasma or adsorbed plasma. Aged serum would not have corrected the APTT.
2. This patient requires infusion of factor VIII concentrate.
3. Adsorbed plasma lacks the vitamin K–dependent fctors (II, VII, IX, X) leaving factors V, VIII, XI, XII, PK, HMWK, and fibrinogen. Aged serum lacks fibrinogen (I), factors II, V, and VIII leaving factors VII, IX, X, XI, XII, HMWK, and PK.

► CASE STUDY 4

A 40-year-old woman was scheduled for an elective surgical procedure. Preadmission testing revealed the following results:

CBC and platelet count	Normal	
PT	18.0 sec	(10–14 sec)
APTT	30.0 sec	(23–36 sec)

After further examination, the patient stated that she had episodes of epistaxis and easy bruising. Additional laboratory testing included:

continued

| PT 1:1 mix | 13.0 sec | (10–14 sec) |
| FVII | 0.30 U/mL | (0.50–1.50 U/mL) |

This patient has factor VII deficiency. Factor VII is not measured by the APTT and is normal, whereas the PT is sensitive to deficiencies of the extrinsic system (factors I, II, V, VII, and X) and is prolonged in these cases.

Questions
1. What material was used to perform the mixing study?
2. What treatment is indicated here?
3. Why was the PT prolonged and the APTT normal in this case?

Answers
1. The mixing study in this case would have been performed with pooled normal plasma or aged serum. Adsorbed plasma would not have corrected the PT.
2. This patient would require fresh frozen plasma or prothrombin-complex concentrate. However, if the deficiency can be attributed to poor diet, liver disease, or warfarin therapy, vitamin K supplementation may be preferable to using blood products.
3. The PT was prolonged because the extrinsic pathway could not proceed normally, caused by the deficiency of factor VII. The APTT was normal because factor VII does not participate in the intrinsic pathway and therefore the test is not sensitive to this defect.

This patient has a lupus anticoagulant with anticardiolipin-antiphospholipid antibodies. These are known to cause recurrent spontaneous abortion, as well as thrombotic events such as stroke, deep vein thromboses, and pulmonary embolism.

Questions
1. What complex is inhibited by LA, causing a prolongation of the clotting time?
2. Why did the PNP correct the APTT in this patient?
3. What form of treatment is indicated here?

Answers
1. The complex which is inhibited by LA is the Prothrombinase complex (factor Xa, V, II, calcium and phospholipid) thereby delaying the formation of fibrin and producing a prolonged clotting time.
2. The high concentration of phospholipid in the PNP bypasses or "neutralizes" the inhibitor thereby allowing the APTT to proceed more normally and produce a shorter or "corrected" value versus the saline.
3. Treatment of a patient with LA would require anticoagulation with warfarin or, in some circumstances, heparin may be used (e.g., in obstetrics; warfarin crosses the placenta and can harm the fetus).

➤ CASE STUDY 5

A 29-year-old woman was seen by her obstetrician for prenatal care. She had three previous pregnancies, two resulting in spontaneous first-trimester miscarriages and the third in fetal demise at 28 weeks' gestation. Laboratory values were as follows:

CBC and platelet count	Normal	
PT	11.5 sec	(10–14 sec)
APTT	45.0 sec	(23–36 sec)
Fibrinogen	375 mg/dL	(160–450 mg/dL)

Further studies included:

APTT 1:1 mix	43.0 sec	(23–36 sec)
dRVVT	33 sec	(< 25 sec)
PNP (PNP versus saline)	32 sec/47 sec	(PNP versus saline < 5 sec)
Anticardiolipin antibodies:	IgG: 55 units	(0–14 units)
	IgA: 5 units	(0–15 units)
	IgM: 12 units	(0–5 units)

➤ CASE STUDY 6

A 25-year-old man was admitted for hernia repair. Admission laboratory data were as follows:

CBC and platelet count	Normal	
PT	12.5 sec	(10–14 sec)
APTT	115 sec	(23–36 sec)
APTT 1:1	32.0 sec	(23–36 sec)
FVIII:C	0.97 U/mL	(0.50–1.50 U/mL)
Factor IX	1.04 U/mL	(0.50–1.50 U/mL)
Factor XI	1.10 U/mL	(0.70–1.30 U/mL)
Factor XII	0.96 U/mL	(0.70–1.40 U/mL)

Interval incubations of the patient's plasma with the APTT reagent, which contained micronized silica as the activator, produced the following results:

5-min incubation	74.0 sec	
10-min incubation	57.0 sec	
15-min incubation	35.0 sec	
Prekallikrein activity	< 0.01 U/mL	(0.30–1.00 U/mL)

This patient was deficient for prekallikrein. Contact system deficiencies (factor XII, HMWK, prekallikrein) do not pose any hemorrhagic risk.

Questions

1. Why was the APTT affected exclusive of the PT?
2. What treatment is indicated here?
3. What materials are appropriate for mixing studies in this deficiency?

Answers

1. The PT measures the extrinsic pathway, in which PK is not involved. Therefore, only the APTT will reflect an abnormal clotting time.
2. No treatment is indicated: there is no associated risk of bleeding.
3. Mixing studies can be performed with pooled normal plasma, adsorbed plasma, and/or aged serum, which all contain PK.

➤ CASE STUDY 7

A 65-year-old woman with liver disease was admitted to the medical intensive care unit. Admission laboratory data were as follows:

PT	14.5 sec	(10–14 sec)
APTT	39.0 sec	(23–36 sec)
Fibrinogen	175 mg/dL	(160–450 mg/dL)
Thrombin time	18 sec	(4–12 sec)

Prolongation of the APTT and thrombin time could be caused by the presence of heparin. This should be ruled out before further testing is performed.

Reptilase time	29 sec	(18–22 sec)

PT and APTT 1:1 mixes showed full correction of the prolongations. Factors VIII:C, IX, XI, and XII were within normal limits.

This patient was not on heparin, as evidenced by the prolonged reptilase time. The combination of a decreased fibrinogen level and prolonged thrombin and reptilase times are indicative of a dysfibrinogenemia, especially in patients with liver disease. Slight prolongation of the PT may also be noted and will not be attributable to any extrinsic factor deficiency. Antigenic assay of fibrinogen usually results in higher values than the functional (clottable) assay.

Questions

1. How can it be known that this patient is not on heparin therapy?
2. Differentiate between the thrombin time and reptilase time with regard to heparin.
3. What treatment is indicated here?

Answers

1. The prolonged thrombin time and reptilase time prove that the patient is not on heparin.
2. Heparin, even in relatively small amounts, will

prolong the thrombin time. The reptilase time, which is unaffected by heparin, will be normal.
3. Treatment for this patient could include anticoagulants if there is evidence of thrombosis.

➤ CASE STUDY 8

A 60-year-old woman was admitted to the emergency department with hemorrhage into the right arm and right breast. No previous history of bleeding or medication was indicated. Laboratory data upon admission were as follows:

PT	12.0 sec	(10–14 sec)
APTT	58.0 sec	(23–36 sec)
Fibrinogen	400 mg/dL	(160–450 mg/dL)
APTT 1:1 mix	40 sec	(23–36 sec)
dRVVT	21 sec	(< 25 sec)
PNP (PNP versus saline)	58 sec/59 sec	(PNP versus saline < 5 sec)

This patient does not have a lupus anticoagulant, but still does not correct on mixing with pooled normal plasma. Further studies must be performed. Incubation of the patient's plasma with pooled normal plasma, in various dilutions for 2 hours at 37°C, indicates the presence of an inhibitor by showing prolongation of the APTT over time. Also, factor analysis indicates decreased activity of a specific factor because of the presence of an inhibitor.

FVIII:C	0.10 U/mL	(0.50–1.50 U/mL)
Factor IX	0.90 U/mL	(0.50–1.50 U/mL)
Factor XI	0.95 U/mL	(0.70–1.30 U/mL)

Factor inhibitor analysis (Bethesda assay) for factor VIII:C produced a titer of 8 Bethesda units of inhibitor activity (normal is less than 0.5 units). One Bethesda unit of inhibitor is equivalent to 50% residual factor activity after incubation at 37°C for 2 hours. This patient developed a spontaneous inhibitor to factor VIII:C that resulted in the massive bleeding into the tissue of her arm and breast.

Questions

1. What material was used to perform the 1:1 ratio mixing study?
2. What test result rules out the presence of a lupus anticoagulant?
3. What treatment is indicated here?

Answers

1. Mixing studies were performed with either pooled normal plasma or adsorbed plasma.
2. The presence of a lupus anticoagulant is ruled out by the negative DRVVT and PNP tests.
3. Treatment of a factor VIII inhibitor can include factor VIII concentrates (human or porcine);

continued

prothrombin-complex concentrates; steroids (alone or in combination); immunosuppressive therapy; cytotoxic agents; or plasmapheresis if the inhibitor titer is very high.

➤ CASE STUDY 9

A 37-year-old man was seen by his physician for a routine physical examination. A full blood workup was drawn and sent to a reference laboratory for analysis. Results were as follows:

CBC and platelet count	Normal	
PT	12.0 sec	(10–14 sec)
APTT	60.0 sec	(23–36 sec)
Thrombin time	4.5 sec	(4–12 sec)

The patient was asymptomatic for any bleeding. Testing was continued and produced the following results:

APTT 1:1 mix	32 sec	(23–36 sec)
FVIII:C	0.90 U/mL	(0.50–1.50 U/mL)
Factor IX	0.77 U/mL	(0.50–1.50 U/mL)
Factor XI	0.45 U/mL	(0.70–1.30 U/mL)

This patient was found to have factor XI deficiency. The initial history revealed that he was of Eastern European–Ashkenazi Jewish background. This factor deficiency is prevalent among this population. The patient's factor level was not depressed enough to produce symptoms, but could have posed a significant surgical risk. Heterozygous factor XI deficiency has a variable presentation and bleeding risk may not correlate with factor levels.

Questions
1. Why was the APTT affected exclusive of the PT in this case?
2. What does the APTT mixing study result indicate?
3. What treatment is indicated here?

Answers
1. The PT measures the extrinsic pathway, in which factor XI is not involved. Therefore, only the APTT will reflect an abnormal clotting time.
2. The APTT mixing study shows a correction of the APTT into the normal range, indicative of a factor deficiency of the intrinsic pathway, most likely factor VIII, IX, XI, XII, HMWK, or PK (a normal PT rules out factor II, V, or X, and a normal TT rules out fibrinogen deficiency).
3. No treatment is necessary for factor XI deficiency unless the patient requires surgery and the factor XI activity is less than 0.20–0.30 U/mL. Fresh, fresh-frozen, or the supernatant plasma after the removal of cryoprecipitate may be used in severe deficiencies to control bleeding.

➤ CASE STUDY 10

A 66-year-old man with a diagnosis of amyloidosis was admitted to the hospital with severe gastrointestinal bleeding. Admission laboratory data included:

CBC	Anemia due to chronic blood loss	
Platelet count	Normal	
PT	45 sec	(10–14 sec)
APTT	95 sec	(23–36 sec)
Fibrinogen	400 mg/dL	(160–450 mg/dL)
Thrombin time	5 sec	(4–12 sec)
PT 1:1 mix	13 sec	(10–14 sec)
APTT 1:1 mix	30 sec	(23–36 sec)
Russell's viper venom time	55 sec	(14–20 sec)
Factor II	0.75 U/mL	(0.50–1.50 U/mL)
Factor V	0.93 U/mL	(0.50–1.50 U/mL)
Factor IX	0.90 U/mL	(0.50–1.50 U/mL)
Factor X	0.05 U/mL	(0.50–1.50 U/mL)

This patient was determined to have factor X deficiency secondary to amyloidosis. Other vitamin K–dependent factors were normal, as was factor V, which ruled out a nutritional deficit or liver involvement.

Questions
1. Why were both PT and APTT prolonged in this case?
2. What test results indicate a factor deficiency as opposed to a circulating anticoagulant?
3. If adsorbed plasma were used in the mixing study, what would you expect the result to be?

Answers
1. Factor X participates in both the intrinsic and extrinsic pathways (also known as the common pathway), which will produce prolongation of both the PT and APTT if deficient.
2. A factor deficiency is present rather than a circulating anticoagulant, demonstrated by the correction of both the PT and APTT on 1:1 mixing and the normal levels of other factors except factor X. The RVVT will be prolonged in factor X deficiency.
3. Adsorbed plasma lacks the vitamin K–dependent factors (II, VII, IX, X) and would therefore not produce a correction on 1:1 mixing studies.

QUESTIONS

1. Which of the following can produce defects that lead to impairment of the coagulation system?
   a. Decreased factor synthesis
   b. Interference of abnormal molecules
   c. Loss, consumption, or inactivation of factors
   d. All of the above

2. Which of the following diseases show decreased activity of factor VIII:C?
   a. Hemophilia A
   b. Hemophilia B
   c. Parahemophilia
   d. Hemophilia C

3. Which coagulation disorder has decreased activity of factor VIII:C, vWF:Ag, and vWFR:Co, and a prolonged bleeding time test?
   a. Hypoprothrombinemia
   b. von Willebrand's disease
   c. Hemophilia A
   d. Hemophilia B

4. The dissolution of a clot with 5-molar urea is an indication of which factor deficiency?
   a. Factor II
   b. Factor XIII
   c. von Willebrand's disease
   d. Lupus anticoagulant

5. The factor defect that has a normal APTT and a prolonged PT is:
   a. Factor I
   b. High-molecular-weight kininogen
   c. Factor VII
   d. Factor X

6. A patient with amyloidosis can have which factor deficiency?
   a. Factor V
   b. Factor X
   c. Factor VIII:C
   d. Factor II

7. The reptilase time will be normal in the presence of:
   a. Heparin
   b. Dysfibrinogenemia
   c. Afibrinogenemia
   d. Hypofibrinogenemia

8. Which of the following is considered a low phospholipid test for LA identification?
   a. Platelet neutralization procedure
   b. Ionophore platelet procedure
   c. Diluted Russell's viper venom time
   d. Kaolin clotting time

9. All of the following statements are true regarding the detection of LA except:
   a. Platelet-poor samples are required.
   b. The APTT is frequently prolonged and is usually the first indication of the presence of LA.
   c. A mixture of patient plasma with pooled normal plasma will correct the prolonged APTT.
   d. The diluted Russell's viper venom time may be used to confirm the presence of LA.

10. Activated protein C resistance:
    a. Is the result of a single point mutation of the factor V gene in 90% of cases
    b. Leads to increased thrombin generation as a result of impaired factor V degradation
    c. Is found in 20% to 60% of the patients with venous thrombosis
    d. All of the above

SUMMARY CHART

➤ Screening tests for coagulation abnormalities should include:
  ➤ **Complete blood count (CBC), platelet count, differential smear**
  ➤ **Prothrombin time (PT)**
  ➤ **Activated partial thromboplastin time (APTT)**
  ➤ **Fibrinogen**
  ➤ **Thrombin time**
  ➤ **Bleeding time**
➤ When the platelet count and morphology are normal, the results of the PT and APTT should be evaluated as follows:
  ➤ **For an abnormal PT with a normal APTT, a mixing study of the PT should be performed using pooled normal plasma; if the PT is corrected, a factor VII deficiency should be considered and subsequent factor assay is indicated.**
  ➤ **For abnormal PTs that do not correct with a mixing study, inhibitors to factors II, V, VII, or X should be considered.**
  ➤ **For a normal PT with an abnormal APTT, a mixing study of the APTT should be performed using pooled normal plasma. If the APTT is corrected, a deficiency of factor(s) VIII:C, IX, XI, XII, prekallikrein (PK), and/or high-molecular-weight kininogen (HMWK) should be considered, with subsequent testing for specific factor assay performed.**
  ➤ **For abnormal APTTs that do not correct with a mixing study, inhibitors to factor(s) VIII:C, IX, XI, XII, PK, and/or HMWK should be considered as well as the presence of the lupus anticoagulant or the anticoagulant heparin.**
  ➤ **The presence of heparin can be ruled out if the thrombin time is normal.**
  ➤ **For specimens that have both an abnormal PT and APTT that corrects with mixing studies, deficiencies of factors I, II, V, and X should be considered.**
  ➤ **If an abnormal PT and APTT does not correct with mixing studies, an inhibitor to factors II, V, or X should be considered.**
➤ The lupus anticoagulants may be IgG, IgA, or IgM in nature and are detected by the platelet neutralization procedure (PNP) and the diluted Russell's viper venom time (dRVVT).
➤ The most common inhibitor to a specific clotting factor is factor VIII:C (FVIII:C); the inhibitor is predominantly IgG and temperature-dependent;

laboratory assays for inhibitors are measured in Bethesda units, where a specimen containing 50% residual FVIII:C activity is considered to contain 1 Bethesda unit.

➤ Laboratory studies for von Willebrand's disease should include a bleeding time, platelet count, PT, APTT, mixing studies, FVIII:C, von Willebrand's factor antigenic component (vWF:Ag), ristocetin cofactor activity (vWFR:Co), ristocetin-induced platelet aggregation, and multimer analysis.

➤ Laboratory findings in patients with hemophilia A include a prolonged APTT, normal PT, and normal bleeding time; mixing studies with normal or adsorbed plasma will correct the APTT.

➤ The thrombin time assesses thrombin-fibrinogen interactions and fibrin polymerization. It will be abnormal in the presence of heparin, hypofibrinogenemia, dysfibrinogenemia, afibrinogenemia, and fibrinogen/fibrin degradation products (FDPs).

ACKNOWLEDGMENTS

The authors gratefully acknowledge the contributions of Judith Brody, MD.

References

1. Rock, G: Defects of plasma clotting factors. In Pittiglio, DH, and Sacher, RA (eds): Clinical Hematology and Fundamentals of Hemostasis, ed 1. FA Davis, Philadelphia, 1987, p 365.
2. Hantgan, RR, et al: Fibrinogen structure and physiology. In Colman, RW, et al (eds): Hemostasis and Thrombosis: Basic Principles and Clinical Practice, ed 3. JB Lippincott, Philadelphia, 1994, p 277.
3. Ibid, p 277.
4. Hirsh J, et al: Approach to the thrombophilic patient. In Colman, RW, et al (eds): Hemostasis and Thrombosis: Basic Principles and Clinical Practice, ed 3. JB Lippincott, Philadelphia, 1994, p 1548.
5. Bommer, W, et al: Kongenitale Afibrinogename. Teil I. Ann Paedlatr 200:46, 1963.
6. Grainick, HR, and Connaghan, W: In Williams, WJ, et al (eds): Hematology, ed 5. McGraw-Hill, New York, 1994, p 1441.
7. Girolami, A, et al: Rarer quantitative and qualitative abnormalities of coagulation. Clin Hematol Coag Dis 14:385, 1985.
8. Hantgan, RR, et al: Fibrinogen structure and physiology. In Colman, RW, et al (eds): Hemostasis and Thrombosis: Basic Principles and Clinical Practice, ed 3. JB Lippincott, Philadelphia, 1994, p 291.
9. Henschen, A, et al: Genetically abnormal fibrinogens—some current characterization strategies. In Haverkate, F, et al (eds): Fibrinogen Structure. Functional Aspects, Metabolism. Walter de Gruyter, Berlin, 1983, p 125.
10. McDonagh, J, et al. In Colman, RW, et al (eds): Hemostasis and Thrombosis: Basic Principles and Clinical Practice, ed 3. Dysfibrinogenemia and Other Disorders of Fibrinogen Structure and Function. JB Lippincott, Philadelphia, 1994, p 321.
11. Reptilase is a registered trademark of Pentapharm Ltd.
12. Latallo, ZS, and Teisseyre, E: Evaluation of Reptilase-R and thrombin clotting time in the presence of fibrinogen degradation products and heparin. Scand J Haematol 13(Suppl):261, 1971.
13. Donati, MB, et al: Fibrinogen degradation in vivo: Effect on the reptilase time and on the thrombin time. Scand J Haematol 13(Suppl):259, 1971.
14. Francis, CW, and Marder, VJ: Physiologic regulation and pathologic disorders of fibrinolysis. In Colman, RW, et al (eds): Hemostasis and Thrombosis: Basic Principles and Clinical Practice, ed 3. JB Lippincott, Philadelphia, 1994, p 1089.
15. Davie, EW, et al: The coagulation cascade: Initiation, maintenance and regulation. Biochemistry 30:10363, 1991.
16. Shapiro, SS, and McCord, IS: Prothrombin. In Spaet, TH (ed): Progress In Hemostasis and Thrombosis, vol IV. Grune & Stratton, New York, 1978.
17. Chong, L-L, et al: A case of "super" warfarin poisoning. Scand J Haematol 36:314, 1986.
18. Jensen, R: Screening and Molecular Diagnosis in Hemostasis. Clin Hemost Rev 13:12, 1999.
19. Poort, SR, et al: A common genetic variation in the 3′-untranslated region of the prothrombin gene is associated with elevated plasma prothrombin levels and an increase in venous thrombosis. Blood 88:3698, 1996.
20. Rosendall, FR, et al: A common prothrombin variant (20210 G to A) increases the risk of myocardial infarction in young women. Blood 90:1747, 1997.
21. DeStefano, V, et al: Prothrombin G20210A mutant genotype is a risk factor for cerebrovascular ischemic disease in young patients. Blood 91:3562, 1998.
22. DeStefano, V, et al: Prevalence of mild hyperhomocysteinaemia and association with thrombophilic genotypes (factor V Leiden and prothrombin G20210A) in Italian patients with venous thromboembolic disease. Br J Haematol 106:564, 1999.
23. DeStefano, V, et al: The risk of recurrent deep venous thrombosis among heterozygous carriers of both factor V Leiden and the G20210A prothrombin mutation. N Engl J Med 341:801, 1999.
24. Owren, PA: The coagulation of blood: Investigation on a new clotting factor. Acta Med Scand (Suppl) 194:1, 1947.
25. Owren, PA, and Cooper, T: Parahemophilia. Arch Intern Med 95:194, 1955.
26. Colman, RW: Factor V. Prog Hemost Thromb 3:109, 1976.
27. Jandl, JH: Blood: Textbook of Hematology. Little, Brown, Boston, 1987.
28. Chiu, HC, et al: Biosynthesis of coagulation Factor V by megakaryocytes. J Clin Invest 75:339, 1985.
29. Nesheim, ME, et al: Isolation and study of acquired inhibitor of human coagulation factor V. J Clin Invest 77:405, 1986.
30. Dahlback, B, et al: Familial thrombophilia due to a previously unrecognized mechanism characterized by poor anticoagulant response to activated protein C: Prediction of a cofactor to activated protein C. Proc Natl Acad Sci USA 90:1004, 1993.
31. Press, RD, and DeLoughery, TG: Thrombotic risk assessment; molecular and conventional testing for a common, treatable genetic disease. Am Assoc Clin Chem Clin Lab News 126:10, 2000.
32. Jensen, R: Screening and molecular diagnosis in hemostasis. Clin Hemost Rev 13:12, 1999.
33. Hall, CA, et al: A clinical and family study of hereditary proconvertin (factor VII) deficiency. Am J Med 37:172, 1964.
34. Dische, FE, and Benfield, V: Congenital factor VII deficiency: Haematological and genetic aspects. Acta Haematol 21:257, 1959.
35. Davie, EW, et al: The coagulation cascade: Initiation, maintenance and regulation. Biochemistry 30:10363, 1991.
36. Owen, CA, Jr, et al: Generation of factor VIII coagulant activity by isolated, perfused neonatal pig livers and adult rat livers. Br J Haematol 43:307, 1979.
37. Shaw, E, et al: Synthesis of procoagulant factor VIII, factor VIII–related antigen and other coagulation factors by the isolated perfused rat liver. Br J Haematol 41:585, 1979.
38. Bloom, AL: The biosynthesis of factor VIII. Clin Haematol 8:53, 1979.
39. Tuddenham, EGD, et al: Response to infusion of proelectrolyte fractionated human factor VIII concentrates in human haemophilia A and von Willebrand disease. Br J Haematol 52:2S9, 1982.
40. Koster, T, et al: Role of clotting factor VIII in effect of von Willebrand factor on occurrence of deep-vein thrombosis. Lancet 345:152, 1995.
41. Miale, JB: Hemostasis and blood coagulation: Hemophilia (factor VIII deficiency) In Miale, JB (ed): Laboratory Medicine: Hematology, ed 6. CV Mosby, St. Louis, 1982, p 823.
42. Ibid.
43. McGlasson, DL: Defects of plasma clotting factors. In Harmening, DM (ed): Clinical Hematology and Fundamentals of Hemostasis, ed 2. FA Davis, Philadelphia, 1992, p 463.
44. Hoyer, LW, and Rick, ME: Implications of immunological methods for measuring antihemophilic factor (factor VIII). Ann NY Acad Sci 240:97, 1975.
45. Ratnoff, OD, and Bennett, B: The genetics of hereditary disorders of blood coagulation. Science 179:1291, 1973.
46. McGlasson, DL: Defects of plasma clotting factors. In Harmening, DM (ed): Clinical Hematology and Fundamentals of Hemostasis, ed 2. FA Davis, Philadelphia, 1992, p 468.
47. Miller, JL: Blood coagulation and fibrinolysis. In Henry, JB (ed): Clinical Diagnosis and Management, ed 17. WB Saunders, Philadelphia, 1984, p 765.
48. Weiss, AE: Circulating inhibitors in hemophilia A and B: Epidemiology and methods of detection. In Brinkhous, KM, and Henker, HC (eds): Handbook of Hemophilia. Excerpta Medica, Amsterdam, 1975, p 29.
49. Shapiro, SS: Hemorrhagic disorders associated with circulating inhibitors. In Ratnoff, OD, and Forbes, CD (eds): Disorders of Hemostasis. Grune & Stratton. Orlando, FL, 1984, p 271.
50. Kasper, CK, et al: A more uniform measurement of factor VIII inhibitors. Thromb Diath Haemorrh 34:869, 1975.
51. Bennett, B, et al: Studies on the nature of antihemophilic factor (factor VIII): Further evidence relating the AHF-like antigens in normal and hemophiliac plasma. J Clin Invest 52:2191, 1971.
52. Montgomery, RR, and Coller, BS: von Willebrand disease. In Colman, RW, et al (eds): Hemostasis and Thrombosis: Basic Principles and Clinical Practice, ed 3. JB Lippincott, Philadelphia, 1994, p 138.
53. Wagner, EE: Immunolocalization of von Willebrand protein in Weibel-Palade bodies of human endothelial cells. J Cell Biol 95:355, 1982.
54. Enbal, A, and Loscalzo, J: Glycocalicin binding to vWf adsorbed onto collagen-coated or polystyrene surfaces. Thromb Res 56:347, 1989.
55. Howard, NA, and Firkin, BG: Ristocetin—a new tool in the investigation of platelet. Thromb Diath Haemorrh 26:362, 1971.
56. Montgomery, RR, and Coller, BS: Von Willebrand disease. In Colman, RW, et al (eds): Hemostasis and Thrombosis: Basic Principles and Clinical Practice, ed 3. JB Lippincott, Philadelphia, 1994, p 141.
57. Ibid, p 138.
58. Ibid, p 146.
59. Ibid, p 144.
60. Coller, BS: Von Willebrand's disease. In Ratnoff, OD, and Farbes, CD (eds): Disorders of Hemostasis. Grune & Stratton, Orlando, FL, 1984, p 241.
61. Holmberg, L, and Nelson, IM: Von Willebrand's disease. Clin Hematol Coag Disord 14:461, 1985.

62. Lombardi, R, et al: Alterations of factor VIII vWf in clinical conditions associated with an increase in its plasma concentration. Br J Haematol 49:61, 1981.

63. Scholtes, MC, et al: The factor VIII ratio in normal and pathological pregnancies. Eur J Obstet Gynecol Reprod Biol 16:89, 1983.

64. Nilsson, IL, et al: The Duke and Ivy methods for determination of bleeding time. Thromb Diath Haemorrh 10:223, 1963.

65. Montgomery, RR, and Coller, BS: Von Willebrand disease. In Colman, RW, et al (eds): Hemostasis and Thrombosis: Basic Principles and Clinical Practice, ed 3. JB Lippincott, Philadelphia, 1994, p 155.

66. Scott, JP, and Montgomery, RR: The rapid differentiation of type IIB von Willebrand's disease from platelet-type (pseudo-) von Willebrand's disease by the "neutral" monoclonal antibody binding assay. Am J Clin Pathol 96:723, 1991.

67. Hedner, U, and Davie, EW: Factor IX. In Colman, RW, et al (eds): Hemostasis and Thrombosis: Basic Principles and Clinical Practice, ed 2. JB Lippincott, Philadelphia, 1987, p 41.

68. Østerud, B, and Rapaport, SI: Activation of factor IX by the reaction product of tissue factor and factor VII: Additional pathway for initiating blood coagulation. Proc Natl Acad Sci USA 74:5260, 1977.

69. DiScipio, RC, et al: Activation of human factor IX (Christmas factor). J Clin Invest 61:1528, 1978.

70. Lindquist, PA, et al: Activation of bovine factor IX (Christmas factor) by factor XIa (activated plasma thromboplastin antecedent) and a protease from Russell's viper venom. J Biol Chem 253:1902, 1978.

71. Hedner, U, and Davie, EW: Factor IX. In Colman, RW, et al (eds): Hemostasis and Thrombosis: Basic Principles and Clinical Practice, ed 2. JB Lippincott, Philadelphia, 1987, p 43.

72. Hultin, M, and Nemerson, Y: Activation of factor X by factors IXa and VIII. A specific assay for factor IXa in the presence of thrombin-activated factor VIII. Blood 52:928, 1978.

73. Biggs, R, and Macfarlane, RG: The reaction of haemophilic plasma to thromboplastin. J Clin Pathol 4:445, 1951.

74. Aggeler, PM, et al: Plasma thromboplastin component (PTC) deficiency: A new disease resembling hemophilia. Proc Soc Exp Biol Med 79:692, 1952.

75. Biggs, R, et al: Christmas disease: A condition previously mistaken for haemophilia. Br Med J 2:1378, 1952.

76. Biggs, R: The inheritance of defects in blood coagulation. In Biggs, R, and Rizza, CR (eds): Human Blood Coagulation, Haemostasis and Thrombosis, ed 3. Blackwell Scientific, Oxford, 1984, p 92.

77. Meyer, D, et al: Cross-reacting material in genetic variants of hemophilia. J Clin Pathol 25:443, 1972.

78. Orstavik, KH, et al: Detection of carriers of hemophilia B. Br J Haematol 42:293, 1979.

79. Nilsson, IM, et al: Hemophilia prophylaxis in Sweden. Acta Paediatr Scand 65:129, 1976.

80. Brinkhous, KM, et al: Prevalence of inhibitors in hemophilias A and B. Thromb Diath Haemorrh 51(Suppl):315, 1972.

81. DiScipio, RG, et al: A comparison of human prothrombin, factor IX (Christmas factor), factor X (Stuart factor), and protein S. Biochemistry 16:698, 1977.

82. DiScipio, RG, et al: Activation of human factor X (Stuart factor) by a protease from Russell's viper venom. Biochemistry 16:5253, 1977.

83. Titani, K, et al: Bovine factor X_1 (Stuart factor): Amino acid sequence of heavy chain. Proc Natl Acad Sci USA 72:3082, 1975.

84. Ichinose, A, and Davie, EW: The blood coagulation factors: Their cDNAs, genes, and expression. In Colman, RW, et al. (eds): Hemostasis and Thrombosis: Basic Principles and Clinical Practice, ed 3. JB Lippincott, Philadelphia, 1994, p 36.

85. Griep, PR, et al: Factor X deficiency in amyloidosis: A critical review Am J Hematol ll:443, 1981.

86. Roberts, HR, and Leflowitz, JB: Inherited disorders of prothrombin conversion. In Colman, RW, et al (eds): Hemostasis and Thrombosis: Basic Principles and Clinical Practice, ed 3. JB Lippincott, Philadelphia, 1994, p 211.

87. Davie, EW, et al: The coagulation cascade: Initiation, maintenance, and regulation. Biochemistry 30:10363, 1991.

88. Thompson, RE, et al: Association of factor XI and high-molecular-weight kininogen in human plasma. J Clin Invest 60:1376, 1977.

89. Kurachi, K, and Davie, EW: Activation of human factor XI (plasma thromboplastin antecedent) by XIIa (activated Hageman factor). Biochemistry 16:5831, 1977.

90. Bouma, BN, and Griffin, JH: Human blood coagulation factor XI: Purification, properties, and mechanism of activation by activated factor XII. J Biol Chem 252:6432, 1977.

91. Fair, BD, et al: Detection by fluorescence of structural changes accompanying the activation of Hageman factor (factor XII) (39773). Proc Soc Exp Biol Med l55:199, 1977.

92. Fujikawa, K, et al: Amino acid sequence of human factor XI, a blood coagulation factor with four tandem repeats that are highly homologous with plasma prekallikrein. Biochemistry 25:2417, 1986.

93. Baglia, PA, et al: Functional domains in the heavy chain region of factor XI: A high-molecular-weight kininogen-binding site and substrate binding site for factor IX. Blood 74:244, 1989.

94. Roberts, HR, and Hoffman, M: Hemophilia and related conditions—inherited deficiencies of prothrombin (factor II), factor V, and factors VII to XII. In Beutler, E, et al (eds): Williams Hematology, ed 5. McGraw-Hill, New York, 1995, p 1433.

95. Seligsohn, U: High gene frequency of factor XI (PTA) deficiency in Ashkenazi Jews. Blood 51:1223, 1978.

96. DeLa Cadena, RA, et al: Contact activation pathway: Inflammation and coagulation. In Colman, RW, et al (eds): Hemostasis and Thrombosis: Basic Principles and Clinical Practice, ed 3. JB Lippincott, Philadelphia, 1994, p 230.

97. Ibid, p 230.

98. Ibid, p 231.

99. Roberts, HR, and Hofman, M: Hemophilia and related conditions—inherited deficiencies of prothrombin (factor II), factor V, and factors VII to XII. In Beutler, E, et al (eds): Williams Hematology, ed 5. McGraw-Hill, New York, 1995, p 1434.

100. Ibid, p 1434.

101. Colman, RW: Surface mediated defense reactions: The plasma contact activation system. J Clin Invest 73:1249, 1984.

102. Meijers, JCM, et al: High levels of coagulation factor XI as a risk factor for venous thrombosis. N Engl J Med 342:696, 2000.

103. Naito, K, and Fujikawa, K: Activation of human blood coagulation factor XI independent of factor XI by thrombin in plasma results in additional formation of thrombin that protects fibrin clots from fibrinolysis. Blood 86:3035, 1995.

104. von dem Borne, PAK, et al: Feedback activation of factor XI by thrombin in plasma results in additional formation of thrombin that protects fibrin clots from fibrinolysis. Blood 86:3035, 1995.

105. von dem Borne, PAK, et al: Thrombin-mediated activation of factor XI results in a thrombin-activatable fibrinolysis inhibitor-dependent inhibition of fibrinolysis. J Clin Invest 99:2323, 1997.

106. Fujikawa, K, and Davie, EW: Human factor XII (Hageman factor). Methods Enzymol 80:198, 1981.

107. Cochrane, CG, et al: Activation of Hageman factor in solid and fluid phases: A critical role of kallikrein. J Exp Med 138:1564, 1973.

108. Loscalzo, J: Pathogenesis of thrombosis. In Beutler, E, et al. (eds): Williams Hematology, ed 5. McGraw-Hill, New York, 1995, p 1527.

109. DeLa Cadena, RA, et al: Contact activation pathway: Inflammation and coagulation. In Colman, RW, et al (eds): Hemostasis and Thrombosis: Basic Principles and Clinical Practice, ed 3. JB Lippincott, Philadelphia, 1994, p 219.

110. Lorand, L, and Kornishi, K: Activation of fibrin stabilizing factor of plasma by thrombin. Arch Biochem Biophys 105:58, 1964.

111. Naski, MC, et al: Characterization of the kinetic pathway for fibrin promotion of α-thrombin-catalyzed activation of plasma factor XIII. Biochemistry 30:934, 1991.

112. Folk, JE, and Finlayson, JS: The epsilon gamma-glutamyl lysine crosslink and the catalytic role of transglutaminases. Adv Protein Chem 31:3, 1977.

113. Colman, RW, et al: Hemostasis and Thrombosis: Basic Principles and Clinical Practice, ed 3. JB Lippincott, Philadelphia, 1994, p 309.

114. Miletich, JP: Factor XIII: Laboratory analysis. In Beutler, E. et al (eds): Williams Hematology, ed 5. McGraw-Hill, New York, 1995, p L91.

115. Bagdasarian, A, et al: Immunochemical studies of plasma kallikrein. J Clin Invest 54:1444, 1974.

116. Mandle, R, Jr, et al: Identification of prekallikrein and high-molecular-weight kininogen as a complex in human plasma. Proc Natl Acad Sci USA 73:4179, 1976.

117. Sollo, DG, and Saleem, A: Prekallikrein (Fletcher factor) deficiency. Ann Clin Lab Sci 15:279, 1985.

118. Hattersley, PG, and Hayse, D: Fletcher factor deficiency: A report of three unrelated cases. Br J Haematol 18:411, 1970.

119. Goodnough, LT, et al: Thrombosis or myocardial infarction in congenital clotting factor abnormalities and chronic thrombocytopenia: A report of 21 patients and a review of 50 previously reported cases. Medicine 62:248, 1983.

120. Currimbhoy, Z, et al: Fletcher factor deficiency and myocardial infarction. Am J Clin Pathol 65:970, 1976.

121. Harris, MG, et al: Multiple cerebral thrombosis in Fletcher factor (prekallikrein) deficiency: A case report. Am J Hematol 19:387, 1985.

122. Saito, H, et al: Defective activation of clotting, fibrinolytic, and permeability-enhancing systems in human Fletcher trait plasma. Circ Res 34:641, 1974.

123. Schiffman, S, and Lee, P: Preparation, characterization, and activation of a highly purified factor XI: Evidence that a hitherto unrecognized plasma activity participates in the interaction of factor XI and XII. Br J Haematol 27:101, 1974.

124. Colman, RW, et al: Regulation of the coagulant activity and surface binding of high molecular weight kininogen. Clin Res 32:551a, 1984.

125. Berrettini, M, et al: Assembly and expression of an intrinsic factor IX activator complex on the surface of cultured human endothelial cells. J Biol Chem 267:19833, 1992.

126. Cheung, PP, et al: Total kininogen deficiency (Williams trait) is due to an Argstop mutation in exon 5 of the human kininogen gene. Blood 78:391a, 1991.

127. Feinstein, DI: Immune coagulation disorders. In Colman, RW, et al (eds): Hemostasis and Thrombosis: Basic Principles and Clinical Practice, ed 3. JB Lippincott, Philadelphia, 1994, p 881.

128. Ibid, p 883.

129. Reece, EA, et al: Spontaneous factor XI Inhibitors: Seven additional cases and review of the literature. Arch Intern Med 144:525, 1984.

130. Poon, MC, et al: A unique precipitating autoantibody against plasma thromboplastin antecedent associated with multiple apparent clotting factor deficiencies in patients with systemic lupus erythematosus. Blood 63:1309, 1984.

131. Feinstein, DI: Acquired disorders of hemostasis. In Colman, RW, et al: Hemostasis and Thrombosis: Basic Principles and Clinical Practice, ed 3. JB Lippincott, Philadelphia, 1994, p 888.

132. Brandt, JT, et al: Spontaneous factor V inhibitor with unexpected laboratory features. Arch Pathol Lab Med 110:24, 1986.

133. McGlasson, DL, et al: Platelet neutralization procedure (PNP): Atypical results seen with a factor V deficiency with and without the presence of an inhibitor. Clin Lab Sci 3:119, 1990.

134. Triplett, DA, and Brandt, JT: Lupus anticoagulants: Misnomer, paradox, riddle. Epiphenomenon. Hematol Pathol 2:121, 1988.

135. Jensen, R: Antiphospholipid antibody syndrome diagnosis. Clin Hemost Rev 10:3, 1996.

136. Ibid.

137. Conley, CL, and Hartmann, RC: A hemorrhagic disorder caused by circulating anticoagulant in patients with disseminated lupus erythematosus. J Clin Invest 31:621, 1952.

138. Loeliger, A: Prothrombin as a co-factor of the circulating anticoagulant in systemic lupus erythematosus. Thromb Diath Haemorrh 3:237, l959.

139. Bonnin, JA, et al: Coagulation defects in a case of systemic lupus erythematosus with thrombocytopenia. Br J Haematol 2:168, 1956.

140. Shapiro, SS, and Thiagarajan, P: Lupus anticoagulants. In Spaet, T (ed): Progress in Hemostasis and Thrombosis, vol 6. Grune & Stratton, New York, 1982, p 263.

141. Shapiro, SS, et al: Mechanism of action of the lupus anticoagulant. Ann NY Acad Sci 370:359, 1981.

142. Thiagarajan, P, et al: Monoclonal immunoglobulin M coagulation inhibitor with phospholipid specificity. Mechanism of a lupus anticoagulant. J Clin Invest 66:397, l980.

143. Harris, EN, et al: Thrombosis, recurrent fetal loss and thrombocytopenia: Predictive value of the anticardiolipin antibody test. Arch Intern Med 146:2153, 1986.

144. Harris, EN, et al: Anticardiolipin antibodies: Detection by radioimmunoassay and association with thrombosis in systemic lupus erythematosus, Lancet 2:1211, 1983.

145. Alving, BM, et al: The dilute phospholipid APTT. A sensitive assay for verification of the lupus anticoagulants. Thromb Haemost 54:709, 1985.

146. Lug, R: Cost-effective and rapid solution to the diagnosis of lupus anticoagulants. Clin Hemost Rev 10:3, 1996.

26

Interaction of the Fibrinolytic, Coagulation, and Kinin Systems; Disseminated Intravascular Coagulation; and Related Pathology

JOHN LAZARCHICK, MD

OBJECTIVES

At the end of this chapter, the learner should be able to:

1. Name the components of the coagulation and fibrinolytic systems.

2. Describe the physiologic interactions of these proteolytic systems.

3. Have an understanding of the clinical and laboratory abnormalities associated with disseminated intravascular coagulation.

4. Understand the laboratory abnormalities associated with primary fibrinolysis versus disseminated intravascular coagulation.

➤ SYSTEMS AND RELATED PATHOLOGY

Normal hemostasis is the result of the balanced interaction of the vascular endothelium and platelets with four biochemical systems[1,2]: the coagulation, the fibrinolytic, the kinin, and, to a lesser extent, the complement systems. The interrelationship between these systems is illustrated in Figure 26–1. The endothelium not only provides procoagulant, fibrinolytic, anticoagulant, and inflammatory functions, but these activities vary among the different vascular beds and in some cases are organ-specific.[3] Detailed discussion of the ever-emerging central role of the vascular endothelium in hemostasis and inflammation is beyond the scope of this chapter and the reader is referred to several excellent reviews on the topic.[4,5] When a stimulus initiates activation of the coagulation system with resultant fibrin formation and the establishment of a hemostatic barrier, a series of enzymes comprising the fibrinolytic system are simultaneously activated to lyse the fibrin thrombus and reestablish vessel lumen integrity and blood flow. This chapter deals with the biochemistry of the components of this fibrinolytic system, its associated pathophysiologic disorders, and laboratory tests available to evaluate individual components and overall function.

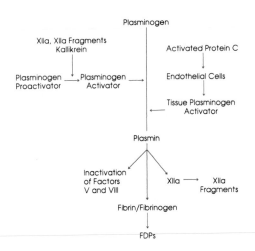

FIBRINOLYTIC SYSTEM

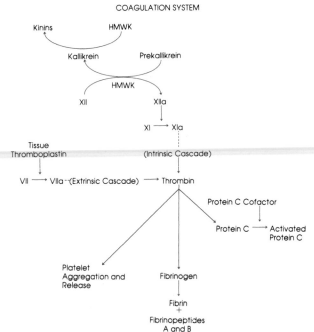

COAGULATION SYSTEM

> **FIGURE 26-1** This schematic summarizes the interaction of the coagulation, fibrinolytic, and kinin systems. High-molecular-weight kininogen (HMWK) and prekallikrein catalyze the activation of factor XII to XIIa. Factor XIIa then promotes the conversion of prekallikrein to kallikrein. The latter liberates kinins from HMWK, thus completing the positive feedback loops of the contact phase of coagulation. Thrombin formed through the extrinsic or intrinsic cascade systems then converts fibrinogen to fibrin and induces platelet aggregation release. Thrombin bound to thrombomodulin on the endothelial surface activates protein C, which can then proteolytically cleave activated factors Va and VIIIa. Direct stimulation of these cells by thrombin leads to release of tissue plasminogen activator and plasminogen activator inhibitor-1 (PAI-1). A second point of interaction between these systems can also result in formation of plasminogen activator. Kallikrein in association with factor XIIa and XIIa fragments convert a plasmin proactivator to its activated state. Through either activating system, plasminogen can be proteolytically cleaved to form plasmin. Plasmin not only lyses fibrin and inactivates factors V and VIII but also degrades factor XIIa to inactivated fragments that are a component of the second plasminogen activator system.

> ## MOLECULAR COMPONENTS: PHYSICOCHEMICAL AND FUNCTIONAL PROPERTIES

The molecular components of the fibrinolytic system consist of (1) the plasma protein plasminogen; (2) its active enzy-

matic form, plasmin; (3) a group of plasminogen activators that convert plasminogen to plasmin; (4) plasmin inhibitors, most prominently α_2-antiplasmin inhibitor; and (5) fibrin/fibrinogen, which serve as substrate for the active enzyme plasmin (Table 26–1).

Plasminogen

Native plasminogen is a single-chain plasma zymogen of approximately 90,000 daltons that circulates in two molecular forms, differing only in their carbohydrate content.[6] It is synthesized by the liver and has a half-life of 2 days. The plasma content is approximately 20 mg/dL. Each form of this molecule has an amino acid terminal glutamic acid (Glu-plasminogen) and is capable of undergoing limited proteolytic cleavage of this region to an incomplete molecule with lysine as the new terminal amino acid (Lys-plasminogen).

> **Table 26-1**
> **COMPONENTS OF THE FIBRINOLYTIC SYSTEM**

	Comments
1. Plasminogen	Circulating zymogen form with molecular weight of 90,000 daltons
2. Plasminogen activators: Tissue plasminogen activator (t-PA)	Endogenous activator liberated from endothelial cells by the action of thrombin
Factor XIIa, kallikrein, factor XIIa fragments, factor XIa	Contact phase activator generated by the initiation of coagulation
Single-chain urokinase	Endogenous activator synthesized in endothelial cells
	Converted to two-chain active form by plasmin and kallikrein
Streptokinase	Bacterial cell product; forms a complex with plasminogen which has intrinsic activating activity
3. Plasminogen activator inhibitor-1 (PAI-1)	Endogenous inhibitor of tissue plasminogen activator; synthesized and secreted by endothelial cells and platelets
4. Thrombin-activatable fibrinolysis inhibitor	Plasma procarboxypeptidase B, activated by thrombin, which suppresses plasminogen binding to fibrin
5. Plasmin	Active serine protease of 70,000 to 75,000 daltons
6. α_2-Antiplasmin inhibitor	Primary inhibitor of plasmin; forms an irreversible complex with plasmin
α_2-Macroglobulin	Serves as a plasmin inhibitor only when α_2-antiplasmin inhibitor binding sites are saturated
7. Fibrinogen, fibrin	Plasmin substrates; proteolytic cleavage results in the generation of degradation products

This latter form is more readily converted to active plasmin by plasminogen activators than the Glu-plasminogen form and is probably of greater physiologic significance.

Plasminogen Activators

The conversion of either form to active plasmin can be initiated through a variety of direct or indirect mechanisms.[7] This group of activating proteins is collectively known as *plasminogen activators*. Regardless of the initiating mechanism, activation of plasminogen to yield plasmin proceeds through the cleavage of the same arginine 560–valine 561 bond in the Glu and Lys forms of plasminogen. These activators are either endogenous or exogenous in origin. Endogenous activators are serine proteases present in the blood and a variety of other tissues, particularly the vascular endothelium. With the initiation of the contact phase of coagulation (see Chap. 23), factor XIa, XIIa fragments, kallikrein, and high-molecular-weight kininogen interact to yield plasminogen-activating ability.[8]

The exact biochemical steps involved in the formation of this intrinsic activator are not completely understood. The activator activity generated by this pathway slowly converts plasminogen to plasmin. The primary source of activators, however, is the vascular endothelium, the site of synthesis of both endothelial cell urokinase, a single-chain precursor, and tissue plasminogen activator (t-PA). The former probably plays a minor role in in vivo fibrinolysis but is the primary activator within the genitourinary system. Single-chain urokinase (scu-PA) is converted to its active form, two-chain urokinase, by either plasmin or kallikrein and is rapidly inhibited by plasminogen activator inhibitor-1 (PAI-1).

t-PA is the primary plasminogen activator within the vascular circulation. Its greater efficiency in thrombolytic therapy and potential for pharmacologic manipulation have led to its widespread use as a therapeutic fibrinolytic agent. This mechanism is probably the major physiologic activator of plasminogen. t-PA is an endothelial cell product with a molecular weight of approximately 68,000 daltons.[9]

Although a number of biochemical stimuli, including histamine, vasopressin, bradykinin, and adrenaline, can induce t-PA release, thrombin generated as result of activation of the coagulation system is the most important release inducer. Thrombin thus serves as a coagulant component (converting fibrinogen to fibrin, aggregating platelets, causing platelet factor V to relocate to the cell surface); as a stimulant to dampen the coagulant process by binding to its endothelial cell receptor, thrombomodulin, thus allowing for the generation of activated protein C; and, finally and paradoxically, as an initiator of fibrinolysis. It is now realized that thrombin, in addition to causing endothelial cell release of PAI-1, also acts to inhibit fibrinolysis through a second mechanism. Thrombin in complex with soluble thrombomodulin fragments activates plasma procarboxypeptidase B, which then binds to the plasminogen binding site on fibrin and thus prevents plasmin formation. This function is termed *thrombin-activatable fibrinolysis inhibitor*.[10]

Activated protein C exerts a negative feedback control on the coagulation process by proteolytically cleaving activated coagulant factors Va and VIIIa, thus limiting further clot formation.[11,12] This latter function of activated protein C is accelerated by its formation of a complex with protein S, which serves as a cofactor. t-PA has a high affinity for fi-brin, and its adsorption to fibrin clots greatly enhances plasminogen conversion to plasmin. Because of a high affinity of both the plasminogen activator and plasminogen for fibrin rather than fibrinogen, the effect of this reaction is accentuated on the surface of and within the clot. Release of t-PA from endothelium is also responsive to a variety of other stimuli, including venous occlusion, strenuous exercise, and treatment with vasoactive drugs, such as the vasopressin derivative DDAVP. t-PA activity is increased several fold under these conditions.[13]

Exogenous activators have been available for clinical use for a number of years. One of these, urokinase, is synthesized by the kidney in addition to the vascular endothelium, as previously mentioned, and is excreted in the urine.[14] It can also be identified in vitro using kidney cell cultures and is a potent direct activator of plasminogen. Its major drawbacks are its expense and its relatively lower affinity for fibrin as compared with t-PA. A consequence of the latter property is that the plasmin generated will not only digest fibrin but also circulating fibrinogen and, therefore, the development of severe hypofibrinogenemia is not uncommon with its use. The other exogenous activator, streptokinase, is a product of beta (β)-hemolytic streptococci. It is not a serine protease and has no intrinsic proteolytic activity but is capable of forming a 1:1 stoichiometric complex with plasminogen. This interaction results in a conformational change of the plasminogen molecule and exposure of its active serine site.[15] The streptokinase-plasminogen complex can then undergo autocatalysis to yield other activators namely, streptokinase-Glu-plasmin and streptokinase-Lys-plasmin. Any of these forms will readily convert free plasminogen to plasmin. Because streptokinase is a bacterial protein, a major limitation with its use in thrombolytic therapy is the induction of an immune response, with resulting antibody development and an inhibition of its activity.

Plasminogen Activator Inhibitor-1

This inhibitor is a member of the family of protease inhibitors that includes antithrombin-III, α_2-macroglobulin, α_1-antitrypsin, and α_2-antiplasmin, and that are collectively referred to as *serpins* (*ser*ine *p*rotease *in*hibitors). PAI-1 is a 53-kd glycoprotein also synthesized by vascular endothelium and released primarily in an inactive, latent state.[16] It is an acute-phase reactant and can be induced by a variety of stimuli, including interleukin-1 (IL-1), endotoxin, and thrombin. Its primary substrate is t-PA. Thus, regulation of fibrinolysis is dependent on the interaction of t-PA with PAI-1. Under basal conditions, most of the t-PA released is bound to PAI-1.

Excess levels of this inhibitor have been associated with thrombotic disease. A common diallelic polymorphism has been described for PAI-1 in which the prevalence of the 4G allele is significantly higher in patients with myocardial infarction who are less than 45 years old.[17]

Plasmin

The pivotal serine protease generated through these complex biochemical processes is plasmin. This protein has a molecular weight of 77,000 to 85,000 daltons, depending on whether Lys-plasmin or Glu-plasmin is formed, and has a transient plasma half-life measured in seconds.[18] Plasmin has the ability to proteolytically degrade both fibrin in clots and native fibrinogen in the circulation into a series of well-characterized end products collectively known as *fibrin/fibrinogen degradation products (FDPs)*. This process results in an asymmetric, progressive breakdown of fibrin and fibrinogen.[19]

The earliest recognized component is fragment X, which is still capable of clotting. A recent finding has been the identification of a small peptide fragment from the B-β chain of fibrinogen, which is released simultaneously with the formation of the X fragment. Measurement by radioimmunoassay of the B-β 15–42 related peptide may prove of value in the documentation of early fibrinolytic states.[20,21] The X fragment undergoes further plasmin attack to yield unclottable Y and D fragments. The Y fragment is further digested to yield an additional D fragment and a single E fragment. It is now realized that the proteolytic cleavage of cross-linked fibrin (i.e., fibrin transaminated through the action of factor XIIIa and calcium) results in other intermediate degradation products (e.g., D2E without the generation of fragment D or E). This proteolytic product is referred to as the D-dimer.

These breakdown products have specific inhibitory effects on the coagulation system and thereby suppress further clot formation. Fragment X is capable of clotting slowly and exerts an anticoagulant effect by competing with fibrinogen for thrombin. It also forms slowly polymerizing complexes with fibrin monomer and inhibits the polymerization step. Fragment D forms abnormal complexes with fibrin monomers as it polymerizes. Fragment E is not known to have any specific anticoagulant effect. In high concentrations (more than 100 μg/mL), the degradation products are capable of inhibiting platelet aggregation and release. Plasmin also exerts a direct limiting effect on the coagulation process by being able to proteolytically cleave and render inactive factors V and VIII, in addition to proteolysing factor XII and platelet glycoprotein Ib, the von Willebrand's factor receptor.

Plasmin Inhibitors

Although plasmin formation characteristically takes place in the area of fibrin deposition with little free plasmin circulating, this enzyme if unchecked by the presence of specific inhibitors, would result in circulating fibrinogen being digested and the blood being rendered unclottable. The primary physiologic inhibitor of plasmin in vivo is α_2-plasmin inhibitor.[22] It rapidly binds to the lysine binding site on plasmin in a 1:1 molar ratio in an irreversible manner. Measurement of these plasmin–α_2-antiplasmin inhibitor complexes has been suggested as an indicator for activation of the fibrinolytic system. Plasmin adsorbed onto fibrin during the fibrinolytic process appears to be protected from this inhibitor because it binds to fibrin through the same lysine binding site. Because this binding site on plasmin is occupied, the inhibitor cannot bind, and clot lysis can proceed. The overall effect is to ensure that plasmin activity is limited to the area of fibrin deposition and to prevent free plasmin from circulating. Other protease inhibitors in plasma include α_2-macroglobulin, C1 inactivator, and α_1-antitrypsin. Of these, only α_2-macroglobulin has a role in plasmin inhibition during normal hemostasis, but it only participates when α_2-antiplasmin inhibitor binding sites for plasmin are saturated.

➤ CONGENITAL ABNORMALITIES

Congenital abnormalities of the fibrinolytic system are rare.[23] Only three cases of an abnormal plasminogen have been reported. In each of these reports, the patient had a history of recurrent thrombotic episodes. Low levels of t-PA activity have been documented in two families and were associated with a similar thrombotic tendency. As mentioned previously, allelic polymorphism has now been documented for PAI-1, with the presence of the 4G allele being associated with premature coronary artery disease.[17] Deficiencies of α_2-antiplasmin inhibitor have been reported in four families to date and, in contrast, are associated with a severe hemorrhagic tendency. Acquired abnormalities of the fibrinolytic system are much more common and are discussed in the next section on disseminated intravascular coagulation and related disorders.

In summary, an integrated system of serine proteases is brought into play once the coagulation process is initiated in response to disruption of blood vessel integrity (Fig. 26–2). The response is balanced so that the same reaction that initiated thrombin formation and fibrin deposition also initiates a series of reactions to lyse the clot. Factor XIIa with other components of the contact phase of coagulation convert plasminogen to plasmin; thrombin stimulates endothelial cells to release t-PA with subsequent plasmin generation. Excess t-PA activity is controlled by the presence of plasminogen activator inhibitor. Because of the high affinity of plasmin for fibrin, most of these fibrinolytic processes are taking place at the site of fibrin deposition within the damaged blood vessel. The presence of plasmin inhibitors further ensures that the proteolytic process is limited to this area.

➤ DISSEMINATED INTRAVASCULAR COAGULATION

Briefly, under normal physiologic conditions when there is damage to the vascular endothelium, platelets adhere to the site of injury, undergo activation, and aggregate. This reaction provides a rich phospholipid environment in which coagulation can proceed. Under most circumstances, the initial coagulant response involves endothelial cell tissue factor (TF) complexing with factor VII or VIIa to form TF-VIIa. This complex then rapidly converts factor X to Xa and factor IX to IXa. The TF-VIIa complex is short-lived because it is quickly inhibited by the naturally occurring inhibitor tissue factor pathway inhibitor (TFPI). The latter forms an inactive quaternary complex of TF–VIIa–Xa–TFPI. Further coagulant response then depends on the formation of IXa-VIIIa through the activation of the intrinsic pathway to convert more factor X to Xa. With the generation of thrombin, fibrinogen is converted to fibrin, factor XIII to its activated form to make the clot insoluble, and further coagulant activity is limited by thrombin converting protein C to its activated form. The latter proteolytically cleaves any factor Va and VIIIa present, resulting in a dampening of further coagulant response. Endothelial cells are stimulated by thrombin to release t-PA and single-chain urokinase to initiate the fibrinolytic process. Excess t-PA and single-chain urokinase are rapidly inhibited by PAI-1, and excess plasmin is bound to α_2-antiplasmin. Thus, further hemorrhage is prevented and vascular repair is initiated to restore normal homeostasis.[24,25]

Consequently, when there is damage to a blood vessel, an ordered, integrated series of reactions involving the coagulation, fibrinolytic, kinin, and complement systems occurs on endothelial cells and platelets at the site of injury, as outlined in the previous chapters, with the initial formation and sub-

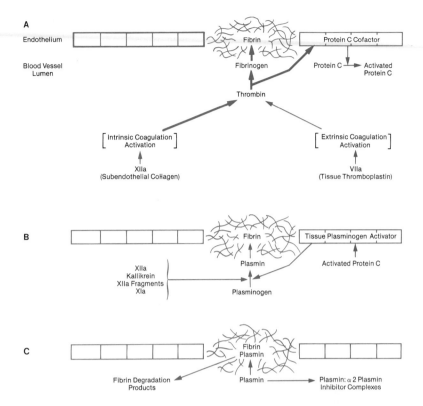

> ➤ **FIGURE 26–2**   *A.* Disruption of endothelial continuity results in platelet adherence, factor XIIa and VIIa formation, and the generation of thrombin to fibrin to reestablish a temporary barrier. Secondarily and simultaneously thrombin complexes with thrombomodulin on the endothelial surface. Protein C once bound to this complex is rapidly converted to its activated state. *B.* Activated protein C proteolytically cleaves factors Va and VIIIa and indirectly causes release of tissue plasminogen activator from endothelial cells, in addition to direct stimulation and release of this glycoprotein by thrombin. *C.* Plasmin-induced proteolysis of the fibrin clot results in the formation of fibrin degradation products. Reendothelialization of the damaged blood vessel begins as clot dissolution is occurring. Excess plasmin is irreversible complexed with its inhibitor, α_2-antiplasmin inhibitor, preventing proteolysis of circulating fibrinogen.

sequent lysis of fibrin deposits. The initial formation of the fibrin clot prevents further hemorrhage and initiates vascular repair. The subsequent clot lysis serves to reestablish blood flow and vascular integrity. This process is normally self-limited and localized. Under certain pathologic stimuli, however, the coagulation response may be accentuated and the normal inhibitory mechanisms overwhelmed. Activation of the coagulation system under these circumstances causes consumption of the coagulation factors and platelets, with subsequent thrombus formation not only at the site of endothelial damage, but in a random manner throughout the microcirculation.[26] This hemorrhagic syndrome has been referred to as *disseminated intravascular coagulation (DIC)*, *defibrination syndrome*, or *consumptive coagulopathy*.

Simultaneous with and secondary to the activation of the coagulation cascade, the fibrinolytic system is activated. Regardless of the nature of the inciting stimulus, the pathophysiologic effect of this process will be reflective of the balance between fibrin deposition (action of thrombin) and fibrinolysis (action of plasmin). The clinical manifestations, thus, can be one of diffuse hemorrhage (Fig. 26–3 and Color Plate 267), owing to depletion of platelets and coagulation factors, ischemic tissue damage caused by vascular occlusion, or the occurrence of both simultaneously in different areas of the microvasculature.

Triggering Mechanisms: Associated Clinical Disorders

The diverse stimuli that are capable of triggering the coagulation cascade in this manner all act through one or more of three mechanisms[27]: (1) activation of the extrinsic coagulation pathway by the release of tissue thromboplastin, (2) activation of the intrinsic coagulation pathway with factor XIIa formation, and (3) direct activation of factors X or II. The exact sequence of intermediary events by which cer-

tain of the stimuli initiate coagulation is well understood, but with other stimuli this process is unknown.

DIC caused by direct activation of factor VII, as seen after massive injury or in certain obstetrical complications, results from release of tissue thromboplastin from the injured tissue or from amniotic fluid entering the circulation. Certain tumors, particularly mucinous adenocarcinomas, are rich in thromboplastin-like material and may act through the same mechanism. The coagulopathy seen with red cell lysis following mismatched blood transfusions may be caused by the release of thromboplastin-like activity from the stroma of these cells. However, evidence would suggest that immune complex formation may be the prime initiator of the coagulant response.[28]

All pathologic stimuli that result in activation of the in-

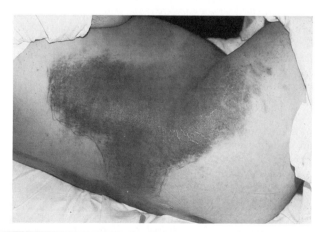

> ➤ **FIGURE 26–3**   Diffuse hemorrhage, a clinical manifestation in a patient with disseminated intravascular coagulation (DIC). Note the multiple cutaneous ecchymoses.

trinsic system probably do so indirectly by means of first inducing endothelial cell damage with subsequent exposure of the subendothelium. Platelet adherence and aggregation and factor XII activation can then occur. This is the proposed mechanism of DIC associated with anoxia, immune complex formation, and sepsis. New experimental insight regarding sepsis now suggests that the mechanism of DIC induced by endotoxins, the lipopolysaccharide constituents of gram-negative organisms, may be more complicated, with endotoxin inducing release of a number of cytokines, including tumor necrosis factor-alpha (TNF-α) and IL-1, and the primary activation of coagulation occurring through the extrinsic (tissue factor–dependent) pathway rather than the intrinsic pathway.[29] TNF-α is capable of inducing tissue factor activity in monocytes and on both the luminal and subendothelial surfaces of endothelial cells. Tissue factor can bind and activate factor VII; the complex of TF-VIIa can then activate factor X, with subsequent thrombin formation. Binding of granulocytes to the endothelial receptors (selectins) induces the release of granulocyte cathepsins and elastases, which then lead to organ damage. Activation of the kinin system, with high-molecular-weight kininogen being converted to kinins, can then cause increased vascular permeability, hypotension, and shock.[25]

Direct activation of coagulation factors can also occur in the presence of proteolytic enzymes. The venoms of certain snakes act through this mechanism (e.g., Russell's viper venom activates factor X whereas venom from the sand rattlesnake causes direct conversion of prothrombin to thrombin). Certain malignancies have also been reported to have either TF- or direct factor X–activating capability, and these properties may account for the DIC seen in these states. A list of clinical conditions associated with these triggering mechanisms is shown in Table 26–2. Although acute promyelocytic leukemia (APL) is included in this list, recent evidence would suggest that the hemorrhagic diathesis associated with APL is a result of primary fibrinolysis rather than DIC. Leukemic promyelocytes are rich in annexin II, a surface phospholipid, which can bind t-PA and plasminogen. Conversion of the plasminogen to plasmin then initiates the fibrinolytic process without thrombin generation.[29]

Clinical Presentation

To a great extent, the clinical presentation depends on which of the proteolytic processes (coagulant or fibrinolytic) is dominant. This allows for a wide spectrum ranging from an acute, severe hemorrhagic disorder to a low-grade disorder with predominantly thrombotic manifestations. A number of factors are important in determining the final clinical picture, including the magnitude and duration of the triggering stimulus; the functional ability of reticuloendothelial system, particularly the liver, to remove from circulation activated coagulation factors, fibrin monomers, fibrin/fibrinogen products, as well as immune complexes; the compensatory ability of the liver and the bone marrow to accelerate clotting factor and platelet production; and, finally, the extent to which any particular organ is involved with hemorrhage or thrombus.[22]

Laboratory Diagnosis

To confirm a laboratory diagnosis of DIC, it has been suggested that there must be confirmation of procoagulant and fibrinolytic component activation, evidence of inhibitor consumption, and biochemical proof of end-organ damage or

> **Table 26-2**
CLINICAL CONDITIONS ASSOCIATED WITH DISSEMINATED INTRAVASCULAR COAGULATION

Thromboplastin Release—Factor VII Activation

Placental abruption

Trauma

Fat emboli syndrome

Mucin-secreting adenocarcinoma

Sepsis*

Promyelocytic leukemia

Retained dead fetus syndrome

Acute intravascular hemolysis*

Amniotic fluid embolus*

Cardiopulmonary bypass surgery

Endothelial Cell Damage—Factor XII Activation

Immune complex disease

Intravascular hemolysis*

Liver disease*

Heat stroke

Sepsis*

Burns

Vasculitis

Anoxia

Acidosis

Factor X/II Activation

Snake venoms

Acute pancreatitis

Liver disease*

Fat emboli syndrome*

*More than one mechanism may be involved.

failure.[25] The laboratory findings in patients with DIC reflect the direct or indirect effects of excess thrombin and plasmin generation (Table 26–3). The constellation of laboratory abnormalities in any particular patient, however, will depend on the nature, magnitude, and duration of the triggering stimulus, the compensatory capacity available, and the underlying disease state. Although the ultimate confirmatory test would be the direct demonstration of fibrin deposition in biopsy material from an involved blood vessel, this is not practical. As a result, a multitude of tests have been utilized by various laboratories to make this diagnosis.[21,30]

It should be pointed out that no single test is diagnostic of DIC; however, in the appropriate clinical setting (patient history and the type of bleeding) a battery of tests can ensure a diagnosis of DIC. Indirect tests that lack specificity for thrombin action include the prothrombin (PT), activated partial thromboplastin (APTT), and thrombin/reptilase clotting times; however, these tests are not always abnormal either individually or as a group. Utilization and degradation of the

> **Table 26–3**
LABORATORY TESTS TO DETECT EXCESS THROMBIN AND/OR PLASMIN ACTIVITY

Excess Protease	Effect	Laboratory Tests
Thrombin	Fibrinogen utilization	Fibrinogen concentration, thrombin/reptilase time, prothrombin and activated partial thromboplastin times
	Utilization/degradation of other coagulation factors	Prothrombin and activated partial thromboplastin times, coagulation factor assays
	Fibrin monomer generation	Soluble fibrin monomer complexes
	Fibrinopeptide A/B release	Fibrinopeptides A and B
	Platelet aggregation/release	Platelet count, β-thromboglobulin, and platelet factor 4
	AT-III complex formation	Thrombin–antithrombin III complexes, AT-III level
Thrombin/plasmin	Proteolysis of fibrinogen/fibrin	Fibrin degradation products, D-dimer concentration, B-β 15–42 peptide assay
	Release/activate	Tissue plasminogen
	Plasminogen activators and inhibitors	Activator level, plasminogen activator inhibitor level
	Soluble fibrin monomer/fibrinogen FDP complexes	Soluble fibrin monomer complexes
Plasmin	Plasminogen utilization	Plasminogen concentration
	Proteolysis of fibrinogen/fibrin	FDPs, thrombin/reptilase times, platelet aggregation and release tests
	Complexes with inhibitor	α_2-Plasmin, inhibitor concentration, α_2-plasmin inhibitor–plasmin complexes
	Proteolysis of factors V/VIII	Factor assays

clotting factors in the DIC process result in prolongation of each of these global tests. Because platelets are also consumed during the coagulation process and their contents released, the finding of thrombocytopenia and elevated plasma levels of the platelet-specific proteins β-thromboglobulin and platelet factor 4 would be expected. The plasma inhibitor, antithrombin III, will complex with thrombin and activated factor X and result in diminished plasma levels of antithrombin III. The presence of thrombin–antithrombin III complexes formed can also be determined using an enzyme-linked immunosorbent assay (ELISA) system. If the fibrin deposition does not completely occlude the lumen of the damaged blood vessel, red cells may undergo a shearing effect as they traverse this area, with resultant fragmentation and the development of a microangiopathic hemolytic anemia (Fig. 26–4 and Color Plate 268).

Conversion of prothrombin to thrombin is the result of cleavage from the parent molecule of a small, inactive peptide referred to as *prothrombin fragment 1.2*. Measurement of this activation peptide has thus far been utilized primarily for diagnosis of a hypercoagulable state; however, it may have equal utility as a molecular marker for DIC.

Specific tests for direct evidence of thrombin activity relate to the action of thrombin on fibrinogen. Other than certain snake venoms, thrombin is the only enzyme that releases the specific peptides fibrinopeptide A (FPA) and B from the fibrinogen molecule. Both ELISA and radioimmunoassays are available commercially to measure each fibrinopeptide.[31] The major drawback to measuring these peptides, paradoxically, is the extreme sensitivity of the assay such that elevated levels can be seen in clinical conditions in which thrombin is only transiently generated. As a consequence of fibrinopeptide release, soluble fibrin monomers are formed that are capable of forming complexes with intact fibrinogen molecules or with fibrin/fibrinogen degradation products. The ability to precipitate these complexes from plasma is the basis for two paracoagulation assays, the ethanol gelation test and the protamine sulfate test. In our laboratory, we are currently measuring soluble fibrin monomer complex formation using a latex agglutination assay for these soluble fibrin monomer complexes. Positive tests for any of these three methods are indirect indications that thrombin was generated; therefore, the coagulation system had to have been activated.

Tests for the secondary activation of the fibrinolytic system

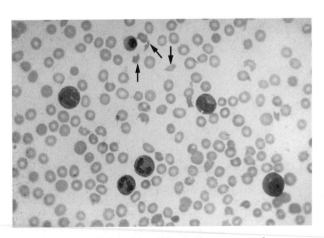

> **FIGURE 26–4**   DIC (peripheral blood). Note presence of schistocytes *(arrows)* and nucleated red cell *(top border)*.

in DIC are primarily directed at demonstrating the action of plasmin on fibrin/fibrinogen. As has already been mentioned, a series of cleavage products are formed, the fibrin/fibrinogen degradation products. The anticoagulant action of these fragments has been noted in the previous section.

A number of immunologic tests are available to measure one or more of the fibrinogen fragments and can yield quantitative information on the degree of fibrinolysis. Because of its ease of performance and specificity (i.e., evidence of plasmin action on cross-linked fibrin), the D-dimer assays are gaining wide popularity as the immunologic assays of choice and automated techniques are now available to quantitate levels. A relatively recent development has been the recognition of an early cleavage product of the B-β chain of the fibrinogen dimer, peptide B-β 15–42.[20] Clinical assessment of the utility of the radioimmunoassay for the B-β 15–42 peptide in diagnosing accelerated fibrinolysis has confirmed its value; however, because it is difficult to perform, it is not recommended for routine evaluation. Direct measurement of the plasminogen concentration in plasma can also be performed, and commercial assays are available.

An indication of increased plasminogen activator activity seen in early stages of DIC can be obtained by performing a euglobulin lysis time.[32] The euglobulin fraction of plasma contains plasminogen, plasminogen activator, plasmin, and fibrinogen. The rapidity of lysis of the fibrin clot is directly related to plasminogen activator levels. The sensitivity of this global assay, however, is limited. As discussed, it is now

possible to directly quantitate each component with commercially available kits. Assays for α_2-antiplasmin inhibitor levels and for circulating plasmin–α_2-antiplasmin inhibitor complexes are under investigation for clinical use.

Table 26–4 summarizes laboratory tests available to diagnose DIC and the constellation of results one can find in this syndrome, depending on the balance between thrombin and plasmin activities and the compensatory capacity of the patient. This table describes three generalized clinical states of DIC, and the typical laboratory abnormalities associated with each.

The decompensated DIC state refers to a condition in which active hemorrhage is evident and in which the consumption of the coagulation factors and platelets exceeds the capacity to increase the synthesis of these components. In the compensated state, laboratory evidence of an accelerated coagulation and fibrinolytic process is evident (increased FPA, soluble fibrin monomer complexes, increased β-thromboglobulin, increased FDPs or D-dimer levels, presence of plasmin–α_2-antiplasmin inhibitor complexes) but the rate of synthesis of the coagulation components is balanced with the rate of destruction. Because of this balance the PT, APTT, thrombin time, and platelet count are usually normal or only mildly abnormal. Confirmation of DIC is then based on finding evidence of coagulation activation peptides (FPA, prothrombin fragment 1.2), complexes of activated coagulant/fibrinolytic components (thrombin–antithrombin III, plasmin–α_2-antiplasmin) in

➤ Table 26-4
LABORATORY TESTS TO DIAGNOSE DIC

Routine Test	Decompensated	Compensated	Hypercoagulable
Prothrombin time	I	N	N
Activated partial thromboplastin	I	N	D
Thrombin time/Reptilase time	I	N/I	N/I
Fibrinogen	D	N	I
Platelet count	D	N/D	N
D-Dimer/fibrin(ogen) Degradation products	I	I	N/I
Euglobulin lysis test	N/I/D	N/D	N
Soluble fibrin monomer Complexes	P	P	Ng
Antithrombin III	D	N/D	N/D

Special Test	Decompensated	Compensated	Hypercoagulable
Coagulation factor levels	D	N/D	I
Fibrinopeptide A	I	I	I
Plasminogen	D	N/D	N
Plasmin–α_2-plasmin Inhibitor complexes	I	I	N
β-Thromboglobulin/platelet factor 4 levels	I	I	I
Thrombin–antithrombin III complexes	I	I	I
Prothrombin fragment 1.2	I	I	I

Abbreviations: I = increased; D = decreased; N = normal; P = positive; Ng = negative

addition to increased fibrin(ogen) degradation products and elevated β-thromboglobulin or platelet factor 4 levels.

The hypercoagulable state is the result of excess thrombin present in the plasma, with a delayed or lessened plasmin response. In this condition, evidence of coagulation activation is apparent (increased levels of FPA, thrombin–antithrombin III complexes, prothrombin fragment 1.2, β-thromboglobulin), but all fibrinolytic activation markers are absent or minimally increased. A characteristic finding in this form of DIC is a shortened APTT. It should be realized that these clinical states are not static and it is not unusual for one to evolve into one of the others, depending on the nature of the underlying disease process and the response to therapy.

Therapy

Therapy for DIC is essentially twofold: treatment or removal of the underlying pathologic stimulus, and maintenance of blood volume and hemostatic function.[26,27] Dramatic improvement in the patient's clinical status with abrupt cessation of bleeding and normalization of the coagulation abnormalities can be seen in certain cases of DIC with removal of the underlying pathologic stimulus alone (e.g., DIC associated with retained dead fetus). In cases of DIC associated with septicemia, appropriate antibiotic therapy is imperative to control the pathologic process (i.e., bacterial or endotoxin-induced vascular damage).

Blood component replacement therapy with transfusion of packed red blood cells, fresh frozen plasma, and platelets to maintain blood volume and to support hemostatic function is indicated in patients with active bleeding or those whose compensatory capacity is limited. In addition to fresh frozen plasma, cryoprecipitate (enriched in fibrinogen, factor VIII, and fibronectin) and prothrombin complex (enriched in vitamin K–dependent clotting factors) are often used as supplemental sources of blood component therapy.

The administration of heparin in DIC has been advocated by a number of investigators, but its use is still controversial.[26,33] On the premise that the underlying pathologic basis for DIC is generation of excess thrombin, and that thrombosis, especially of small vessels, is the process that most affects morbidity and mortality, heparin should theoretically be indicated to slow or stop the coagulation process by complexing with antithrombin III to inhibit thrombin or Xa. This ameliorating effect has been noted with the use of subcutaneous low-dose heparin therapy in mild to moderate DIC.[21] Its use can result in increased bleeding, and because heparin itself affects a number of coagulation tests, it is often difficult to monitor the effect of conventional therapy. Heparin should be utilized and is most effective in cases of DIC that present with clinical evidence of a hypercoagulable state with evident vascular thrombosis.

When major peripheral vessels are occluded as part of the hypercoagulable process, the use of fibrinolytic agents (recombinant t-PA, streptokinase, or urokinase) may be indicated as an initial management choice with subsequent heparinization, but clinical experience with this form of therapy is minimal. Table 26–5 summarizes the previously described profile of DIC.

► RELATED DISORDERS

Primary fibrinolysis is an unusual situation in which plasmin is formed in the absence of coagulation taking place. The clinical presentation in this disorder is similar to DIC, with diffuse hemorrhage occurring as a result of increased plasma fibrinolytic activity. Several mechanisms can initiate this process. The presence of proteolytic enzymes in plasma that are capable of either directly or indirectly converting plasminogen into plasmin can occur in certain disease states. The genitourinary system is enriched in urokinases, which can enter the systemic circulation following various urologic procedures. The fibrinolytic state seen with metastatic prostatic carcinoma is another example of this mechanism.

The basis for the hemorrhagic state seen following cardiopulmonary bypass surgery is complex, with platelet dysfunction and hemodilution of coagulant proteins as the primary defects; activation of the plasminogen-plasmin system with increased fibrinolytic activity is also well documented.

The failure of the hepatic clearance mechanism to remove plasminogen activator accounts for the increased fibrinolytic activity seen in a variety of hepatic disorders, particularly cirrhosis. Under normal circumstances the hepatic reticuloendothelial system removes not only activated clotting proteins, but also plasminogen activator from the systemic circulation. When this function is impaired because of hepatic disease or in patients who have portocaval shunting procedures, the removal of plasminogen activator is less than adequate and hyperplasminemia occurs, with resultant hemorrhage. Increased fibrinolytic activity can also be seen in patients undergoing liver transplantation, especially during the reperfusion phase following reanastomosis of vessels.

The occurrence of DIC with secondary fibrinolysis is well documented in patients with acute promyelocytic leukemia, although as previously discussed, this disorder clearly causes primary fibrinolysis through surface membrane annexin II binding of t-PA and plasminogen. It is now recognized, however, that the coagulopathy these patients develop may also result from a primary fibrinolysis. The mechanism(s) is unsettled but may involve direct activation by the leukemic cells with release of a urokinase-type or tissue-type plasminogen activator.[34]

The coagulation abnormalities seen in these fibrinolytic disorders are similar to those in DIC, with prolonged PT, APTT, and thrombin times. These defects result from the hypofibrinogenemic state induced by the proteolytic cleavage of fibrinogen by excess plasmin, in addition to the catabolic effect of this enzyme on factors V and VIII. FDP concentrations are increased and, as previously noted, will further interfere with coagulation by acting as antithrombins. With the excess plasmin activity, the euglobulin lysis time is typically shortened. Because thrombin is not generated during this pathologic process, several laboratory tests can serve to readily distinguish primary fibrinolysis from DIC. The platelet count is typically normal, fibrinopeptides A and B levels are not elevated, and circulating fibrin monomer complexes and elevated D-dimer levels are absent in primary fibrinolysis in contrast to the results in DIC.

Thrombotic thrombocytopenic purpura is the syndrome of unknown etiology in which fibrin and platelet thrombi are formed diffusely throughout the microvasculature in contrast to the localized thrombus formation seen in DIC.[35] The clinical picture consists of a pentad of findings: (1) fever, (2) microangiopathic hemolytic anemia, (3) thrombocytopenia, (4) azotemia, and (5) vacillating neurologic deficits. Despite fibrin and platelet deposition, this disorder is not typically associated with excessive activation of the coagulation system.

➤ **Table 26-5**
PROFILE DIC

Synonyms	Conditions Associated with DIC	Suggested Triggering Mechanisms	Clinical Manifestations	Clinical Laboratory Findings	Sequential Therapy

1. Consumptive coagulopathy
 	
2. Defibrination syndrome
	Obstetric accidents
	
	Intravascular hemolysis
	
	Septicemia
	
	Viremia (varicella)
	
	Leukemias:
	  Acute
	    Promyelo-cytic
	  Other
	
	Solid malignancy
	
	Acidosis alkalosis
	
	Burns
	
	Crush injury and tissue necrosis
	
	Vascular disorders
		Amniotic fluid, which posses-ses thrombo-plastic activity
		
		Retained fetus, which posses-ses thrombo-plastic activity
		
		By-product of red cell hemolysis (phospholipid)
		
		Antigen/antibody complexes
		
		Endotoxin release
		
		Chronic stasis
		
		Complement activation
			1. *General signs:* significant hemorrhaging (usually from 3 unrelated sites: melena and hematemesis, epistaxis, or hemoptysis) fever, hypotension, acidosis, hypoxia, proteinuria, hematuria
			
			2. *Specific signs:* petechiae, purpura, gangrene, wound bleeding, venipuncture bleeding, subcutaneous hematomas
			
			3. *Microthrombi*
			
			4. *End-organ dysfunction*
				Hypofibrinogene-mia
				
				Abnormal PT
				
				Abnormal PTT
				
				Abnormal thrombin time
				
				Abnormal platelet count
				
				Abnormal tourniquet test
				
				Abnormal clot retraction
				
				Abnormal factors V and VIII
				
				Positive fibrin(ogen)-split products
				
				Positive prota-mine sulfate test
				
				Positive ethanol gelatin test
				
				AT-III consumption
				
				Leukocytosis
				
				Schistocytosis
				
				Thrombocyto-penia
				
				Reticulocytosis
					1. Remove or treat triggering process
					
					2. Stop or slow coagulation process
					  a. Miniheparin
					  b. Heparin
					  c. Antiplatelet drugs
					  d. AT-III con-centrates
					
					3. Blood component replacement
					  a. Platelets
					  b. Cryopre-cipitate
					  c. Prothrombin complex
					
					4. Antifibrinolytic therapy*
					  a. Epsilon aminocap-roic acid (EACA)

*Sequential therapy used only after clotting is stopped (3% of patients may require this therapy).
Abbreviations: PT = prothrombin time; PTT = partial thromboplastin time; AT-III = antithrombin III

➤ **Table 26-6**
OTHER CAUSES OF FIBRINOLYTIC ACTIVATION

Clinical Condition	Mechanism	Clinical Manifestation	Other Hemostatic Alterations

1. Chronic liver disease	Abnormal fibrinolytic inhibitor (α_2-macroglobulin)
	
	Abnormal hepatic clearance of plasminogen activators
		Often fulminant hemor-rhage with massive he-moptysis, hematachezia, melena, or epistaxis
		
		May also demonstrate petechiae, purpura, spider telangiectasia, ecchymoses
			1. Hypofibrinogenemia (due to lysis)
			2. Elevated FDP (X, Y, D, and E)
			  a. Defective fibrin monomer/ polymerization
			  b. Platelet dysfunction
			3. Proteolysis of factors V, VIII, IX, XI
			4. Platelet defects
			  a. Thrombocytopenia
			  b. Platelet dysfunction (FDP, PF3)
			5. Coagulation protein defects
			  a. Decreased synthesis of factors II, VII, IX, and X
			  b. Decreased synthesis of Fletcher factor
			  c. Decreased or dysfunc-tional synthesis of AT-III

> **Table 26-6**
OTHER CAUSES OF FIBRINOLYTIC ACTIVATION (*Continued*)

Clinical Condition	Mechanism	Clinical Manifestation	Other Hemostatic Alterations

2. Cardiopulmonary bypass (CPB)	Unclear; possibly direct activation of fibrinolysis by the oxygenation system of pump-induced accelerated flow rates may alter endothelial plasminogen	Hemorrhage; hematuria, petechiae/purpura, and oozing from intravenous site in conjunction with increased chest tube loss	1. Hyperfibrinolysis results in
			  a. Elevated FDP
			  b. Hypofibrinogenemia
			  c. Low factors V and VIII
			2. Functional platelet defect
			  a. CPB-induced
			  b. Drug-induced
			3. Thrombocytopenia
			4. Hyperheparinemia-heparin rebound(?)
			5. DIC(?)

3. Malignancy	Poorly understood; in several instances tumor extracts possess the ability to activate directly or indirectly the fibrinolytic system (e.g., gastric carcinoma, sarcomas, and prostatic carcinoma	Thrombosis/hemorrhage	1. Thrombocytopenia 2. Platelet function defects 3. Elevated FDP 4. Decreased AT-III 5. DIC(?)

4. Acute promyelocytic leukemia	Release of urokinase-type and tissue-type plasminogen activators from leukemic cells	Severe hemorrhage	1. Hypofibrinogenemia (due to fibrin(ogen) lysis
			2. Marked elevation of FDP (X, Y, D, and E)
			  a. Defective fibrin monomer/polymerization
			  b. Platelet dysfunction
			3. Proteolysis of factors V, VIII, XI, XII
			4. Decreased plasminogen
			5. Plasmin–α_2-antiplasmin complexes

Abbreviations: FDP = fibrin/fibrinogen degradation products; PF3 = platelet factor 3; AT-III = antithrombin III

Supportive evidence that this syndrome represents an abnormality of the fibrinolytic system is suggested by the finding of diminished or absent fibrinolytic activity, particularly of t-PA, in plasma and blood vessels affected with microthrombi. Therapy has not been standardized, but antiplatelet drugs (e.g., aspirin or dipyridamole), plasmapheresis, and exchange transfusion have been used either singularly or in combination with variable success (see Chap. 24). Table 26–6 summarizes the other causes of fibrinolytic activation.

➤ CASE STUDY

A 32-year-old white woman, gravida 3, para 2, in her 36th week of gestation noted the sudden onset of lower abdominal pain and profuse vaginal bleeding. She was rushed to the emergency department. On examination she was noted to be hypotensive, with a blood pressure of 70/40 and marked tachycardia. Large ecchymoses and continuous oozing of blood from venipuncture sites were evident. A fetal heart tone was barely audible. Births of her other children were uncomplicated, and the family history was negative for a hemorrhagic diathesis.

Initial coagulation studies revealed PT of 26 sec (normal is 11 to 13 sec); APTT of 84 sec (normal is 24 to 30 sec); platelet count of 20,000/μL (normal is 140,000 to 440,000/μL); fibrinogen, 85 mg/dL (normal is 145 to 350 mg/dL); FDPs, greater than 40 μg/mL (normal is less than 10 μg/mL); and protamine sulfate test, positive (normal is negative). A blood smear showed numerous red cell fragments present.

A diagnosis of DIC was made based on the patient's clinical presentation and the supportive laboratory data. The patient was placed on intravenous fluids to maintain her blood pressure and was given 2 units of fresh frozen plasma and 10 units of platelets. She was taken to the operating room and underwent a caesarean section. Her bleeding abated postoperatively and all coagulation parameters returned to normal within 36 hours.

This case is illustrative of an obstetric complication, placental abruption, that resulted in an acute DIC syndrome. Several triggering mechanisms have been postulated as an explanation for the underlying coagulopathy in this disorder, including the release of thromboplastin-like material from the amniotic fluid and tissue necrosis in the area of the retroperitoneal hemorrhage. The laboratory parameters are consistent with a consumptive coagulopathy and secondary fibrinolysis. With the delivery and removal of the placenta, the source of the triggering mechanism was removed and the pathologic process stopped. Restoration of normal hemostatic parameters occurs within hours postoperatively and usually no further blood component replacement therapy is required.

QUESTIONS

1. D-Dimer formation is the result of the action of plasmin on:
   a. Fibrin monomer
   b. Fibrinogen
   c. Cross-linked fibrin
   d. FDPs

2. Inactivation of factors Va and VIIIa is caused by:
   a. Thrombin
   b. Protein S
   c. t-PA
   d. Activated protein C

3. In primary fibrinolysis, which of the following laboratory tests will be abnormal?
   a. Platelet count
   b. D-Dimer level
   c. Fibrinopeptide A level
   d. Thrombin time

4. In DIC presenting clinically as a hypercoagulable state, it is not unusual for which of the following coagulation times to be paradoxically shortened?
   a. Reptilase time
   b. Euglobulin lysis time
   c. APTT
   d. Thrombin time

5. The primary inhibitor of the fibrinolytic system is:
   a. Antithrombin III
   b. α_2-Antiplasmin
   c. Protein C
   d. α_2-Macroglobulin

SUMMARY CHART

- ➤ Normal hemostasis is the result of the balanced interaction of the vascular endothelium and platelets with four biochemical systems: coagulation, fibrinolytic, kinin, and complement systems.
- ➤ The molecular components of the fibrinolytic system consist of plasminogen, plasmin, plasminogen activators, plasmin inhibitors, and fibrin(ogen).
- ➤ Native plasminogen is a single-chain plasma zymogen of approximately 90,000 daltons that circulates in a lysine and glutamic acid form.
- ➤ Plasminogen activators include tissue plasminogen activator (t-PA), urokinase, and streptokinase.
- ➤ Thrombin complexed with soluble thrombomodulin fragments activates procarboxypeptidase B, which binds to the plasminogen binding site on fibrin, preventing plasmin formation; this is known as thrombin-activatable fibrinolysis inhibitor.
- ➤ Plasmin is a serine protease that has the ability to degrade fibrin in clots and native fibrinogen in circulation into a series of well-characterized end products known as fibrin/fibrinogen degradation products (FDPs).
- ➤ The primary physiologic inhibitor of plasmin in vivo is α_2-antiplasmin; it binds to the lysine binding site on plasmin in a 1:1 molar ratio in an irreversible manner.
- ➤ Disseminated intravascular coagulation (DIC) occurs when the coagulation response has been accentuated and the normal inhibitory mechanisms are overwhelmed and cannot stop thrombus formation; coagulation factors and platelets are consumed with subsequent thrombus formation throughout the microcirculation.
- ➤ Triggering mechanisms of DIC may include activation of the extrinsic coagulation pathway by release of tissue thromboplastin, activation of the intrinsic coagulation pathway with factor XIIa formation, or direct activation of factor X or II.
- ➤ The decompensated DIC state refers to a condition in which active hemorrhage is evident and in which the consumption of the coagulation factors and platelets exceeds the capacity to increase the synthesis of these components.
- ➤ The compensated state of DIC refers to laboratory evidence of accelerated coagulation and fibrinolysis; however, the rate of synthesis of the coagulation components is balanced with the rate of destruction.
- ➤ The hypercoagulable state of DIC is the result of excess thrombin present in the plasma, with a delayed or weakened plasmin response.
- ➤ Therapy for DIC is aimed at treatment or removal of the underlying pathologic stimulus and maintenance of blood volume and hemostatic function.
- ➤ Primary fibrinolysis is a condition in which plasmin is formed in the absence of coagulation processes; prothrombin time (PT), activated partial thromboplastin time (APTT), thrombin time, and FDP are increased, and euglobulin lysis time is shortened.
- ➤ The FDP fragment X is capable of clotting and exerts an anticoagulant effect by competing with fibrinogen for thrombin; fragments D and Y are unclottable.
- ➤ Clinical conditions associated with DIC may include placental abruption, trauma, sepsis, promyelocytic leukemia, cardiopulmonary bypass, immune complex disease, burns, anoxia, liver disease, and snake bites.

References

1. Kaplan, AP, et al: Interaction of the clotting, kinin forming, complement and fibrinolytic pathways. NY Acad Sci 389:25, 1982.
2. Sundsmo, JS, and Fan, DS: Relationships among the complement, kinin, coagulation and fibrinolytic systems. Springer Semin Immunopathol 6:231, 1983.
3. Rosenberg, RD, and Aird, WC: Vascular-bed-specific hemostasis and hypercoagulable states. N Eng J Med 340:994, 1999.
4. Benedict, CR, et al: Endothelial-dependent procoagulant and anticoagulant mechanism. Tex Heart Inst J 21:86, 1984.
5. Esmon, CT: Cell mediated events that control blood coagulation and vascular injury. Ann Rev Cell Biol 9:1, 1993.
6. Castellino, FJ: Recent advances in the chemistry of the fibrinolytic systems. Chem Rev 81:431, 1981.

7. Miller, JL: Normal fibrinolysis. In Henry, JB (ed): Clinical Diagnosis and Management by Laboratory Methods, ed 17. WB Saunders, Philadelphia, 1984, p 769.

8. Mandle, RJ, and Kaplan, AP: Hageman factor-dependent fibrinolysis: Generation of fibrinolytic activity by the interaction of human activated factor XI and plasminogen. Blood 54:850, 1979.

9. Bachman, F, and Kruithof, IEKO: Tissue plasminogen activator: Chemical and physiological aspects. Semin Thromb Hemost 10:6, 1984.

10. Hosaka, Y, et al: Thrombomodulin in human plasma contributes to inhibit fibrinolysis through acceleration of thrombin-dependent activation of plasma procarboxypeptidase. Thromb Haemost 79:371, 1998.

11. Owen, WG: The control of hemostasis. Arch Pathol Lab Med 106:209, 1982.

12. Owen, WG, and Esmon, CT: Functional properties of an endothelial cell cofactor for thrombin-catalyzed activation of protein C. J Biol Chem 256:5532, 1981.

13. Prowse, CV, and Cash, JD: Physiologic and pharmacologic enhancement of fibrinolysis. Semin Thromb Hemost 10:51, 1984.

14. Rickli, EE: The activation mechanism of human plasminogen. Thromb Diath Haemorrh 34:386, 1975.

15. Brogden, RN, et al: Streptokinase: A review of its clinical pharmacology, mechanism of action and therapeutic uses. Drugs 5:357, 1973.

16. Edelberg, JM, et al: Vascular regulation of plasminogen activator inhibitor-1 activity. Semin Thromb Hemost 20:319, 1994.

17. Vaughn D: Update on plasminogen activator inhibitor-1. Can J Cardiol. 14(suppl D):14, 1998.

18. Gonzalez-Gronow, M, et al: Purification and some properties of the glu- and lys-human plasmin heavy chains. J Biol Chem 252:2175, 1977.

19. Marder, VJ, et al: High molecular weight derivatives of human fibrinogen produced by plasmin. I. Physicochemical and immunologic characterization. J Biol Chem 244:2111, 1969.

20. Kudryk, B, et al: Measurement in human blood of fibrinogen/ fibrin fragments containing the B-beta 15–42 sequence. Thromb Res 25:277, 1982.

21. Ockelford, A, and Carter, J: DIC: Application and utility of diagnostic tests. Semin Thromb Hemost 8:198, 1982.

22. Aoki, N, and Harpel, PC: Inhibitors of the fibrinolytic enzyme system. Semin Thromb Hemost 10:24, 1984.

23. Kwaan, HC: Disorders of fibrinolysis. Med Clin N Amer 56:163, 1972.

24. Carey, MJ, and Rodgers, GM: Disseminated intravascular coagulation: Clinical and laboratory aspects. Am J Hematol 59:65, 1998.

25. Bick, RL: Disseminated intravascular coagulation: Pathophysiological mechanisms and manifestations. Semin Thromb Hemost 24:3, 1998.

26. Bick, RL: Disseminated intravascular coagulation: Objective criteria for clinical and laboratory diagnosis and assessment of therapeutic response. Clin Appl Thromb Hemost 1:3, 1995.

27. Muller-Berghaus, G: Pathophysiology of generalized intravascular coagulation. Semin Thromb Hemost 3:209, 1977.

28. Levi, M, et al: Pathogenesis of disseminated intravascular coagulation in sepsis. JAMA 270:975, 1993.

29. Menell, J, et al: Annexin II and bleeding in acute promyelocytic leukemia. N Eng J Med. 340:994, 1999.

30. Fareed, J, et al: Impact of automation on the quantitation of low molecular weight markers of hemostatic defects. Semin Thromb Hemost 9:355, 1983.

31. Hirsh, J: Blood tests for the diagnosis of venous and arterial thrombosis. Blood 57:1, 1981.

32. Buckell, H: The effect of citrate on euglobulin methods of estimating fibrinolytic activity. J Clin Pathol 11:403, 1958.

33. Mant, MJ, and King, EG: Severe, acute disseminated intravascular coagulation. A reappraisal of its pathophysiology, clinical significance and therapy based on 47 patients. Am J Med 47:557, 1979.

34. Tallman, MS, et al: New insights into the pathogenesis of coagulation dysfunction in acute promyelocytic leukemia. Leuk Lymph 11:27, 1993.

35. Bukowski, RM: Thrombotic thrombocytopenic purpura: A review. Prog Hemost Thromb 6:287, 1982.

27 Introduction to Thrombosis and Anticoagulant Therapy

Aamir Ehsan, MD

Julie A. Plumbley, MD

OBJECTIVES

At the end of this chapter, the learner should be able to:

1. Name natural anticoagulants and inhibitors present in plasma.
2. Understand the role of endothelium in thrombogenesis.
3. Understand the mechanism of thrombin/thrombomodulin.
4. Understand the protein C and protein S systems.
5. List the inherited causes of thrombophilia in order of frequency of occurrence.
6. Name the risk factors and acquired conditions leading to thromboembolism.
7. Name the laboratory tests to evaluate patients with hypercoagulable states.
8. Understand the issues in laboratory testing in patients with thrombosis.
9. Name laboratory tests for evaluation of lupus anticoagulant and antiphospholipid syndrome.
10. Understand the mechanism of heparin-induced thrombocytopenia.
11. Name laboratory tests for evaluation of heparin-induced thrombocytopenia.
12. Explain the mechanism of action and understand the conditions in which heparin, oral anticoagulant, and thrombolytic agents are used.
13. Name the most common laboratory tests to monitor oral anticoagulant therapy.
14. Name laboratory tests to monitor heparin therapy.

It has been estimated that more than 600,000 individuals in the United States suffer from pulmonary embolism (PE) each year and that among these more than 150,000 are fatal. These pulmonary emboli arise from almost innumerable deep venous thromboses (DVTs). PE complicating venous thrombosis is one of the most common causes of death in the United States. When one considers the thrombotic complications of arterial disease as manifested in stroke, myocardial infarction (MI), peripheral vascular disease, and PE, thrombosis is by far the most common mechanism of death encountered in the western countries.

More than 150 years ago, Virchow called attention to the fundamental processes involved in the pathogenesis of thrombosis. These included (1) the role of the blood vessel, (2) the flow of the blood within the vessel, and (3) the chemistry of the blood itself. Clinicians and the public alike have become well versed regarding risk factors for the arterial vascular disease of atherosclerosis that, particularly in the western countries, manifests primarily as stroke and MI. Stroke and MI often have thrombosis as the final mechanism of occlusion, usually secondary to the primary atherosclerotic vascular lesion. The thrombogenic surface of the vessel, the altered (turbulent) flow, as well as the blood itself all contribute to thrombus formation in this setting.

Altered flow within the blood vessel is also a well-recognized problem, particularly in the diseased vessel as previously described and in the sedentary or postoperative patient. It is not uncommon, when added to other risks of thrombophilia, that the slowing of blood flow by prolonged sitting as in long airline or driving trips (or writing a book chapter on hypercoagulable states) can precipitate thrombosis in the venous circulation.

This chapter concerns itself primarily with thrombophilia caused by abnormalities in the plasma and the laboratory identification of abnormalities. Up until the middle part of the 1980s, the laboratory had little to offer in the identification of etiologic or risk factors in patients who suffered from thrombosis. Initial interest in these states of risk dates back to the 1960s with the identification of the relationship of lupus anticoagulant to thrombosis and has proceeded to the understanding of the molecular aspects of several of these conditions. These are addressed in the discussion of inherited and acquired thrombophilia later.

Since the first description by Egeberg[1] in 1965 of a Norwegian family with congenital deficiency of antithrombin III (AT-III) and a thrombotic diathesis, understanding of the existing connections between alteration of coagulation inhibitors and thromboembolism progressed rapidly. Abnormalities of hemostasis, as observed in venous thrombosis, primarily reflect disturbances in two regulatory mechanisms, the physiologic coagulation inhibitors and the fibrinolytic system. Hereditary deficiencies in activated protein C resistance, prothrombin gene G20210 mutation, AT-III, protein C (PC), protein S (PS), and defects of the fibrinolytic system, as well as the existence of antiphospholipid antibodies, are the abnormalities most directly associated with thromboembolic disease in patients under 40 years of age. In patients over 40, cancer may be another cause of thromboembolic disease.[2]

In the discussion that follows, these risk factors for thromboses are addressed individually; however, the reader is encouraged to recall that the development of thrombosis[3] is a complex process involving the vessel wall, the flow of the blood, as well as procoagulants and anticoagulants. Inherited and acquired risk factors often "collaborate" in the evolution of the disease.

► REGULATION OF COAGULATION AND FIBRINOLYSIS

The regulation of hemostasis is complex and involves interaction of many components of the coagulation system. In a normal, healthy person, procoagulant and anticoagulant systems are in equilibrium. This balance may be tipped in either direction by a change in clinical circumstances. Because the levels of regulatory and procoagulant proteins vary, a patient may vacillate among a thrombotic, a prothrombotic, and a balanced state. Platelets, endothelial cells, subendothelial structures, and plasma components play important roles. The expression of these functions will be either a thrombotic factor or an antithrombotic reaction during the occurrence of thrombosis.

The Role of Endothelium

The endothelium plays a key role in the regulation of hemostasis. As arteries become smaller in their path into the tissue, the ratio of the surface area to the volume of the blood contained therein rises remarkably. The peak of this activity is reached in the capillary bed where, at a vessel diameter as small as 4 μ, the surface area-to-volume ratio approaches 1000 mM^2/μL[4,5] (Fig. 27–1). More graphically, this is the same as spreading 1 mL of liquid uniformly over the surface of an average game table. No cell or molecule passes through a capillary without having contact with an endothelial cell. This provides a fertile ground for ligand receptor interaction and endothelial cell activation.

Endothelial cells play a key role in the hemostasis-coagulation sequence. They possess both prothrombotic as well as antithrombotic properties.

Prothrombotic Properties

Endothelial cell injury leads to adhesion of platelets to the subendothelial collagen and thus platelet activation. En-

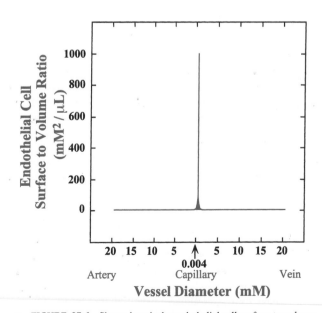

► FIGURE 27–1 Shown here is the endothelial cell surface-to-volume ratio and vessel diameter.

dothelial cells also secrete von Willebrand's factor (vWF), which is essential for platelet and collagen adhesion. Procoagulant properties can be explained by the release of tissue factors from endothelial cells, resulting in activation of the extrinsic pathway. In addition, endothelial cells express binding sites for activated factors IXa and Xa. Lastly, endothelial cells produce inhibitor of tissue plasminogen activator (t-PA), which suppresses fibrinolysis.

Antithrombotic Properties

Intact endothelium prevents the adherence of the platelets to underlying collagen and thus prevents one mode of platelet activation. Even if the platelets are activated, the endothelial cells release prostacyclin (PGI$_2$) and nitric oxide, which are potent inhibitors of platelet aggregation. The PGI$_2$ molecule is the product of arachidonic acid metabolism in the endothelium and is the most potent natural inhibitor of platelet function. The anticoagulant properties of the endothelial cell are mediated by thrombomodulin and heparin cofactor II (described later). Lastly, endothelial cells synthesize t-PA, which promotes fibrinolytic activity and degrades fibrin deposits from endothelial surfaces.

Thrombotic Factors

The Platelets

Thrombin generation in plasma is greatly accelerated by the presence of platelets. Indeed, the activated platelets have an enhanced capacity to catalyze interactions between the activated coagulation factors. This capacity is caused by a rearrangement of the phospholipid structure of the platelet membrane that accompanies the platelet shape change, which offers support for the surface-dependent activation process of coagulation. The platelet release reaction also contributes to the thrombogenesis because when platelets are exposed to various stimuli (e.g., thrombin), the alpha (α) granule contents are released. These granules contain the platelet-specific proteins, platelet factor 4 (PF4), beta (β)-thromboglobulin, platelet-derived growth factor, and a variety of other proteins, including fibrinogen, factor V, and vWF, which provide platelet aggregation, thrombin generation, and local platelet adhesion.

Procoagulant Factors and Generation of Thrombin

Endothelial cells can be induced by various cytokines and endotoxins to produce tissue factor, the activator of the factor VII and the initiator phase of coagulation pathway. In addition, endothelial cells express binding sites for activated factors IXa and Xa. Thrombin is one of the most fascinating enzymes in the coagulation system (Table 27–1). Among the various activities of thrombin are the following:

1. It proteolytically cleaves fibrinogen to produce two molecules of fibrinopeptide A and two molecules of fibrinopeptide B from the Aα and Bβ fibrinogen chains, respectively. This results in conversion of fibrinogen to fibrin monomer. The released fibrin monomers may polymerize to form fibrin thrombi.
2. It converts plasma and platelet factor XIII to an active transglutaminase, which, in turn, cross-links fibrin with covalent amide bonds that render the fibrin insoluble.

> ### Table 27-1
> ### ROLE OF THROMBIN
>
> 1. Cleaves fibrinogen to form fibrinopeptides A and B and fibrin monomers
> 2. Activates factors V, VIII, XI, and XIII and protein C
> 3. Activates platelets to aggregate and secrete granule contents, generating platelet procoagulant activity
> 4. Induces endothelial release of platelet-activating factor, prostacyclin, von Willebrand's factor, interleukin-1, thrombospondin, tissue plasminogen activator, and plasminogen activator inhibitor-1
> 5. Induces granulocyte chemotaxis and adherence to endothelial monolayers to macromolecules
> 6. Depresses reticuloendothelial clearance of activated products of coagulation

3. It can activate the procoagulant factors, factors V, VIII, and XI, to participate in amplifying its own generation.
4. It also binds to platelets at low concentration and initiates shape change, aggregation, and secretion. This includes inducing platelets to make PF3 available on the surface, which facilitates the generation of thrombin by the prothrombin complex.

Thrombin/Thrombomodulin Interaction

Thrombomodulin is critical for the regulation of coagulation. When thrombin is generated at a remote location and is released into the circulation, it will pass to the first capillary bed where it will bind quantitatively to the thrombomodulin on the surface of the endothelium.[6,7] When bound, it changes its enzymatic specificity, no longer recognizing fibrinogen as substrate. Paradoxically, it acts on a circulating zymogen, PC, generating activated protein C (APC). APC cleaves factors Va and VIIIa in the presence of its cofactor, PS. APC also contributes to fibrinolysis by inactivating plasminogen activator inhibitor-1 (PAI-1). Working in concert with its cofactor, PS, the APC proteinase complex constitutes, on a molar basis, the most active inhibitor of plasma coagulation identified and this factor Va–protein C pathway plays a significant role in the regulation of thrombus formation (Fig. 27–2). Therefore, thrombin indirectly possesses antithrombotic activities, limiting the extent of its own generation. In addition to binding thrombin, other activated serum proteases make their way to the capillary bed and bind to antithrombin that is associated with the heparinoids that are located on the surface of the endothelium membrane.

Antithrombotic Factors

Normal plasma contains a sophisticated system of serine protease inhibitors capable of inhibiting many of the activated proteases generated during coagulation and thereby opposing the generation of thrombin (Fig. 27–3). Three types of natural anticoagulants are present in the plasma: (1) AT-III and heparin cofactor II (HC-II), which are serine-protease inhibitors; (2) PC, which, when activated becomes APC which is then capable of degrading factor Va and VIIIa in the presence of its cofactor PS; and (3) a recently described inhibitor of the tissue factor pathway referred to as tissue factor pathway inhibitor (TFPI).

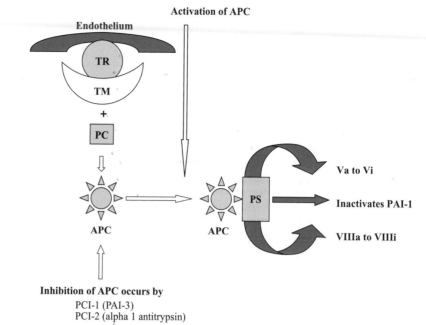

> **FIGURE 27–2** Thrombin binds to thrombomodulin on the surface of endothelial cell. Thrombin/thrombomodulin complex acts on protein C, resulting in the formation of activated protein C (APC). APC cleaves factors Va and VIIIa in the presence of its cofactor, protein S. APC also inactivates plasminogen activator inhibitor-1 (PAI-1). Inhibition of APC occurs by PCI-1 and PCI-2. Abbreviations: TR = thrombin; TM = thrombomodulin; PC = protein C; PS = protein S; PCI = protein C inhibitor.

Antithrombin (Antithrombin-III)

According to the current international nomenclature, AT-III is renamed antithrombin (AT). Therefore, from here onward, the term *AT* will be used instead of AT-III. AT, a heparin cofactor, is an α_2-glycoprotein with a molecular weight of 58,000 daltons (d). It is composed of a single chain of 432 amino acids. Its in vivo half-life is about 2 to 3 days. It is synthesized in the liver and belongs to the serine protease inhibitor superfamily. AT is a major inhibitor of thrombin and factor Xa. Other coagulation factors such as XIIa, XIa, and IXa are also inhibited but to a lesser extent.

Normally, AT is a relatively weak inhibitor of the serine proteases, but it may be activated by various glucosaminoglycans—in particular, heparin and the heparin sulfates. Heparin, which is highly negatively charged, interacts with a domain in the AT molecule containing a high density of basic amino acids, particularly lysine. As a result of the conformational changes in the AT molecule, arginine is made readily available to the active site residue of throm-

bin and other serine proteases. A complex that possesses no enzymatic and no inhibitor activity is formed between AT and the serine protease. As the complex forms, the heparin molecule falls off and is ready to react on another AT molecule. Therefore, heparin administered even in small doses converts AT from a slow, relatively ineffective inhibitor to a fast, effective one. Thus, by inducing a conformational change in the AT molecule, heparin can increase the inhibitory effects of AT by 1000 to 10,000-fold.

Heparin Cofactor II

HC-II was first identified by Birginshaw in 1974[8] and isolated by Tollefsen in 1981.[9] The primary amino acid structure of HC-II is quite distinct from that of AT. The specificity of HC-II is narrowly restricted to thrombin. It does not inhibit other coagulation factors. HC-II also possesses an affinity for heparin that is significantly less than that of AT. Therefore, a higher concentration of heparin is necessary to accelerate thrombin inhibition by this cofactor. The other mucopolysaccharides such as dermatan sulfate are able to accelerate dramatically the action of this protease inhibitor. Indeed, it appears likely that the observed anticoagulant effects of mucopolysaccharides other than heparin are primarily a result of interactions with HC-II. HC-II probably plays a minimal role when heparin is used clinically as an anticoagulant. Tollefsen has suggested that HC-II may function as a second-line inhibitor of thrombin after its activation by dermatan sulfate present on the surface of the vessel wall. It has also been suggested that HC-II is present in a functional active form in human platelets and that platelet HC-II could play a role in the regulation of thrombin generated on the platelet surface.

The Protein C and S System

PC is a vitamin K–dependent zymogen that, once activated by thrombin, proteolytically degrades factors VIIIa and Va, two of the major cofactors involved in thrombin generation.[10] PC has a molecular weight of 62,000 d. It is a glycoprotein with heavy and light chains linked by a disulfide

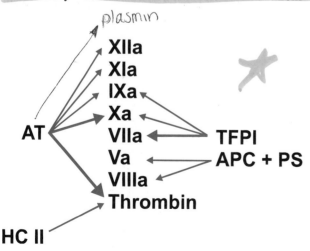

> **FIGURE 27–3** Physiologic inhibitors of coagulation. Abbreviations: AT = antithrombin; APC = activated protein C; XIIa = activated factor XII; HC-II = heparin cofactor II; PS = protein S; TFPI = tissue factor pathway inhibitor.

bond. The anticoagulant role of PC is also described under thrombin/thrombomodulin interaction, earlier, and is depicted in Figure 27–2.

Thrombin activation of PC in the presence of thrombomodulin is modulated by activated factor V (Va). High factor Va concentrations, which can be generated on and bound to endothelial cell surfaces, enhance the activation rate, whereas low concentrations of factor Va inhibit PC activation. This mechanism provides a feedback control on the activation process of PC. PC function is significantly enhanced in the presence of its cofactor (PS) and phospholipids. In the absence of adequate quantities of PS, PC function is inadequate to control the generation of thrombin.

PS is a vitamin K–dependent protein that is produced in the liver as well as in megakaryocytes and endothelial cells. PS is synthesized and released as a single chain with a molecular weight of 69,000 to 84,000 d. It is unique among the vitamin K–dependent coagulation proteins in that it is not the zymogen of a serine protease. Plasma PS circulates in two forms: one form is bound to the C4b-binding protein (C4bBP) from the complement system, the other is free. Only the free form of PS functions as PC cofactor. Platelets also contain PS. Therefore, activation of platelets provides not only a surface for procoagulant reactions, but also a surface and a cofactor for eventual control of the thrombin generation.

Two PC inhibitors have been described. The first is protein C inhibitor-1 (PCI-1), which is identical to plasminogen activator inhibitor-3 (PAI-3). PCI-1 forms a complex with PC, and this complex formation is enhanced in the presence of heparin. More recently, a second inhibitor of PC has been described. This PCI-2, unlike PCI-1 is believed to be heparin-independent and has a relatively high concentration.[11] The amino acid analysis revealed that PCI-2 is identical to α_1-antitrypsin.

Tissue Factor Pathway Inhibitor

More recently described is an inhibitor of the tissue factor pathway referred to as TFPI. TFPI circulates and is associated with a lipoprotein that inhibits plasma coagulation in two ways: (1) it serves to bind the activated form of either factor X or factor IX, thereby inhibiting their enzymatic activity; and (2) when bound to TFPI, the complex of factor X or IX binds to the factor VII tissue factor complex on a membrane, competitively inhibiting further activation of factor X or factor IX at the site.[12] These actions are depicted in Figure 27–4.

Regulation of Fibrinolysis

Physiologic fibrinolysis results in the proteolytic degradation of polymerized fibrin. The central reaction in this system is the conversion of a proenzyme, plasminogen, to the proteolytic enzyme plasmin. Plasminogen is a 90,000-d glycoprotein synthesized in the liver. Its half-life is 2 to 3 days. Plasminogen circulates free or bound to histidine-rich glycoprotein (HRGP), to α_1-antiplasmin, and to fibrinogen. The physiologic activation of plasminogen is achieved by the extrinsic pathway initiated by the t-PA released from the endothelial cells after stimulation, and by the intrinsic pathway through a factor XIIa–dependent activator and urokinase.

A specific group of inhibitors has been described that controls the fibrinolytic process in the plasma. These serine pro-

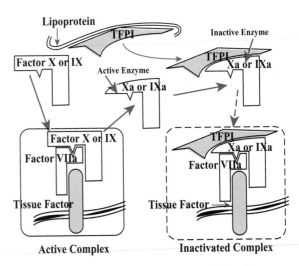

> FIGURE 27–4   Shown here is the interaction of tissue factor pathway inhibitor (TFPI) with factors VII, IX, and X.

tease inhibitors are members of the protein superfamily called *serpins*. They are structurally homologous to many inhibitors of the serine proteases of the coagulation system (Table 27–2). Plasmin activity is regulated and inhibited by a number of plasma proteins such as α_2-antiplasmin, α_2-macroglobulin, α_1-antitrypsin, AT (especially in the presence of heparin), and C1 esterase inhibitor. Physiologically, α_2-antiplasmin is the main plasmin inhibitor. α_2-Antiplasmin is a 60,000-d glycoprotein circulating in the plasma at a concentration of a 1 micromolar. Its properties include the immediate inhibition of plasmin, interference with the absorption of plasminogen to fibrin, and susceptibility to factor XIII catalyzed cross-linking to fibrin. The combined effects of these three characteristics render α_2-antiplasmin much more specific and effective in inhibition of fibrinolysis than any of the other major inhibitors.

Plasminogen activators (PAs) are inhibited by a number of specific proteins. In recent years, research has revealed the existence of at least three different inhibitors of the ex-

> ► Table 27-2
> **INHIBITORY EFFECT OF THE SERINE-PROTEASE INHIBITORS**

Serpin	Inhibitory Effects
α_2-Antiplasmin	Plasmin
α_2-Macroglobulin	Thrombin, plasmin, kallikrein
α_1-Antitrypsin	Thrombin, trypsin, chymotrypsin, factor XIa, elastase, activated protein C
AT	Thrombin; factors Xa, XIIa, IXa, and XIa; plasmin; kallikrein
C1 inhibitor	Kallikrein, plasmin, factors XIIa and XIa, C1 esterase
Antichymotrypsin	Chymotrypsin
HC-II	Thrombin
Protein C inhibitor	Activated protein C
PAI-1 and PAI-2	Plasminogen activators

trinsic system: PAI-1, PAI-2, and PAI-3, identified in plasma and urine (Table 27–3). PAI-3 has also been described as one of the APC inhibitors, PCI-1. The most important inhibitor is PAI-1, a 50-kd plasma glycoprotein that is the primary fast-acting inhibitor of t-PA and a member of the serpin protein superfamily. The physiologic plasma concentration of PAI-1 varies widely from 0 to 60 ng/mL, with an average range of 5 to 20 ng/mL. The physiologic fibrinolytic activity seems to result primarily from the balance between t-PA and its first inhibitor.

The fibrinolytic system is as complex as the coagulation system. The cause-and-effect relationship between the frequency of deficiencies in the physiologic fibrinolytic system and the occurrence of thromboembolism is not fully understood. However, it seems that the most common abnormality is the presence of an excess of PAI-1 leading indirectly to a decreased functional availability of the t-PA.

➤ INHERITED THROMBOPHILIA

Inherited thrombophilia is a group of congenital hematologic disorders that includes a variety of thrombophilic (hypercoagulable) states that usually present clinically as venous and/or arterial thrombosis. Hypercoagulability is usually defined as an alteration of the blood coagulation mechanism that predisposes to thrombosis.

Before proceeding, it is useful to point out that the molecular basis for disease can manifest in two fundamentally different ways. If one thinks about the example of classic hemophilia, one can see that a single mutation in a gene can lead to the phenotype of a distinct clinical disease in the patient. This type of transmission is referred to as a *single gene disorder*. Alternatively, it is possible for the mutation to occur in a gene and, rather than generate the phenotype of the disease process, the lesion increases the risk that a disease will occur. The classical examples of this are the inherited risk for atherosclerosis and many of the conditions that have been identified with thrombosis. Exceptions, of course, would be the homozygous presentation of PC and PS deficiency in which virtually all affected neonates suffer from purpura fulminans in the perinatal period. In contrast, the heterozygous condition is widely variable in the expression of thrombosis. There is little question that these conditions impart a risk; however, the majority of people who carry heterozygous mutations that have been associated with thrombosis do not manifest a thrombotic disease. These molecular as well as acquired disorders all constitute risk factors. In order for thrombosis to manifest clinically, more than one and presumably several of these risk factors need to be present simultaneously to overcome the natural inhibitory processes in the blood that normally protect against thrombosis.

Activated Protein C Resistance — Factor V Leiden

When thrombin is generated at a remote location and is released into the circulation, it passes to the capillary bed where it will bind quantitatively to the thrombomodulin on the surface of the endothelium. This mechanism is described earlier and is depicted in Figure 27–2.

Deficient anticoagulant response of plasma to the addition of APC is called APC resistance (APC-R). This concept of resistance to APC was first described by Dahlback and associates in 1993.[13] Decreased ability of APC to inactivate factor Va results in a thrombophilic state. Possible mechanisms of APC-R include inhibitors to APC (autoantibodies), functional PS deficiency, and mutated forms of factors V and VIII molecules. In the majority of cases, this APC-R is the result of a genetic defect. A defect in factor V gene involving the point mutation at codon 506 of exon 10 (arginine 506 to glutamine 506 or factor V Leiden or FV:Q^{506}) is most often the cause of APC-R.[14] This is the site where APC cleaves and inactivates the procoagulant factor Va. The mutated factor Va thus cannot be inactivated by APC and results in persistence of procoagulant activity. Therefore, it increases risk of venous thrombosis. Recently, mutations at the arginine 306 residue in factor V, the second APC site, have been reported.[15] No genetic abnormalities in the factor VIII gene have been identified to cause APC-R in humans.

APC-R is the most common risk factor associated with inherited venous thrombosis among Caucasians. It can be detected in 20% to 60% of patients with recurrent venous thrombosis and shows autosomal-dominant inheritance. The heterozygous state is relatively common in western countries and accounts for approximately 6%[16] of the general population.[17,18] The prevalence in Hispanic, African-American, Asian, and Native American populations appears to be low. The thrombotic risk for patients carrying heterozygous factor V mutation is increased five to ten times, while the risk for homozygous patients is 50 to 100 times.

➤ Table 27–3
TPA INHIBITORS

	PAI-1	PAI-2	PAI-3
Origin	Plasma	Placenta	Urine
	Platelets	Leukocytes	Plasma
	Endothelial cell	Macrophages	
	Granulocytes		
MW (daltons)	54,000	47,000	50,000
Inhibitory effect	TPA	TPA	UK
	UK	UK	APC
Concentration	0–1.3 nM	2 µM (3rd trimester)	—

Abbreviations: UK = urokinase; APC = activated protein C; MW = molecular weight; nM = nanomoles; µM = micromoles

Factor V Leiden–associated thrombotic risk appears to be dependent on the underlying clinical setting. Although oral contraceptives and pregnancy significantly increase the risk for venous thrombosis in women with the mutation, the increased thrombotic risk in patients with preexistent cancer or recent surgery cannot be demonstrated.[16] There are no convincing data that factor V Leiden mutation confers an increased risk for arterial thrombosis. Recent data for factor V Leiden, as an independent risk factor for myocardial infarction is controversial.

Most of the screening tests for APC resistance are functional activated partial thromboplastin time (APTT)–based assays. The APTT is performed with the addition of calcium chloride ($CaCl_2$) in the presence and absence of a standardized amount of APC, and two clotting times are converted into an APC ratio (Fig. 27–5). In a normal person, the addition of APC to plasma induces a prolonged clotting time. This occurs because APC cleaves and inactivates factors Va and VIIIa. In patients with APC resistance, the clotting time is shortened. Factor Va is not cleaved and, therefore, not activated. The test results can be interpreted by comparing the ratio to the normal range, or by normalizing it to the APC resistance ratio obtained using normal pooled plasma. By diluting the patient's plasma with an excess of factor V–deficient plasma, the sensitivity and specificity of the APTT-based APC-R assay can be increased. The addition of factor V–deficient plasma normalizes the concentrations of other plasma proteins involved in the formation and regulation of thrombin and, thus, allows the analysis of plasma from patients who are taking oral anticoagulants or have other factor deficiencies. The limitation of this APTT-based functional assay is that the results are unreliable when the test is performed on patients that are given heparin or have an underlying inhibitor (lupus anticoagulant), because these conditions could prolong the baseline APTT. The test, however, may be performed during an acute thrombotic episode.

The genetic test for FV:Q[506] mutation is often referred to as the factor V Leiden assay. In this test, the genomic deoxyribonucleic acid (DNA) is isolated from blood mononuclear cells. A 267-base pair region of the factor V gene surrounding codon 506 is amplified using polymerase chain reaction (PCR). After digestion with a restriction enzyme (*Mnl* I), the sample DNA is then sized by electrophoresis in agarose gel stained with ethidium bromide. The gel is photographed using an ultraviolet illumination, and the band pattern and size are analyzed allowing specific genotypes to be identified (normal, heterozygous, or homozygous).

The genetic test is usually performed to confirm the factor V Leiden mutation and has several advantages over plasma-based functional assays. The genetic test is not affected if the patient is receiving anticoagulants or has plasma inhibitors (such as lupus anticoagulant). It does not have a threshold range such as the functional plasma-based assays, and it can differentiate between heterozygous and homozygous states.

At present the most cost-effective approach in diagnosing patients with factor V Leiden is to perform an APTT-based functional assay for APC-R. Patients with low APC-R ratios (results may vary among different laboratories) should be genotyped for the factor V mutation. For example, in our coagulation laboratory at University Hospital at San Antonio, a ratio of less than 0.9 is considered abnormal. Even in laboratories in which there is an excellent concordance between APC-R assays and the results of factor V Leiden mutation assays, some patients with a low APC-R ratio and negative genetic results can still be identified. The significance of this finding is uncertain and may be related to mutation other than FV:Q[506].

Protein C Deficiency

Hereditary deficiency of PC is autosomal dominant. The prevalence for inherited PC deficiency among patients with inherited venous thrombosis is estimated to be 6% to 10%. The frequency of the heterozygous state varies between 1/300 and 1/1000, and the frequency of the homozygous state is estimated to be 1/50,000.[19] The homozygotes have a marked tendency for recurrent venous thrombosis and PE, neonatal purpura fulminans, and warfarin-induced skin necrosis.

Warfarin-induced skin necrosis has been associated in patients with PC deficiency. It occurs during the first few days of warfarin therapy. Warfarin ingestion results in a decrease in vitamin K–dependent factors. Because of the short half-life of PC as compared to other vitamin K–dependent factors, the decrease in PC level occurs before the decrease in factor II and X levels. This causes a temporary imbalance between procoagulant and anticoagulant factors, resulting in a transient hypercoagulable state that leads to thrombosis.

Infants with inherited homozygous PC deficiency may

APC-V RATIO: $$\dfrac{\text{Patient Clot time APC/CaCl}_2}{\text{Patient Clot time CaCl}_2}$$

Normal ratio: more than 1.0

Case 1: $\dfrac{84\ \text{sec}}{35\ \text{sec}}$

The APC-V ratio in this case is 2.4, the test is negative for APC resistance, therefore no genetic test is needed.

Case 2: $\dfrac{31\ \text{sec}}{35\ \text{sec}}$

The APC-V ratio is less than 0.9, the test is positive for APC resistance and therefore this patient should be tested for Factor V Leiden mutation by PCR.

Note: The test result can be interpreted by comparing the ratio to the normal range or by normalizing it to the APC resistance ratio obtained using normal pooled plasma.

➤ **FIGURE 27–5** Data on the functional assay for activated protein C are shown here. This is an APTT-based assay and the APC-V ratio can be calculated by measuring the patient clot time with and without activated protein C (APC) in the presence of $CaCl_2$. In a normal person, the ratio is more than 0.9. In case 1, the ratio is 2.4 and thus the test is negative for activated protein C resistance (APC-R). In case 2, the ratio is less than 0.9 and the test for APC-R is positive. In case 2, therefore, the patient should be tested for factor V Leiden mutation by polymerase chain reaction (PCR).

Abbreviation: APC-V = activated protein C-factor V ratio

develop thrombosis of small capillaries including that of cerebral vessels, bacterial sepsis, and laboratory evidence of disseminated intravascular coagulation (DIC). The condition is usually fatal and is called *neonatal purpura fulminans*. It is also important to note that the physiologic level of PC in a newborn is low and may be near zero in the sick preterm infant, but usually rises rapidly after birth.

The functional assay is used as the screening assay for inherited deficiency. The antigenic assay is used to determine the mechanism of the deficiency (decreased production or abnormal protein) and is rarely necessary in diagnosis. Based on immunologic and functional assays, two subtypes of heterozygous PC deficiency have been described. Type I deficiency is the most common subtype, which involves a reduction in both the activity and antigen of PC (to approximately 50% of normal). Type II deficiency is less frequent; the affected individuals have normal antigenic levels but reduced functional activity of PC (as a result of molecular or genetic defects).[20,21]

The procedures used for immunologic assays are enzyme-linked immunosorbent assay (ELISA), electroimmunodiffusion (Laurell rocket electrophoresis), and radioimmunoassay. The commonly used Laurell rocket test is performed in a 1% agarose gel medium containing antiserum specific for PC. Electrophoresis is used to migrate the proteins into the antibody field after the plasma wells are applied to the wells in the agarose. A rocket-shaped precipitate pattern forms along the axis of migration, the length of which is proportional to the antigen concentration.

In the simpler functional assay, PC is activated in the presence of the specific activator extracted from *Agkistrodon contortrix* venom. The resulting APC inhibits the factors V and VIII, and thus prolongs the APTT. The enzyme's anticoagulant activity can be measured in a clotting assay or its amidolytic activity can be measured using a chromogenic assay. Using both the clotting and amidolytic assays, useful information regarding the nature of molecular defect in type II PC deficiency may be detected. The cases have been described with normal PC antigen level but reduction in PC anticoagulant activity and normal amidolytic activity by chromogenic assay. For this reason, clot-based PC assays are preferred (Table 27–4).

Acquired PC deficiency can be seen in a number of conditions (Table 27–5) that include liver disease, DIC, warfarin therapy, severe infection/septic shock, adult respiratory distress syndrome, postoperative states, acute thrombotic episode and secondary to chemotherapy (L-asparaginase, methotrexate, cyclophosphamide, and 5-fluorouracil).

Protein S Deficiency

PS is a vitamin K–dependent plasma glycoprotein that is synthesized mainly in the liver and endothelial cells. PS exists in

an active free form (cofactor for APC) and inactive bound form complexed to complement binding protein C4bBP. The active free form accounts for 40% of the total PS.[21]

PS deficiency is inherited as an autosomal-dominant disorder. The prevalence of PS deficiency in the general population is 1 in 33,000. The incidence of PS deficiency in patients with venous thrombosis is 6% to 10%. The heterozygotes have a strong tendency to develop DVT, PE, cerebral and mesenteric thrombosis, superficial thrombophlebitis, and arterial thrombosis and may also develop warfarin-induced skin necrosis. Patients with homozygous PS deficiency are severely affected and may develop neonatal purpura fulminans just after birth, similar to that seen with PC deficiency.

Both immunologic and functional methods are available that can measure PS. The reliable measurements of total PS antigen are by radioimmunoassay, ELISA and electroimmunodiffusion (Laurell rocket electrophoresis). The Lau-

> **Table 27–5**
CAUSES OF ACQUIRED DEFECTS OF COAGULATION INHIBITORS

Inhibitors	Causes of Acquired Defects
AT	DIC
	Liver disease
	Nephrotic therapy
	Oral contraceptives
	L-Asparaginase
Protein C	Oral anticoagulant treatment
	DIC
	Vitamin K deficiency
	After plasma exchange
	Postoperative state
	L-Asparaginase
	Liver disease
Protein S	Oral anticoagulant treatment
	Pregnancy
	Oral contraceptives
	Vitamin K deficiency
	Liver disease
	Diabetes type I
	Acute inflammation
	Newborn infants

> **Table 27–4**
CLASSIFICATION OF HEREDITARY PC DEFICIENCIES

Subtypes	Antigen	Anticoagulant Activity	Amidolytic Activity
I	Low	Low	Low
IIa	Normal	Low	Low
IIb	Normal	Low	Normal

rell rocket test is performed in a 1% agarose gel medium containing antiserum specific for PS. Electrophoresis is used to migrate the proteins into the antibody field after the plasma wells are applied to the wells in the agarose. A rocket-shaped precipitate pattern forms along the axis of migration, the length of which is proportional to the total antigen concentration. The addition of polyethylene glycol (PEG) to plasma causes the C4bBP complex but not the free PS to precipitate and, thus, correlation of free PS antigen with functional free PS activity can be made.

Functional assays are performed for the quantitative measurement of the free functional PS level based on the ability of PS to serve as a cofactor for the anticoagulant effect of APC inhibition of factor Va. This inhibition is reflected by the prolongation of the clotting time of a system that is enriched with factor Va, a physiologic substrate for APC.

Based on the immunologic and functional assays described earlier, three subtypes of PS deficiency have been noted (Table 27–6). The most common type I deficiency is associated with low antigenic level of total and free PS levels and low activity level of PS. In type IIa deficiency, total PS is normal; however, the free and functional PS activity is low. In type IIb deficiency, total and free antigen levels are normal, but activity level of PS is low.

Acquired PS deficiency can be seen in liver disease, DIC, pregnancy, oral contraceptive use, vitamin K deficiency, during an acute thrombotic event, and in therapy with warfarin and L-asparaginase (see Table 27–5). C4bBP is an acute-phase reactant. Therefore, the amount of free PS may decrease in inflammatory conditions such as systemic lupus erythematosus (SLE), inflammatory bowel disease, pregnancy, and acquired immunodeficiency syndrome (AIDS).

Antithrombin Deficiency

The prevalence of AT deficiency in the general population has been estimated at 1/2000 to 1/5000. The prevalence of AT deficiency in patients with inherited venous thrombosis is 3% to 5%.[22] The pattern of inheritance is autosomal dominant. The majority of affected individuals are heterozygous with AT levels between 40% and 70% of normal. Homozygous individuals have extremely low levels of AT levels. The initial clinical manifestations may occur spontaneously in half of the patients and are characterized by thrombosis of the deep veins of the lower extremities, mesenteric veins, and PE. In the other half of the patients, the clinical manifestations may be related to pregnancy, use of oral contraceptive pills, surgery, or trauma.

Various methods have been described for the measurement of AT. Immunologic assays such as radial immunodiffusion are available that measure the antigen levels but cannot be used to detect dysfunctional molecules. To detect the qualitative abnormality of the AT molecules, two functional assays have been developed. The first is the AT-heparin cofactor assay, in which thrombin is added to patient's plasma containing AT in the presence of heparin. This test measures the ability of heparin to bind to lysyl residues on the AT and catalyze the neutralization of coagulation enzymes such as thrombin or factor Xa, or both. Residual thrombin is then determined with a thrombin-specific chromogenic substrate. The concentration of AT is inversely proportional to residual thrombin activity. The second test is the progressive AT activity assay, which measures the capacity of AT to neutralize the enzymatic activity of thrombin in the absence of heparin. The AT-heparin cofactor assay detects all the different subtypes of the deficiency states and is, therefore, the best single laboratory screening test for this disorder.

Based on immunologic and functional assays, two types of AT deficiency can be distinguished phenotypically. In the common type I deficiency (quantitative defects) there is a proportionate decrease in both antigen and function of AT. It is due to genetic mutations producing silent alleles. Approximately 80 distinct mutations have been described in patients with a type I deficiency.[23,24] The type II deficiency (qualitative or dysfunctional defects) is associated with point mutations. It can be further subdivided into three subtypes: (1) those characterized by abnormalities primarily affecting the serine protease inhibition site for thrombin/Xa, (2) those affecting the heparin-binding site, and (3) those with pleiotropic effects on both protease inhibition and heparin binding. Table 27–7 summarizes the classification of hereditary AT deficiencies.

Based on functional assays, the prevalence of thrombosis appears to be different in heterozygous patients with type II defects. Individuals with low plasma AT heparin cofactor activity and normal progressive AT activity (heparin-binding site defects) have infrequent thrombotic episodes. In contrast, heterozygous type II patients with both diminished progressive AT activity and AT-heparin cofactor activity (thrombin-binding site defects) sustain venous thrombosis as often as type I patients.

Acquired AT deficiency can be seen in liver disease, DIC, pregnancy, eclampsia, or preeclampsia, use of oral contraceptives, nephrotic syndrome, after major surgery, during acute thrombotic episode, and secondary to heparin and L-asparaginase therapy (see Table 27–5).

Prothrombin Nucleotide G20210A Mutation

Prothrombin (coagulation factor II) is a vitamin K–dependent factor that is converted to thrombin by factor Xa in the presence of factor Va, Ca^{2+}, and phospholipids. The combination of factor Va, Xa, Ca^{2+}, and phospholipid is called *prothrombinase complex*. Hereditary disorders of prothrombin synthesis may result in quantitative defects (decreased production) and qualitative defects (dysfunctional prothrombin molecule). Clinically both of these defects may result in a bleeding diathesis.

A 21-kb long gene present on chromosome 11 codes for the prothrombin molecule. This gene consists of 14 exons and 13 introns. A mutation in the prothrombin gene has been recently described.[25] Presence of a single guanine (G) to adenine (A) mutation at nucleotide position 20210 has been shown to be associated with an elevated prothrombin level and an increased risk of DVT.

> ## Table 27-6
> ## CLASSIFICATION OF HEREDITARY PS DEFICIENCIES

Subtypes	Total PS	Free PS	PS Activity
I	Low	Low	Low
IIa	Normal	Low	Low
IIb	Normal	Normal	Low

> **Table 27-7**
CLASSIFICATION OF HEREDITARY AT DEFICIENCIES

| Subtypes | AT Antigen | ACTIVITY | |
		AT-Heparin Cofactor	Progressive AT
I	Low	Low	Low
IIa	Normal	Low	Low
IIb	Normal	Low	Normal
IIc	Normal	Normal	Low

The heterozygous G20210A mutation is found in 2% of healthy controls, 6% and 7% of venous thrombosis patients, and 18% of selected thrombophilia patients with positive family history. The relative risk for venous thrombosis in heterozygotes is approximately threefold.[26] Carriers of this mutation have higher plasma prothrombin levels than the controls with normal 20210 genotype. A high level of prothrombin alone is not a reliable marker of disease predisposition, whereas detection of the mutation by genetic testing appears to be a reliable prognostic factor.

At present, the PCR test for G20210A mutation is available in clinical laboratories. In this test, DNA is isolated from blood mononuclear cells and a 506-bp region of the prothrombin gene is amplified using PCR. The amplified product is digested with restriction endonuclease enzyme *Hin*d III. After digestion with *Hin*d III, the sample DNA is then sized by electrophoresis in agarose gel stained with ethidium bromide. The gel is photographed using ultraviolet illumination and the band pattern and size are analyzed, allowing identification of specific genotypes (normal, heterozygous, or homozygous). Among the Dutch population, the prothrombin gene mutation is the second most common genetic defect (the most frequent being the factor V Leiden mutation). Because of the high prevalence of APC resistance (FV:Q[506]) and of the prothrombin gene mutation (G20210A), combinations of genetic defects are relatively common. Patients with both mutations (double heterozygotes) may have a high risk of thrombosis. However, more studies are needed to improve our understanding of the ethnicity-specific variability of the factor V Leiden and prothrombin gene mutations.

Hyperhomocysteinemia

Homocysteine is an amino acid derived from metabolic conversion of methionine. Homocysteine is usually metabolized within the cells to methionine (via remethylation pathway) and to cysteine (via transulfuration pathway). Remethylation to methionine involves two pathways. In the first remethylation pathway, homocysteine accepts a methyl group from betaine. In the second remethylation pathway, homocysteine accepts a methyl group from 5-methyltetrahydrofolate, with vitamin B_{12} acting as a cofactor. This pathway is catalyzed by methionine synthase. The transulfuration pathway is catalyzed by cystathione β-synthetase with vitamin B_6 as a cofactor[27] (Fig. 27–6).

Hyperhomocysteinemia (an elevated plasma level of homocysteine) is a risk factor for the development of early atherosclerotic vascular disease and venous thrombosis. Some investigators include hyperhomocysteinemia under acquired disorders, whereas recent studies suggest that these should be included among the list of inherited causes of thrombophilia.

Hyperhomocysteinemia can be inherited or acquired. Inherited forms have genetic defects that involve (1) the remethylation pathway, as a result of a deficiency of methylene tetrahydrofolate reductase (MTHFR); and (2) the transulfuration pathway, owing to deficiency of cystathione β-synthetase. The mutation of *MTHFR* gene (alanine substitution to valine at amino acid 677) is more common. This mutation can vary from 1.5% to 15%, depending on the population studied.[28] The frequent causes of acquired hy-

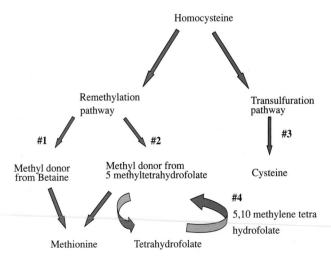

> FIGURE 27–6 Homocysteine can be metabolized to methionine (via remethylation) and to cysteine (via transulfuration). The numbers represent the enzymes involved in the reactions: (*1*) Betaine homocysteine methyltransferase; (*2*) methionine synthase in the presence of cofactor vitamin B_{12}; (*3*) cystathione β-synthetase in the presence of cofactor vitamin B_6; (*4*) methylene tetrahydrofolate reductase (MTHFR).

perhomocysteinemia are secondary to deficiencies of folate, vitamin B_{12} and/or vitamin B_6, which are cofactors in homocysteine metabolism.

Possible mechanisms by which hyperhomocysteinemia acts as a thrombogenic and atherogenic risk factor includes vascular smooth muscle proliferation, inhibition of endothelial cell growth and intimal thickening, activation of factor V, and inhibition of PC activation. Severe hyperhomocysteinemia is secondary to genetic defects and characterized by mental retardation, premature atherosclerosis, venous thromboembolism, and skeletal abnormalities. Mild to moderate hyperhomocysteinemia can be secondary to genetic or acquired conditions and is an independent risk factor for stroke, MI, and peripheral vascular disease. Levels of homocysteine can be measured by high-pressure liquid chromatography. A PCR-based genetic test is now available to detect the common Ala 677 Val mutation in the *MTHFR* gene.

Tissue Factor Pathway Inhibitor (TFPI) Deficiency

TFPI may play a significant role in preventing thrombus formation; however, deficiency of this inhibitor is yet to be associated with thromboembolic disease. Evidence suggests that TFPI neutralizes two proteases simultaneously; and the inhibitory actions of TFPI occur through three domains.[29] The first domain inhibits factor VIIa/tissue factor (TF) complex, whereas the second domain inhibits factor Xa. The function of the third domain is unclear. TFPI can be found in endothelial cells, plasma, and platelets. The endothelial cell pool represents the majority of the TFPI. Most of the plasma pool is complexed with various lipoproteins, whereas only 10% of the TFPI is present as a free form and is biologically active.

Recombinant TFPI is now available and has been evaluated in a few studies, with results showing a possible role of TFPI in the interruption of thrombus formation. Whether or not there is a congenital deficiency of this inhibitor leading to thromboembolic conditions is not yet known.

Factor XII Deficiency

Factor XII is one of the contact factors that initiate the intrinsic pathway of coagulation in vitro. It is also known as Hageman factor; named after the patient in whom its deficiency was identified in Cleveland in 1955. Patients with factor XII deficiency have a prolongation of APTT but no bleeding diathesis. Instead, a number of cases with venous thromboembolism and myocardial infarction have been described in factor XII–deficient patients. Mr. Hageman himself died of a PE. Because factor XIIa is involved in activating plasminogen, the thrombophilic tendency in factor XII deficiency patients has been attributed to reduced plasma fibrinolytic activity. The incidence of thrombosis in patients with heterozygous or homozygous factor XII deficiency in the absence of other thrombotic risk factors is uncertain and, thus, an increased thrombotic risk associated with factor XII deficiency remains to be well defined.

Heparin Cofactor II Deficiency

Heparin cofactor II is a single-chain glycoprotein present in human plasma that inhibits only thrombin but does not inhibit other coagulation factors. The affinity of heparin cofactor II for heparin is lower than that of AT and requires a higher concentration of heparin to affect in vitro testing (more than the therapeutic concentration (i.e., more than 1 U/mL of heparin). Therefore, heparin cofactor II probably plays an insignificant role in the clinical setting.[30] On the contrary, the activity of heparin cofactor II can be increased several folds by dermatan sulfate, which has no effect on the activity of AT. The clinical manifestations of hereditary heparin cofactor II deficiency range from asymptomatic patients to arterial and venous thrombosis. More studies are needed to determine the significance of this deficiency.

Dysfibrinogenemia

Dysfibrinogenemia is defined as a condition in which there is a structural or functional abnormality of the fibrinogen molecule, or both. If congenital, the inheritance is autosomal dominant. The clinical presentation is variable. Sixty percent of the patients are asymptomatic, bleeding diathesis can be seen in 20% of cases, and 20% of cases may present with recurrent arterial or venous thromboembolism, or both.[31]

A number of functional and biochemical defects of the fibrinogen molecule have been described. These include abnormality in binding of thrombin to fibrinogen, release of abnormal fibrinopeptides, defective fibrin polymerization and cross-linking, decreased activation of plasminogen, and resistance to lysis by plasmin. These abnormalities are reflected in the routine coagulation assays as prolongation of PT, APTT, reptilase time, and thrombin time. The fibrinogen concentration by functional assay is low, but is normal when measured immunologically. An important point to consider is that the abnormal fibrinogen may not be incorporated into the clot, and the soluble molecules that remain in the serum can be mistaken for fibrinogen degradation products, in some assays, leading to the misdiagnosis of active fibrinolysis and thus DIC.

Dysfibrinogenemia can be seen in acquired conditions such as severe liver disease, as a part of paraneoplastic syndrome in hypernephroma, and secondary to paraproteinemia.[32] Acquired dysfibrinogenemia is rarely symptomatic and thrombotic complications have not been described.

Elevated Plasma Factor VIII Coagulant Activity

The significance of elevated plasma factor VIII coagulant levels as a risk factor for thrombosis (elevated functional and antigenic levels) has been studied in a selected population. This abnormality could not be attributed to inflammation, because less than 10% of the patients with factor VIII:C levels of greater than 150% had elevations in acute-phase reactant (such as C-reactive protein, fibrinogen, and erythrocyte sedimentation rate [ESR]). However, additional data are required to determine the association of elevation of factor VIII:C and thrombosis.

Lipoprotein a (Lpa) and Thrombosis

Lpa represents a low-density lipoprotein (LDL)–like particle having a protein moiety apoprotein B-100 linked by a disulfide bridge to a glycoprotein called apolipoprotein a (Apo a). Elevated levels of Lpa are under genetic control and have been recognized as an atherothrombogenic factor. But the underlying mechanisms for this pathogenicity are not well understood. There is a structural homology of Apo a with plasminogen, and laboratory studies have shown that Lpa inhibits fibrinolysis. It effectively competes with plasminogen for binding to fibrin or endothelial cells. It also binds t-PA and may also stimulate the release of PAI-1 from endothelial cells. Although some studies do show evidence of Lpa in atherogenesis/thrombogenesis and association with chronic heart disease, more prospective studies are required to evaluate the exact role of Lpa as an independent risk factor for arterial thrombosis.[33–35]

➤ ACQUIRED THROMBOTIC DISORDERS

Lupus Anticoagulant/ Antiphospholipid Syndrome

Antiphospholipid (aPL) syndrome is one of the acquired thrombotic disorders. The clinical features of aPL syndrome include thrombosis and recurrent pregnancy loss and sometimes thrombocytopenia or hemolytic anemia.[36] The thrombosis may be arterial or venous and tends to recur in the same site. aPL syndrome is considered secondary when it occurs in association with another disorder, and primary when unassociated with any identified underlying disorder. Secondary aPL syndrome is most frequently associated with SLE or other autoimmune disease, but has occasionally been seen after exposure to certain pharmaceuticals (such as phenothiazines, quinidine, hydralazine, procainamide) and in patients with underlying malignancies. The overall prevalence of aPL syndrome is difficult to determine because of variations in laboratory techniques and diagnostic criteria. In spite of this, prevalence of aPL syndrome in SLE patients has been examined by many researchers. The frequency of lupus anticoagulant (LA) and anticardiolipin (aCL) in nearly 2000 SLE patients reported in the literature is 31% and 40%, respectively. Patients with SLE and aPL antibodies had a 30% to 40% risk of thrombosis.[37]

Laboratory evidence of aPL antibodies can be in the form of either immunologically demonstrated aPL antibodies; ELISAs for aCL antibodies being the most frequently used LA, or both. The term *lupus anticoagulant* refers specifically to the laboratory phenomenon of prolongation of phospholipid-dependent coagulation assays such as the APTT not attributable to a specific factor deficiency.

The presence of aPL antibodies, either demonstrated by LA or detected immunologically, is not sufficient for the diagnosis of aPL syndrome. The clinical features must also be present (Table 27–8). aPL antibodies may be present in the absence of aPL syndrome. In particular, infection-associated aPL antibodies are usually transient and rarely associated with thrombotic complications.[38,39] Most aPL antibodies detected in children are of this type; however, aPL syndrome rarely occurs in children.

History of Antiphospholipid Syndrome

The term *antiphospholipid antibody* is actually inaccurate. A more accurate term would be *antiphospholipid-protein antibodies*. This is because the antibodies have specificities for certain proteins when those proteins are bound to phospholipids or other surfaces such as microtiter plates. "Lupus anticoagulant" is also not entirely accurate because the phenomenon is not always associated with SLE and causes thrombosis in vivo even though it behaves as an anticoagulant in vitro. However, for historical reasons, the terms aPL antibody and LA are well embedded in the literature.

In 1963, Bowie and colleagues published a paper calling

> ➤ **Table 27-8**

CRITERIA FOR DIAGNOSIS OF "DEFINITE" ANTIPHOSPHOLIPID ANTIBODY SYNDROME

A minimum of one clinical and one laboratory feature should be present.

Clinical

- Confirmed vascular thrombosis

- Pregnancy morbidity, to include one of the situations described below:

  - ≥ 1 unexplained death at ≥ 10 week EGA

    Morphologically normal neonate

  - ≥ 1 premature birth at ≤ 34 week EGA

    Due to severe pre-eclampsia, eclampsia, or severe placental insufficiency

    Morphologically normal neonate

  - ≥ 3 unexplained consecutive spontaneous abortions at < 10 weeks EGA

    Maternal and paternal chromosomes normal

    No maternal anatomic or hormonal abnormality

Laboratory

- Medium to high titer IgG and/or IgM aCL antibody in blood on ≥ 2 occasions, ≥ 6 weeks apart measured by standardized ELISA for β2GPI-dependent aCL antibodies

- LA in plasma on ≥ 2 occasions, ≥ 6 weeks apart detected per ISTH guidelines

Abbreviations: EGA = estimated gestational age; LA = lupus anticoagulant; β2GPI = β_2-glycoprotein I; ISTH = International Society on Thrombosis and Haemostasis

Source: Adapted from the International Consensus Statement on Preliminary Classification Criteria for Definite Antiphospholipid Syndrome. Post-conference workshop, October 10, 1998, Eighth International Symposium on Antiphospholipid Antibodies.[34]

---

attention to a syndrome they had observed in patients with SLE.[40] The syndrome, still unnamed, consisted of recurrent venous or arterial thrombosis accompanied by paradoxical prolongation of clotting times in phospholipid-dependent clotting assays. This phenomenon of prolonged clotting times in the absence of specific factor inhibitors or deficiencies came to be known as lupus anticoagulant. As in many SLE patients, some of these patients were observed to have a false positive venereal disease research laboratory test (VDRL). The VDRL is a serologic screening test for syphilis that uses a mixture of cardiolipin (an acidic phospholipid found in beef heart), lecithin, and cholesterol. Given the coexistence of the LA phenomenon and the antiphospholipid antibodies demonstrated by a positive VDRL, it seemed likely that LA antibodies were nonspecific antibodies that reacted with both platelet and reagent phospholipids. The interference of such antibodies with phospholipid-dependent coagulation reactions could prolong clotting times. How these antibodies promote coagulation in vivo was not understood and is still unproven, but eventually the concept of an aPL syndrome proposed by Harris in 1987 took hold and the terms are still with us.[41]

Immunology

In 1983, Harris and colleagues developed a solid-phase radioimmunoassay (RIA) for aCL antibodies.[42] Recall that cardiolipin is one of the components of the VDRL. High titers of these antibodies correlated well with the presence of LA, thrombosis, and thrombocytopenia. The aCL assay, now usually done by ELISA rather than by RIA, is the most frequently used immunologic assay for the identification of aPL antibodies.[43] Over the years it has been shown that aPL antibodies can be detected by using various phospholipids, including phosphatidylinositol, phosphatidic acid, and phosphatidylserine. In addition, investigators have shown that LAs and aCL antibodies in a given patient can often be separated. In 1990, three groups working independently found that the majority of aCL antibodies bind phospholipid-bound β_2-glycoprotein I (β2GPI).[44-46] β2GPI, also known as apolipoprotein H, is a 50-kd plasma protein present at a concentration of approximately 200 mg/mL that appears to have anticoagulant properties, although its physiologic role is uncertain. Some LAs have also been shown to bind in a β2GPI-dependent manner.[47] In addition, a large proportion of LAs and some aCL antibodies bind prothrombin.[48-50] These antibodies usually do not deplete plasma levels of β2GPI and prothrombin because they bind only when these antigens are attached to phospholipid surfaces. Occasionally, patients with SLE have reduced prothrombin levels and a resulting hemorrhagic diathesis. Other phospholipid-binding proteins may also be targets of thrombogenic aPL antibodies.

Mechanism of Thrombosis

It would be reasonable to question whether aPL antibodies are causative in aPL syndrome or merely an epiphenomenon that is of importance in diagnosis. It is likely that multiple perturbations of hemostatic mechanisms are required to bring about thrombophilia. It would be reasonable to assume that, if they were part of the etiology, they would affect phospholipid-dependent reactions in vivo and in vitro. In vitro evidence of such effects have been reported and include inhibition of activated protein C, inhibition of antithrombin-dependent anticoagulant mechanisms, inhibition of fibrinolysis, induction of increased soluble tissue factor, inhibition of prostacyclin secretion, promotion of platelet activation, interference with the anticoagulant properties of β2GPI, and displacement of annexin V from trophoblast.[51] Annexin V is a protein that has potent anticoagulant properties in vivo and that may modulate thrombosis on the surfaces of cells lining placental and systemic vasculatures. Interference with the function of annexin V may play a role in aPL syndrome in which there is recurrent pregnancy loss.[52]

The Laboratory's Contribution to the Diagnosis of aPL Syndrome

Overall, the presence of LA is a better predictor of thrombosis and pregnancy loss than the presence of high-titer anticardiolipin antibodies.[53] However, some patients with aPL syndrome do not have both LA and aCL antibodies. Therefore, the laboratory diagnosis of aPL syndrome should include both coagulation assays for LA and immunologic assays for aPL antibodies. Some authors have suggested that a broad panel of aPL antibodies should be included when investigating aPL syndrome as a possible cause for recurrent fetal loss.[54] In the following discussion, we concentrate on the hematology laboratory's role in working up a suspected case of aPL syndrome.

As in most diagnostic algorithms, initial assays with broad sensitivity are performed and, if positive, they are followed by confirmatory assays that are more specific (Table 27–9). The Subcommittee on Lupus Anticoagulant/Antiphospholipid Antibody of the Scientific and Standardization Committee of the International Society on Thrombosis and Haemostasis has recommended criteria, paraphrased here, for the diagnosis of LA[55] (Table 27–10).

1. *Prolongation of at least one phospholipid-dependent clotting assay.* Examples of such assays include the APTT, dilute PT (dPT), kaolin clotting time (KCT), and the dilute Russell's viper venom time (dRVVT) and colloidal silica clotting time.[56-59] Because of the heterogeneity of these antibodies, no single screening test will detect all of them. A minimum of two "screening" assays should be available in a laboratory offering LA testing. Having three screening tests available is optimal.
2. *Evidence of inhibition of clotting is demonstrated by mixing studies.* This involves mixing the patient's plasma and pooled normal plasma and repeating the phospholipid-dependent clotting assay in which the prolongation of clotting time was observed. If the prolongation disappears ("corrects") with mixing, this usually indicates that there is a factor deficiency.
3. If the results of the mixing study suggest an LA, then *evidence of phospholipid-dependence* is required for confirmation. Confirmatory assays

> **Table 27-9**
SCREENING AND CONFIRMATORY ASSAYS THAT CAN BE USED IN LA TESTING

If This Screening Assay Is Positive . . .	One of These Techniques Should Be Used as a Confirmatory Test
APTT-based assay	Platelet neutralization procedure Hexagonal phase phospholipid test (e.g., Staclot LA) Phospholipid dilutions
Dilute Russell's viper venom (dRVV) time	dRVV confirm Platelet vesicles Platelet neutralization procedure
Taipan snake venome time	Platelet neutralization procedure
Dilute prothrombin time (thromboplastin inhibition test)	Phospholipid dilutions of same
Kaolin clotting time *or* Silica clotting time	Platelet vesicles Inosithin Bovine phospholipids

Screening assays detect a prolonged clotting time. Confirmatory assays demonstrate whether or not the prolongation is decreased by phospholipids capable of neutralizing the LA antibody.

Source: Horbach, DA, et al: Lupus anticoagulant is the strongest risk factor for both venous and arterial thrombosis in patients with systemic lupus erythematosis. Thromb Haemostas 76:916, 1966.

> **Table 27-10**
> # CRITERIA FOR LUPUS ANTICOAGULANTS

A Tested Sample Should Show Each of the Following:

1. Prolongation of at least one phospholipid-dependent clotting test

2. Evidence of inhibitory activity shown by the effect of patient plasma on pooled normal plasma

3. Evidence that inhibitory activity is dependent on phospholipid

4. Satisfactory exclusion of another coagulopathy that could give similar laboratory results

Source: Horbach, DA, et al: Lupus anticoagulant is the strongest risk factor for both venous and arterial thrombosis in patients with systemic lupus erythematosis. Thromb Haemostas 76:916, 1996.

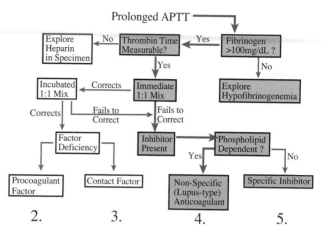

> **FIGURE 27–7** In the hematology laboratory, detection of LA usually begins with an elevated APTT. This figure is a flowchart that illustrates an approach to the diagnosis of LA. The shaded boxes show the typical abnormalities that can be seen when LA is present in the sample.

demonstrate phospholipid-dependence by demonstrating a reversal of the LA effect when excess phospholipid is added to the test mixture. This can be in the form of platelets, platelet vesicles or hexagonal (II) phase phospholipids. The excess phospholipid binds and neutralizes the LA, leaving enough phospholipid to provide a surface on which coagulation reactions can proceed.[60,61] A confirmatory assay that corresponds to the initial type of assay and mixing study that were positive should be used. Solid-phase assays for aPL antibodies, such as the aCL assay, should not be considered confirmatory for LA activity.

4. In addition, *absence of clinical or laboratory evidence of a specific inhibitor of any one coagulation factor* may also be necessary, because specific factor inhibitors can cause mixing studies to remain uncorrected. The clinical presentation is very important and may be informative. Patients with factor inhibitors have a bleeding diathesis rather than thrombosis.

These steps can be carried out in various ways, using various discrete assays or by using integrated systems for the diagnosis of LA that incorporate an initial assay, mixing study, and a procedure that confirms phospholipid-dependence into a single kit. Table 27–9 lists screening and confirmatory assays that have been used, and Figure 27–7 illustrates an approach to the diagnosis of LAs.[55]

In addition to the requirements for diagnosis already mentioned, several other elements are crucial to arriving at the correct diagnosis in cases suspicious for aPL syndrome, as follows: (1) Care should be taken to use properly prepared platelet-poor plasma in order to avoid false-negative results caused by the neutralization of LA by platelet membrane phospholipids.[62] (2) Immunologic assays for antiphospholipid antibody should also be done. (3) Testing should be repeated after a minimum of 6 weeks to demonstrate persistence of the LA. Transient aPL antibodies do not appear to be associated with the clinical complications of aPL syndrome. (4) Finally, the diagnosis of aPL syndrome should make sense based on the patient's history and clinical findings.

Laboratory testing for LA is currently hindered by the lack of standardized controls. Laboratories have no option other than to use patient plasmas that have proved positive

for LA. Trials of potential standardized controls containing monoclonal anti-β2GPI and antiprothrombin antibodies are ongoing.[63,64]

A Walk Through the Algorithm

In the hematology laboratory, detection of aPL antibodies usually begins with the APTT. In this discussion, we trace the laboratory diagnosis of an LA as depicted in Figure 27–7.[65] In many, but not all, patients with aPL antibodies the APTT is prolonged. Some APTT assays are more sensitive to LA than others and, therefore, they vary in their value as initial tests.[66,67] Remember that prolongation of the APTT also occurs with heparin therapy, heparin contamination, insufficient volume of blood for the amount of anticoagulant in the sample tube, DIC, factor deficiencies, and antibody against specific coagulation factors in the intrinsic and common pathways. Clinical history elucidates the cause of some prolonged APTTs and, depending on the clinical situation, other assays such as the thrombin time and fibrinogen level may be employed to identify heparin contamination or DIC. If the prolonged APTT is unexpected or not explained by the causes mentioned earlier, laboratory investigation for LA is warranted, especially in a patient with a history of thrombosis or other findings indicating aPL syndrome.

If the APTT is prolonged and investigation of a possible LA is indicated, the next step is to perform an APTT using a 1:1 mix of the patient's plasma and normal pooled plasma. If the APTT does not correct, then either antibody to a phospholipid in the test system or antibody to a specific coagulation factor is responsible. Correction can be defined in different ways, but probably the most useful approach is to consider an APTT corrected when it returns to within 5 seconds of the APTT of the pooled normal plasma.[68] If the APTT does not correct in the 1:1 mix, then confirmatory testing is indicated, as discussed earlier.

If the APTT does correct, then the abnormality is attributable to coagulation factor deficiency or a time-dependent antibody. Specific coagulation factor inhibitors are usually time-dependent. It has also been observed that up to 30% of LAs are time dependent.[68,69] An incubated 1:1 mix allows for detection of a time-dependent inhibitor. Interpretation of incubated mixing studies can be challenging. The incubated mix should be used only if the immediate mix corrects. The incubated mix helps to detect inhibitors, but cannot be used to determine their etiology. The use of unmixed incubation controls, as shown in Figure 27–8, is suggested.[65] Assays for specific coagulation factors can detect factor deficiencies, and serial dilutions are helpful in detecting antibodies to specific coagulation factors.

Therapy and Monitoring

Because LA can prolong coagulation tests, it may interfere with the usual tests (APTT and prothrombin time [PT]) used to monitor anticoagulation. Unfractionated heparin therapy, in the acute event or in pregnancy, may require heparin assay to monitor therapy. Warfarin therapy is monitored by the PT assay, with an international normalized ratio (INR) of 2.5 being the usual target. However, this is a complex issue for two reasons: (1) there is controversy regarding the optimal degree of anticoagulation, and (2) some thromboplastins are more sensitive to the effects of LAs than others. Monitoring therapy with a PT using one of these thromboplastins can be misleading even if the baseline INR of the patient with an LA is within the reference range. During anticoagulation, the INR may be prolonged by the LA and appear to be within therapeutic range, although the patient is actually insufficiently anticoagulated.

The effect of LA on the PT is not predictable, creating problems when determining the appropriate INR to use for oral anticoagulation. Because of the variable effect, it would be prudent to determine the therapeutic INR for each patient with LA who receives oral anticoagulant therapy. The goal of therapy is to reduce the functional level of vitamin K–dependent factors in the plasma; therefore, an assay of one of the factors to confirm the therapeutic effect should be done after the patient is receiving a stable dose of anticoagulant. The assay of factor X is the most frequently used, with a target of 20% to 25% activity. The LA can also affect clot-based assays, so the assay for factor X needs to be an assay that uses a chromogenic substrate in a reaction that is not phospholipid-dependent. Once the factor X is confirmed to be in the therapeutic interval, the corresponding INR can be used for monitoring, if the INR is in a sensitive range (i.e., less than 6.0). For the rare patient whose LA has a profound effect on the INR, precluding its use, periodic assay of factor X may be necessary. In aPL syndrome associated with recurrent fetal loss, subcutaneous unfractionated heparin or low-molecular-weight heparin plus aspirin are often used.[70]

Features of aPL syndrome include venous or arterial thrombosis, recurrent pregnancy loss, and thrombocytopenia. The aPL antibodies, manifesting as LA or detected by immunologic tests such as the aCL ELISA, may be seen in the setting of aPL syndrome or be incidental and without apparent ill effect. The aPL syndrome can be associated with SLE and other autoimmune disorders as well as with drugs. It can also occur in the absence of a known underlying disease process. Laboratory diagnosis of aPL antibodies is complex and requires an approach that takes into account the heterogeneity of the antibodies. Laboratories offering testing for LAs should have a systematic approach that ensures that an adequate investigation takes place when there is clinical concern regarding aPL syndrome.

Heparin-Induced Thrombocytopenia

Heparin-induced thrombocytopenia (HIT) is another seemingly paradoxical antibody-mediated cause of venous and arterial thrombosis. Studies have shown that between 1% and 5% of hospital patients exposed to heparin for 1 to 2 weeks develop HIT. Of patients diagnosed with HIT, approximately one-third will develop overt thrombosis and of these, about one-third will suffer amputation or death. Hence, the overall chance of serious morbidity or mortality as a result of a course of heparin therapy is about 3 per 1000.[71,72] Early recognition and appropriate treatment may reduce these numbers.

Heparin is a widely used anticoagulant that can be administered intravenously (IV) or subcutaneously (SC) both to prevent thrombosis in high-risk patients and to limit progression of established thrombosis. It is also used as a flush to keep IV lines open. Heparin is often used to prevent clotting in extracorporeal circulation such as that in heart-lung bypass machines, in which case it can be infused or the tubing coated with heparin.

HIT is characterized by a sudden unexplained decrease in platelet count, occurring five or more days after the initiation of heparin therapy. This lag is consistent with an immune response related to heparin administration.

Nomenclature seen in the literature regarding this syndrome can be confusing. Over the years, various names have been used for this syndrome, such as HITTS (heparin-induced thrombocytopenia with thrombosis syndrome), and HIT type II. These terms have been used to distinguish immune-mediated HIT from the mild, nonimmune-mediated thrombocytopenia, which may occur within the first few days of heparin administration. This nonimmune (also called HIT type I) thrombocytopenia resolves spontaneously and does not increase risk for thrombosis. For the rest of this chapter, when the term *HIT* is used, it signifies the immune-mediated disorder in which there is a risk of thrombosis.

Clinical Manifestations

Although HIT may present with simultaneous thrombocytopenia and thrombosis, or occasionally with thrombosis preceding thrombocytopenia, the first manifestation of HIT is usually a sudden unexplained decrease in platelet count of 30% to 50% or to less than 100×10^9/L, occurring 5 or more days (usually 5 to 8 days) after the initiation of he-

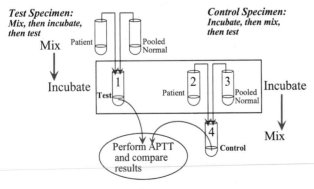

Incubated Mixing Study:
1:1 Mixture of the Patient plasma with Pooled Normal Plasma

Test Specimen:
Mix, then incubate, then test

Mix   Patient   Pooled Normal

Incubate

Test   1

Control Specimen:
Incubate, then mix, then test

Patient   2   3   Pooled Normal

Incubate

4   Control

Mix

Perform APTT and compare results

▶ **FIGURE 27–8** Incubated mixing study can be performed as shown in this figure. For details, refer to the accompanying text.

parin therapy. The platelet count rarely decreases to 15×10^9/L or less. The mean nadir has been reported to be approximately 60×10^9/L.[71]

HIT can cause both venous and arterial thrombosis, but venous thrombosis occurs about four times more often. DVT, PE, lower limb arterial thrombosis, and coronary arterial thromboses may occur.[71,73] Other sequelae can also be seen. Thromboses may be multiple. The occurrence of multiple arterial thromboses is sometimes referred to as "white clot syndrome," because the thrombi formed in high-flow vessels have a high platelet and fibrin content and relatively few red blood cells.

Accurate diagnosis of HIT requires a high degree of suspicion on the part of the physician caring for the heparin-exposed patient. Recommendation for monitoring platelet counts vary, but it seems prudent to check a baseline platelet count at the initiation of heparin therapy and to repeat platelet counts at intervals of several days. Because of the timing of the onset of HIT, particular vigilance around day 4 after initiation of heparin (day 0 being the first day of heparin administration) and for 10 days thereafter is particularly crucial. Patients who have had previous exposure to heparin may have an anamnestic response and develop HIT rapidly after repeat heparin exposure. Many other things can cause decreases in the platelet count; among these are fever, splenomegaly, and medications. These should be considered before concluding that HIT is the cause. In spite of their thrombocytopenia, HIT patients rarely have a bleeding diathesis.

If suspicion of HIT is high, all sources of heparin exposure should be discontinued immediately. Continued heparin exposure greatly increases the risk of thrombosis. Assays are available to assist in the diagnosis of HIT, but discontinuation of heparin should not wait for these results. Alternative anticoagulant therapy (hirudin analogs or danaparoid, usually) should be considered because of the high risk of thrombosis even after heparin is discontinued. Platelet counts often rise rapidly after the discontinuation of heparin. The return of the platelet count to normal within 5 to 7 days of discontinuation of heparin is consistent with a diagnosis of HIT, although some patient's platelet counts have been observed to take up to a month to recover completely. As with most immune reactions, heparin antibodies may remain in the plasma for extended periods of time. However, testing should occur within 6 weeks of a thrombocytopenic event.

The risk of HIT appears to be greater in patients exposed to large amounts of heparin, such as when systemic anticoagulation is required. However, patients with exposures to very small amounts of heparin, such as that used to keep IV lines from clotting when not in use, have also developed HIT.[74]

Mechanism

Heparin complexed with PF4 is the antigen usually responsible for initiating HIT[75–77] (Fig. 27–9). PF4 is present in the α granules of platelets and is released when heparin or other agonists activate them. Antibodies to these heparin-PF4 (H-PF4) complexes form in some patients. IgM, IgA, and IgG specific for H-PF4 antigen have all been detected in patients with HIT, although IgG is most common.[78] When the H-PF4-antibody immune complex is bound by platelet FcγRIIa receptors (a subtype of receptor found on platelets that binds the constant portion of immunoglobulin molecules), two things

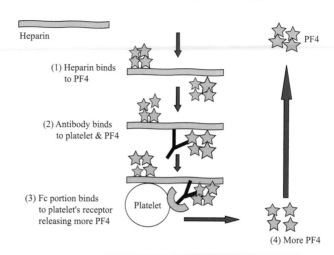

> **FIGURE 27–9**   Heparin complexed with PF4 is the antigen usually responsible for initiating HIT (*1*). An antibody is formed against heparin-PF4 complexes (*2*). The antibody complexes with heparin-PF4 and the Fc portion of the antibody binds to the platelet FcγRIIa receptor (*3*), resulting in platelet activation and release of more PF4 (*4*), which then binds to more heparin.

may happen.[79] Firstly, splenic macrophages may remove the platelets, as they are now coated with Ig attached to the platelet Fc receptors, resulting in thrombocytopenia, and secondly, the attachment of the immune complex to the Fc receptor can result in platelet activation. The activated platelets release substances that attract and activate more platelets. Levels of thrombin increase, which along with platelet-derived microparticles can ultimately result in thrombosis. Endothelial cell damage or activation probably also plays a role in the development of thrombosis.[80]

Many patients who do not develop HIT form these antibodies.[81] This suggests that other factors are required for the development of HIT besides H-PF4 antibodies. One fascinating and controversial possibility is that the His[131] polymorphism in the gene for the platelet FcγRIIa receptor may increase susceptibility to HIT.[78,82–84]

Unfractionated heparin (UH), still the most commonly used heparin, is the major culprit in causing HIT. HIT occurs less often with porcine UH than with bovine UH. Low-molecular-weight heparin, although less antigenic than UH, can also cause HIT.[85]

Laboratory Diagnosis

Two types of assays are commonly used to assist in the diagnosis of HIT: functional assays and antigen assays. The antigen assays are ELISAs that use the H-PF4 complex as the target antigen to detect HIT-type immunoglobulin in the patient's serum. Functional assays may simply look for platelet aggregation or may be a variation on a platelet aggregation method that detects products of the platelet release reaction, such as serotonin or adenosine triphosphate (ATP). These assays use the patient's serum, heparin, and donor platelets. Either bovine or porcine heparin may be used in the assays. There is no need for the laboratory to determine whether the patient has received bovine or porcine heparin. It is important to use platelets from donors whose platelets are known to be reactive to HIT sera. It is unknown why some donors' platelets are reactive and others are not. Occasional combinations of known HIT sera and known reactive HIT-reactive platelets do not aggregate. Therefore, it has been suggested that platelets from two donors whose platelets are known to react to HIT sera should be used. If platelet aggregation occurs or if there is evidence of the release reaction only at a low concentration of heparin (0.1 U/mL), this is evidence that the patient's serum contains antibodies that activate and aggregate platelets in the presence of a therapeutic concentration of heparin.

In any of these functional assays, it is important to use appropriate controls to exclude the presence of non–heparin-induced aggregation. In addition to using a control that lacks heparin, the use of a control containing a high concentration of heparin (100 U/mL) is included (Fig. 27–10). When HIT serum is tested using a high concentration of heparin, aggregation should not occur. It is reasonable that this might be caused by antigen (heparin) excess, but nonspecific inhibition of platelet aggregation in response to other agonists (collagen, adenosine diphosphate [ADP], and epinephrine) has also been observed. In any case, aggregation of platelets at both low and high concentrations of heparin is considered to be evidence that the aggregation is caused by a mechanism other than that of HIT.[86–89]

One of the functional assays is the serotonin release assay (SRA). It is currently the primary comparison procedure because most of the available data on clinical outcomes has been gathered in studies using this assay. Donor platelets are incubated with ^{14}C-serotonin, to allow its uptake into their dense bodies. These platelets are then washed, removing free ^{14}C-serotonin that has not become incorporated. They are then exposed to the serum of the patient to which is added a therapeutic concentration of heparin. If the patient's serum contains H-PF4 antibodies capable of activating platelets, then the radioactively labeled serotonin will be released from the dense granules. The test specimen is then centrifuged and the supernatant tested for ^{14}C activity.[87] This assay is regarded by some as the most specific HIT assay. However, it is time-consuming and requires the use of radioisotopes.

Another commonly used functional assay takes advantage of the release of ATP from platelet dense granules when H-PF4 antibodies stimulate the release reaction.[90] The indicator reagent contains both luciferin and luciferase. The substrate luciferin is converted to a product by luciferase in an ATP-dependent reaction that emits photons. Therefore, if the platelet release reaction occurs, the ATP from the platelets will result in a detectable light emission. This is referred to as lumi-aggregometry. This technique is also used to test for platelet secretion (release reaction) in response to a variety of agonists. The same controls as used in the SRA are also appropriate for this method. This assay is somewhat less labor intensive than the SRA because it can be done with platelet-rich plasma rather than washed platelets, and radioisotopes are not used.

Flow cytometric methods for diagnosing HIT have also been developed. These employ fluorescent antibodies against platelet glycoproteins and forward angle light scatter (indi-

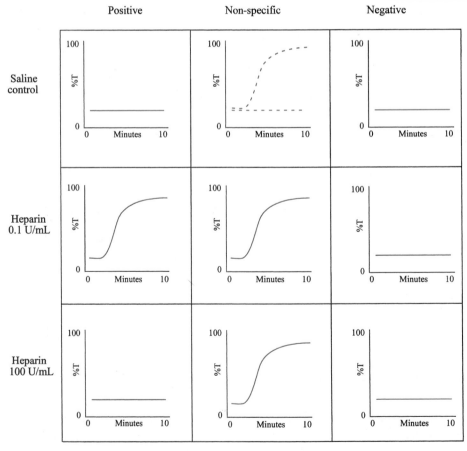

▶ **FIGURE 27–10**   Interpretation of samples for HIT assays by platelet aggregometry is shown here. The test is positive when aggregation or ATP release is seen with a low concentration of heparin (0.1 U/mL). The test is negative when no aggregation or ATP release is seen with the low concentration of heparin. The test is nonspecific when aggregation or ATP release is seen with both low and high concentrations of heparin or with saline control, or both.

cating cell size) to detect platelet microparticles generated when donor platelets are exposed to patient sera which are able to cause platelet aggregation in the presence of therapeutic concentrations of heparin. Adequate data comparing the results of flow cytometry assays with clinical outcomes are not available, but these methods seem promising in their ease of performance, and have been observed to correlate well with the SRA.[88,91]

The clinical diagnosis of HIT often remains unconfirmed by any of these laboratory techniques. Sensitivities and specificities reported for these assays vary, but overall are suboptimal. No single technique is reliable enough to be considered a gold standard for the diagnosis of HIT.[88] Sensitivity and specificity can be improved by using more than one methodology to test for heparin-associated antibodies, including one H-PF4 ELISA. In cases suspicious for HIT, repetition of the assays every few days may provide confirmation. Clinical decision making should be based predominantly on clinical impression. However, laboratory evidence of HIT is often helpful in supporting the decision to discontinue heparin and use an alternative anticoagulant.

Therapy and Monitoring

Stopping all heparin exposure is the most important step in preventing or limiting thrombosis in patients with HIT. However, even after cessation of heparin, the patient still has a risk of approximately one in three for developing thrombosis. Therefore, the use of other anticoagulants should be considered. In addition, the substitution of another anticoagulant may be beneficial in patients with an established thrombus.

Because of the risk of venous limb gangrene, distal ischemic necrosis that is present despite palpable or Doppler-identifiable arterial pulses, the oral anticoagulant warfarin sodium should not be used in a patient with HIT unless the patient is also adequately anticoagulated by another non-heparin anticoagulant for the first few days.[92] The early warfarin-induced reduction of functioning protein C in the presence of increased thrombin generation seen in HIT, puts the patient at very high risk for this and other thrombotic complications.

Low-molecular-weight heparin (LMWH) is also not recommended for the treatment of HIT. Although it is less likely to induce HIT once a patient has a heparin-induced antibody, exposure to LMWH carries a risk of thrombosis.[85]

Ancrod, a defibrinogenating snake venom, has been used to treat HIT, but is problematic because it increases thrombin generation. In addition, there is a risk of thrombosis with rapid injection, so it must be administered slowly, over 12 to 24 hours. It cannot be used for rapid anticoagulation, a disadvantage compared to danaparoid and hirudin.[93]

Anticoagulants available for use in HIT patients include heparinoids such as danaparoid and thrombin inhibitors such as hirudin and argatroban. The adjunctive use of medications that limit platelet function is also under investigation. Examples include glycoprotein IIb/IIIa (GPIIb/IIIa) inhibitors such as GPI 562 and ADP receptor antagonists, clopidogrel and ticlopidine.[94]

Danaparoid, a heparinoid, is a mixture of the glycosaminoglycans heparan sulfate, dermatan sulfate, and chondroitin sulfate. Its anticoagulant effect is primarily owing to catalysis of the inactivation of factor Xa. It also has some antithrombin (anti-IIa) effects and interacts with heparin cofactor II. It can be administered subcutaneously or intravenously.

Because of somewhat predictable distribution and metabolism, dosing can be based on the patient's weight. Although recent publications suggest that monitoring is not necessarily required during treatment unless the patient is very large (more than 90 kg) or very small (less than 55 kg) or has some degree of renal failure, it seems prudent to monitor danaparoid therapy, particularly if the required assay is available. Danaparoid therapy can be monitored using the anti-Xa activity assay (target range is 0.5 to 0.8 anti-Xa U/mL). This requires the use of a standard curve prepared with danaparoid. H-PF4 antibodies may cross-react with danaparoid in vitro but do not appear to have a negative effect on patient outcome.[93,95,96]

Hirudin, an anticoagulant produced in the salivary glands of leeches, is a direct thrombin inhibitor. It has no structural similarity to heparin and so does not cross-react with heparin-dependent antibodies. A hirudin derivative known as lepirudin and recombinant hirudin are available for treatment of HIT. Hirudin therapy is commonly monitored using the APTT, with a target value of 1.5 to 3.0 times the median of the normal range. However, variable responses of APTT reagents to hirudin can be problematic. Early data show promising results for the Ecarine clotting time (a snake venom–derived assay); however, clinical outcome data are still being gathered. Daily monitoring is recommended because hirudin is predominantly cleared by the kidneys. Therefore, monitoring is especially important in patients with impaired renal function.[93,95,96]

Argatroban is a synthetic thrombin inhibitor that functions similarly to hirudin but that is cleared normally even in patients with moderate to severe renal failure. As of this writing, results of clinical trials are pending.[93]

➤ OTHER ACQUIRED CONDITIONS ASSOCIATED WITH THROMBOSIS

Thrombosis with Pregnancy and Use of Oral Contraceptives

There is a sixfold increased risk of thromboembolism during pregnancy. The puerperium (6-week period after delivery) is associated with a higher risk of thrombosis than pregnancy. The presence of coexistent inherited thrombophilia during pregnancy represents a significant added risk. In a Swedish population, approximately 50% of women with venous thrombosis had APC-R and 65% to 75% of the thrombotic events occurred during pregnancy.[97,98] Thrombosis during pregnancy is attributable to the following conditions: (1) venous stasis in the lower extremities, caused by the gravid uterus; (2) trauma to pelvic veins during delivery; (3) the placenta, which is rich in tissue factor, may produce increased thrombin, and also releases plasminogen activator–2, reducing fibrinolytic activity; (4) increased levels of most coagulation proteins (fibrinogen can be increased to 600 mg/dL); (5) a significant decline in plasma levels of free and total PS; and (6) elevated D-dimer level during the third trimester. Although PC and AT levels remain normal during pregnancy, both are decreased during preeclampsia.

The risk of venous or arterial thrombosis secondary to oral contraceptives is related to estrogen dose. Most oral contraceptives prescribed in the United States contain low-dose estrogen. However, even the use of low-dose estrogen contraceptives confers a fourfold increased risk of thrombosis when compared with nonusers. This risk may become significant if the women also have an inherited thrombophilia. The exact mechanism of the prothrombotic state is not well understood, but it is thought that these medications may cause an acquired APC-R–like state.[99]

Thrombosis and Nephrotic Syndrome

Nephrotic syndrome is characterized by heavy proteinuria (more than 3.5g/day), hypoalbuminemia, severe edema, and hyperlipidemia. Thrombosis of both venous and arterial systems is seen. The renal vein is the most common site involved. Renal vein thrombosis is present in approximately one-third of patients.[100] The incidence of thrombosis varies depending on the severity of the disease. Depending on the complex interaction between hepatic protein biosynthesis and the severity of renal disease, the following changes of coagulation parameters can be seen: AT levels are often decreased; PC and S are increased; factors V, VII, VIII, X, and XIII are increased; whereas factors XI and XII are decreased. In addition, platelet hyperactivity can also be seen in these patients.

Thrombosis and Medications

L-Asparaginase, used as a part of induction chemotherapy for acute lymphoblastic leukemia (ALL), may cause venous thrombosis (intracranial thrombosis is observed most frequently). The incidence of venous thrombosis has been estimated to be 1.2%.[101] This drug causes a significant reduction in hepatic synthesis of both procoagulant (factors V, VII, VIII, IX, X, XI, and fibrinogen) and anticoagulant proteins (AT, PC, and PS). The alteration in the hemostatic balance in a particular patient determines the risk of thrombosis or bleeding. There may be a prolongation of PT, APTT, and thrombin time. These transient abnormalities resolve within 1 to 2 weeks after cessation of the drug. Recent studies indicate that, in children with ALL, L-asparaginase is a risk factor for thrombosis, but that those who develop thrombi have additional risk factors. Some consideration should be given to the evaluation of other risk factors for thrombophilia prior to beginning the medication. If other risk factors are present, prophylaxis may be indicated.

Increased risk of thrombosis has also been described in women with breast cancer who are receiving chemotherapy.[102] The basis of thrombogenicity among these patients is not well understood, and possible causes include low-grade DIC, impairment of vitamin K metabolism, and altered hepatic protein synthesis.

Thrombosis and Other Conditions

Microangiopathic hemolytic anemia (MAHA), disseminated intravascular coagulation (DIC), thrombotic thrombocytopenic purpura (TTP), and hemolytic uremic syndrome (HUS) could lead to formation of platelet and fibrin microthrombi, occluding the capillaries and arterioles most frequently in the kidneys, heart, brain, spleen, and adrenal glands. The occurrence of thrombosis in patients with malignancy can be caused by cancer itself or occur secondary to chemotherapy (mitomycin D, L-asparaginase). The most common sites of cancer predisposing to thrombosis are the gastrointestinal and genitourinary tracts and lungs. The possible causes for thrombosis include activation and production of procoagulants by tumor cells, and low-grade DIC. None of the clotting tests currently available are specific for cancer. Recurrent thrombosis in the presence of adequate anticoagulation raises the possibility of underlying occult malignancy.

Myeloproliferative disorders predispose patients to venous or arterial thrombosis, especially when the platelet count and hematocrit are not controlled by therapy. Increased blood viscosity and activation of platelets may be the cause for thrombosis. In patients with paroxysmal nocturnal hemoglobinuria (PNH), there is a predilection for thrombosis in intraabdominal and cerebral vessels. A diagnosis of PNH should be suspected in patients with pancytopenia, elevated reticulocyte count, low iron studies, and negative family history of thrombosis.

Thrombosis and Major Trauma

DVT and PE are common complications after major trauma. Five independent risk factors for DVT following major trauma have been defined. These include older age, blood transfusion, surgery, fracture of the femur or tibia, and spinal cord injury. In one study in which prophylaxis was not used, 58% of patients admitted to the trauma unit developed lower extremity DVTs.[103] Therefore, effective prophylaxis is necessary in patients with major trauma.

➤ DIAGNOSTIC APPROACH AND ISSUES IN LABORATORY TESTING IN PATIENTS WITH THROMBOSIS

The purpose of detecting hypercoagulable states is to predict and prevent thromboembolic disease and its complications, identify risk factors, modify treatment regimens, and discover underlying diseases that might be amenable to treatment (Tables 27–11 through 27–15). The diagnostic evaluation of patients with thrombotic diathesis initially involves consideration of two things: (1) whether the disorder is inherited or acquired, and (2) whether the thrombosis involves primarily the veins or arteries (Table 27–16). For example, a young person with recurrent DVT is most likely to have an inherited defect of one or more of the anticoagulant proteins. On the other hand, the hypercoagulable state in an elderly bedridden person is most likely to be acquired. Therefore, the knowledge of the coagulant, anticoagulant, and fibrinolytic systems; complete history and physical examination; ethnic background (factor V Leiden is very rare in African Americans and Asians); and identification of the risk factors are the basic but very important steps that need to be considered before one orders assays for inherited disorders.

Specific laboratory tests of interest in patients with thrombophilia have been addressed in other sections of this chapter. There are, however, some issues that deserve consideration when approaching the laboratory evaluation of a patient who has suffered from thrombosis. These issues are summarized in Table 27–17 and are addressed briefly below.

Complete History and Physical Examination

A complete personal, family, and drug history is extremely important in evaluating patients with acute, recurrent, or remote thrombosis. The patient should be carefully questioned about all the possible risk factors for thrombosis. A significant family history of thrombosis strongly suggests the possibility of inherited thrombophilia. If the patient is female, history of oral contraceptive use and obstetric history is im-

> **Table 27–11**
DIFFERENTIAL DIAGNOSIS OF HYPERCOAGULABLE STATES

Hereditary Conditions

1. Factor V Leiden mutation
2. Prothrombin gene mutation
3. AT-III deficiency
4. Protein C deficiency
5. Protein S deficiency
6. Heparin cofactor II deficiency
7. TFPI deficiency
8. Elevated lipoprotein a
9. Homocysteinemia
10. Factor XII deficiency
11. Elevated factor VIII levels
12. Plasminogen deficiency
13. Increased plasminogen activator inhibitor

Acquired Conditions

1. Antiphospholipid antibodies
2. Heparin-induced thrombocytopenia
3. Malignancy
4. Autoimmune disorders
5. Nephrotic syndrome
6. Myeloproliferative disorders/PNH
7. Behçet's syndrome
8. Microangiopathic hemolytic anemia (DIC, TTP, HUS)

> **Table 27–12**
RISK FACTORS FOR VENOUS THROMBOEMBOLISM

Pregnancy

Oral contraceptives

Obesity

Surgery

Trauma

General anethesia

Malignancy

Immobility

Varicose veins

Infection

Congestive heart failure

Advancing age

Infusion of prothrombin complex concentrates

Diabetes mellitus and hyperlipidemia

Treatment related:

L-Asparaginase

Mitomycin

portant. Presence of constitutional symptoms, hemoptysis, melena, or hematuria may suggest underlying occult malignancy. Recurrent thrombosis despite anticoagulation therapy may suggest underlying malignancy. Atherosclerotic vascular disease and renal disease (nephrotic syndrome) can lead to arterial or venous thromboembolism.

Ethnic background is also important in evaluating patients with inherited thrombophilia. The factor V Leiden mutation is common in people of European descent and extremely rare in African-American, Native-American, or Asian populations. Physical examination should be specifically directed to examining vascular system, skin, extremities, heart, chest, and abdomen.

Do Not Test During the Acute Event
Thrombotic events, whether on the arterial or venous side of the circulation, are capable of consuming naturally occurring coagulation inhibitors (PC, PS, AT) that are of interest for testing. In addition, a number of these components are either positive or negative acute phase reactants. Anticoagulant therapy also affects these concentrations variably. For these reasons, testing during the acute event and during anticoagulant therapy will produce both false positive and false negative results.

Conditions That Can Interfere with Test Results
A number of physiologic and pathologic states as well as medications may affect plasma levels of PC, PS, and AT. One of the most common problems is the interpretation of these assays under inappropriate conditions. Levels of PC, PS, and AT are physiologically low in newborns, during pregnancy (PC may be high), and in the early postpartum states. Pathologic decreases in levels of PC, PS, and AT can be seen in postthrombotic states, the postoperative states, severe liver disease, and DIC. In nephrotic syndrome, PS and AT levels are decreased while PC levels may be increased.

PC and PS are vitamin K–dependent proteins, and both

> **Table 27–13**
EVALUATION OF A PATIENT WITH SUSPECTED THROMBOPHILIA (HEREDITARY/ACQUIRED)

1. Age of onset
2. Any underlying associated risk factors
3. Number of events (initial or recurrent)
4. Site of thrombosis
5. Any documented evidence of pulmonary embolism or DVT
6. Whether recurrent thromboembolism occurred despite therapeutic anticoagulation
7. Any history of recurrent fetal loss, MI, or stroke
8. Any medications that can lead to thrombosis (oral contraceptives, chemotherapy)
9. Family history of venous thromboembolism

> **Table 27-14**

SUGGESTED EVALUATION CRITERIA FOR INHERITED THROMBOPHILIA

1. Thrombosis at any age especially in younger patients*
2. Recurrent thrombosis
3. Significant family history of thrombosis
4. Thrombosis at unusual sites (other that deep veins of legs)

*Studies have demonstrated that the yield in detecting inherited risk factors for thrombophilia in the aged occurs at the same rate and would have the same value in guiding clinical management.

functional and antigenic levels will be reduced during oral anticoagulation therapy. Warfarin has on rare occasion elevated AT levels in patients with a hereditary defect of this coagulation inhibitor. Heparin therapy may falsely lower AT activity. Heparin therapy will not affect plasma levels of PC and PS but will interfere with APTT-based activity assays. For these reasons, it is a good practice to test for these deficiency states at least 2 weeks after completing the initial 3- to 6-month course of oral anticoagulant therapy. Deficiency states for PC, PS, and AT may be excluded if the levels for these proteins are normal during the acute thrombotic episode. But finding a low level of these proteins during this period will need to be confirmed by repeat testing after anticoagulation is discontinued. The first-

> **Table 27-15**

TESTING FOR INHERTIED THROMBOPHILIA

Plasma Coagulation Screening

PT

APTT

Thrombin and reptilase times

Anticoagulant System

APC resistance assay (APTT-based assay)

Protein C (functional and antigenic)

Protein S (functional and antigenic)

AT (functional and antigenic)

Fibrinolytic System

Fibrinogen (functional and antigenic)

Factor XII activity

Plasminogen (functional)

Genetic tests

Factor V (FV:Q^{506}) Leiden mutation

Prothrombin gene mutation (nucleotide G20210A)

MTHFR gene mutation

Additional Tests

Homocysteine level

Lipoprotein a level

> **Table 27-16**

COAGULATION DEFECTS AND SITES OF THROMBOSIS

Defects	Venous	Arterial
Factor V Leiden*	+ +	−
Prothrombin gene mutation	+ +	?
PC deficiency†	+ +	−
PS deficiency	+ +	−
AT deficiency	+ +	−
Hyperhomocysteinemia	+	+ +
Lipoprotein a	−	+ +
Antiphospholipid syndrome	+ +	+ +
Heparin-induced thrombocytopenia	+ +	+ +

*Women who smoke and take oral contraceptives have an increased risk of myocardial infarction.
†A slight increased risk of stroke has been reported.

degree relatives can be investigated to document the inherited nature of the deficiency. Confirmation of the deficiency state of PC and PS can be done after temporary discontinuation of oral anticoagulant therapy for 2 weeks while treating with injectable heparin at therapeutic doses.

The conditions that can alter the baseline APTT can interfere with the interpretation of APTT-based assays. For example, the presence of lupus anticoagulant, warfarin, or heparin therapy and factor deficiencies or factor inhibitors can increase the ratios determined in APTT-based assays and may give false negative results. The use of added factor V–deficient plasma in the APC-R assay eliminates many of the preanalytic variables.

Because most patients hospitalized for thrombosis are in the acute postthrombotic state and are receiving anticoagulant therapy or have illnesses that may interfere with testing, the tests for PC, PS, and AT levels are generally better suited to the outpatient setting and have a limited role in the diagnosis of thrombophilia in the hospitalized patient.

The genetically based tests, including factor V Leiden

> **Table 27-17**

ISSUES IN LABORATORY TESTING IN PATIENTS WITH THROMBOSIS

- Ensure a complete history and physical examination is obtained.
- Do not test during the acute event.
- Consider conditions that can interfere with test results.
- Test in the appropriate clinical setting.
- Use functional assays when possible.
- In arterial thrombosis, consider the additional evaluation of hyperhomocysteinemia and lipoprotein a.
- Repeat testing prior to diagnosis.
- Ensure that the yield in performing testing is high, making evaluation worthwhile.

mutation, prothrombin gene mutation, and MTHFR mutation, are not affected by physiologic or pathologic states and anticoagulation therapy. Therefore, the genetic tests and not the functional assays can be performed in these settings.

Test in the Appropriate Clinical Setting

This is a complex issue that extends beyond the scope of this chapter. However, there are a few points to remember. The development of a thrombus, regardless of the clinical setting, requires the accumulation of more than one inherited or acquired risk factor. Venous thrombosis in almost any clinical setting would merit a comprehensive evaluation. For some time, it was thought that evaluation for inherited thrombophilia should be limited to the "young" patient with thrombosis. Studies have demonstrated that the yield in detecting inherited risk factors for thrombophilia in the aged occurs at the same rate and would have the same value in guiding clinical management.

Functional Assays

Many of the molecules of interest in thrombophilia can be assayed using functional or antigenic assays. Whenever quality functional assays are available, they should be the first assays to be performed. In general, if the assay is within the reference range, further testing would not be indicated. In contrast, if the functional assay is below the reference range, evaluation by antigenic assay is needed to determine if a normal amount of abnormally functioning molecule is being produced.

In Arterial Thrombosis, Consider the Additional Evaluation of Hyperhomocysteinemia and Lipoprotein A

The usefulness of testing for thrombophilia in patients with arterial disease, particularly MI and stroke, continues to be discussed in the literature. A consensus has not evolved regarding the usefulness of laboratory testing in these settings. Risks in relation to hyperhomocysteinemia and Lpa have been well demonstrated. LA and HIT can cause either venous or arterial thrombosis. The absence of exposure to heparin or related compounds eliminates the need to consider HIT.

Repeat Testing Prior to Diagnosis

Virtually all of the assays involved in the evaluation of thrombophilia are influenced by a variety of factors in both the preanalytic and analytic phases. Because of this, false positive testing is a common problem. Therefore, positive tests should be confirmed before the patient is labeled as having a deficiency state.

Performing Testing and Making Evaluation Worthwhile

These assays are not indicated as a routine preoperative evaluation if the aim is to detect the risk of thrombosis in the absence of a known personal or family history of thrombosis. Also, there is no valid indication for these tests if the patient is over 70 years of age and has a risk factor for venous thromboembolism. Patients who present with thrombosis and who are comprehensively evaluated will have more than a 50% probability of having a thrombophilic risk factor identified. The usefulness of determining thrombophilic risk factors continues to evolve. At the time of this writing, only

the finding of antiphospholipid antibody or lupus-type anticoagulant tends to direct clinicians to modify therapy. It is very likely that, as clinical studies evolve, treatment strategies will also evolve that will be directed by one or more of the thrombophilic risk factors.

➤ ANTICOAGULANT THERAPY

Patients with venous thrombosis are most frequently treated with unfractionated heparin acutely, followed by long-term oral anticoagulants.[104,105] This is done to prevent propagation of the thrombus, to reduce the risk of embolus, and to allow for natural resolution. Because of difficulties with appropriate monitoring, the use of LMWH is becoming more popular; however, these medications are still considerably more expensive than unfractionated heparin. Patients who are in a clinical setting (i.e., perioperative) that creates a high risk of thrombosis are also treated with low doses of anticoagulants to prevent thrombus formation.

Unfractionated Heparin Therapy

Heparin is an unbranched polysaccharide that is heavily sulfated, making it anionic. Commercial preparations are made by extracting these molecules from bovine lungs or porcine intestines. Therefore, the heparins that are extracted are variable in size (4000 to 35,000 d; averaging 12,000 to 13,000 d). The nature and degree of sulfation and the size of the molecule influence the biologic activity.

The anticoagulant activity of heparin is to function as a cofactor. When heparin is added to purified activated coagulation factors, the coagulation factor is not inhibited. Heparin acts by accelerating the rate at which AT is capable of binding to the activated serine protease, irreversibly inhibiting its activity. In the absence of heparin, neutralization of thrombin or factor Xa will occur in a time frame of approximately 15 minutes. In the presence of heparin, the same reaction occurs more rapidly than it is possible to make the first measurement.

Administration and Monitoring

Unfractionated heparin must be administered parenterally, most frequently intravenously but it can also be used subcutaneously.[106] Clearance of heparin is primarily by cellular clearance (reticuloendothelial cells) and renal filtration. At usual doses, the clearance is by the reticuloendothelial cells and provides an average half-life of approximately 60 to 90 minutes. At higher doses, renal filtration becomes a factor when the reticuloendothelial system is saturated. This may be an explanation for the varying half-life of heparin with increasing dose.

The dose of heparin is determined by the weight of the patient. It is given as a bolus dose followed by continuous IV infusion. Because of the length of the half-life of the drug, monitoring should not occur until equilibrium is reached at about 6 hours or longer after beginning or changing therapy. Once within the therapeutic interval, daily monitoring is sufficient.

When used for therapeutic purposes, heparin has a very narrow therapeutic interval. The goal, of course, is to prevent thrombosis without causing hemorrhage. If the drug is given in inadequate doses and serum concentrations are below effective levels, the consequence can be thrombosis and embolism, causing significant morbidity and even mortality.

When concentrations are elevated, the anticoagulant properties will cause hemorrhage. It is the obligation of the laboratory to inform clinicians of the method that the laboratory recommends for monitoring heparin and the therapeutic interval.

Heparin therapy can be monitored by one of two strategies. The first strategy involves monitoring the effect of heparin on the patient's coagulation system. This is done most frequently using the APTT. The second is the target concentration strategy in which the concentration of heparin in the blood is determined. Both of these strategies have been demonstrated to be effective in monitoring populations of patients receiving unfractionated heparin. Unfortunately, when the two are compared directly, there is very poor correlation between the concentration of heparin and the resulting APTT.

The APTT has been used for the monitoring of heparin since the 1950s. The general "rule of thumb" is a therapeutic interval of one-and-a-half to two-and-a-half times the upper limits of the reference range for the APTT. Problems in the monitoring of heparin are based on (1) variable drug, (2) variable response of the patient, (3) variable response of the reagent in the test, and (4) variability in the instrument used.[107] It is necessary for each laboratory to determine the responsiveness of the instrument/reagent method for the APTT to heparin in the patients' specimens. This process needs to be done each time there is a change in the reagent or instrument used in the laboratory.

The concentration of heparin in the blood can be reflected by assays that take advantage of the neutralization of the activity of thrombin or factor Xa. These assays can use either a clot endpoint or chromogenic substrate with a spectrophotometric endpoint. The assays provide the enzyme (thrombin or activated factor X), the inhibitor (antithrombin), and a marker (fibrinogen in the plasma or chromogenic substrate). The rate or amount of conversion of the substrate is inversely proportional to the concentration of heparin present in the specimen.

Another assay for quantifying the amount of heparin in the blood uses protamine sulfate, an antagonist to heparin. Protamine sulfate binds to heparin in a stoichiometric fashion, neutralizing its activity. Assays, based on the thrombin time, can be constructed using known concentrations of protamine sulfate, thereby judging the amount of heparin by the amount of protamine sulfate required to neutralize heparin.

All of these approaches to monitoring heparin therapy have their advantages and disadvantages. The dominating methods being used at the present time are the APTT and the chromogenic assay, which uses the inhibition of factor Xa. The APTT has the advantage of being inexpensive (one-tenth the cost of the Xa inhibitory assay), it can be rapidly and easily performed by many different technologists in the laboratory, is available at all hours, and reflects the anticoagulant activity of heparin in the patient's specimen. Its significant disadvantage is the wide variability resulting from the variables described earlier.

The heparin assay has the advantage of being reproducible with more precise therapeutic intervals, making clinical management less problematic. Its disadvantages are that the test is somewhat technically demanding and difficult to provide at all times, and is significantly more expensive than the APTT. Some clinicians are also concerned that target concentration may lead to over- or underanticoagulation because of the numerous variables influencing individual patient response.

With the advent of better-defined heparin products with more predictable patient responses, it is likely that assay of heparin will move toward the target concentration strategy.

Low-Molecular-Weight Heparin

LMWH is prepared from unfractionated heparin by fractionation or depolymerization, producing heparins of a more uniform molecular weight (ranging from 1000 to 12,000 d; averaging 5000 d) and function. These molecules function through the same mechanism as unfractionated heparin. They tend to have a greater impact on the inhibition of factor Xa than on other enzymes. A significant advantage of LMWH is that it is administered subcutaneously and, in many patients, it does not require therapeutic monitoring. Dosing is generally once or twice daily and can be administered by patients, similar to the way diabetic patients can administer their own insulin.

It appears that LMWH will replace unfractionated heparin in many clinical circumstances where heparin is required. These products are still not satisfactory for use in extracorporeal circulation (cardiopulmonary bypass, extracorporeal membrane oxygenation). In addition, despite the fact that many patients do not require monitoring, those of unusually low or high body weight, patients with renal failure, pediatric patients, and patients with other complicating medical conditions that may influence heparin metabolism require careful ongoing evaluation. Monitoring of LMWH requires the target concentration strategy because the therapeutic concentrations do not influence the APTT or other coagulation tests in a dose-dependent way. These tests may, however, be prolonged during therapy.

A final comment is warranted regarding some preanalytic issues in monitoring heparin therapy. A natural inhibitor of heparin, called PF4, is released from platelets. The presence of platelets in the specimen or the activation of platelets during collection can thus lead to a false lowering of heparin assayed in the specimen. Therefore, care should be taken to collect a high-quality specimen, and its preparation should include assuring that the specimen has a very low platelet count.

Oral Anticoagulation

As described in the synthesis of coagulation factors in Chapter 23, vitamin K plays a key role in the postribosomal modification of many of the serine proteases. Vitamin K is a cofactor for a carboxylase that inserts an additional carboxyl group on the glutamic acid residues in the amino terminal end of coagulation factors II, VII, IX, and X in addition to PC and PS. This process is a kinetic one in which the vitamin K, through two enzymatic steps, is recycled and can be reused for the carboxylation of multiple molecules.

A coumarin compound, ultimately named warfarin, that was capable of inhibiting the recycling of vitamin K was identified, isolated, and synthesized and first given to patients in 1941. Warfarin acts by interfering with the recycling of vitamin K after it has performed its carboxylation function. This makes warfarin interesting in two respects: (1) Warfarin is not truly an anticoagulant; it leads to the production of coagulation factors that have reduced anticoagulant function. Adding warfarin to a tube of blood does not inhibit coagulation. (2) Warfarin functions by changing the action of vitamin K in the synthesis of coagulation factors from a kinetic one to a stoichiometric one; that is, one vitamin K molecule produces one change in the glutamic acid molecule rather than a single vitamin K molecule being able to modify several through a cycling process.

Because warfarin functions by altering the synthesis of coagulation factors, and because of the half-life, the synthetic rate of coagulation factors is variable. In most patients it takes 5 to 7 days of warfarin therapy before a stable anticoagulant effect can be achieved.

Anticoagulant therapy with warfarin has the same problem that was described earlier with heparin. The drug has a narrow therapeutic interval and less than optimal tests to monitor the drug. Since 1935, when Armand Quick described the prothrombin time, and in 1941, when the first patient was treated with warfarin, the PT has been used to monitor therapy. As with the problem of heparin and the APTT, it was discovered in the late 1970s that there was a wide degree of variability in the response of thromboplastin reagents and instruments that were used for the PT when evaluating patients who were receiving warfarin therapy. It has been possible to overcome some of the difficulties with this variability by normalizing the responses of thromboplastin reagents against an international standard. This process is referred to as the *international normalized ratio (INR)*. The INR is described by the following formula:

$$INR = \left\{ \frac{PT_{pat}}{PT_n} \right\}^{ISI}$$

in which the INR is the international normalized ratio, PT_{pat} is the patient's prothrombin time, PT_n is the prothrombin time that reflects the mean of the reference range, and ISI is the international sensitivity index. The ISI needs to be developed for each thromboplastin reagent and instrument combination used in performing prothrombin times and calculation of the INR. It is now understood that ideal reagents for performing the INR are those that have ISIs below 1.7. Some reagents are exquisitely sensitive, having an ISI of 1 or less, leading to other problems with accuracy and precision in specimens with high INR. The optimal reagent would have an ISI of 1.3 to 1.5.

When monitoring patients who are taking oral anticoagulant therapy, the INR is maintained between 2 and 3. The exceptions to this therapeutic interval include patients who have a complicating lupus anticoagulant in whom higher ISIs may be indicated (2.5 to 3.5) and patients who have cardiac valves in whom the INR is recommended to be 2.5 to 3.5.

The greatest difficulty in managing oral anticoagulation in patients with thrombosis is the large number of medications and other factors that can increase or decrease the metabolism of warfarin. These drug interactions are important considerations for clinicians who are treating patients.

Alternative Anticoagulants

Because some patients cannot tolerate heparin, there are other anticoagulants that are now being used in a limited way. The first of these includes analogs of hirudin, a small protein found in the leech that has a potent inhibitory effect on thrombin. Hirudin has been used effectively in a variety of clinical settings as an anticoagulant. However, monitoring of hirudin therapy continues to be difficult. It is recommended that hirudin therapy be monitored using the APTT. As one might expect, however, the problem of the variability of the APTT (instrument/reagent combinations) creates difficulties in monitoring similar to the problems encountered with heparin. A newer method, the ecarin clotting time, uses snake venom. Although it shows some promise as a better method for monitoring hirudin, outcome studies are not complete.

Another compound called danaparoid, which is similar to LMWH, has been developed. Danaparoid, rather than being a heparin, is a collection of heparanoids including chondroitin sulfate, dermatan sulfate, and others. Its anticoagulant effects are directed primarily at the factor Xa with lesser effects on other serine proteases. When used for the purpose of prophylaxis to prevent thrombosis, it does not require monitoring. However, when needed to therapeutically treat patients with thrombosis, the drug requires monitoring using the Xa inhibitory assay. Thrombin-based assays are not effective. This drug has the disadvantage of having no antidote (protamine sulfate, which can neutralize unfractionated heparin and LMWH in the event of overdose, has no effect on danaparoid). In addition, the drug has a long half-life (approximately 18 hours).

Antiplatelet Agents

Used alone or in combination with other anticoagulants, a number of antiplatelet function agents have been developed. By far the most commonly used agent is aspirin. It functions by inhibiting prostaglandin synthesis. Its action has been well recognized for over 20 years, and its use (in low doses) for prophylaxis to prevent stroke and MI has been well characterized. Aspirin has been used in combination with heparin or LMWH in the therapy of patients with lupus-type anticoagulants who are pregnant and have suffered from recurrent spontaneous abortion. They are also used together in some patients who have arterial thrombotic events.

Vascular surgeons and cardiologists are becoming more and more adept at using thrombolytic agents, lysing clots that are formed in coronary arteries and other vessels. The site of these thrombi can then be stented with devices that hold the lumen of the artery open and allow recirculation beyond the previous occlusion. The difficulty that has occurred with these therapies has been the prevention of rethrombosis of the vessel. The most promising of the agents used in this postthrombolytic and stenting situation have been inhibitors of platelet function with or without heparin. Those used are ones that prevent platelet aggregation by binding to the $\alpha_2\beta_1$ receptor (GPIIb/IIIa) on the surface of the platelet. In addition, there are new agents that bind specifically to the ADP receptor on the surface of the platelet, preventing activation of the platelet.

Other antiplatelet agents are likely to be developed in the near future. Their effectiveness is gradually increasing, as clinicians become more accustomed to their application. In general, these antiplatelet agents have not required laboratory monitoring.

Thrombolytic Therapy

If a thrombus has been formed and has been in place in situ for a short period of time, precluding organization, logic would dictate that accelerating the lysis of the clot may help preserve function in the vascular bed served by the vessel. Thrombolytic therapy using urokinase and streptokinase has been available for more than two decades. More recently, other thrombolytic agents have become available.

The medications that convert plasminogen to plasmin without fibrin as a cofactor may be classified in two categories: (1) agents that activate directly plasminogen to plasmin, and (2) agents that are fibrin specific. In the former group are streptokinase or urokinase. The latter group includes t-PA.

Because the goal to be achieved is the lysis of fibrin clots, agents that are specific for fibrin would logically be preferred. Streptokinase and urokinase cause a hypofibrinogenemia secondary to fibrinogenolysis in virtually all patients, even when the medication is given by a catheter into the specific artery containing the clot. In practice, the magnitude of this hypofibrinogenemia tends not to be clinically significant with regard to hemorrhage, although hemorrhagic complications can occur. The advantage of the fibrin-specific agents is that it is feasible to administer these agents systemically rather into the vessel containing the thrombus in a catheter-directed fashion. It would be incorrect to assume that generalized fibrinogenolysis is precluded by fibrin specificity. In fact, t-PA can bind to circulating fibrin degradation products, activate plasmin, and cleave fibrinogen. Therefore, although less frequent and less severe, fibrin-specific agents can be complicated by hypofibrinogenemia.

The thrombolytic activity in thrombolytic therapy, in general, is not monitored. However, prior hemostatic evaluation is of value. Firstly, evaluation of hemostasis can be helpful in predicting which patients are at the greatest risk for bleeding when thrombolytic therapy is used. Secondly, those patients who have had thrombolytic therapy that need to be followed by a surgical procedure, such as coronary artery bypass, need to have their hemostatic mechanism evaluated prior to the surgical procedure. Evaluation in this case would include the usual initial tests of hemostatic evaluation: PT, APTT, fibrinogen assay, thrombin time, and platelet count. Frequently these patients are receiving therapeutic heparin, complicating the evaluation. Should evaluation still be considered necessary, heparin effect can be neutralized by adding heparinase to the specimen submitted to the laboratory.

➤ CASE STUDY 1

A 40-year-old man presented to the emergency department with a swollen, painful right leg of 3 days' duration and shortness of breath for the past 12 hours. He also had sharp pain in the left side of his chest when he took a deep breath.

Pertinent History

Past Illnesses: Had pneumonia 8 years ago with full recovery.

Occupation: Cross-country truck driver.

Social Habits: Drinks alcohol occasionally on a social basis. Has smoked a pack of cigarettes a day for 22 years.

Family History: Mother died of "clots in her lungs." Father and siblings are alive and well. One sister had a "clot in her leg" after she delivered her only child.

Pertinent Physical Findings

Vital Signs: Blood pressure, 110/75 mm Hg; respirations, 20/min; pulse, 72/min and regular; temperature, 38°C; weight, 130 kg.

Chest: Distant breath sounds on the left with dullness to percussion. Heart examination is not remarkable.

Bones, Joints, and Muscle: Right leg, ankle, and foot are slightly edematous. There is a positive Homans' sign on the right (abruptly flexing the right ankle produces pain in the calf and behind the knee).

Laboratory Findings

Hgb, 14.5g/dL; WBC, 12,000/μL ($\uparrow$); differential WBC: Neutrophils, 9100/μL ($\uparrow$); lymphocytes, 2200/μL; monocytes 500/μL; eosinophils, 200/μL; platelet count 220,000/μL

PT, 12 sec; INR, 1.0; APTT, 22 sec; fibrinogen, 269 mg/dL; thrombin time, 18 sec; D-dimer, 500 ng/mL ($\uparrow$)

Cholesterol, 230 mg/dL ($\uparrow$), HDL, 25 mg/dL ($\downarrow$)

Questions

1. What is the differential diagnosis?
2. What diagnostic procedures may be of value?
3. What laboratory tests may be helpful in determining the etiology of the condition?
4. What risk factors are present in this patient?
5. What therapy is indicated?
6. How is the therapy monitored?

Answers

1. This is most likely venous thrombotic episode (VTE). Swelling in the leg could be lymphatic obstruction from infection or tumor. Chest pain has several possibilities in the cardiac and pulmonary areas. Both together in this sequence require excluding VTE.
2. Ventilation perfusion scan of the lungs, chest x-ray, and Doppler imaging of the deep veins of the upper legs and, possibly, pulmonary angiogram. V/Q and Doppler scans were positive in this case. Chest x-ray showed an effusion on the right.
3. Activated protein C resistance, factor V Leiden by PCR, prothrombin gene mutation 20210 by PCR, MTHFR by PCR, possibly anticardiolipin. After recovery and conclusion of anticoagulation, protein C, protein S, AT. All of these were performed, and the patient was found to be heterozygous for factor V Leiden, only.
4. Obesity, factor V Leiden, occupation. Cigarette smoking is strongly associated with arterial, but not venous, thrombosis. The same is true for the patient's lipid studies.
5. Parenteral anticoagulation (unfractionated heparin or LMWH) followed by oral anticoagulation.
6. APTT and PT/INR.

► CASE STUDY 2

A 28-year-old gravida 2, para 0 woman desires to have children. She comes to you for advice because she has miscarried two prior pregnancies and is concerned about her ability to have a successful pregnancy.

Current Medications: Patient reports taking aspirin for headaches but otherwise takes no medications.

Family History: Parents and siblings are alive and well.

Pertinent History

Hematopoietic: No history of anemia, bleeding disorder, jaundice, or easy bruising. Two years ago she had a clot in her left leg that was treated with anticoagulants for 6 months. The leg has a small amount of swelling by the end of the day. She has never received a blood transfusion.

Menstrual History: Unremarkable menstrual cycle, although somewhat irregular. Last menstrual period: 39 days ago.

Pertinent Physical Findings

Vital Signs: Blood pressure, 125/80 mm Hg; respirations, 16/min; pulse, 72/min, and regular.

Skin: Mild livedo reticularis is noted on distal arms and legs.

Pelvic and Rectal Examination: The cervix is parous and soft.

Bones, Joints, and Muscle: No edema is apparent in the left leg at the time of the examination.

Laboratory Findings

Hgb, 13.5 g/dL; WBC, 8000/μL; differential WBC: Neutrophils, 5100/μL; lymphocytes, 2200/μL; monocytes, 500/μL; eosinophils, 200/μL; platelet count, 100,000/μL.

PT, 12 sec; INR, 1.0; APTT, 70 sec ($\uparrow$); fibrinogen, 269 mg/dL; thrombin time, 18 sec.

Questions

1. What is the initial test that should be ordered to evaluate the patient's prolonged APTT? What can this test tell you about the clotting abnormality?
2. An equal mix of the patient's plasma with normal plasma demonstrates an APTT of 62 seconds. What can you conclude regarding the cause of the prolongation of her APTT?
3. Further laboratory testing reveals a prolonged dilute Russell's viper venom time, which normalizes when excess phospholipid is added to the plasma. Based on the results of these tests, what is the probable cause of her prolonged APTT?

Answers

1. The 1:1 mixing study with normal plasma; the test will differentiate between a coagulation inhibitor or factor deficiency.

2. The 1:1 mixing study fails to completely correct the APTT, indicating the presence of an inhibitor.
3. She has a lupus anticoagulant and history consistent with the antiphospholipid syndrome (recurrent spontaneous abortion, mild thrombocytopenia, and deep venous thrombosis).

QUESTIONS

1. Which characteristic of endothelial cells suppresses fibrinolysis?
   a. Platelet adhesion
   b. Production of t-PA inhibitor
   c. Secretion of von Willebrand's factor
   d. Release of tissue factors

2. Which of the following statements concerning warfarin is true?
   a. It inhibits production of contact coagulation factors.
   b. It decreases the function of vitamin K–dependent factors.
   c. It interferes with cyclic vitamin K prior to carboxylation.
   d. It will inhibit coagulation in a standard tube of blood.

3. Which cell plays a key role in the regulation of hemostasis?
   a. Endothelial cell
   b. Neutrophil
   c. Fibroblast
   d. Eosinophil
   e. Erythrocyte

4. A 28-year-old man suffered from recurrent deep venous thrombosis and pulmonary embolus. Studies in the laboratory show that his plasma is unable to inhibit factors VIIIa and Va, indicating the plasma is deficient in which naturally occurring inhibitor/anticoagulant?
   a. Protein C
   b. Antithrombin
   c. High-molecular-weight kininogen
   d. Ferrochelatase
   e. Fibronectin

5. A 28-year-old woman with known systemic lupus erythematosus presents with a swollen painful left leg. She had had one prior deep venous thrombosis. She has no children but has had two spontaneous abortions. Which laboratory test do you expect to be often abnormal?
   a. Prothrombin time
   b. Activated partial thromboplastin time
   c. Assay for protein C
   d. Assay for plasminogen
   e. Assay for antithrombin

6. A 25-year-old woman presents with a thrombus in her right leg. She had a similar event 2 years ago in the left leg. Her mother, a paternal uncle, and her sister have all had episodes of thrombosis, and one of these was a pulmonary thromboembolus. Any of the following are potential etiologies; which is the most likely?
   a. Protein S deficiency
   b. Antithrombin deficiency
   c. Hyperhomocysteinemia
   d. Factor V Leiden
   e. Factor XI deficiency

SUMMARY CHART

➤ Endothelial cells function to facilitate platelet adhesion and platelet activation at the site of injury, secrete von Willebrand's factor, and secrete an inhibitor of tissue plasminogen, which suppresses fibrinolysis.

➤ Natural anticoagulants in plasma include antithrombin (AT), heparin cofactor II (HC-II), protein C (PC), protein S (PS), and tissue factor pathway inhibitor (TFPI).

➤ Antithrombin is a major inhibitor of thrombin and factor Xa.

➤ Protein C is a vitamin K–dependent zymogen that, once activated by thrombin, proteolytically degrades factors VIIIa and Va, two of the major cofactors involved in thrombin generation.

➤ TFPI inhibits plasma coagulation by (1) binding the activated form of either factor X or factor IX, and (2) inhibiting further binding of factor X or factor IX via the TFPI-X-IX membrane complex.

➤ Inhibitors of plasmin include α_2-antiplasmin, α_1-antitrypsin, α_2-macroglobulin, AT, and C1 esterase inhibitor.

➤ Inhibitors of plasminogen include plasminogen activator inhibitor-1 (PAI-1), PAI-2, and PAI-3, with PAI-1 being the most significant inhibitor of tissue plasminogen activator (t-PA).

➤ Inherited thrombophilia is a group of congenital hematologic disorders that includes a variety of hypercoagulable states that usually present as venous or arterial thrombosis, or both.

➤ Activated protein C resistance (APC-R) can be defined as deficient anticoagulant response of plasma to the addition of APC. Causes of APC-R include inhibitors to APC, functional PS deficiency, and mutated forms of factor V and VIII molecules; factor V Leiden is the most common cause of APC-R.

➤ The prothrombin nucleotide G20210A mutation can be described as a single guanine to adenine mutation at nucleotide position 20210 and is associated with increased risk of deep vein thrombosis and elevated prothrombin levels.

➤ Antiphospholipid (aPL) syndrome is an acquired thrombotic disorder. Laboratory evidence of aPL antibodies can be in the form of either immunologically demonstrated aPL antibodies; enzyme-linked immunosorbent assay (ELISA) for anticardiolipin antibody, and/or lupus anticoagulant.

➤ The APTT may be prolonged in heparin therapy or contamination, insufficient volume of sample, disseminated intravascular coagulation (DIC), factor deficiencies, and antibodies directed against factors in intrinsic or common pathways.

➤ Heparin-induced thrombocytopenia is described as a sudden decrease in the platelet count 5 days after heparin therapy is initiated and is caused by the interaction of platelet factor 4 (PF4) on the platelet membrane.

➤ Unfractionated heparin is an unbranched polysaccharide that is prepared from bovine lungs or porcine intestines with a range of molecular weight from 4000 to 35,000 daltons. It acts by accelerating the rate at which AT is capable of binding thrombin. Heparin therapy is monitored by the APTT, with a target value of one-and-a-half times the upper limits of the reference range for the APTT.

➤ Low-molecular-weight heparin (LMWH) is prepared from unfractionated heparin by fractionation or depolymerization, producing heparins of 1000 to 12,000 daltons. They inhibit factor Xa more efficiently and do not require therapeutic monitoring.

➤ Vitamin K is a cofactor for a carboxylase that inserts an additional carboxyl group on the glutamic acid residues in the amino terminal end of coagulation factors II, VII, IX, and X.

➤ Warfarin therapy or oral anticoagulation therapy acts by interfering with the recycling of vitamin K and depressing the activities of factors II, VII, IX, and X; PC; and PS.

➤ Warfarin therapy is monitored by the prothrombin time (PT) and international normalized ratio (INR); the INR is maintained between 2 and 3 for patients on anticoagulant therapy.

➤ Thrombolytic agents include t-PA, urokinase, and streptokinase. Hemostatic evaluation includes PT, APTT, fibrinogen assay, thrombin time, and platelet count.

ACKNOWLEDGMENT
The authors wish to express their deep gratitude to John D. Olson, MD, PhD, for his assistance in preparing this chapter. His knowledge of and commitment to the subject were inspiring and invaluable. Without his guidance this work would not have been possible.

References
1. Egeberg, O: Inherited antithrombin deficiency causing thrombophilia. Thromb Diath Hemorrh 13:516, 1965.
2. Nordstrom, M, et al: Deep venous thrombosis and occult malignancy: An epidemiological study. Br Med J 308:891, 1994.
3. Stump, D, and Mann, KG: Mechanisms of thrombus formation. Ann Emerg Med 17:1138, 1988.
4. Olson, JD: Mechanisms of hemostasis: Effect on intracerebral hemorrhage. Stroke 24(Suppl 12):109, 1993.
5. Olson, JD: Hemostasis and thrombosis. Considerations in pregnancy. In Loftus, CM (ed): Neurosurgical aspects of pregnancy. Am Ass Neuro Surg 1996.
6. Walker, FJ: Structural and functional properties of protein C. In Hoyer, LW, and Drohan, WN (eds): Recombinant Technology in Hemostasis and Thrombosis. Plenum Press, New York, 1991, p 81.
7. Rosenberg, RD, and Bauer, KA: Prothrombinase generation and the regulation of coagulation. In Loscalzo, J (ed): Thrombosis and Hemorrhage. Blackwell Scientific, Boston, 1994, p 21.
8. Birginshaw, GF, and Shanberg, JN: Identification of two distinct cofactors in

human plasma. Inhibition of thrombin and activated factor X. Thromb Res 4:463, 1974.

9. Tollefsen, DM, et al: Heparin cofactor II: Purification and properties of a heparin-dependent inhibitor of thrombin in human plasma. J Biol Chem 257:2161, 1982.

10. Neumann, CB, et al: Protein C and protein S: Methodological and clinical aspects. In Shearer, MJ (ed): Vitamin–Dependent Protein: Analytical, Physiological, and Clinical Aspects, CRC Press, Boca Raton, FL, 1993, p 144.

11. Hieb, MJ, et al: Inhibition of activated protein C by recombinant alpha-1 antitrypsin variant with substitution of arginine for leucine for methionine. J Biol Chem 265:2365, 1990.

12. Sandset, PM, and Abildgaard, U: Extrinsic pathway inhibitor—the key to feedback control of blood coagulation initiated by tissue thromboplastin. Haemost 21:219, 1991.

13. Dahlback, B, et al: Familial thrombophilia due to a previous unrecognized mechanism characterized by poor anticoagulant response to activated protein C: Prediction of a cofactor to activated protein C. Proc Natl Acad Sci USA 90:1004, 1993.

14. Bertina, RM, et al: Mutation in blood coagulation factor V associated with resistance to activated protein C. Nature 369:64, 1994.

15. Williamson, D, et al: Factor V Cambridge: A new mutation (Arg 306 Thr) associated with resistance to activated protein C. Blood 91:1140, 1998.

16. Ridker, PM, et al: Mutation in the gene coding for coagulation factor V and the risk of myocardial infarction, stroke, and venous thrombosis in apparently healthy men. N Engl J Med 332:912, 1995.

17. Dahlback, B: Inherited thrombophilia: Resistance to activated protein C as a pathogenic factor of venous thromboembolism. Blood 85:607, 1995.

18. Dahlback, B, et al: Resistant to activated protein, the FV:Q 506 allele, and venous thrombosis. Ann Hematol 72:166, 1996.

19. Tait, RC, et al: Prevalence of protein C deficiency in the healthy population. Thromb Haemost 73:87, 1995.

20. D'Angelo, SV, et al: Relationship between protein C antigen and anticoagulant activity during oral anticoagulation and in selected disease states. J Clin Invest 77:416, 1986.

21. Engesser, L, et al: Hereditary protein C deficiency: Clinical manifestations. Ann Intern Med 106:677, 1987.

22. Comp, PC: Congenital and acquired hypercoagulable states. In Hull, R, and Pineo, GF (eds): Disorders of Thrombosis. WB Saunders, Philadelphia, 1996, p 339.

23. Sheffield, WB, et al: Antithrombin structure and function. In High, KA, and Roberts, HR (eds): Molecular Basis of Thrombosis and Hemostasis. Dekker, New York, 1995, p 355.

24. Menache, D, et al: Antithrombin III: Physiology, deficiency, and replacement therapy. Transfusion 32:580, 1992.

25. Poort, SR, et al: A common genetic variation in the 3′-untranslated region of the prothrombin gene is associated with elevated plasma prothrombin levels and an increase in venous thrombosis. Blood 88:3698, 1996.

26. Kapur, RK, et al: A prothrombin gene mutation is significantly associated with venous thrombosis. Arterioscler Thromb Vasc Biol 17:2875, 1997.

27. De Stefano, V, et al: Inherited thrombophilia: Pathogenesis, clinical syndromes, and management. Blood 87:3531, 1996.

28. D'Angelo, A, and Selhub, J: Homocysteine and thrombotic disease. Blood 90:1, 1997.

29. Jensen, R, and Ens, GE: Tissue factor pathway inhibitor. Clin Hemost Rev 6:1, 1992.

30. Tollefsen, DM: Laboratory diagnosis of antithrombin and heparin cofactor II deficiency. Semin Thromb Hemost 16:162, 1990.

31. Ebert, RF: Index of Variant Human Fibrinogens. CRC Press, Boca Raton, FL, 1991.

32. Dawson, NA, et al: Acquired dysfibrinogenemia. Am J Med 78:682, 1985.

33. Scanu, AM: Atherothrombogenicity of lipoprotein (a): The debate. Am J Cardiol 82:26Q, 1998.

34. Djurovic, S, and Berg, K: Epidemiology of Lp(a) lipoprotein: Its role in atherosclerotic/thrombotic disease. Clin Genet 52:281, 1997.

35. Marcovina, SM, and Koschinsky, ML: Lipoprotein (a) as a risk factor for coronary artery disease. Am J Cardiol 82:57U, 1998.

36. Wilson, WA, et al: International consensus statement on preliminary classification criteria for definite antiphospholipid syndrome: Report of an international workshop. Arthritis Rheum 42:1309, 1999.

37. McNeil, HP, et al: Immunology and clinical importance of antiphospholipid antibodies. Adv Immunol 49:193, 1991.

38. Triplett, DA, et al: The relationship between lupus anticoagulants and antibodies to phospholipid. JAMA 259:550, 1988.

39. Male, C, et al: Clinical significance of lupus anticoagulants in children. J Pediatr 134:199, 1999.

40. Bowie, EJW, et al: Thrombosis in systemic lupus erythematosus despite circulating anticoagulants. J Lab Clin Med 62:416, 1963.

41. Harris, EN: Syndrome of the black swan. Br J Rheumatol 26:324, 1987.

42. Harris, EN, et al: Anticardiolipin antibodies: Detection by radioimmunoassay and association with thrombosis in systemic lupus erythematosus. Lancet 2:1211, 1983.

43. Loizu, S, et al: Measurement of anticardiolipin antibodies by enzyme-linked immunosorbent assay: Standardization and quantitation of results. Clin Exp Immunol 62:738, 1985.

44. Galli, M, et al: Anticardiolipin antibodies (ACA) directed not to cardiolipin but to a plasma cofactor. Lancet 335:1544, 1990.

45. Matsuurra, E, et al: Anticardiolipin cofactor(s) and differential diagnosis of autoimmune disease. Lancet 336:177, 1990.

46. McNeil, HP, et al: Antiphospholipid antibodies are directed against a complex antigen that includes a lipid binding inhibitor of coagulation: β2Glycoprotein I (apolipoprotein H). Proc Natl Acad Sci USA 87:4120, 1990.

47. Oosting, JD, et al: Lupus anticoagulant activity is frequently dependent on the presence of Beta2-Glycoprotein I. Thromb Haemostas 67:499, 1992.

48. Bevers, EM, et al: Lupus anticoagulant IgG's (LA) are not directed to phospholipids only, but to a complex of lipid-bound human prothrombin. Thromb Haemostas 66:629, 1991.

49. Permpikul, P, et al: Functional and binding studies of the roles of prothrombin and Beta2Glycoprotein I in the expression of lupus anticoagulant activity. Blood 83:2878, 1994.

50. Galli, M, et al: Different anticoagulant and immunological properties of antiprothrombin antibodies in patients with antiphospholipid antibodies. Thromb Haemostas 77:486, 1997.

51. Roubey, RAS: Autoantibodies to phospholipid-binding plasma proteins: A new view of lupus anticoagulants and other "antiphospholipid" autoantibodies. Blood 84:2854, 1994.

52. Rand, JH, and Wu, X: Antibody-mediated disruption of the annexin-V antithrombotic shield: A new mechanism for thrombosis in the antiphospholipid syndrome. Thromb Haemostas 82:649, 1999.

53. Horbach, DA, et al: Lupus anticoagulant is the strongest risk factor for both venous and arterial thrombosis in patients with systemic lupus erythematosus. Thromb Haemostas 76:916, 1996.

54. Coulam, CB, et al: American Society for Reproductive Immunology report of the committee for establishing criteria for diagnosis of reproductive autoimmune syndrome. Am J Reprod Immunol 41:121, 1999.

55. Brandt, JT, et al: Criteria for the diagnosis of lupus anticoagulants: An update. Thromb Haemostas 74:1185, 1995.

56. Arnout, J, et al: Optimization of the dilute prothrombin time for the detection of the lupus anticoagulant by use of a recombinant tissue thromboplastin. Br J Haematol 87:94, 1994.

57. Thiagarajan, P, et al: The use of the dilute Russell viper venom time for the diagnosis of lupus anticoagulants. Blood 68:869, 1986.

58. Exner, T, et al: A sensitive test demonstrating lupus anticoagulant and its behavioral patterns. Br J Haematol 40:143, 1978.

59. Norbis, F, et al: Diluted Russell's viper venom time and colloidal silica clotting time for the identification of the phospholipid-dependent inhibitors of coagulation. Thromb Res 85:427, 1997.

60. Triplett, DA, et al: A hexagonal (II) phase phospholipid neutralization assay for lupus anticoagulant identification. Thromb Haemostas 70:787, 1993.

61. Triplett, DA, et al: Laboratory diagnosis of lupus inhibitors: A comparison of the tissue thromboplastin inhibition procedure with a new platelet neutralization procedure. Am J Clin Pathol 79:678, 1983.

62. Sletnes, KE, et al: Preparation of plasma for the detection of lupus anticoagulants and antiphospholipid antibodies. Thromb Res 66:43, 1992.

63. Arnout, J, et al: Lupus anticoagulant testing in Europe: An analysis of results from the first European concerted action on thrombophilia (ECAT) survey using plasmas spiked with monoclonal antibodies against human β2-Glycoprotein I. Thromb Haemostas 81:929, 1999.

64. Arnout, J, and Vermylen, J: Lupus anticoagulant: Influence on the international normalized ratio [letter to the editor]. Thromb Haemostas 81:847, 1999.

65. Olson, JD: Addressing clinical etiologies of a prolonged aPTT. CAP Today13:28, 1999.

66. Adcock, DM, and Marlar, RA: Activated partial thromboplastin time reagent sensitivity to the presence of the lupus anticoagulant. Arch Pathol Lab Med 116:837, 1992.

67. Brandt, JT, et al: The sensitivity of different coagulation reagents to the presence of lupus anticoagulants. Arch Pathol Lab Med 111:120, 1987.

68. Brandt, JT, et al: Laboratory identification of lupus anticoagulants: Results of the second international workshop for identification of lupus anticoagulants. Thromb Haemostas 74:1597, 1995.

69. Lazarchick, J, and Kizer, J: The laboratory diagnosis of lupus anticoagulants. Arch Pathol Lab Med 113:177, 1989.

70. Lockshin, MD: Pregnancy loss in the antiphospholipid syndrome. Thromb Haemostas 82:641, 1999.

71. Warkentin, TE: Clinical presentation of heparin-induced thrombocytopenia. Semin Hematol 35(Suppl 5):9, 1998.

72. Nand, S, et al: Heparin-induced thrombocytopenia with thrombosis: Incidence, analysis of risk factors, and clinical outcomes in 108 consecutive patients treated at a single institution. Am J Hematol 56:12, 1997.

73. Warkentin, TE, and Kelton, JG: A 14-year study of heparin-induced thrombocytopenia. Am J Med 101:502, 1996.

74. Chong, BH: Heparin-induced thrombocytopenia. Br J Haematol 89:431, 1995.

75. Van Cott, EM: How to diagnose and manage heparin induced thrombocytopenia. CAP Today March:50, 1997.

76. Amiral, J, et al: Platelet factor 4 complexed to heparin is the target for antibodies generated in heparin-induced thrombocytopenia. Thromb Haemostas 68:95, 1992.

77. Amiral, J, et al: Presence of autoantibodies to interleukin-8 or neutrophil-activating peptide-2 in patients with heparin-associated thrombocytopenia. Blood 88:410, 1996.

78. Suh, J-S, et al: Characterization of the humoral immune response in heparin-induced thrombocytopenia. Am J Hematol 54:196, 1997.

79. Kelton, JG, et al: Heparin-induced thrombocytopenia: Laboratory studies. Blood 72:925, 1988.

80. Cines, DB, et al: Immune endothelial-cell injury in heparin-associated thrombocytopenia. N Eng J Med 316:581, 1987.

81. Amiral, J, et al: Generation of antibodies to heparin-PF4 complexes without thrombocytopenia in patients treated with unfractionated or low-molecular-weight heparin. Am J Hematol 52:90, 1996.

82. Brandt, JT, et al: On the role of platelet FcγRIIa phenotype in heparin-induced thrombocytopenia. Thromb Haemostas 74:1564, 1995.

83. Burgess, JK, et al: Single amino acid mutation of Fcγ receptor is associated with the development of heparin-induced thrombocytopenia. Br J Haematol 91:761, 1995.

84. Arepally, G, et al: FcτRIIa polymorphism, subclass-specific IgG anti-heparin/PF4 antibodies and clinical course in patients with heparin-induced thrombocytopenia and thrombosis. Blood 88(Suppl 1, abstr):281a, 1996.

85. Warkentin, TE, et al: Heparin-induced thrombocytopenia in patients treated with low-molecular-weight heparin or unfractionated heparin. N Eng J Med 332:1330, 1995.

86. Isenhart, CE, and Brandt, JT: Platelet aggregation studies for the diagnosis of heparin-induced thrombocytopenia. Am J Clin Pathol 99:324, 1993.

87. Sheridan, D, et al: A diagnostic test for heparin-induced thrombocytopenia. Blood 67:27, 1986.

88. Walenga, JM, et al: Laboratory tests for the diagnosis of heparin-induced thrombocytopenia. Semin Thromb Hemostas 25(Suppl 1):43, 1999.

89. Walenga, JM, et al: Laboratory tests for heparin-induced thrombocytopenia: A multicenter study. Semin Hematol 36(Suppl 1):22, 1999.

90. Stewart, MW, et al: Heparin-induced thrombocytopenia: An improved method of detection based on lumi-aggregometry. Br J Haematol 91:173, 1995.

91. Lee, DH, et al: A diagnostic test for heparin-induced thrombocytopenia: Detection of platelet microparticles using flow cytometry. Br J Haematol 95:724, 1996.

92. Warkentin, TE, et al: The pathogenesis of venous limb gangrene associated with heparin-induced thrombocytopenia. Ann Intern Med 127:804, 1997.

93. Warkentin, TE, and Barkin, RL: Newer strategies for the treatment of heparin-induced thrombocytopenia. Pharmacotherapy 19:181, 1999.

94. Haas, S, et al: Heparin-induced thrombocytopenia: The role of platelet activation and therapeutic implications. Semin Thromb Hemostas 25(Suppl 1):67, 1999.

95. Warkentin, TE: Heparin-induced thrombocytopenia: Pathogenesis, frequency, avoidance and management. Drug Safety 5:325, 1997.

96. Laposata, M, et al: College of American Pathologists conference XXXI on laboratory monitoring of anticoagulant therapy: The clinical use and laboratory monitoring of low-molecular weight heparin, danaparoid, hirudin and related compounds, and argatroban. Arch Pathol Lab Med 122:799, 1998.

97. Hellgren, M, et al: Resistance to activated protein C as a basis for venous thromboembolism associated with pregnancy and oral contraceptives. Am J Obstet Gynecol 173:210, 1995.

98. Bokarewa, MI, et al: Arg 506-Gln mutation in factor V and risk of thrombosis during pregnancy. Br J Haematol 92(2):473–478, 1996.

99. Olivieri, O, et al: Resistance to activated protein C in healthy women taking oral contraceptives. Br J Haematol 91:465, 1995.

100. Harris, RC, and Ismail, N: Extrarenal complications of the nephrotic syndrome. Am J Kidney Dis 23:477, 1994.

101. Priest, JR, et al: A syndrome of thrombosis and hemorrhage complicating L-asparaginase therapy for childhood acute lymphoblastic leukemia. J Pediatr 100:984, 1982.

102. Goodnough, LT, et al: Increased incidence of thromboembolism in stage IV breast cancer treated with a five-drug chemotherapy regimen. Cancer 54:1264, 1984.

103. Geerts, WH, et al: A prospective study of venous thromboembolism after major trauma. N Engl J Med 331:1601, 1994.

104. Brandt, JT (ed): College of American Pathologists Consensus Conference XXXI on Laboratory Monitoring of Anticoagulant Therapy. Arch Path Lab Med 122:765, 1998.

105. Dalen, JE, and Hirsh, J (eds): Fifth American College of Chest Physicians Consensus Conference on Antithrombotic Therapy. Chest 114(Suppl):439S, 1998.

106. Doyle, DJ, et al: Adjusted subcutaneous heparin or continuous intravenous heparin in patients with acute deep venous thrombosis. A randomized trial. Ann Intern Med 107:441, 1987.

107. Basu, D, et al: A prospective study of the value of monitoring heparin treatment with the activated partial thromboplastin. N Engl J Med 287:324, 1972.

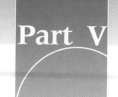

28 Routine Hematology Methods

JANIS WYRICK-GLATZEL, MS, MT(ASCP)
VIRGINIA C. HUGHES, MS, MT(ASCP)

OBJECTIVES

At the end of this chapter, the learner should be able to:

1. Calculate a manual white blood cell count, red blood cell count, and platelet count.

2. Calculate a percentage of reticulocytes and an absolute/corrected reticulocyte count.

3. Calculate a reticulocyte production index.

4. List errors in the performance of a centrifugal microhematocrit determination.

5. Calculate the mean corpuscular volume, mean corpuscular hemoglobin, and mean corpuscular hemoglobin concentration.

6. Identify factors that affect the erythrocyte sedimentation rate.

7. Identify hemoglobins separated at alkaline and acid pH in hemoglobin electrophoresis.

8. Name a method for quantifying hemoglobin A_2 and hemoglobin F.

9. Describe the differential solubility test for hemoglobin S.

10. Describe a procedure for detecting Heinz bodies.

11. Identify conditions that show increased and decreased osmotic fragility.

12. Describe the basic principle for the Ham's test and the sugar water test for paroxysmal nocturnal hemoglobinuria.

13. Explain the basic principle of the cyanmethemoglobin method for hemoglobin determination.

14. Describe the effects of a lipemic specimen on hemoglobin determinations.

15. Calculate a corrected white blood cell count for a peripheral blood smear containing more than 10 nucleated red blood cells per 100 white blood cells.

16. Differentiate between a venipuncture and capillary puncture.

17. Identify the appropriate site for capillary puncture on an infant.

Our goal in this chapter is to present the student with basic hematologic procedures. Emphasis is placed on interpretation as well as on procedure. At the end of some procedures, we have included a comment section that serves as a potpourri, highlighting general points of information concerning the procedure, its limitations, and its interpretations.

As technology and automation have expanded, some procedures have become antiquated. We believe, however, that an understanding of the basic procedures will serve as a sound building block for the application of more advanced technology.

➤ COLLECTION OF BLOOD SPECIMENS

Blood collection for hematologic studies can be performed via venipuncture (blood collected from a vein) or by capillary puncture (blood collected from the heel, finger, earlobe, or toe). The anticoagulant used most often in routine hematology methods, excluding coagulation analysis, is ethylene diaminetetraacetic acid (EDTA).

There are many preanalytic steps to follow in the process of blood collection, such as patient identification, requisition verification of laboratory orders, and biohazard safety, to name a few. These items, as well as venipuncture and capillary puncture methodology, are discussed here.

Patient Identification

Hospitalized Patients

Hospitalized patients wear a wristband with the following information: (1) patient's first and last name, and middle initial; (2) hospital number; (3) date of birth or age; (4) gender; (5) name of physician; and (6) location or room number. All of this information should be cross-checked with the laboratory requisition form or laboratory orders for each patient. If the patient is not wearing wristband, a nurse should be notified to verify patient identification.

Outpatients

For outpatients who have blood collected, the phlebotomist should ask the patient to recite his or her full name, address, social security number, and date of birth. The phlebotomist must check this information with the laboratory requisition form or physician's record of laboratory orders.

Safety

Universal precautions should be in practice at all times when collecting blood specimens. This means that all specimens should be handled as if they were infected with the hepatitis B virus or human immunodeficiency virus (HIV).

Such safety precautions include wearing a new pair of latex gloves for each patient, washing hands between patients, and disposing of needles and contaminated supplies in a puncture-resistant biohazard container (sharps).

Verification of Laboratory Requisitions

With each request for blood collection and laboratory analysis there must be a laboratory requisition that is either written or contained in the laboratory information system (LIS). Information contained on the requisition is outlined in Table 28–1. The phlebotomist needs to verify that the patient information on the requisition form or specimen label is correct before blood is collected. He or she should be aware of the appropriate anticoagulants for the tests being performed as well as the volume of blood required.

Labeling the Blood Specimen

A properly labeled specimen is essential to patient care. The consequences of a patient being treated based on another patient's results can be detrimental and sometimes fatal, depending on the situation. Many hospitals and laboratories have implemented preprinted patient labels that contain the following information: (1) patient's first and last name, (2) age, (3) gender, (4) hospital number, (5) test ordered, (6) unique bar code, (7) type of tube required, (8) social security number, (9) patient location, and (10) name of physician. An example of a patient label is illustrated in Figure 28–1.

The tubes in which blood is collected should be labeled after the blood is collected and not before; this alleviates labeling another tube if blood cannot be collected success-

> ### ➤ Table 28-1
> ### INFORMATION PRESENT ON LABORATORY REQUISITION

Patient's full name
Age of patient
Social security number
Hospital number
Date/time of collection
Physician's name
Accession or specimen number
Location where order was placed
Ordered tests

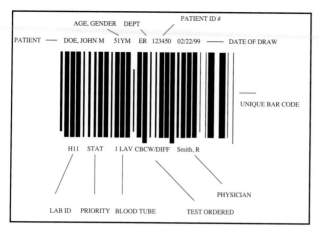

> ➤ **FIGURE 28–1** Example of a specimen label with bar code.

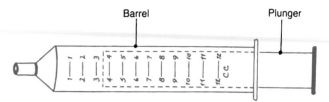

> ➤ **FIGURE 28–3** The syringe consisting of a barrel and plunger. (From Wedding, ME, and Toenjes, SA: Medical Laboratory Procedures. FA Davis, Philadelphia, 1998, p 97, with permission.)

fully on the first venipuncture. If preprinted labels are not available, the patient's first and last name and social security number should be on the tube of blood.

Venipuncture Methodology

Principle Venipuncture can be performed via syringe or by using the more popular evacuated tube system.[1] Syringes have become somewhat antiquated in the blood collection scenario because of multisample availability with the evacuated tube system. However, this technique is still available and used on patients with small veins, in blood culture collection, and in arterial blood gas collection. Briefly, once the needle (attached to the syringe) enters the vein, blood will appear in the hub of the syringe (Fig. 28–2). The phlebotomist controls the volume of blood being collected by pulling up on the plunger (Fig. 28–3). Once the syringe is filled, the phlebotomist releases the tourniquet and withdraws the needle. The blood collected must be placed into the correct tubes as soon as possible to avoid coagulation (clotting) of the specimen.

The evacuated tube system offers the benefit of multisample blood collection. This means that more than one tube of blood can be collected with one needlestick. An evacuated tube system usually consists of a disposable sterile needle, a needle holder, and an evacuated tube (Fig. 28–4).

Briefly, the multisample needle is pointed at both ends (Fig. 28–5). The end covered with a rubber sheath is screwed into the needle holder; the other end is inserted into the vein. The most common vein entered is the median cubital vein (Fig. 28–6) located in the antecubital fossa of the forearm; other veins used include the cephalic and basilic veins. The application of the rubber tourniquet is depicted in Figure 28–7. Once the vein is entered, tubes can be inserted into the body of the needle holder, puncturing the rubber sheath to withdraw the blood. Additional tubes can be filled in this manner. This apparatus alleviates the transfer of blood from the syringe to appropriate collection vials, which subjects the specimen to hemolysis because of the speed at which blood from the syringe is ejected. The reader should refer to any phlebotomy textbook for the actual procedure.

Capillary Puncture Methodology

In hematologic studies, blood collected by capillary puncture is most often performed on the pediatric population

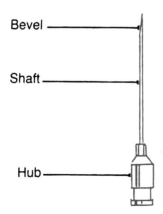

> ➤ **FIGURE 28–2** The hypodermic needle consisting of the bevel, shaft, and hub. The hub attaches to the syringe. (From Wedding, ME, and Toenjes, SA: Medical Laboratory Procedures. FA Davis, Philadelphia, 1998, p 97, with permission.)

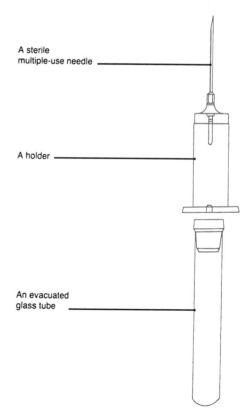

> ➤ **FIGURE 28–4** The evacuated tube system consisting of a double-pointed needle, a plastic holder, and a vacuum tube with a rubber stopper. (From Wedding, ME, and Toenjes, SA: Medical Laboratory Procedures. FA Davis, Philadelphia, 1998, p 95, with permission.)

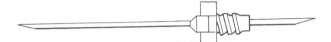

> FIGURE 28–5   The multisample needle, pointed at both ends with one end insulated in a rubber sheath. (From Wedding, ME, and Toenjes, SA: Medical Laboratory Procedures. FA Davis, Philadelphia, 1998, p 95, with permission.)

and, to a lesser extent, on elderly patients and those whose veins are collapsed or indiscriminate to the phlebotomist. The most common site for a capillary puncture in infants is the plantar surface of the heel perpendicular to the big toe or perpendicular to the fourth or fifth toe on the opposite side of the foot (Fig. 28–8). In older infants and the elderly population, the palmer (fleshy) surface of the distal phalanx of the middle or ring finger may be punctured, with the middle finger being the first choice.[2] Briefly, the site of puncture is warmed to enhance blood flow, cleansed with isopropyl alcohol, and punctured with a sterile lancet. The first drop is wiped away and the appropriate volume of blood is collected into either microhematocrit tubes (heparinized) or microtainers that contain EDTA. (Refer to any phlebotomy textbook for the actual procedure.)

➤ MANUAL BLOOD CELL COUNTS

Hemacytometer

The *hemacytometer* counting chamber is used for cell counting. It is constructed so that the distance between the bottom of the *coverslip* and the surface of the counting chamber is 0.1 mm (Fig. 28–9). The surface of the chamber contains two square-ruled areas separated by an H-shaped moat. These two squares are identical, allowing the tech-

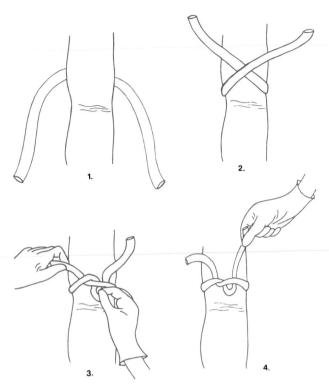

> FIGURE 28–7   Application of the rubber tourniquet. (From Wedding, ME, and Toenjes, SA: Medical Laboratory Procedures. FA Davis, Philadelphia, 1998, p 102, with permission.)

nologist to duplicate the cell count. Each has a total area of 9 mm^2 (3 mm on each side). These squares are divided into nine primary squares (Fig. 28–10), each with an area of 1 mm^2 (1 mm on each side). The four corner primary squares are used when counting leukocytes. These four corner primary squares are further divided into 16 smaller secondary squares, each with an area of 0.04 mm^2. The four corner and center secondary squares of the center primary square (see Fig. 28–10) are used to count erythrocytes. All 25 secondary squares of the center primary square are used to count platelets, and each of these 25 squares is further divided into 16 smaller tertiary squares (see Fig. 28–10).

The boundary lines of the central primary square are either double or triple. When the boundary line is double, all the cells within the square and those touching the innermost line are counted. If the boundary line is triple, all of the cells within the squares and those touching the middle line inward are counted.

Hemacytometers and coverslips should meet the specifications of the National Bureau of Standards and are so

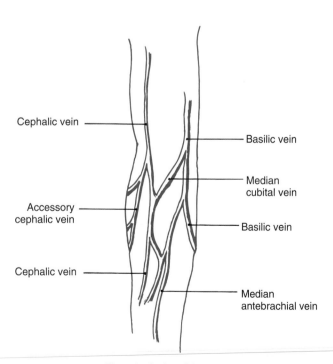

> FIGURE 28–6   The path of veins of the arm. (From Wedding, ME, and Toenjes, SA: Medical Laboratory Procedures. FA Davis, Philadelphia, 1998, p 100, with permission.)

Cephalic vein

Basilic vein

Median cubital vein

Accessory cephalic vein

Basilic vein

Cephalic vein

Median antebrachial vein

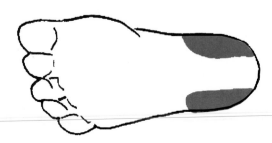

> FIGURE 28–8   Infant heel. Dark areas indicated by arrows represent recommended areas for infant heel puncture.

HEMACYTOMETER

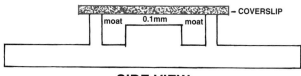

SIDE VIEW

➤ **FIGURE 28–9** Hemacytometer, side view.

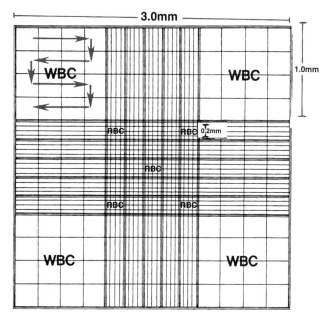

➤ **FIGURE 28–10** Spencer Bright-Line double counting system with improved Neubauer ruling. This represents an enlarged view of one of the two ruled squares of the hemacytometer. The four corner primary squares are used for counting white blood cells. The arrows in the upper left corner square represent the suggested counting pathway of cells. Five secondary squares (labeled RBC) of the center primary square are used for counting red blood cells. In platelet enumeration, all 25 squares of the center primary square are counted. (From Wedding, ME, and Toenjes, SA: Medical Laboratory Procedures. FA Davis, Philadelphia, 1998, p 277, with permission.)

marked by the manufacturer. A standardized coverslip should be used that has been ground to fit the specifications of the hemacytometer, ensuring a uniform depth and, therefore, a constant volume (see Fig. 28–9). A regular coverslip must not be used.

With the introduction of sophisticated electronic equipment such as the Coulter Counter (Beckman-Coulter) and the Cell-Dyn (Abbott Diagnostics) into the field of hematology, there is diminished need for manual cell counting. However, knowledge of this method is still important. Manual cell counts are often performed in patients with extreme cases of thrombocytosis, thrombocytopenia, leukocytosis, and leukopenia. Perhaps the most clear-cut use for manual cell counts is for measuring body fluids such as cerebral spinal fluid (CSF) and pleural fluid, as these can be counted only by manual methods.

Blood Dilution Vials

Dilution of blood samples may be performed by using prepackaged blood dilution vials available from manufacturers, such as the Unopette kit by Becton-Dickinson Vacutainer System (Fig. 28–11). Each vial is filled with premeasured diluent and capillary pipets appropriate for the necessary dilutions. A wide variety of test vials are available, including those for white blood cells (WBCs), platelets, red blood cells (RBCs), eosinophils, and hemoglobin. With the implication of infectious disease such as hepatitis and acquired immunodeficiency syndrome (AIDS), mouth suctioning pipets (Thoma pipets) are no longer advocated as proper procedure for making blood dilutions. Any changes in dilution factors that may vary with the manufacturer must be kept under consideration. Once the dilutions are made, the manual counts may be performed as described next.

Red Blood Cell Counts Using the Unopette System (see Fig. 28–11)

The Unopette system of red cell enumeration is an easier and less tedious procedure than the Thoma diluting pipet. The correct volume of diluent is contained in the Unopette reservoir, which eliminates "overshooting" the diluent with a manual diluting pipet.

Specimen Free-flowing capillary or well-mixed anticoagulated venous blood is obtained. EDTA is the anticoagulant of choice.

Principle Venous or capillary blood samples are drawn by capillary action at a specific volume into the Unopette reservoir containing RBC diluent. The reservoir is then mixed by inversion several times and charged onto the hemacytometer to be counted microscopically.

Equipment

Unopette reservoir No. 5851 containing 1.99-mL diluting fluid

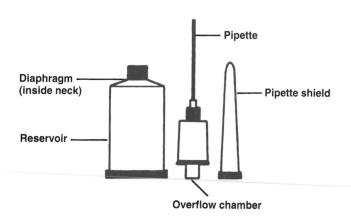

➤ **FIGURE 28–11** Unopette system, consisting of a reservoir containing a diluent, a pipet used to deliver the specimen, a reservoir, and a pipet shield used to puncture the plastic seal on reservoir, and as a cap for the pipet to prevent evaporation. (From Wedding, ME, and Toenjes, SA: Medical Laboratory Procedures. FA Davis, Philadelphia, 1998, p 234, with permission.)

Sodium chloride, 8.5 g

Sodium azide, 0.1 g

Distilled water, 1000 mL

Capillary pipet (10 μL)

Hemacytometer and coverslip

Microscope

Hand counter

Petri dish lined with moist filter paper

Procedure

1. Using the protective shield on the capillary pipet, puncture the diaphragm of the reservoir (Fig. 28–12A).
2. Remove the shield from the pipet assembly by twisting.
3. Holding the pipet almost horizontally, touch the tip of the pipet to the blood. Pipet will fill by capillary action (Fig. 28–12B). Filling will cease automatically when the blood reaches the end of the capillary bore in the neck of the pipet.[3]
4. Wipe the outside of the capillary pipet to remove excess blood that would interfere with the dilution factor.
5. Squeeze reservoir slightly to force out some air while simultaneously maintaining pressure on the reservoir.
6. Cover the opening of the overflow chamber of the pipet with index finger and seat the pipet securely in the reservoir neck (Fig. 28–12C).
7. Release pressure on the reservoir. Then remove finger from the pipet opening. At this time, negative pressure will draw blood into the reservoir.
8. Squeeze the reservoir gently two or three times to rinse the capillary bore, forcing diluent up into, but not out of, the overflow chamber, releasing pressure each time to return mixture to the reservoir.
9. Place index finger over the upper opening and gently invert several times to thoroughly mix blood with diluent (Fig. 28–12D).
10. Let mixture stand 10 minutes before charging the hemacytometer.
11. To charge the hemacytometer, convert to dropper assembly by withdrawing the pipet from the reservoir and reseating securely in reverse position (Fig. 28–13).
12. Invert the reservoir and discard the first 3 or 4 drops of mixture.
13. Clean the hemacytometer and its coverslip with an alcohol pad and let dry.
14. Carefully charge the hemacytometer with diluted blood by gently squeezing the sides of the reservoir to expel contents until the chamber is properly filled (Fig. 28–14).
15. Place the hemacytometer in a moist Petri dish for 10 minutes to allow red cells to settle. (Moistened filter paper retains evaporation of diluted specimen while standing.)
16. Mount the hemacytometer on the microscope and lower its condenser.
17. Procedure for counting RBCs:
    a. Cells are scanned under a 10× objective to ensure even distribution.
    b. Use a 40× objective (high-dry) to count the erythrocytes in the five squares labeled RBC of the center primary square (see Fig. 28–10). This

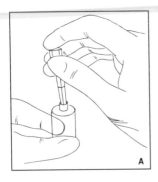
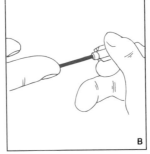
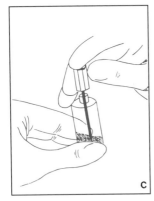
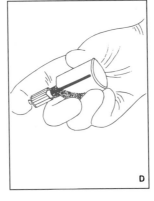

► **FIGURE 28–12** Schematic for using Unopette system. *A.* Using shield of capillary pipet, puncture diaphragm of reservoir. *B.* Fill capillary with sample from fingerstick or venous blood specimen. *C.* Transfer sample to reservoir by squeezing reservoir slightly to force out some air. Do not expel any liquid. Cover opening of overflow chamber with index finger. Maintain pressure until pipet is secured in reservoir neck. Squeeze reservoir several times to rinse capillary bore without expelling any liquid. *D.* Place index finger over upper opening and gently invert several times to thoroughly mix sample with diluent. (From Wedding, ME, and Toenjes, SA: Medical Laboratory Procedures. FA Davis, Philadelphia, 1998, p 235, with permission.)

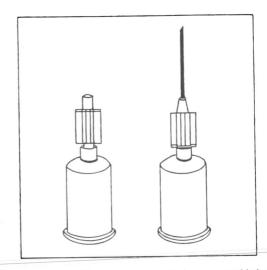

► **FIGURE 28–13** Unopette conversion to dropper assembly by withdrawing pipet from reservoir and securing it in reverse position. (From Wedding, ME, and Toenjes, SA: Medical Laboratory Procedures. FA Davis, Philadelphia, 1998, p 236, with permission.)

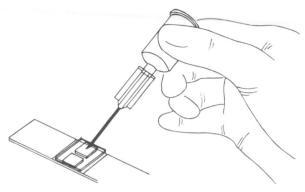

➤ FIGURE 28–14 Charging of hemacytometer by Unopette inversion of reservoir dropper assembly. The first 3 or 4 drops are discarded before hemacytometer is loaded. (From Wedding, ME, and Toenjes, SA: Medical Laboratory Procedures. FA Davis, Philadelphia, 1998, p 236, with permission.)

counting procedure is repeated on the opposite side of the hemacytometer.

c. To count the cells in the tertiary squares, use the following pattern:

(1) Count cells starting in the upper left corner square, continue to the right-hand square, drop down to the next row; continue counting from the right-hand square to the left square (see Fig. 28–10). Continue counting in this fashion until the total area in that secondary square has been counted.

(2) Count all cells that touch any of the upper and left lines; do not count any cell that touches a lower or right line (Fig. 28–15).

(3) The difference between the highest and lowest number of cells of the 10 squares should be no greater than 25.

Note: Diluted blood samples can be kept at room temperature for about 6 hours, although is it best to use the sample immediately.[4]

Calculations The basic formula for the calculation of the number of RBCs per cubic millimeter of diluted blood is as follows:

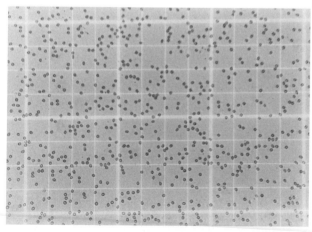

➤ FIGURE 28–15 Photography of erythrocytes loaded onto a Neubauer hemacytometer at $100\times$ magnification. These squares represent 6 of 25 secondary squares of the center primary square.

No. of cells/mm³

$$= \frac{\text{No. of cells} \times \text{Depth factor} \times \text{Diluting factor}}{\text{Area}}$$

$$= \frac{\text{No. of cells} \times 10 \times 200}{0.2 \times 0.2 \times 5}$$

Note: Depth factor equals depth of chamber, which is 0.1 mm. This must be multiplied by 10 to obtain 1 mm³. A factor of 10,000 may be employed for simplification, which is the result of:

$$\frac{\text{Depth factor} \times \text{Dilution factor}}{\text{Area}} \text{ or } \frac{10 \times 200}{0.2} = 10,000$$

Conversion to SI Units To convert this number to SI units (system of internationalized units) or 10^{12} RBCs/L, a factor of 10^6 is used, so that 5.0×10^6 RBCs/mm³ $\times 10^6 = 5.0 \times 10^{12}$/L. This factor of 10^6 represents a conversion in the total volume of the five squares counted, which is 1.00 µL converted to liters.

Interpretation

Normal Values

Newborn	4.4–5.8×10^{12}/L
Infant/child	3.8–5.5×10^{12}/L
Adult male	4.7–6.1×10^{12}/L
Adult female	4.2–5.4×10^{12}/L

Errors in RBC Enumeration

Erroneous results in RBC counting may be the result of an incorrect dilution, faulty equipment, technique, or nature of the sample.

The blood sample must be free of clots and thoroughly mixed. The technologist must pay close attention when filling the chamber, because overfilling would change the depth factor while raising the coverslip and underfilling would produce falsely decreased red cell counts.

White Blood Cell and Platelet Counts Using the Unopette System

Principle Free-flowing capillary or well-mixed anticoagulated venous blood is added to a diluent at a specific volume in the Unopette reservoir. The diluent lyses the erythrocytes but preserves leukocytes and platelets. The diluted blood is added to the hemacytometer chamber. Cells are allowed to settle for 10 minutes before leukocytes and platelets are counted. (Refer to manufacturer's instructions for the procedure.)

Equipment

Unopette reservoir no. 5854/5855 (1.98 mL of diluent)

Ammonium oxalate, 11.45 g

Sorensen's phosphate buffer, 1.0 g

Thimerosal, 0.1 g

Purified water, qs to 1000 mL

Unopette capillary pipet, 20-µL capacity

Hemacytometer and coverslip

Microscope

Lint-free wipe

Alcohol pads

Hand counter

Petri dish lined with moist filter paper

Specimen Free-flowing capillary or well-mixed anticoagulated venous blood is obtained. EDTA is the anticoagulant of choice.

Procedure

1. Puncture the diaphragm of the Unopette reservoir and add sample using a 20-μL capillary pipet as described earlier for the RBC count using the Unopette system.
2. Let the diluent-blood mixture stand 10 minutes to allow the RBCs to hemolyze. This mixture can stand for up to 3 hours.
3. Charge the hemacytometer as described for the RBC counts using the Unopette system.
4. Place the hemacytometer in a Petri dish lined with moist filter paper and let sit for 10 minutes to allow cells to settle.

Count and Calculations A *leukocyte count* is performed with a Neubauer hemacytometer as follows:

1. Under 100× magnification, leukocytes are counted in all nine large squares of counting chamber.
2. Total WBC/mm³ = No. of WBCs × 10 × 100/9, or one can more easily determine the total cell count by adding 10% of count to total number of cells counted, and then multiplying this figure by 100 to get total leukocyte count. This is a simplification of the general formula described in other sections, which involves multiplying the cells counted by 10 to correct the depth of chamber and dividing by the number of squares enumerated.[5]

Example: If an average of 60 cells is counted on both sides of chamber, add 10%, or 6, to 60 and multiply by 100 to get 6600 leukocytes/mm³ This number can then be multiplied by a factor of 10^6 to derive SI units of 6.6×10^9/L.

A *platelet count* is performed with a Neubauer hemacytometer as follows:

1. Under 400× magnification using bright-light or phase microscopy, platelets are counted in all 25 small squares within the large center square (see Fig. 28–10). Duplicate counts on a sample (e.g., both sides of a hemacytometer) should agree within 10% for counts to be valid.
2. Multiply the average number of platelets counted on both sides of chamber by 1000 to get total platelet count/mm³. Multiply this number by a factor of 10^6 to have the platelet count in SI units or 10^9/L. This step of multiplying by 1000 simplifies multiplication of dilution factor (100) and depth (10) which is equal to 1000.[6]

Example: An average of 230 platelets were enumerated on both sides of the hemacytometer using the Unopette system for platelet determinations.

$$\text{Platelets/mm}^3 = 230 \times 1000 = 230,000/\text{mm}^3 \times 10^6$$
$$= 230 \times 10^9/\text{L}$$

Comments

1. Diluent and blood should be properly mixed before filling the hemacytometer.
2. The hemacytometer must be properly filled to avoid erroneous results in manual cell counting.
3. If the chamber is overfilled, as indicated by the presence of excess fluid in the moat of the hemacytometer, clean the hemacytometer and recharge the chamber. As with all manual counts, the diluent sample must be thoroughly mixed before charging the hemacytometer, which must be properly filled.
4. A highly elevated leukocyte or platelet count may make accurate counting difficult. In either instance, a secondary dilution should be made. When calculating the total count, adjust the formula to allow for secondary dilution. There are physiologic variations to consider when performing WBC counts. Higher counts are seen following exercise, emotional stress, anxiety, and food intake. Blacks generally show slightly lower WBC counts than whites.
5. Platelets appear as dense, dark bodies and can be round, oval, or rodlike, sometimes showing dendritic processes (Fig. 28–16). Their internal granular structure and pearlescent sheen allow the platelets to be distinguished from debris, which is often refractile. RBCs appear as ghost cells. Use caution when RBCs have inclusions present, so as not to confuse the inclusion with platelets.
6. If platelet clumping is observed, redilute the count. If clumping is still present, obtain a fresh specimen. Because of the adhesive property of platelets, fingerstick specimens are least desirable.
7. The phase platelet determination should be compared with a review of the blood film for correction of count and morphology.
8. EDTA is the anticoagulant of choice when performing phase platelet counts. The student should be aware of "platelet satellitosis" when using this anticoagulant.[7] Platelet satellitosis appears as neutrophils ringed with adhesive platelets. Obtain correct platelet counts by collecting a fresh specimen with sodium citrate as the anticoagulant. When sodium citrate is used as an anticoagulant, make the correction for the dilution by multiplying by 1.1.
9. Ordinary light microscopy may be used; however, in this method differentiation and enumeration are more difficult.

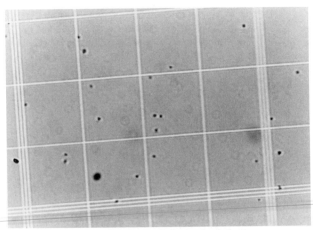

➤ **FIGURE 28–16** Photograph of platelets loaded onto a hemacytometer using a 40× objective (phase contrast). The platelets appear as dense, refractile, dark bodies that can be round, oval, or rod-shaped with a diameter of approximately 2 to 4 μm.

Interpretation

Normal Values (WBC)

Newborn	$9.0–30.0 \times 10^9$/L
1 week	$5.0–21.0 \times 10^9$/L
1 month	$5.0–19.5 \times 10^9$/L
6–12 months	$6.0–17.5 \times 10^9$/L
2 years	$6.2–17.0 \times 10^9$/L
Child/adult	$4.8–10.8 \times 10^9$/L

Normal Values (Platelets)
$130–400 \times 10^9$/L

Reticulocyte Counts

Reticulocytes are immature RBCs that contain remnant cytoplasmic ribonucleic acid (RNA) and organelles such as mitochondria and ribosomes. Reticulocytes are visualized by staining with vital dyes (such as new methylene blue) that precipitate the RNA and organelles, forming a filamentous network of reticulum. The reticulocyte count is a means of assessing the erythropoietic activity of the bone marrow. A number of new methods have been devised to improve the reproducibility and accuracy among medical technologists who perform such counts and are discussed next.

Reticulocyte Count Using the Miller Disc

Principle The Miller disc allows the medical technologist to isolate and enumerate reticulocytes in a large square, while counting mature red cells in a smaller square (Fig. 28–17).

Reagents New methylene blue: Dissolve 10.0 g of new methylene blue (NMB) and 8.9 g of NaCl (0.152 mol/L) in 1000 mL of distilled water. Filter through Whatman No. 1 filter paper before use. Store at room temperature.

Equipment

Miller ocular disc

Whole blood anticoagulated with EDTA

Microscope slides

10×75 mm test tubes

6-inch capillary tubes

Hand counter

Procedure

1. Add an equal number of drops of thoroughly mixed EDTA-anticoagulated blood and NMB mixture to a glass 10×75 mm tube.
2. Make a conventional wedge smear and let air-dry. Do not counterstain with Wright stain.
3. Use a $100\times$ objective and a $10\times$ ocular secured

with a Miller disc (see Fig. 28–17), and choose a section of the smear where the cells are close to each other but not touching or overlapping. Count a total of 20 fields.

4. In each field, count RBCs in the smaller square and reticulocytes in the larger square.

Calculations Calculate the percentage of reticulocytes per the following formula:

$$\% \text{ Reticulocytes} = \frac{\text{Total reticulocytes in larger square} \times 100}{\text{Total RBCs in smaller square} \times 9}$$

This calculation is usually based on a total of 1000 erythrocytes counted. (*Example:* 10 reticulocytes and 900 RBCs.)

$$\% \text{ Reticulocytes} = \frac{10}{900 \times 9} \times 100 = 0.12\%$$

Interpretation

Normal Values

Newborn (0–2 weeks)	2.5%–6.0%
Adult	0.5%–2.0%

The Absolute Reticulocyte Count The absolute reticulocyte count is calculated according to the following formula:

$$\text{Absolute reticulocyte count} = \frac{\% \text{ Reticulocyte count} \times (\text{RBC count}) (10^{12}/\text{L})}{100}$$

The absolute reticulocyte count expresses the number of reticulocytes in 1 mm^3 of whole blood: it is not a percentage of RBCs. The normal range is $24–84 \times 10^9$/L. Higher reticulocyte counts have been reported in normal persons living at an altitude greater than 60,000 feet above sea level, with significantly higher values in women than in men.[8] The reticulocyte count is most often expressed as a percentage of total red cells. In states of anemia, the reticulocyte percentage is not a true reflection of reticulocyte production. A correction factor must be used so as not to overestimate marrow production, because each reticulocyte is released into whole blood containing few RBCs—a low hematocrit (Hct)—thus relatively increasing the percentage. The corrected reticulocyte count may be calculated by the following formula:

$$\text{Corrected reticulocyte count} = \frac{\text{Reticulocyte \%} \times \text{Patient Hct \%}}{45 \text{ (average normal Hct)}}$$

For example, if a patient presenting with a reticulocyte count of 12% and a hematocrit of 24%, the corrected reticulocyte count would be 12% times (24/45), or 6.4%. In other words, the patient who presents with a reticulocyte count of 12% and a hematocrit of 24% would have the equivalent of a reticulocyte count of 6.4% in a patient with a hematocrit of 45%.

Estimating the RBC production by using the corrected reticulocyte count may yield erroneously high values in patients when there is a premature release of younger reticulocytes from the marrow (owing to increased erythropoietin stimulation). The premature reticulocytes are called "stress

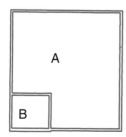

► **FIGURE 28–17** The visible field of the Miller ocular disc. In each field reticulocytes are counted in the larger square (*A*) and red blood cells are counted in the smaller square (*B*). The area of square B is one-ninth that of square A.

or shift" reticulocytes. These result when the reticulocytes of the bone marrow are shifted to the circulation pool to compensate for anemia. The younger stress reticulocytes present with more filamentous reticulum. The mature reticulocyte may present with granular dots representing reticulum. Normally, reticulocytes lose their reticulum within 24 to 27 hours after entering the peripheral circulation. The premature stress reticulocytes have increased reticulum and require 2 to 2.5 days to lose their reticulum, resulting in a longer peripheral blood maturation time (Table 28–2).

The peripheral smear should be carefully reviewed for the presence of many polychromatophilic macrocytes, thus indicating stress reticulocytes and the need for a correction for both the RBC count and the presence of stress reticulocytes. The value obtained is called the *reticulocyte production index (RPI)*. To calculate the RPI, the following formula is used:

$$RPI = \frac{\text{Reticulocyte count \% } \times \text{ Patient Hct/45 (normal Hct)}}{2 \text{ (Stress reticulocyte maturation time at 25\% Hct)}}$$

so that if a patient has a corrected reticulocyte count of 12% and a hematocrit of 25%, the RPI is 12/2, or 6. An RPI equal to or greater than 3 represents an adequate response to anemia by the bone marrow, whereas an RPI of less than 2 is considered an inadequate response of erythropoiesis by the bone marrow to a state of anemia (Fig. 28–18).

Comments The reticulocyte count is elevated (1) in patients with hemolytic anemia, (2) in those with hemorrhage (acute and chronic), (3) following treatment of iron-deficiency anemia and the megaloblastic anemias, and (4) in patients with uremia.

The reticulocyte count is decreased in cases of (1) aplastic anemia, (2) aplastic crises of hemolytic anemias, and (3) ineffective erythropoiesis as seen in thalassemia, pernicious anemia, and sideroblastic anemia.

Reticulocytopenia in the presence of a suggested hemolytic anemia may often make diagnosis difficult. The diagnosis of hemolytic anemia can be made because the combination of both hemolysis and reticulocytopenia results in a rapidly falling hemoglobin and hematocrit.

By convention, singly dotted reticulocytes are not counted. A reticulocyte must contain two or more discrete blue granules. The granular reticulum of the reticulocyte may be confused with Heinz bodies. Heinz bodies stain as light bluish-green granules present at the periphery of the red cell.

According to the pattern of reticulum and the degree of maturation, reticulocytes can be divided into four categories from the youngest to the most mature.

> ### ➤ Table 28–2
> ### THE MATURATION TIME FOR RETICULOCYTES

Maturation Time	Hematocrit (%)
1 day	45
1.5 days	35
2 days	25
3 days	15

Manual Reticulocyte Count without the Miller Disc

Procedure
1. Mix equal amounts of blood with NMB staining solution in a test tube.
2. Draw the blood-dye mixture up into a capillary tube. Allow the mixture to stand for 10 minutes at room temperature.
3. Prepare thin wedge smears of blood-dye mixture using 1 small drop. Let air-dry. Do not fix or counterstain slides with Wright's stain.
4. Under oil-immersion magnification, count all red cells in each field where the cells do not overlap, inclusive of reticulocytes.
5. Count 1000 red cells in consecutive oil immersion fields. Record the number of reticulocytes seen.

Calculations Calculate the percentage of reticulocytes as follows:

$$\% \text{ Reticulocytes} = \frac{\text{Reticulocyte count} \times 100}{1000 \text{ RBCs}}$$

Note: Counting 1000 red cells is sufficient for normal or increased reticulocyte counts. However, for decreased reticulocyte counts, 2000 or more red cells should be counted. A proper quality control sample should be run in parallel to verify accurate reporting; such samples are available through manufacturers and contain known reticulocyte values.

There is a high degree of inaccuracy in the manual reticulocyte count owing to error ($\pm2\%$ in low counts and $\pm7\%$ in high counts) and lack of reproducibility among technologists. However, these inaccuracies have been overcome with the application of reticulocyte enumeration by flow cytometry.

➤ AUTOMATED RETICULOCYTE COUNTS

Reticulocyte Count by Flow Cytometry

The reticulocyte count is one of the most important diagnostic indicators of erythropoietic activity. Its usage in the clinical laboratory is paramount to the diagnosis and monitoring of the hemolytic anemias, blood loss, and inherent erythropoietic response of the bone marrow. The measurement of reticulocytes by flow cytometry has alleviated many of the inaccuracies associated with manual methods, such as standard error with low and high counts, lack of reproducibility among medical technologists, and inconsistent use of the Miller disc. Figure 28–19 illustrates "gating" of RBCs in a flow cytometry analysis of reticulocyte enumeration. Refer to Chapter 30 for a detailed description of flow cytometry and its applications.

Reticulocyte Count Using Coulter Instrumentation

Principle Retic Prep[9] reagent contains two solutions that effectively precipitate basophilic RNA from red blood cells and remove hemoglobin from the erythrocyte, leaving the precipitate complex intact. The total RBC population is then measured using the VCS concept of volume, conductivity, and light scatter on Coulter reticulocyte instrumentation.

INITIAL SEPARATION OF ANEMIA
Reticulocyte Index

>3   <2

HEMOLYTIC
ANEMIA

TEST	HYPOPROLIFERATIVE	MATURATION ABNORMALITY
Smear-Indices		
Cell Size	Normal	Microcytic or Macrocytic
Fragmentation	Absent	Present
LDH	Normal	Increased
Bilirubin	Low-normal	Normal-elevated
Marrow		
M/E ratio	Normal-Low	High
Morphology	Normal	Megaloblastic / Defect in hemoglobinization

➤ **FIGURE 28–18** The initial separation of anemia. Anemia may be broadly classified on the basis of the reticulocyte index as hemolytic (index > 3) or impaired production, either a hypoproliferative or maturation abnormality (index < 2). Further tests are required to separate the latter two functional defects as shown. LDH = lactate dehydrogenase; M:E = myeloid-to-erythroid ratio.

Reagents and Equipment Coulter Retic Prep reagent kit:

Reagent A: NMB in buffered solution 0.06%

Reagent B: Sulfuric acid with stabilizers, stored at room temperature, 0.08%

Coulter instrumentation with reticulocyte capability

2-μL and 50-μL air displacement pipets

Pipet tips

12 × 75 mm disposable test tubes

STAT-MATIC Repetitive Dispenser, Model 5819 or equivalent timer

Note: Refer to specific instrument protocol for sampling procedures

Specimen Whole blood collected by venipuncture or fingerstick methodology is placed into EDTA collection tubes.

Procedure
1. Collect blood as described.
2. Prime the STAT-MATIC dispenser to fill outlet and inlet tubing of reagent B, making sure no bubbles are present in tubing.
3. Label two 12 × 75 test tubes. Mark one A and one B.
4. Dispense 4 drops of reagent A into the tube labeled A while positioning the bottle in a vertical direction (angled position will change prepared dilution).
5. Into the tube marked A, dispense 50 μL of thoroughly mixed whole blood or quality control specimen. Be careful not to let blood adhere to side of tube. Gently mix by inversion and allow it to

stand for 5 minutes at room temperature, but no longer than 60 minutes.
6. Transfer 2 μL of the blood-stain mixture from tube A into the bottom of tube B.
7. Position the tube marked B containing the blood-stain mixture at a 30-degree angle under the tip of the reagent B dispenser. Press down on the STAT-MATIC dispenser plunger, releasing 2 mL of reagent B into tube B. Do not mix; wait 30 seconds before aspirating the sample into the instrument.

Note: To ensure that no bubbles occur when dispensing reagent B, let it run down the side of tube at a rapid speed to ensure mixing with blood-stain solution.

Comments
1. Sample preparation should be carried out at room temperature.
2. Other dyes that utilize flow cytometry techniques for reticulocyte enumeration, such as thiazole orange, may produce falsely high counts when red blood cell inclusions are present in increased numbers.[10]

➤ RED BLOOD CELL INDICES

The values obtained for the erythrocyte count, hematocrit, and hemoglobin concentration can be further used to calculate RBC indices, which define the size and hemoglobin content of the average RBC in a given specimen of blood. The values for the RBC indices are useful tools in the classification of anemias.

The three most commonly used RBC indices are (1) mean corpuscular volume (MCV), (2) mean corpuscular hemoglobin (MCH), and (3) mean corpuscular hemoglobin concentration (MCHC) (Fig. 28–20).

Mean Corpuscular Volume

This is the average volume of the RBC, in cubic microns (μ^3) or femtoliters (fL). Normal erythrocytes have an MCV of 80 to 100 fL (replaces old units, μ^3). Results lower than 80 fL indicate a smaller-than-normal MCV; that is, the cells are on the average microcytic. Similarly, an MCV of greater than 100 fL indicates the cells are macrocytic.

It is imperative to interpret the value for MCV along with a careful inspection of the peripheral blood smear, because the MCV is only a mean volume measurement. It is possible, for example, to have a wide variation in cell size—from

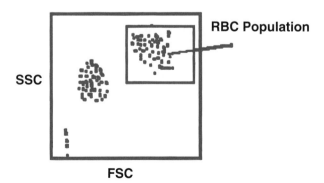

RBC Population

SSC

FSC

➤ **FIGURE 28–19** "Gating" of RBCs in a flow cytometry analysis of reticulocyte enumeration. Platelets, noise, and other debris are excluded from count. FSC = forward scatter; SSC = side scatter.

MMC HEMATOLOGY		☐ RETIC	
		☐ PLATELET	
☒ CBC ☐ HGB ☐ HCT ☐ WCB ☐ DIFF			

06 / 18 / 84   TEST NO.

	SA	OP CODES	
White blood cell count	11.6	WBC × 10³	7.8 ± 3
	3.09	RBC × 10⁶	M 5.4 ± 0.7 F 4.8 ± 0.6
Hemoglobin and hematocrit	9.5	HGB gm	M 16.0 ± 2 F 14.0 ± 2
	28.3	HCT %	M 47 ± 5 F 42 ± 5
Mean red cell indices	91.5	MCV μ³	M 87 ± 7 F 90 ± 9
	30.7	MCH μμg	29 ± 2
	33.5	MCHC %	35 ± 2
Red cell distribution width	11.7	RDW	M – F 10 ± 1.5
Platelet count and platelet volume	125.	PLT × 10³	M – F 140 – 440
	12.8	MPV μm³	M – F 8.9 ± 1.5

➤ **FIGURE 28–20**   The results of blood cell counts and indices. (From Hillman, RS, and Finch, CA: Red Cell Manual, ed 7. FA Davis, Philadelphia, 1996, p 43, with permission.)

cells that are microcytic to some that are macrocytic—and still have an MCV within the normal range. This may be true if there are a large number of reticulocytes in the peripheral blood because reticulocytes usually have a larger volume than do adult cells.

$$MCV = \frac{Hematocrit\ (\%) \times 10}{RBC\ count\ (millions/mm^3)}$$

or

$$MCV = \frac{Hematocrit\ (L/L) \times 10^{15}\ fL/L}{RBC\ count\ (\times 10^{12}/L)}$$

or

$$MCV = \frac{Hct\ (L/L) \times 10^3\ fL}{RBC\ count/L}$$

where 1 fL = 10^{15}/L. This value is reported in fL (μ^3) to the nearest whole number. Normal values for MCV are 80 to 94 fL for males and 81 to 100 fL for females.

Example: Hematocrit = 42% or 0.42 L/L, RBC = 5.7 × 10^{12}/L.

$$MCV = \frac{42\% \times 10}{5.7\ RBC/mm^3}$$

$$MCV = 74\ fL$$

Mean Corpuscular Hemoglobin

This is the average weight of hemoglobin, in absolute units, in the RBC. The result gives the average content of hemoglobin per erythrocyte in picograms (pg). The MCH value is usually higher in newborns and infants because their MCV is higher than that of adults.

$$MCH = \frac{Hemoglobin\ (g/100\ mL) \times 10}{RBC\ count\ (millions/mm^3)}$$

or

$$MCH = \frac{Hemoglobin\ (g/100\ mL) \times 10^{13}\ pg/L}{RBC\ count\ (10^{12}/L)}$$

or

$$MCH = \frac{Hemoglobin\ g/L\ pg}{RBC/L}$$

Note: Multiplying by 10^{13} is a conversion to picograms (Hgb g/100 mL × 10 × 10^{12}). 1 g = 10^{12} pg.

Example: Hemoglobin = 14.0 g/100 mL, RBC count = 5.2 × 10^{12}/L.

$$MCH = \frac{14.0\ (g/100\ mL) \times 10^{13}\ pg/L}{5.2 \times 10^{12}/L}$$

$$MCH = 27\ pg$$

Normal values for MCH = 27 to 31 pg.

Mean Corpuscular Hemoglobin Concentration

This is the average concentration of hemoglobin in each individual RBC. It is a ratio of the weight of hemoglobin to the volume of the RBC.

$$MCHC = \frac{Hemoglobin\ (g/100\ mL) \times 100}{Hematocrit\ (\%)}$$

or

$$MCHC = \frac{Hemoglobin\ (g/100\ mL)}{Hematocrit\ (L/L)}$$

Example: Hemoglobin = 15 g/100 mL. Hematocrit = 45%. The MCHC is calculated as:

$$MCHC = \frac{15\ g/100\ mL \times 100}{45\%}$$

$$MCHC = 33.3\%$$

This value is reported to the nearest 10th of a percent. Normal values for MCHC = 32.0% – 36.0%.

Comments   Determination of the MCV, MCH, and MCHC gives valuable information that helps to characterize RBCs. According to the MCV, erythrocytes may be classified as normocytic, microcytic, or macrocytic. Based on the

MCHC, erythrocytes may be classified as normochromic or hypochromic (Table 28–3). The MCH only expresses the mean weight of hemoglobin per erythrocyte.

RBC Distribution Width (RDW)

This is the coefficient of variation of the red cell volume distribution. It is provided by automated hematology instruments and is used as an indication of anisocytosis. An elevated RDW may be seen on blood smears with varying degrees of anisocytosis. This parameter is useful in distinguishing iron-deficiency anemia (increased) from the hemoglobinopathies (normal).[11]

$$RDW = \frac{\text{Standard deviation of RBC volume} \times 100}{\text{Mean MCV}}$$

Normal values for RDW = 11.5% to 14.5%.

Mean Platelet Volume (MPV)

The MPV represents the average size of platelets. It is determined from the arithmetic mean of the platelet histogram provided by the hematology analyzer. The normal values may range from 7.4 to 10.4 fL. The MPV may be increased in idiopathic thrombocytopenic purpura (ITP) and in hypoxic states of chronic obstructive pulmonary disease (COPD).[12]

➤ OTHER ROUTINE HEMATOLOGY METHODS

Erythrocyte Sedimentation Rate (ESR)

The ESR test measures the settling of erythrocytes in diluted human plasma over a specified time period.[13] This numeric value is determined (in millimeters) by measuring the distance from the bottom of the surface meniscus to the top of erythrocyte sedimentation in a vertical column containing diluted whole blood that has remained perpendicular to its base for 60 minutes. Various factors affect the ESR, such as RBC size and shape, plasma fibrinogen, and globulin levels, as well as mechanical and technical factors.

The ESR is directly proportional to the RBC mass and inversely proportional to plasma viscosity. In normal whole blood, RBCs do not form rouleaux; the RBC mass is small and, therefore, the ESR is decreased (cells settle out slowly). In abnormal conditions when RBCs can form rouleaux, the RBC mass is greater, thus increasing the ESR (cells settle out faster).

Historically, there have been two methods of performing the ESR: the Westergren method,[14] and the Wintrobe and Landsberg method.[15]

Westergren Determination

This method is preferred by National Committee for Clinical Laboratory Standards (NCCLS) because of its simplicity and greater distance of sedimentation measured in the longer Westergren tube. The straight tube is 30 cm long, 2.5 mm in internal diameter, and calibrated in millimeters from 0 to 200. Approximately, 1 mL of blood is required.[16] In addition, the tubes negate the process of pipetting whole blood directly into the tube with a glass Pasteur pipet; instead, a solution of sodium citrate or sodium chloride is mixed with 1 mL of blood. The Westergren tube is then plunged vertically into the blood mixture, and blood fills by capillary action to the top of the tube. A Westergren rack is also provided (Fig. 28–21).

Reagents and Equipment

Westergren tubes

Westergren rack

Disposable pipets

0.5 mL of sodium citrate or sodium chloride in puncture-ready vials

EDTA-anticoagulated whole blood

Procedure

1. Collect whole blood anticoagulated with EDTA.
2. Dilute whole blood with 0.5 mL of 3.8% sodium citrate or 0.85% sodium chloride.
3. Mix the blood-diluent solution by inversion.
4. Insert the Westergren tube into the plungeable vial cap of the diluent mixture. Let blood draw to the top of the tube by capillary action. Place the tube in the Westergren rack in a vertical position and leave undisturbed for 1 hour.

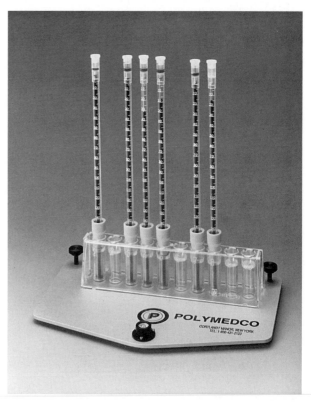

➤ **FIGURE 28–21** Westergren methodology for ESR. (Courtesy of Polymedco, Inc., Cortlandt Manor, NY.)

➤ Table 28–3
CLASSIFICATION OF ANEMIA

MCV (fL)	MCHC (%)	Classification
80–100	32–36	Normocytic, normochromic
< 80	< 32	Microcytic, hypochromic
> 100	32–36	Macrocytic, normochromic

5. After 1 hour has passed, record the distance in millimeters from the top of the column of red cells to the plasma–red cell interface. The buffy coat should not be included in this measurement.

Interpretation
Normal Values

Adult men	0–15 mm/h
Adult women	0–20 mm/h

Comments The ESR is not a very specific or diagnostic test. Despite the time constraints and the lack of specificity among disorders that can cause an abnormal ESR, however, the test is still used in many institutions as a screening test for inflammation.

Perhaps the usefulness of this test lies in its ability to differentiate among diseases with similar symptoms or to monitor the course of an existing disease. For example, early in the course of an uncomplicated viral infection, the ESR is usually normal, but it may rise later with a superimposed bacterial infection. Within the first 24 hours of acute appendicitis, the ESR is not elevated, but in the early stage of acute pelvic inflammatory disease or ruptured ectopic pregnancy, it is elevated. The ESR is elevated in established myocardial infarction but normal in angina pectoris. Table 28–4 lists disorders associated with an increased ESR.

Factors That Affect the ESR
Plasma Factors Increased plasma concentration of fibrinogen, along with immunoglobulin, will result in rouleaux formation and an increased ESR. It can, therefore, be expected that disease states that are characterized by hyperfibrinogenemia or elevated immunoglobulin levels will result in an increased ESR.

RBC Factors When rouleaux formation cannot occur, owing to the shape or size of the RBC, a decreased or low ESR is expected. This is observed with sickle cells, acanthocytes, and spherocytes. The ESR is of little diagnostic value in severe anemia or in hematologic states evidenced by poikilocytosis. Table 28–5 lists factors that influence the ESR.

Anticoagulants Sodium citrate or EDTA can be used without an effect on the ESR. Sodium or potassium oxalate can cause RBC shrinkage. Heparin causes only a slight amount of shrinkage, but a falsely elevated ESR. Our anticoagulant of choice is EDTA because of its routine use in the hematology laboratory.

Mechanical Factors Different normal values are given for various methods owing to variations in the caliber of the tube and the height of the column of blood. For example, in

> **Table 28-4**
> ## DISEASES ASSOCIATED WITH AN ELEVATED ESR

Rheumatoid arthritis	Malignant neoplasms
Multiple myeloma	Paraproteinemias
Cryoglobulinemia	Macroglobulinemia
Temporal arteritis	Hyperfibrinogenemia
Inflammatory diseases	Chronic infections
Pregnancy	Collagen disease
Anemia	Polymyalgia rheumatica

> **Table 28-5**
> ## FACTORS AFFECTING THE ESR

Increase	Decrease
Rouleaux formation	Microcytes
Fibrinogen (elevated)	Sickle cells
Immunoglobulin (excess)	Spherocytes

the Wintrobe ESR method, tubes range from 0 to 100 mm and have different normal values than that of the Westergren method.

Automated Mini-Ves ESR
The MINI-VES is an automated benchtop analyzer designed to measure the ESR in 20 minutes instead of 1 hour. The MINI-VES consists of a central processing unit, an optical reading assembly, a reading assembly motor, and a keyboard. The 20-minute reading correlates to the 1-hour Westergren ESR,[17] by means of an automated analyzer and specially designed collection tubes (VACU-TEC or VES-TEC) which standardize readings and are designed to fit any standard-sized collection tube holder. One milliliter of sample is drawn up into a solution of 0.109 mol/L sodium citrate. The tube is placed into one of the four positions of the MINI-VES at an 18-degree angle with respect to the vertical axis, which causes an acceleration of red cell sedimentation, rendering results comparable to Westergren. The instrument first records an initial ESR reading via its optical assembly. A second reading is performed 20 minutes later to yield ESR results that correlate with the Westergren method. The MINI-VES also has the capability of a 40-minute reading, which corresponds to a 2-hour Westergren ESR.

Hematocrit

Centrifugal Microhematocrit Method
Principle Hematocrit is defined as the volume occupied by erythrocytes (RBCs) in a given volume of blood and is usually expressed as a percentage of the volume of the whole blood sample.

The hematocrit is usually determined by spinning a blood-filled capillary tube in a centrifuge. The Coulter Counter series of analyzers provides an indirect measurement of hematocrit (see the earlier section on automated cell counting).

Reagents and Equipment
Capillary tubes, heparinized or plain (75 mm)

Microhematocrit centrifuge (Fig. 28–22)

Microhematocrit rotor (Fig. 28–23)

Microhematocrit reader (Fig. 28–24)

Procedure
1. Draw venous blood from an antecubital vein and into potassium EDTA. Take care to avoid tourniquet stasis, as this can elevate venous hematocrit results. Carefully mix the blood, preferably on a mechanical rotator. The blood specimen may also be obtained through capillary puncture using a heparinized capillary tube to collect the specimen.
2. Once adequately mixed, place the unmarked end of

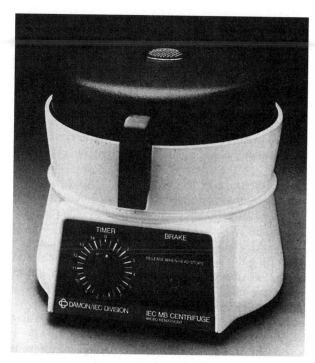

> ➤ FIGURE 28–22 Microhematocrit centrifuge. (Photo courtesy of International Equipment Co.) (From Wedding, ME, and Toenjes, SA: Medical Laboratory Procedures. FA Davis, Philadelphia, 1998, p 220, with permission.)

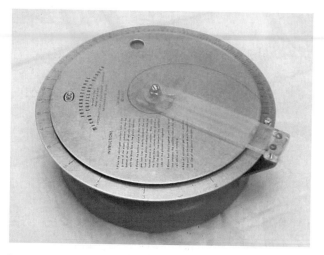

> ➤ FIGURE 28–24 Microhematocrit reader. (Photo courtesy of International Equipment Co.)

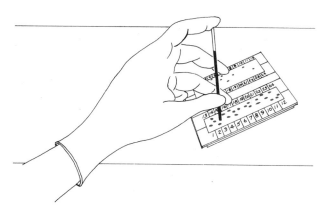

> ➤ FIGURE 28–25 Securing the capillary tube with sealing clay. (From Wedding, ME, and Toenjes, SA: Medical Laboratory Procedures. FA Davis, Philadelphia, 1998, p 220, with permission.)

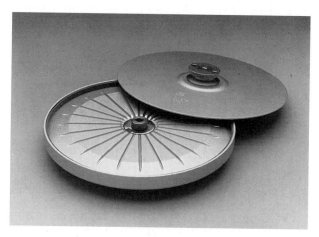

> ➤ FIGURE 28–23 Microhematocrit rotor. (Photo courtesy of International Equipment Co.)

a plain capillary tube in the blood and let it fill rapidly to approximately three-quarters of its length. Tipping the tube horizontally will speed filling. Then remove the tube from the blood and wipe it clean of excess blood.

3. Seal the capillary tubes by placing the dry end into the tray with sealing compound at a 90-degree angle (Fig. 28–25). Rotate the capillary tube slightly and remove it from the tray. The sealant plug should be from 4 to 6 mm long. Inspect the seal carefully for a perfectly flat bottom, perpendicular to the length axis.[18]

4. Secure the filled capillary tubes in the microhematocrit centrifuge with the sealed end toward the periphery. This should be done in duplicate at end-to-end positions. Make sure to record the numbers where tubes are seated in the centrifuge.

5. Centrifuge for 5 minutes at a set speed (force is approximately 14,500 rpm). This separates RBCs from plasma and leaves a band of buffy coat consisting of WBCs and platelets at the interface (Fig. 28–26).

6. Allow the centrifuge to stop on its own; *do not handbrake.*

7. Read the hematocrit as the percentage of whole venous blood occupied by RBCs. Using a constant-bore capillary tube, obtain a distance ratio on a microhematocrit reader. Set the reader first with the clay–red cell interface at 0%. Next, shift the ruled scale or etched line to 100% and align it with the plasma meniscus. Read down to the percent spiral line that intersects with the RBC-WBC interface. This percentage is the hematocrit value. Do not include the buffy coat layer in this value. If the buffy coat layer exceeds 2%, it should be recorded and noted as volume of packed WBCs.

8. Results should duplicate within 1%.

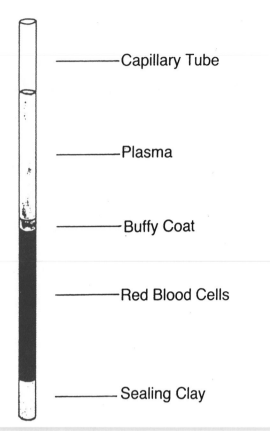

- Capillary Tube
- Plasma
- Buffy Coat
- Red Blood Cells
- Sealing Clay

➤ **FIGURE 28–26**   Diagram of a centrifuged microhematocrit tube of whole blood. (From Wedding, ME, and Toenjes, SA: Medical Laboratory Procedures. FA Davis, Philadelphia, 1998, p 220 with permission.)

Interpretation
Normal Values

	Percent	SI Units (L/L)
Newborn	53–65	0.53–0.65
Infant/child	30–43	0.30–0.43
Man	42–52	0.42–0.52
Woman	37–47	0.37–0.47

Comments
1. Incomplete sealing of the capillary tubes will give falsely low results because, in the process of spinning, RBCs and a small amount of plasma will be forced from the tube.
2. If the buffy coat is included in the RBCs when reading the result, the hematocrit will be falsely elevated.
3. The microhematocrit centrifuge should never be forced to stop by applying pressure to the metal coverplate. This will cause the RBC layer to "sling" forward, and will result in a falsely elevated value.
4. The hematocrit is usually three times the hemoglobin value.
5. The Standard International (SI) unit (L/L) of reporting expresses the hematocrit as the volume of packed RBCs in relation to volume of the whole blood.

➤ PREPARATION OF BLOOD SMEARS AND GROSS EXAMINATION

Peripheral Blood
The preparation and examination of a peripheral blood smear is one of the most frequently requested tests in the hematology laboratory. This procedure is requested not only for the diagnosis of hematologic disease but also to provide information for the diagnosis of nonhematologic diseases, for indicating side effects in chemotherapy, and for monitoring patient therapy. Reasons such as these make it essential that a blood smear be prepared correctly and examined in such a way as to provide the physician with an accurate interpretation.[17]

Two methods are routinely used to prepare blood smears:

1. Slide-to-slide or "push" smears
2. Automatic spinner[19]

Blood smears are prepared with EDTA-anticoagulated blood to minimize degenerative changes in the blood cells. The collection tube must contain the appropriate amount of blood so that it can mix with the anticoagulant. If there is an excess of anticoagulant, artifacts will occur. To ensure good preservation of cellular morphology, differential smears should be made as soon as possible and no later than 3 hours after collection.[20]

Slide-to-Slide Method

Principle A small drop of blood is placed near the frosted end of a clean glass slide. A second slide is used as a spreader. The blood is streaked in a thin film over the slide (Fig. 28–27). The slide is allowed to air-dry and is then stained.

Equipment

Glass slides, 3 × 1 inch (precleaned with frosted edge)

Capillary tubes, plain

Procedure
1. Fill a capillary tube three-quarters full with the anticoagulated specimen.
2. Place a drop of blood, about 2 mm in diameter, approximately 1/3 inch from the frosted area of the slide.
3. Place the slide on a flat surface, and hold the narrow side of the nonfrosted edge between your left thumb and forefinger.
4. With your right hand, place the smooth clean edge of a second (spreader) slide on the specimen slide, just in front of the blood drop.
5. Hold the spreader slide at a 30-degree angle, and draw it back against the drop of blood.
6. Allow the blood to spread almost to the edges of the slide.

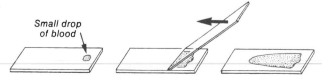

Small drop of blood

➤ **FIGURE 28–27**   Preparation of a peripheral blood smear, slide-to-slide technique.

7. Push the spreader slide forward with one light, smooth, and fluid motion. A thin film of blood in the shape of a bullet with a feathered edge will remain on the slide.
8. Allow the blood film to air-dry completely before staining.

Comments

1. A good blood film preparation will be thick at the drop end and thin at the opposite end.
2. The blood smear should occupy the central portion of the slide and should not touch the edges.
3. The thickness of the spread when pulling the smear is determined by the (1) angle of the spreader slide (the greater the angle, the thicker and shorter the smear),[16] (2) size of the blood drop, and (3) speed of spreading.
4. This is one of the easiest and most popular methods for producing a blood smear, but it does not produce quality smears. The WBCs are unevenly distributed and RBC distortion is seen at the edges. Smaller WBCs such as lymphocytes tend to reside in the middle of the feathered edge. Large cells such as monocytes, immature cells, and abnormal cells can be found in the outer limits of this area.

Automatic Spinner Technique

Principle Although there are several automatic slide spinners on the market, their basic principle remains the same. A small quantity of patient blood is placed in the middle of a 3 × 1 inch glass slide. The slide is held in a horizontal position by a platen. The motor of the spinner is activated and accelerates rapidly to a predetermined speed. When the slide has spun for its predetermined time, the motor quickly stops.

A slide with a monolayer of cells is produced, suitable for evaluation. An even distribution of cells over the entire slide makes this preparation ideal for performing differentials on samples with low WBC counts, as well as normal specimens. One disadvantage is that the slides must be extremely clean to prevent the shearing and spreading of cells as they are spun. The main disadvantage to this method is the hazard of blood aerosols from the spinner. Biohazard safety gear must be worn (goggles, gloves, lab coat).

Romanowsky Blood Stains

Principle A Romanowsky stain is any stain combination consisting of eosin Y or eosin B with methylene blue and/or any of its oxidation products. Such stains produce the typical purple coloration of leukocyte nuclei and neutrophilic granules as well as the numerous blues and pinks found in other cell types.[21] Methyl alcohol is used as both a solvent and fixative in this procedure.

Reagents and Equipment

Stain:

Powdered commercial Wright stain, 9 g

Powdered commercial Giemsa stain, 1 g

Glycerin, 90 mL

Absolute anhydrous methyl alcohol, 2910 mL

Note: Ingredients are mixed in a brown bottle 1 month before use. Mixture should be thoroughly shaken and filtered before staining smears.

15 M phosphate buffer, pH 6.4

Procedure

1. Align blood-smeared slides on the horizontal rack so that smears are facing upward.
2. Cover the entire smear for 1 minute with prepared stain.
3. Carefully add buffer in same quantity as stain and mix by maneuvering the slide. Do not let the stain mixture spill off slides.
4. Rinse the stain with neutral distilled water until the stained area appears pink.
5. Allow the slide to air-dry.

Comments

1. Insufficient washing, alkaline stain, or prolonged staining may lead to bluish-red cells and dark blue nuclei.
2. Inadequate staining, prolonged washing, or stain that is too acidic may lead to red cells that have stained too red and pale grayish-blue nuclei.
3. Precipitates present on slides may be caused by insufficient washing, allowing stain to dry on slides, or by using dirty slides.[21] Only precleaned slides should be used for staining blood smears.
4. Table 28–6 describes the characteristic staining patterns of Romanowsky-like stains on the cellular components of hematologic cells.

The Hema-Tek Automated Slide Stainer

Principle The Hema-Tek slide stainer (Fig. 28–28) is a fully automated bench-top instrument capable of housing up

► **Table 28–6**
ROMANOWSKY STAINING PATTERNS OF HEMATOLOGIC CELLS

Cellular Constituent	Color
Nuclei	Purple
Myeloblast cytoplasm	Blue
Promyelocyte cytoplasm	Blue
Myelocyte cytoplasm	Pink
Metamyelocyte cytoplasm	Pink
Neutrophil cytoplasm	Pink
Lymphocyte cytoplasm	Blue
Monocyte cytoplasm	Gray-blue
Erythroblast cytoplasm	Dark blue
Erythrocyte	Pink
Basophilic granules	Purple-black
Neutrophilic granules	Pink-purple
Platelet granules	Pink-purple
Azurophilic granules	Red or purple
Auer bodies	Purple
Döhle bodies	Blue
Howell-Jolly bodies	Purple
Cabot rings	Pink-purple

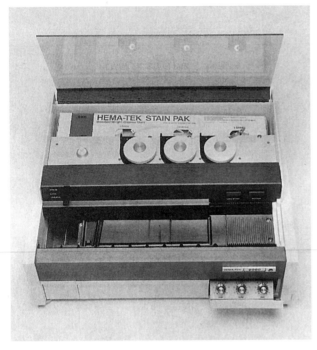

➤ **FIGURE 28–28** The Hema-Tek Slide Stainer and Stain-Pak. (Courtesy of the Bayer Corporation, Tarrytown, NY.)

to 25 slides. These slides are pulled along a metal platen and stained at a rate of one slide per minute. This instrument has delivered uniform reproducibility and is nearly maintenance-free. The stain is contained in a "stain-pak" that sits within the instrument connected by stylets and tubing and consists of Wright-Giemsa stain, buffer, and rinse. These stains are triggered to pump and deliver a certain amount of solution to the slide via capillary space on the instrument.

Once the slide has been stained and rinsed, it passes through a final panel on the metal platen to be air-dried. The slides then drop into a separate compartment where they can sit until the differential is performed. For further inquiries, the reader is referred to the Ames Hema-Tek operation manual.[22]

Examination of the Peripheral Blood Smear

There are several necessary steps in the examination of the peripheral blood smear, as described next.

Low-Power (10×) Scan

1. Determine the overall staining quality of the blood smear.
2. Determine if there is a good distribution of the cells on the smear.
   a. Scan the edges and center of the slide to be sure there are no clumps of RBCs, WBCs, or platelets.
   b. Scan the edges for abnormal cells.
3. Find an optimal area for the detailed examination and enumeration of cells.
   a. The RBCs should not quite touch each other.
   b. There should not be areas containing large amounts of broken cells or precipitated stain.
   c. The RBCs should have a graduated central pallor.

High-Power (40×) Scan

1. Determine the WBC estimate.
   a. The WBC estimate is performed under high

power (400× magnification) according to the values given in Table 28–7.
2. Correlate the WBC estimate with the WBC counts per mm³.
3. Evaluate the morphology of the WBCs and record any abnormalities, such as toxic granulation or Döhle bodies.

Oil Immersion (100×) Examination

1. Perform a 100 WBC differential count.
   a. All WBCs are to be included.
2. Evaluate RBC anisocytosis, poikilocytosis, hypochromasia, polychromasia, and inclusions.
3. Perform a platelet estimate and evaluate platelet morphology.
   a. Count the number of platelets in 10 oil immersion fields.
   b. Divide by 10.
   c. Multiply by 15,000/mm³ if the slide was prepared by an automatic slide spinner; multiply by 20,000/mm³ for all other blood smear preparations.
4. Correct any total WBC count per mm³ that has greater than 10 nucleated red blood cells (NRBCs) per 100 WBCs.
   a. When performing the WBC differential, do not include NRBCs in your count, but report them as the number of NRBCs per 100 WBCs.
   b. Use the following formula to correct a WBC count:

$$\text{Corrected WBCs/mm}^3 = \frac{\text{WBC/mm}^3 \times 100}{100 + \text{No. of NRBCs/100 WBCs}}$$

The examination of the peripheral blood smear is performed as part of the hematologic laboratory workup called the complete blood count (Fig. 28–29).

Buffy Coat Preparation for Decreased WBC Counts

Principle The WBC:RBC ratio contained with an EDTA tube is increased by centrifugation and removal of the top layer of cells. Albumin and normal saline are added to the tube to prevent cell overcrowding. Aliquots of the cell suspension are cytocentrifuged onto slides and stained with Wright-Giemsa stain for WBC classification.[23]

Specimen EDTA-anticoagulated venous blood is the specimen of choice.

➤ **Table 28–7**
ESTIMATION OF TOTAL WBC COUNT FROM THE PERIPHERAL BLOOD SMEAR

No./High Power Field	Estimated Total WBC Count/mm³
2–4	4000–7000
4–6	7000–10,000
6–10	10,000–13,000
10–20	13,000–18,000

➤ **FIGURE 28–29** Hematology laboratory report sample form illustrating the complete blood count (CBC).

Procedure

1. Centrifuge the blood sample for 5 minutes at 2000 rpm.
2. Transfer the top layer of cells (approximately 0.5 mL) to a Wintrobe hematocrit tube. This layer will contain red cells.
3. Centrifuge the Wintrobe tube for 5 minutes at 2000 rpm.
4. Carefully remove the plasma without disturbing the cells.
5. Transfer the top layer of cells (approximately 0.03 mL) to a 20-mL plastic vial.
6. Prepare a 1% to 2% RBC suspension with normal saline in the plastic vial.
7. Add 3 drops of 22% bovine albumin to a 10-mL RBC suspension.
8. Add 6 drops of the suspension to the cytocentrifuge holders.
9. Centrifuge the specimen for 5 minutes at 1400 rpm.
10. Allow the slides to air-dry before staining with Wright-Giemsa stain.

Comments

1. This method of buffy coat preparation alleviates the tedious counting of a low number of WBCs on the peripheral blood smear and misrepresentation of a 100 white cell differential.
2. The amount of albumin added may vary depending on the presence of artifacts on the blood smear. If there is an excess of albumin, the cells will appear too dark.

➤ TESTS FOR HEMOGLOBINS

Hemoglobinometry

Principle Hemoglobin, the main component of the RBC, transports oxygen to and CO_2 from the body's tissues. Hemoglobin in circulating blood is a mixture of hemoglobin, oxyhemoglobin, carboxyhemoglobin, and minor amounts of other forms of this pigment. It is necessary to prepare a stable derivative involving all forms of hemoglobin in the blood in order to measure this compound accurately. The cyanmethemoglobin (HiCN) derivative can be conveniently and reproducibly prepared and is widely used for hemoglobin determination. All forms of circulating hemoglobin are readily converted to HiCN except for sulfhemoglobin, which is rarely present in significant amounts. Cyanmethemoglobin can be measured accurately by its absorbance in a colorimeter.

The basic principle of the cyanmethemoglobin (HiCN, hemoglobin-cyanide method) is that blood diluted in a solution of potassium ferricyanide yields oxidation to the ferric state (Fe^{3+}) to form methemoglobin (Hi-hemoglobin). This solution reacts with potassium cyanide to form stable cyanmethemoglobin, which is read on a spectrophotometer at 540 nm.

Procedure Automated hematology analyzers routinely perform hemoglobin determinations. The reader is referred to manufacturer instructions for specific methodology.

Interpretation

Normal Values (g/100 mL)

Man	14–18
Woman	12–16
Newborn	17–23
3-month-old	9–14
10-year-old	12–14.5

Hemoglobin Electrophoresis

Principle Electrophoresis is defined as the movement of charged particles in an electric field. The different normal and abnormal hemoglobins show different mobilities of migration patterns in an electric field at a fixed pH. The usual support medium is cellulose acetate at an alkaline pH of 8.5. The procedure that follows is from Helena Laboratories, and all reagents and apparatus are available through their organization.[24]

Reagents

Hemolysate reagent

Controls A_1FSC; normal A_1A_2 patient

Buffer: Supre-Heme buffer (one envelope is dissolved in distilled water and diluted to 980 mL tris-EDTA-boric acid buffer, pH 8.4)

Ponceau S stain

Destain: 5 mL of glacial acetic acid per 100 mL distilled water, a 5% solution

MGH FORM NO. 7-406 R 8/82

Dehydrating agent: Absolute methanol

Clearing solution: 150 mL of glacial acetic acid, 350 mL of absolute methanol, and 20 mL of Clear aid

Titan III-H cellulose acetate plates

Equipment

Cliniscan

Helena Titan power supply

Incubator-oven-dryer

Electrophoresis chamber

Super Z sample well plate

Super Z aligning base

Applicator

Zip-zone chamber wicks

Procedure

1. Preparation of hemolysate: Spin EDTA blood for 20 minutes at 3000 rpm to pack the RBCs. Remove the plasma and buffy coat. Add 6 drops of hemolysate reagent to 1 drop of packed RBCs. Let stand for 1 minute; then vortex for 1 minute. Hemolysate may be frozen and then thawed to ensure complete hemolysis.

2. Preparation of electrophoretic chamber: Pour 100 mL of buffer into each outer compartment. Soak a wick in each compartment, and then drape it over the bridge, making sure it contacts the buffer. Cover the chamber.

3. Preparation of cellulose acetate plates: Number the plates on the bottom right of the glossy side. Wet the plates by slowly lowering the rack into a container of buffer. Allow them to soak for at least 5 minutes.

4. Preparation of sample well plates: Clean with distilled water and dry each well with a cotton swab. Prepare two rinse plates by filling the wells with distilled water. Prepare the patient samples by using a 5-lambda (λ) microdispenser to fill the wells on clean dry plates. Patient samples should be run in duplicate, and a normal A_1A_2 and A_1FSC control should be run on each plate. Cover with glass slide to prevent evaporation.

5. Loading the cellulose acetate plates:
   a. Prime the applicator by depressing several times into the same well plate and then depressing once on a blotter.
   b. Remove the cellulose acetate plate from the buffer; blot once firmly and place on the aligning base with the number at the bottom left.
   c. Load the applicator by depressing three times into the sample well plate; then transfer the applicator to the aligning base, and depress the bar firmly for 5 seconds.
   d. Place the plate, glossy side up, across the bridge in the electrophoresis chamber.

6. Electrophoresis at 350 volts for 25 minutes.

7. Staining:
   a. Apply Ponceau S for 5 minutes. Drain for 5 to 10 seconds.
   b. Four successive washes of 5% glacial acetic acid are used to destain. Leave in each for 2 minutes, draining for 5 seconds between each wash.
   c. Use two successive washes of absolute methanol to dehydrate. Leave for 2 minutes in each, draining for 5 seconds between each wash.
   d. Apply clearing solution for 5 minutes.
   e. Dry vertically for 1 to 2 minutes.
   f. Dry in the oven for 3 to 4 minutes, acetate side up.

8. Scan the plate with the Cliniscan using a 525-nm filter, slit size 5, and optics filter wheel V-2 O.D.

9. Label the plate and store in a plastic envelope as a permanent record.

Results Variant hemoglobins are reported in relative percentages.

Hemoglobin A_1 (HbA$_1$)	95%–97%
Hemoglobin A_2 (HbA$_2$)	2%–3%
Hemoglobin F (HbF)	
Birth	60.0%–90.0%
After 1 year	1.0%–2.0%

Comments At an alkaline pH, hemoglobins S and D have the same mobility, as do hemoglobins A_2, C, E, and O_{Arab}. These hemoglobins may be separated by electrophoresing on citrate agar at an acid pH (Fig. 28–30). Hemoglobin A_2 may also be quantitated by column. HbF separates from HbA in this system and migrates slightly closer to the origin. However, cellulose acetate electrophoresis is not recommended as an initial screening test during the neonatal period because large amounts of HbF form a heavy band overlapping the adjacent bands of HbA or HbS.[25] The procedure for separation and quantitation of HbF is based on acid or alkali resistance, or both (see Acid Elution Test for HbF).

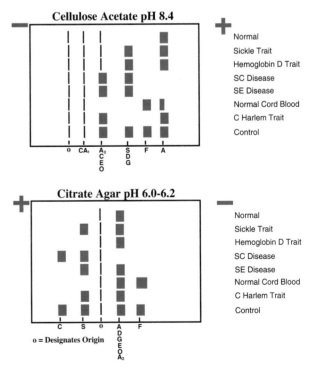

➤ FIGURE 28–30 Comparative hemoglobin electrophoresis. Hemoglobin electrophoresis on cellulose acetate and citrate agar, indicating patterns of mobility. The width of the band is not indicative of hemoglobin concentration.

Citrate Agar Hemoglobin Electrophoresis

Principle As mentioned earlier, electrophoresis is the movement of charged particles in an electric field. Using citrate agar at an acid pH facilitates the separation of hemoglobins that migrate together on other media (cellulose acetate) at a different pH (alkaline). The following procedure is that of Helena Laboratories, and all reagents and apparatus are available from their organization.

Reagents

Hemolysate reagent

Controls A_1FSC; normal A_1A_2

Buffer: Citrate buffer. Dissolve one package in distilled water and dilute to 1 L.

Stain:

10 mL of 5% glacial acetic acid

5 mL of toluidine in methanol

1 mL of sodium nitroferricyanide in water

1 mL of 3% hydrogen peroxide

Note: Prepare fresh on day of use

Titan IV citrate agar plates

Equipment

Helena Titan power supply

Electrophoresis chamber

Sample well plate

Aligning base

Applicator

Sponge wicks

Procedure

1. Preparation of hemolysate: Spin EDTA blood for 20 minutes at 3000 rpm to pack the red cells. Remove the plasma and buffy coat. Add 10 drops of hemolysate reagent to 1 drop of packed RBCs. Let stand for 1 minute, then vortex for 1 minute. Hemolysate may be frozen and then thawed to ensure complete hemolysis.
2. Preparation of electrophoresis chamber: Pour 100 mL of buffer into each outer compartment. Soak a sponge wick in each compartment, then place it so that the top of the sponge protrudes over the inner ridge of the compartment. Cover the chamber.
3. Preparation of sample well plates: Clean all wells with distilled water and dry with cotton swabs. Prepare the patient samples by using a 5-λ microdispenser to fill the wells. Patient hemolysates should be run in duplicate, plus an A_1FSC and an A_1A_2 control should be run on each plate. Cover the plate with a glass slide to prevent evaporation.
4. Loading of citrate agar plates:
   a. Prime the applicator by pressing several times into the sample well plate, and then dispensing once on a blotter.
   b. Place the Titan IV citrate agar plate on the aligning base.
   c. Load the applicator by pressing three times into the sample well plate; then transfer the applicator to the aligning base.
   d. Depress the applicator onto the gel surface using

no pressure, and allow hemolysate to absorb for 1 minute.
6. Place the plate gel side down across the inner ridges of the electrophoresis chamber with the application point near the anode.
7. Electrophorese for 40 minutes, at 40 mA per plate and 50 V per plate.
8. Staining:
   a. Place the plate in a staining dish and puddle the stain over the surface. Let stand for 5 to 10 minutes.
   b. Rinse with distilled water for 10 minutes.
   c. Cover with another gel plate and seal with tape to store.

Results With this procedure, hemoglobin S and D can be separated. Hemoglobin D, instead of migrating with HbS as in an alkaline buffer, will migrate with HbA. This procedure also separates hemoglobins A_2 and E from HbC, as hemoglobins A_2 and E will migrate with HbA, leaving HbC by itself. The pattern from cathode to anode is hemoglobin C–hemoglobin S–hemoglobin A_1–hemoglobin A_2–hemoglobin D–hemoglobin E–hemoglobin F (see Fig. 28–30).

Hemoglobin A_2 by Column Chromatography

Principle This is an anion-exchange chromatography method. The anion exchange resin is a preparation of cellulose covalently coupled to small, positively charged molecules, which will attract negatively charged molecules. Hemoglobins have positive or negative charges, owing to properties of their component amino acids. Here buffer and pH favor net negatively charged hemoglobins, which are attracted and bound to the resin. Once bound, the hemoglobins can be selectively eluted and measured on a spectrophotometer. This procedure (the Sickle-Thal column method) is that of Helena Laboratories.

Reagents

Control: Quik column control

Sickle-Thal Quik Column

Hemoglobin A_2 developer

Hemoglobin S developer

Hemolysate reagent C

Note: All are available from various manufacturers.

Equipment

Column rack and collection tubes

Spectrophotometer

Procedure

1. Preparation of hemolysate: Add 50-μL EDTA blood plus 200-μL hemolysate reagent C to a small test tube. Vortex vigorously and allow to stand 5 minutes before use.
2. Preparation of columns:
   a. Allow to come to room temperature.
   b. Turn each column upside down twice, place it in the rack, remove top cap, and resuspend with a pipet.
   c. Remove the bottom cap and allow the buffer to drain out.
   d. After the resin repacks, remove any buffer

remaining at the top, being careful not to disturb the resin.

3. Slowly apply 100 μL of patient hemolysate to the column and allow it to absorb into the resin.

4. Put 100 μL of patient hemolysate in a large collection tube and quantity sufficient (Q.S.) to 15 mL with distilled water. Label this tube "total fraction."

5. Elution of HbA_2:
   a. Slowly apply 3 mL of HbA_2 developer and allow it to pass through the column into the small collection tube (approximately 30 minutes).
   b. Q.S. the tube to 3 mL with distilled water.

6. Elution of HbS (optional):
   a. Slowly add 10 mL of HbS developer to the column in aliquots of 3 mL, 3 mL, and 4 mL.
   b. Allow it to pass through the column into a large collection tube (approximately 1.5 to 2 hours).
   c. Q.S. the tube to 15 mL with distilled water.

7. Using the spectrophotometer at 415 nm, record the absorbance of the HbA_2 eluate, the HbS eluate, and the total fraction.

Results

$$\% \ HbA_2 = \frac{OD \ HbA_2 \ eluate \times 100}{5 \times OD \ total \ fraction}$$

$$\% \ HbA_2 = \frac{OD \ HbS \ eluate \times 100}{OD \ total \ fraction}$$

where OD = optical density.

The HbS eluate is optional, as it can be picked up on alkaline electrophoresis. The normal range for HbA_2 is 1.5% to 4.0%. This can be used to separate HbA_2 and HbC or HbE. Elevated levels of HbA_2 may be useful in diagnosing beta (β)-thalassemia. Be careful not to underload or overload the column with the hemolysate. Overloading the column may cause incomplete separation of the HbA_2. Underloading the column may make visual collection of the HbA_2 fraction impossible.[26]

Solubility Test for Hemoglobin S

Principle Sickling hemoglobin, which is defined as any hemoglobin that causes erythrocytes to sickle under conditions of low oxygen tension, in a deoxygenated state will form a precipitate when exposed to a high-molarity phosphate buffer solution.[27] This precipitation is the result of tactoids forming from deoxygenated hemoglobin molecules, producing a turbid solution. This turbidity is qualitatively determined from the inability to visualize black type lines on a white background. This procedure utilizes packed RBCs.

Reagents and Equipment

12 × 75 mm disposable glass or plastic test tubes

Reading card with 14-point or 18-point black type in straight lines on a white background approximately 0.5 cm apart (see Fig. 11–11)

Centrifuge (1500–2000 g)

Stock solution:

Dibasic potassium phosphate, anhydrous (1.24 mol), K_2HPO_4, 216 g

Monobasic potassium phosphate, crystals (1.24 mol), KH_2PO_4, 169 g

Saponin, 10 g

Distilled water, qs to 1 L

Note: Reagent should be stored at 4°C for approximately 1 month and should be checked against a known positive and negative control. There are many commercial kits available that mimic this procedure (i.e., Sickle-quik, General Diagnostics), and each new reagent should be checked with known positive and negative controls.

Working Solution Sodium hydrosulfite (dithionite) $Na_2S_2O_4$ (5 mg/mL of stock reagent) is added on the day of testing.

Procedure

1. Pipet 2 mL of working solution into a labeled 12 × 75 mm test tube.
2. Allow the working solution to warm to room temperature.
3. Centrifuge whole blood (EDTA) at 1500 to 2000 g for 5 minutes to remove buffy coat and plasma.
4. Add 10 μL of packed erythrocytes.
5. Mix and wait 5 minutes.
6. Hold the tube approximately 2.5 cm in front of the white card with black lines.
7. Read for qualitative determination of turbidity.

Results A negative result (indicating no sickling hemoglobins) occurs when the black lines are visible through the test solution.

A positive result (indicating the presence of a sickling hemoglobin) is indicated by a very turbid solution in which the black lines cannot be seen through the test solution (see Fig. 11–11). Other sickling hemoglobins may be present; therefore, this test is not specific for hemoglobin S. Table 28–8 depicts hemoglobins that can be present from negative and positive results of this test. Both positive and negative controls must be run for each solubility test performed.

Comments

1. Erroneous results may be seen in normal blood transfused to an anemic patient whose native blood contains sickling hemoglobin, or in transfused blood that contains a sickling hemoglobin.
2. Cold reagent may cause inaccurate results; the same holds true when whole blood is used instead of packed cells, the latter because of excess gamma globulins, extreme leukocytosis, or hyperlipidemia.[25]

▶ **Table 28–8**
HEMOGLOBINS PRESENT POSITIVE/NEGATIVE SOLUBILITY TESTS

Positive	Negative
HbC_{Harlem}	HbA
HbS	HbF
HbS_{Travis}	HbC
$HbC_{Ziguinchor}$	HbD
	HbG
	HbE
	Hb Lepore
	HbA_2

Acid Elution Test for Hemoglobin F

Principle The passage of erythrocytes from an Rh-positive fetus into the circulation of an Rh-negative mother results in the formation of specific Rh antibodies. In subsequent pregnancies, the Rh antibodies formed in the blood serum of the Rh-negative mother are readily transmissible through the placenta into the circulation of the fetus. The action of the antibodies on the Rh-positive cells of the fetus may result in a disease entity recognized as isohemolytic disease, or erythroblastosis.[28] The acid elution procedure will detect fetal red blood cells in maternal circulation based on the properties of adult hemoglobin and fetal hemoglobin. Adult hemoglobin (HbA) will dissolve out of solution, whereas fetal hemoglobin (HbF) will be resistant to the acid medium and stain pink. This procedure is performed on Rh-negative mothers who have been sensitized to the Rh factor as a consequence of giving birth to an Rh-positive fetus. Mothers are administered specific gamma globulin containing anti-Rh_o(D) to suppress the immune response. The amount of Rh immune globulin (RhIg) administered is calculated by assessing the magnitude of fetal/maternal hemorrhage.

Reagents

Red Cell Fixing Solution, Product No. 101–10 (Sure-Tech Diagnostics Inc.): Ethanol 80% v/v denatured

Citrate/Phosphate buffer, Product No. 101–20 (Sure-Tech Diagnostics): 0.2 mol/L

Hemoglobin Staining Solution, Product No. 101–30 (Sure-Tech Diagnostics, Inc): Erythrosin, 0.1%

Note: Reagents are stored at room temperature and are stable for the period indicated on the label. Do not pour used reagents back into original containers.

Specimen Maternal blood collected with EDTA or oxalate should be used. Samples should be stored at 2°C to 8°C until assayed. Blood-EDTA mixtures have been reported to be satisfactory for use up to 2 weeks when stored under refrigeration It is recommended that specimens be tested as soon as possible.

Quality Control A high-positive control may be prepared by adding 0.1 mL of cord blood to 0.9 mL adult blood. A low-positive control may be prepared by adding 0.05 mL of the same cord blood to 0.95 mL of the same adult blood. These spiked controls are then diluted with saline and assayed in the same manner as the patient sample. Normal adult blood may serve as the negative control.

Procedure

1. Mix the blood sample by gentle inversion.
2. Place 3 drops of 0.85% saline and 2 drops of blood into a glass test tube, and mix gently.
3. Place 1 drop of diluted blood on a glass slide near one end. Prepare a smear by drawing the edge of another slide through the drop and across the slide.
4. Air-dry the slide at room temperature.
5. Place the slide in a Coplin jar containing sufficient Red Cell Fixing Solution to cover the smear. Raise and lower the slide 2 or 3 times for even distribution of the fixing solution, and allow the slide to remain in the solution at room temperature for 5 minutes.
6. Remove the slide from the fixing solution, rinse thoroughly with deionized water, and air-dry.
7. Place the dry slide in a Coplin jar containing sufficient Citrate/Phosphate buffer to cover the smear. Raise and lower the slide 2 or 3 times for even distribution of the buffer and allow the slide to remain in solution at room temperature for 10 minutes.
8. Remove the slide from the buffer solution, rinse briefly with deionized water, and blot excess water from the edges.
9. Place the wet slide in a Coplin jar containing sufficient Hemoglobin Staining Solution to cover the smear. Raise and lower the slide 2 or 3 times for even distribution of the stain and allow the slide to remain in the stain at room temperature for 3 minutes.
10. Remove the slide from the Hemoglobin Staining Solution, rinse thoroughly with deionized water, and allow it to dry at room temperature.
11. Slides must be examined by using oil immersion. Fetal cells will stain a dark reddish-pink whereas adult cells will appear white to light pink with a slightly darker center (Fig. 28–31).

Calculations Results may be expressed as either % fetal cells or fetal/adult RBC ratio.

% Fetal Cells The percentage of erythrocytes containing fetal hemoglobin may be determined in several ways. The American Association of Blood Banks (AABB) recommends the following be used[29]:

1. Count the total number of adult red and fetal erythrocytes in as many fields as required to give a total count of at least 2000 cells.
2. Calculate % fetal cells in the total counted.

Example:

Total RBCs counted = 2150

Total fetal RBCs counted = 10

% Fetal cells = $10/2150 \times 100 = 0.46$

Fetal/Adult RBC Ratio

1. Count the total number of adult and fetal erythrocytes in as many fields as required to give a total count of at least 2000 cells.
2. Divide the total number of fetal cells by the total number of adult cells to obtain a ratio.

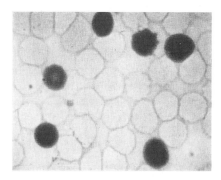

➤ **FIGURE 28–31** Kleihauer-Betke stain of blood from a newborn. Red-staining cells contain hemoglobin F; clear-staining cells contain hemoglobin A. (From Diggs, LW: Hematology. In Listen, Look and Learn. Health and Education Resources, Inc., Bethesda, MD, with permission.)

Example:

Total adult RBCs counted = 2150

Total fetal RBCs counted = 10

Fetal/adult RBC ratio = 20/2150 = 0.0046

RhIg Dosage The number of vials of RhIg necessary to protect against Rh immunization is based on the volume of fetomaternal hemorrhage and may be calculated using % fetal cells or fetal/adult RBC ratio.

Fetal Cells

Volume of fetomaternal hemorrhage (FMH) = % fetal cells × 50

Doses of RhIg required = FMH/30

Example:

If % fetal cells = 0.80; FMH = 0.80 × 50 = 40 mL

Doses of RhIg required = 40/30 = 1.3 doses (give 2 doses)

Note: when the number to the right of the decimal point is less than 5, round down and add one dose of RhIg. When the number to the right of the decimal point is 5 or greater, round up to the next number and add one dose of RhIg; for example, 2.9 doses (calculated) requires 4 doses.

Fetal/Adult RBC Ratio

Fetal/Adult RBC Ratio	Volume of FMH	No. of Vials
0.0–0.0045	up to 15 mL	1
0.0046–0.0090	15–30 mL	2
0.0091–0.0135	30–45 mL	3
0.0136–0.0180	45–60 mL	4
0.0181–0.0225	60–75 mL	5

Note: For each ratio interval of .0045, one additional vial of RhIg is indicated. If the dose calculation results in a fraction, administer the next number of whole vials of RhIg.

Staining for Heinz Bodies

Principle Heinz bodies are denatured hemoglobin precipitated in the RBC and attached to the RBC membrane. They are not visible with Wright's stain but show up with supravital staining (crystal violet) and phase microscopy (see Color Plate 83).

Reagents and Equipment

Crystal violet solution: 1.0 g of crystal violet dissolved in 50 mL of a 0.85% saline solution, which is shaken for 5 minutes and filtered before storage

Methyl violet solution: 0.5 g of methyl violet dissolved in 100 mL of a 0.85% saline solution, which is shaken for 5 minutes and filtered before storage

Glass slides and coverslip

Microscope

Procedure

1. Mix equal volumes of EDTA blood and stain in a small test tube. Either stain may be used.
2. Incubate for 20 minutes at room temperature.
3. Remix the blood-stain solution and transfer 1 drop to a slide.
4. Place a coverslip on the slide and examine for Heinz bodies under oil immersion.

Results Heinz bodies appear as irregular, refractile, purple inclusions, 1 to 3 μm in diameter, located on the periphery of the cell. They may even seem to be outside the cell. Reticulocytes are not stained by this technique.[30]

➤ TESTS FOR HEMOLYTIC ANEMIAS

Osmotic Fragility

Principle Whole blood is added to a series of saline dilutions. Exposure to hypotonic solution causes water to be drawn into the erythrocyte through osmosis. This eventually leads to swelling of the erythrocyte, leaking, and bursting of the cell. Once the cell bursts, hemoglobin is released and can be measured with a spectrophotometer. The presence or absence of hemolysis is an effective measure of erythrocyte susceptibility to hypotonic damage. This test is more than just an index of cell shape; it is also a measure of the surface-to-volume ratio. When an RBC's membrane surface decreases and its volume remains the same or increases, the cell becomes more turgid and less deformable. This is because the RBC membrane is flexible but not elastic. The result of this loss of surface-to-volume ratio is similar to what happens to a small plastic bag that is filled with more and more water.

Spherocytes, which have a decreased surface-to-volume ratio, demonstrate an increased osmotic fragility. This is because of their inability to swell in a hypotonic medium before leaking hemoglobin. Sickle cells, target cells, and other poikilocytes are relatively resistant to osmotic change and therefore demonstrate a decreased osmotic fragility.

Reagents and Equipment

Twenty-four 12 × 75 mm test tubes

Two 5-mL serologic pipets (TD), one 3-mL pipet

Parafilm squares

One heparinized normal control sample

One heparinized patient sample

Linear graph paper

1% NaCl solution:

  Weigh 1.0 g NaCl crystals on an analytic balance.

  Place crystals in a 100-mL volumetric flask and fill to the mark with distilled water.

  Stir to completely dissolve NaCl.

Spectrophotometer

Note: Procedure can also be performed using Unopette Erythrocyte Fragility Test Kit by Becton Dickinson Vacutainer Systems. When using this kit, note that saline dilutions are prepackaged in individual reservoirs.

Procedure

1. Arrange two series of 12 tubes in the rack. Label both sets of tubes 1 through 12. The first series of tubes 1 through 12 is for the patient and the second series is for the control.
2. With a 5-mL pipet and 1% NaCl solution, and with the other 5-mL pipet, add distilled water into the series of patient tubes according to the following scheme:

Tube	1% NaCl(mL)	DI Water (mL)	NaCl%
1	4.25	0.75	0.85
2	3.50	1.50	0.70
3	3.25	1.75	0.65
4	3.00	2.00	0.60
5	2.75	2.25	0.55
6	2.50	2.50	0.50
7	2.25	2.75	0.45
8	2.00	3.00	0.40
9	1.75	3.25	0.35
10	1.50	3.50	0.30
11	1.25	3.75	0.25
12	0.75	4.25	0.15

3. Thoroughly mix the contents of each tube by covering with parafilm and inverting several times.
4. With a 3-mL pipet, transfer 2.5 mL of solution from the first set of tubes to the corresponding second set. Only one pipet is necessary if you start to transfer with the most dilute solution.
5. Draw blood into a tube containing heparin. Immediately add 50 μL of blood into each tube of the first set. The blood should drop directly into the solution. Do not allow the blood to drop onto the sides of the tube.
6. Add 50 μL of known normal blood, collected in the same manner, to each tube in the second set.
7. Let the tubes sit at room temperature for half an hour.

8. Mix gently and centrifuge at 2000 rpm for 5 minutes.
9. When interpreting results, note which tubes show initial and complete hemolysis. Initial hemolysis is recognized by a faintly pink supernatant and a cell button at the bottom of the tube. Complete hemolysis is seen as a red supernatant with possibly a button of cell stroma at the bottom of the tube.
10. This test may be quantitated by measuring each tube on a spectrophotometer. To do this, two additional tubes are necessary. This first is a blank containing 50 μL of blood to which 2.5 mL of 0.9% NaCl is added, which will result in no hemolysis. The second blank is complete (100%) hemolysis and is obtained by adding 50 μL of blood to 2.5 mL of distilled water.
11. These blanks are run in parallel with the other tubes.
12. After centrifugation, the supernatant of each tube is removed, and its optical density (OD) is read in a spectrophotometer using a 540-nm filter.[31] The percentage of hemolysis in each tube is calculated using the following equation:

$$\% \text{ Hemolysis} = \frac{\text{OD}\,(x) - \text{OD}\,0.85\%}{\text{OD}\,(0) - \text{OD}\,0.85\%}$$

where OD (x) represents absorbance of sample solution of NaCl concentration and OD (0) represents a sample blank; NaCl concentration (0.00%). An osmotic fragility curve may be drawn by plotting the percentage of hemolysis in each tube against the corresponding concentration of NaCl solution, as shown in Figure 28–32. It is helpful to plot the

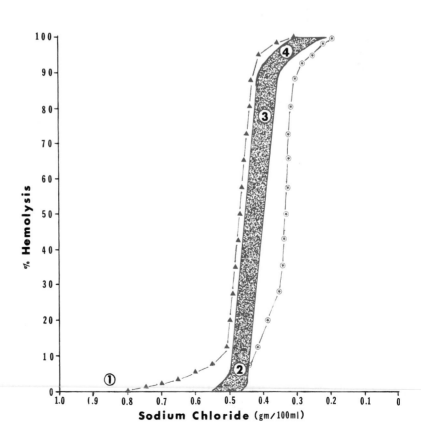

➤ FIGURE 28–32 Comparative osmotic fragility curve (⊛, sickle cell anemia; ▲, hereditary spherocytosis). Normal range is shaded. 1 = normal biconcave disc; 2 = disc-to-sphere transformation; 3 = disc-to-sphere transformation; 4 = lysis.

normal control with the patient's values so that any difference can be seen more clearly.

Interpretation

1. Patient values are always reported with the value of the control. With the normal samples, initial hemolysis is generally around 0.45%, with complete hemolysis occurring at 0.30% or 0.35%.
2. Examples of initial and complete hemolysis in various conditions follow:

	Initial Hemolysis (% NaCl)	Complete Hemolysis (% NaCl)
Normal	0.45	0.35
Hereditary spherocytosis	0.65	0.45
Acquired hemolytic anemia	0.50	0.40
Hemolytic disease of the newborn	0.55	0.40
Thalassemia	0.35	0.20
Sickle cell anemia	0.35	0.20

It may be necessary in some cases to incubate the patient's heparinized blood for 24 hours at 37°C. This will enhance increased osmotic fragility, which may reveal a subtle but abnormal osmotic fragility not apparent upon initial testing.

Comments

1. Fresh heparinized blood is recommended, but defibrinated blood may be used. Oxalate, EDTA, or citrate should not be used because of the additional salts present.
2. Perform this test immediately, because cell shape and osmotic conditions change with time.
3. Osmotic fragility can be altered by pH and temperature.
4. If the plasma is significantly jaundiced, replace the plasma with isotonic saline before testing to prevent interference.
5. Hemolytic organisms in a blood specimen can cause erroneous results owing to hemolysis, which is not attributed to test conditions.
6. If the patient has a low hemoglobin level, wash the patient and control cells once with isotonic saline and resuspend with equal volumes of RBCs and saline for both specimens. This will correct for the anemia.
7. In some anemias, when poikilocytosis accompanies a low hemoglobin level, decreased osmotic fragility may be seen. This may be the result partly of decreased hemoglobin concentration and not of the presence of poikilocytes.

Acidified Serum Test (Ham's Test) for Paroxysmal Nocturnal Hemoglobinuria

Principle Confirmation of diagnosis of paroxysmal nocturnal hemoglobinuria (PNH) is dependent on a positive acidified serum test result. The RBCs of patients with PNH are complement-sensitive. In this test, complement will affix to the RBCs at a slightly acidic pH, become activated by the alternative pathway, and result in lysis of the RBCs.[32]

Reagents and Equipment

Venous patient specimen

Venous normal control (ABO compatible)

Five 12 × 75 mm test tubes

0.2 N HCl

1-mL serologic pipets

Two Erlenmeyer flasks

Glass beads

Procedure

1. Collect venous specimens from patient and control in a plastic syringe and defibrinate by swirling in an Erlenmeyer flask that contains glass beads.
2. Centrifuge the defibrinated blood and separate serum from cells. Save the normal control serum, the patient's serum, and RBCs.
3. Wash the RBCs from the patient and control three times with isotonic saline, and dilute to a 50% cell suspension.
4. Label test tubes 1 through 5.
5. Add the reagents to the five tubes in numerical order, as shown below:

	Tubes				
Reagents	1	2	3	4	5
Patient serum	0.5 mL	0.5 mL			
Normal serum			0.5 mL	0.5 mL	0.5 mL
0.2 N HCl	0.5 mL		0.5 mL		0.05 mL
Patient's RBCs (50%)	1 drop	1 drop	1 drop	1 drop	
Normal RBCs (50%)					1 drop

6. Cover with parafilm and incubate all tubes for 1 hour at 37°C.
7. Centrifuge and examine supernatant for hemolysis.

Interpretation

1. Patients with PNH will demonstrate hemolysis in tubes 1 and 3. Tube 3 was run in the event that the patient had decreased complement levels.
2. Little or no hemolysis will be seen in tubes 2 and 4.
3. No hemolysis should be seen in the control, tube 5.

Comments

1. The optimum pH for this test is 6.5 to 7.0.
2. Blood containing a large number of spherocytes, as seen in hereditary spherocytosis (HS), may result in a false-positive result.
3. The test result may be positive also in hereditary erythroblastic multinuclearity with positive acidified serum (HEMPAS) test. There are, however, two differentiating features; in HEMPAS the RBCs are not lysed by the patient's own acidified serum, and the sugar water test result is negative for patients with this condition.

Sugar Water Test for Paroxysmal Nocturnal Hemoglobinuria

Principle In patients with PNH, the sucrose solution provides a low ionic strength environment that allows complement proteins to bind to the RBCs. These abnormal cells are extremely complement-sensitive, which results in complement-mediated lysis.

Reagents and Equipment

Stock sucrose solution:

Dissolve 486 g sucrose and 5.1 g sodium barbital in 500 mL distilled water.

Adjust the pH to 7.3 to 7.4 with HCl and water to reach 1 L.

Store at 4°C.

Working sucrose solution: Mix 20 mL stock solution with 80 mL water.

Test tubes, 12 × 75 mm

1-mL serologic pipets

Spectrophotometer

Procedure

1. Prepare a 50% blood suspension from EDTA-anticoagulated whole blood. Determine the ABO blood group.
2. Access type-compatible fresh normal serum or serum from an AB donor. Serum can be stored at −20°C for up to 1 week.
3. Prepare the following mixtures using 12 × 75 mm test tubes:

Test Tube	1	2	3	4
Sucrose, mL	0.90	0.95	0.95	
Cells, mL	0.05	0.05		0.05
Serum, mL	0.05		0.05	
0.01 M NH$_4$OH, mL				0.95

4. Incubate mixtures for 60 minutes at room temperature.
5. After incubation, add 4 mL of 0.15 M NaCl and centrifuge to remove residual cells for 1 to 2 minutes at 3400 rpm.
6. Take absorbance readings of the supernatant against a water blank at 540 nm.

Calculations The % lysis is calculated by the following formula:

% Lysis
$$= \frac{\text{OD tube 1} - (\text{OD tube 2} + \text{OD tube 3}) \times 100}{(\text{OD tube 4} - \text{OD tube 2})}$$

Comments

1. Although this test does not always accurately reflect complement-sensitive cells, a percent lysis value of greater than 10 is considered diagnostic for PNH.[32]
2. Other disease states may yield less than 5% lysis, such as megaloblastic anemia and autoimmune hemolytic anemia, causing false-positive results.
3. Fresh samples should be used to retain potent complement activity on PNH cells.

Autohemolysis Test

Principle When defibrinated blood is incubated at 37°C for 48 hours, only minimal hemolysis will occur. In patients with hereditary spherocytosis (HS), autohemolysis is increased. The addition of glucose or adenosine triphosphate

(ATP) to the incubation state will decrease the percentage of the abnormal hemolysis seen in the spherocytes of HS patients.

Reagents and Equipment

Ammonia water: Add 0.4 mL concentrated ammonium hydroxide to 1 L of deionized water.

0.239 M ATP:

Weigh out 121 mg of ATP, dilute with 1 mL saline, and carefully neutralize to pH 7.5 to 8.0 with 1 M NaOH.

This solution must be sterilized through to a 0.45-μm pore filter unit syringe.

Sterile 10% dextrose in 0.85% NaCl solution.

Sterile 125-mL Erlenmeyer flasks with approximately 25 glass beads (4 mm)

Sterile polypropylene tubes with caps (12 × 75 mm)

Sterile 5-mL pipets

Sterile 3-mL syringes

Spectrophotometer set to read at 540 nm

Assorted volumetric flasks, test tubes, and Pasteur pipets

Procedure

Day 1

1. Draw 25 mL of blood from the patient, and carefully defibrinate by swirling blood in a sterile 125-mL Erlenmeyer flask with glass beads. Repeat the same procedure for a control sample.
2. Prelabel six sterile 12 × 75 mm polypropylene tubes for each patient, and control and dispense the appropriate reagents as follows:

Tubes	1	2	3	4	5	6
10% dextrose in saline (mL)			0.1	0.1		
0.239 M ATP (mL)					0.1	0.1

*Tubes 1 and 2 remain plain

3. Add 2 mL of the appropriate defibrinated blood to each tube and gently rotate to mix.
4. Incubate for 24 hours in a 37°C incubator.
5. Prepare a 1:100 dilution of defibrinated blood by pipetting 0.5 mL of whole blood into a 50-mL volumetric flask, and bring it to volume with ammonia water. This is done for both the control and the patient blood.
6. Centrifuge remaining defibrinated blood, and remove serum.
7. Prepare a reagent blank by making a 1:10 dilution of serum with 4.5 mL ammonia water. This is done for both the control and the patient serum.
8. Refrigerate serum for use on day 3.
9. Read the OD of the whole blood dilutions against the serum blanks at 540 nm. Record these results.

Day 2

1. Rotate incubated samples gently, and reincubate for an additional 24 hours.

Day 3

1. Gently mix incubated samples, and pool pairs.
2. Perform a spun hematocrit on each sample (total

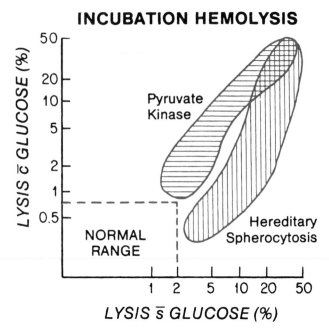

INCUBATION HEMOLYSIS

> ➤ **FIGURE 28–33** Incubation hemolysis test. This test provides a further measure of cell resistance to hemolysis. Pyruvate kinase–deficient blood demonstrates an abnormal rate of hemolysis that is independent of the presence or absence of glucose in the incubation media. In contrast, the blood from a patient with hereditary sphero-cytosis shows more marked hemolysis when glucose is absent (s). (From Hillman, RS, and Finch, CA: Red Cell Manual, ed 7. FA Davis, Philadelphia, 1996, p 124, with permission.)

three hematocrits per patient and control). Record results.
3. Pour each sample into a tube, and centrifuge for 5 minutes at 2500 rpm.
4. Remove the serum from each tube, and prepare a 1:10 dilution of each serum with ammonia water (0.5 mL serum with 4.5 mL ammonia water).
5. Make a 1:10 dilution of original serum saved from day 1. This will be your serum blank.
6. Read the OD of the serum samples made in step 4 at 540 nm using the sample prepared in step 5 as the reagent blank.

Calculations The percentage of hemolysis for each tube is calculated as shown here:

% Hemolysis
$$= \frac{(100 - \text{Hct of tube}) \times \text{OD of serum sample}}{\text{OD of whole blood} \times 10}$$

Normal Values	Lysis at 48 Hours
Without added dextrose	0.2%–2.0%
With added dextrose	0–1.0%
With added ATP	0–0.8%

Comments When normal blood is incubated for 48 hours under sterile conditions, the amount of hemolysis is relatively small. If dextrose or ATP is added, hemolysis is further slowed. Increased autohemolysis occurs in many types of hemolytic anemia. The patterns that may be observed, according to Dacie and Lewis,[33] are as follows:

- *Type I:* Patients whole red cells show slight autohemolysis, corrected by dextrose, as seen in glucose-6-phosphate dehydrogenase (G6PD) deficiency, hexokinase deficiency, and acquired nonspherocytic hemolytic anemia.
- *Type II:* Patients with moderate autohemolysis without dextrose and in whom correction with dextrose does not take place, as seen in pyruvate kinase deficiency and acquired spherocytic hemolytic anemia.
- *Type III:* Patients with marked autohemolysis without dextrose correction, seen in HS and triose phosphate isomerase deficiency (Fig. 28–33).

The autohemolysis test is no longer used in the differential diagnosis of nonspherocytic congenital hemolytic anemia, because specific enzymatic assays are now available that are considerably more accurate. It is, however, a useful screening test for some RBC enzyme deficiencies in the detection of hemolysis.

QUESTIONS

1. Twenty microliters of blood are drawn into a Unopette system for a WBC count. Fifty cells are counted on one side and 52 on the other side of the hemacytometer (4 large squares). Calculate the WBC count.
   a. 12.5×10^9/L
   b. 12.7×10^9/L
   c. 12.0×10^9/L
   d. 3.0×10^9/L

2. If a patient has a reticulocyte count of 8% with a hematocrit of 18%, what is the corrected reticulocyte count?
   a. 20%
   b. 2.3%
   c. 3.2%
   d. 8%

3. Which of the following errors will cause falsely elevated results for a centrifugal microhematocrit?
   a. Reading of buffy coat with red cells
   b. Incomplete sealing of capillary tubes
   c. Allowing the centrifuge to stop without breaking
   d. All of the above

4. Which of the following factors affect(s) the ESR?
   a. Increased fibrinogen
   b. Extreme poikilocytosis
   c. Use of heparin as an anticoagulant
   d. All of the above

5. What type of hemoglobin electrophoresis would be best to separate hemoglobins S and D?
   a. Cellulose acetate at alkaline pH
   b. Citrate agar at acid pH
   c. Either cellulose acetate or citrate agar may be used

6. What is the principle for the acid elution test for HbF?
   a. HbF is resistant to acid elution; it can be precipitated and stained

b. HbF is susceptible to acid elution; it can be dissolved and measured photometrically

c. HbF is resistant to acid elution; it can be separated by aspirating the acid from the remaining hemoglobin

d. HbF is susceptible to acid elution; it can be destroyed and the denatured hemoglobin can be detected by a color reaction

7. Which condition shows increased osmotic fragility?
   a. Hereditary spherocytosis
   b. Sickle cell anemia
   c. Acquired hemolytic anemia
   d. Hemolytic disease of the newborn

8. What is the basic principle of both the Ham test and the sugar water test for PNH?
   a. Complement-mediated RBC lysis
   b. Precipitation of abnormal RBCs
   c. Vital staining of affected RBCs
   d. Differential agglutination of RBCs

9. Calculate the corrected WBC count for a smear containing 20 NRBCs (WBC count = 4500/μL).
   a. 4500/μL
   b. 375/μL
   c. 4480/μL
   d. 3750/μL

10. What is the principle of the cyanmethemoglobin method in the colorimetric determination of hemoglobin?
    a. Potassium ferricyanide oxidizes hemoglobin to methemoglobin; potassium cyanide converts methemoglobin to cyanmethemoglobin
    b. Potassium cyanide oxidizes hemoglobin to methemoglobin; potassium ferricyanide converts methemoglobin to cyanmethemoglobin
    c. Potassium ferricyanide oxidizes hemoglobin to cyanmethemoglobin; cyanmethemoglobin degenerates to form potassium cyanide
    d. Potassium cyanide reduces hemoglobin to cyanmethemoglobin

11. Electrophoresis can be defined as:
    a. Movement of large particles through a column
    b. Movement of small particles through a column
    c. Movement of charged particles in an electric field
    d. Tagging of a small molecule with a fluorescent protein

12. If five white blood cells are counted under 400× magnification, what is the estimated white blood cell count?
    a. 4000–7000/mm³
    b. 7000–10,000/mm³
    c. 10,000–13,000/mm³
    d. 13,000–18,000/mm³

13. Hematocrit can be defined as:
    a. Volume occupied by white blood cells in a given volume of blood expressed as a percentage
    b. Volume occupied by platelets in a given volume of blood expressed as a percentage
    c. Volume occupied by red blood cells in a given volume of blood expressed as a percentage
    d. Volume occupied by stromal cells in a given volume of blood expressed as a percentage

14. A patient presents with an MCV of 78 fL and an MCHC of 33%. How would this anemia be classified?
    a. Microcytic, normochromic
    b. Normocytic, normochromic
    c. Microcytic, hypochromic
    d. Normochromic, hyperchromic

15. What effect do sickle cells have on the ESR?
    a. Increased
    b. Decreased
    c. Normal

SUMMARY CHART

➤ The evacuated tube system methodology for venipuncture has advantages over the syringe method by utilizing a multisample needle so that more than one evacuated tube may be drawn.

➤ The most common site for a capillary stick in infants is the plantar surface of the heel.

➤ The hemacytometer counting chamber is used for manual cell counts. The counting chamber has a total area of 9 mm²; the four corner primary squares are used for counting leukocytes, the center square for platelets, and the four corner and center square of the primary square for counting erythrocytes.

➤ The Unopette system for manual cell counts consists of a reservoir containing diluent, a pipet to deliver the specimen, and a pipet shield to puncture the reservoir.

➤ The normal platelet value is 150 to 350 × 10⁹/L.

➤ Reticulocytes are immature RBCs that contain remnant cytoplasmic RNA and can be visualized by supravital stains such as new methylene blue.

➤ A corrected reticulocyte count is derived by multiplying the % reticulocytes by the patient's hematocrit, and dividing by the normal hematocrit (45%).

➤ The normal range for adult reticulocytes counts is 0.5% to 2.0%.

➤ A reticulocyte production index (RPI) of 3 or greater represents an adequate response to anemia by the bone marrow; an RPI of less than 2 is considered an inadequate response of erythropoiesis by the bone marrow to states of anemia.

➤ The red cell distribution width (RDW) is a measure of anisocytosis and is calculated by the standard deviation of RBC volume × 100 divided by mean MCV.

➤ The erythrocyte sedimentation rate (ESR) measures the settling of erythrocytes in diluted human plasma

- over a specified time period and may be affected by plasma, red cell, and mechanical factors.
- ➤ Hematocrit is defined as the volume occupied by erythrocytes in a given volume of blood and is usually expressed as a percentage of the volume of the whole blood sample.
- ➤ The normal hematocrit for men is 42% to 52%; for women, it is 37% to 47%.
- ➤ The hematocrit is usually three times the hemoglobin value.
- ➤ A Romanowsky stain is any stain combination consisting of eosin Y or eosin B with methylene blue or any of its oxidation products.
- ➤ A corrected white blood cell count is calculated by multiplying the WBC/mm^3 by 100, and dividing by 100 plus the number of nucleated RBCs per 100 WBCs.
- ➤ The cyanmethemoglobin method for the determination of hemoglobin is based on the principle of blood diluted in a solution of potassium ferricyanide yields oxidation to the ferric state (Fe^{3+}) to form methemoglobin; this solution reacts with potassium cyanide to form stable cyanmethemoglobin, which is read at 540 nm on a spectrophotometer.
- ➤ The normal hemoglobin value for a man is 14 to 18 g/dL; for a woman, it is 12 to 16 g/dL.
- ➤ Electrophoresis is defined as the movement of charged particles in an electric field; hemoglobin electrophoresis relies on the premise that abnormal hemoglobins migrate at a fixed pH.
- ➤ The solubility test for hemoglobin S is based upon the deoxyhemoglobin properties of HbS; when exposed to high-molarity phosphate buffer, HbS will precipitate out of solution.
- ➤ The acid elution test for hemoglobin F is based on the principle that the HbF is resistant to acid elution and will retain the pink stain; hemoglobin A will be eluted from the red cell and appear colorless (ghost cells).
- ➤ Heinz bodies are denatured hemoglobin precipitated in the RBC and attached to the red cell membrane; they are visible by utilization of supravital stains such as crystal violet.
- ➤ The osmotic fragility test is a measure of the surface-to-volume ratio of the red cell; whole blood is added to a series of saline dilutions, which causes water to be drawn into the erythrocyte through the process of osmosis. Eventually, the red cell bursts, releasing hemoglobin, which can then be measured on a spectrophotometer.
- ➤ The acidified serum test (Ham's test) is diagnostic for the diagnosis of paroxysmal nocturnal hemoglobinuria (PNH) and involves the addition of normal serum, patient serum, acidified serum, patient red cells, and normal red cells to a series of tubes; the red cells of patients with PNH are complement-sensitive and will lyse when exposed to acidified serum.
- ➤ In the sugar water test, PNH red cells are exposed to a sucrose solution, which provides a low ionic strength environment that allows complement proteins to bind to the red cells, resulting in complement-mediated cell lysis.
- ➤ The autohemolysis test is based on the premise that red cells from patients with hereditary spherocytosis will lyse at a faster rate than normal red cells when incubated at 37°C for 48 hours; the addition of ATP or glucose will decrease the hemolysis in patients with hereditary spherocytosis; in contrast, patients with pyruvate kinase deficiency demonstrate increased hemolysis independent of glucose or adenosine triphosphate.
- ➤ The mean corpuscular volume (MCV) is equal to the hematocrit (%) multiplied by 10 and divided by the RBC count.
- ➤ The mean corpuscular hemoglobin (MCH) is equal to the hemoglobin (g/dL) multiplied by 10 and divided by the RBC count.
- ➤ The mean corpuscular hemoglobin concentration (MCHC) is equal to the hemoglobin (g/dL) divided by the hematocrit (%), and multiplied by 100.

References

1. Stockbower, JM, et al: Procedures for the Collection of Diagnostic Blood Specimens by Venipuncture, ed. 3. NCCLS H3-A3. Villanova, PA, July 1991, p 13.
2. McCall, RE, and Tankersley, CM: Phlebotomy Essentials, ed 2. Lippincott, Philadelphia, 1998 p 241.
3. The Unopette System for RBC Determinations, Becton Dickinson, Rutherford, NJ, 1991.
4. Palko, T, and Palko, H: Laboratory Procedures for the Medical Office. McGraw-Hill, New York, 1996, p 286.
5. The Unopette System for WBC/Platelet Determinations, Becton-Dickinson, Rutherford, NJ, 1991, p 8.
6. Palko, T, and Palko, H: Laboratory Procedures for the Medical Office. McGraw-Hill, New York, 1996, p 347.
7. Dale, NL, and Schumacher, HR: Platelet satellitism—new spurious results with automated instruments. Lab Med 13:5, 1982.
8. Finch, CA, et al: Method for Reticulocyte Counting. NCCLS H16-P. Villanova, PA, 1985, vol 5, no 10, p 226.
9. Coulter Retic-Prep, Coulter Corporation, Miami, FL, PN 7507938-C, October 1993.
10. Morris, MW, and Davey, FR: Basic examination of blood. In Henry, JB (ed): Clinical Diagnosis and Management by Laboratory Methods, ed 19. WB Saunders, Philadelphia, 1996, p 574.
11. Williams, WJ, et al: Hematology, ed 4. McGraw-Hill, New York, 1990, p 15.
12. Onder, I, et al: Platelet aggregation size and volume in chronic obstructive Pulmonary disease. Mater Med Pol 29(1–4):11, 1997.
13. Koepke, JA, et al: Reference Procedure for the Erythrocyte Sedimentation Rate (ESR) Test. NCCLS H2-A2, ISSN 3099–0273. Villanova, PA, 1988, vol 8, no 3.
14. Westergren, A: Die Senkungsreaction. Ergeb Inn Med Kinderheikd 5:531, 1924.
15. Wintrobe, MM, and Landsberg, JW: A standardized technique for blood sedimentation test. Am J Med Sci 189:102, 1935.
16. Henry, JB: Clinical Diagnosis and Management by Laboratory Methods, ed 19. WB Saunders, Philadelphia 1991, p 590.
17. Diesse Diagnostics, MINI-VES Insert, Smithfield, RI, 1999.
18. van Assendelft, OW, et al: Procedure for Determining Packed Cell Volume by the Microhematocrit Method. NCCLS, H7-A. Villanova, PA, 1985, vol 5, no 5, p 107.
19. Morris, MW, and Davey, FR: Basic examination of blood. In Henry, JB (ed): Clinical Diagnosis and Management by Laboratory Methods, ed 19. WB Saunders, Philadelphia, 1996, p 575.
20. Wedding, ME, and Toenjes, SA: Medical Laboratory Procedures. FA Davis, Philadelphia, 1992, p 273.
21. Morris, MW, and Davey, FR: Basic examination of blood. In Henry JB (ed): Clinical Diagnosis and Management by Laboratory Methods, ed 19. WB Saunders, Philadelphia, 1996, p 576.
22. Ames Hema-Tek Operational Manual, ed 2. Miles Laboratories, Elkhart, IN, 1980.
23. DeNunzio, J: Buffy coat preparation for leukopenic specimens. Lab Med, 16:497, 1985.
24. Helena Laboratories, Method for Hemoglobin Electrophoresis, Beaumont, TX, 1985.
25. Kim, HC, et al: Separation of hemoglobins. In Williams, WJ, et al (eds): Hematology, ed 4. McGraw-Hill, New York, 1990, p 1711.
26. Schneider, RG: Chromatographic (Microcolumn) Determination of Hemoglobin A$_2$. NCCLS H9-A. Villanova, PA, 1989, vol 9, no 17, p 935.

27. Schneider, RG, et al: Solubility Test for Confirming the Presence of Sickling Hemoglobins. NCCLS H10-A. Villanova, PA, 1986, vol 6, no 10, p 209.
28. Fetal Hemoglobin Procedure No. 101, Sure-Tech Diagnostics Associates, Inc, St Louis, MO, 1996.
29. Vengelen-Tyler, V (eds): Technical Manual, ed 13. American Association of Blood Banks, Bethesda, MD, 1999, p 507.
30. Beutler, E: Heinz body staining. In Williams, WJ, et al (eds): Hematology, ed 4. McGraw-Hill, New York, 1990, p 1701.

31. Beutler, E: Osmotic fragility. In Williams, WJ, et al (eds): Hematology, ed 4. McGraw-Hill, New York, 1990, p 1717.
32. Elghetany, MT, and Davey, FR: Erythrocytic disorders. In Henry, JB (ed): Clinical Diagnosis and Management by Laboratory Methods, ed 19. WB Saunders, Philadelphia, 1996, p 635.
33. Dacie, JV, and Lewis, SM: Practical Hematology, ed 4. Grune & Stratton, New York, 1968.

29

Principles of Automated Differential Analysis

ELLEN HOPE KEARNS, MS, SH(ASCP)H
LEE A. LAMONICA, BS, MT(ASCP), CLS(NCA)

OBJECTIVES

At the end of this chapter, the learner should be able to:

1. Discuss principles of advanced hematology analyzers with blood cell histogram/scattergram differentials.

2. Explain the main use of automated blood cell histogram/scattergram differentials.

3. Describe when to accept an automated histogram/scattergram differential or perform a conventional manual differential.

4. Determine the correct action to be taken when a result is flagged.

5. Interpret patient data generated by advanced hematology analyzers, including the hemogram parameters, red cell histograms, platelet histograms, and leukocyte histograms/scattergrams.

6. Identify current trends in automated differential analysis.

7. Describe the importance of quality control and quality assurance measures for automated differential analysis.

8. Explain circumstances that could contribute to spurious or artifactual results and appropriate actions to be followed.

The differential analysis of peripheral blood smears consists of the examination and identification of leukocyte/white blood cell subpopulations, an evaluation of red blood cell morphology, and an estimation of platelet quantity. It used to represent one of the most frequently ordered and most time-consuming hematology test procedures. Differential analysis of peripheral blood was considered the single laboratory test from which the most information regarding patient disease status could be derived.[1] Examination of peripheral blood smears, for example, can reveal hematologic abnormalities such as anemia and leukemia, aid in the identification of infectious conditions including infectious mononucleosis and parasitemia, monitor the progress of disease, and follow a patient's response to therapy.[2]

In the past two decades, the demands of the laboratory marketplace have led to mergers of a number of leading hematology instrument manufacturers. At the same time, advanced technologies have enhanced automated methods for analyzing peripheral blood cell populations.[3–7] In addition to providing complete blood count (CBC) parameters such as white blood cells (WBCs), red blood cells (RBCs), hemoglobin (Hgb), hematocrit (Hct), platelets (PLTs), and RBC indices, current instruments also differentiate and quantify WBC subpopulations, and identify samples with abnormalities for further review. Many instruments also determine parameters such as red cell and platelet distribution widths (RDW and PDW), and mean platelet volume (MPV). A number of advanced hematology analyzers perform automated reticulocyte counting as well.

The automated leukocyte analysis eliminates statistical variations associated with 100- or 200-cell manual differential counts based on the increased number of cells (several thousand) that are analyzed. This has also contributed to the increased sensitivity of automated leukocyte differentials to abnormalities such as the clumping of platelets and the presence of nucleated red blood cells (NRBCs) and leukemic blasts.[8,9] Moreover, a number of studies suggest that the automated differential is more efficient and cost-effective than the manual procedure.[10–12] Despite advantages of using the automated differential to evaluate hematologically normal patients, further studies are required before automated methods totally replace the manual procedure, particularly in evaluating blood samples from oncology patients,[13–16] and neonatal intensive care populations.[17]

Automated differential analysis is currently based on the quantitation and evaluation of cell volume, cell light scattering, and cytochemistry, used alone or in combination. Applications of cell volume analysis will be illustrated by the Coulter (Model S Plus IV) three-part screening differential, which provides information about granulocytes, lymphocytes, and mononuclear cell fractions.[18,19] Coulter's newer VCS technology (Models STKS, MAXM, and GEN S) combines volume, conductivity, and light scatter in a single integrated system that enumerates neutrophils, eosinophils, basophils, monocytes, and lymphocytes illustrated in a three-dimensional scatterplot of cell populations and subpopulations.[20] Applications of VCS technology are illustrated by the Coulter Model STKS. The corporate name of Coulter Electronics changed recently to Beckman Coulter, Inc. The leukocyte differential, available from Technicon H-1 system within the Bayer Corporation, Diagnostics Division, demonstrates cell analysis based on light-scattering events and cytochemistry.[21] The Sysmex (SE-Series) hematology analyz-

ers from Sysmex Corporation use a combination of technologies for identifying and separating leukocyte cell populations and subpopulations, including the electronic resistance detection principle with radiofrequency signals for recognizing cell density characteristics of leukocyte populations. These instruments generate a WBC scattergram and red cell and platelet histograms.[22] The CELL-DYN hematology analyzers from Abbott Laboratories, Inc., use advanced technologies, including high-resolution flow cytometry optical WBC, platelet, and RBC analyses.

➤ EVALUATION OF BLOOD SPECIMENS BY CELL VOLUME ANALYSIS: THE COULTER MODEL S PLUS SERIES

The third-generation Coulter Model S Plus Series (S Plus II, S Plus III, S Plus IV, S Plus V, S Plus VI) and the STKR (pronounced "stacker") instruments generate three histograms representing WBCs, RBCs, and platelet volume distributions, expressed in femtoliters (fL). Histograms of WBCs, RBCs, and platelets are displayed simultaneously with CBC information.

Leukocyte Histogram Analysis

The leukocyte histogram analysis should be used as a screening tool to detect the presence of hematologic disease. Leukocytes in ethylene diaminetetraacetic acid (EDTA)–anticoagulated peripheral blood are separated into three major cell fractions by cell volume analysis (Fig. 29–1). Using an isotonic saline solution and lysing reagent to dilute and differentially shrink WBCs, the instruments differentiate between lymphocytes (lymphocytes and atypical lymphocytes), granulocytes (segmented neutrophils, bands, metamyelocytes, eosinophils, and basophils), and mononuclear cells (monocytes, promyelocytes, myelocytes, plasma cells, and blasts) based on differences in nuclear size and cytoplasmic complexity. Cells with a volume of approximately 35 to 90 fL are defined as lymphocytes. Those with volumes ranging from 160 to 450 fL are classified as granulocytes, and those ranging from 90 to 160 fL are identified as mononuclear cells. Results are expressed in absolute and relative numbers for each cell category.[5]

To highlight results that are out of range, the Coulter instrument backlights the offending number. Backlighting occurs in the presence of abnormal cells or interferences to alert the operator to the possibility of erroneous or abnormal results. Region flag indicators, or R flags (R1, R2, R3, R4), indicate the specific location(s) of abnormalities in the WBC size distribution (Fig. 29–2). They may also denote overlapping of two or more of the cell populations at the four desig-

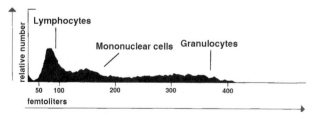

➤ **FIGURE 29–1**   Coulter leukocyte histogram differential. (From Significant Advances in Hematology, Coulter Electronics, Hialeah, FL, 1983, p 8, with permission.)

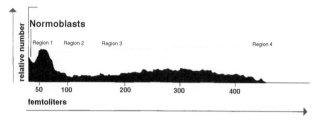

> **FIGURE 29–2**   Region flags (R flags) superimposed on Coulter S Plus IV WBC histogram. (From Significant Advances in Hematology, Coulter Electronics, Hialeah, FL, 1983, p 9, with permission.)

nated threshold/valley regions (35, 90, 160, and 450 fL) of the WBC size distribution histogram. Common abnormalities associated with each flag[23] are listed in Table 29–1.

The presence of backlighting and/or flagging of the results suggest that a manual differential count or careful microscopic scanning of a stained peripheral blood smear is indicated. The decision to perform a manual differential should be based on the individual laboratory's established criteria for manual review of automated histogram differential analysis. Examples of criteria for manual review and reference values for the automated histogram differential, established at a tertiary care hospital, appear in Tables 29–2 and 29–3, respectively.

Red Cell Histogram Analysis

Particles with a volume of greater than 36 fL and less than or equal to 360 fL are identified as RBCs. The RBC histogram displays particles with a volume greater than 24 fL, but the mean corpuscular volume (MCV) is calculated from the area under the curve of the RBC histogram, depicted in

> **Table 29–1**
> **ABNORMALITIES ASSOCIATED WITH SPECIFIC FLAGGING REGIONS OF THE COULTER MODEL S PLUS SERIES WBC HISTOGRAM**

R Flat	Region	Abnormality
R1	Far left	Erythrocyte precursors Cryoglobulins Nonlysed erythrocytes Giant and/or clumped platelets
R2	Between lymphocytes and monocytes	Blasts Basophilia Eosinophilia Plasma cells Abnormal/variant lymphocytes
R3	Between monocytes and granulocytes	Abnormal cell populations Eosinophilia Immature granulocytes
R4	Far right	Increased absolute granulocytes
RM		Multiple flags

Source: Pierre, RV: Seminar and Case Studies: The Automated Differential. Coulter Electronics, Hialeah, FL, 1985, p 9, with permission.

> **Table 29–2**
> **CRITERIA FOR MANUAL REVIEW OF THE COULTER HISTOGRAM DIFFERENTIAL ESTABLISHED AT A TERTIARY CARE HOSPITAL**

WBC count: $< 4.0 \times 10^9/L$
$> 15.0 \times 10^9/L$

Monocytes: $> 15.0\%$

Lymphocytes: $> 50\%$

Granulocytes: $< 50\%$

All backlighting

All R flags

All incomplete computations

> **Table 29–3**
> **REFERENCE VALUES FOR SELECTED BLOOD CELL PARAMETERS ESTABLISHED AT A TERTIARY CARE HOSPITAL**

Granulocytes	50%–75%
Lymphocytes	25%–40%
Monocytes	4%–10%

Figure 29–3. Deviations in the shape and position of the RBC histogram indicate changes in RBC size or shape, or both. An RBC distribution that is shifted to the left indicates the presence of microcytosis. Conversely, when the curve is shifted to the right, such as in folic acid deficiency, macrocytosis is indicated.

The availability of red cell parameters such as RBC, Hgb, Hct, MCV, mean corpuscular hemoglobin (MCH), and mean corpuscular hemoglobin concentration (MCHC), in conjunction with information derived from RBC histograms, may provide valuable information for assessing erythrocytic disorders. The RDW represents a parameter that quantifies relative anisocytosis. It is calculated as the coefficient of variation (CV) of the MCV (Table 29–4). Its usefulness in the early detection of iron-deficiency anemia and in distinguishing between iron-deficiency anemia (increased RDW) and beta (β) thalassemia (normal RDW) has been suggested.[24]

Platelet Histogram Analysis

The platelet histogram displays native platelet size. Particles with volumes ranging from 2 to 20 fL are counted. The raw data are fit to a log-normal distribution (Fig 29–4), from which the reported platelet count is calculated.

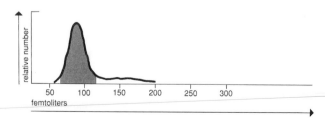

> **FIGURE 29–3**   Normal Coulter RBC histogram. (From Significant Advances in Hematology, Coulter Electronics, Hialeah, FL, 1983, p 11, with permission.)

> ### Table 29-4
> ### CALCULATION OF THE RDW AS DETERMINED BY COULTER

$$RDW = \frac{SD}{Mean} \times 100$$

Normal range = 11.5%–14.5%

Source: Pierre, RV: Seminar and Case Studies: The Automated Differential. Coulter Electronics. Hialeah, FL, 1985, p 38, with permission.

The MPV and PDW are additional parameters describing platelet size. The MPV is equivalent to the MCV and is inversely proportional to the platelet count (Fig 29–5).[25] The PDW measures uniformity of platelet size and is equivalent to the RDW. In combination with the platelet histogram, the MPV and PDW provide greater distinction between normal and abnormal platelet populations.

➤ ADVANCES IN THE COULTER LEUKOCYTE DIFFERENTIAL ANALYSIS: VCS TECHNOLOGY

Coulter Models STKS, MAXM, and GEN S

The Coulter WBC differential has been expanded to include enumeration of eosinophils and basophils, by com-

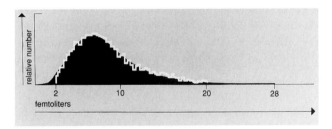

> ➤ FIGURE 29–4 Normal Coulter platelet histogram. (From Significant Advances in Hematology, Coulter Electronics, Hialeah, FL, 1983, p 13, with permission.)

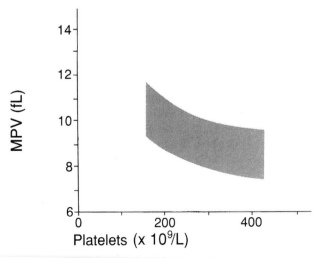

> ➤ FIGURE 29–5 Coulter MPV normogram. (From Significant Advances in Hematology, Coulter Electronics, Hialeah, FL, 1983, p 14, with permission.)

bining measurements of cell volume with conductivity and light-scatter data (Table 29–5). The Coulter VCS technology (Models MAXM and GEN S) is a single-channel analysis method that uses three independent energy sources to probe approximately 8000 cells in their near-native state. Cell volume is based on the Coulter principle of electrical impedance to measure the size of the cells. Light-scattering characteristics provide additional information about cell structure and shape. This technology is particularly useful for identifying eosinophils. Conductivity measurements are made using a high-frequency electromagnetic probe and reflect the nuclear, granular, and chemical properties of cells. Conductivity measurements aid in differentiating between cells of similar size, such as lymphocytes and basophils, which differ in internal structure.

The VCS technology has been enhanced on the Coulter GEN S system by utilizing two new features. These features include Intellikenetics, a software and hardware management tool to assist in the control of fluctuations in the laboratory environment, such as ambient temperature and Accu-Gate, which allows for an improved level of flagging abnormalities. The Coulter Model GEN S offers a 33-parameter CBC, including the quantitative, five-part differential with online reticulocyte analysis. The Coulter Model MAXM offers a 26-parameter CBC, including a quantitative five-part differential.

The Coulter Model STKS (pronounced "stack-S") system appears in Figure 29–6. An example of this model's leukocyte analysis is provided in Figure 29–7. Individual cells are depicted as points on a scatterplot, reflecting cell volume and light-scattering characteristics. Clusters of cells are identified as lymphocytes, monocytes, neutrophils, and eosinophils based on their relative position on the scatterplot. Separate scatterplots comparing cell volume and conductivity properties are generated to quantify basophils.

> ### Table 29-5
> ### MEASUREMENTS ASSOCIATED WITH COULTER'S VCS TECHNOLOGY

Volume (V)	Using direct current (DC) impedence, the VCS module measures the volume of each cell.
Conductivity (C)	As radiofrequency (RF) penetrates the cell, information is gathered about the size and internal structure of the cells.
Scatter (S)	When an unstained cell is struck by a laser beam, scattered light spreads out in every direction. Then median-angle light-scatter signals, using a proprietary new detector, are collected to obtain information about cell surface structure and cellular granularity.
VCS	A single-channel analysis method that uses three independent energy sources to probe approximately 8000 cells in their near-native state.

Source: Adapted from The Coulter MAX and MAXM AL with Reticulocytes Hematology Flow Cytometry Systems. Coulter® Corporation, 1996, with permission.

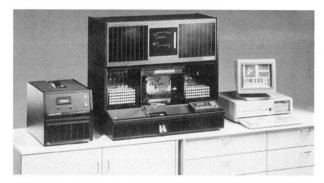

➤ **FIGURE 29-6**   Coulter STKS Hematology System. (Courtesy of Coulter Corporation, Miami, FL.)

Floating discriminators examine areas between different cell populations. Abnormalities are identified by specific region flags. The STKS flagging system is enhanced by providing specific alphanumeric codes and three types of messages, including suspect, definitive, and condition messages. Common abnormalities associated with each flagging message appear in Table 29-6. Suspect messages flag abnormal cell populations or distributions such as certain red cell abnormalities, platelet clumping, variant lymphocytes, and immature granulocytes. These messages appear in the cell classification window on the sample analysis display, and abnormalities should be confirmed by a microscopic review. Definitive messages flag decreases and increases for all test parameters based on numeric limits set by the laboratory. A message appears in the cell classification window on the sample analysis display if the results of the sample exceed preset limits. Condition messages indicate whether the white cell, red cell, and platelet populations are abnormal or normal. In addition to flagging messages, data from cell counts, white cell scatter plots, and size-distribution histograms are sent to a data management system (DMS).

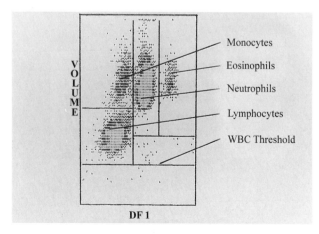

➤ **FIGURE 29-7**   White blood cell analysis by Coulter VCS technology. (From Coulter VCS Technology Casebook, Coulter Electronics, Hialeah, FL, 1989, p 62, with permission.)

➤ EVALUATION OF BLOOD SPECIMENS BY LIGHT SCATTERING AND CYTOCHEMICAL ANALYSIS: THE TECHNICON H-1 AND BAYER ADVIA 120 HEMATOLOGY SYSTEMS

Technicon H-1 System

Although the Advia 120 has replaced the Technicon series of hematology systems, a significant number of Technicon H-1's are still in operation throughout the United States. As a result, a brief description of this technology will be presented. Enumeration and identification of blood cells by the Technicon H-1 system (Fig. 29-8) is based on optical flow cytometry, cytochemistry, and light scattering. The instrument's sampling mechanism divides blood samples into aliquots that are treated in four separate reaction chambers; the red cell and platelet reaction chamber, hemoglobin reaction chamber, basophil/lobularity reaction chamber, and peroxidase reaction chamber. Cells are counted as they pass through a flow cell. A laser beam is located on one side of the flow cell. As the cells pass in front of the beam, they are counted by a light-scatter detector.

Red Cell and Platelet Histogram Analysis

Red cells and platelets are identified on the basis of light-scattering properties. A buffered reagent isovolumetrically fixes and spheres platelets and red cells, while light scattered at high and low angles concurrently measures cell volume and optical density. Red cell and platelet histograms are generated based on light-scatter measurements translated into cell volume. Additional parameters such as red cell distribution width (RDW) and platelet cell volume (PCV) are derived from these histograms. The instrument's interpretive report identifies and grades (1+ to 4+) various RBC abnormalities, including microcytosis, macrocytosis, hypochromia, hyperchromia, and anisocytosis.

The Technicon H-1 system's RDW reference range of 10.2% to 11.8 % is different from the Coulter analyzer's range of 11.5% to 14.5 %.[17] The difference is likely a result of each instrument's individualized mathematical trimming of the data. Because the absolute value reported for the CV of RBC size is variable based on the program of each standardized analyzer, each laboratory should determine its own normal ranges.

Leukocyte Analysis

WBCs are fixed with formaldehyde and stained with peroxidase in the peroxidase reaction chamber. The chamber is heated to a relatively high temperature, which lyses platelets and RBCs and causes the WBCs to be fixed and dehydrated. Narrow forward-angle light-scatter and tungsten light optics are used to measure WBC size and peroxidase activity, respectively. Myeloperoxidase is a granulocyte enzyme marker that is present to varying degrees in neutrophils, eosinophils, and monocytes but absent from basophils, lymphocytes, and blasts.[26] A peroxidase scattergram depicting peroxidase staining intensity on the abscissa and cell size on the ordinate is generated (Fig 29-9). Each point in the scattergram characterizes the peroxidase activity and size of a single cell. Clusters of points represent distinct leukocyte subpopulations.

➤ Table 29-6
SUMMARY OF FLAGGING MESSAGES GENERATED BY THE COULTER VCS DIFFERENTIAL

Population	Suspect	Condition	Definitive
White cells	Immature granulocytes	Normal WBC population	Leukocytosis
	Variant lymphocytes	Abnormal WBC population	Leukopenia
	Blasts	No message	Neutrophilia
	Review slide	Edited data	Neutropenia
		Full clog	Monocytosis
		Partial clog 1	Lymphocytosis
		Partial clog 2	Lymphopenia
			Basophilia
			Eosinophilia
Red cells	Dimorphic RBC population	Normal RBC population	Anemia
	Microcytic RBCs	Abnormal RBC population	Microcytosis
	RBC fragments	Abnormal RBC population	
	RBC agglutination	No message	Macrocytosis
		Edited data	Anisocytosis
			Poikilocytosis
			Hypochromia
			Pancytopenia
			Erythrocytosis
Platelets	Giant platelets	Normal platelet, population	
	Thrombocytosis		
	Platelet clumping	Abnormal platelet, population	Thrombocytopenia
		No message	Large platelets
			Small platelets

Source: Adapted from Pierre, R: Seminar and Case Studies: The Automated Differential. Coulter Electronics, Inc., Hialeah, FL, July 1991, p 75, with permission.

A specific basophil count is determined separately in the basophil/lobularity chamber. Whole blood is exposed to an acid buffer that selectively lyses all cells except basophils.

The resulting particles are subsequently sorted, and their forward angle and light-scattering properties quantified.

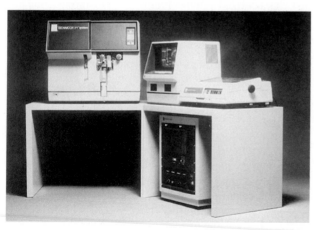

➤ **FIGURE 29–8** Technicon H-1 System. (Courtesy of Bayer Corporation, Diagnostic Division, Tarrytown, NY.)

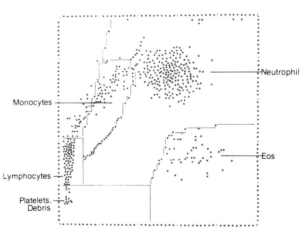

➤ **FIGURE 29–9** Technicon H-I WBC/peroxidase scattergram. Cell size is indicated on the y axis, peroxidase activity on the x axis. (From Brown, BA: Hematology: Principles and Procedures, ed 6. Lea & Febiger, Philadelphia, 1993, p 373, with permission.)

Because basophils are resistant to lysis, they appear larger than the bare nuclei of other leukocytes, scatter more light, and appear higher on the vertical axis of the scattergram (Fig 29–10). A fixed horizontal threshold separates the nuclei of other WBCs from basophils.

The WBC differential report generated by the Technicon H-1 system not only indicates the relative percentages and absolute values for neutrophils, lymphocytes, monocytes, eosinophils, and basophils, but also provides additional interpretative data to signal the presence of abnormalities. The differential report defines the proportion of leukocytes with high myeloperoxidase content, designated the HPX fraction, and the percentage of large unstained cells (LUCs). Increased myeloperoxidase activity may be associated with reactive states, megaloblastic anemia, or hyperproliferative granulopoiesis, whereas increased numbers of LUCs may reflect the presence of atypical lymphocytes or blasts. Normal ranges of 0% to 3.7% for LUCs and 0% to 5.4% for HPX have been established.[21]

ADVIA 120 Hematology System

The ADVIA 120 Hematology System from the Bayer Corporation, Diagnostics Division (Tarrytown, NY) uses Unifluidics technology and consists of an analytic module, along with an optional autosampler and a data manager (Fig. 29–11). This analyzer has a throughput of 120 samples per hour and can perform the following blood counts:

(1) complete blood counts (CBC), (2) CBC plus white cell differential counts, and (3) reticulocyte counts.

The ADVIA 120 hematology analyzer uses two separate and independent flow cytometers to count and identify blood cells. The operator is able to sample via automated closed tube, manual closed tube, and manual opened tube. The minimum sample volume required is 157 μL. The autosampler consists of a rack-style apparatus able to hold a capacity of 150 sample tubes (15 racks of 10 tubes). The autosampler automatically transports, mixes, identifies via barcode reader, and aspirates samples in closed tubes. A manual bar-code reader is available for manual aspiration.

The Unifluidics Technology

Once a sample is aspirated, it is delivered into a ceramic shear valve, where it is divided into separate aliquots for analysis. Reagents and aliquots are subsequently drawn into respective reaction chambers: (1) hemoglobin reaction chamber, (2) basophil reaction chamber, (3) RBC reaction chamber, (4) reticulocyte reaction chamber, (5) peroxidase reaction chamber, (6) shear valve, and (7) reagent pump. The Unifluidics block is made up of eight acrylic blocks with directional pathways for the sample to flow for analysis. Once testing is completed, the sample and reagent mixture is directed to the waste container, a subcomponent of the analyzer, and appropriate rinsing of reaction chambers takes place. The following sections outline specific details about RBC, reticulocyte, platelet, and WBC analyses, and morphology flagging.

Red Blood Cell Analysis

The RBC reaction chamber provides measurements for the RBC count, RBC indices, hemoglobin concentration, and platelet counts. Once a constant volume of sample has passed through the chamber both low-angle (2 to 3) and high-angle (5 to 15) light scatter is measured. An RBC scatter cytogram is graphically illustrated by instrument software, where the high-angle light scatter is plotted on the x axis and the low-angle light scatter on the y axis.

Hemoglobin concentration is measured by absorbance at 546 nm and graphically illustrated on the volume/hemoglobin concentration (V/HC) cytogram. In this case, the hemoglobin concentration is plotted along the x axis and cell volume along the y axis. Red blood cells are further characterized as hypochromic, normochromic, and hyperchromic, with the addition of hemoglobin markers set at 28 g/dL and 41 g/dL. RBCs with a hemoglobin concentration less than the former are characterized as hypochromic, and cells with a hemoglobin concentration greater than 41 g/dL are characterized as hyperchromic. Values within the range of 28 and 41 g/dL are normochromic. Figure 29–12 illustrates an RBC hemoglobin concentration histogram of a hyperchromic sample. Cell markers for RBC volume are also used to assess microcytic, normocytic, and macrocytic cells. The RBC markers used are set at 60 fL and 120 fL. RBCs with a volume less than the former are characterized as microcytic, and red cells with a volume greater than 120 fL are characterized as macrocytic. Values within the range of 60 and 120 fL are normocytic.

The RBC volume histogram provides for the MCV and RDW measurements. The histogram has a range of 0 to 200 fL. Samples with normal values exhibit a bell-shaped curve between 60 and 120 fL. The MCV is the mean of the

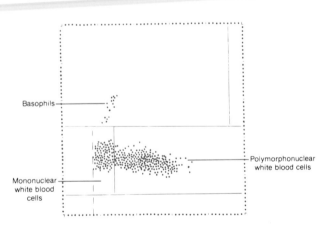

Basophils

Mononuclear white blood cells

Polymorphonuclear white blood cells

➤ **FIGURE 29–10**   Technicon H-1 cytogram for basophil/lobularity. (From Brown, BA: Hematology: Principles and Procedures, ed 6. Lea & Febiger, Philadelphia, 1993, p 374, with permission.)

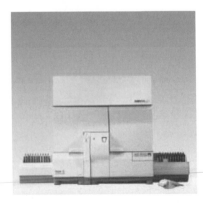

➤ **FIGURE 29–11**   Bayer ADVIA 120 System. (Courtesy of Bayer Corporation, Diagnostic Division, Tarrytown, NY.)

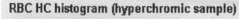

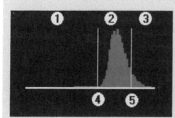

RBC HC histogram (hyperchromic sample)

① ② ③

1 Hypochromic region
2 Normochromic region
3 Hyperchromic region
4 28 g/dL marker
5 41 g/dL marker

④ ⑤

➤ **FIGURE 29–12** Bayer ADVIA 120 RBC hemoglobin concentration histogram demonstrating hyperchromia. (Courtesy of Bayer Corporation, Diagnostics Division, Tarrytown, NY.) Abbreviation: HC = Hemoglobin concentration

RBC volume histogram. In the case of a decreased MCV with increased numbers of microcytic red cells, the histogram will be skewed to the left, indicating red cells with volumes less than 60 fL. Conversely, in the case of an increased MCV, the histogram will be skewed to the right, indicating the presence of macrocytic red cells with volumes greater than 120 fL. The RDW is a measurement of anisocytosis and is calculated from the CV of the red cell population. The RDW will be flagged when the value exceeds 16%.

Reticulocyte Analysis

The respective aliquot for reticulocyte enumeration travels from the retic reaction chamber through the flow cell, where low-angle light scatter (2 to 3), high-angle light scatter (5 to 15), and absorption measurements take place. The two former measurements are proportional to cell size and hemoglobin concentration, respectively, and the latter measurement (light absorption) is proportional to ribonucleic acid (RNA) content in that stained reticulocytes absorb more light than mature red cells. The results of these three parameters are plotted on a retic volume histogram by cell size only, with a range of 0 to 200 fL.

Platelet Analysis

Platelet enumeration takes place in the RBC reaction chamber. The respective aliquot of sample passes through the flow cell, where low-angle and high-angle light scatter are detected and electronically amplified. In the case of platelets, low-angle light scatter is amplified 30 times, and high-angle light scatter is amplified 12 times. Using the Mie theory[27] of light scattering for homogenous spheres, the low-angle and high-gain (amplified signals) scatter is converted into cell volume and high-angle and high-gain scatter is converted to a refractive index. The ADVIA 120 produces a platelet scatter cytogram that plots the data respective to cell volume and refractive index, and a platelet map grid that lists ranges for cell volume (0 to 30 fL) and refractive index (1.3500 to 1.4000). The actual platelet count comprises both normal-sized platelets and large platelets. Other cellular debris, such as RBC fragments and ghost cells, is excluded from the count.

White Blood Cell Analysis

The total WBC count is measured from two reaction chambers, the peroxidase chamber and the BASO/lobularity chamber. In the peroxidase chamber, a constant volume of sample passes through the flow cell (Fig. 29–13), where ab-

Peroxidase Flowcell

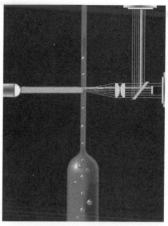

Peroxidase Cytogram

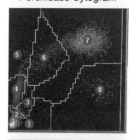

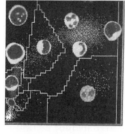

1 Noise
2 Nucleated Red Blood Cells
3 Platelet Clumps
4 Lymphocytes and Basophils
5 Large Unstained Cells
6 Monocytes
7 Neutrophils
8 Eosinophils

➤ **FIGURE 29–13** Bayer ADVIA 120 peroxidase sheath depicts the sample stream as two fluids pass through the flow cell. (Courtesy of Bayer Corporation, Diagnostics Division, Tarrytown, NY.)

sorption and forward light scattering are measured. The former is a measurement of peroxidase staining of WBCs (the cells absorb light proportional to the amount of peroxidase stain present), and the latter measures WBC size. The instrument produces a PEROX cytogram, which is divided into 100 counting channels on each axis. Light absorption is depicted on the x axis, and forward scatter on the y axis. This results in distinct populations of clusters of cells that can further be categorized by position, area, and density on the cytogram (see Fig. 29–13).

In the BASO/lobularity reaction chamber, a specific aliquot of sample is passed through the flow cell, where low-angle light scatter and high-angle light scatter are measured. The size of the cell or nucleus and nuclear configuration (nuclear shape and cell density) are analyzed. The BASO cytogram consists of 50 channels on each axis. High-angle light scatter or nuclear configuration is plotted on the x axis and low-angle light scatter or cell size is plotted on the y axis. As a result, distinct clusters of cells are formed and analyzed respective of the cells position, area, and density on the cytogram. The number of cells or nuclei, or both, are then enumerated in each cluster.

Morphology Flagging

Morphology flags on the ADVIA 120 Analyzer are programmed based on flagging algorithms for the purpose of alerting laboratory personnel to suspect or abnormal samples. When a flag is triggered, the operator should perform the prescribed corrective action before results are reported. Flagging is divided into three entities: suspect morphology, flag, and triggering criteria. Table 29–7 gives examples of morphology flagging by the ADVIA 120 analyzer.

➤ EVALUATION OF BLOOD SPECIMENS BY ELECTRONIC RESISTANCE DETECTION WITH HYDRODYNAMIC FOCUSING TECHNIQUE: THE SYSMEX SE-SERIES

Sysmex instruments produced a comprehensive series of multiparameter hematology analyzers including, but not limited to, the following: the NE-Series (NE-8000/7000/6000/5500/4500), the SE-Series (SE-9000/9500), and automated reticulocyte analyzers (R-3500/R-500), released in 1988, 1995, and 1998, respectively.[28–30] Both SE-Series analyzers are tabletop automated instruments capable of mixing blood sample tubes, scanning sample barcode identification labels, and sampling from blood collection tubes using a cap-piercing, closed tube sampling apparatus. The instruments contain two major components: the main unit, and the data management system. Each instrument contains two communication ports for interfacing with a laboratory information system (LIS) computer and data printers. The primary difference between the SE-9000 and the SE-9500 is that the SE-9000 focuses on samples analyzed within 24 hours post–sample collection, whereas the SE-9500 permits analysis of blood samples from 24 to 72 hours post–sample collection and may be configured to include an optional automated reticulocyte analyzer, the RAM-1. The Sysmex RAM-1 succeeded the previous models of automated reticulocyte analyzers (R-1000, R-3000 and R-3500). In 1999, Sysmex released two more technically advanced, computerized, fully automated hematology instruments: the Sysmex™ XE-2100 and SF-3000. The XE-2100 is a compact, benchtop hematology analyzer that provides more functions and more reportable parameters than those instruments previously released by Sysmex. The XE-2100 analyzer reports a total of 32 analytic parameters, including the routine CBC and five-part WBC differential, an NRBC count, and reticulocyte analysis. The SF-3000 is designed to provide accurate analytic results on 23 parameters and to detect the presence of hematologic abnormalities in the blood samples.

The following is a brief discussion of the Sysmex SE-9000 model (Fig. 29–14). The SE-9000 provides test results for 21 parameters composed of CBC parameters, analytic platelet and red cell parameters, WBC differential parameters, a WBC scattergram, and histograms. Relative percentages and absolute values for neutrophils, monocytes, lymphocytes, basophils, and eosinophils are reported, and additional interpretive reports provide comprehensive information for each test sample. Interpretive comments are very useful in assessment of data analysis and identification of abnormal samples.[31]

Red Cell and Platelet Histogram Analysis

The SE-series instrument generates RBC and platelet histograms along with the following associated parameters: RBC distribution width by standard deviation (RDW-SD), RBC distribution width by coefficient of variation (RDW-CV) and mean platelet volume (MPV). Red cell histograms are generated in a manner similar to that used for platelets. The principal differences occur in the methods used to eliminate interferences of small red cells on the platelet count and histogram and in the particle selection for generating the histogram.

To size and count the red cells and platelets, the direct current (DC) electrical impedance blood cell counting method is enhanced by hydrodynamic focusing with sheath flow technology. The DC method enhanced by hydrodynamic focusing eliminates problems known to be associated with the

---

➤ Table 29-7
EXAMPLES OF MORPHOLOGY FLAGGING BY THE ADVIA 120 HEMATOLOGY ANALYZER

Suspect Morphology	Flag	Triggering Criteria
Anisocytosis	ANISO	RDW ≥ 16%
Atypical lymphocytes	ATYP	% LUC ≥ 4.5 and % LUC ≥ (% BLASTS plus 1.5)
Blasts	BLAST	% BLASTS 1.5% to 5% and % LUC ≥ 4.5%, or % BLASTS ≥ 5% WBCB
Hemoglobin concentration variation	HCVAR	HDW ≥ 3.4 g/dL
Hyperchromia	HYPER	% HYPER ≥ 4%
Hypochromia	HYPO	% HYPO ≥ 4%
Immature granulocytes	IG	((% NEUT + % EOS) − % PMN) ≥ 5%
Large platelets	LPLT	% LPLT > 10% PLT
Macrocytosis	MACRO	% MACRO ≥ 2.5%
Microcytosis	MICRO	% MICRO ≥ 2.5%
Platelet clumps	PLT-CLM	Clumps count > 300

Abbreviations: RDW = red cell distribution width; LUC = large unstained cells; HDW = hemoglobin distribution width; NEUT = neutrophils; EOS = eosinophils; PMN = polymorphonuclear cell; LPLT = large platelet

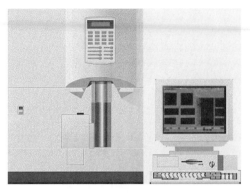

➤ **FIGURE 29–14** Sysmex SE-9000 System. (Courtesy of Sysmex™ Reagents America, Inc, Los Alamitos, CA, with permission.)

DC detection method, such as inconsistent sizing, coincidence, and recirculating cells. Sysmex SE Series systems obtain hemoglobin values by use of a cyanide-free, nontoxic reagent (Sulfolyser). Hemoglobin values are determined by absorption measurements at 555 nm using a diode light source and detector. The Sysmex SE-9000 uses a separate channel for the WBC count and utilizes the DC electrical impedance particle counting method. Electronic discriminators, also known as gates, float between cell populations and unwanted debris, such as red cell stroma and platelets.

Leukocyte Analysis

The principles used in generating the WBC differential scattergram include simultaneous measurements of WBCs by radiofrequency (RF) and DC detection methods for identifying and delineating WBC populations. There are separate detector channels for the determination of cell populations. The RF method detects and sizes lyse-treated cells based on density and nuclear size, whereas the DC method sizes the entire cell, nucleus, and cytoplasm. The first DC-RF detection channel determines lymphocytes, monocytes, and granulocytes. These results plus eosinophil and basophil determinations result in the five-part WBC differential. The second channel is used with a special reagent for detecting and dis-

criminating the presence of immature (IMI) WBCs, such as shift to the left, blasts, and platelet clumping.

Flagging

Flagging of abnormal samples is provided in two areas of each sample report. The presence of a NEGATIVE flag indicates the sample analysis successfully passed all criteria used for analyzing results and is free from any instrument detectable abnormalities. A POSITIVE flag, however, is an indication that one or more abnormalities have been detected by the instrument. Consequently, the laboratory must review the results and apply the appropriate established protocol.

Flagging messages are divided into three separate codes: MORPH, DIFF, and COUNT. MORPH flags refer to the cell distribution analysis within the DIFF and IMI scattergrams and histograms; DIFF flags are related to the numerical expression of the WBC differential analysis; and COUNT flags are messages related to numerical expression of the blood cell count and associated values. Table 29–8 depicts examples of flagging messages in a WBC analysis.

The Sysmex R-3500 Reticulocyte Analyzer

The R-3500 can process 120 samples in 1 hour and is compatible with the SE-Series hematology analyzer for high automation capabilities. This instrument is compact and provides for three modes of operation: (1) sampler mode, (2) manual mode, and (3) capillary mode. The sampler mode automatically mixes and samples the specimen by use of a cap-piercing device and requires 25 μL of blood. The manual mode is sampled from an opened tube for single sample analysis and requires 100 μL of blood. The capillary mode accommodates prediluted samples and requires 40 μL of blood.

Technology for the R-3500 utilizes an argon laser and flow cytometry as well as a fluorescent dye, auramine-O. Red cells are stained with the fluorescent dye and illuminated by the argon laser. This produces a specific wavelength intensity or forward fluorescence directly proportional to a quantity of RNA in each cell. Electronic signals are generated by

➤ **Table 29-8**
EXAMPLES OF FLAGGING MESSAGES GENERATED BY SYSMEX ASSOCIATED WITH WBC ANALYSIS

Message	Display	Primary Triggers	Code
Neutropenia	Neutro ↓	Neut#	DIFF
Neutrophilia	Neutro ↑	Neut#	DIFF
Lymphopenia	Lymph ↓	Lymph#	DIFF
Lymphocytosis	Lymph ↑	Lymph#	DIFF
Monocytosis	Mono ↑	Mono#	DIFF
Eosinophilia	Eo ↑	Eo#	DIFF
Basophilia	Bas ↑	Bas#	DIFF
Leukocytopenia	Leuko ↓	WBC#	COUNT
Leukocytosis	Leuko ↑	WBC#	COUNT
Wbc Abn Scatt	Wbc Abn Scatt	Scattergram	MORPH

Abbreviations: Neut = neutrophil; Eo = eosinophil; WBC = white blood cell; Wbc Abn Scat = abnormal white blood cell scattergram; Lymph = lymphocyte

the scattered light and fluorescent intensity and plotted on a two-dimensional scattergram. The red cell population is separated into mature erythrocytes, reticulocytes, and platelets. Forward fluorescence is plotted on the x axis and forward scatter (cell size) on the y axis. Results are reported as red cell count, reticulocyte number (RET#), and reticulocyte percent. Additionally, this analyzer has a unique feature of dividing the reticulocyte population into three subpopulations: low fluorescence ratio (LFR), middle fluorescence ratio (MFR), and high fluorescence ratio (HFR). The reticulocyte maturation can be assessed from these subpopulations, whereby the youngest reticulocytes are associated with the HFR and the most mature with the LFR.

➤ EVALUATION OF BLOOD SPECIMENS BY MULTIANGLE POLARIZED SCATTER SEPARATION (M.A.P.S.S.) TECHNOLOGY: THE CELL-DYN DIFFERENTIAL (ABBOTT CELL-DYN MODELS 3200, 3500R, AND 4000)

CELL-DYN is the brand name for hematology systems developed and manufactured by Abbott Laboratories, Abbott Park, Illinois, U.S.A. The CELL-DYN analyzers include the CELL-DYN 3200, 3500R, and 4000, among others. CELL-DYN uses its proprietary Multi-Angle-Polarized-Scatter-Separation (M.A.P.S.S.) technology to identify and count the five white cell subpopulations, red blood cells, and platelets.

The CELL-DYN 3200 automated hematology analyzer uses two independent measurement channels for analysis of blood specimens. The optical channel is used for determining the WBC, nuclear optical count (NOC), and RBC/PLT data. A second, separate channel is used for hemoglobin (HGB) determination. The analyzer aspirates the sample and separates it into three separate, diluted volumes to analyze for (1) WBC, (2) RBC/PLT, and (3) HGB. WBC and RBC/PLT are analyzed in the optical flow cell (Fig. 29–15).

When the sample suspension is injected into the faster-moving cell-free liquid (sheath fluid), the cells are forced into single file by a process known as *hydrodynamic focusing*. The cells are passed through the flow cell where the light scatter from the cell is measured. The light source is a vertically polarized helium neon laser. The instrument measures both types of forward-angle light scatter (0 and 10 degrees, or narrow angle) and both types of orthogonal (side) light scatter (90 degrees) and depolarized (90 degrees D; Fig. 29–16). Different cell types scatter the light at varying angles, giving information about cell size, internal structure, granularity, and surface morphology. The analyzer uses M.A.P.S.S. technology, which provides a WBC optical count (WOC).

WBC Optical Count/WBC Differential
The CELL-DYN 3200 enumerates WBCs that scatter light at 0 degrees. Light scattered at 0, 10, 90, and 90 degrees D differentiate the WBCs into five subpopulations (neutrophils, monocytes, lymphocytes, eosinophils, and basophils). Briefly, data from the complexity (10) and granularity (90) channels are used to classify each cell as mononuclear. This would include degranulated basophils or polymorphonuclear cells. Next, the eosinophils are separated from the neutrophils

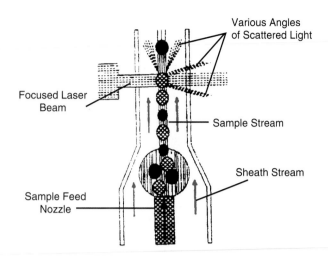

➤ FIGURE 29–15 A drawing of the CELL-DYN 3200 optical flow cell. In the flow cytometer, a cell suspension is transferred from the mixing chamber through a sample tube into a special flow chamber with a minute opening at the tip. Then, the suspension is injected into a stream of rapid-moving, cell-free liquid known as sheath fluid. The two liquids travel at different rates of speed and do not intermingle. The special geometry of the flow cell and flow rate of the sheath forces the cells into a single file. This process is called hydrodynamic focusing. (From CELL-DYN 3200 Operator's Manual, Section 3, Principles of Operation Flow Cytometry, pp 3–9, 91401818-November 1997. Abbott Laboratories, Inc, Abbott Park, IL, with permission.)

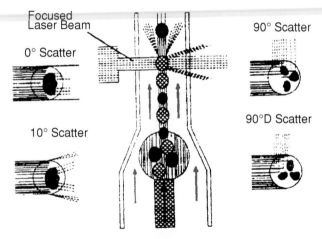

➤ FIGURE 29–16 A drawing illustrating the measurement of light scattered during the WBC optical measurement process. The WBC count is measured by enumerating the number of occurrences found above a hardware threshold in the 0° channel. The white cell data, presented graphically as a scatterplot, differentiates WBCs into five subpopulations: neutrophils, lymphocytes, monocytes, basophils, and eosinophils. (From CELL-DYN 3200 Operator's Manual, Section 3, Principles of Operation Flow Cytometry, pp 3–12, 91401818–November 1997. Abbott Laboratories, Inc, Abbott Park, IL, with permission.)

using data from the 90D channel. Then, the mononuclear cells are separated into lymphocytes, monocytes, and basophils using the size (0) and complexity (10) measurements. Finally, all of the data are combined and displayed on a "dot plot," or scattergram, where the instrument assigns a specific color to each of the aforementioned cell types, thus allowing for easy interpretation of the WBC differential results.

Nuclear Optical Count
It is difficult to accurately measure samples containing fragile WBCs because of the rapid breakdown of cells dur-

ing the measurement process. In this case, an alternative method of testing these samples is the nuclear optical count (NOC). Instead of using the WOC, when fragile WBCs are suspected, the HGB sample segment is transferred to the optical flow cell instead of being sent to a waste chamber. While in the HGB flow cell, the HGB reagent lyses the cytoplasmic membrane of the WBCs, but allows the nuclear membrane to remain intact. This results in a greater stability of the WBCs in the sample.

RBC and Platelet Measurements

The RBC count and distribution from the 0-degree channel are used to determine the MCV. The total platelet count is taken from the 10-degree channel.

Hemoglobin Measurement

The HGB channel is used for the colorimetric determination of hemoglobin. A light-emitting diode (LED) with a wavelength of 540 nm is the light source used. A photo detector measures the light that is transmitted through the sample.

CELL-DYN 3500R

The CELL-DYN 3500R uses four independent measurement channels for blood sample analysis. Like the CELL-DYN 3200, one channel is the optical channel for determining the WOC and a separate hemoglobin channel is used for determining HGB concentration. Two additional impedance channels are used for determining the WBC impedance count (WIC) and RBC/PLT data.

Dual WBC Analysis

The CELL-DYN 3500R uses the same WOC and NOC methodologies as does the CELL-DYN 3200. An additional impedance channel is used for determining the WIC. WIC and WOC results are compared by the instrument. If there is a statistically significant difference, a warning flag will be displayed. Differences may be caused by the presence of abnormal cells such as fragile WBCs, nucleated RBCs, and lyse-resistant RBCs. By using these combined methodologies, abnormal cells can be better detected.

RBC/PLT Analysis

RBCs and PLTs are sized and counted by the aperture impedance method. This method measures the electrical pulse generated by particles suspended in a conductive liquid as they pass through the aperture. The sample is first diluted in a fluid that conducts electricity. The cells are then drawn through a small opening or aperture. With an electrode situated on each side of the aperture, an electrical current is passed between the two electrodes. As each cell passes through the aperture, the current flow between the two electrodes decreases, producing an electrical pulse whose amplitude is proportional to the size of the cell.

Hemoglobin Analysis

After the WIC count is completed, samples from WIC dilutions are transferred to an HGB flow cell. In the flow cell, light is reflected from an LED source and the absorbance of the samples is read at 540 nm. The absorbance is directly proportional to the concentration of HGB in the sample.

CELL-DYN 4000

The CELL-DYN 4000 incorporates all of the technologies used in the CELL-DYN 3200 and 3500R models together

with fluorescence flow cytometry in one platform. This merger of technology created the possibility for new additional parameters. For example, DNA and RNA fluorescence can now be used to distinguish NRBCs from viable and nonviable WBCs. RNA fluorescence can also measure reticulocytes and the immature reticulocyte fraction (IRF). Optional random access tests are available for both reticulocyte and immunologic platelet counts. A hydrodynamically focused impedance method is employed for primary erythrocyte counts, secondary platelet counts, and erythrocyte and platelet size distribution analysis.

▶ QUALITY CONTROL AND QUALITY ASSURANCE MEASURES FOR AUTOMATED SCREENING DIFFERENTIAL INSTRUMENTS

Quality control measures for the automated screening differential consist of performing daily, monthly, and annual instrument maintenance procedures as specified by the manufacturer, and evaluating instrument and precision on a daily or per-shift basis with stabilized controls for which target values/mean standard deviation (SD) have been established.[32] Usually three levels of control material are analyzed to evaluate instrument performance over the spectrum of clinically relevant values.[33] In addition, establishing action limits for manual review of automated results is essential. Separate criteria for review of automated results should be established by each laboratory for adult and pediatric patient populations, as well as for oncology, acquired immunodeficiency syndrome (AIDS), and transplantation patients. Action limits on RDW, Hgb, and RBC count and indices may be included to trigger a morphological evaluation of blood films for RBC abnormalities. Similarly, action limits on platelet counts should be established to verify manually low automated platelet counts.

Participation in external quality assurance programs provided by manufacturers of quality control materials and the College of American Pathologists (CAP) Survey Program should be included in a comprehensive quality control program.[34] Participation is essential for meeting the requirements of accrediting and regulatory agencies such as Joint Commission on Accreditation of Hospitals (JCAHO) and the Clinical Laboratory Improvement Amendments of 1988 (CLIA '88). Comparison of laboratory performance with that of other laboratories evaluating aliquots of the same specimen by the same method (intralaboratory quality control) provides an independent assessment of instrument accuracy. Comparison of laboratory values with those reported by other institutions should include not only a comparison of the test result, but also, when applicable, a comparison of the SD. An increased SD may indicate problems in instrument performance, comprehensive instrument control, or maintenance, and problem logs can provide valuable information.

In an era of managed care and since the inception of diagnosis-related groups (DRGs) in 1983, modern hematology laboratories have needed to implement significant cost-containment measures. To reduce operating costs, laboratory managers have reevaluated their laboratories' current instrumentation and procedures, attempted to decrease the number of labor-intensive tests performed by laboratory personnel, and scrutinized laboratory productivity and performance capabilities. The results of cost-effectiveness studies have supported the selective process of replacing labor-intensive, routine clinical hematology procedures such as the manual leukocyte differential counts with automated three-part or five-part WBC histogram/scattergram differentials. Current trends point to increased hematology testing, requiring automated specimen processing, multitest analysis, and advances in data processing. Thus, in addition to the improved accuracy and precision of automated whole blood differential analysis, new advances in hematology analyzers are directed at improving laboratory safety, productivity, efficiency, and work flow. Because current automated analyzers with histogram differential capabilities generate comprehensive interpretive reports containing detailed information about abnormalities, careful evaluation of the data can provide an efficient screening tool. A review of the literature suggests that the newer hematology analyzers have become increasingly sophisticated and the chances of advanced automated blood cell analyzers missing a significant abnormality are small. Nevertheless, despite advanced technologies currently in use, artifactual and spurious results may still exist in hematologic test results even though in some cases, the utility of the automated differential for screening and monitoring patients has outperformed the routine manual differential in detecting hematologic abnormalities such as increased presence of NRBCs, eosinophilia, high percentages (more than 30%) of WBC blasts, and monocytosis.[35–37] In addition, the automated histogram/scattergram differential has reduced the statistical variability associated with the microscopic WBC differential method (200-cell count) based on the increased number of cells (more than 8000 cells) that are analyzed by automated differential analysis.[28] However, a number of research reports underscore the importance of the smear differential for confirming and reviewing automated results.[3–5] As such, the authors reaffirm the notion that each individual laboratory needs to establish appropriate criteria for manual review of automated differentials for pathologic samples.

Confirmatory evaluation of blood smears to identify abnormalities can be considerably more efficient and less labor-intensive with the help of automated differential results. Automated results can direct the technologist to focus on specific problems and troubleshoot for spurious and artifactual results that may arise in either quantitative or qualitative parameters. Artifactual hematologic abnormalities in laboratory test results can lead to serious complications as a result of an incorrect diagnosis and inappropriate treatment based on undetected, technically induced errors.[37,38] Improved features such as user-friendly computer software and enhanced software capabilities in terms of improved cell population separation, automated CD4 and CD8 counts, and automated reticulocyte counts are new features of the Coulter GEN S system.[20] In addition to the aforementioned improved features, bar-code sample identification, closed tube sampling, and greater sample throughput enhance overall laboratory safety, efficiency, and productivity. Moreover, these advanced features contribute to cost-effective laboratory operations and efforts to preserve quality patient care in the managed care environment. In the past, automated hematologic analysis of bone marrow aspirates and body fluids was not feasible because of limitations associated with samples containing very low cell counts, the presence of microclots and extraneous debris, decreased sample vol-

ume, and interferences by heparin anticoagulants. However, recent advances in hematology instrumentation have overcome such obstacles, and automated procedures for analyzing body fluids and bone marrow specimens are currently available.[39]

Whenever a hematologic disorder is suspected in a patient, the authors strongly suggest that clinical hematology laboratories continue to offer a microscopic examination of blood cells as an optional alternative to the automated method, regardless of the cost and labor-intensity factors associated with the manual procedure. As laboratory professionals, we need to be mindful that the automated laboratory services that we provide are valuable and effective in terms of minimizing the overall cost and maximizing the quality of patient care.[40] Finally, one's awareness of instrument limitations and clinical applications of automated hematology test results may prevent clinicians from ordering inappropriate test patterns and incorrect treatment of patients with suspected hematologic disorders.

➤ CASE STUDIES: LEUKOCYTE HISTOGRAM/SCATTERGRAM ANALYSIS

The following cases illustrate automated differential analysis of whole blood samples derived from Coulter (S Plus IV and STKS), Technicon (H-1), Abbott (CELL-DYN 4000), Sysmex (SE-9000), and Bayer (ADVIA 120) instruments. Although examples in this case studies section include the aforementioned Coulter, Technicon, Sysmex, Bayer, and Abbott hematology systems, a number of other automated hematology analyzers perform CBCs and histogram/scattergram differentials. Some of them include the HC-1020 (Danam, Dallas, TX); and the ABX series (ABX, Horsham, PA). The authors do not endorse any particular model. Owing to the abundance of advanced hematology analyzers and publication delay factors, it is not feasible to identify and individually discuss all of these systems. Information, instrument manuals, and descriptions of upgraded models are usually available from the manufacturers.

➤ CASE STUDY 1: GRANULOCYTOSIS/NEUTROPHILIA

Sysmex SE 9000 WBC scattergram (Fig. 29–17) illustrates a large granulocyte population, a small lymphocyte population, and a number of immature granulocytes. Along with an elevated WBC count, this illustration is consistent with a shift to the left.

Neutrophilia
Coulter STKS WBC scatterplot depicts neutrophilia (Fig. 29–18). WBCs, 30.5×10^9/L; 91% neutrophils. The manual differential analysis revealed 48% neutrophils, 24% bands, 10% metamyelocytes, 6% myelocytes, and 12% lymphocytes.

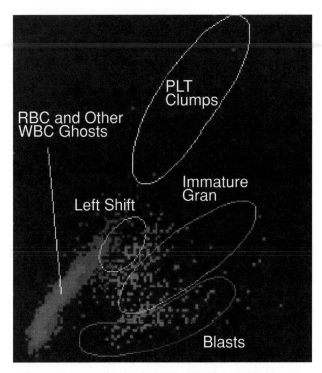

➤ **FIGURE 29–17** Sysmex SE 9000 graphic illustration of a scattergram depicting immature granulocytes and neutrophilia consistent with a shift to the left. (From Sysmex Reagents America, Inc, Los Alamitos, CA, with permission.)

➤ **CASE STUDY 2: ACUTE LYMPHOBLASTIC LEUKEMIA**

Examination of Coulter S Plus IV WBC histogram (Fig. 29–19) reveals a single WBC peak spanning the region between 50 and 150 fL. The shaded area represents the normal WBC distribution. An R2 flag alerts the operator to the skewed patient WBC distribution to the right of the normal lymphocyte peak. The R3 flag reflects the absence of a normal granulocyte peak. The manual differential analysis revealed the presence of 11% lymphoblasts, 50% lymphocytes, 32% neutrophils, 1% metamyelocytes, and 6% myelocytes.

Acute Lymphoblastic Leukemia

Coulter STKS WBC scatterplot (Fig. 29–20) demonstrates the presence of lymphoblasts at the top of the scatterplot, overlapping areas that would contain normal monocytes and neutrophils. A suspect blast flag was generated by the instrument. Manual differential showed 18% lymphocytes, 49% blasts, 23% neutrophils, and 10% monocytes.

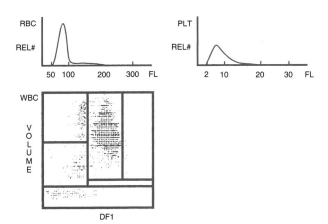

➤ **FIGURE 29–18** Coulter STKS WBC scatterplot depicting neutrophilia. WBC 30.5 × 10⁹/L, 91% neutrophils.

➤ **CASE STUDY 3: CHRONIC LYMPHOCYTIC LEUKEMIA**

Coulter STKS WBC scatterplot (Fig. 29–21) illustrates a case of chronic lymphocytic leukemia. Note the predominance of a lymphocytic population. Manual differential revealed 72% lymphocytes, 12% atypical lymphs, and 16% neutrophils.

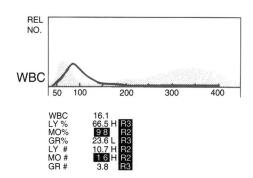

WBC	16.1		
LY %	66.5	H	R3
MO%	9.8		R2
GR%	23.6	L	R3
LY #	10.7	H	R2
MO #	1.6	H	R2
GR #	3.8		R3

➤ **FIGURE 29–19** Coulter S Plus IV histogram depicting acute lymphoblastic leukemia. The shaded area represents the normal WBC distribution. (From Pierre, RV: Section One: WBC case studies. In Pierre, RV (ed): Seminar and Case Studies: The Automated Differential. Coulter Electronics, Hialeah, FL, 1985, p 16, with permission.)

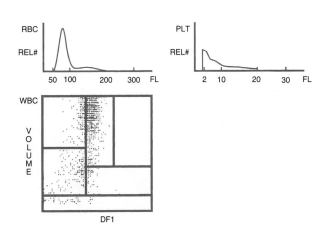

➤ **FIGURE 29–20** Coulter STKS WBC scatterplot demonstrating the presence of lymphoblasts at the top of the scatterplot overlapping areas that would contain normal monocytes and neutrophils. A suspect blast flag was generated by the instrument.

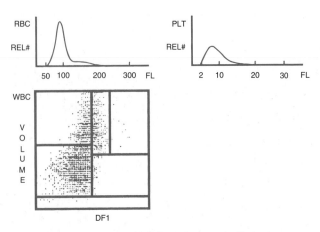

> **FIGURE 29–21**   Coulter STKS WBC scatterplot illustrating a case of chronic lymphocytic leukemia. Note the predominance of a lymphocytic population.

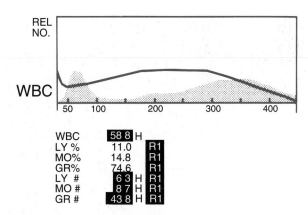

WBC	58 8	H	
LY %	11.0		R1
MO%	14.8		R1
GR%	74.6		R1
LY #	6 3	H	R1
MO #	8 7	H	R1
GR #	43 8	H	R1

> **FIGURE 29–23**   Coulter S Plus IV histogram illustrating a case of chronic myelocytic leukemia. The shaded area represents the normal WBC distribution. (From Pierre, RV: Section One: WBC case studies. In Pierre, RV (ed): Seminar and Case Studies: The Automated Differential. Coulter Electronics, Hialeah, FL, 1985, p 25, with permission.)

► CASE STUDY 4: ACUTE MYELOBLASTIC LEUKEMIA

Bayer ADVIA 120 WBC/peroxidase and basophil cytograms (Fig. 29–22) from the sample of a patient with acute myeloblastic leukemia. The instrument triggered an IG flag because the percentage of neutrophils plus eosinophils minus the total percentage of polymorphonuclear cells was greater than 5.0%.

► CASE STUDY 5: CHRONIC MYELOCYTIC LEUKEMIA

Coulter S Plus IV WBC histogram (Fig. 29–23) demonstrates a broadened curve extending through the mononuclear and immature granulocyte regions, and an elevation at the right of the normal lymphocyte peak. This irregularity is characteristic of the lymphopenia and granulocytosis associated with granulocytic immaturity, often seen in chronic myeloproliferative disorders. An R1 flag suggests the presence of nucleated RBCs and/or clumped platelets.

► CASE STUDY 6: CHRONIC MYELOCYTIC LEUKEMIA IN BLAST CRISIS

Coulter STKS WBC scattergram (Fig. 29–24) illustrates a case of chronic myelogenous leukemia in blast crisis. A suspect blast flag was generated by the instrument. A manual differential showed 35% blasts, 1% promyelocytes, 4% myelocytes, 1% metamyelocytes, 5% bands, 36% neutrophils, 10% basophils, 5% monocytes, and 3% lymphocytes. Note the presence of cells with increased volume overlapping regions normally containing monocytes and neutrophils.

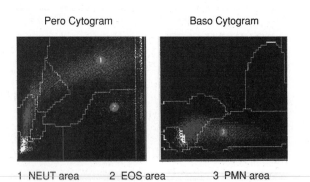

Pero Cytogram   **Baso Cytogram**

1 NEUT area   2 EOS area   3 PMN area

> **FIGURE 29–22**   Bayer ADVIA 120 peroxidase and basophil cytograms depicting a case of acute myeloblastic leukemia. (From Bayer Corporation, Diagnostics Division, Tarrytown, NY, with permission.)

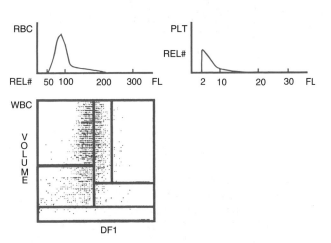

> **FIGURE 29–24**   Coulter STKS WBC scatterplot illustrating a case of chronic myelocytic leukemia in blast crisis. A suspect flag was generated by the instrument. Note the presence of cells with increased volume overlapping regions normally containing monocytes and neutrophils.

➤ CASE STUDY 7: INFECTIOUS MONONUCLEOSIS

The Coulter S Plus IV WBC histogram (Fig. 29–25) reveals an abnormal WBC distribution with a lymphocyte peak that was shifted to the right of normal, suggesting the presence of an abnormal lymphocyte/mononuclear population. The R2 flag is consistent with the presence of large atypical lymphocytes.

➤ CASE STUDY 8: MONOCYTOSIS

Coulter STKS WBC scatterplot (Fig. 29–26) depicts monocytosis. Note the increased concentration of cells in the monocyte region. Scan of the corresponding stained peripheral blood smear confirmed the presence of 24% monocytes.

➤ CASE STUDY 9: EOSINOPHILIA

Coulter STKS WBC scatterplot (Fig. 29–27). Note the increased number of cells in the eosinophil region. Manual differential analysis confirmed the presence of 10% eosinophils.

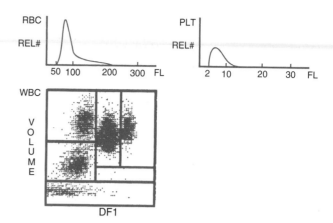

➤ **FIGURE 29–27** Coulter STKS WBC scatterplot. Note the increased number of cells in the eosinophil region.

➤ CASE STUDY 10: NUCLEATED RED BLOOD CELLS

By analyzing this graphic illustration of the Sysmex SE-9000 WBC scattergram, a large number of NRBCs are displayed (Fig. 29–28). Coulter STKS WBC scatterplot (Fig. 29–29) depicts an increase in particles appearing below the WBC threshold in a specimen containing NRBCs and Howell-Jolly bodies. Manual differential revealed 2% NRBCs, and occasional Howell-Jolly bodies.

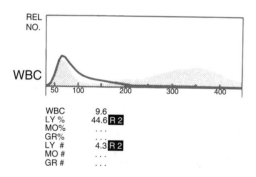

➤ **FIGURE 29–25** Coulter S Plus IV histogram depicting infectious mononucleosis. The shaded area represents the normal WBC distribution. (From Pierre, RV: Section One: WBC case studies. In Pierre, RV (ed): Seminar and Case Studies: The Automated Differential. Coulter Electronics, Hialeah, FL, 1985, p 12, with permission.)

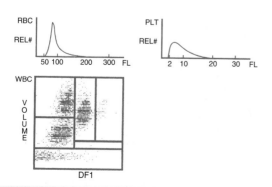

➤ **FIGURE 29–26** Coulter STKS WBC scatterplot depicting monocytosis. Note the increased concentration of cells in the monocyte region.

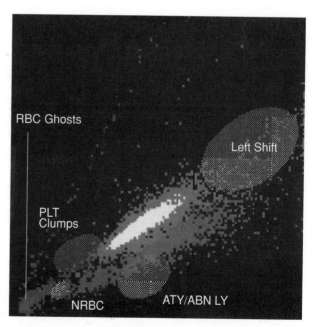

➤ **FIGURE 29–28** Sysmex SE-9000 graphic illustration of a scattergram depicting abnormalities associated with the presence of nucleated RBCs. (From Sysmex Reagents America, Inc, Los Alamitos, CA, with permission.)
Abbreviations: ATY/ABN LY = atypical abnormal lymphocytes; NRBC = nucleated red blood cell; PLT = platelet

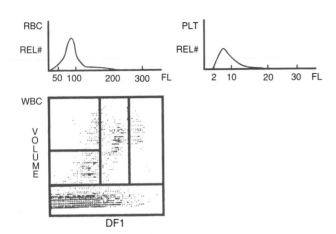

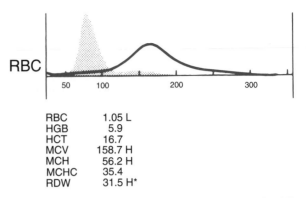

> **FIGURE 29–29**   Coulter STKS WBC scatterplot depicting an increase in particles appearing below the WBC threshold in a specimen containing nucleated red blood cells and Howell-Jolly bodies.

RBC	1.05 L
HGB	5.9
HCT	16.7
MCV	158.7 H
MCH	56.2 H
MCHC	35.4
RDW	31.5 H*

> **FIGURE 29–31**   Coulter S Plus IV RBC histogram depicting folic acid deficiency. The shaded area represents normal RBC volume distribution. (From Pierre, RV: Section One: WBC case studies. In Pierre, RV (ed): Seminar and Case Studies: The Automated Differential. Coulter Electronics, Hialeah, FL, 1985, p 45, with permission.)

➤ CASE STUDIES: RED CELL AND PLATELET ANALYSIS

The following histograms/cytograms represent case studies that depict some of the more frequently encountered RBC and platelet abnormalities.

➤ CASE STUDY 11: IRON-DEFICIENCY ANEMIA

Bayer ADVIA 120 RBC cytogram and histograms (Fig. 29–30) are consistent with iron-deficiency anemia. The instrument triggered the morphology flag HYPO that stands for hypochromia. When a flag is triggered, the operator should review the results and take the recommended action.

➤ CASE STUDY 12: FOLIC ACID DEFICIENCY

The Coulter S Plus IV RBC histogram (Fig. 29–31) demonstrates an abnormal shift to the right, suggesting macrocytosis. Note the extremely elevated MCV and RDW, reflecting marked macrocytosis and anisocytosis, respectively.

➤ CASE STUDY 13: COLD AGGLUTININS

The Coulter S Plus IV RBC histogram (Fig. 29–32) appears relatively normal except for a slight elevation at the far right of the curve. Red cell indices, however, are flagged with the letter "H," emphasizing marked elevations in the MCH and MCHC. In addition, RBC parameters show discrepancies among the RBC count, Hgb, and Hct, which normally differ by a factor of 3.[28] The Hct and the RBC count are disproportionately low, which is characteristic of cold agglutinins.

➤ CASE STUDY 14: SICKLE THALASSEMIA

The Coulter S Plus IV RBC histogram (Fig. 29–33) demonstrates an abnormal shift to the left of the RBC volume distribution, representing a moderate microcytosis. The RBC parameters are consistent with microcytic anemia (decreased MCV) and anisocytosis (increased RDW). In addition to iron deficiency, an increased RDW has been reported in patients with hemoglobin SS, hemoglobin SC, and sickle β thalassemia.[31]

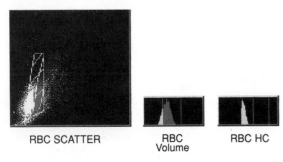

RBC SCATTER   RBC Volume   RBC HC

> **FIGURE 29–30**   Bayer ADVIA 120 cytogram and histograms illustrating a case of iron-deficiency anemia. A HYPO flag was triggered because the percent HYPO was greater than 4.0%. (From Bayer Corporation, Diagnostics Division, Tarrytown, NY, with permission.) Abbreviation: HC = hemoglobulin concentration

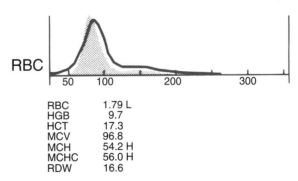

RBC	1.79 L
HGB	9.7
HCT	17.3
MCV	96.8
MCH	54.2 H
MCHC	56.0 H
RDW	16.6

> **FIGURE 29–32**   Coulter S Plus IV RBC histogram depicting abnormalities associated with the presence of cold agglutinins. The shaded area represents normal RBC volume distribution. (From Pierre, RV: Section One: WBC case studies. In Pierre, RV (ed): Seminar and Case Studies: The Automated Differential. Coulter Electronics, Hialeah, FL, 1985, p 55, with permission.)

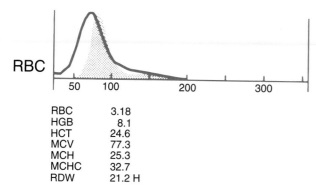

> ➤ **FIGURE 29–33** Coulter S Plus IV RBC histogram depicting a case of sickle thalassemia. The shaded area represents normal RBC volume distribution. (From Pierre, RV: Section One: WBC case studies. In Pierre, RV (ed): Seminar and Case Studies: The Automated Differential. Coulter Electronics, Hialeah, FL, 1985, p 45, with permission.)

RBC	3.18
HGB	8.1
HCT	24.6
MCV	77.3
MCH	25.3
MCHC	32.7
RDW	21.2 H

➤ CASE STUDY 15: POST-RBC TRANSFUSION

The Coulter STKS RBC histogram (Fig. 29–34) depicts a dimorphic RBC population in a patient who had received an RBC transfusion. Distinct microcytic and normocytic RBC populations are apparent.

➤ CASE STUDY 16: PLATELET CLUMPING

The Coulter S Plus IV PLT histogram (Fig. 29–35) appears normal. A PLT count, however, is not computed, based on disagreement among simultaneous independent automated PLT count determinations. The WBC histogram depicts interference of approximately 35 fL. This is confirmed by an R1 flag. Careful examination of the peripheral blood smear reveals the presence of PLT clumps. The RBC histogram is unremarkable.

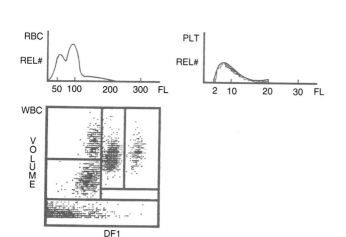

> ➤ **FIGURE 29–34** Coulter STKS RBC histogram depicting a dimorphic RBC population.

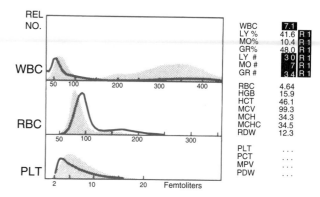

> ➤ **FIGURE 29–35** Coulter S Plus IV RBC histogram depicting abnormalities associated with platelet clumping. The shaded area represents normal platelet volume distribution. (From Pierre, RV: Section One: WBC case studies. In Pierre, RV (ed): Seminar and Case Studies: The Automated Differential. Coulter Electronics, Hialeah, FL, 1985, p 71, with permission.)

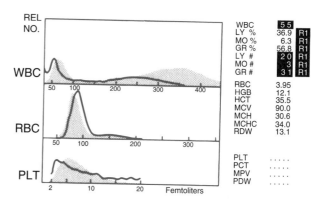

> ➤ **FIGURE 29–36** Coulter S Plus IV RBC histogram reflecting the presence of giant platelets. The shaded area represents normal platelet volume distribution. (From Pierre, RV: Section One: WBC case studies. In Pierre, RV (ed): Seminar and Case Studies: The Automated Differential. Coulter Electronics, Hialeah, FL, 1985, p 73, with permission.)

➤ CASE STUDY 17: GIANT PLATELETS

The Coulter S Plus IV PLT histogram (Fig. 29–36) is grossly abnormal and fails to return to baseline near 20 fL. The R1 flag reflects the high left shoulder of the WBC histogram. Examination of a stained peripheral blood film reveals the presence of giant platelets. The RBC histogram is unremarkable.

QUESTIONS

1. What is the main use of the leukocyte histogram differential?
   a. Diagnostic laboratory test for hematologic diseases
   b. Research tool for the routine hematology laboratory
   c. Replacement for the conventional manual differential
   d. Screening tool for hematologic diseases.

2. What should be the basis for the decision to accept an automated leukocyte histogram differential or to perform a conventional manual differential?
   a. Each individual laboratory's established criteria for manual review of automated differential analysis
   b. Availability of qualified technologists
   c. Laboratory workload
   d. Manufacturer's recommendation

3. A 47-year-old woman was admitted to the hospital for elective surgery. Her bleeding history was unremarkable. Results from her admission CBC revealed normal RBC parameters, an increased WBC count, and a decreased PLT count. The Coulter WBC histogram revealed a large shoulder to the left of the lymphocyte region accompanied by an R1 flag. The letter "H" appeared next to the WBC count. What should be done first, to verify these results?
   a. Examine the patient's blood smear for the presence of blasts and immature granulocytes, shift to the left.
   b. Request another sample from the patient and repeat the automated CBC and differential on the new sample.
   c. Notify the hematologist.
   d. Examine the patient's stained peripheral blood smear for platelet clumps and/or NRBCs.

4. An RBC histogram that shows an RBC distribution curve that is shifted to the left is characteristic of which of the following?
   a. Macrocytosis
   b. Anisocytosis
   c. Microcytosis
   d. Spherocytosis

5. In the WBC differential report generated by Technicon instruments, increased numbers of LUCs can include:
   1. Variant lymphocytes
   2. Promyelocytes
   3. Blasts
   4. Rubricytes
      a. 1, 2, 3
      b. 1, 3
      c. 2, 4
      d. 4 only

6. Which of the following best describes the principle of the Coulter Model STKS?
   a. Laser and light scatter
   b. Volume, cell size, and cytochemistry
   c. Volume, conductivity, and light scatter
   d. Laser and immunofluorescence

7. The RDW represents a parameter that quantifies relative:
   a. Macrocytosis
   b. Anisocytosis
   c. Platelet size
   d. Microcytosis

8. The MPV and PDW are parameters describing:
   a. White cell size
   b. Red cell size
   c. Platelet size
   d. Multiple cell size

9. Region flags or R flags indicate which of the following:
   1. A decreased RBC count
   2. Specific locations of abnormalities in the WBC size distribution
   3. Erroneous results
   4. Overlapping of two or more of the cell populations at the four threshold areas of the WBC size distribution histogram
      a. 1, 2, 3
      b. 1, 3
      c. 2, 4
      d. 4 only

10. Which of the following best describes the principle of the Technicon H-6000 and H-1?
    a. Electrical impedance, volume, and conductivity
    b. Flow cytometry, cytochemistry, and light scatter
    c. Chemiluminesence and laser cell counting
    d. Cell volume and light scatter

11. The Coulter Model S Plus IV differentiates lymphocytes, granulocytes, and mononuclear cells based on differences in:
    a. Overall cell size
    b. Cytoplasmic size
    c. Nuclear size and cytoplasmic complexity
    d. Nuclear size

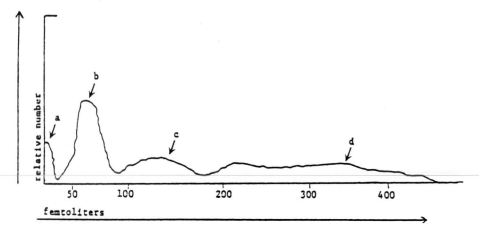

See question 12.

12. Which area of the cell size distribution WBC histogram from a Coulter analyzer illustrated on page 612 is appropriate for a mononuclear population curve?
    a. a
    b. b
    c. c
    d. d

13. Where does platelet enumeration take place in the Bayer ADVIA 120 hematology analyzer?
    a. Peroxidase reaction chamber
    b. RBC reaction chamber
    c. Hemoglobin reaction chamber
    d. Basophil reaction chamber

14. Which fluorescent dye is used to stain reticulocytes in the Sysmex R-3500?
    a. Fluorescein isothionate
    b. Propidium iodide
    c. Auramine-O
    d. Phycoerythrin

technique to size and count red blood cells and platelets.
➤ CELL-DYN hematology analyzers from Abbott Laboratories use multiangle polarized scatter separation technology (M.A.P.S.S.).
➤ Quality control procedures should be established according to each institution's criteria.
➤ Establishing criteria for review of automated results should be established for each institution.
➤ Criteria to detect spurious results should be established by each individual laboratory to prevent the reporting of erroneous results.

ACKNOWLEDGMENTS

The authors would like to acknowledge and thank the Bayer Corporation, Sysmex Corporation of America, and Abbott Laboratories for their contributions to this chapter.

References

1. Hyun, BH, et al: Practical Hematology. WB Saunders, Philadelphia, 1975, p 193.
2. O'Connor, BH: A Color Atlas and Instruction Manual of Peripheral Blood Cell Morphology. Williams & Wilkins, Baltimore, MD, 1984, p 1.
3. Watson, JS, and Davis, RA: Evaluation of the Technicon H-1 hematology system. Lab Med 18:316, 1987.
4. Miers, MK, et al: Evaluation of the Coulter S Plus IV three-part differential as a screening tool in a tertiary care hospital. Am J Clin Pathol 87:745, 1987.
5. Girswold, DJ, and Champagne, VD: Evaluation of the Coulter S-Plus IV three-part differential in an acute care hospital. Am J Clin Pathol 84:49, 1985.
6. Greendyke, RM, et al: A comparison of differential white blood cell counts using manual technique and the Coulter S-Plus IV. Am J Clin Pathol 84:348, 1985.
7. Van Hove, L: Which hematology analyzer do you need? Lab Hematol 4:32, 1998.
8. Bowen, KL, et al: Platelet clumps, nucleated red cells, and leukocyte counts: A comparison between the Abbott CELL-DYN 4000 and Coulter STKS. Lab Hematol 4:7, 1998.
9. Bolinger, P: The Technicon H-1 hematology analyzer: Sensitivity and specificity of blast identification in peripheral blood. In Simson, E, et al (ed): Proceedings of the Technicon H-1 Hematology Symposium. Technicon Instruments Corp, New York, 1985, p 39.
10. Kalish, RJ, and Becker, K: Evaluation of the Coulter S-Plus IV three-part differential in a community hospital, including criteria for its use. Am J Clin Pathol 86:751,1986.
11. Gauvin, GP, et al: Evaluation of the SYSMEX CC-800/PDA-410 system with trimodal histogram for white cell differential analysis. Lab Med 18:373, 1987.
12. Buttarello, M, et al: Evaluation of four automated hematology analyzers: A comparative study of differential counts (imprecision and inaccuracy). Am J Clin Pathol 97:345, 1992.
13. Lai, AP, et al: Automated leukocyte differential counts in acute leukemia: A comparison of the Hematolog D, H600 and Coulter S-Pus IV. Clin Lab Haematol 8:33, 1986.
14. Dwewinko, B: Utility of the Technicon H-1 system in malignant disease. In Simson, E, et al (ed): Proceedings of the Technicon H-1 Hematology Symposium, Technicon Instruments Corp, New York, 1985, p 23.
15. Hoyer, J, et al: Detection and classification of acute leukemia by the Coulter STKS hematology analyzer. Am J Clin Pathol 91:352, 1996.
16. Hope, E: A study to evaluate the accuracy and reliability of the Coulter histogram differential for monitoring human oncology samples. State University of New York at Stony Brook, Stony Brook, NY, December 1987 (unpublished report).
17. Nelson L, et al: Laboratory evaluation of differential white blood cell count information from the Coulter S-Plus IV and Technicon H-1 in patient populations requiring rapid "turnaround" time. Am J Clin Pathol 91:563, 1989.
18. Payne, BA, and Pierre, RV: Using the three-part differential: Part I, investigating the possibilities. Lab Med 17:459, 1986.
19. Payne, BA, and Pierre, RV: Using the three-part differential: Part II. Implementation of the system. Lab Med 17: 517, 1986.
20. Kessler, C, et al: Performance of the COULTER GENS System's white cell differential on an abnormal specimen data set. Lab Hematol 3:32, 1997.
21. Ross, DW, and Bentley, SA; Evaluation of an automated hematology system (Technicon H-1). Arch Pathol Lab Med 110:803, 1986.
22. Besson, I, et al: Differential leukocyte count (DLC) performance evaluation of the Sysmex SE-9000 hematology workstation. Lab Hematol 2:22, 1996.
23. Pierre, RV: Section One: WBC case studies. In Pierre, RV (ed): Seminar and Case Studies: The Automated Differential. Coulter Electronics, Hialeah, FL, 1985, p 7.
24. Bessman, JD: Red cells. In Bessman, JD (ed): Automated Blood Counts and Differentials. John Hopkins University Press, Baltimore, MD, 1988, pp 9–20.
25. Bessman, JD: Platelets. In Bessman, JD (ed): Automated Blood Counts and Differentials. John Hopkins University Press, Baltimore, MD, 1988, pp 57–65.
26. Perkins, ML, and DeSantis, DE: Special stains and cytochemistry. In Har-

SUMMARY CHART

➤ Automated differential analysis is an important screening tool in the laboratory but does not replace the necessity for the manual procedure.
➤ Automated differential analysis is currently based on cell volume and characteristics in cell light scattering and cytochemistry.
➤ Coulter VCS technology uses three independent energy sources, including electrical impedance to measure volume, light-scattering characteristics for determination of cell structure and shape, and conductivity (RF) for differentiation of white blood cell subpopulations.
➤ Leukocyte histogram differentials quantify and separate white blood cell subpopulations.
➤ Red cell histograms quantitate red blood cells and calculate cell size (MCV) and red cell distribution width (RDW) as well as measure hemoglobin, including mean corpuscular hemoglobin (MCH) and mean corpuscular hemoglobin concentration (MCHC).
➤ Platelet histograms quantitate and display parameters involving size and uniformity of platelets.
➤ Region flags, backlighting, and suspect message flags alert the technologist to areas in need of further review.
➤ Technicon automated blood analyzers are based on principles of optical flow cytometry, cytochemistry, and light scattering.
➤ Bayer ADVIA 120 hematology analyzer uses Unifluidics technology.
➤ Sysmex automated blood analyzers use direct current (DC) and a hydrodynamic focusing

mening, DM (ed): Clinical Hematology and Fundamentals of Hemostasis. FA Davis, Philadelphia, 1992, p 645.

27. Villarreal, C, et al: Mie scattering and the physical mechanisms of sonoluminescence. Phys Rev E Stat Phys Plasma Fluids Relat Interdiscip Topics 61:403, 2000.

28. Thalheimer-Scherrer, R, et al: Automated five-part white blood cell differential counts: Efficiency of software-generated white blood cell suspect flags of the hematology analyzers Sysmex SE-9000, Sysmex NE-8000, and Coulter STKS. Arch Pathol Lab Med 121:573, 1997.

29. Lamb, AA, et al: Performance Characteristics of the Sysmex NE-8000 Automated Hematology Analyzer. A Hematology Monograph. Baxter Diagnostics, McCaw Park, IL, 1990, pp 1–14.

30. Butterello, M, et al: Sysmex SE-9000 hematology analyzer: Performance evaluation on leukocyte differential counts using an NCCLS H20-A protocol. Am J Clin Pathol, 108:674, 1997.

31. Automated Hematology Analyzer SE-9000, No. 461–2455-9. Kobe, Japan, Toa Medical Electronics Co. Ltd, 1994 (operator's manual).

32. Rodak, BF: Diagnostic Hematology. WB Saunders, Philadelphia, 1995, p 45.

33. Ward, PG, et al: Standardization for routine blood counting—the role of interlaboratory trials. In Cavill, I (ed): Methods in Hematology Quality Control. Churchill-Livingstone, New York, 1982, p 102.

34. Rickets, C: Intralaboratory quality control using control samples. In Cavill, I (ed): Methods in Hematology Quality Control. Churchill-Livingstone, New York, 1982, p 151.

35. Cox, CJ, et al: Evaluation of the Coulter Counter Model S-lus IV. Am J Clin Pathol 84:297, 1985.

36. Payne, BA, and Pierre, RV. Using the three-part differential: Part II. Implementation of the system. Lab Med, 17:517, 1986.

37. Brigden, ML, and Dalal, BI: Morphologic abnormalities, pseudosyndromes, and spurious test results. Lab Med 30:397, 1999.

38. Brigden, ML, and Dalal, BI: Cell counter-related abnormalities. Lab Med 30:325, 1999.

39. D'Onofrio, G, et al: Automated analysis of bone marrow: Routine implementation and differences from peripheral blood. Lab Hematol 4:71, 1998.

40. Kisabeth, R: The future of laboratory hematology: Bleak or bright? Lab Hematol 4:106, 1998.

30

Applications of Flow Cytometry to Hematology and Hemostasis

Donna M. Gandour, PhD

BASIC CONCEPTS OF FLOW CYTOMETRY
 Sample Preparation
 Cytometer Operation
 Data Analysis

APPLICATIONS OF FLOW CYTOMETRY
 Lymphocyte Subsetting and CD4 T-Cell Enumeration
 Leukemia and Lymphoma Immunophenotyping
 Leukemia and Lymphoma DNA Content Analysis
 Hematopoietic Progenitor Cell Enumeration
 Flow Crossmatching
 Detection of Paroxysmal Nocturnal Hemoglobinuria
 Reticulocyte Enumeration
 Detection of Fetomaternal Hemorrhage
 Platelet Studies
 Emerging Applications for Antigen Quantitation
 Emerging Assays for Soluble Factors

OBJECTIVES

At the end of this chapter, the learner should be able to:

1. Define flow cytometry.
2. Define the four main tasks required for flow cytometric analysis.
3. Name the three main systems of the flow cytometer.
4. Define the parameters measured by flow cytometry.
5. Name four common fluorochromes used in flow cytometry.
6. Define the criteria used in the CD (cluster of differentiation) group classification.
7. Describe three different analysis methods for obtaining population percentages.
8. Describe how absolute counts are calculated using reference beads.
9. Define the DNA cell cycle phases measurable by flow cytometry.
10. Define the antibodies used for enumerating T helper cell populations.
11. Describe how flow cytometry is used for analyzing leukemias and lymphomas.
12. Describe the assay for stem cell enumeration.
13. Describe the assay for reticulocyte enumeration.
14. Describe an assay for platelet function.
15. Describe flow crossmatching.
16. Describe the assay used to detect paroxysmal nocturnal hemoglobinuria.
17. Describe the assay used to detect fetomaternal hemorrhage.
18. Describe emerging assays and applications.

Flow cytometry is a technology that provides rapid measurements (-metry) of physical characteristics of cells (cyto-) suspended in a moving fluid stream (flow). These measurements are made on a per-cell basis at rates of up to 10,000 cells per second. Because most hematologic tissues are easily prepared as cell suspensions, they are excellent candidates for flow cytometric analysis. Accordingly, results from a survey of 94 clinical flow cytometry laboratories revealed that the largest percentage (38%) were affiliated with the hematopathology division.[1] For the remainder of the flow labora-tories, 22% were affiliated with immunopathology, 25% were independent, and 15% were associated with other departments. This chapter presents basic concepts of flow cytometry and focuses on applications related to hematology.

➤ BASIC CONCEPTS OF FLOW CYTOMETRY

Flow cytometric analysis can be broken down into four main tasks: preparing samples, operating the cytometer, analyzing data, and interpreting results. In clinical laboratories, these tasks can be performed by one to four individuals, depending on the organization of the laboratory and the expertise of the personnel. In many instances, the fourth task requires the expertise of a specialty physician. Attention to detail for each task, however, is critical for obtaining meaningful results. The next sections present general information related to these tasks. Specific details will be provided later as each application is discussed.

Sample Preparation

Because flow cytometry measures cellular characteristics, it is important that the sample handling and preparation methods preserve these characteristics. The cellular characteristics measured are surface area, granularity and internal complexity, and fluorescent colors. The fluorescent colors usually result from reactions with staining reagents. Cellular characteristics can be affected by specimen collection factors including the anticoagulant, the storage temperature, and the specimen age.

Specimen Collection and Handling

Specimen collection requirements vary based on the application. For example, for enumeration of leukocyte subpopulations, blood and marrow are usually collected in K_3-ethylene diaminetetraacetic acid (EDTA), stored at room temperature, and analyzed within 24 hours of collection. In contrast, for assays of cell function, sodium heparin is usually the anticoagulant of choice. Thus, it is important that each laboratory verify conditions for specimen stability for each type of assay performed.

Lymphoid tissue specimens are also analyzed by flow cytometry. The tissue is harvested and placed in a sterile container containing cold tissue culture medium. Next, it is disaggregated into a single-cell suspension by gentle teasing with forceps, followed by filtration through a 50-micron (μ) mesh. If needed, erythrocytes can be removed with lysing reagents such as ammonium chloride or by using density gradients. Cell suspensions prepared from lymphoid tissues should be processed quickly for analysis to avoid artifacts caused by nonviable cells. A common density gradient medium used for blood, marrow, and lymphoid tissue is ficoll-hypaque. After underlaying a volume of blood or cell suspension with the medium and then centrifuging, erythrocytes, dead cells, and myeloid cells pellet to the bottom of the tube while viable mononuclear cells remain at the gradient/plasma interface. It is always prudent, especially with pathologic samples, to verify that the populations of interest are not also being removed.

Once the specimen is in single-cell suspension, aliquots are stained. Staining reagents provide additional information about a cell, and different reagents provide different pieces of information. For example, one reagent might bind in proportion to the amount of deoxyribonucleic acid (DNA) present, whereas another might bind in proportion to the number of specific receptor sites present. Factors that can affect staining results include the temperature at which the staining is done, the amount of fluorescent light present, as well as the pH and tonicity of wash buffers. Accordingly, recommendations by the reagent manufacturers regarding staining conditions should be followed, and exposure of stained samples to direct fluorescent light should be minimized.

Staining with Fluorescent Dyes

There are two approaches to staining cells. The first is to use special fluorescent dyes as staining reagents. These dyes have affinities for specific cell constituents. For example, propidium iodide and thiazole orange bind to nucleic acids, while PKH-26 binds to membrane lipids. Some dyes, such as propidium iodide, require cell membrane permeabilization for the dye to reach its target, whereas other dyes, such as thiazole orange, can diffuse through the cell membrane. In addition, some dyes are equilibrium dyes, meaning that staining is only measurable when the cell is suspended in the dye, whereas other dyes require that unbound dye be washed off. Figure 30–1 illustrates a general staining scheme using fluorescent dyes. Table 30–1 presents commonly used dyes.

Staining with Antibodies

In the second approach, the staining reagents are antibodies that have been chemically linked or conjugated to fluorescent dyes known as *fluorochromes*. This staining approach is called *immunophenotyping*. "Immuno-" refers to the use of antibodies and "phenotyping" refers to characterizing an organism or cell; therefore, immunophenotyping utilizes antibodies for characterizing cells. Only cells expressing the molecule or antigen recognized by the antibody will be stained with the fluorochrome. The antigen can be located on the cell surface or it can be intracellular.

Both polyclonal antibodies purified from antisera and monoclonal antibodies produced from cloned, immortalized B-cell cultures are used for immunophenotyping. Generally, monoclonal antibodies are preferred because they are homogeneous, highly specific, and well characterized. As shown in Table 30–1, several colors of fluorochromes are available for use with standard cytometers. Many vari-

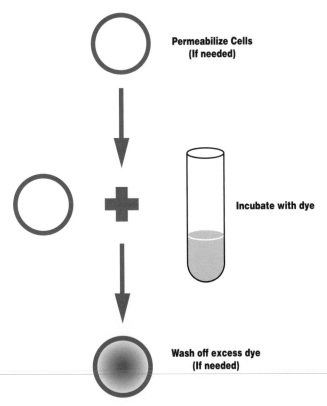

Permeabilize Cells (If needed)

Incubate with dye

Wash off excess dye (If needed)

➤   FIGURE 30–1   General staining scheme using fluorescent dyes.

➤ **Table 30-1**
COMMON FLUORESCENT DYES AND FLUOROCHROMES USED IN FLOW CYTOMETRY

Application	Dye/Fluorochrome	Target	Emission (nm)
DNA Content			
Propidium iodide (PI)	D	Double-stranded (DS) nucleic acids	575, 630
7-Aminoactinomycin D (7-AAD)	D	DNA	660
Acridine orange (AO)	D	DS nucleic acids	650
		Single-stranded nucleic acids	530
Reticulocytes			
Thiazole orange (TO)	D	RNA	525
Pyronin Y	D	RNA	575
Cell Physiology			
Fluo-3-cell activation	D	Ca^{2+}	525
SNARF-1-pH	D	H^+	575
DCFH-DA-oxidative burst	D	H_2O_2	525
Rhodamine 123-drug efflux	D	Mitochrondria	525
PKH-26-proliferation	D	Membrane lipids	525
Immunophenotyping			
Fluorescein isothiocyanate (FITC)	F	Antigen (via antibody linked to fluorochrome)	525
Phycoerythrin (PE)	F	Antigen (via antibody linked to fluorochrome)	575
Peridinin chlorophyll protein (PerCP)	F	Antigen (via antibody linked to fluorochrome)	670
PE-Texas red (PE-TxR)	F	Antigen (via antibody linked to fluorochrome)	630
PE-carbocyanin-5 (PE-Cy5)	F	Antigen (via antibody linked to fluorochrome)	670
Allophycocyanin (APC)	F	Antigen (via antibody linked to fluorochrome)	660

ations of staining protocols exist for immunophenotyping. Figure 30–2 illustrates a general staining scheme for immunophenotyping of leukocytes for surface antigens.

Because cells from different lineages or subpopulations bear unique combinations of antigens, populations can be identified using appropriate antibody combinations. To do this, antibodies of different specificities are conjugated to different fluorochromes and then combined. T-cell subsetting is an example that illustrates the power of using antibody combinations. Using a triple antibody combination, it is possible to detect five populations at once (Fig. 30–3). Details regarding the antibodies used in the example are discussed in a following section.

Standard antibody combinations are available for most routine applications from the major reagent manufacturers. To provide consistency for identifying monoclonal antibodies from different manufacturers, a classification system has been devised. The system identifies antibodies based on their reactivity with antigens, rather than by the name given by the manufacturer. With this classification, different antibodies binding the same antigen, as determined by flow cytometry and gel electrophoresis, are classified in the same "cluster of differentiation," or CD group. The CD groups are numbered, and antibodies within the same group bind the same antigen. New CD groups are added during the International Workshop on Human Leukocyte Differentiation Antigens, when new antibodies are identified. As of the Sixth Workshop held

in 1996, there were 166 CD groups.[2] Table 30–2 presents antibodies commonly used for hematology applications.

Cytometer Operation

Five procedures are required for cytometer operation. They include startup, quality control, optimization, data collection, and shutdown.

Startup

Each cytometer manufacturer provides a startup procedure. Startup includes turning on the cytometer and computer, filling and emptying sheath and waste reservoirs, respectively, and priming fluidics.

Quality Control

Quality control (QC) procedures are performed to monitor instrument performance and to assure consistency from day to day. For this purpose, the manufacturers provide a QC software program that is used in conjunction with fluorescent beads. The beads are run under standard conditions, and measurements are made. Because the beads are very stable, any major fluctuations in these measurements indicate a possible cytometer problem. Additional QC procedures may be required depending on the application.[3]

Optimization

During optimization the operator adjusts the cytometer settings so that cell populations in the sample can be properly

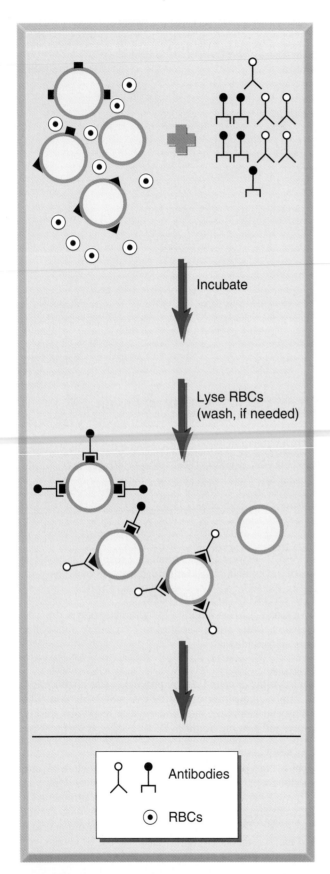

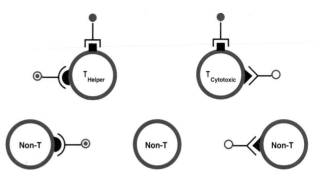

➤ **FIGURE 30–3**   Detection of five T-cell populations using three-color staining.

put on the stage, then the lighting, optics, and stage position are adjusted so that the cells can be seen. Similarly, optimization entails running a sample from a normal donor and adjusting the cytometer settings to bring the populations of interest on scale. It is important to use a normal donor for this purpose because patient samples may lack certain populations. To understand which settings can be adjusted, it is important to understand how a cytometer functions. The next section combines an overview of cytometer function with explanations of the electronic controls whose settings can be adjusted during optimization.

Cytometer Overview

All flow cytometers consist of three systems—the fluidics, optics, and electronics—in addition to a computer. The fluidics consists of pressurized air and saline sheath fluid that, together, carry the sample into the cytometer, through the flow cell, and then to waste (Fig. 30–4). The sample flow rate and the cell concentration are adjusted so that while in the flow cell, each cell passes through a laser beam, one at a time. As a cell passes through the laser beam, multiple characteristics (parameters) are measured rapidly and simultaneously. The parameters measured are forward-scattered laser light (FSC), side-scattered laser light (SSC), and up to four colors of fluorescent light (FL1, FL2, FL3, and FL4).

FSC and SSC parameters are based on the physical characteristics of a cell. The larger the cell, the greater is the FSC signal, and the more internal complexity or granularity, the greater the SSC signal. The number of colors measured depends on the staining reagents used and whether or not the cell bound any reagents. The standard laser used in clinical systems is a 488-nm blue argon ion laser; therefore, the fluorescent dyes used must absorb this wavelength to produce fluorescent light. A dual laser system is illustrated (see Fig. 30–4). The addition of a 635-nm red diode laser expands the repertoire of fluorescent dyes that can be used.

As signals are emitted from the cell, the optical system separates and routes the different colored light to the appropriate photodetectors using strategically placed optical filters and mirrors. These mirrors and filters transmit, reflect, absorb, or block specific wavelengths of light. A dedicated photodetector measures the signal intensity for its respective parameter. Typically, the optical system is set up to detect green (515- to 545-nm) signal in FL1, orange (564- to 606-nm) signal in FL2, and two shades of red signals, one (greater than 670 nm) in FL3 and other (653 to 669 nm) in FL4.

➤ **FIGURE 30–2**   General staining scheme for staining leukocytes with antibodies. RBCs = red blood cells.

analyzed. This is analogous to what is done to prepare for examining a specimen on a microscope slide. The slide is

> **Table 30–2**
USEFUL ANTIBODIES FOR HEMATOLOGY APPLICATIONS

CD	Antigen	Cell Targets	IM	AL	LDb	LDtf	Misc
				APPLICATIONS			
CD1a	Gp49	Cortical and mature thymocytes, Langerhans' cells	−	+S	−	−	
CD2	LFA-2 receptor	Thymocytes, NK cells, T cells	−	+C	+S	+S	
CD3	T-cell receptor	Pan–T-cell marker	+	+S	+C	+S	
CD4	MHC class II receptor	T-cell subset (helper T), monocytes, early myeloid progenitors	+	+S	+C	+S	
CD5	Gp67	T cells, B-cell subset	−	+S	+C	+C	
CD7	Gp40	T cells, NK-cell subset, progenitor cell subset	−	+C	+C	+S	
CD8	MHC class I receptor	T-cell subset (cytotoxic T), NK-cell subset	+	+S	+C	+S	
CD10	CALLA, neutral endopeptidase	Pro– and pre–B cells, granulocytes	−	+C	+C	+C	
CD11c	p150, 95	Neutrophils, monocytes, NK cells	−	−	+S	+S	
CD13	Aminopeptidase N	Granulocytes, monocytes	−	+C	−	+S	
CD14	LPS receptor	Monocytes, macrophages, neutrophils	+	+C	−	−	
CD15	Lewis^x, X-hapten	Granulocytes, monocytes, progenitor cell subset, mast cells	−	+S	−	−	
CD16	FcγRIII receptor	Granulocytes, NK cells, monocytes	+	+S	+S	+S	
CD19	Gp95	Pan–B-cell marker	+	+C	+C	+C	
CD20	p35	B cells	−	+S	+C	+C	
CD22	BL-CAM	B cells	−	+S	+S	+S	
CD23	Fcε receptor	Eosinophils, B-cell subset	−	−	+S	+C	
CD25	IL-2 receptor	T cells	−	−	+S	−	
CD32	FcγRII receptor	Granulocytes, monocytes, B-cell subset	−	−	−	−	
CD33	Gp67	Monocytes	−	+C	−	+S	
CD34	Gp116	Progenitor cells	−	+C	−	−	PCE
CD38	ADP-ribosyl cyclase	Subsets in all hematopoetic lineages	−	+S	+S	+S	
CD41	GPIIb	Megakaryocytic cells, platelets	−	+S	−	−	
CD42b	GPIbα	Megakaryocytic cells, platelets	−	+S	−	−	
CD45	LCA	All leukocytes	+	−	+C	+C	PCE
CD55	Decay-accelerating factor	Erythrocytes, granulocytes					PNH
CD56	N-CAM	T-cell subset, NK cells	+	−	+S	+S	
CD57	Oligosaccharide	T-cell subset, NK-cell subset	−	−	+S	+S	
CD59	Membrane inhibitor of reactive lysis	Erythrocytes, granulocytes					PNH
CD61	GPIIIb	Megakaryocytic cells, platelets	−	+S	−	−	
CD64	FcγRI receptor	Myelomonocytic cells, activated neutrophils	−	+S	−	−	
CD65	Ceramide 12-saccharide		−	−	−	−	
CD71	Transferrin receptor	Upregulated on proliferating cells	−	+S	−	−	
CD103	αE integrin subunit	T cells, monocytes, hairy-cell leukemia	−	−	+S	−	
CD117	c-kit, stem cell factor receptor	Stem cells	−	+S	−	−	

continued

> **Table 30-2**
USEFUL ANTIBODIES FOR HEMATOLOGY APPLICATIONS (*Continued*)

| | | | APPLICATIONS | | | | |
CD	Antigen	Cell Targets	IM	AL	LDb	LDtf	Misc
FMC7		B cells	–	–	+S	+S	
HLA-DR	MHC class II	T-cell subsets, monocytes, all B cells, NK cells, progenitor cells	–	+C	–	–	
IgM/D/A	Ig heavy chains	B cells	–	–	–	+S	
Kappa/Lambda	Ig light chains	B-cell subset, all cells with Fc receptors	–	+C	+C	+C	
GlyA	Glycophorin A	Erythroid cells	–	+S	–	–	
HgbF	Hemoglobin F	Fetal erythrocytes					FMH
TdT	Terminal deoxytransferase	Pro– and pre–B cells, cortical thymocytes	–	+S	–	–	
MPO	Myeloperoxidase	myeloid cells	–	+S	–	–	

Abbreviations: AL= acute leukemia; IM = immunophenotyping; LDb = lymphoproliferative disease (blood and bone marrow); LDtf = lymphoproliferative disease (tissue and fluids); NK = natural killer; +C = core panel; +S = supplemental panel; PNH = paroxysmal nocturnal hemoglobinuria, PCE = progenitor cell enumeration; FMH = fetomaternal hemorrhage
  Antibody data from reference 2.
  Core and supplemental panel information from reference 18.

Threshold

Measurements are not made on every particle that passes through the laser beam. For a particle to be recognized by the system, it must first register above the threshold. The threshold (also known as trigger) parameter is used to limit what is analyzed by the cytometer. For example, if a sample contained many small debris particles, the operator could eliminate them from the analysis by setting a threshold limit on size (FSC). In this case, the cytometer will only assign a particle an event number and display its corresponding parameter values if the particle's FSC signal is above the threshold limit. This helps assure that when data are collected and stored, they will represent cells in the sample, not debris. Different applications utilize different threshold parameters and settings. For example, in leukocyte analysis assays, it is useful to add CD45-PerCP, a pan-leukocyte marker, to each sample and threshold on FL3. Under these conditions, leukocyte data are included in the data file, whereas data from red-cell stroma and platelets are not. Regardless of what parameter is used, however, it is important not to set the threshold limit too high to avoid excluding the population of interest.

Photodetectors

Photodetectors convert the light signals into electrical signals called voltage pulses. In Figure 30–4, the pulse shown for each parameter represents the signal intensity as the cell passes through the laser beam. The stronger the signal becomes, the higher the pulse is. The electronics measures the height of each pulse, and then converts this information to a number ranging from 0 to 1023. Accordingly, the stronger the signal, the higher the number.

The sensitivity of a detector can be increased by increasing the voltage supplied to it. Using green fluorescence as an example, the amount of voltage applied to the FL1 detector depends on the sample. If the signal is weak, as with a dimly staining population, the voltage must be increased to detect the population. If the signal is very bright, the voltage can be lower. During optimization, the operator ensures that both bright and dim populations are on scale.

Amplification

For samples in which the signal range can be greater than 10-fold for a given parameter, logarithmic amplification must be used for that parameter. Logarithmic amplifiers basically manipulate the signal conversion so that very bright and very dim signals can both be displayed on the 1024-channel scale.[4] Most cytometers use a four-decade log scale, meaning that the signals are converted to numbers between 1 and 10,000, or 10^0 to 10^4.

Leukocyte immunophenotyping assays generally require logarithmic amplification for the fluorescence parameters and linear amplification for the scatter parameters. This is because cells can exhibit very dim to very bright staining, whereas cell size and granularity measurements are confined to smaller range. In contrast, for whole blood analyses of platelets and erythrocytes, logarithmic amplification of FSC is required to distinguish these two populations from one another.

Fluorescence Compensation

Many fluorescent dyes used in flow cytometry emit a wide array of wavelengths after absorbing laser light. The optical filters help assure that the appropriate wavelengths reach the correct detector; however, some FL2 dyes emit some green light, which is detected by the FL1 detector, and vice versa. This spectral bleed-over also occurs with some FL3 and FL4 dyes. Fluorescence compensation is an electronic control that, when properly set, removes the effect of this bleed-over so that each detector only measures signal for the appropriate fluorescent dye. Details for how this is done electronically can be found elsewhere.[4,5] For multicolor applications, compensation must be correctly set to assure that each detector is reporting the correct information. Otherwise, the

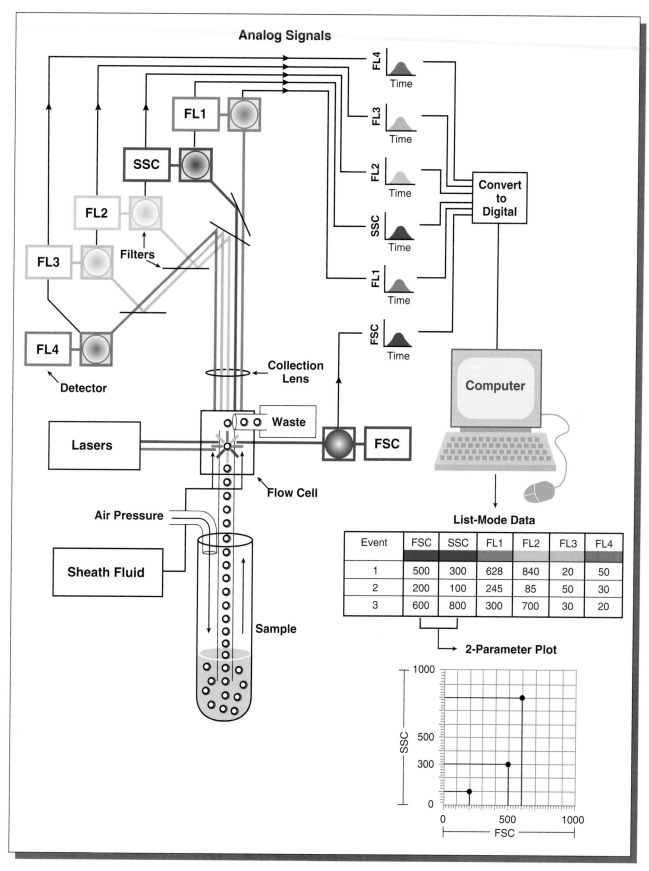

Analog Signals

Event	FSC	SSC	FL1	FL2	FL3	FL4
1	500	300	628	840	20	50
2	200	100	245	85	50	30
3	600	800	300	700	30	20

List-Mode Data

2-Parameter Plot

➤ FIGURE 30–4 Schematic of cell analysis using a two-laser flow cytometer.

data will be suspect. Methods for adjusting and checking compensation are provided by the cytometer manufacturers and are also available from other sources.[3,5]

Data Collection

After optimization is complete, the operator activates features in the software to store data for each sample in separate list-mode data files. The software allows the operator to input sample information, such as the number of events to analyze, the file name, the patient identification number, and the reagents used to prepare each sample. As the sample is run, the parameter measurements for each event are stored in a list that continues to grow until the number of events to be analyzed has been reached. The data are stored in the list-mode file along with sample information entered by the operator. Figure 30–4 depicts a file containing data for three events, but typical list-mode files contain information for 10,000 events.

Shutdown

A shutdown procedure is provided by the cytometer manufacturer. It consists of cleaning and decontaminating the cytometer, and then turning the power off. Depending on the dyes used for an assay, it may be necessary to perform a short cleaning procedure between assays. This avoids possible dye carryover to subsequent samples. For example, some dyes, such as propidium iodide, which is used for DNA analysis assays, can cause erroneous results by elevating FL2 and FL3 signals if introduced into immunophenotyping samples. To avoid this artifact, a cleaning procedure must be performed after the DNA samples are run.

Data Analysis

There are basically two objectives for performing data analysis. One objective is to obtain statistics on the parameters measured. Population percentages, absolute cell counts, and fluorescence intensity measurements are statistics typically reported. The other objective is to identify abnormal populations based on light scatter or staining patterns, or both. The prerequisite for performing this type of analysis, of course, is to be able to identify normal populations using the same parameters.

Identifying Populations

Because most hematologic samples contain multiple cell populations, it is necessary to first identify the population of interest for further analysis. This is done by visual inspection of the data in a plot. The three dots displayed in the FSC/SSC plot represent the three events in the data file (see Fig. 30–4). The x and y coordinates of each dot represent the event's FSC and SSC measurements; therefore, the location of each dot is very informative. With only three events, however, it is impossible to determine if multiple populations exist.

Figure 30–5A displays a similar plot displaying data from a list-mode file containing 10,000 events. This data was collected from a blood sample that was stained and then lysed to remove erythrocytes. With this large data set, it is possible to visualize multiple populations. Three cell populations are displayed and color-coded for clarity. Lymphocytes are small and contain no granules; therefore, the FSC and SSC values are low compared to those for the monocytes and neutrophils. Monocytes are larger and contain more vacuoles than lymphocytes; as a result, the FSC and SSC values are higher. Fi-

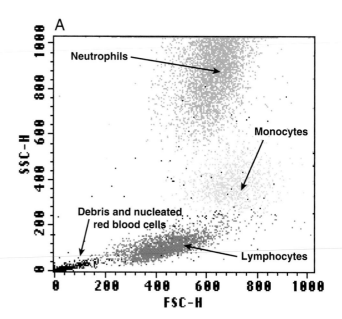

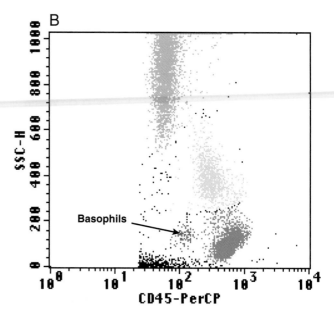

➤ **FIGURE 30–5** Leukocyte populations discernible in lysed whole blood. *A.* FSC/SSC display. *B.* CD45/SSC display. Note how in *B,* debris and basophils can be resolved from the lymphocyte population.

nally, neutrophils contain many granules yet they are similar in size to monocytes; therefore, their FSC values are similar, but their SSC values are much higher than monocytes.

In Figure 30–5B, the same file is displayed with CD45-PerCP on the x axis rather than FSC. This plot illustrates the utility of CD45 for resolving leukocyte populations. Using the CD45/SSC plot, it is now possible to resolve debris, nucleated red cells, and basophils from lymphocytes. Although the FSC/SSC plots are useful, CD45/SSC plots are being used more frequently for leukocyte analysis, especially for bone marrow samples in which interfering nucleated red cells are more frequent.

Whole blood is commonly used for platelet and erythrocyte assays. Figure 30–6 displays the location of platelet, erythrocyte, and leukocyte populations in whole blood. For some applications, other parameter combinations are used for

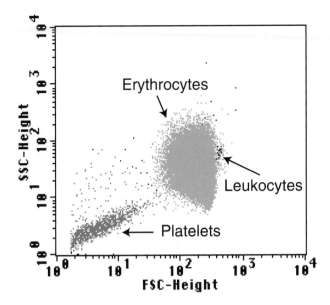

> ➤ **FIGURE 30–6** Populations discernible in whole blood.

identifying populations. They will be discussed, when relevant.

Gating

Most analyses focus on a single population. Gating is a software feature used to restrict analysis to a particular population. A gate is created by drawing a graphic boundary around a population.

In Figure 30–7A, a gate has been drawn around the lymphocytes. Figures 30–7B and 30–7C compare the effect of using no gate or using the lymphocyte gate to display the fluorescein isothiocyanate (FITC) and allophycocyanin (APC) fluorescence values from the data file. With no gate, the fluorescence of monocytes, neutrophils, and debris is displayed along with the lymphocyte fluorescence, making it impossible to obtain statistics on lymphocytes alone. The lymphocyte gate restricts the fluorescence data, making statistical calculations possible for a particular population. Next we will see how these calculations are done.

Quadrant Statistics

Quadrant markers divide two-parameter plots into four sections called *quadrants*. The quadrants are used to distinguish negative, single-positive, and double-positive populations from one another. Using Figure 30–7C as an example, negative events are represented by dots with low FL1 (FITC) and FL4 (APC) values, single-positive events are represented by dots with either high FL1 and low FL4 values or low FL1 and high FL4 values, and double-positive events are represented by dots with high FL1 and FL4 values.

Quadrant markers are set to encompass the negative population within the lower left (LL) quadrant (Fig. 30–7C). For applications in which it is difficult to distinguish the negative population from the single-positive populations, a replicate sample stained with a subclass control reagent is used. This control reagent contains an antibody of the same immunoglobulin subclass as the staining reagent, conjugated to the same fluorochrome, but specific for an antigen not found in humans. These staining conditions produce a negative population appropriate for setting quadrants.

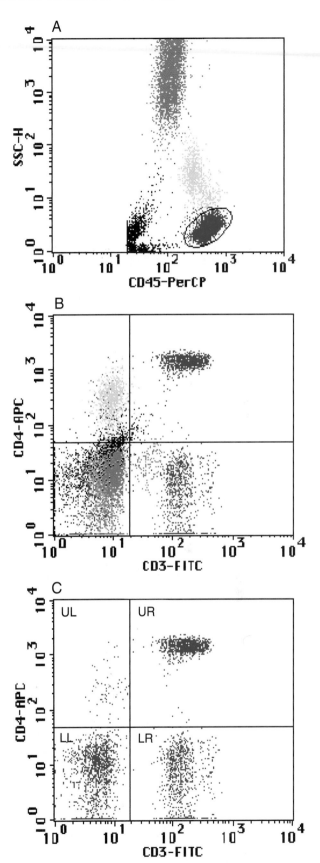

> ➤ **FIGURE 30–7** The effect of a lymphocyte gate *(A)* on fluorescence. Fluorescence events in *B* (ungated) and *C* (gated data) are color-coded to their respective populations in *A*. Using a gate provides a means for analyzing one population at a time.
> Abbreviations: UL = upper left; UR = upper right; LL = lower left; LR = lower right

Gated Events: 3484
Total Events: 10000

Quad	Events	% Gated	% Total
UL	72	2.07	0.72
UR	1184	33.98	11.84
LL	1321	37.92	13.21
LR	907	26.03	9.07

➤ **FIGURE 30–8** Quadrant statistics from Figure 30–7C. UL = upper left; UR = upper right; LL = lower left; LR = lower right.

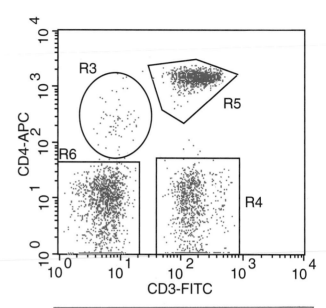

Percentages are calculated based on the number of events within each quadrant. The statistics for Figure 30–7C are shown (Fig. 30–8). Events falling in the upper right (UR) quadrant are double-positive and, according to the statistics, this quadrant contains 1184 events. The % Gated statistic reflects the percentage of lymphocytes that are double-positive. It was calculated by dividing the number of events in UR by the number of events in the lymphocyte gate [(1184 ÷ 3484) × 100 = 33.98]. To calculate the events in UR as a percentage of the total events (% Total), the total event number is used as the denominator [(1184 ÷ 10,000) × 100 = 11.84]. The % Gated statistics are used most frequently because they are based on the population of interest.

Region Statistics

Regions can also be used to partition a two-parameter plot for analysis. Although four regions are displayed (Fig. 30–9), at least eight are usually available with the current software packages. This is useful when there are more than four populations on a plot. Regions can also be drawn in various shapes to fit each population. The % Gated and % Total statistics are calculated as in quadrant statistics, except that the number of events in each region is used as the numerator. Figure 30–9 displays the same data shown in Figure 30–7C; thus, the region R5 statistics are comparable to the UR statistics in Figure 30–8. In region analysis, the operator usually has to readjust the regions from donor to donor even though the samples were stained with the same reagents. This is necessary because there are small shifts of populations that occur from one donor to the next.

A newer variation of region analysis uses elliptical-shaped regions that are linked to a cluster analysis algorithm. This algorithm directs each region to move to encompass its target population as each new data file is analyzed. These self-adjusting regions are called Attractors™.

Single-Parameter Histogram Statistics

For some applications, statistical information from one parameter is sufficient. Figure 30–10 displays the FITC data shown in Figure 30–9. The FL1 values are displayed on the x axis, and the number of events expressing each value is displayed on the y axis. Markers are set so that events with FL1 values higher than those of the negative population can be measured. As with quadrants, if the negative population is difficult to distinguish from the positive population, a

Gated Events: 3484
Total Events: 10000

Region	Events	% Gated	% Total
R2	3484	100.00	34.84
R1	62	1.78	0.62
R3	68	1.95	0.68
R4	908	26.06	9.08
R5	1171	33.61	11.71
R6	1322	37.94	13.22

➤ **FIGURE 30–9** Analysis using regions.

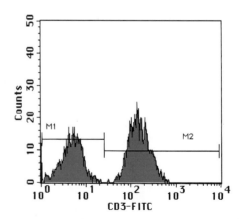

Gated Events: 3484
Total Events: 10000

Marker	Left, Right	Events	% Gated	% Total	Median
All	1, 9910	3484	100.00	34.84	95.17
M1	1, 26	1384	39.72	13.84	5.09
M2	26, 9140	2086	59.87	20.86	148.55

➤ **FIGURE 30–10** Analysis using a single-parameter histogram with markers.

subclass control sample can be used to determine where to set the markers. Percentages are calculated using the number of events between the markers as the numerator and the gated events or total events for the denominator. In this example, 59.87% of the lymphocytes were positive for CD3.

Histograms displaying cellular DNA content measurements (Fig. 30–11) require the use of specialized algorithms for calculating population percentages. In DNA analysis, cells are stained with a fluorescent dye that binds in proportion to the amount of DNA present. Analysis of proliferating cells stained with DNA dyes reveals three populations: those with the normal complement of DNA, those with a double complement of DNA, and those in between. These populations are referred to as G_0/G_1-phase cells, G_2+M-phase cells, and S-phase cells, respectively. Figure 30–11 illustrates the location of these populations and the percentages, as computed using a DNA analysis program.

Absolute Cell Counts

So far, methods for obtaining percentage statistics have been presented. In many applications, the absolute count, which is reported as the number of cells per microliter of specimen, is more useful. In flow cytometry there are two ways to obtain this statistic without relying on hematology analyzer information. The first requires that the cytometer analyze a fixed volume of sample. That way, the number of events for the population of interest can be expressed per microliter of sample, and this can be extrapolated back to the volume of specimen used to prepare the sample. For example, if the there are 3000 events of the population of interest in 20 μL of sample, and the sample contains 1:10 dilution of whole blood, then the absolute count is calculated as:

$$\frac{3000 \text{ events}}{20\text{-}\mu L \text{ sample}} \times 10 = 1500 \text{ events/}\mu L \text{ blood}$$

Because few cytometer models can measure fixed volumes of sample, the more common way to obtain absolute counts utilizes fluorescent reference beads.[6] In this approach, a known number of reference beads is added to the sample,

which also contains a known volume of specimen. A data file is collected, and region statistics are used to measure the number of cell population events and the number of bead events. The ratio of these two numbers is determined and the absolute count is calculated using the formula:

$$\frac{\text{No. cell population events}}{\text{No. bead events}} \times \frac{\text{No. beads per sample}}{\mu L \text{ specimen per sample}}$$

$$= \text{No. cells/}\mu L \text{ specimen}$$

Fluorescence Intensity Measurements

For some applications, population percentages and absolute counts are not useful. Instead, the amount of staining reagent bound is informative, so the fluorescence intensity is measured. The median is the statistic most commonly reported for this purpose, because it best represents the average fluorescence per cell in a population. Using the median, it is also possible to make relative comparisons of antigen expression among populations. For example, if the staining reagent is an antibody, then the fluorescence intensity is related to the number of antigens present. Reviewing Figure 30–10, if a ratio of the medians of the positive and negative populations is calculated (148.55/5.09) the positive cells appear to bear approximately 30 times more antigen than the negative cells. This is only a relative measurement; however, and the actual number of antigen molecules present cannot be quantitated without additional information.

New methods exist for converting the fluorescence intensity into standardized measurements, such as antibodies bound per cell (ABC) or molecules of equivalent soluble fluorochrome (MESF).[7] These methods utilize calibrated beads. This makes it possible to compare results from different cytometers. It also brings the investigator closer to determining the number of reagent binding sites per cell.

The simplest method for converting fluorescence intensity to ABC is as follows. The cell sample is run on the cytometer and the electronic settings are optimized to bring the population of interest on scale. Next, calibrated fluorescent beads are analyzed. The calibrated beads contain at least four populations, each bearing different standardized amounts of fluorochrome per bead. This information is used along with specialized software to convert the fluorescence measurements, which usually range from 1 to 10,000, into molecules of fluorochrome (Fig. 30–12). Next, the sample is analyzed. If the antibody was manufactured to contain one fluorochrome molecule per antibody, then the number of fluorochrome molecules per cell equals the ABC. Based on what is known about the antibody binding characteristics, the number of antigen molecules per cell can be determined. For example, if one antibody binds one antigen molecule, then the number of antigen molecules per cell equals the ABC. Likewise, if one antibody binds two antigens, then the number of antigens is twice the ABC.

► APPLICATIONS OF FLOW CYTOMETRY

In the survey cited earlier,[1] more than 80% of the clinical flow laboratories reported that they routinely perform CD4 enumeration and leukemia and lymphoma analyses. Approximately 50% performed stem cell enumeration, DNA analysis, and immunophenotyping for myelodysplasia; and less than 23% performed reticulocyte enumeration, neu-

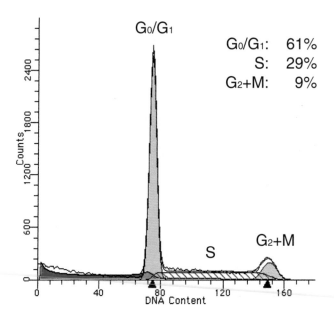

► **FIGURE 30–11** Analysis of DNA data using a single-parameter histogram and software modeling.

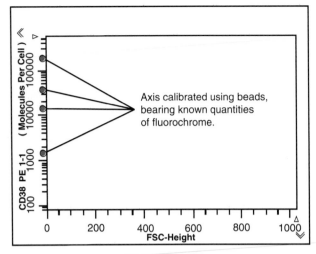

Axis calibrated using beads, bearing known quantities of fluorochrome.

> **FIGURE 30–12**   Calibration of fluorescence intensity into fluorochromes per cell using calibration beads.

> **Table 30-3**

PANELS FOR LYMPHOCYTE SUBSETTING ANALYSES

Tube	Three-Color
A	CD3/CD4/CD45
B	CD3/CD8/CD45
C	CD3/CD19/CD45
D	CD3/CD16+CD56/CD45
Four-Color	
A	CD3/CD8/CD45/CD4
B	CD3/CD16+CD56/CD45/CD19

Data from reference 10.

trophil function tests, and platelet function tests. The next section presents typical applications, as well as some with potential clinical relevance.

Lymphocyte Subsetting and CD4 T-Cell Enumeration

These assays are used in evaluating immunodeficiency disease states. The lymphocyte subsets measured are the T cytotoxic, T helper, B, and natural killer (NK) cells. In acquired immunodeficiency syndrome (AIDS), the human immunodeficiency virus (HIV) infects and kills the CD4 helper T lymphocytes; therefore, a decrease in this subset is related to disease progression. Current guidelines from the Centers for Disease Control and Prevention (CDC) recommend monitoring CD4 counts in HIV-positive individuals every 3 to 4 months. Antiviral treatment is initiated based on the CD4 count and on viral ribonucleic acid (RNA) levels. If the count is below 500 per cubic millimeter; or if the viral RNA level is either greater than 10,000 copies by the branched DNA method or greater than 20,000 copies by reverse-transcriptase polymerase chain reaction, then treatment is initiated.[8]

Lymphocyte subsetting is also used to evaluate other immunodeficiency diseases. For example, in thymic hypoplasia T cells are markedly reduced, whereas in X-linked hypogammaglobulinemia, B cells are frequently absent. In severe combined immunodeficiency syndrome, both B and T cells are markedly reduced or absent.[9]

Sample Preparation

Extensive guidelines for lymphocyte subsetting and CD4 T-cell enumeration in HIV-positive patients have been published by the CDC[10] and the National Clinical Committee for Laboratory Standards.[11] A similar method is followed for evaluating other immunodeficiencies. Briefly, if the blood will be processed within 30 hours, it can be collected in K_3EDTA, heparin, or acid citrate dextrose (ACD). If it will be processed in 30 to 48 hours, it should be collected in either heparin or ACD. Aliquots of blood are stained with a CDC-recommended panel listed in Table 30–3. If absolute counts are required, reference beads are included in each staining tube. After staining, a lysing fixative is added

to lyse erythrocytes, inactivate pathogens, and preserve the leukocytes. Samples are stored in the dark and analyzed within 24 hours. Method control cells are used to assure that the reagents are performing properly. The control cells consist of fixed cells with known percentages and absolute counts of subpopulations. Blood from a healthy donor is also an acceptable control.

Cytometer Operation

Instrument settings are optimized while running samples from a healthy subject. Both FSC and SSC amplifiers are set to linear amplification while fluorescence amplifiers are set to logarithmic amplification. The threshold is set to FL3 so that the predominant data will be collected on leukocytes (CD45-PerCP positive cells) rather than the numerous particles of erythrocyte stroma present in the sample. Enough events are collected so that at least 2500 lymphocytes can be analyzed. For a sample from a healthy donor, collecting 10,000 events yields the requisite number of lymphocytes for analysis.

Data Analysis

Results from a CD3/CD8/CD45/CD4-stained sample from a healthy subject are shown (Fig 30–13). An applications-specific software program was used to analyze the data for population percentages and absolute counts using the elliptical Attractors™ regions described earlier. The three T-cell subset percentages are displayed along with the absolute counts for each population, the absolute lymphocyte count (CD45), and the TH/S ratio (CD4:CD8 ratio). Each laboratory must determine its own normal reference range using healthy subjects; however, reference ranges are available from the manufacturers to use as an initial guide. Typical ranges for lymphocyte subset percentages for adults, expressed as percent of lymphocytes, are 56% to 86% for CD3, 33% to 58% for CD4, 13% to 39% for CD8, 5% to 26% for CD16+56, and 5% to 22% for CD19 lymphocytes. A normal range for absolute CD4 counts is 404 to 1612 cells per microliter.[12] The normal range for the TH/S ratio is typically between 1 and 1.5. The TH/S ratio is not as useful now that absolute counts are readily available.

The second sample in this two-tube panel was stained with CD3/CD16+56/CD45/CD19 to enumerate T cells, B cells and NK cells, but the results are not shown. This tube is mainly for quality control because the sum of the subset

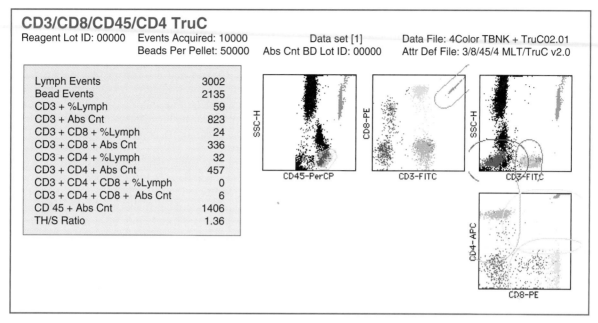

CD3/CD8/CD45/CD4 TruC

Reagent Lot ID: 00000 | Events Acquired: 10000 | Data set [1] | Data File: 4Color TBNK + TruC02.01
Beads Per Pellet: 50000 | Abs Cnt BD Lot ID: 00000 | Attr Def File: 3/8/45/4 MLT/TruC v2.0

Lymph Events	3002
Bead Events	2135
CD3 + %Lymph	59
CD3 + Abs Cnt	823
CD3 + CD8 + %Lymph	24
CD3 + CD8 + Abs Cnt	336
CD3 + CD4 + %Lymph	32
CD3 + CD4 + Abs Cnt	457
CD3 + CD4 + CD8 + %Lymph	0
CD3 + CD4 + CD8 + Abs Cnt	6
CD 45 + Abs Cnt	1406
TH/S Ratio	1.36

➤ **FIGURE 30–13** Four-color lymphocyte subset analysis using Attractors™ regions.

counts should be equivalent to the CD45 lymphocyte count. The second tube is also useful for evaluating the other immunodeficiencies described earlier.

It is important to note the quantity of information obtainable from one tube using four-color analysis. One study compared the four-color two-tube method with the original two-color six-tube method. The study revealed that the although both methods yielded comparable results, using the four-color method resulted in a 15% decrease in the cost per test and a 50% reduction in time expenditure by the technologist.[13]

Leukemia and Lymphoma Immunophenotyping

Leukemia is a term used to denote a malignancy that occurs at any step in the differentiation from a blast in the bone marrow to a mature leukocyte in the peripheral blood. Acute leukemias are malignancies of the immature cells within the bone marrow, whereas chronic leukemias are primarily malignancies of mature cells in the peripheral blood. Leukemias may be lymphoid or myeloid in origin. *Lymphomas* are malignancies of the lymphoid system.

Immunophenotyping is used to detect, characterize, and monitor the abnormal cell population. Characterizing the malignancy can be useful for directing therapy and for determining prognosis. Flow cytometry can be used to establish diagnosis for pre-B acute lymphocytic leukemia (ALL), T-ALL, B chronic lymphocytic leukemia (CLL), small lymphocytic lymphoma, acute myelocytic leukemia (AML), and hairy-cell leukemia; and it can assist in the diagnosis of follicular center non-Hodgkin's lymphoma (NHL), mantle cell lymphoma, large-cell B-NHL, Burkitt's lymphoma, large granular lymphocyte disorders, and plasma cell disorders.[14] Of course, the optimal utilization of flow cytometric data in patient care includes the integration of clinical, morphological, and other data.[15]

Once the immunophenotype of the neoplastic population is known, the size of the population can be tracked to de-termine the effectiveness of the treatment, to monitor for minimal residual disease during clinical remission, and to detect relapse. Minimal residual disease detection is considered "rare event analysis," because a detectable neoplastic population can be as low as 1 in 10,000 bone marrow cells. This analysis requires a complex methodology too detailed to present here but available elsewhere.[16]

Sample Preparation

Recommendations for processing and preparing leukemia and lymphoma samples have been published by the U.S.-Canadian consensus group and should be consulted for details.[17,18] Specimens include peripheral blood, marrow, lymphoid biopsies, and fine-needle aspirates. Sodium heparin is the anticoagulant of choice for blood and marrow processed within 48 hours of collection. ACD is acceptable for peripheral blood samples processed 48 to 72 hours after collection, but it is not recommended for bone marrow because the large anticoagulant-to-specimen ratio may cause viability problems as a result of fluctuations in pH.[16] Tissue specimens and fine-needle aspirates should be processed immediately into single-cell suspensions and stored in cold isotonic medium to maintain high viability. Because flow cytometric analysis for this application relies on the detection of abnormal staining patterns, it is critical to maintain high viability because necrotic cells can cause staining artifacts, making the results difficult to interpret.

The U.S.-Canadian consensus group published recommendations of monoclonal antibodies to use in core and supplemental panels (see Table 30–2), but they did not recommend specific antibody combinations.[18] Thus, unlike T-cell subsetting, there are no fixed panels, nor normal ranges for results. It is up to each laboratory to devise the combinations of reagents, and to construct panels. Owing to the complexity of disease, the U.S.-Canadian consensus group recommends using two-color combinations at a minimum, although in many instances three- and four-color combinations are preferable.[19] The reagents used in these panels are designated by the manufacturers as "analyte-specific reagents" (ASRs) in accordance with the guidelines from the Food and Drug Administration (FDA). Manufacturers provide basic information on ASRs such as CD number, antibody concentration, and staining volume per fixed number of normal leukocytes; but the burden of establishing performance characteristics of ASRs in "home brew" tests is strictly the responsibility of the testing laboratory.[20]

Before samples are stained, cell counts are performed and each specimen is adjusted to a standardized cell concentration. A typical staining method is to incubate one million leukocytes with each monoclonal antibody combination, lyse the erythrocytes, then wash and fix the samples. A peripheral blood sample from a healthy subject should also be processed and stained to confirm that the reagents are working. For antigens not normally found on peripheral blood cells, such as CD34, it may be necessary to use a cell line bearing the antigen of interest as a positive control. It is also useful to prepare an unstained sample from each donor that has been processed along with the stained samples. This negative control can be used to determine if elevated autofluorescence, perhaps resulting from chemotherapy, is a factor that must be taken into consideration during optimization or data analysis. Samples should be stored in the dark until analyzed, preferably within 24 hours.

Cytometer Operation

Instrument settings are optimized using samples from a healthy subject; however, owing to the abnormal nature of neoplastic cells, it is likely that the FSC and SSC settings may need to be adjusted from patient to patient to visualize all populations. FSC is set to linear amplification and SSC can be either in linear or log, depending on the laboratory protocol. Fluorescence parameters are measured with logarithmic amplification. FSC is typically the threshold parameter. A minimum of 10,000 to 20,000 events is collected per sample. As the patient undergoes therapy, it may be necessary to collect a larger number of events to adequately analyze the neoplastic population.

Data Analysis

Data analysis for this application consists mainly of visual inspection to detect abnormal scatter or staining patterns, or both. As mentioned earlier, this requires a firm knowledge of the staining patterns of normal cells. The CD45/SSC plot is very useful for detecting abnormal populations. Once the abnormal population is detected, a gate is set on it and then the population is examined for expression of additional antigens. Region statistics can be used to estimate the percentage of the abnormal population relative to the rest of the cells in the sample. The U.S.-Canadian consensus group advises against setting quadrant markers and determining percent positivity of the neoplasm for a particular antigen. Instead, the abnormal population should be characterized as being negative, dim, or bright for an antigen.[19] Based on the antigenic profile of the abnormal population, the lineage and sometimes the subtype of the leukemia can be defined. This analysis process requires extensive practice under the supervision by an expert. An extremely useful CD-ROM containing case studies and tutorials is available for training purposes.[21]

A hallmark of neoplastic leukocytes is the abnormal expression of antigen, also known as *antigen infidelity*. This includes over- and underexpression; asynchronous expression, meaning that the antigen is expressed during a maturation phase in which it is usually absent; and aberrant expression. Aberrant expression refers to the coexpression of antigens normally found on different lineages.[22]

Figures 30–14A and 30–14B display data collected on bone marrow from a healthy subject and from one with AML, respectively. The abnormal population is readily observed based on its underexpression of CD45 and low SSC. The normal lymphocyte population is highlighted in color for reference.

Data from the same two subjects are also shown in Figures 30–14C and 30–14D, respectively. This is an example of asynchronous antigen expression because CD34 is found on immature myeloid cells whereas CD15 is found on mature myeloid cells. From Figure 30–14C it is clear that the two antigens are not normally coexpressed.

Figures 30–15A and 30–15B display data collected on peripheral blood from a healthy donor and from one with B-CLL, respectively. Quadrant markers were drawn to emphasize the difference in the staining patterns rather than for calculating statistics. This is an example of aberrant antigen expression because CD5 is a T-lineage antigen, whereas CD19 is a B-lineage antigen. Data from the same two subjects are also shown in Figures 30–15C and 30–15D, respectively. The plots display data from CD19-positive lymphocytes. The clonal nature of the B-cell malignancy is apparent based on kappa (κ) and lambda (λ) expression. Typically, there are twice as many κ-bearing B-cells as λ-bearing. In this case, the malignant clone is κ-positive and it has overgrown to such an extent that the λ-positive cells are not detectable.

A wealth of information has been published regarding the antigenic profiles and classification strategies for specific types and subtypes of leukemias and lymphomas.[19,23,24] These publications are easily available in most medical libraries, or copies can be ordered via the Internet.[25]

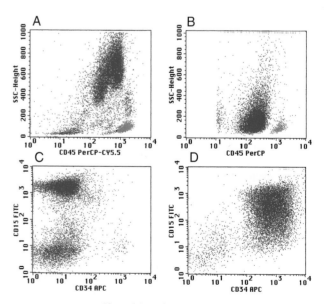

➤ **FIGURE 30–14** Normal (*A* and *C*) and abnormal (*B* and *D*) scatter and staining patterns in bone marrow. The abnormal sample is from a patient with acute myelocytic leukemia. The normal lymphoid population is colored for reference. In *B* the abnormal population is apparent because of its low SSC and dim CD45 staining, and in *D* owing to the coexpression of CD15 and CD34. These two antigens are normally expressed in different maturation phases.

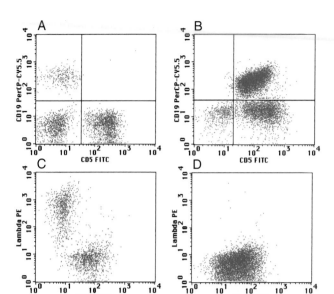

➤ **FIGURE 30–15**   Normal (*A* and *C*) and abnormal (*B* and *D*) staining in peripheral blood. The abnormal sample is from a patient with chronic lymphocytic leukemia. In *B*, the abnormal population is apparent because of the coexpression of CD5 and CD19, two antigens normally found on different lineages. In *D*, where there are usually twice as many kappa cells as lambda cells, it is apparent that the abnormal clone has overgrown and replaced the normal population.

Leukemia and Lymphoma DNA Content Analysis

DNA content analysis provides an additional way to characterize malignant cells. In contrast to immunophenotyping, which can provide diagnostic information, DNA content analysis mainly provides prognostic information. As described earlier, the percentages of cells in each phase of the cell cycle are estimated based on the amount of DNA present in each cell. The cell-cycle phase percentage most often monitored is the S-phase percentage (%S-phase) because S-phase cells are replicating DNA, which is related to proliferation. The assumption is that the higher the S phase, the more rapidly the population is proliferating and the more aggressive the malignancy. Owing to the complexity of the neoplastic process, this assumption is not always valid. To date, S-phase analysis has been shown to be of prognostic value only in NHL,[26] multiple myeloma,[27] and primary plasma cell leukemia.[28] The latter two studies combined immunophenotyping with DNA analysis to specifically monitor the DNA content of plasma cells.

Another role for S-phase analysis in leukemia and lymphoma is for determining the effectiveness of cytokine therapy in increasing the proliferative rate of tumor cells.[26] Some malignancies, such as CLL and low-grade NHL, exhibit low proliferative rates that are thought to make them less susceptible to cytostatic chemotherapy.[29] Monitoring % S phase provides a way to determine when to start chemotherapy after cytokine treatment.

DNA ploidy is also monitored in some leukemias. DNA ploidy measurements indicate whether the cells in a population contain normal or abnormal amounts of DNA compared to a normal reference population. Cells with an abnormal content are designated as *DNA aneuploid*, whereas those with a normal content are designated as *DNA diploid*.

The only instance in which ploidy measurements have consistently been of prognostic value is pediatric ALL; there, DNA aneuploidy is associated with increased long-term remissions.[26]

Sample Preparation

The specimens analyzed are the same as those described under the immunophenotyping section. The fluorescent dye typically used by clinical laboratories for DNA analysis is propidium iodide (PI). Gloves should be worn while handling PI because it is carcinogenic. If DNA content alone is to be analyzed, then the simplest procedure consists of lysing erythrocytes with ammonium chloride, washing out the lyse solution and debris, then incubating approximately 1 million cells in a detergent-based PI solution containing RNAse A.[30] This method produces free nuclei. The samples must remain in the PI solution while they are analyzed on the cytometer, otherwise DNA staining is lost if the dye is washed out or diluted. For a method control, ficolled peripheral blood mononuclear cells (PBMCs), obtained from a healthy subject are processed in parallel with patient samples. Finally, if ploidy is to be assessed, a second aliquot of the patient specimen is spiked with 0.2×10^6 normal PBMCs. The PBMCs are noncycling (G_0 phase), making them ideal for use as a diploid reference standard.

If immunophenotyping is combined with DNA analysis, the cell membrane must be preserved. To accomplish this, a different procedure is required. One million leukocytes are first stained with an FITC-conjugated antibody, washed, and then permeabilized with absolute ethanol followed by staining in a detergent-free PI solution.[31] For instrument setup purposes, processed, unstained (no antibody, no PI), FITC-only stained, and PI-only stained samples are also prepared.

All samples are filtered through 30-μ mesh to remove aggregates. Samples are stored at 4°C in the dark until analyzed. Nuclei preps should be analyzed within 4 hours, whereas whole-cell preps can be held overnight.

Cytometer Operation

Instrument setup for DNA analysis differs in many ways from that for immunophenotyping. Because the range of signals detected is only two- to fourfold, linear amplification is used for the DNA fluorescence parameter. If FITC staining is also being measured, the FL1 amplifier is set to log. Either FL2 or FL3 can be used to detect PI fluorescence. Whichever parameter is used to measure DNA, it is also used as the threshold parameter. For this example, we assume DNA is measured in FL2, so the threshold parameter would be set to FL2. Instead of measuring the height of the pulse detected by the FL2 detector as in immunophenotyping, the area of the pulse (also called the integral) is measured. This provides better quantitation of the fluorescence per nucleus or cell analyzed. Finally for increased resolution, the sample flow rate on the cytometer is set to low (approximately 12 μL/min).

Additional QC measures are required for DNA applications. Because DNA analysis algorithms utilize assumptions about where the various cell-cycle phase populations are located, the linearity of amplifier used to measure PI fluorescence must be verified. For example, because PI fluorescence intensity is proportional to the DNA content, then G_2+M phase cells should be twice as bright as those in G_1, and the mean of G_2+M peak should be twice the mean of the G_1 peak. If the amplifier is not linear, then this relationship does not hold true and the statistics calculated by the algorithm will be inaccurate. To verify linearity, chicken erythrocyte nuclei are stained with PI and run under standardized settings. These nuclei are processed to form singlets and doublets. A single-parameter FL2 histogram of the population reveals at least two peaks: the dimmest one is the singlets and the one to the right of it, the doublets (Fig. 30–16). If the amplifier is linear, the ratio of the doublet mean to the singlet mean should fall between 1.95 and 2.05. In addition, for the best resolution, the coefficient of variation (CV) of the singlet peak should be less than or equal to 3.0%. The CV relates to the width of the peak. The narrower the peak, the more accurate are the statistics calculated by the algorithm. Specifications for linearity and CV are provided by the cytometer manufacturers. The specifications cited earlier were for a BD FACSCalibur™ using the DNA QC Kit.

Optimization entails running the PBMC diploid control sample, and adjusting the FL2 voltage to place the G_0/G_1 population at channel 200 on a 1023 scale. If dual FITC/PI-stained samples are to be analyzed, the unstained control is run with the threshold on FSC because the sample contains no PI, and the FL1 detector voltage is adjusted to bring the population on scale. Next, compensation is set while running the FITC-only sample, then the PI-only stained sample. Scatter parameters are set to linear amplification and adjusted to bring the populations on scale.

Data are collected with the threshold set to FL2 and set low enough to collect some debris. This ensures that no populations are accidentally eliminated. The DNA consensus group recommends acquiring a minimum of 10,000 events, not including debris or aggregates, per list mode data file.[32] After running the samples, it is important to clean the sample introduction port because PI cross-contamination of immunophenotyping samples can falsely elevate the FL2 and FL3 values. The same cleaning procedure that is used before shutdown works well for this purpose.

Data Analysis

The data file from the patient sample alone is used for calculating cell cycle percentages, and the data file from the patient sample spiked with normal PBMCs is used for calculating ploidy. Even when not spiked with normal PBMCs, histograms from patient samples may reveal two G_0/G_1 peaks because both normal and malignant leukocytes are present. Usually the leftmost population is the normal diploid component.

Automated software packages are used for DNA histogram analysis. They report cell-cycle phase percentages; CVs; the background, aggregates, and debris percentage (BAD); the % diploid; % aneuploid; the number of events modeled; and the DNA index (DI) (Fig. 30–17). The sample used for the figure was a leukemic cell line spiked with PBMCs. When the sample preparation is adequate, the CV of the PBMC G_0 peak should be less than 2.5%.[26] In this example it was 1.5%.

For accurate S-phase analysis using single-color analysis, the DNA consensus group recommends that the tumor population comprise at least 15% of the sample. If dual-color staining is used to allow gating on the tumor population, then the tumor cell percentage can be lower.[32] The DNA histogram analyzed from the gated population, however, should still contain at least 10,000 events. Reviewing the statistics in the example, these requirements were met.

The DNA consensus group recommends not reporting % S-phase results from histograms if the debris and aggregates statistic is greater than 20%.[32] It is also up to each laboratory to determine its own ranges for low, medium, and high % S phase based on their own analyses, and to define separate ranges for each type of malignancy examined.[32] In contrast to the example shown, clinical samples typically have S phases less than 20%.

Ploidy is reported as the DI. The DI is calculated by dividing the tumor G_0/G_1 peak mean by the diploid control G_0/G_1 peak mean. A DI of 1.0 denotes diploidy and a DI

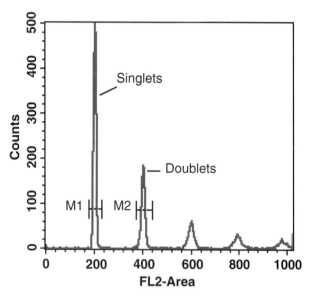

➤ **FIGURE 30–16** Quality control of the FL2-A amplifier using chicken erythrocyte nuclei stained with propidium iodide. Amplifier linearity is measured using the ratio of the doublet population mean to the single population mean. It should range between 1.95 and 2.05. Resolution is determined by measuring the coefficient of variation (CV) of the singlet peak. It should be less than 3%.

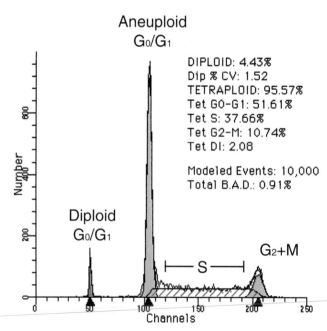

➤ **FIGURE 30–17** A DNA histogram of a leukemic T-cell line spiked with peripheral blood mononuclear cells (first peak). The statistics were calculated using software modeling.

other than 1.0 denotes aneuploidy.[32] The DI of 2.0 in the example indicates that the tumor line is aneuploid, more specifically, tetraploid.

Hematopoietic Progenitor Cell Enumeration

Hematopoietic progenitor cells (HPCs), sometimes called *hematopoietic stem cells,* are CD34-positive leukocytes found primarily in the bone marrow and cord blood, and in low numbers (0.01%) in the peripheral blood. They can replace failed marrow in various anemias, and more recently are being used to rescue cancer patients from the fatal aplasia that results from high-dose chemotherapy.[33] In the past, bone marrow samples were harvested either from the patient before chemotherapy, or from a human leukocyte antigen (HLA)–matched donor. This method was laborious and painful for the donor. With the advent of HPC mobilization techniques, it has become possible to obtain large numbers of peripheral blood progenitor cells (PBPCs) through apheresis. Mobilization techniques consist of administering various combinations of drugs and growth factors, then harvesting after a given period of time. Progenitor cell enumeration assays provide a way to monitor donors on mobilization protocols. With this information, there is more certainty that the requisite number of PBPCs will be obtained the first time the donor is apheresed. More importantly, during the apheresis a PBPC count can be obtained and, based on this information, it can be decided whether to continue until the target number has been reached or whether to have the donor return later for an additional apheresis procedure.[33]

Sample Preparation

Two methods predominate for HPC enumeration. The first is a lyse and wash method,[34] the second is lyse-no-wash.[35] The first method can be used on peripheral blood, cord blood, and bone marrow samples, but it contains more steps and some studies show that cell loss can occur during the washes.[36] The second method is intended for use with peripheral blood or leukopheresis samples, but not with bone marrow. The second method also contains fewer steps and is compatible with an automated software analysis program. Because PBPC enumeration is more prevalent than HPC analysis of bone marrow, the second method is described here.

Peripheral blood is collected in EDTA, and leukapheresis samples are collected in ACD. Fifty-microliter aliquots are stained with a two-tube panel consisting of a CD34 tube and control tube. The CD34 tube contains a nucleic acid dye (FL1), CD34-PE, and CD45-PerCP, and the control tube contains nucleic acid dye, IgG subclass control-PE, and CD45-PerCP. Both tubes contain reference count beads for determining absolute counts. Control cells containing known numbers of CD34-positive cells are available and should be processed in parallel with the patient samples. After a 15-minute incubation, a lysing fixative is added; the samples are then analyzed on the cytometer after 30 minutes.

Cytometer Operation

The cytometer is set up with FSC and SSC in linear amplification, and FL1, FL2, and FL3 in log amplification. The threshold is set to FL1 to collect mainly nucleated cells. A minimum of 60,000 events is required for accurate enumeration because the target population is typically less than 5%.

Data Analysis

Results from an analysis are shown (Fig. 30–18). This is a type of rare event analysis; therefore, multiple parameters and gating strategies are used to discriminate the CD34 cells from background. The automated algorithm applies sequential gates to isolate and enumerate the population. The control tube is analyzed to correct for background events falling within the gates shown on final two plots.

Flow Crossmatching

Flow crossmatching is used to determine if a recipient contains alloantibodies against cells from a potential donor. The test assists in identifying transplantation recipients with a high risk for rejection, and it can also aid in monitoring for rejection posttransplantation. For example, in bone marrow transplantation even low concentrations of alloantibodies can be responsible for engraftment failure.[37] The crossmatch is performed in much the same way it is done for blood transfusions except that the class I and class II HLAs are the alloantigens. The donor cells used for targets are lymphocytes from peripheral blood, spleen, or lymph nodes, because lymphocytes bear both classes of HLA. T lymphocytes bear primarily class I, whereas B lymphocytes bear both classes I and II, making it possible to test the recipient for both types of alloantibodies. Anti–class I antibodies of the IgG isotype appear to be the most detrimental with respect to graft survival. Generally, a negative flow crossmatch means that the transplantation can proceed, whereas a positive crossmatch means that additional tests must be performed.[37]

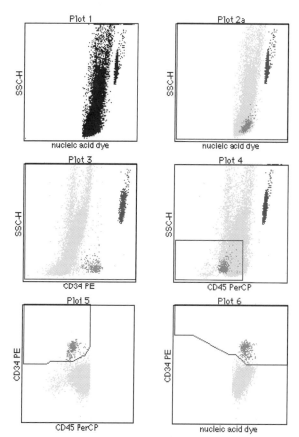

Absolute CD34 cell count: 277.9 /µL (CY = 4.5 %)   Dilution Factor: 1.00

➤ **FIGURE 30–18** Enumeration of hematopoietic progenitor cells using an automated, sequential gating algorithm.

Sample Preparation

Extensive details for this procedure are available.[38] Briefly, PBMCs or lymphocytes prepared from donor spleen or lymph node are suspended in buffered saline containing newborn calf serum. Next, aliquots of 2.5×10^5 cells are placed in three separate tubes. A positive control serum (PPS) is added to the first tube, a negative control serum (NHS) is added to the second, and the recipient serum is added to the third. Typically 20 to 50 μL of serum is added per tube. After a 30-minute incubation at 4°C, the samples are washed three times with cold buffered saline, then a combination of anti-human IgG-FITC, CD19-PE, and CD3-PerCP is added to each tube. The samples are incubated at 4°C for 20 minutes, then washed another three times, and fixed in cold 2% paraformaldehyde. Finally, they are held in the dark at 4°C and analyzed within 1 week. The samples are kept cold during the staining procedure to maintain high viability. Otherwise, they may nonspecifically bind antibodies making the results difficult to interpret.

Several factors are critical for performing this assay. They include using an anti-human IgG that is Fc-specific, and that is composed of only F(ab′)$_2$ fragments to reduce nonspecific binding. This antibody must also be titered for this assay. The PPS positive control serum is pooled from several donors known to have high concentrations of anti-HLA antibodies. It should also be titered so that on a 1024-channel scale, the staining intensity is approximately 100 to 200 channels brighter than the NHS sample. The NHS serum is pooled from several donors lacking alloantibodies. To confirm that this serum is truly negative, it should be screened against several donors before use as a control.[38]

Cytometer Operation

The cytometer is set up for basic three-color immunophenotyping. FSC and SSC are set to linear, the threshold is set to FSC, and FL1, FL2, and FL3 are set to log amplification. Typically, 10,000 events are collected per list mode data file.

Data Analysis

A gate is set on the T lymphocytes, then the FL1 fluorescence is viewed on a histogram. Although the FL1 parameter was set to log during data collection, some laboratories prefer to display the data on a 1024-channel scale[37] as shown in this example (Fig. 30–19). The figure displays histograms for an NHS serum sample (left) and a PPS serum sample (right). A positive crossmatch would exhibit a staining intensity with a median somewhere between the two controls. Each laboratory must determine its own cutoff for a positive crossmatch.[38] The method for determining the cutoff is published, but basically it entails running the NHS on several donors of different HLA types, determining the median fluorescence value for each donor, then determining the mean of all these values. The cutoff for a positive crossmatch is the channel value that is two standard deviations above the mean.[38] Separate cutoffs should be defined for T- and B- cell populations. The significance of the results from the B-cell population is not clear.

Detection of Paroxysmal Nocturnal Hemoglobinuria

Paroxysmal nocturnal hemoglobinuria (PNH) is a rare acquired clonal disorder of hematopoietic stem cells caused by a somatic mutation of the X-linked *PIG-A* gene, which is in-

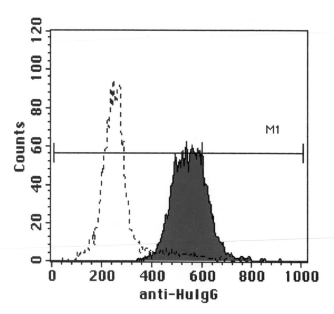

➤ FIGURE 30–19   Flow cytometry crossmatching. The negative (NHS) control (*dotted*) and positive control (*solid*) are shown. (List mode data courtesy of Dr. Robert Bray, Emory University, Atlanta, GA.)

volved in the synthesis of glycosyl phosphatidyl inositol (GPI), an anchor molecule that attaches proteins to the cell membrane.[39] This leads to a diminished expression of GPI-linked proteins, two of which are responsible for the susceptibility of erythrocytes to lysis by complement. They are CD55 and CD59, decay-accelerating factor (DAF) and membrane inhibitor of reactive lysis (MIRL), respectively.[40] Two patterns of PNH have been described, cases that present as a progressive pancytopenia with marrow failure, and those with primary aplastic anemia in which PNH appears later in the disease.[39] The mainstays for diagnosis of PNH, such as the Ham test, rely on the lysis of affected erythrocytes by complement. Flow cytometric assays provide a more sensitive and quantitative means for establishing a diagnosis of PNH. In fact, granulocytes and monocytes appear to be the first cells affected at a time when erythrocytes appear normal and Ham test negative.[39] In addition to being useful as a diagnostic tool, serial monitoring of the clone size is possible through flow cytometry. Studies are currently being conducted to determine if this information will help predict an individual's clinical course.[41]

Sample Preparation

A basic protocol is presented. Peripheral blood is collected in EDTA and processed within 6 hours. If the specimen is not processed by then, it should be stored at 4°C. For erythrocyte staining, two 5-μL aliquots of whole blood are stained, one with fluorochrome-conjugated subclass control antibody and the other with fluorochrome-conjugated CD59. After staining, the samples are washed and fixed. Similarly, for granulocyte staining, two 50-μL aliquots of blood are stained, one with a subclass control and one with CD59, except that after staining, the erythrocytes are lysed, then the samples are washed and fixed. In addition, normal control samples of stained erythrocyte and granulocyte samples are prepared from a healthy donor. For clearest results it is recommended that antibodies to two GPI-dependent antigens be used, such as CD55 and CD59. This also adds specificity in analyzing patients with isolated deficiencies of either CD55 (Inab blood group phenotype) or CD59 (congenital 20kdHRF deficiency).[40] Adding a lineage-specific antibody to GPI-independent antigens, such as CD15, can also be useful for gating purposes.[41]

Cytometer Operation

The cytometer is set up with FSC and SSC set to log amplification for samples stained for erythrocytes, and linear amplification for samples stained for granulocytes. Fluorescence parameters are set to log amplification, and the threshold is set to FSC. Erythrocyte samples are run with the flow rate set to low, because of the high cell number. Ten thousand events are collected per list mode data file.

Data Analysis

Using FSC and SSC, a gate is set on erythrocytes or neutrophils. The most common way to analyze fluorescence staining is to use a single-parameter histogram to evaluate CD59 staining intensity. The purpose of data analysis is to detect type I, type II, and type III populations. Type I populations represent normal staining. The normal control sample is analyzed, and markers are set to delineate where type I populations will fall. The solid lines in Figures 30–20A and 30–20B labeled R1 represent type I staining. Type III populations are completely deficient in CD59 expression. The patient's subclass control sample is analyzed, and markers are set to delineate where type III populations will fall. The dotted lines in Figure 30–20A and 30–20B labeled R3 represent type III staining. Type II populations are partially deficient in CD59 expression, and they display

staining intensities between those of type I and type III. Cells with intermediate staining intensity will fall in the area labeled R2. The patient sample is analyzed, and the percentage of type I, II, and III populations is determined for erythrocytes and for neutrophils[40] (Figs. 30–20C and 30–20D). Flow cytometric analyses of PNH patients have helped clarify the classification of PNH into two types: (1) hemolytic PNH, characterized by overt episodes of intravascular hemolysis, typically with large clones, and (2) hypoplastic PNH, dominated by cytopenia with no overt hemolysis and small, mainly type II, erythrocyte clones.[41]

Reticulocyte Enumeration

Reticulocytes are immature erythrocytes, newly emerged from the bone marrow. They are characterized by the trace amounts of intracellular RNA. They circulate in the peripheral blood for approximately 2 days before all RNA is lost, and they become mature erythrocytes.[42] Reticulocyte enumeration is used for evaluating anemias, for monitoring the effectiveness of erythropoietin therapy for dialysis patients, for monitoring bone marrow function after chemotherapy, and for monitoring engraftment after bone marrow transplantation.[42]

Sample Preparation

Reticulocytes are detected by flow cytometry based on the presence of RNA. Coriphosphine-O and thiazole orange are two dyes commonly used. Guidelines on the preparation and analysis of reticulocytes by a variety of methods are available.[43] The thiazole orange method is presented here. Blood is collected in EDTA. For accurate counts it should be processed immediately because the reticulocytes continue the maturation process in the specimen tube. Five microliters of blood is added to 1 mL of 1% thiazole orange in buffered saline. If the data will be analyzed manually, a control tube is prepared by adding 5 μL of blood to 1 mL of buffered saline. After a 30-minute incubation in the dark, at room temperature, the samples are analyzed. Method control cells containing known numbers of reticulocytes are available, and a control sample is processed in parallel with the patient samples.

Cytometer Operation

FSC, SSC, and FL1 are set to log amplification; all compensation circuits are set to zero; and the threshold is set to FSC. The flow rate is set to low, and 10,000 events are collected per list mode data file.

Data Analysis

The results from the analysis of an automated reticulocyte enumeration software program are shown (Fig. 30–21). A gate is set around the erythrocyte population to exclude platelets, and FL1 fluorescence of the gated population is displayed. The marker that separates negative from positive events is set by the algorithm. The percentage statistic for the positive region is calculated along with the mean fluorescence intensity. Normal values for adults range from 0.5% to 2.0%.[44] If a red blood cell count is supplied, the absolute count is calculated by multiplying the count by the % Reticulocytes statistic. Normal counts range from 33 to 137 cells/μL. The mean fluorescence (Mean FL1) of the population is related to its maturity, and it is used to calculate the immature reticulocyte fraction (IRF). The IRF is

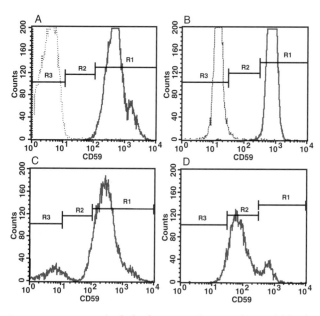

➤ FIGURE 30–20 Analysis of paroxysmal nocturnal hemoglobinuria data. Normal staining patterns for erythrocytes (A) and neutrophils (B) are shown in solid lines. Background staining is represented by the fluorescence from the patient's subclass control sample and displayed as dotted lines. These controls are used for drawing regions to denote type I, II, and III populations (R1, R2, and R3, respectively). Patient data for erythrocytes (C) and neutrophils (D) reveal the presence of type II and type III populations for both cell types. (List mode data courtesy of Dr. Jonni Moore, Hospital of the University of Pennsylvania, Philadelphia, PA.)

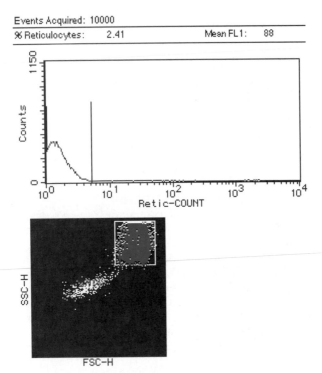

Events Acquired: 10000
% Reticulocytes: 2.41   Mean FL1:   88

> **FIGURE 30–21** Reticulocyte enumeration using thiazole orange. Absolute counts are calculated by the software by multiplying the % Retics by the RBC count entered by the operator. The FL1 mean is related to the maturity of the population.

similar in concept to the concept of estimating left-shifted granulocytes. It is useful for assessing reticulocyte responsiveness to various treatments and conditions.[42]

Manual data analysis is performed by first analyzing the gated erythrocyte population of the unstained control sample, and setting the markers to delineate positive staining. Next, the stained sample is analyzed using the same markers, and the percentage of events with fluorescence intensities higher than the control sample is calculated. If the mean fluorescence intensity is required, the geometric mean statistic is utilized.

Detection of Fetomaternal Hemorrhage

The detection of circulating fetal erythrocytes in maternal blood is key for the obstetric management of blood group Rh-negative women carrying an Rh-positive fetus, and for assessing placental injury after trauma. Through flow cytometry, it is possible to detect as low as 0.02% fetal erythrocytes in maternal blood, making this assay a type of rare event analysis.[45]

Sample Preparation

Fetal erythrocytes are identified by the presence of hemoglobin F (HgbF), an intracellular antigen. Blood is collected in EDTA, and 5 mL is fixed in 1 mL 0.05% glutaraldehyde in buffered saline. After 10 minutes, the blood is washed three times with buffered saline and the cell pellet is resuspended in 0.5 mL buffered saline containing Triton-X 100 detergent to permeabilize the cells. After 3 minutes, the cells are washed and resuspended to 0.5 mL. Ten microliters is stained with anti-HgbF-FITC for 15 minutes, then washed twice and resuspended in 0.1% formaldehyde in

buffered saline. Controls are also processed in parallel with patient samples. They include a negative control consisting of blood from a nonpregnant donor, and two levels of positive controls consisting of the negative control specimen spiked with 1% and 5% cord blood, respectively.[45]

Cytometer Operation

FSC, SSC, FL1, and FL2 are set to log amplification. Standard two-color compensation is performed. The threshold is set to FSC, and 50,000 events are collected per list mode data file.[45]

Data Analysis

Leukocytes display autofluorescence that interferes with the analysis. To eliminate leukocytes from the analysis, a plot of SSC/FL2 is created and a gate is set around the FL2 dim population (Fig. 30–22B). The FL1 fluorescence of the gated population is displayed on an FL1 histogram. The negative control is run and markers are set so that brighter events can be quantitated. The marker placement is verified by analyzing both positive controls and obtaining histogram statistics for the bright population. The 1% positive control is shown (Fig. 30–22C). Finally, the patient samples are analyzed and the percentage of anti-HgbF cells is calculated. The clinically relevant range of HgbF-positive cells is 0 to 5.4%, with 0.02% being the average for nonpregnant donors, and 0.6% or greater being a decision point for additional dosing for Rh immune globulin.[45]

Platelet Studies

A variety of flow cytometry assays exist for platelet studies. They include assays to measure platelet activation status, platelet activation function, platelet-bound immunoglobulin, and platelet production.[46] This information is useful for evaluating patients with coronary artery disease to determine if anticoagulant therapy is sufficient, for studying congenital platelet disorders, and for evaluating thrombocytopenias.[46–48] The following presentation focuses on platelet activation function studies.

Sample Preparation

Whole blood is collected in heparin or sodium citrate. Immediately after collection, 100 μL is fixed in 1 mL of 2% paraformaldehyde in buffered saline. This is the resting control. Within 5 minutes of collection, two 0.45-mL aliquots of blood are placed in two tubes. One tube is incubated for 5 minutes at room temperature in 5 μM adenosine diphosphate (ADP). The second tube is the negative control, incubated with buffered saline. After the incubation, 50 μL from each tube is pipeted into two new tubes containing 1 mL of paraformaldehyde to stop the activation. The samples are fixed for 30 minutes and stored in the cold until stained. For staining, the samples are washed in Tyrode's buffer to remove fixative and lyse erythrocytes, then stained with CD41-FITC, a pan-platelet marker, and CD62P-PE, which detects P-Selectin, a platelet activation antigen.[47] After staining, the samples are washed and then resuspended in 1 mL of Tyrode's buffer. A healthy donor specimen is also processed in parallel with patient samples as a method control. In addition, subclass control, CD41-FITC–only, CD62P-PE–only stained samples are also prepared from the normal donor for cytometer setup purposes.

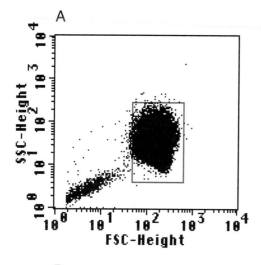

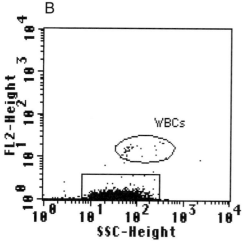

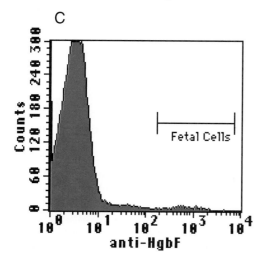

➤ **FIGURE 30–22** Analysis of data to detect fetomaternal hemorrhage using anti-hemoglobin F (HgbF) staining. Interference by autofluorescent leukocytes is removed by gating on the FL2 dim population *(B)*. A control sample spiked with 1% cord blood is shown. (List mode data courtesy of Viki Mosiman and Marina Gever, BD Biosciences, San Jose, CA.)

Cytometer Operation

The cytometer is set up with FSC, SSC, FL1, and FL2 in log amplification. The subclass control sample is used to adjust the FL1 and FL2 autofluorescence signal to the first

decade on an FL1/FL2 plot. Compensation is adjusted using the single-stained samples. The threshold is set to FL1 to collect primarily platelet data. Ten thousand platelet events are collected.

Data Analysis

Using the subclass control data file, a gate is drawn on the platelets on a CD41/SSC plot, then the gated events are displayed on an FSC/CD62P plot. Quadrant markers are set to encompass the population LL quadrant. The normal and patient files are analyzed using these markers. Data from a resting (Fig. 30–23A) and an activated (Fig. 30–23B) sample are shown. The activated platelets exhibit a larger size because of aggregation and increased CD62P intensities.[49] Both UR and UL quadrant statistics are summed to estimate the percentage of activated platelets.

Emerging Applications for Antigen Quantitation

Antigen quantitation provides a standardized way to express fluorescence intensities. The standardization is achieved by running samples of beads bearing standardized amounts of fluorochrome on the cytometer after the settings have been optimized for the samples. This makes it possible to convert observed fluorescence intensities from relative units (1 to 10,000) to fluorochromes per cell. Results can be compared among different cytometers, as long as the beads have also been run. One example of the potential use of this information is as a prognostic indicator in the management of AIDS.[50,51] The CD38 expression on CD8-positive cells can be evaluated, and it appears that when examining samples from patients with similar CD4 counts, an elevated CD38 expression correlates with a worse outcome.[50] Examples of results from patients expressing normal (Fig. 30–24A) and elevated (Fig. 30–24B) CD38 expression are shown. The calibration points from running the standardized beads are shown on the y axis.

Another application for antigen quantitation is in the detection of neutrophil activation. One research group has shown that CD64 expression is elevated in patients who later became septic as detected by microbiologic techniques.[52] The CD64 elevation was not observed in patients with other types of inflammation. In addition, CD64 expression was activated in patients receiving interferon-gamma treatment. Thus, CD64 expression may be an effective way to determine, early on, if dosing is appropriate. Similar promise has been shown in using neutrophil expression of CD11b/CD18 to monitor effectiveness of cytokine therapy in patients receiving granulocyte colony-stimulating factor.[53]

Finally, another application for antigen quantitation is for assisting in delineating normal cells from leukemic cells. For example, one study has shown that quantitation of CD16 expression is useful for a differential diagnosis of chronic myelogenous leukemia (CML) from other chronic myeloproliferative diseases. In this study, the CML cells exhibiting depressed CD16 expression were compared to neutrophils from healthy donors, and patients with bacterial infections, polycythemia, and thrombocythemia.[54]

Emerging Assays for Soluble Factors

The utility of flow cytometry is expanding the detection of soluble factors. These assays use sandwich techniques

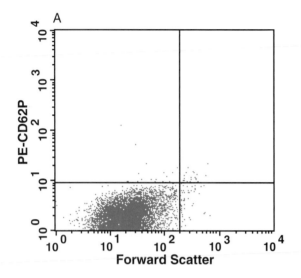

Gated Events: 9748

Quad	Events	% Gated
UL	23	0.24
UR	29	0.30
LL	9633	98.82
LR	63	0.65

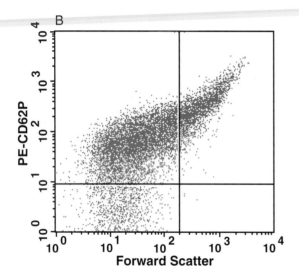

Gated Events: 9818

Quad	Events	% Gated
UL	6466	65.86
UR	2247	22.89
LL	1101	11.21
LR	4	0.04

➤ FIGURE 30–23   Staining pattern of resting (A) and ADP-activated (B) platelets. Note the increase in size and CD62P staining. The size increase is a result of aggregation.

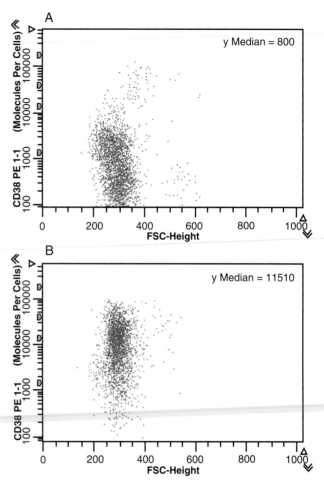

➤ FIGURE 30–24   CD38 expression of CD8-positive cells from two individuals with HIV infections and similar CD4 counts. Studies have shown that individuals with normal staining (A) experience less severe disease progression compared with individuals with elevated expression (B).[50] (List mode data courtesy of Dr. David Miller, Broward Community Blood Center, Fort Lauderdale, FL.)

whereby a capture molecule, usually an antibody, is attached to a bead population. The test fluid containing the antigen of interest is incubated with the beads, the beads are washed, and a fluorochrome-conjugated reporter antibody is added to detect antigen bound to the bead. The reporter antibody is specific for a different antigenic determinant than the capture antibody.[55]

One group assayed plasma for von Willebrand's factor (vWF) using collagen-coated beads for capture and rabbit anti-human vWF followed by goat anti-rabbit Ig-FITC for the reporter antibody. Quantitation of this factor is performed in evaluating von Willebrand's disease, which is a heterogeneous disorder exhibiting numerous variants and subtypes. The flow results correlated with the standard ristocetin cofactor assay, with the flow assay exhibiting less interassay variability than the standard assay.[56]

A final example illustrates the utility of mixing multiple bead populations, each conjugated to a different capture reagent, together to assay for several factors at once. This is accomplished using beads of different colors for each analyte.[55,57] For example, one group devised an assay that used a mixture of 15 capture bead populations, each specific for a different cytokine. In this assay, the bead populations were distinguishable from one another based on the FL2/FL3 fluorescence, and the reporter molecule was FITC conjugated. Thus, the bead population is gated on an

FL2/FL3 plot, then the FITC intensity evaluated for each analyte.[57] This assay shows great potential for monitoring patients undergoing cytokine therapy, and for evaluating patients with various types of inflammatory diseases.

QUESTIONS

1. Which of the four main tasks related to flow cytometric analysis often requires the expertise of a specialty physician?
   a. Sample preparation
   b. Cytometer operation
   c. Data analysis
   d. Results interpretation

2. Antibodies binding the same antigen are classified in the same:
   a. Isotype
   b. ABO group
   c. CD group
   d. HLA group

3. Which characteristics apply to monoclonal antibodies?
   a. Purified from antisera
   b. Derived from cloned, immortalized B-cell cultures
   c. Highly specific and well characterized
   d. High background staining

4. Which is not a major system in a flow cytometer?
   a. Threshold
   b. Fluidics
   c. Optics
   d. Electronics

5. Which parameter is typically used to measure green fluorescence?
   a. FL2
   b. FL3
   c. FL1
   d. FL4

6. An FSC/SSC plot displays two populations, A and B. Population A is to the left of population B. Based on this information, which statement is true?
   a. Cells of population B are more granular than those in A.
   b. Cells of population A are larger than those in B.
   c. Cells of population A are smaller than those in B.
   d. Cells in population A are more granular than those in B.

7. This is used to restrict the data analysis to one population.
   a. Compensation
   b. Linear amplification
   c. Gating
   d. Logarithmic amplification

8. Reviewing Figures 30–7C and 30–8, what is the percentage of CD3-positive/CD4-negative lymphocytes?

   a. 9.07
   b. 37.92
   c. 26.03
   d. 13.21

9. Reviewing Figures 30–7C and 30–8, which two quadrant statistics must be summed to obtain the percentage of CD3-positive lymphocytes?
   a. UL and UR
   b. UR and LR
   c. UL and LL
   d. LL and LR

10. Reviewing Figure 30–9, which region statistic would be used to measure the percentage of lymphocytes that is CD3-negative/CD4-positive?
    a. R3, % Gated
    b. R3, % Total
    c. R4, % Gated
    d. R4, % Total

11. Reviewing Figure 30–10, what is the percentage of CD3-negative lymphocytes?
    a. 5.09
    b. 13.84
    c. 39.72
    d. 59.87

12. In comparing cell-cycle phases within a cell population, which of the following expressions are true with respect to DNA content?
    a. S phase $> G_2+M$ phase
    b. G_2+M phase $>$ S phase
    c. G_2+M phase $> G_0/G_1$ phase
    d. S phase $< G_0/G_1$ phase

13. Which terms relate to fluorescence intensity measurements?
    a. Molecules of equivalent soluble fluorochrome
    b. Median fluorescence
    c. % Gated
    d. Antibodies bound per cell

14. A sample contains 50 µL of blood and 40,000 reference beads. A 10,000-event data file is collected and analyzed using region statistics. The following information was obtained: There were 1500 events for cell population X, and 1000 bead events in the data file. Calculate the absolute count per microliter of blood for population X.
    a. 533
    b. 1200
    c. 8000
    d. 120

15. What is monitored in HIV-positive individuals to determine if antiviral treatment should begin?
    a. CD3 percentages
    b. CD8 absolute counts
    c. CD8 percentages
    d. CD4 absolute counts

16. Which disease is not characterized by a reduction of T lymphocytes?
    a. Severe combined immunodeficiency
    b. X-linked hypogammaglobulinemia
    c. Thymic hypoplasia
    d. Acquired immunodeficiency disease syndrome

17. Which statements are true regarding DNA content analysis?
    a. It is used as a diagnostic test.
    b. It has prognostic value for a limited number of hematologic malignancies.
    c. It has prognostic value for a wide range of hematologic malignancies.
    d. None of the above.

18. Which antibodies are used for hematopoietic progenitor cell enumeration?
    a. CD34
    b. CD25
    c. CD10
    d. CD45

19. Anti-HgbF is used to detect:
    a. Reticulocytes
    b. Fetal erythrocytes
    c. Platelets
    d. Leukemias

20. Reticulocytes are detected using:
    a. Anti-HgbF
    b. Thiazole orange
    c. Phycoerythrin
    d. Propidium iodide

21. Paroxysmal nocturnal hemoglobinuria is detected by:
    a. A decrease in CD59 staining intensity on erythrocytes
    b. An increase in CD59 staining intensity on neutrophils
    c. A decrease in CD59 staining intensity on neutrophils
    d. A decrease in CD45 staining intensity on erythrocytes

22. Flow crossmatching detects:
    a. Alloantibodies in the donor's serum
    b. Alloantibodies in the recipient's serum
    c. Cytotoxic T cells in the donor's blood
    d. a and b

23. Which statements are not true?
    a. CD38 staining intensity on CD4 lymphocytes has prognostic value in AIDS.
    b. Increased CD64 staining intensity on neutrophils shows promise as an early indicator for sepsis.
    c. Increased CD11/CD18 staining intensities on neutrophils are related to neutrophil activation.
    d. Measuring CD64 staining intensity may be useful for monitoring gamma-interferon therapy.

SUMMARY CHART

➤ Flow cytometry is a technology that provides rapid measurements of physical characteristics of cells suspended in a moving fluid stream.

➤ Flow cytometric analysis can be broken down into four main tasks: preparing samples, operating the cytometer, analyzing data, and interpreting results.

➤ The cellular characteristics measured in flow cytometry include surface area, granularity and internal complexity, and fluorescent colors.

➤ For enumeration of leukocyte subpopulations, blood and marrow are usually collected in ethylene diaminetetraacetic acid (EDTA), stored at room temperature, and analyzed within 24 hours of collection.

➤ Preparation for lymphoid tissue analysis involves harvesting of tissue into a sterile container containing cold tissue medium followed by disaggregation into a single-cell suspension, filtration, and staining of target cell population.

➤ Immunophenotyping utilizes fluorochrome-conjugated antibodies to identify target populations.

➤ Monoclonal antibodies are preferred over polyclonal antibodies in immunophenotyping; they are homogeneous, highly specific, and well characterized. These antibodies are produced from cloned B-cell cultures.

➤ Antibodies within a CD (cluster of differentiation group) bind the same antigen or epitope.

➤ The five procedures that define flow cytometer operation are startup, quality control, optimization, data collection, and shutdown.

➤ Optimization involves running a sample from a normal subject and adjusting the cytometer settings to bring the cell populations of interest on scale.

➤ Forward scatter (FSC) is related to the size of the cell whereby the larger the cell is, the greater the FSC signal.

➤ Side scatter (SSC) is related to the internal complexity or granularity of the cell.

➤ The parameters FL1, FL2, FL3, and FL4 represent measurements of four different fluorochromes.

➤ The threshold parameter of the flow cytometer is used to limit what is analyzed by the instrument and what is not analyzed.

➤ The photodetectors of the flow cytometer convert light signals into electrical signals called voltage pulses, whereby the higher the pulse is, the stronger the signal.

➤ Fluorescence compensation is an electronic control that corrects for bleed-over of fluorescent dyes so that each detector measures signals corresponding to the appropriate fluorescent dye.

➤ The objectives of data analysis in flow cytometry include obtaining statistics on populations percentages, absolute cell counts, and fluorescence intensity measurements; and identifying abnormal populations based on light scatter or staining patterns, or both.

➤ Gating is a software feature that allows the operator to focus on a single population of cells.

➤ Quadrant statistics are used to distinguish negative, single-positive, and double-positive cell populations.

➤ A subclass control reagent contains an antibody of the same immunoglobulin subclass as the staining reagent, conjugated to the same fluorochrome, but specific for an antigen not found in humans.

➤ In DNA analysis, cells are stained with a fluorescent dye that binds in proportion to the amount of DNA present; the G_0/G_1 represent the normal complement of DNA, the G_2+M represents a double complement of DNA, and the S-phase cells are intermediate.

➤ In acquired immunodeficiency syndrome (AIDS), the human immunodeficiency virus infects and kills the CD4 helper T lymphocytes and therefore results in a decrease in the CD4 subset on flow analysis.

➤ Typical ranges for lymphocyte subset percentages in adult donors are CD3 (56% to 86%), CD4 (33% to 58%), CD8 (13% to 39%), CD16+56 (5% to 26%), and CD19 (5% to 22%).

➤ Leukemia refers to a malignancy that occurs at any step in the differentiation from a blast in the bone marrow to a mature leukocyte in the peripheral blood.

➤ Flow cytometry can be used to diagnose pre-B acute lymphocytic leukemia (ALL), T-ALL, B chronic lymphocytic leukemia (CLL), small lymphocytic leukemia, acute myelocytic leukemia (AML), hairy-cell leukemia, non-Hodgkin's lymphoma (NHL), mantle cell lymphoma, large-cell B-NHL, Burkitt's lymphoma, large granular lymphocyte disorders, and plasma cell dyscrasias.

➤ In analyses for leukemia and lymphoma, specimens include peripheral blood, marrow, lymphoid biopsies, and fine-needle aspirates. Sodium heparin is the anticoagulant of choice, and blood and marrow and should be processed within 48 hours of collection.

➤ Asynchronous expression refers to the abnormal expression of antigen in leukemia wherein the antigen is expressed during a maturation phase in which it is normally absent.

➤ Hematopoietic progenitor cells are CD34-positive leukocytes found primarily in the bone marrow and cord blood, and in low numbers in the peripheral blood.

➤ Flow crossmatching is used to determine if a recipient contains alloantibodies against cells from a potential donor, with HLA classes I and II serving as alloantigens.

➤ The monoclonal antibodies used to detect paroxysmal nocturnal hemoglobinuria are antibodies to the glycosyl phosphatidyl inositol (GPI)–linked proteins, CD55 and CD59.

➤ Enumeration of reticulocytes in flow cytometry utilizes coriphosphine-O or thiazole orange to detect the presence of RNA in these cells.

➤ The sensitivity in the detection of a fetomaternal hemorrhage using flow cytometry is as low as 0.02%, with 0.6% defined as a decision point for administering Rh immune globulin.

➤ Platelet studies via flow cytometry includes platelet activation status, platelet activation function, platelet-bound immunoglobulin, and platelet production.

ACKNOWLEDGMENTS

Attractors and FACSCalibur are trademarks of Becton, Dickinson and Company. Many thanks to Dr. Raul Braylan, Dr. Tom Frey, Ms. Betty Eastham, Ms. Susan Zanjani, Ms. Sue Merrill, Mr. Antonio Mele, and Ms. Maria Quist, for their contributions.

References

1. McCoy, JP, and Kern, DF: Current practices in clinical flow cytometry. A practice survey by the American Society of Clinical Pathologists. Am J Clin Pathol 111:161, 1999.
2. Kishimoto, T, et al: Leukocyte Typing VI: White Cell Differentiation Antigens. Garland Publishing, New York, 1997.
3. Owens, MA, and Loken, MR: Flow Cytometry Principles for Clinical Laboratory Practice. Quality Assurance for Quantitative Immunophenotyping. Wiley-Liss, New York, 1995.
4. Melamed, MR, et al: Flow Cytometry and Sorting. Wiley-Liss, New York, 1990.
5. Givan, AL: Flow Cytometry: First Principles. Wiley-Liss, New York, 1992.
6. Nicholson, JK, et al: Evaluation of alternative CD4 technologies for the enumeration of CD4 lymphocytes. Immunol Methods 177:43, 1994.
7. Schwartz, A, et al: Standardizing flow cytometry: A classification system of fluorescence standards used for flow cytometry. Cytometry 33:106, 1998.
8. Centers for Disease Control and Prevention: Report of the NIH Panel to define principles of therapy of HIV infection and guidelines for the use of antiretroviral agents in HIV-infected adults and adolescents. MMWR 47(No. RR-5):70, 1998.
9. Adelman, DC, and Abba, T: Allergic and immunologic disorders. In Tierney, LM, et al (eds): Current Medical Diagnosis and Treatment. Appleton & Lange, Stamford, CT, 1998, p 755.
10. Centers for Disease Control and Prevention: 1997 revised guidelines for performing CD4+ T-cell determinations in persons infected with human immunodeficiency virus (HIV). MMWR:46(No. RR-2):8, 1997.
11. National Committee for Clinical Laboratory Standards (NCCLS): Clinical applications of flow cytometry: Quality assurance and immunophenotyping of lymphocytes; approved guideline. NCCLS document H42-A, 1998.
12. Hilerio, F, and Niesler, HM: FACS® MultiSET™ system. Productivity and performance in CD4 monitoring with 4-color MultiTEST™/TruCOUNT™ technology. BD Biosciences, San Jose, 1998. White paper.
13. Kutok, JL, et al: Four-color flow cytometry immunophenotypic determination of peripheral blood CD4+ T-lymphocyte counts. Am J Clin Pathol 110:465, 1998.
14. Ward, MS: The use of flow cytometry in the diagnosis and monitoring of malignant hematological disorders. Pathology 31:382, 1999.
15. Davis, BH, et al: U.S.-Canadian consensus recommendations on the immunophenotypic analysis of hematologic neoplasia by flow cytometry: Medical indications. Cytometry 30:249, 1997.
16. Campana, D, and Coustan-Smith, E: Detection of minimal residual disease in acute leukemia by flow cytometry. Cytometry 38:139, 1999.
17. Stelzer, GT, et al: U.S.-Canadian consensus recommendations on the immunophenotypic analysis of hematologic neoplasia by flow cytometry: Standardization and validation of laboratory procedures. Cytometry 30:214, 1997.
18. Stewart, CC, et al: U.S.-Canadian consensus recommendations on the immunophenotypic analysis of hematologic neoplasia by flow cytometry: Selection of antibody combinations. Cytometry 30:231, 1997.
19. Borowitz, MJ, et al: U.S.-Canadian consensus recommendations on the immunophenotypic analysis of hematologic neoplasia by flow cytometry: Data analysis and interpretation. Cytometry 30:236, 1997.
20. Mahon, K: Regulating analyte-specific reagents: How it works. Lab Med 30:442, 1999.
21. Borowitz, MJ, and Silberman, MA. Cases in flow cytometry. [Interactive CD-ROM]. Carden Jennings Publishing, Charlottesville, 1999. Available: http://www.cjp.com.
22. Terstappen, LW, et al: Flow cytometric characterization of acute myeloid leukemia. Part II. Phenotypic heterogeneity at diagnosis. Leukemia 6:70, 1992.
23. Tbakhi, A, et al: Flow cytometric immunophenotyping of non-Hodgkin's lymphomas and related disorders. Cytometry 25:113, 1996.
24. Harris, NL, et al: A revised European-American classification of lymphoid neoplasms: A proposal from the international lymphoma study group. Blood 84:1361, 1994.
25. http://www.ncbi.nlm.nih.gov:80/entrez/query/static/citmatch.html
26. Duque, RE, et al: Consensus review of the clinical utility of DNA flow cytometry in neoplastic hematopathology. Cytometry 14:492, 1993.
27. San Miguel, JF, et al: A new staging system for multiple myeloma based on the number of S-phase plasma cells. Blood 85:448, 1995.

28. Garcia-Sanz, R, et al: Primary plasma cell leukemia: Clinical, immunophenotypic, DNA ploidy, and cytogenetic characteristics. Blood 93:1032, 1999.

29. Brown, PD: S-phase induction by interleukin-6 followed by chemotherapy in patients with chronic lymphocytic leukemia and non-Hodgkin's lymphoma. Leuk Lymphoma 34:325, 1999.

30. Robinson, JP: Handbook of Flow Cytometry Methods. Wiley-Liss, New York, 1993, p 97.

31. Robinson, JP: Handbook of Flow Cytometry Methods. Wiley-Liss, New York, 1993, p 100.

32. Hedly, DW, et al: DNA cytometry consensus conference—special reports. Cytometry 19:295, 1995.

33. Chapman, B: Transplanting hematopoietic progenitor cells. CAP Today Feb 1999, p 48.

34. Sutherland, DR, et al: The ISHAGE guidelines for CD34+ cell determination by flow cytometry. J Hematotherapy 5:213, 1996.

35. McNiece, I, et al: Minimization of CD34+ cell enumeration variability using the ProCOUNT standardized methodology. J Hematotherapy 7:499, 1998.

36. Menendez, P, et al: Comparison between a lyse-and-then-wash method and a lyse-non-wash technique for the enumeration of CD34+ hematopoietic progenitor cells. Cytometry 34:264, 1998.

37. Scornik, JC: Detection of alloantibodies by flow cytometry: Relevance to clinical transplantation. Cytometry 22:259, 1995.

38. Bray, RA: Flow cytometry crossmatching for solid organ transplantation. Methods Cell Biol 41:103, 1994.

39. Socie, G, et al: Late clonal diseases of treated aplastic anemia. Semin Hematol 37:91, 2000.

40. Pui, JC, et al: Flow cytometric diagnosis of paroxysmal nocturnal hemoglobinuria. In Parker, J, and Stewart, C (eds): Purdue Cytometry CD-ROM. Clinical Edition, vol 3. Purdue University Cytometry Laboratories, West Lafayette, IN, 1997.

41. Hillmen, P, and Richards, SJ: Implications of recent insights into the pathophysiology of paroxysmal nocturnal haemoglobinuria. Br J Haematol 108:470, 2000.

42. Koepke, JA: Update on reticulocyte counting. Lab Med 30:339, 1999.

43. National Committee for Clinical Laboratory Standards (NCCLS): Methods for reticulocyte counting (flow cytometry and supravital dyes); approved guideline. NCCLS document H44-A, 1997.

44. Nicoll, CD: Appendix: Therapeutic drug monitoring and laboratory reference ranges. In Tierney, LM, et al (eds): Current Medical Diagnosis and Treatment. Appleton & Lange, Stamford, CT, 1998, p 1536.

45. Davis, BH: Detection of fetal red cells in fetomaternal hemorrhage using a fetal hemoglobin monoclonal antibody by flow cytometry. Transfusion 38:749, 1998.

46. Rinder, HR: Platelet function testing by flow cytometry. Clin Lab Sci 11:365, 1998.

47. Ault, KA, et al: Platelet activation in patients after an acute coronary syndrome: Results from the TIMI-12 trial. J Am Coll Cardiol 33:634, 1999.

48. Ault, KA: Reticulated platelets: The birth of a new test for thrombopoiesis. Clin Immunol Newsletter 17:1, 1997.

49. Ault, KA, and Mitchell, JA: Analysis of platelets by flow cytometry. Methods Cell Biol 42:275, 1994.

50. Liu, Z, et al: Elevated relative fluorescence intensity of CD38 antigen expression on CD8+ T cells is a marker of poor prognosis in HIV infection: Results of 6 years of follow-up. Cytometry 26:1, 1996.

51. Iyer, SB, et al: Quantitation of CD38 expression using QuantiBRITE_ beads. Cytometry 33:206, 1998.

52. Davis, BH: Quantitative neutrophil CD64 expression: Promising diagnostic indicator of infection or systemic acute inflammatory response. Clin Immunol Newsletter 16:121, 1996.

53. Falanga, A, et al: Neutrophil activation and hemostatic changes in healthy donors receiving granulocyte colony-stimulating factor. Blood 93:2506, 1999.

54. Kabutomori, O, et al: CD16 antigen density on neutrophils in chronic myeloproliferative disorders. Hematopathology 107:661, 1997.

55. Fulton, RJ, et al: Advanced multiplexed analysis with the FlowMetrix system. Clin Chem 43:1749, 1997.

56. Kempfer, AC, et al: Binding of von Willebrand factor to collagen by flow cytometry. Am J Pathol 111:418, 1999.

57. Carson, R, and Vignali, D: Simultaneous quantitation of fifteen cytokines using a multiplexed flow cytometric assay. J Immunol Meth 227:41, 1999.

31 Special Stains/ Cytochemistry

Joan Steiner-Adler, EdD, MT(ASCP) CLS(NCA)
Mary Loring Perkins, MS, MT(ASCP)SH

OBJECTIVES

At the end of this chapter, the learner should be able to:

1. Define cytochemistry and discuss historical development.

2. Perform cytochemical enzyme and nonenzyme stain methods.

3. Discuss the clinical applications of cytochemical staining methods.

4. Interpret the score of leukocyte alkaline phosphatase staining and relate the score to a probable clinical diagnosis.

5. Compare and contrast methods in regard to cells identified and diagnostic applications.

6. Identify the types of cells that are stained by myeloperoxidase, Sudan black B, and chloroacetate esterase.

7. Identify the types of cells that are stained by the specific esterase stain.

8. Discuss nonspecific esterase staining in regard to cells identified and the diagnostic value of sodium fluoride inhibition studies.

9. Discuss the diagnostic value of the tartrate-resistant acid phosphatase stain.

10. Describe the clinical applications of periodic acid–Schiff staining.

11. Discuss the clinical applications of the terminal deoxynucleotidyl transferase test.

12. Diagram a flowchart to summarize the workup of a patient.

► DEFINITION AND HISTORICAL BACKGROUND OF CYTOCHEMISTRY

Cytochemistry is defined as the microscopic study of chemical constituents in cells. Proper clinical management depends on an accurate diagnosis of the proper subtype classification and evaluation of the extent of hematologic neoplasms, which is added by cytochemical markers. The hematology technologist routinely evaluates Wright-stained peripheral blood smears and bone marrow preparations in order to identify and characterize erythrocytes, leukocytes, and hematologic disorders. Before 1980, this type of morphological evaluation was already common. However, for hematologic neoplasms, these morphological studies provide the initial step for diag-

nosis, whereas enzymatic and nonenzymatic cytochemical studies can often provide accurate classification and evaluation of the extent of the disease (see Chap. 16). The most popular enzymatic markers involve cytochemical or histochemical reactions. These types of reactions have the advantage of directly observing the cells containing markers. These techniques are generally performed in the traditional hematology or histology laboratory.

Today, the diagnosis of hematologic disorders continues to evolve. With refinement of immunocytochemistry and better monoclonal antibodies, more is known about hematologic neoplasm diagnosis. Newer laboratory disciplines including flow cytometry, cytogenetics, and molecular biology further enhance diagnosis. Despite these new changes, the basic approach for diagnosis has not changed. The basic approach is still morphological evaluation followed by cyto-chemical and immunologic studies. Flow cytometry (see Chap. 30), cytogenetics, and molecular biology studies are performed to provide additional information or to confirm diagnosis. This chapter is devoted to cytochemical methods. Figure 31–1 illustrates a cytochemical approach to acute leukemias.

Technical Considerations

The technologist needs to be alert to the technical problems of performing cytochemical studies. The specimens of choice are fresh blood smears or imprints of peripheral blood, bone marrow, lymph node, and spleen tissue sections. Specimens may be stored, but the storage time is determined either by the stability of the biologic material or the sensitivity of the cytochemical reagents. If using air-dried smears, lower storage temperature better preserves the enzymatic material. However, if unfixed air-dried smears are kept in the refrigerator, the condensation can hemolyze the red blood cells and cause distortion of the morphology of nucleated cells. To prevent distortion and hemolysis, storage at 4°C to 10°C should take place in a desiccator or slides should be wrapped in moisture-absorbing paper or cotton.

Fixatives can affect the results of the cytochemical stain. The composition of the fixative should be determined by the cytochemical studies being performed. An unfixed air-dried smear is generally the preferred specimen. The type of specimen is often determined by the disease suspected.

In the diagnosis of leukemias, smears from blood and marrow specimens are often available. Imprints and tissue sections are used for diagnosis of lymphomas. Blood smears and imprints stained with Wright's or Giemsa stain are used for light microscopy morphology studies. Tissue sections can be stained with hematoxylin and eosin (H & E) or Giemsa stains.

➤ CYTOCHEMICAL ENZYME STAINS

Leukocyte Alkaline Phosphatase Stain

Purpose In some laboratories, the majority of the cytochemical methods are performed in the histology rather than the hematology section. However, the leukocyte alkaline phosphatase (LAP) is generally always performed in the hematology section of the laboratory.

The LAP enzyme is located in the tertiary or microvesicular granules of segmented neutrophils, bands, and some metamyelocytes. LAP activity increases with stages of neutrophil maturity. The enzyme is combined with a substrate at an alkaline pH to form a colored precipitate at sites of hydrolysis.

This cytochemical procedure is primarily relied on to distinguish chronic myelogenous leukemia (CML) from leukemoid reactions and myeloproliferative disorders such as polycythemia vera (PV) or myelofibrosis. One-hundred consecutive mature neutrophils and bands are counted on an LAP-stained blood smear. Table 31–1 shows how the reaction is graded from 0 (none) to 4+ (brilliant intensity). Scoring should be performed on an area of the slide where the cell distribution is most suitable for differential counting. The edges of the smear or areas of cell overlapping should be avoided. Two technologists should perform counts because the scoring method is somewhat subjective. The two counts should match by approximately 10%. Because score values vary for different disease states as well as with technical bias, each laboratory must establish its own normal values.

Principle The LAP within the neutrophil hydrolyzes the substrate naphthol-AS-BI phosphate. The hydrolyzed substrate then couples with the dye (fast red-violet salt LB) and precipitates out at the site of enzyme activity. The degree of staining noted is proportional to enzymatic activity.

Specimen Fingerstick specimens are acceptable; however, fresh heparinized samples of whole blood are routinely used. The use of ethylene diaminetetraacetic acid (EDTA)–anticoagulated blood is not recommended because it inhibits LAP activity. If staining is to be delayed, fix slides and store at −20°C within 2 hours of specimen collection. Optimally, smears should be thin.

LAP Control Establishing limits for LAP control:

1. Obtain a fresh heparinized sample from an individual with an elevated LAP score. Samples from a pregnant woman in the last trimester or a woman taking oral contraceptives are suitable. The control is usually stable for 12 months.
2. Prepare smears, allow to dry, fix with LAP fixative, and rinse. Allow fixed smears to air-dry, then store at −20°C.

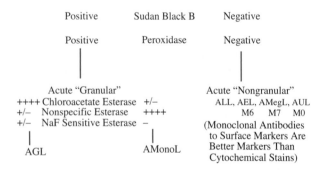

Acute Leukemia

| Positive | Sudan Black B | Negative |
| Positive | Peroxidase | Negative |

Acute "Granular"
++++ Chloroacetate Esterase +/−
+/− Nonspecific Esterase ++++
+/− NaF Sensitive Esterase −

AGL

AMonoL

Acute "Nongranular"
ALL, AEL, AMegL, AUL
M6   M7   M0
(Monoclonal Antibodies to Surface Markers Are Better Markers Than Cytochemical Stains)

➤ **FIGURE 31–1** Cytochemical approach to the diagnosis of acute leukemias.
Abbreviations: AGL = acute granulocytic leukemia; NaF = sodium fluoride; AMonoL = acute monocytic leukemia; ALL = acute lymphoblastic leukemia; AEL = acute erythroleukemia; AmegL = acute megakaryoblastic leukemia; AUL = acute null cell leukemia.

➤ **Table 31–1**
LEUKOCYTE ALKALINE PHOSPHATASE SCORING

LAP SCORING SCALE AND CHARACTERISTICS

Grade	Stain Intensity	Granulation
0	None	None
1+	Fine/diffuse	Occasional
2+	Moderate	Moderate
3+	Strong	Many
4+	Brilliant	Nucleus obscured

Source: Mary Jo Fackler, BSc, MT (ASCP), SH, with permission.

3. Prepare and read a series of slides from the new control and the old control. A minimum of five slides for each control is recommended. Calculate the mean LAP score with a control range of ±15.

Reagents Control: Heparinized blood with score of approximately 200. Fix and store at −20°C.

1. Fixative: Store at room temperature. Reagent expires in 90 days; pH 4.2 to 4.55.
   Sodium citrate (formula weight [FW] 294.10), 0.282 g
   Citric acid (FW 210.14), 1058 g
   Deionized water, 200 mL
   Acetone, 300 mL
   Allow dry reagents to dissolve in water before adding acetone.
2. Substrate solution: Aliquots of 45 mL are stored at −20°C. Reagent expires in 8 months.
   2-amino-2-methyl-1,3-propanediol, 13.15 g
   0.1 N HCl, 125 mL
   Check the pH (9.5 to 9.7) before adding 0.2 g naphthol-AS-BI phosphate dissolved in 10 mL N,N-dimethylformamide. Add sufficient quantity (QS) with deionized water to 2500 mL.
3. Dye: 40-mg aliquots of fast red-violet salt LB are stored at −20°C.
4. Mayer's hematoxylin counterstain

Procedure

1. Allow the smears to dry for 30 minutes. (This helps to keep the cells from washing off slides when rinsing after fixation.)
2. Fix the smears in fixative for 30 seconds at room temperature.
3. Rinse with distilled water.
4. Thaw the substrate solution to room temperature (22°C to 24°C); check with a thermometer.
5. Add dye to the substrate solution, gently agitate, filter, and use immediately.
6. Place the slides, including control, in mixture for 15 minutes at room temperature.
7. Rinse the slides in distilled water.
8. Counterstain with Mayer's hematoxylin for 2 minutes.
9. Rinse the slides in distilled water.
10. Air-dry and mount with synthetic medium.

Interpretation One-hundred mature neutrophils and bands are counted and graded according to the scale 0 to 4+

presented in Table 31–2. To calculate the LAP score, the grade of staining is multiplied by the number of neutrophils counted for that grading. The final LAP score is obtained by adding together the value of each grade score. An example of LAP score calculation is provided in Table 31–2.

Report the patient score if the control is within established limits. Each laboratory must establish its own normal values. The normal LAP scores recommended for this method range between 11 and 95.

LAP activity is decreased in patients with CML, paroxysmal nocturnal hemoglobinuria (PNH), sickle cell anemia, sideroblastic anemia, and hereditary hypophosphatasia. Increased activity is seen in leukemoid reactions, myeloproliferative disorders such as polycythemia vera (PV), and myelofibrosis (Table 31–3). As previously noted, increased values are also noted during the third trimester of pregnancy.

Comments

1. Thin blood smears should be prepared so that the white blood cells (WBCs) do not touch erythrocytes (RBCs). Thick smears may falsely elevate results.
2. Only segmented and band-form neutrophils are scored. Do not include other cells. Monocytes and eosinophils do not stain.
3. LAP slides need to be scored as quickly as possible because the dye tends to fade.
4. The staining procedure should be carried out with the slides protected from direct light as much as possible.
5. The substrate should be between 18°C and 26°C for optimal staining.

Myeloperoxidase Stain

Purpose Myeloperoxidase (MPO) can be found in neutrophils, eosinophils, and monocytes but not in lymphocytes. The enzyme in eosinophils is different from that in other cells because it remains active in an acidic environment. Peroxidase enzyme is found in the primary (or azurophilic) granules of cells in the myeloid lineage and plays a central role in effective microbial killing during phagocytosis. The peroxidase in these granules is referred to as *myeloperoxidase,* which distinguishes it from other peroxidases such as eosinophilic peroxidase and platelet peroxidase. Primary granules are present from the promyelocyte stage (late blast) to the neutrophilic stage of maturation. Accordingly, promyelocyte, myelocytes, metamyelocytes, bands, and segmented neutrophils are strongly positive for MPO. These granules are described as being absent in myeloblasts; however, limited MPO activity

> **Table 31-2**
LAP SCORE CALCULATION

Grade	Number of Cells Counted	Calculation	LAP Score
0	60	0 × 60 = 0	0
1+	20	1 × 20 = 20	20
2+	14	2 × 14 = 28	28
3+	5	3 × 5 = 15	15
4+	1	4 × 1 = 4	4
Total	100		67

Source: From procedures by Mary Loring Perkins, MT (ASCP), SH, and Joe Marty, MS, MT (ASCP).

> **Table 31-3**
LAP REACTIVITY IN VARIOUS DISORDERS

	Leukemoid Reaction	Chronic Granulocytic Leukemia	Acute Granulocytic Leukemia	Polycythemia Rubra Vera (PRV)	Myelofibrosis	Paroxysmal Nocturnal Hematuria	Pregnancy
Leukocyte alkaline phosphatase score	↑	↓	Varies	↑	Varies	↓	↑

Source: From procedures by Mary Loring Perkins, MT(ASCP), SH, and Joe Marty, MS, MT(ASCP).

is demonstrated at the sites of future primary granule synthesis with staining methods. This characteristic of myeloblasts is most useful for differentiating blast cells in acute myelogenous leukemias (AML) such as FAB subclasses M1, M2, and M3 from blast cells in acute lymphoblastic leukemia (ALL).

Principle The peroxidases are enzymes capable of catalyzing the oxidation of substances by hydrogen peroxide. The oxidized substance indicates the presence of peroxidized activity within a cell. Benzidine is no longer used as the indicator for this cytochemical reaction because of its carcinogenic potential. Another substance that serves as an indicator is 3-amino-9-ethylcarbazole. Accordingly, in the presence of MPO, hydrogen peroxide oxidizes the substrate, 3-amino-9- ethylcarbazole (AEC), which will form a blue-black precipitate that may be easily identified as coarse granulation under light microscopy (Fig. 31–2 and Color Plate 269).

The peroxidase activity in leukocytes is derived from a group of isoenzymes. Therefore, there are cytochemical methods available for a single to several isoenzymes. Other alternative methods are (1) peroxidase and cyanide-resistant peroxidase (cyanide-resistant peroxidase is positive only in eosinophils), and (2) pseudoperoxidase for hemoglobin (the hemoglobin in RBCs and late erythroblasts stains dark brown).

Specimen Blood smears or bone marrow touch imprints may be used. A fresh capillary sample is preferred for smears; however, EDTA, heparinized, or oxalated specimens are acceptable. Fresh samples are required because peroxidase activity decreases with exposure to light and heat or on prolonged storage.

Reagents
1. Fixative (buffered formalin acetone, pH 6.6). Stored at 4°C to 10°C, reagent has a shelf-life of 90 days.
   Na_2HPO_4 anhydrous (FW 141.96), 0.2 g
   KH_2PO_4 anhydrous (FW 136.09), 1.0 g
   Deionized water, 300 mL
   Add 250 mL of reagent-grade formalin 37%.
   Add 450 mL of reagent-grade acetone.
   The pH should be 6.6. If necessary, adjust the pH with appropriate buffer salt.
2. 0.02 *M* acetate buffer, pH 5.2. Stored at 4°C to 10°C, reagent has a shelf-life of 90 days.
   Distilled water, 900 mL
   Sodium acetate (FW 136.08), 2.72 g
   Adjust the pH to 5.2 with dilute acetic acid.
   Bring the volume to 1000 mL with distilled water.
3. Hydrogen peroxide (30%)
4. 3-amino-9-ethylcarbazole (AEC substrate)
5. Dimethylsulfoxide (DMSO)
6. Mayer's hematoxylin

Procedure
1. Fix the smears or bone marrow touch preparations for 15 seconds.
2. Rinse with deionized water.
3. Incubate the smears for 8 minutes at room temperature in a freshly made filtered mixture containing the following:
   AEC, 10 mg
   DMSO, 6 mL
   Acetate buffer, 50 mL
   Hydrogen peroxide (30%), 0.005 mL
4. Rinse with deionized water.
5. Stain with Mayer's hematoxylin for 2 minutes.
6. Rinse in deionized water.
7. Air-dry and mount with a coverslip.

Interpretation
1. A positive reaction for MPO is indicated by the presence of bluish-black granules. Most cells in the myelocytic series demonstrate strongly positive peroxidase activity indicated by coarse blue-black granulation (see Fig. 31–2 and Color Plate 269). Only the enzyme activity of the blasts should be assessed. A positive reaction of the blasts in blood indicates myeloblastic or myelomonocytic leukemia. Reactivity in mature granulocytes is not of diagnostic importance, but it indicates the stain is working.
2. Positive staining is also noted in eosinophils and monocytes. Monocytes demonstrate weakly positive or diffuse staining with only a few peroxidase-positive granules present. Monoblasts noted in acute monocytic leukemia are usually negative, whereas

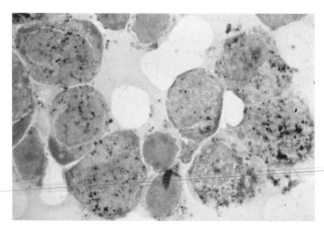

> **FIGURE 31-2**   Myeloperoxidase positivity in acute myelogenous leukemia (M2).

monoblasts in acute myelomonocytic leukemia may demonstrate weak reactivity. Eosinophils reveal strong peroxidase activity. Only RBCs and erythroblasts stain positive after methanol treatment.

3. Because Auer rods are strongly peroxidase-positive, MPO staining is useful for demonstrating their presence.

4. Early myeloblasts, erythroblasts, lymphocytes, mature basophils, and plasma cells are generally negative for myeloperoxidase.

5. The enzyme activity present in human megakaryocytes, platelets, and the hairy cells of hairy-cell leukemia is visible only by electron microscopy, not by light microscopy.

Comments

1. Because peroxidase enzymes are sensitive to light, smears should be stained immediately and stored in the dark. Smears that are older than 2 weeks at room temperature or that have been exposed to excessive light or fixed in formaldehyde should not be reported as peroxidase-negative. If smears are to be stained at a later date, they should be fixed, air-dried, and stored properly protected in the freezer.

2. Permount should not be used for mounting. Color usually fades before microscopic observation can be made. In addition, xylene should not be used to clean unmounted slides.

3. A positive control may be obtained from healthy individuals.

4. One indicator of overincubation is positive peroxidase activity in RBCs.

Alternative Method— Myeloperoxidase Stain

Purpose MPO staining methods are useful for identifying myelocytic leukemias because granulocytes and their precursors stain positive, whereas cells of the lymphoid and erythroid lineage stain negative. In some cases, enzyme activity is not visible by light microscopy, but is visible by electron microscopy or immunochemical techniques. If the standard MPO methods do not stain blasts that are still suspected to be of myeloid origin, an alternative method can be used. As noted, the MPO enzyme is present in the primary granules of myeloid cells. They first appear in the early promyelocyte stage and persist through subsequent stages of maturation. Limited MPO activity is noted in myeloblasts. This method is particularly useful for identifying blasts in poorly differentiated forms of AML, such as FAB subclass M1.

Principle In the presence of MPO, hydrogen peroxide oxidizes the substrate, benzidine dihydrochloride, which forms a black precipitate. The oxidized substrate essentially appears at the site of the enzyme activity and is interpreted as a positive marker for the presence of MPO.

Specimen Smears or bone marrow touch preparations can be used. A fresh capillary sample is preferred for smears; however, EDTA, heparinized, or oxalated specimens are acceptable. Fresh samples are required, because peroxidase activity decreases with exposure to light and heat or after prolonged storage.

Reagents

1. Fixative (stored at room temperature, reagent has a shelf-life of 90 days).

Formaldehyde (37%), 10 mL
Absolute ethyl alcohol, 190 mL

2. Zinc sulfate solution:
Zinc sulfate ($ZnSO_4$, $7H_2O$), 0.38 g
Deionized water, 10 mL

3. Substrate solution: Filtered and stored at room temperature, reagent expires in 6 months. Add the following reagents in order, mixing well after each addition:
Ethyl alcohol (30%), 100 mL
Benzidine dihydrochloride, 0.3 g
Zinc sulfate solution, 1.0 mL
Sodium acetate (F.W. 136.1), 1.0 g
Hydrogen peroxide (30%), 0.005 mL
Sodium hydroxide (1.0 N), 1.5 mL
Safranin O, 0.2 g

Note: Benzidine is a potential carcinogen, and the following precautions should be taken when handling the reagent or its solutions:

- Wear protective clothing, including gloves, laboratory coat, and mask when weighing out powders.
- Use mechanical aids for all pipetting.
- Clean up spills immediately.
- Wash hands after completion.
- Weigh benzidine in a hood.
- The 30% alcohol may be warmed with hot tap water to facilitate dissolving of the benzidine.

Procedure

1. Fix the smears or bone marrow touch preparations for 60 seconds.
2. Rinse with deionized water.
3. Incubate for 30 seconds in a substrate solution at room temperature.
4. Rinse with deionized water.
5. Air-dry and mount with a coverslip.

Interpretation Positive staining for peroxidase activity is indicated by the presence of black granulation. Enzyme activity noted in blasts is of the most diagnostic importance, whereas positive reactions in mature granulocytes provide limited diagnostic value.

Cyanide-Resistant Peroxidase for Eosinophils

Purpose To differentiate eosinophils and their precursors from monocytes and granulocytes.

Reagents

1. Fixative: Cold buffered formol acetone
2. 3,3-diaminobenzidine tetrahydrochloride
3. 0.05 M Tris buffer, pH 7.6
4. Hydrogen peroxide (3%)
5. Sodium cyanide
6. 1 N HCl
7. 1 N sodium hydroxide
8. Synthetic mounting medium
9. Counterstains:
   a. Mayer's hematoxylin
   b. Giemsa stain
10. Incubating medium:
    a. Dissolve 5.0 mg of 3,3-diaminobenzidine tetrahydrochloride in 10 mL 0.05 Tris buffer.

b. Add 0.05 mL (1 drop) of 3% hydrogen peroxide.
c. Add 5.0 mg of sodium cyanide and mix well.
d. Adjust pH to 7.6 with HCl solution or sodium hydroxide solution.
e. Use immediately.

Procedure

1. Fix the smears in cold buffered formol acetone for 30 seconds, wash with tap water, and air-dry.
2. Stain the smears with the cyanide-containing incubation medium for 15 minutes at room temperature.
3. Wash in water.
4. Counterstain with hematoxylin or Giemsa stain for 5 minutes.
5. Wash in water, dry, and mount in a synthetic mounting medium.

Interpretation   Eosinophils and their precursors stain dark brown. Monocytes and granulocytes other than eosinophils are negative for this stain.

Comment   The reagent 3,3-diaminobenzidine tetrahydrochloride may be a carcinogen. Use *with* caution.

➤ CYTOCHEMICAL ESTERASES

Esterases are a group of enzymes that are found in a variety of tissues and hematopoietic cell lines. Esterases are known to hydrolyze aliphatic or aromatic ester bonds in an acid or neutral pH. In regard to hematopoietic cells, they are capable of splitting naphthol and naphthol derivatives from their esters. A strong granular positivity can be found in acute promyelocytic leukemia (M3), with occasional staining of Auer rods. In some patients with erythroleukemia, erythroblasts are positive.

Certain esterases have been demonstrated in leukocytes that have been separated into nine subtypes or isoenzymes. These isoenzymes may be classified as either specific or nonspecific, depending on the particular substrate hydrolyzed, the optimum pH for enzyme activity, and time of reaction.

Isoenzymes 1, 2, 7, 8, and 9 are referred to as specific (or chloroacetate) esterases (SE) because they are found in all stages of myelocytic maturation and mast cells. Accordingly, specific esterases are valued as a marker for early cells of myeloid lineage. The specific esterase (SE) enzymes hydrolyze the substrate naphthol-AS-D chloroacetate (NASDA) at a neutral or slightly alkaline pH and are resistant to sodium fluoride treatment.

Nonspecific esterases (NSE) comprise isoenzymes 3, 4, 5, and 6, which are found in a variety of cell types such as monocytes, plasma cells, megakaryocytes, and certain T-lymphocyte subsets. Depending on the nonspecific esterase, either alpha (α)-naphthyl butyrate or α-naphthyl acetate is hydrolyzed at a slightly acid pH. The nonspecific esterase activity of monocytes and monoblasts may be distinguished from the nonspecific esterase activity of other cells with the addition of an inhibitor such as sodium fluoride to the incubation medium. The NSE activity of monocytes and macrophages is inhibited or abolished, whereas the activity of other cells remains unaffected (Figs. 31–3 and 31–4, and Color Plates 270 and 271). The NSE reaction is often used as a specific marker for early monocytes and macrophages.

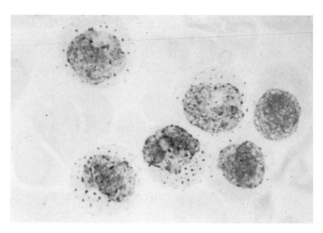

➤ **FIGURE 31–3**   Nonspecific esterase α-naphthyl acetate positivity in acute monocytic leukemia (M5b).

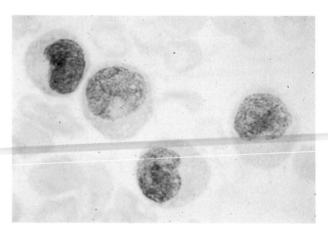

➤ **FIGURE 31–4**   Nonspecific esterase stain with sodium fluoride inhibition in acute monocytic leukemia (M5b).

A third group of esterases uses aminocaproic esters as a substrate. This group is confined to human mast cells.

Cytochemical esterase staining is used as a tool for differentiating cells in the myeloid series from cells in the monocytic series. The results of staining have been relied on to distinguish precursor cells in acute myelogenous leukemia (FAB subclasses M2 and M3) from precursor cells in acute myelomonocytic leukemia (FAB subclass M4) and acute monocytic leukemia (FAB subclass M5).

Specific Esterase

Naphthol-AS-D Chloroacetate Esterase

Purpose   Specific esterase staining with naphthol-AS-D chloroacetate esterase (CAE) is valued as a marker for early cells of myeloid lineage and is used most often to identify immature granulocytic cells in acute leukemias. If found in blasts, this marker is considered evidence of myeloid origin. Specific esterase is present in the primary granules of myeloid cells. Table 31–4 shows the cytochemical staining patterns related to acute nonlymphocytic leukemias. Demonstration of this stain is also useful for diagnosing granulocytic sarcoma and extramedullary hematopoiesis.

Principle   The specific esterase enzyme within granulocytes hydrolyzes the substrate naphthol chloroacetate. The hydrolyzed substrate then couples with the diazonium salt

➤ **Table 31-4**
CYTOCHEMISTRY MARKERS FOR SUBCLASSIFICATION OF NONLYMPHOCYTIC LEUKEMIA

	M1 AML	M2 AML	M3 APL	M4 AMML	M5 AMoL	M6 EL	M7 MegL	AEoL
MPO	+	+	+	+	+/−	−*	−	+
SBB	+	+	+	+	+/−	−*	−	+
CAE	+/−	+	+	+	−	−*	−	−
NSE	−	−	+/−	+	+	+/−	+/−	−
AcP	−	−/+	+	+	−	−	−	−
PAS	+/−	−/+	+/−	+/−	+/−	+	+	−
CrP	−	−	−	−	−	−	−	+

*Negative reaction is for erythroblasts only; myeloblasts present will stain positive with MPO and SBB.
Abbreviations: MPO = myeloperoxidase; SBB = Sudan black B; CAE = chloroacetate esterase; NSE = nonspecific esterase; AcP = acid phosphatase; PAS = periodic acid–Schiff; CrP = cyanide-resistant peroxidase; AML = acute myeloblastic leukemia; APL = acute promyelocytic leukemia; AMML = acute myelomonocytic leukemia; AMoL = acute monocytic leukemia; EL = erythroleukemia; MegL = megakaryoblastic leukemia; AEoL = acute eosinophilic leukemia

(hexazotized pararosaniline). The diazo dye precipitates out at the site of enzymatic activity. Positive activity is easily identified under light microscopy by the presence of highly colored granulation.

Specimen Paraffin sections, smears, and bone marrow touch preparations are used. Fresh capillary samples are preferred for smears; however, EDTA- or heparin-anticoagulated blood is acceptable. Activity can be demonstrated after long periods of storage, even in paraffin sections.

Reagents

1. Esterase fixative, pH 6.6; stored at 4°C, reagent expires in 90 days:
   a. In 120 mL of deionized water dissolve:
      Na_2HPO_4 (FW 141.96), 0.08 g
      KH_2PO_4 (FW 136.09), 0.40 g
   b. Add formaldehyde (37%), 100 mL
      Acetone, 180 mL
   c. Adjust pH to 6.6 if necessary with appropriate buffer salt.
2. Phosphate buffer, 0.1 *M*, pH 6.5; stored at 4°C, reagent expires in 90 days. Discard if mold develops.
   a. In 1000 mL of deionized water dissolve:
      NaH_2PO_4 H_2O (FW 137.99), 9.45 g
      Na_2HPO_4 (FW 141.96), 4.47 g
   b. Check pH and adjust to 6.5 if necessary with appropriate buffer salt solution.
3. Substrate solution. Store in glass (not plastic) stoppered bottle at 4°C. Reagent expires in 30 days.
   a. Dissolve 100 mg of naphthol-AS-D chloroacetate in 10 mL of *N,N*-dimethylformamide (FW 73.1).
4. Pararosaniline solution: Store in brown bottle at 4°C to 10°C. Expires in 3 months. *Caution:* Pararosaniline is a potential carcinogen.
   a. Dissolve 1.0 g pararosaniline HCl (FW 323.8) in 20 mL distilled water plus 5 mL concentrated HCl. Solution may be gently heated to dissolve pararosaniline.
   b. Filter.
5. Sodium nitrite solution (*must be prepared daily*):
   a. Dissolve 1.0 g $NaNO_2$ (FW 69.0) in distilled water to a volume of 25 mL.
6. Mayer's hematoxylin

7. Acid alcohol working solution
   Ethanol (70%), 5 mL
   Deionized water, 995 mL
   Concentrated HCl, 0.05 mL
8. Bluing agent
   $NaHCO_3$, 1 g
   Deionized water, 100 mL

Procedure

1. Deparaffinize and hydrate the sections. The fixative B5 may be used if the fixation time is short and if the mercury precipitate is not removed with iodine.
2. For blood smears and imprints, fix in esterase fixative and wash well with deionized water at 4°C for 30 seconds.
3. Incubate the slides in the "incubation mixture" for 30 minutes. The incubation mixture is prepared as follows:
   a. To 40 mL of buffer, add 1.0 mL of substrate solution.
   b. In a separate test tube, add 0.1 mL of sodium nitrite solution to 0.1 mL of pararosaniline solution. Wait 1 minute and add the buffer substrate solution.
   c. Filter.
4. After 30 minutes at room temperature, check the control slide microscopically. If the reacting cells are not red enough, refilter the solution and replace the slides for 15 to 30 minutes.
5. Wash the slides in running tap water for 5 minutes.
6. Counterstain for 2 minutes in Mayer's hematoxylin.
7. Rinse well with deionized water.
8. Dip in the bluing solution until the counterstain turns from purple to blue (approximately 10 dips).
9. Wash, dry, and mount the smears with Permount. Tissue sections must be rehydrated and cleared in xylene before mounting.

Interpretation The cytoplasm of granulocytes and tissue mast cells show sites of activity as bright red granulation. Nuclei are counterstained blue in cells of the granulocytic series (Fig. 31–5 and Color Plate 272). Activity is weak or absent in monocytes and lymphocytes. When found in blasts, this is evidence of myeloid origin.

Comments Esterase activity is inhibited to varying de-

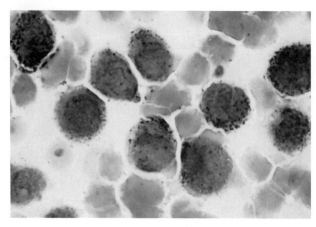

➤ **FIGURE 31-5** Specific esterase naphthol-AS-D chloroacetate positivity in acute promyelocytic leukemia (M3)

grees by mercury, acid solutions, heat, and iodine. False-negative reactions may occur under the following conditions:

1. Slides overheated during the drying process.
2. Mercury crystals removed from tissues with an iodine solution.
3. Tissues fixed in an acid fixative such as Zenker's (formalin or acetic) or Bouin's fixative.
4. Tissues decalcified in an acid solution.
5. Solutions used that are too old.

Nonspecific Esterase (Fluoride Resistant)

α-Naphthyl Butyrate, α-Naphthyl Acetate

Purpose The nonspecific esterase (NSE) stain is used primarily to differentiate monocytic leukemias from granulocytic leukemias. α-Naphthyl acetate esterase is a marker for monocytes, megakaryocytes, plasma cells, and platelets. α-Naphthyl butyrate esterase is a marker for monocytes, promonocytes, and monoblasts. To detect cells of monocytic lineage, the staining process is repeated with sodium fluoride and then evaluated for a lack of activity. The lack of activity with the addition of sodium fluoride distinguishes monoblastic leukemias from myeloblastic leukemia. NSE is used most often to identify precursor cells in the acute myelomonocytic (FAB subclass M4) and acute monocytic leukemias (FAB subclass M5). Acute promyelocytic (FAB subclass M3) and erythroblastic leukemia (FAB subclass M6) may stain weakly positive.

Principle The NSEs are a group of enzymes capable of hydrolyzing various aliphatic and aromatic short-chain esters. If using α-naphthyl butyrate as a substrate and hexazonium pararosaniline as a coupler, normal monocytes show a strong, cytoplasmic, diffuse staining pattern. Approximately 80% of cells show a sensitive reaction with the addition of sodium fluoride. In the other 20%, the reaction shows a weak granular staining.

Specimen Blood or bone marrow smears, tissue touch preparations, and cytocentrifuge preparations may be used. A fresh capillary sample is preferred; however, EDTA or heparinized specimens are acceptable.

Reagents
1. Esterase fixative, pH 6.6; stored at 4°C, reagent expires in 90 days.

   a. In 300 mL of deionized water, dissolve:
   Na_2HPO_4 (FW 141.96), 0.2 g
   KH_2PO_4 (FW 136.09), 1.0 g
   Formaldehyde (37%), 250 mL
   Acetone, 450 mL
   b. Adjust the pH to 6.5 if necessary with appropriate buffer salt. (*Note:* pH of the fixative has a tendency to increase if allowed to sit. If the pH is near 6.5, allow the fixative to stand overnight, and then test the new fixative on a known positive.)
2. Phosphate buffer, 0.15 *M*, pH 6.3; stored at 4°C, reagent expires in 90 days. Discard if mold growth is observed.
   NaH_2PO_4, H_2O (FW 137.99), 8.02 g
   Na_2HPO_4 (FW 141.96), 2.4 g
   Deionized water, 1000 mL
   Check the pH and adjust to 6.3 if necessary with appropriate buffer salt.
3. Substrate solution: Store in glass-stoppered bottle at 4°C to 10°C. Good for 1 month. Dissolve 250 mg α-naphthyl butyrate in 12.5 mL ethylene glycol monomethyl ether (Eastman Kodak). If α-naphthyl butyrate is in liquid form, then use 0.225 mL per 12.5 mL of solvent.
4. Sodium nitrite solution (prepare daily):
   a. Dissolve 1.0 g $NaNO_2$ (FW 69.0) in distilled water to a volume of 25 mL.
5. Pararosaniline solution (this is a possible carcinogen; see note under Comments, later). Stored in a brown bottle at 4°C to 10°C, reagent has a shelf-life of 90 days.
   a. Dissolve 1.0 g pararosaniline HCl (FW 323.8) in 20 mL distilled water plus 5 mL concentrated HCl. Solution may be gently heated to dissolve pararosaniline.
6. Mayer's hematoxylin
7. Acid alcohol working solution:
   Ethanol (70%), 15 mL
   Deionized water, 995 mL
   Concentrated HCl, 10.05 mL
8. Bluing agent:
   $NaHCO_2$, 1 g
   Deionized water, 100 mL

Procedure
1. Fix the smears for 30 seconds at 4°C to 10°C in the esterase fixative.
2. Wash three times with deionized water.
3. Air-dry the smears and place in a Coplin jar.
4. Incubate the smears for 45 minutes at room temperature in the following mixture:
   a. To 40 mL of buffer (pH 6.3), add 2 mL of substrate solution.
   b. In a separate container, add 0.2 mL sodium nitrite solution to 0.2 mL pararosaniline solution. Wait 1 minute and add to the buffer substrate solution.
   c. Filter into a Coplin jar.
5. Wash well with deionized water.
6. Counterstain with hematoxylin for 2 minutes.
7. Wash well with deionized water.
8. Place the slides in bluing reagent for 30 seconds.
9. Wash well with deionized water.
10. Air-dry and mount with Permount.

Interpretation The use of sodium fluoride is recommended because only monocytes show the strongest reaction that can be inhibited. The brick-red precipitate staining disappears (see Figs. 31–3 and 31–4 and Color Plates 270 and 271). Staining of granulocytes, lymphocytes, and early erythroblasts is not inhibited by sodium fluoride.

Two different substrates are available; α-naphthyl butyrate is the most specific for monocyte lineage and α-naphthyl acetate is more sensitive. If α-naphthyl acetate is used as a substrate in an acidic medium with prolonged incubation, a subset of T lymphocytes shows an intense dotlike activity. Immunologic studies indicate that this enzyme is present in the helper subset of T lymphocytes. It is not a marker for T-cell ALL. It is a useful marker of T-lymphocytic leukemia and T-cell lymphomas, including mycosis fungoides, Sézary cell leukemia, and hairy-cell leukemia. Monocytes, without the addition of sodium fluoride, exhibit diffuse, strong cytoplasmic staining.

Comments

1. Pararosaniline is a possible carcinogen, and the following precautions should be taken when handling the reagent or its solutions.
   a. Wear protective clothing: gloves, laboratory coat, smock. Wear a mask when weighing out powders.
   b. Use mechanical pipetting aids for all pipetting.
   c. Immediately clean up all spills.
   d. Wash hands after completion.
2. A control must be run to be sure reagents are working.
3. Hexazotized reagents are unstable and must be used immediately.
4. Fixation keeps the enzyme from washing out of the cell during staining and improves the morphological preservation of the cells.
5. Smears should be fixed after drying, even if staining is to be performed at a later date.
6. Since this method depends on an enzymatic reaction, care must be taken to preserve enzyme activity by avoiding exposure to light and heat as well as prolonged storage. Store fixed smears in freezer.
7. For sodium fluoride inhibition studies, add NaFl, 1.5 mg/mL, to incubation mixture.
8. When the incubation time is increased to 2 hours, the enzyme activity in the lymphocytes can be demonstrated.

Combined Esterase

Purpose Combined esterase studies are used to evaluate the ratio of myelocytic and monocytic cells on a smear. This staining method is most often relied on to differentiate acute myelomonocytic leukemia (FAB subclass M4) from acute monocytic leukemia (FAB subclasses M5a and M5b). The combined esterase approach is especially valuable when a limited number of smears are available.

Principle The esterase enzymes within cells hydrolyze the substrate α-naphthyl butyrate and naphthol-AS-D chloroacetate. The hydrolyzed substrate then couples with the dye, fast-blue BB, or pararosaniline, and the colored complex formed precipitates out at the site of enzymatic activity.

Specimen This may be a fresh smear or a bone marrow touch preparation. For smears, fresh capillary samples are preferred; however, anticoagulated specimens are acceptable.

Reagents

1. Esterase fixative, pH 6.6. Stores at 4°C, reagent expires in 3 months.
   a. In 120 mL of deionized water dissolve:
      Na$_2$HPO$_4$ (FW 141.96), 0.08 g
      KH$_2$PO$_4$ (FW 136.09), 0.40 g
   b. Formaldehyde (37%), 100 mL
   c. Acetone, 180 mL
   d. Adjust pH to 6.6 if necessary with appropriate buffer salt.
2. Phosphate buffer, pH 7.4. Stored at 4°C, reagent expires in 90 days. Discard if any mold is observed.
   a. NaH$_2$PO$_4$ H$_2$O (FW 137.99), 1.67 g
   b. Na$_2$HPO$_4$ (FW 141.96), 7.74 g
   c. Deionized water, 1000 mL
   d. Adjust pH to 7.4 if necessary with appropriate buffer salt solution.
3. Naphthol-AS-D chloroacetate. Store at 0°C.
4. Substrate solution. Stored at 4°C in glass stoppered bottle; reagent expires in 30 days.
   a. Naphthol-AS-D chloroacetate, 20 mg
   b. N,N-dimethylformamide (FW 73.1), 10 mL
5. Fast-blue BB salt. Store at 0°C.
6. Mayer's hematoxylin
7. Bluing agent:
   a. NaHCO$_3$, 1 g
   b. Deionized water, 100 mL
8. Refer to the earlier NSE procedure for reagents needed for step 1 of this combined esterase procedure.

Procedure

1. Perform as for an NSE procedure, but do not counterstain.
2. Incubate the slides in the following filtered mixture for 20 minutes at room temperature:
   a. Buffer, 38 mL
   b. Substrate solution, 2 mL
   c. Fast-blue BB, 20 mg
3. Wash well with deionized water.
4. Counterstain with hematoxylin for 2 minutes.
5. Wash well with deionized water.
6. Place the slides in bluing reagent for 30 seconds.
7. Wash, air-dry, and mount with a coverslip.

Interpretation Monocytes and macrophages demonstrate diffusely brown-red staining. T lymphocytes usually stain with punctate red granules. Mast cells, early promyelocytes, and later granulocytes demonstrate a granular blue staining (Fig. 31–6 and Color Plate 273).

Comments

1. The cytoplasmic CAE activity, as demonstrated by this method, may not be entirely specific.
2. Weak enzyme activity in the blood cells should be made with caution.

➤ OTHER STAINS

Acid Phosphatase Stain/Tartrate-Resistant Acid Phosphatase

Purpose Acid phosphatase is a lysosomal enzyme that is present in many tissues and all hematopoietic cells. In humans, these enzymes can be classified as erythrocytic and nonerythrocytic. The erythrocytic enzymes have a limited substrate specificity. The nonerythrocytic enzymes are often

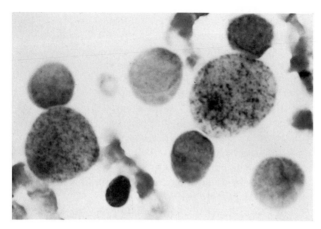

➤ **FIGURE 31–6**   Combined esterase positivity in acute myelomonocytic leukemia (M4).

tissue- or cell-specific. Seven isoenzymes have been classified as nonerythrocytic, with isoenzymes 2 and 4 being noted in neutrophils and monocytes; isoenzyme 3 in lymphocytes and platelets; and isoenzyme 5 in the hairy cells seen in leukemic reticuloendotheliosis (hairy-cell leukemia). The findings of acid phosphatase staining alone are of limited diagnostic value unless run in conjunction with tartrate inhibition studies. With the addition of tartrate to the incubation medium, the acid phosphatase activity of all isoenzymes is abolished, with the exception of isoenzyme 5. Because isoenzyme 5 is specific to hairy cells, the finding of tartrate resistance on a smear supports the diagnosis of hairy-cell leukemia (Fig. 31–7 and Color Plate 274).

Acid phosphatase activity has been shown to be higher in T lymphocytes than in B lymphocytes and is, therefore, useful for identifying lymphoblasts in many cases of acute T-lymphocytic leukemia. If present in T cells, the activity is localized in the Golgi area and assumes a dotlike appearance. This presentation is not specific to T lymphocytes and may be noted in other cells such as activated macrophages, lymphocytes, Gaucher cells, and histiocytes, but these are tissue cells. Additional cytochemical markers should be evaluated before making a diagnosis of acute T-lymphocytic leukemia.

Principle   The acid phosphatase within the white cell hydrolyzes the substrate naphthol-AS-BI phosphoric acid. The hydrolyzed substrate then couples with the dye (hexazotized pararosaniline) and precipitates out at the site of en-

zymatic activity. The addition of tartrate to the incubation medium inhibits all acid phosphatase isoenzyme activity with the exception of the enzyme fraction found in hairy-cell leukemia (isoenzyme 5).

Specimen   Blood smears, bone marrow touch preparations, lymph node and spleen imprints, or frozen sections may be used. Fresh capillary samples are preferred; however, EDTA or heparinized specimens are acceptable.

Reagents

1. Acid phosphatase fixative, pH 5.4; stored at 4°C to 10°C, reagent expires in 90 days. Discard if RBC morphology is poor.
   a. Dissolve 0.63 g of citrate acid (FW 210.14) in 30 mL of deionized water.
   b. Add 10 mL of methanol and 60 mL of acetone.
   c. Mix and adjust the pH to 5.4 with concentrated NaOH solution.
2. 0.1 N acetate buffer, pH 5.2; stored at 4°C, reagent expires in 90 days.
   a. Distilled water, 600 mL
   b. Sodium acetate (FW 136.1), 13.6 g
   c. Adjust the pH to 5.2 with 1.0 M acetic acid. Bring the volume to 1000 mL with distilled water.
3. Tartrate sodium acetate buffer, pH 5.2; stored at 4°C to 10°C, reagent expires in 3 months.
   a. Dissolve 3.75 g of l-(+)-tartaric acid in 490 mL of 0.1 N acetate buffer.
   b. Adjust the pH to 5.2 with concentrated NaOH.
   c. Bring the volume to 500 mL with distilled water.
4. 0.1 M acetic acid
   a. Distilled water, 200 mL
   b. Glacial acetic acid (F.W. 60.05, 16N), 1.25 mL
5. l-(+)-tartaric acid
6. Substrate solution: Stored in a glass stoppered bottle at 4°C to 10°C, reagent has a shelf-life of 30 days. Discard if it turns pink.
   a. Dissolve 100 mg of naphthol-AS-BI phosphoric acid in 10.0 mL N,N-dimethylformamide.
   b. When used infrequently, make up fresh by adding 10 mg naphthol-AS-BI phosphoric acid in 1.0 mL N,N-dimethylformamide.
7. Sodium nitrate solution (4%) (prepare daily):
   a. Dissolve 1.0 g NaNO$_2$ (FW 69.0) in distilled water to a volume of 25 mL.
8. Pararosaniline solution (4%) (possible carcinogen; see comments under NSE staining, earlier). Stored in brown bottles at 4°C to 10°C, reagent has a shelf-life of 90 days.
   a. Dissolve 1.0 g of pararosaniline HCl (FW 323.8) in 20 mL distilled water plus 5 mL concentrated HCl. Solution may be gently heated to dissolve pararosaniline. Filter.
9. Mayer's hematoxylin
10. Acid alcohol solution
    a. Concentrated HCl, 0.05 mL
    b. Ethanol (100%), 3.5 mL
    c. Deionized water, 996.5 mL
11. Bluing reagent:
    a. NaHCO$_3$, 1 g
    b. Deionized water, 100 mL

Procedure

1. Fix the smears, touch preparations, or frozen section for 30 seconds with cold fixative.

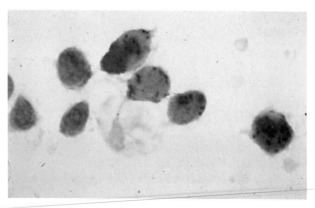

➤ **FIGURE 31–7**   Tartrate-resistant acid phosphatase (TRAP) stain of peripheral blood showing positivity in hairy cells and no staining in neutrophils.

2. Wash three times with deionized water. Air-dry.
3. Incubate the smears or imprints at 37°C in the appropriate filtered mixture:
    a. Acid phosphatase stain:
        Acetate buffer, 50 mL
        Stock substrate solution, 2 mL
        In a separate container, add 0.2 mL of 4% sodium nitrate solution to 0.2 mL of 4% pararosaniline solution. Wait 1 minute and then add to the buffer substrate solution.
    b. Tartrate-resistant acid phosphatase (TRAP) stain:
        Acetate-tartrate buffer, 50 mL
        Stock substrate solution, 2 mL
        In a separate container, add 0.2 mL of 4% sodium nitrate solution to 0.2 mL of 4% pararosaniline solution. Wait 1 minute and then add to the buffer substrate solution.
4. Incubate for 60 minutes at 37°C.
5. Wash three times in tap water.
6. Counterstain with hematoxylin for 2 minutes.
7. Rinse well with deionized water.
8. Place in the bluing solution for 30 seconds.
9. Wash. dry, and mount with Permount. Frozen tissue sections must be dehydrated and cleared in xylene before mounting.

Interpretation Acid phosphatase activity is demonstrated by the presence of an orange-red precipitate with pararosaniline. Myelogenous cells, lymphocytes, plasma cells, monocytes, and platelets have a positive reaction. The test result is considered positive when two or more cells exhibit strong (4+) activity or more than 40 dark red or purple granules. The presence in the blood of strong enzyme activity that is tartrate resistant is highly suggestive of hairy-cell leukemia. The presence of lymphoblasts may be indicated if acid phosphatase staining is present in a focal dotlike pattern at the sites of Golgi bodies. Increased activity has occasionally been observed in myeloma cells.

Comments

1. A control must be run along with patient samples to ensure that the reagents are working properly.
2. Because hexazotized reagents are unstable, they must be used immediately.
3. Fixation prevents the enzyme from washing out of the cell during staining and improves the morphological preservation of the cells.
4. Enzyme activity may be extended by avoiding exposure to light and heat as well as prolonged storage.
5. Smears may be kept at room temperature for at least 2 weeks at −20°C without apparent loss of enzymatic activity.
6. After a few weeks, reaction products may precipitate out (salting-out phenomenon) and be confused with true positive staining.
7. Controls should be fixed, air-dried, and stored at −20°C.
8. Increasing the temperature beyond 37°C causes inactivation of the enzyme and decomposition of the azo dye, resulting in nonspecific precipitation.
9. Mayer's hematoxylin as a counterstain gives a light gray tint to the cytoplasm of the leukocytes, which may mask weak enzymatic activity. In contrast, methyl green may give poor nuclear detail, but weak enzymatic activity if the cytoplasm is not masked.

Terminal Deoxynucleotidyl Transferase Test

Purpose Terminal deoxynucleotidyl transferase (TdT) is valued as a marker for primitive lymphoid populations. This nucleus-derived enzyme is observed in pre-B cells and T lymphoblasts, but is absent in B lymphocytes. TdT activity is elevated in FAB classes L1 and L2, which include T-cell, null cell, and sometimes pre–B-cell leukemias. Furthermore, 90% of ALL and lymphoblastic lymphoma patients demonstrate strong TdT activity. TdT is regarded as specific for primitive cells of lymphoid lineage; however, exceptions have been noted in a significant number of patients presenting with acute undifferentiated leukemia and CML blast crisis. TdT methods are generally relied on to differentiate ALL from acute myelogenous leukemia (AML) when morphological classification is uncertain. TdT may be assayed by immunofluorescence and immunoperoxidase techniques, as well as by radioimmunoassay.

Principle TdT is classified as a deoxyribonucleic acid (DNA) polymerase immunoperoxidase that is present in lymphocytic cells. Fluorescein isothiocyanate (FITC)–labeled goat anti-rabbit antibody is incubated with the sample. TdT activity in the nucleus is indicated by the presence of fluorescence in cells.

Specimen A nonheparinized bone marrow aspirate or one in which the cells have been separated and washed three times with culture media (RPMI-1640) and 2% fetal calf serum may be used. Peripheral blood samples may be used; however, special specimen collection is required. Slides should be stored at 4°C in the dark and stained within a few days of preparation.

Reagents

1. Antiserum, Kit No. 9311 SB (Bethesda Research Laboratories)
2. Rabbit anti-calf TdT, affinity-purified IgG
3. Goat anti-rabbit IgG, FITC conjugated
    a. The endpoint of antibody activity should be determined each time a new batch of antiserum is received.
    b. Dilute antiserum to the optimum ratio using diluting media. An 8- to 10-fold dilution is recommended for the rabbit anti-calf TdT, and a 70- to 100-fold dilution for the goat anti-rabbit TdT.
    c. Store anti-TdT at 4°C. Aliquot anti-rabbit antiserum (20 lambda) and store at −20°C.
4. Diluting media: RPMI with 2% fetal calf serum and 0.1% sodium azide.
5. Phosphate buffered solution (PBS), pH 7.4:
    $NaH_2PO_4 \cdot H_2O$, 0.4 g
    Na_2HPO_4, 1.6 g
    NaCl, 8.0 g
6. Controls:
    a. Prepare cytopreps from a known ALL patient with a positive TdT.
    b. Air-dry cytopreps.
    c. Wrap with plastic wrap.
    d. Freeze and store at −70°C.
    e. Bring to room temperature before unwrapping.
    f. Follow test procedure and treat as an unknown sample.

g. A negative control may be prepared from mouse serum and a phosphate buffer solution.

Procedure

1. Circle an area rich in nucleated cells on the side with a diamond scribe. Fix slides in methanol at 4°C for 30 minutes.
2. Rinse well in PBS to remove all fixative. Do not air-dry.
3. Hydrate the fixed slides in PBS for 5 minutes at room temperature.
4. Carefully wipe off all of the sample on the slide outside the circle. Apply 10 μL of primary antibody (anti-calf TdT) onto this area and distribute it over the circle. Incubate for 30 minutes at room temperature in a humid chamber. It is very important that the slide does not dry out.
5. Wash slides with three changes of PBS over a period of 15 minutes to remove excess antibody. Wipe off all of the excess PBS around the circle, being especially careful not to let the sample dry out.
6. Apply 15 μL of secondary antibody (FITC F[ab']$_2$ goat anti-rabbit IgG) to the circled area of the slide and incubate for 30 minutes at room temperature in a humid chamber.
7. Repeat the wash procedure as in step 5.
8. Apply a small drop of mounting medium and cover with a coverslip.
9. Examine the nuclei for fluorescence at 495-nm excitation with a barrier filter. Record the intensity of fluorescence, 0 to 4+, and the percentage of cells that are positive. The preparation can be stored in the dark in the refrigerator for several days.

Interpretation Most patients with T-cell and precursor B-cell ALL and lymphoma have positive TdT activity. Although it may help distinguish ALL from AML, 5% of AML patients exhibit TdT activity. In addition, 50% of patients with acute undifferentiated leukemia and 30% of patients in CML blast crisis also exhibit TdT activity. In summary, TdT is valued as a marker for identifying primitive lymphoid cells.

Comments

1. Peripheral blood, bone marrow aspirate smears, or touch preparations may be examined for TdT activity. The slides should be stored for no longer than 7 days at room temperature. Optimally, staining should be carried out as soon as possible.
2. A control slide should be run with patient samples as well as with each new lot number of reagents.

➤ NONENZYME STAINS

Sudan Black B Stain

Purpose Sudan black B (SBB) is a fat-soluble dye. It is used to differentiate myelogenous and myelomonocytic leukemias (FAB subclasses M1, M2, and M3) from ALL; therefore, staining patterns correlate closely with the patterns observed with MPO and CAE methods. SBB stains lipids present in the granulocytes and monocytes (Fig. 31–8 and Color Plate 275). The intensity and coarseness of staining increases with the stages of myelocytic maturation. The

term *sudanophilic* has been applied as a characteristic of cellular structures that are stained by SBB. In comparison with MPO reactions, all cellular structures that demonstrate MPO activity also demonstrate sudanophilia. One advantage of SBB methods over MPO methods is the increased stability of SBB-stained smears when exposed to sunlight or heat and when stored for prolonged periods.

Principle SBB stains phospholipids, neutral fats, and sterols. The mechanism by which the SBB reaction demonstrates the presence of phospholipid is not clearly understood, but it is believed to be based on the ability of fat-soluble dye to disassociate from its solvent and penetrate lipoprotein complexes. Phospholipids are concentrated in the primary, secondary, and tertiary granules of neutrophils and, to a lesser extent, in the lysosomal granules of monocytes and macrophages. Lymphocyte and lymphocyte precursors are generally negative with SBB; however, rare exceptions of SBB positivity have been noted in Burkitt's lymphoma and in the blast crisis associated with chronic lymphocytic leukemia (CLL).

Specimen Smears or bone marrow touch preparations may be used. A fresh capillary sample is preferred for smears; however, EDTA, heparinized, or oxalated specimens are acceptable.

Reagents

1. Polyvinyl pyrrolidone (K-29–33)
2. Phosphate buffer, pH 7.2
   0.15 *M* Na$_2$HPO$_4$ (21 g/L), 7.0 mL
   0.15 *M* Na$_2$H$_2$PO$_4$ H$_2$O (20.7 g/L), 3.0 mL
   Distilled water, 30.0 mL
3. Fixative, pH 5.5; store at room temperature in amber bottle; expires in 90 days:
   a. Dissolve 10 g of Plasdone in 400 mL of absolute ethanol.
   b. Add 75 mL of 37% formaldehyde.
   c. Add 10 mL of phosphate buffer, pH 7.2.
   d. Add 15 mL of liquefied phenol.
4. SBB solution expires in 1 year:
   a. Dissolve 1.5 g of SBB in 500 mL of absolute ethanol.
   b. Stir with a magnetic stirrer for 60 minutes; filter before use.
5. Phosphate: Phenol buffer expires in 6 months:
   a. Dissolve 0.48 g of anhydrous Na$_2$HPO$_4$ (FW 141.96) in 400 mL of distilled water.

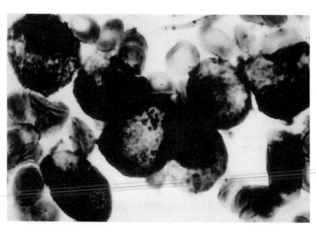

➤ **FIGURE 31–8**   Sudan black B positivity in acute promyelocytic leukemia (M3).

b. Dissolve 64 g of crystalline phenol (or 72.8 mL of liquefied phenol) in 120 mL of absolute ethanol and mix with the phosphate.

6. Nuclear counterstain expires in 1 year:
   a. Aqueous cresol violet (1%)
7. Background stain expires in 1 year:
   a. Aqueous light green (0.2%) to which 2 drops of glacial acetic acid have been added

Procedure

1. Fix the smears or touch preparations for 60 seconds.
2. Rinse three times with tap water.
3. Incubate the slides in the following mixture for 60 minutes (prepare daily):
   a. Phosphate-phenol buffer, 20 mL
   b. SBB solution, 30 mL
   c. A filtering solution is not necessary.
4. Rinse in 70% ethanol.
5. Air-dry.
6. Counterstain for 10 seconds in 1% violet. Wash three times in tap water. Air-dry.
7. Counterstain for 10 seconds in 0.2% light green. Wash three times in tap water. Air-dry and mount with a coverslip.

Interpretation

1. Positive staining for SBB is indicated by the presence of brownish-black cytoplasmic granules. Positive staining is found in mature and immature granulocytes and many myeloblasts (see Fig. 31–8 and Color Plate 275).
2. Positive staining is also noted in eosinophils and monocytes. Monocytes demonstrate weakly positive or diffuse staining. Eosinophils reveal strong SBB reactivity that is described by distinct staining of an outer shell with a clear or an unstained center.
3. Early myeloblasts, lymphocytes, erythroblasts, mature basophils, megakaryocytes, and platelets are generally negative for SBB staining.

Comments

1. Mayer's hematoxylin or Giemsa stain may be used as counterstains.
2. Normal blood smears should always be run as a positive control.

Periodic Acid–Schiff Reaction

Purpose Periodic acid–Schiff (PAS) stains cytoplasmic glycogen, glycoproteins, mucoproteins, and high-molecular-weight carbohydrates, which are present in a variety of hematopoietic cells. Because many cell lines exhibit PAS positivity, evaluation of the pattern and intensity of staining may be useful for differentiating cell lines. Lymphocytes, granulocytes, monocytes, and megakaryocytes all demonstrate positive reactivity with varying intensity and pattern. Platelets exhibit a strong stain. Generally, early granulocytes stain in a light, diffuse pattern, with increasing intensity and coarseness noted with stages of maturation. Eosinophil granules do not take up the stain, but the background cytoplasm stains positively. In CML and PV, PAS staining is diffuse in the neutrophils. Lymphocyte staining is more granular and coarse. Lymphoblasts in ALL (FAB subclasses L1 and L2) have been known to exhibit "block" staining. Lymphocytes

in Burkitt's type ALL (FAB subclass L3) stain negative with PAS. In CLL, Hodgkin's disease, and lymphosarcoma, the lymphocytes show positive granules. One important clinical application of PAS staining is for supporting the diagnosis of DiGuglielmo's disease or erythroleukemia (FAB subclass M6). Normal erythrocytes and erythrocyte precursors will present with negative reactivity, whereas erythrocyte precursors in erythroleukemia demonstrate intense PAS granular pattern. Occasionally, a positive stain is found in the anemias, including iron-deficiency, pernicious, aplastic, and hemolytic types. Positive PAS reactions have been noted in infectious mononucleosis and chronic renal disease or in any disturbance of glycogen metabolism. Although still popular in many clinical laboratories, PAS methods have largely been replaced by more specific cytochemical markers that are capable of establishing more definitive diagnoses.

Principle PAS oxidizes complex carbohydrates such as glycogen to aldehydes. The aldehydes react with Schiff's reagent to release a colored product. Basic fuchsin is a frequently used dye that imparts a magenta color (Fig. 31–9 and Color Plate 276).

Specimen Smears or bone marrow touch preparations may be used. Anticoagulants do not inhibit activity. Paraffin tissue sections may also be used, but sections must first be hydrated.

Reagents

1. Fixative: Stored at room temperature, reagent has a shelf-life of 1 year.
   Reagent-grade formalin (37%), 50 mL
   Absolute ethanol, 450 mL
2. Periodic acid (1%): Stored at room temperature, reagent has a shelf-life of 3 months:
   Periodic acid, 5 g
   Deionized water, 500 mL
3. Schiff's reagent: Stored at 4°C, reagent has a shelf-life of 3 months:
   Basic fuchsin Cl 42500, 2.5 g
   Deionized water, 500 mL
   Sodium metabisulfite, 5 g
   1 N HCl, 50 mL
   Stir all ingredients for 2 hours, or until the solution turns yellow (light amber). Add 4.0 g of activated charcoal. Filter until all charcoal is removed from the solution. Do not use the solution if it turns pink.
4. Sodium metabisulfite ($Na_2S_2O_5$) (0.5%): Stored at

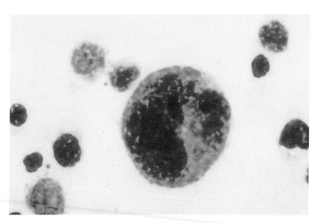

▶ **FIGURE 31–9** Periodic acid–Schiff positivity in erythroleukemia (M6).

room temperature, reagent has a shelf-life of 3 months:
Sodium metabisulfite, 2.5 g
Deionized water, 500 mL
5. Hematoxylin
6. Acid alcohol solution: Stored at room temperature, reagent expires in 6 months:
HCl (1%) in ethanol (70%), 2.5 mL
Deionized water, 497.5 mL
7. Sodium bicarbonate solution (1%). At room temperature, reagent has a shelf-life of 6 months:
Sodium bicarbonate, 5 g
Deionized water, 500 mL

Procedure

1. Fix the smears for 15 minutes. Paraffin tissue sections must be hydrated if they have already been fixed.
2. Rinse *gently* in deionized water. Vigorous rinsing may lead to the loss of cells or tissue from the slides.
3. Place in periodic acid for 10 minutes.
4. Rinse in deionized water and dry.
5. Place the dried smears in Schiff's reagent for 30 minutes.

6. Place in three 10-minute changes of metabisulfite solution.
7. Wash in deionized water for 10 minutes.
8. Counterstain with hematoxylin for 2 minutes.
9. Rinse in deionized water.
10. Place in sodium bicarbonate (bluing) solution for 30 seconds.
11. Rinse in deionized water, dry (tissue needs to be dehydrated), and mount with Permount.

Interpretation Cellular structures that stain positive for PAS appear bright magenta. Lymphocytes, granulocytes, monocytes, and megakaryocytes may demonstrate positive reactivity with varying intensity and pattern. Neutrophils present on the smear may serve as a suitable positive control. Normal erythrocytes and erythrocyte precursors are negative. In erythroleukemia (FAB subclass M6), the erythrocyte precursors usually stain intensely positive; however, early RBCs may occasionally be positive in sideroblastic anemia, iron deficiency, and thalassemia. Lymphoblasts in Burkitt's type ALL stain PAS-negative. The findings of PAS staining should not be used to distinguish the leukemias because staining patterns are variable.

Cytochemical stains are summarized in Table 31–5.

➤ Table 31–5
SUMMARY OF CYTOCHEMICAL STAINS

Stain	Purpose	Interpretation	Cells Stained	Comments	Color Plates
Leukocyte alkaline phosphatase (LAP)	To distinguish CML from leukemoid reactions and myeloproliferative disorders	Decreased LAP score: CML, PNH, sickle cell anemia, sideroblastic anemia, hereditary hypophosphatasia. Increased LAP score: Leukemoid reactions, polycythemia vera, pregnancy.	(+) Neutrophils (+/−) B lymphocytes Count 100 cells and grade from 0 to 4 (+) (see Table 31–1)	Use fresh heparinized blood (EDTA can inhibit LAP activity). Can store at −20° C. Blood from a pregnant woman in the last trimester makes a suitable positive control.	277 278
Myeloperoxidase (MPO)	To distinguish myeloblastic or myelomonocytic leukemia from acute lymphoblastic leukemia	If only blasts are assessed, a positive reaction indicates myeloblastic or myelomonocytic leukemia.	MPO is found in the primary granules and Aüer rods of late myeloblasts through the neutrophils, as well as eosinophils and monocytes, but not lymphocytes.	Fresh specimens are required. All myeloperoxidases are sensitive to heat and to methanol, and are somewhat sensitive to storage.	279
Cyanide-resistant peroxidase	To distinguish eosinophils and their precursors from monocytes and granulocytes	Eosinophils and their precursors stain dark brown. Monocytes and granulocytes are negative.	Stains eosinophils and their precursors, only.	As for all peroxidase stains, use fresh capillary blood for smears or bone marrow touch preparations. EDTA, heparinized, or oxalated specimens are acceptable.	280
Sudan black B (SBB)	To distinguish myeloblastic or myelomonocytic leukemia from lymphoblastic leukemia	Dark brownish-black granules indicate a positive reaction and the myeloid series.	Neutrophil precursors and granulocytes are strongly stained; monocytes have weak staining.	Smears do not have to be fresh, an advantage over MPO stain. Results parallel MPO. Stains lipids; it is not an enzyme stain.	281 282

➤ **Table 31-5**

SUMMARY OF CYTOCHEMICAL STAINS (*Continued*)

Stain	Purpose	Interpretation	Cells Stained	Comments	Color Plates
Specific esterase (naphthol-AS-D chloroacetate esterase (CAE))	To distinguish myeloblastic or myelomonocytic leukemia from lymphoblastic leukemia	A positive reaction is indicated by bright red granules found in the cytoplasm of mature and immature granulocytes (except eosinophils) with blue nuclei.	Neutrophil precursors with differentiation, granulocytes, and mast cells have a positive reaction; monocytes have weak staining.	Can use paraffin-embedded tissue. Reaction is less sensitive than MPO. Results parallel peroxidase and SBB stains.	283
Nonspecific esterase (NSE) α-naphthyl butyrate or α-naphthyl acetate	To distinguish monocytic leukemia from granulocytic leukemia when sodium fluoride is added and the positive reaction is inhibited	Monocyte precursors and monocytes stain bright reddish-brown. Monocyte lineage is confirmed if the color is inhibited when sodium fluoride is added.	Stains monocytes, monocyte precursors, plasma cells, and macrophages. Megakarocytes give a positive reaction with α-naphthyl acetate. Subsets of T lymphocytes show punctate staining.	Fresh capillary blood specimens are preferred; however, anti-coagulated specimens are acceptable, as are bone marrow touch preparations.	284 285
Combined esterase (both substrates)	To differentiate acute myelo-monocytic leukemia (M4) from acute monocytic leukemia (M5a and b)	A dark brownish-red color indicates monocytes or macrophages. T lymphocytes show punctate red granules. A granular blue staining indicates mast cells, early promyelocytes, and late granulocytes	Stains monocyte precursors, monocytes, mast cells, macrophages, early promyelocytes, and late granulocytes.	If the number of blood smears is limited, do a combined stain, which can differentiate between M4 and M5a or M5b.	286
Acid phosphatase	Useful for identifying lymphoblasts in acute T-cell lymphocytic leukemia	If present in T lymphocytes, the activity is located in the Golgi area and has a dotlike appearance. A positive reaction in other cells is an orange-red precipitate at the site.	Stains all hematopoietic cells and many tissues; lymphocytes, activated macrophages, plasma cells, platelets, Gaucher cells, and histiocytes.	Before making a diagnosis of T-cell lymphocytic leukemia, other markers should be performed. Blood smears, bone marrow, lymph node, spleen imprints, or frozen sections are acceptable.	287 288
Tartrate-resistant acid phosphatase (TRAP)	If positive stain is tartrate-resistant, it is highly suggestive of hairy-cell leukemia.	There is strong enzyme activity in the blood when tartrate is added to incubation medium; all acid phosphatase is inhibited except isoenzyme 5, found in hairy-cell leukemia.	Specific for hairy cells.	Fresh blood smears are preferred, also lymph node and spleen implants. Air-dry two smears, one patient and one control. If necessary, slides can be stored at −20° C for 2 weeks, wrapped.	289
Periodic acid–Schiff (PAS)	To differentiate different cell lines; i.e., lymphoblasts (L1 and L2) from early granulocytes, and from Burkitt's (L3); to	Lymphoblasts in ALL (L1 and L2) exhibit block staining. Early granulocytes show light diffuse staining.	Stains many hematopoietic cells (except pronomoblasts), early and late granulocytes, lymphocytes,	Stains cytoplasmic glycogen, mucoproteins and high-molecular-weight carbohydrates. Many cells are positive.	290 291

continued

> **Table 31-5**
SUMMARY OF CYTOCHEMICAL STAINS (*Continued*)

Stain	Purpose	Interpretation	Cells Stained	Comments	Color Plates
	support a diagnosis of erythroleukemia (M6); aids in diagnosis of some ALL and subtypes of AML	Erythrocyte precursors in erythroleukemia demonstrate intense PAS (bright red) positivity. In CML and polycythemia vera, PAS staining is diffuse in the neutrophils. L3 is negative.	megakaryocytes, and erythrocyte precursors in certain conditions; found in any disturbed glycogen metabolism	Blood smears or bone marrow preparations may be used. If using paraffin sections, hydrate first. May need more specific cytochemical markers to confirm a diagnosis.	
Terminal deoxynucleotidyl transferase (TdT)	To differentiate ALL from AML; used as a marker for primitive lymphoid populations; increased in L1 and L2	Presence of green fluorescence indicates TdT activity	Stains T lymphoblasts and pre-B cells; TdT marker is not found in mature B lymphocytes	Nucleus-derived enzyme can be assayed by immunofluorescence, immunoperoxidase, and radioimmunoassay. Nonheparized bone marrow aspirates and peripheral blood may be used. Wash cells three times in culture media. Store slides at 4°C in the dark. Stain within a few days.	292

Abbreviations: CML = chronic myelogenous leukemia; PNH = paroxysmal nocturnal hematuria; EDTA = ethylene diaminetetraacetic acid; ALL = acute lymphocytic leukemia; AML = acute myelogenous leukemia

QUESTIONS

1. A 66-year-old woman presents with an LAP score of 8. What is a possible clinical correlation for this score?
   a. Normal
   b. Leukemoid reaction
   c. Chronic granulocytic leukemia
   d. Pregnancy

2. A 57-year-old woman has an LAP score of 52. What is a possible clinical correlation for this score?
   a. Normal
   b. Leukemoid reaction
   c. Chronic granulocytic leukemia
   d. Pregnancy

3. In which condition would the majority of cells stain positive with myeloperoxidase and Sudan black B?
   a. Acute lymphocytic leukemia
   b. Acute myelogenous leukemia
   c. Chronic lymphocytic leukemia
   d. Erythroleukemia

4. Which of the following cells would demonstrate positive staining with Sudan black B?
   a. Lymphocyte
   b. Basophil
   c. Promyelocyte
   d. Erythroblast

5. Which of the following cells would stain positive using the specific esterase stain?
   a. Megakaryocytes
   b. Macrophages
   c. Neutrophils
   d. Lymphocytes

6. Staining of which of the following cell lines would be inhibited by the addition of sodium fluoride to nonspecific esterase methods?
   a. Megakaryocyte
   b. Plasma cell
   c. Lymphocyte
   d. Monocyte

7. For which of the following disease states would the acid phosphatase/TRAP stain have diagnostic value?
   a. Erythroleukemia
   b. Hairy-cell leukemia
   c. Chronic lymphocytic leukemia
   d. Burkitt's lymphoma

8. For which of the following disease states would periodic acid–Schiff staining have diagnostic value?
   a. Erythroleukemia
   b. Hairy-cell leukemia
   c. Chronic lymphocytic leukemia
   d. Myelomonocytic leukemia

9. Which enzyme stain is a marker for primitive lymphoid populations?
   a. Nonspecific esterase
   b. Sudan black B

c. Chloroacetate esterase

d. Terminal deoxynucleotidyl transferase

10. Which staining procedure utilizes both α-naphthyl butyrate and naphthol-AS-D chloroacetate?

a. Sudan black B

b. Acid phosphatase

c. Periodic acid–Schiff

d. Combined esterase

11. Myeloperoxidase is sensitive to all of the following except:

a. Heat

b. Storage

c. Heparin

d. Methanol

12. What two stains parallel each other in separating acute granulocytic leukemia from acute lymphocytic leukemia?

a. Acid phosphatase and alkaline phosphatase

b. Nonspecific esterase and specific esterase

c. Periodic acid–Schiff and Prussian blue

d. Peroxidase and Sudan black B

13. A medical technologist sees blasts on a peripheral blood smear that she cannot identify with confidence. Peroxidase and Sudan black B stains are performed, and both contain a few positive granules. The nonspecific esterase stain using α-naphthyl butyrate esterase as the substrate is strongly positive. The reaction is inhibited with the addition of sodium fluoride. This would indicate that the type of leukemia is:

a. Acute lymphocytic leukemia

b. Acute erythroleukemia

c. Acute monocytic leukemia

d. Chronic lymphocytic leukemia

14. Which cytochemical stain is used to stain glycogen granules? (Positive is a bright red color.)

a. Nonspecific esterase

b. Acid phosphatase

c. Peroxidase

d. Periodic acid-Schiff

 SUMMARY CHART

➤ Leukocyte alkaline phosphatase (LAP) distinguishes chronic myelogenous leukemia (CML) from leukemoid reactions and myeloproliferative disorders. A decreased LAP score is present with CML, paroxysmal nocturnal hematuria, sickle cell anemia, sideroblastic anemia, and hereditary hypophosphatasia. An increased LAP score is found with leukemoid reaction, polycythemia vera, and pregnancy. Stains neutrophils (+) and B lymphocytes (+/−). Fresh heparinized blood should be used.

➤ Myeloperoxidase (MPO) staining distinguishes myeloblastic or myelomonocytic leukemia from acute lymphoblastic leukemia (ALL). If only blasts are assessed; a positive reaction indicates myeloblastic or myelomonocytic leukemia. MPO stains peroxidase enzyme found in the primary granules and Aüer rods; does not stain lymphocytes. Fresh specimens are required.

➤ Cyanide-resistant peroxidase staining distinguishes eosinophils from monocytes and granulocytes. Eosinophils and their precursors stain dark brown. Monocytes and granulocytes stain negative. Fresh capillary blood for smears or bone marrow touch preparations should be used.

➤ Sudan black B (SBB) staining distinguishes myeloblastic or myelomonocytic leukemia from lymphoblastic leukemia. Dark brownish-black granules indicate a positive reaction. Neutrophil precursors and granulocytes are strongly stained. SBB stains lipids; it is not an enzyme stain. Results parallel MPO.

➤ Specific esterase (naphthol-AS-D chloroacetate esterase [CAE]) staining distinguishes myeloblastic or myelomonocytic leukemia from lymphoblastic leukemia. Bright red granules found in the cytoplasm of granulocytes indicates a positive reaction. Embedded tissue in paraffin can be used.

➤ Nonspecific esterase (NSE) staining distinguishes monocytic leukemia from granulocytic leukemia when sodim fluoride is added and the positive reaction is inhibited. Monocyte precursors and monocytes stain bright reddish-brown and color is inhibited with the addition of sodium fluoride. Fresh capillary blood specimens are preferred.

➤ Combined esterase (both substrates) staining differentiates acute myelomonocytic leukemia (M4) from acute monocytic leukemia (M5a and b). Dark brownish-red color indicates monocytes or macrophages. T lymphocytes show punctate red granules.

➤ Acid phosphatase staining is useful for identifying lymphoblasts in acute T-cell lymphocytic leukemia. T lymphocytes demonstrate a dotlike appearance if present. A positive reaction in other cells is an orange-red precipitate. Blood smears, bone marrow, lymph node, spleen imprints, or frozen sections are acceptable.

➤ If positive acid phosphatase is resistant to addition of tartrate, it is highly suggestive of hairy-cell leukemia. All acid phosphatase is inhibited except isoenzyme 5, found in hydrochloric acid (HCl). Fresh blood smears are preferred; lymph node and spleen implants may also be used. Air-dried smears are accepted.

➤ Periodic acid–Schiff (PAS) staining differentiates different cell lines (e.g., lymphoblasts [L1 and L2] from early cell lines) and from Burkitt's and is particularly useful in the diagnosis of erythroleukemia. Lymphoblasts in ALL exhibit block staining. Early granulocytes show light diffuse staining. Erythrocyte precursors in erythroleukemia demonstrate intense PAS (bright red) positivity.

➤ Terminal deoxynucleotidyl transferase (TdT) staining differentiates ALL from AML. The presence of green fluorescence indicates TdT activity. TdT stains T lymphoblasts and pre-B cells, but not mature B lymphocytes. Nucleus-derived enzyme may be assayed. Nonheparinized bone marrow aspirates and peripheral blood may be used.

See the bibliography for this chapter at the back of the book.

32 Coagulation

Cynthia S. Johns, MSA, MT(ASCP)SH
Gordon E. Ens, MT(ASCP)

OBJECTIVES

At the end of this chapter, the learner should be able to:

1. Explain the diagnostic use of a bleeding time.
2. Correlate platelet aggregation results with clinical conditions.
3. Explain the use of the activated partial thromboplastin time and prothrombin time.
4. Explain the use of the thrombin time and reptilase time.
5. List conditions having low and high fibrinogen levels.
6. Relate clinical conditions to measurements of von Willebrand factor antigen.
7. Identify methods for laboratory diagnosis of protein C and protein S deficiencies.
8. Identify an activated partial thromboplastin time result in conjunction with mixing studies that indicates presence of circulating anticoagulants.
9. List criteria for the laboratory diagnosis of lupus anticoagulants.
10. Identify various endpoint detection methodologies employed by coagulation instrumentation.

➤ GENERAL POINTS REGARDING COAGULATION PROCEDURES

1. Most coagulation procedures are performed on plasma, thereby requiring the addition of calcium in order to perform the tests because the anticoagulant used, sodium citrate, binds free calcium.

2. Testing is performed at 37°C ± 1°.

3. Each laboratory should develop its own normal values reflecting the methodology, reagents, instrumentation, and patient population.

4. The technique used in obtaining and processing the patient's blood sample and the conditions under which samples are stored or transported determine the integrity of the final test result. Traumatic venipuncture may result in activation of coagulation factors, and improper storage conditions may result in the deterioration or (in the case of the factor VII) activation of coagulation factors. Appropriate procedures for the collection of blood for coagulation testing include the following:

   a. Collect blood by clean venipuncture technique using 1 part buffered sodium citrate plus 9 parts of whole blood. Blue-top evacuated tubes with buffered sodium citrate may be used if a discard tube is drawn first and then the blue top is filled to the proper amount. Mix by gentle inversion.

   b. Centrifuge blood as soon as possible for 10 minutes at 2500 × g.

   c. Remove platelet-poor plasma immediately into a plastic tube and refrigerate for no more than 4 hours before testing.

   d. Freeze plasma at −70°C if unable to perform test within 4 hours.

   e. Immediately before testing the plasma, rapid thawing in a 37°C water bath is recommended to prevent denaturation of fibrinogen.

5. Sodium citrate is the anticoagulant used for routine coagulation procedures. Either 3.2% (0.109 M) or 3.8% (0.129 M) are acceptable, although 3.2% is preferred.[1] Other anticoagulants such as ethylene diaminetetraacetic acid (EDTA), heparin, or oxalate are unacceptable.

6. The ratio of blood to anticoagulant should be 9:1. A disproportion of blood to anticoagulant is seen in patients with polycythemia.[1] When the hematocrit is higher than 55%, the amount of sodium citrate used should be adjusted (decreased) according to the following calculation:

$$C = 1.85 \times 10^{-3} \times (100 - H) \times V$$

   where C = volume of sodium citrate in milliliters,
   H = hematocrit in percent, and
   V = volume of whole blood in milliliters.

7. Immunologic assays are currently available for a number of coagulation factors, inhibitors, and proteins involved in fibrinolysis. Because these assays determine the presence or absence of proteins and not their biologic activity, functional testing should be performed in addition, when possible.

8. Enzyme-specific synthetic substrates: In the past, evaluation of hemostasis has relied on traditional procedures based on the detection of clot formation.

The innovation of enzyme-specific synthetic substrates has had a great impact on the field of hemostasis. The knowledge of molecular structures for different enzymes and the cleavage points of their corresponding substrate factors has led to the development of synthetic substrates that are cleaved by a single factor enzyme. Synthesis of synthetic substrates occurs when the amino acids of the substrate on the molecule fit into the active sites and the binding sites of the enzyme. All synthetic substrates rely on cleavage of the peptide by their specific enzymes, releasing a chromogenic complex such as paranitroaniline or a fluorogenic complex such as aminoisophthalic acid dimethyl ester (AIE), which may be detected and measured by means of a spectrophotometer or fluorimeter. Various synthetic chromogenic and fluorogenic assays exist for the evaluation of plasmin, plasminogen activator, alpha-2 (α)$_2$-antiplasmin, kallikrein, antithrombin (AT-III), factor Xa, thrombin, and several other serine proteases, making these assays applicable for routine laboratory testing. Procedures using synthetic substrates have certain advantages over the traditional clot formation techniques. They can be performed rapidly, are sensitive, allow a greater degree of standardization, require smaller sample volumes, and are well suited for automation. Synthetic substrates facilitate measuring the activity of clotting factors and their inhibitors. Often, individual stages of a reaction can be assayed without having to observe the entire cascade of the clotting process. As the field of blood coagulation continues to undergo major technical advancement, the use of synthetic substrates will gain increasing significance and may replace some of the time-honored clotting tests currently used in the routine clinical laboratory.

➤ PLATELET FUNCTION TESTS

Platelet function studies measure or monitor the platelet's ability to adhere and aggregate, and have historically presented a challenge for the clinical laboratory because of the lack of reliable, accurate, and easy-to-perform testing methodologies. In the past, platelet function has been assessed by the bleeding time and platelet aggregation studies. However, both methods are time-consuming, cumbersome, and lack correlation to bleeding risk.[2,3] Because evaluation of platelet function can be of critical importance in the hemostatic management of a patient, especially for those undergoing surgical procedures in which there is a history of clinically significant bleeding,[4] improved ability to assess platelet function in a timely and efficient manner is essential.

The platelets' contribution to the hemostatic mechanism is through adhesion and aggregation, which is known as *primary hemostasis*. Adhesion is defined as the platelet's ability to stick to a surface, such as subendothelial collagen. Aggregation assesses the platelets' ability to stick to each other. For this to occur, platelets must be able to secrete the contents of their organelles (α granules, dense bodies), which contributes to additional platelet activation and aggregation. In the laboratory, the bleeding time has been used to measure platelet adhesion, whereas aggregation studies have been used to observe platelet secretion and the ability to stick to each other.

Bleeding Time

Principle Bleeding time is defined as the time taken for a standardized skin wound to stop bleeding. On vessel injury, platelets adhere and form a homeostatic platelet plug. Bleeding time measures the ability of these platelets to arrest bleeding and, therefore, measures platelet number and function. Capillary contractility and both the intrinsic and extrinsic systems of coagulation function in a minor capacity in the bleeding time. Bleeding time is measured as a screening procedure used to detect both congenital and acquired disorders of platelet function. The bleeding time assesses in vivo platelet function.

Several devices are available for making standardized incisions when performing a bleeding time. *Caution:* Each patient should be informed that, with any bleeding time procedure, the possibility of faint scarring exists. Keloid formation, although rare, may occur in certain patients.

Reagents and Equipment

Sterile bleeding time device

Stopwatch, with seconds available

Sphygmomanometer

Filter paper disc (Whatman No. 11)

Alcohol swab

Butterfly bandage and covering bandage

Procedure Before a bleeding time is measured, it is important that a platelet count be obtained within the past 24 hours. The bleeding time is directly influenced by platelet number if the patient's platelet count is less than 100,000 per μL.[5]

1. Place the patient's arm on a steady support with the muscular area over the lateral aspect of the forearm exposed. The preferred site for the procedure is 5 cm below the antecubital crease. Take care to avoid surface veins, scars, and bruises. If the patient has a notable amount of hair, lightly shave the area first.
2. Place the sphygmomanometer at 40 mm Hg. The time between the inflation of the cuff and the incision should be between 30 and 60 seconds. This pressure should be maintained for the duration of the test.
3. Cleanse the arm with an alcohol swab and allow it to air-dry.
4. Remove the device from the package, being careful not to contaminate the instrument by touching or resting the blade-slot end on any unsterile surface.
5. Remove the safety clip.
6. Hold the device securely between thumb and middle finger.
7. Gently rest the device on the patient's forearm and apply minimal pressure so that both ends of the instrument are lightly touching the skin. The incision may be made either parallel or perpendicular to the antecubital crease of the patient's arm. However, the bleeding time may vary, depending on the direction of the incision. Therefore, normal ranges should be established and the procedure performed using one consistent direction.
8. Push the trigger and start the stopwatch simultaneously. The blade will make an incision of a standardized length and depth, the size of which is dependent on the device utilized.
9. Remove the device from the patient's forearm immediately after making the incision.
10. After 30 seconds, blot the excess flow of blood with filter paper. Bring the filter paper close to the incision, but do not touch the paper directly to the incision so as not to disturb the formation of a platelet plug.
11. Blot the excess blood every 30 seconds thereafter until blood no longer stains the paper. Stop the timer. This is the patient's bleeding time. Bleeding times are determined to the nearest 30 seconds.
12. If the bleeding continues after 15 minutes, terminate the test and apply pressure to the incision site. Report the bleeding time as greater than 15 minutes.
13. Remove the blood pressure cuff and carefully cleanse around the incision site with alcohol. Apply a butterfly bandage across the cut and keep in place for 24 hours to prevent scarring. Apply covering bandage.

Interpretation Normal values are approximately 2.5 to 9.5 minutes but may vary with the direction, length, and depth of the incision. Owing to variations in technique and patient population, it is recommended that each laboratory establish its own "normal" values. Prolonged bleeding times are found in the following situations:

- Thrombocytopenia[5] (platelet count less than 50,000 per μL)
- Inherited platelet dysfunction
- Following administration of aspirin or aspirin-containing drugs
- Following administration of other drugs that inhibit platelet function such as antihistamines

Comment If the incision fails to bleed or if a small vein is cut, disregard the bleeding time of the incision and repeat the test. In older patients, bleeding may only occur subcutaneously (under the skin). Obtaining an accurate bleeding time in these patients may not be possible.

The bleeding time should be measured as part of a diagnostic workup of a quantitative or qualitative platelet disorder, not for the evaluation of a coagulation factor deficiency.

The bleeding time increases in proportion to the decrease in platelet count. The use of aspirin, aspirin-containing drugs, and antihistamines causes a prolonged bleeding time. The patient should be instructed not to take any aspirin or drugs containing aspirin for 1 week before the test is performed.

Platelet Aggregation

Principle Platelets function in primary hemostasis by forming an initial platelet plug at the site of vascular injury. The phenomenon occurs partly through the ability of platelets to adhere to one another, a process known as *aggregation*. Substances that can induce platelet aggregation include collagen, adenosine diphosphate (ADP), epinephrine, thrombin, serotonin, arachidonic acid, the antibiotic ristocetin, snake venoms, antigen-antibody complexes, soluble fibrin monomer complexes, and fibrin(ogen) degradation products (FDPs). These aggregating agents induce platelet aggregation or cause platelets to release endogenous ADP, or both.

Platelet aggregation is an essential part of the investigation of any patient with a suspected platelet dysfunction.

Platelet aggregation is studied by means of a platelet aggregometer, a photo-optical instrument connected to a chart recorder. Platelet-rich plasma, which is turbid in appearance, is placed in a cuvette, warmed to 37°C in the heating block of the instrument, and stirred by a small magnetic bar. Baseline light transmittance through the platelet-rich plasma is recorded. The addition of an aggregating agent causes the formation of larger platelet aggregates with a corresponding increase in light transmittance, because of a clearing in the platelet-rich plasma. The change in light transmittance is converted to electronic signals and recorded as a tracing by the chart recorder.

Note: There are some basic requirements for platelet aggregation as an in vitro means of evaluating platelet function:

1. In performing platelet aggregation studies, a clean venipuncture is crucial. Hemolyzed samples should not be utilized because red blood cells contain ADP, which can prematurely activate platelets.
2. Plasma from fasting patients is preferred for testing. Lipemic samples may obscure changes in optical density during platelet aggregation.
3. Sodium citrate is the anticoagulant used in aggregation studies. Keep in mind that in vitro aggregation is dependent on the presence of calcium ions, and sodium citrate's mechanism to prevent coagulation in the sample is by binding calcium ions. However, the concentration of calcium after anticoagulation with sodium citrate should still be sufficient for aggregation to occur.
4. Fibrinogen must be present in the test sample for aggregation to occur.
5. The plasma sample should not come in contact with a glass surface unless the surface is siliconized, because glass will cause platelet activation and adhesion to its surface.
6. Aggregation studies should be performed at 37°C at a pH of 6.5 to 8.5. To help maintain pH values, all samples, once collected, should be capped to prevent CO_2 loss. The presence of CO_2 helps to maintain the pH of the sample.
7. Test samples should be maintained at room temperature during processing. Cooling inhibits the platelet aggregating response. Just before performing the test, the plasma is incubated at 37°C in the heat block of the aggregometer.
8. Platelet-rich plasma samples should be allowed to stand for approximately 30 minutes prior to performing aggregation testing. This is necessary for the platelets to regain their responsiveness after undergoing the preparation procedure.
9. All aggregation studies should be performed within 3 hours of sample collection.
10. Stirring is necessary to bring the platelets in close contact with one another to allow aggregation to occur.
11. Aggregating agents should be prepared fresh daily and brought to room temperature before use. They must have known potency and be added in small volumes.
12. Control tests using platelet-rich plasma from a known normal donor must be performed at the same time as the patient samples.
13. It is essential that the patient refrain from taking any anti-inflammatory drugs at least 1 week before testing. These drugs inhibit the platelets' release reaction.
14. Thrombocytopenia makes evaluation of the aggregation responses difficult.

Reagents and Equipment

Control and patient platelet-rich plasma

Aggregometer and cuvettes

Magnetic stirring bar

Pipets

Normal saline

Sodium metabisulphite

Aggregating agents (agonists):

Adenosine-5′-phosphate (ADP): Prepare appropriate dilutions in normal saline.

Collagen: Prepare appropriate working concentrations in normal saline.

Ristocetin: Prepare appropriate working solutions in deionized water.

Arachidonic acid: Prepare appropriate dilutions in deionized water (if needed).

Epinephrine: Prepare appropriate dilutions in 0.1% sodium metabisulphite.

Procedure

1. Collect 10 to 20 mL of blood into plastic tubes containing 3.2% (0.109 *M*) or 3.8% (0.129 *M*) sodium citrate. Be careful to maintain a 9:1 blood to anticoagulant ratio. Centrifuge the citrated venous blood sample at room temperature (18°C to 25°C) at 150 to 200 × g for 10 to 15 minutes. Perform a platelet count on the platelet-rich plasma. Dilute the platelet-rich plasma with platelet-poor plasma to obtain a platelet count of 250×10^9/L. Plasma may be left at room temperature in capped plastic tubes for up to 2 hours before testing. Repeat procedure for control sample.
2. The aggregometer should be warmed to 37°C prior to use according to the manufacturer's recommendations.
3. Pipet the appropriate volume of platelet-rich plasma into an appropriate aggregometer cuvette and place in the 37°C heat block for 1 minute to warm the test plasma.
4. Pipet the appropriate volume of platelet-poor plasma into a separate cuvette if required by the individual aggregometer. This is used as a plasma "blank" to adjust the baseline optical density reading to correct for the effects of lipemia, icterus, or hemolysis in the patient sample.
5. Place a magnetic stirring bar into the cuvette. Platelets must be constantly stirred throughout the testing procedure to allow them to come into contact with each other in order to observe the adhesion and aggregation process.
6. Pipet the recommended volume of aggregating agent to the plasma. Observe the aggregation curve for a defined period of time (i.e., 3 to 5 minutes).

7. Tests are usually performed with various dilutions of ADP, collagen, arachidonic acid, ristocetin and epinephrine for patient and normal control plasma samples.

Interpretation Platelet aggregation occurs as a two-step process, known as *primary* and *secondary waves of aggregation*. The primary wave of aggregation is observed when platelets adhere to one another in the presence of an external agent (agonist) such as ADP, epinephrine, or ristocetin. Secondary aggregation is characterized as the aggregation that occurs after the platelets have been stimulated to secrete the substances contained in their organelles. It should be noted that some agonists will stimulate primary aggregation and some will stimulate secondary aggregation. Others will stimulate both primary and secondary aggregation, yielding a "biphasic" aggregation curve (Fig. 32–1). In addition, different concentrations of the same agonist can produce varying patterns of primary and secondary aggregation. For example, low concentrations of ADP induce biphasic aggregation (i.e., both a primary and a secondary wave of aggregation); very low concentrations of ADP induce a primary wave followed by disaggregation; and high concentrations of ADP induce a single, broad

wave of aggregation[6] (Fig. 32–2). A biphasic aggregation response to ADP will not be seen in patients with platelet release disorders. Patients with Glanzmann's thrombasthenia show incomplete aggregation with ADP regardless of the final concentration.

Platelet aggregation induced by collagen is characterized by a lag period before aggregation, followed by only a single wave of aggregation. A biphasic aggregation response is seen with the antibiotic ristocetin; however, often only a single broad wave of aggregation will occur. Platelet aggregation induced with arachidonic acid causes a rapid secondary wave of aggregation. Biphasic aggregation is observed with epinephrine. One-third to one-half of normal, healthy patients only produce a primary wave of aggregation with epinephrine.[7] The aggregating agent thrombin induces a biphasic wave of aggregation. Platelet aggregation induced by serotonin normally produces a primary wave of aggregation with a maximum of 10% to 30% transmittance followed by disaggregation[7] (see Fig. 32–1).

In patients with severe von Willebrand disease, aggregation to ristocetin is characteristically absent. Decreased to normal aggregation to ristocetin can be seen in patients with mild von Willebrand disease. Correction of the abnormal ristocetin aggregation curves can be seen by the addition of normal, platelet-poor plasma to the patient's platelet-rich plasma. Abnormal ristocetin-induced platelet aggregation may also occur in patients with Bernard-Soulier syndrome, platelet storage pool defects, and idiopathic thrombocytopenic purpura (ITP).

Comment In evaluating patients with suspected platelet disorders, the aggregating agents most commonly used are ADP in varying concentrations, collagen, epinephrine, and ristocetin. Aspirin, aspirin compounds, and anti-

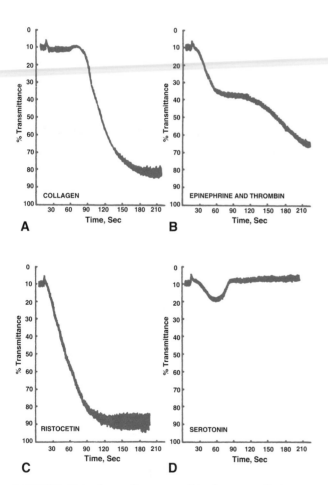

➤ **FIGURE 32–1** Aggregation curves with various aggregating agents. *A.* Aggregation curve induced by collagen. Note the lag time before aggregation followed by a single wave of aggregation. *B.* Aggregation curve induced with epinephrine and thrombin. Note the biphasic wave of aggregation. *C.* Aggregation curve induced by ristocetin. A biphasic wave of aggregation as well as a single wave of aggregation may be seen. *D.* Aggregation curve induced by serotonin. Generally a single wave of aggregation followed by disaggregation is seen.

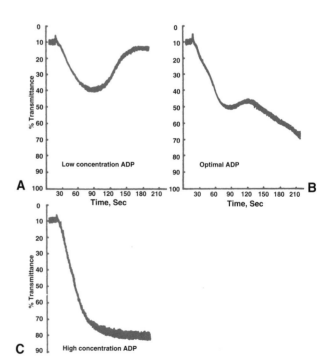

➤ **FIGURE 32–2** Aggregation curves induced with various concentrations of adenosine diphosphate (ADP). *A.* Very low concentrations of ADP induce a primary wave of aggregation followed by disaggregation. *B.* The optimal concentration of ADP induces a biphasic wave of aggregation. *C.* High concentrations of ADP induce a broad wave of aggregation.

inflammatory drugs inhibit the secondary wave of aggregation by inhibiting the release reaction of the platelet. Reduced or absent aggregation as well as disaggregation curves may be observed in patients taking medication containing aspirin. Other medications or substances have also been identified as inhibiting platelet function, such as ibuprofen, red wine, and a variety of herbs. Patients should be questioned carefully about possible ingestion of these substances prior to interpreting abnormal aggregation results.

The intensity of platelet aggregation may be estimated by recording the change in absorbances as a percentage of the difference in absorbance between platelet-rich and platelet-poor plasma. This has limited usefulness because absorbance is dependent on the size and density of platelet clumping and the number of platelets that aggregate. A more complex analysis of aggregation related to the rate of aggregation may also be obtained. However, visual interpretation of the aggregation curves suffices and can establish whether aggregation is abnormal or normal.

➤ TESTS TO MEASURE THE INTRINSIC SYSTEM

Activated Partial Thromboplastin Time

Principle The activated partial thromboplastin time (APTT) is a screening test used to evaluate the intrinsic pathway of coagulation, or more precisely, to measure all the plasma coagulation factors with the exception of factors VII and XIII and platelet factor 3 (PF3). The formation of fibrin occurs at a normal rate only if the factors involved in the intrinsic pathway (factors VIII, IX, XI, and XII) and the common pathway (factors I, II, V, and X) are present in normal concentrations. Optimal activation is achieved by the addition of a platelet phospholipid substitute, which eliminates the test's sensitivity to platelet number and function, as well as the addition of activators such as kaolin, celite, micronized silica, and ellagic acid, which eliminates the variability of activation by glass contact. The APTT is also used to screen for inhibitors of the intrinsic pathway such as the lupus-like anticoagulant, and to monitor heparin therapy.

Reagents and Equipment

Coagulation analyzer (automated or semiautomated)

Commercial activated partial thromboplastin reagent

Note: Because commercial APTT reagents vary in the type of activator used, they will have different requirements for optimal contact activation time between the reagent and plasma during the testing process. The manufacturer's recommendations should be followed and the incubation time on the coagulation analyzer set accordingly. Failure to adhere to correct incubation times for the specific reagent used may yield erroneous results.

Procedure

1. Collect the blood by clean venipuncture technique according to the recommended procedures previously described.
2. Process and store the plasma samples following recommended guidelines.
3. Reconstitute the activated partial thromboplastin reagent according to the manufacturer's directions.

4. Perform APTT according to the manufacturer's package insert.
5. Record the time for fibrin formation (clotting time).
6. Testing on control and test plasma may be performed once or in duplicate. If using single-sample testing, studies should be performed to verify that the analyzer's precision is within acceptable limits. Report results to the nearest 0.1 seconds. If performing testing in duplicate, calculate the mean clotting time before reporting. (*Note:* As a rule, duplicate results should agree within ± 5% of each other.)

Interpretation Each laboratory should develop its own normal range based on the type of analyzer, reagent, and patient population. The test result is abnormal in patients with deficiencies of any factor involved in the intrinsic or common pathway. The APTT may be prolonged when factor levels are less than 30% to 40% of normal, depending on reagent sensitivity. Hypofibrinogenemia (levels less than 100 mg/dL) will prolong the APTT. When the APTT is used to monitor heparin therapy, it is typically considered to be in the therapeutic range if it is prolonged 1.5 to 2.5 times the patient's baseline level.

Comment Both the APTT and the prothrombin time (PT) should be performed as screening procedures, because together they evaluate the intrinsic, extrinsic, and common pathways of coagulation.

➤ TESTS TO MEASURE THE EXTRINSIC SYSTEM

One-Stage Prothrombin Time (Quick)[8]

Principle The PT is the time required for the formation of a fibrin clot when plasma is added to a thromboplastin-calcium mixture. The test is a measure of the extrinsic pathway of coagulation involving factors II, V, VII, and X (as well as fibrinogen). Tissue thromboplastin activates factor VII, which proceeds through the cascade, ultimately generating thrombin. The thrombin thus formed converts fibrinogen to fibrin. The rate of fibrin formation depends on the level of factors II, V, VII, and X and fibrinogen. Therefore, the PT can be used as an indicator of the overall activity of these factors.

The test is a valuable screening procedure used to indicate possible factor deficiencies of the extrinsic or common pathway. The PT test is sensitive to the vitamin K–dependent factors of the extrinsic (factor VII) and common pathways (factors II and X) and is, therefore, used as a means of monitoring oral anticoagulant therapy. *Note:* The fourth vitamin K–dependent factor, factor IX, is measured by the APTT.

Reagents and Equipment

Coagulation analyzer (automated or semiautomated)

Commercial thromboplastin

Note: Commercial thromboplastins differ in the source of thromboplastin utilized (i.e., rabbit brain, rabbit brain-lung combination, recombinant human), leading to differences in reagent sensitivity, and, therefore, greater variations in the PT results obtained. Reagent sensitivity is indicated by the International Sensitivity Index (ISI), which is a comparison of the reagent performance to the gold standard thromboplastin used by the World Health Organization

(WHO).[9] The WHO thromboplastin has been assigned an ISI value of 1.0. Commercial thromboplastins are calibrated using the WHO standard and assigned an ISI value that reflects their sensitivity. Thromboplastins with a low ISI (close to 1.0) are considered to be extremely sensitive. The higher the ISI, the lower the sensitivity of the reagent. Keep in mind that the lower the ISI, the greater the prolongation of the PT that is observed.

Procedure

1. Collect blood by clean venipuncture technique according to recommended procedures previously described.
2. Process and store the plasma samples following recommended guidelines.
3. Reconstitute the thromboplastin/CaCl$_2$ reagent according to the manufacturer's directions.
4. Perform the PT procedure according to the manufacturer's package insert.
5. Record the time for fibrin formation (clotting time).
6. Testing on control and test plasma may be performed in duplicate or singly. If using single testing, studies should be performed to verify that the analyzer's precision is within acceptable limits. Report results to the nearest 0.1 second. If performing testing in duplicate, calculate the mean clotting time before reporting. (*Note:* As a rule, duplicate results should agree within ±5% of each other.)
7. The international normalized ratio (INR) should be reported along with the PT results, using the ISI of the thromboplastin. Most coagulation analyzers have the capability of calculating the INR in addition to the PT results. The calculation is performed as follows:

$$INR = \left\{ \frac{\text{Patient PT}}{\text{Mean of normal range}} \right\}^{ISI}$$

Interpretation The normal range for PTs is approximately 10 to 13 seconds. This range varies with the type of thromboplastin employed in the testing process. Each laboratory must develop its own "normal" range based on the type of analyzer, reagent, and patient population.

The PT is prolonged in individuals with a factor deficiency involving a single factor (i.e., patients with a congenital deficiency) or involving multiple factors (i.e., patients with acquired deficiencies such as liver disease, oral anticoagulant therapy, or patients with vitamin K deficiency). The PT may also be prolonged in the presence of circulating anticoagulants such as FDPs and heparin.

In patients with polycythemia, the PT is prolonged as a result of a change in the ratio of anticoagulant to plasma. For coagulation testing, the blood to sodium citrate ratio should always be maintained at 9:1. Elevated hematocrits greater than 55% (such as in polycythemia) yield a smaller amount of plasma in the collection tube, thereby increasing the proportion of anticoagulant in the plasma. Increased citrate will bind the calcium chloride added to the system during the testing process, causing a prolongation of the PT. In this case, the amount of citrate should be adjusted (decreased) prior to specimen collection to compensate for the elevated hematocrit, as previously described. PT results will be shortened when the plasma is stored for longer than 4 hours at 4°C because of cold activation of factor VII.

➤ COAGULATION FACTOR ASSAYS

One-Stage Quantitative Assay Method for Factors II, V, VII, and X

Principle The prothrombin time is the basis of this test system, with specific factor-deficient plasmas being added to the patient plasma. The percentage of factor activity is determined by the amount of correction detected when specific dilutions of patient plasma are added to the factor-deficient plasma. These results are obtained from an activity curve made using clotting times of dilutions of normal reference plasma and specific factor-deficient plasma.

Reagents and Equipment

Commercial thromboplastin

Specific factor-deficient plasma (II, V, VII, and X)

Note: It is recommended that the factor-deficient plasma utilized be verified as having less than 1% activity for the specific factor being measured.

Imidazole buffered saline, pH 7.3 ± 0.1

Normal reference plasma (commercial reference plasma with known factor levels)

Instrument: Same as that used for PT assay

Procedure

1. Preparation of the activity curve:
   a. Prepare 1:10, 1:20, 1:40, 1:80, 1:160, 1:320, 1:640, and 1:1280 serial dilutions of the normal reference plasma with imidazole-buffered saline. The 1:10 dilution is considered 100% factor activity. It is recommended that at least five dilutions be used to prepare the factor activity curve, although it is common to use seven or eight dilutions (Table 32–1).
   b. Warm thromboplastin to 37°C.
   c. Perform the following test procedure on each dilution. *Note:* These steps may be performed either manually or by an automated coagulation analyzer.
      (1) Add 0.1 mL of specific factor-deficient plasma to 0.1 mL of the diluted normal reference plasma and warm to 37°C for the allotted time based on the manufacturer's specifications.
      (2) Add 0.2 mL of commercial thromboplastin to the sample and determine the clotting time.
      (3) Testing may be performed either singly or in duplicate. If performing duplicate testing, repeat steps 1 and 2 on the duplicate sample and average results.
   d. Plot results on 2 × 3 cycle log graph paper, with percent factor activity on the x axis and seconds on the y axis. Draw a best-fit line. The curve will demonstrate a plateau at the least concentrated dilutions and should be plotted as such, demonstrating the end of sensitivity for the assay. If using an automated analyzer, the curve is generally constructed internally and stored for a specified length of time.
2. Procedure for testing patient plasma:
   a. Warm thromboplastin to 37°C.
   b. Prepare a 1:10 and 1:20 dilution of citrated

> ## Table 32-1
> ### PREPARATION OF TEST DILUTIONS FOR REFERENCE PLASMA IN THE ONE-STAGE ASSAY FOR FACTORS

Tube No.	Amount of Plasma	Imidazole Buffered Saline	Dilution	% of Factor
1	0.1 mL	0.9 mL	1:10	100.00
2	0.5 mL of Tube No. 1	0.5 mL	1:20	50.00
3	0.5 mL of Tube No. 2	0.5 mL	1:40	25.00
4	0.5 mL of Tube No. 3	0.5 mL	1:80	12.50
5	0.5 mL of Tube No. 4	0.5 mL	1:160	6.25
6	0.5 mL of Tube No. 5	0.5 mL	1:320	3.13
7	0.5 mL of Tube No. 6	0.5 mL	1:640	1.56
8	0.5 mL of Tube No. 7	0.5 mL	1:1280	0.78

patient plasma with imidazole-buffered saline. It is important to keep samples and dilutions refrigerated until they are to be tested.

c. Add 0.1 mL of specific factor-deficient plasma to 0.1 mL of diluted patient plasma.

d. Add 0.2 mL of thromboplastin to the sample and determine the clotting time.

e. Testing may be performed either singly or in duplicate. If performing duplicate testing, repeat steps c and d on the duplicate sample and average the results.

f. Repeat steps c, d, and e on the 1:20 dilution of patient plasma. The results of the 1:10 and 1:20 dilution should agree within 20%. Report the average of the two results. *Note:* Nonspecific inhibitors will often have a "dilutional" effect, demonstrating nonparallel curves with increasing dilutions. This should be considered if the results of the 1:10 and 1:20 dilutions do not agree within 20%. In this case, results should *not* be averaged, but further dilutions performed to determine the correct factor activity result.

g. Read the percent activity directly from the activity curve (Fig. 32–3). From this curve, a result of 35 seconds on a 1:10 dilution of patient plasma would be interpreted as 8.3% activity. If the curve was generated using an automated coagulation analyzer, the results will automatically be read from the curve and printed out. *Note:* Specific volumes required for adding

factor-deficient plasma, diluted patient plasma, and thromboplastin reagent may vary depending on the automated analyzer used. The volumes previously recommended may be used if performing the test manually.

Interpretation An approximate range of 50% to 150% is considered normal. Each laboratory should define its own normal range based on instrument, reagent, and patient population.

One-Stage Quantitative Assay Method for Factors VIII, IX, XI, and XII

Principle The APTT is the basis of this test system. This method is also based on the ability of patient plasma to correct specific factor-deficient plasma. Results in percent activity are obtained from an activity curve.

Reagents and Equipment

APTT reagent

0.025 M CaCl$_2$

Specific factor-deficient plasma (VIII, IX, XI, and XII)

Normal reference plasma (commercial reference plasma with known factor levels)

Imidazole-buffered saline, pH 7.3 $\pm$ 0.1

Instrument for APTT assay

Procedure

1. Preparation of activity curve:

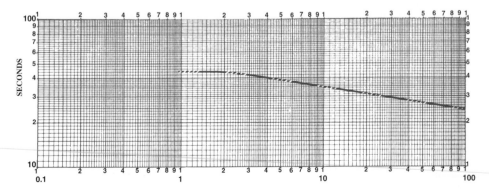

> FIGURE 32–3 Factor V activity curve.

a. Prepare 1:10, 1:20, 1:40, 1:80, 1:160, 1:320, 1:640, and 1:1280 serial dilutions of the normal reference plasma with imidazole-buffered saline (see Table 32–1). The 1:10 dilution is considered 100% factor activity.

b. Prewarm the $CaCl_2$ and APTT reagent to 37°C.

c. Perform the following test procedure on each dilution. *Note:* These steps may be performed either manually or by an automated coagulation analyzer.

   (1) Add 0.1 mL of specific factor-deficient plasma and 0.1 mL of diluted normal reference plasma to 0.1 mL APTT reagent. Mix well and incubate for the specified time according to reagent manufacturer's instructions.

   (2) Add 0.1 mL $CaCl_2$ into the mixture at the end of the incubation time and determine the clotting time.

   (3) Testing may be performed either singly or in duplicate. If performing duplicate testing, repeat steps 1 and 2 on the duplicate sample and average the results.

d. Plot results on 2 × 3 cycle log graph paper, with percent factor on the x axis and seconds on the y axis. Draw a best-fit line. The curve will demonstrate a plateau at the least concentrated dilutions and should be plotted as such, demonstrating the limit of sensitivity for the assay.

2. Procedure for testing patient plasma:

   a. Prewarm $CaCl_2$ and APTT reagent to 37°C.

   b. Prepare a 1:10 and 1:20 dilution of citrated patient plasma with imidazole-buffered saline. It is important to keep samples and dilutions refrigerated until they are to be tested.

   c. Add 0.1 mL of specific factor-deficient plasma and 0.1 mL of diluted patient plasma to 0.1 mL APTT reagent. Mix well and incubate for the recommended time.

   d. Add 0.1 mL $CaCl_2$ into the mixture at the end of specified time and determine the clotting time.

   e. Testing may be performed either singly or in duplicate. If performing duplicate testing, repeat steps c and d on the duplicate sample and average the results.

   f. Repeat steps c, d, and e on the 1:20 dilution of patient plasma. The results of the 1:10 and 1:20 dilution should agree within 20%. Report the average of the two results.

      Note: Nonspecific inhibitors will often have a "dilutional" effect demonstrating nonparallel curves with increasing dilutions. This should be considered if the results of the 1:10 and 1:20 dilutions do not agree within 20%. In this case, results should *not* be averaged, but further dilutions performed to determine the correct factor activity result.

   g. Read the percent activity directly from the activity curve (similar to that displayed in Fig. 32–3). If using an automated analyzer, the results may be automatically read from the curve and printed out.

      Note: Specific volumes required for adding factor-deficient plasma, diluted patient plasma, and APTT reagent may vary depending on the automated analyzer used. The volumes previously recommended may be used if performing the test manually.

Interpretation An approximate range of 50% to 150% is considered normal. Each laboratory must define its own normal range based on instrument, reagent, and patient population.

Comment

1. If the result from the 1:20 dilution is greater than the highest curve point (i.e., 1:10), prepare additional dilutions of the patient sample with buffered saline until results fall within the linearity range of the curve. If the result from the 1:10 dilution is lower than the lowest curve point (i.e., 1:1280), report the factor activity as less than 0.8%.

2. To calculate the percent activity for additional dilutions tested, multiply the result by the dilution factor for the percent activity of the patient sample.

3. These tests require the same considerations as the APTT and PT assay in regard to quality control, specimen handling, reagent preparation, and points of procedural importance. The assay should be performed on the same equipment and in the same manner as all other coagulation assays in the laboratory.

➤ TESTS TO MEASURE FIBRIN FORMATION

Thrombin Time

Principle The thrombin time (TT) is the time required for thrombin to convert fibrinogen to an insoluble fibrin clot. Fibrin formation is triggered by the addition of thrombin to the specimen and, therefore, bypasses prior steps in the coagulation cascade. The TT does not measure defects in the intrinsic or extrinsic pathways. The test is affected by abnormal levels of fibrinogen, dysfibrinogenemia, and the presence of circulating anticoagulants (antithrombins) such as heparin and FDPs.

Reagents and Equipment

Coagulation analyzer

Commercial thrombin reagent

Normal control plasma

Procedure

1. Collect blood by clean venipuncture technique according to recommended procedures previously described.

2. Process and store plasma samples following recommended guidelines.

3. Reconstitute thrombin reagent according to the manufacturer's instructions.

4. Incubate 0.1 mL of control or patient plasma at 37°C for 2 minutes.

5. Add 0.05 mL of prewarmed thrombin reagent.

6. Measure the clotting time.

7. Perform the test in duplicate and average the results.

8. If the patient's average clotting time greatly exceeds the average control time, the test should be repeated

using a 1:1 mixture of the patient's plasma and normal or control plasma (see Interpretation).

Interpretation The normal value is approximately 10 to 15 seconds. The TT is prolonged in patients with hypofibrinogenemia (usually less than 100 mg/dL), dysfibrinogenemia, and in the presence of circulating anticoagulants such as heparin or FDPs. If the 1:1 mixing study results in a clotting time that approximates that of the control plasma, a deficiency or a molecular abnormality of fibrinogen is most likely indicated. If the mixing study fails to correct the TT, the presence of a circulating inhibitor is indicated.

Reptilase Time

Principle The reptilase time is similar to the TT except that the clotting sequence is initiated with the snake venom enzyme, reptilase. Reptilase is thrombinlike in nature and hydrolyzes fibrinopeptide A from the intact fibrinogen molecule. This is in contrast to thrombin, which hydrolyzes fibrinopeptide A and B from fibrinogen. The clot that forms due to the action of reptilase on fibrinogen is more fragile than that formed by thrombin's action on fibrinogen. The advantage of the reptilase time is that it is not inhibited by heparin. There is only a minimal effect on the reptilase time by FDPs.

Reagents and Equipment

Coagulation analyzer

Reptilase reagent

Platelet-poor citrated plasma (control or test plasma)

Procedure

1. Collect blood by clean venipuncture technique according to the recommended procedures previously described.
2. Process and store plasma samples following recommended guidelines.
3. Reconstitute the reptilase reagent according to the manufacturer's instructions.
4. Test the control or patient plasma with the reptilase reagent according to the manufacturer's instructions.
5. Measure the clotting time.
6. Perform testing in duplicate; calculate the average clotting time, and report results to the nearest tenth of a second. Duplicate results should agree ± 0.5 seconds.

Interpretation Normal values are approximately 15 to 20 seconds. Except for fibrinogen$_{Oklahoma}$ and fibrinogen$_{Oslow}$, all the congenital dysfibrinogenemias have an infinite reptilase time. The reptilase time is also infinitely prolonged in cases of congenital afibrinogenemia. In states of

hypofibrinogenemia, the reptilase time may be variable, depending on the levels of fibrinogen present. The reptilase time is moderately prolonged in the presence of FDPs and is unaffected by heparin (Table 32–2).

Comment In the presence of heparin, thrombin is inhibited through the interaction of antithrombin (AT-III). However, heparin does not interfere with reptilase's ability to cleave fibrinopeptide A from fibrinogen. A comparison of both TT and reptilase time will aid in detecting the presence of thrombin inhibitors such as heparin.

Fibrinogen Activity

Principle Fibrinogen can be quantitatively measured by a modification of the TT because the thrombin clotting time of dilute plasma is inversely proportional to the concentration of fibrinogen. This method involves testing dilutions of both patient plasma and control plasma with an excess of thrombin. Results are calculated from a calibration curve.

Reagents and Equipment

Coagulation analyzer

12×75 test tubes

Commercial fibrinogen determination kit:

Thrombin, 100 National Institutes of Health (NIH) units per mL, bovine lyophilized

Fibrinogen standard: Fibrinogen concentration is standardized by the macro-Kjeldahl method. Reconstitute according to manufacturer's directions. Mix by gentle inversion; do not shake.

Owren's Veronal buffer, pH 7.35

Control (with a known fibrinogen concentration)

Procedure

1. Collect blood by clean venipuncture technique according to recommended procedures previously described.
2. Process and store plasma samples following recommended guidelines.
3. Reconstitute the thrombin reagent according to the manufacturer's directions.

Preparation of Calibration Curve

1. Make dilutions of the fibrinogen standard with Owren's Veronal buffer as follows: 1:5, 1:15, and 1:40. Make all transfers from the first test tube.
   a. 1:5 dilution (first tube): 1.6 mL buffer plus 0.4 mL of fibrinogen standard
   b. 1:15 dilution (second tube): 0.8 mL of buffer plus 0.4 mL of mixture from the first test tube

> **Table 32–2**
TEST COMPARISON

Thrombin Time	Reptilase Time	Defect
Infinitely prolonged	Infinitely prolonged	Dysfibrinogenemia
Infinitely prolonged	Infinitely prolonged	Afibrinogenemia
Prolonged	Equally prolonged	Hypofibrinogenemia
Prolonged	Normal	Heparin
Prolonged	Slightly to moderately prolonged	FDPs

c. 1:40 dilution (third tube): 2.8 mL of buffer plus 0.4 mL of mixture from the first test tube

2. Perform duplicate determinations on each dilution of the fibrinogen standard as follows:

a. Incubate 0.2 mL of fibrinogen standard dilution at 37°C for at least 2 minutes but no more than 5 minutes.

b. Add 0.1 mL of thrombin reagent.

c. Measure the clotting time. Average the results of the duplicate determinations.

Calibration Curve Using the graph paper furnished, plot the clotting time in seconds on the vertical (y) axis versus the concentration of fibrinogen standard dilutions on the horizontal (x) axis. Draw a best-fit line.

Note: A fibrinogen calibration curve should be prepared with each new lot of reagent. It is not necessary to prepare a curve each time the procedure is run. If using an automated analyzer, the curve is generally constructed internally and stored for a specified length of time.

Sample Assay

1. Make a 1:10 dilution of the patient plasma or control with Owren's Veronal buffer, using 0.1 mL of plasma and 0.9 mL of buffer.

2. Perform duplicate determinations on each as follows. These steps may be performed either manually or by an automated analyzer.

a. Incubate 0.2 mL of the patient dilution at 37°C for at least 2 minutes but no more than 5 minutes.

b. Add 0.1 mL of thrombin reagent.

c. Measure the clotting time. Average the results of the duplicate determinations.

3. Read results from calibration curve and record in mg/dL (Fig. 32–4). If using an automated analyzer, the results may be automatically read from the curve and printed out.

Interpretation Normal values range from approximately 200 to 400 mg/dL. Prolonged clotting times may indicate either a low fibrinogen concentration or the presence of inhibitors such as heparin or circulating FDPs. The effect of heparin may be excluded by performing a TT using reptilase instead of thrombin, because reptilase is unaffected by heparin. A comparison of clotting times using both TT and reptilase time may help to distinguish a fibrinogen deficiency from a dysfibrinogenemia.

Low fibrinogen levels are seen in infants and children and in those with congenital afibrinogenemia or hypofibrinogenemia. Acquired deficiencies are seen in liver disease, disseminated intravascular coagulation (DIC), and fibrinolysis.

High fibrinogen levels are seen during pregnancy and in women taking oral contraceptives. Fibrinogen is considered an acute-phase reactant, and, therefore, high levels may be seen in states of acute infection, neoplasms, collagen disorders, nephrosis, and hepatitis.

Comment If a prolonged clotting time is obtained using a 1:10 dilution of patient plasma, this may indicate low fibrinogen levels of 50 mg/dL or less. Retest the sample using a 1:5 or 1:2 dilution with buffered saline and divide the results by 5 or 2, respectively, to obtain the final results. If a short clotting time is obtained using a 1:10 dilution of patient plasma, this may indicate high fibrinogen levels of 400 mg/dL or more. Retest the sample using a 1:20 dilution and multiply the results by 2 to obtain the final results.

A number of automated instruments are available that measure fibrinogen concentrations based on change in optical density as part of the PT determination. This is known as a PT-derived fibrinogen. Fibrinogen activity determined by this methodology is more susceptible to interfering substances such as increased levels of FDPs, which may cause unreliable results.

Fibrinogen antigen levels may also be assayed by means of radial immunodiffusion (RID) or nephelometry. This is a measure of the total amount of fibrinogen protein present, compared to fibrinogen activity, which is a measure of its functional ability. Determination of both fibrinogen antigen and activity levels is useful in evaluating dysfibrinogenemias, which will show abnormal fibrinogen activity with normal antigen levels.

Factor XIII Screening Test

Principle Stabilization of the fibrin clot depends on plasma factor XIII, which converts hydrogen bonds to covalent bonds by transamination. In the absence of factor XIII, the hydrogen-bonded fibrin polymers are soluble in 5 *M* urea or 1% monochloroacetic acid.

Reagents and Equipment

5 *M* urea or 1% monochloroacetic acid

Bovine thrombin (200 NIH units/mL)

0.15 NaCl

Patient plasma

37°C water bath

Procedure

1. Add 0.5 mL of the patient plasma and 0.1 mL of thrombin reagent to a 12 × 75 mm glass test tube.

2. Incubate at 37°C for 30 minutes.

3. Remove the clot from the test tube with a glass rod.

4. Wash the clot with cold saline.

5. Place the clot in a clean 12 × 75 mm test tube containing 1 mL of 5 *M* urea or 1% monochloroacetic acid.

6. Incubate the tube at room temperature for 24 hours.

Interpretation After 24 hours, the presence of a formed clot indicates a plasma factor XIII concentration of greater than 1% to 2%. Patients who present with a homozygous deficiency of factor XIII show dissolution of a fibrin clot, usually within 1 hour. This is indicative of factor XIII levels of less than 1%, which is significant because these are usually the only patients who exhibit hemorrhagic tendencies.[10]

Comment A deficiency of factor XIII is not detected by other coagulation tests; therefore, hemostatic evaluation is not complete without a factor XIII assay. Because the minimum required level of factor XIII is about 5%, this assay will reliably detect those individuals with a rare factor XIII deficiency. It should be noted that factor XIII can also be assayed by newer chromogenic techniques, which will quantitate factor XIII activity levels.[11]

► TESTS FOR VON WILLEBRAND DISEASE

von Willebrand Factor Antigen

Principle von Willebrand factor antigen (vWF:Ag) can be quantitated using enzyme-linked immunosorbent assay

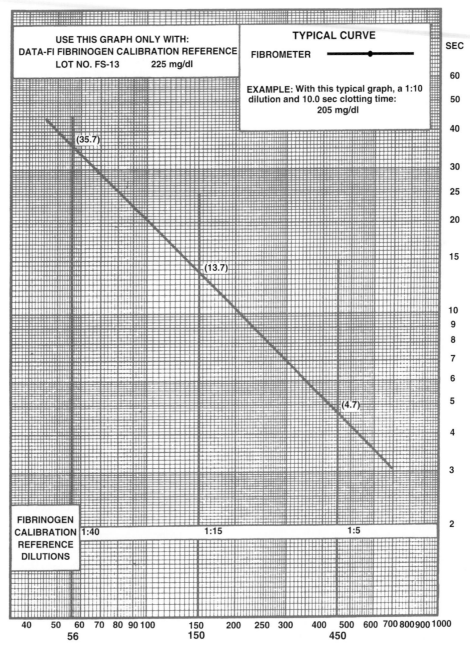

USE THIS GRAPH ONLY WITH:
DATA-FI FIBRINOGEN CALIBRATION REFERENCE
LOT NO. FS-13   225 mg/dl

TYPICAL CURVE
FIBROMETER

EXAMPLE: With this typical graph, a 1:10
dilution and 10.0 sec clotting time:
205 mg/dl

FIBRINOGEN CALIBRATION REFERENCE DILUTIONS

Fibrinogen in mg/dL

> FIGURE 32–4 Fibrinogen calibration curve.

(ELISA), Laurell rocket electrophoresis, or latex immunoassay (LIA). These methods measure total von Willebrand factor protein, independent of its ability to function. An enzyme immunoassay is most commonly used for the quantitative determination of von Willebrand factor (vWF) and is usually assayed by the sandwich technique, also known as ELISA (Fig. 32–5).

A microtiter plate coated with specific rabbit anti-human vWF antibodies captures the vWF to be measured. Rabbit anti-vWF antibody coupled with peroxidase binds to the remaining free antigenic determinants of vWF, forming the "sandwich." The bound enzyme peroxidase is then detected by its activity on the substrate orthophenylenediamine in the presence of hydrogen peroxide. The reaction is stopped with a strong acid. The intensity of the color produced is di-

rectly related to the vWF concentration present in the plasma sample and is read from a standard curve.

The vWF molecule is composed of low-molecular-weight and high-molecular-weight portions. The low-molecular-weight portion of the vWF molecule is responsible for the procoagulant activity, and reacts with homologous antibodies that appear in certain polytransfused type A hemophiliacs. The other entity is high molecular weight, composed of several monomers, each having a molecular weight of 850,000 daltons. These monomers aggregate to form polymers, with a total a molecular weight as high as 20 million daltons. This structure is the support of the von Willebrand activity or "ristocetin cofactor." The monomer itself is composed of subunits, each of molecular weight about 200,000 daltons, linked with one another by disulfide bridges and

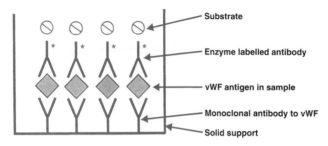

➤ FIGURE 32–5 Principle of the sandwich enzyme-linked immunosorbent assay (ELISA) test for von Willebrand factor antigen (vWF:Ag). (Modified from Constantine, N, et al: Retroviral Testing, Essentials for Quality Control and Laboratory Diagnosis. CRC Press, Boca Raton, FL, 1992, p 71, with permission.)

composing a carbohydrate portion. The vWF:Ag is synthesized by the endothelial cells and is also present in platelets.

Reagents and Equipment

Optical density reader with 492-nm filter

Vortex

Multiple adjustable pipet and tips

12 × 75 plastic tubes

3 M H_2SO_4

Hydrogen peroxide (H_2O_2) (30%)

Reference plasma

Normal and abnormal controls

Commercial ELISA vWF kit

Procedure

1. Collect blood by clean venipuncture technique according to recommended procedures previously described.
2. Process and store the plasma samples following recommended guidelines.
3. Perform the assay according to the manufacturer's recommendations.

Note: Newer methods are now available for use on automated analyzers.

Interpretation The vWF antigen is an acute-phase reactant, and levels increase above normal during pregnancy, use of birth control pills, physical exercise, and stress. They also rise with age. Elevated vWF antigen levels may also be observed when there is injury to the vascular endothelium, such as cancer, fever, in hepatic or renal disorders, during the postoperative period, or with thrombosis and myocardial infarction.

The vWF antigen level is decreased in von Willebrand disease.

von Willebrand Factor Activity von Willebrand factor activity (vWF:RCo, ristocetin cofactor) is produced in the endothelial cells and is composed of large and small multimers. It is the property of the factor VIII/vWF complex that is responsible for agglutination of platelets in the presence of ristocetin. Decreased or increased amounts of agglutination are becoming very important in diagnosis and prognosis of several disease states. In von Willebrand disease, the amount of agglutination is usually decreased, with the exception of type IIB and "pseudo" or "platelet-type" von Willebrand deficiency. Levels of vWF activity are determined by the ability

of the test plasma to induce agglutination of a standardized platelet suspension in the presence of ristocetin.

Principle In this test, normal reconstituted lyophilized platelets are mixed with dilutions of control or test plasma. Ristocetin is added, and the rate of aggregation is quantitated. The rate of aggregation is proportional to vWF factor activity.[12] The activity of unknown test samples is extrapolated from a reference graph obtained by testing dilutions of normal pooled plasma.

Reagents and Equipment

Platelet aggregometer

Aggregometer cuvettes

12 × 75 mm plastic test tubes with caps

Plastic centrifuge tubes

Micropipets

Lyophilized platelets

Ristocetin reagent

Normal pooled plasma

Reference plasma

Procedure

1. Collect blood by clean venipuncture technique according to recommended procedures previously described.
2. Process and store the plasma samples following recommended guidelines.
3. Prepare dilutions of reference plasma in normal saline as follows: 1:2, 1:4, 1:8, and 1:16. The 1:2 dilution represents 100% activity.
4. Prepare 1:2 and 1:4 dilutions of the control and patient's plasma in normal saline.
5. Prepare the reference blank by mixing 0.25 mL of reconstituted platelets plus 0.25 mL of normal saline in an aggregometer cuvette.
6. To a second aggregometer cuvette, pipet 0.4 mL of reconstituted platelets. Add 0.05 mL of the 1:2 reference plasma dilution. Incubate at 37°C for 2 minutes in the aggregometer.
7. Add a magnetic stirring bar to the cuvette.
8. Set the baselines for 0% and 100% on the aggregometer.
9. When the 0% baseline has stabilized, add 0.05 mL of ristocetin. Note the point of ristocetin addition on the chart paper.
10. Observe aggregation until the point of completion (usually 4 to 5 minutes).
11. Repeat steps 6 through 10 on each dilution of reference plasma.
12. Repeat steps 6 through 10 on each dilution of patient plasma.

Calculation

1. Draw a slope along the steepest linear portion of the agglutination curve, being sure the line intersects the chart baseline.
2. From the point of intersection at the baseline, measure over 2 cm. At the 2 cm point, draw a perpendicular line that intersects the slope line.
3. Read the slope value off the chart paper.
4. Prepare a standard curve by plotting the slope value of each dilution of reference plasma on semi-log

graph paper, with the percentages on the x axis and the slope value on the y axis. Draw a best-fit line.

5. Read the slope value of each control and patient plasma off of the standard curve. Multiply by the appropriate dilution factor. Report as percent of normal.

Note: Newer methods are now available for use on automated analyzers.

Interpretation Normal values are approximately 50% to 150% activity (compared with normal pooled plasma as reference). Patients with von Willebrand disease range from 0% to 50% activity. There is a good degree of correlation between the activity of vWF in vitro and its activity in vivo, as assayed by means of the bleeding time.[12] The results typically correlate well with vWF:Ag. vWF activity may become normal in individuals with von Willebrand disease during inflammation or pregnancy, or following transfusion with components rich in factor VIII, despite the prolonged bleeding times.[13,14] Patients who present with a variant form of von Willebrand disease may show prolonged bleeding times in the face of decreased to normal vWF levels but increased activity to ristocetin.[13]

Normal or increased levels of vWF are found in patients with hemophilia A and Bernard-Soulier syndrome. Certain disease states such as diabetes mellitus, hyperthyroidism, liver disease, chronic renal failure, pregnancy, endothelial cell damage, and disorders of the myeloproliferative syndrome may cause an increase in the level of vWF activity. Because of these variations, it is suggested that two or three separate assays be performed before making a diagnosis.

➤ TESTS FOR NATURAL AND PATHOLOGIC CIRCULATING ANTICOAGULANTS

Antithrombin Assays

Antithrombin (AT-III) is a naturally occurring inhibitor of blood coagulation and plays an important role in maintaining blood in the fluid state. It is an α_2-globulin that is synthesized in the liver and circulates in the plasma. It is the major plasma inhibitor responsible for neutralizing the activity of thrombin, factors IXa, Xa, XIa, and XIIa, and plasmin. Antithrombin slowly, progressively, and irreversibly inhibits the action of thrombin by forming a 1:1 stoichiometric complex with thrombin. This complex forms when the active serine site of thrombin binds with the arginine site of antithrombin. The inhibition of thrombin by antithrombin is greatly accelerated by heparin.

Antithrombin activity and antigen can be measured by a variety of techniques. The most frequently used assays are (1) chromogenic substrate assays, (2) Laurell rocket immunoelectrophoresis, (3) Mancini radial immunodiffusion, and (4) microlatex particle immunologic assay (LIA).

Antithrombin Functional Assay (Activity)

Synthetic Substrate Assay

Principle Chromogenic antithrombin assays measure the functional levels of antithrombin in plasma by an amidolytic method using a synthetic substrate. Plasma containing antithrombin is diluted in the presence of heparin and incubated with excess thrombin, forming an antithrombin-thrombin-heparin complex. The remaining thrombin catalyzes the release of p-nitroaniline (pNA) from the chromogenic substrate. The release of pNA is measured by either an endpoint or kinetic method at 405 nm. The absorbance obtained is inversely proportional to the concentration of antithrombin in the sample and may be quantitated by interpolation from a calibration curve.

Reagents and Equipment

Instrument reader or automated analyzer at 405 nm

Chromogenic substrate

Multiple pipets and tips

Reference plasma

Normal and abnormal controls

Buffered saline

Procedure

1. Collect blood by clean venipuncture technique according to recommended procedures previously described.
2. Process and store the plasma samples following recommended guidelines.
3. Perform testing according to the manufacturer's recommendations.

Antithrombin Immunologic Assays (Antigen)

Radial Immunodiffusion Assay (RID)

Principle RID plates contain monospecific antibody in agarose gel. Samples are diluted and added to precut wells in the gel. The samples are allowed to diffuse into the gel for 48 to 72 hours until precipitin rings are formed. The diameter of the rings is measured and can be read from a standard curve prepared from serial dilutions of reference plasma or a reference table provided by the manufacturer.

Reagents and Equipment

Antithrombin reagent kit with RID plates

Control and patient plasma

Reference plasma

Procedure

1. Collect blood by clean venipuncture technique according to recommended procedures previously described.
2. Process and store the plasma samples following recommended guidelines.
3. Prepare serial dilutions of reference plasma according to the manufacturer's recommendations.
4. Prepare dilutions of the control and patient plasma according to the manufacturer's recommendations.
5. Pipet each dilution of reference plasma, control plasma, and patient plasma into separate wells on the RID plate. Record the location of each.
6. Allow the plate to sit in a humid chamber on a flat surface at room temperature for a specified length of time.

Calculation

1. Measure the precipitin ring diameters to the nearest 0.1 mm using a calibrated eyepiece.

2. Read the antithrombin concentrations corresponding to each ring diameter from the standard curve or reference table.

Microlatex Particle Immunologic Assay (LIA)

Principle A beam of monochromatic light is allowed to traverse a suspension of microlatex particles to which specific antibodies have been attached by covalent bonding. If the light is of a wavelength that is much greater than the diameter of the latex particles, it can pass through the latex suspension unabsorbed. However, in the presence of the antigen being tested, the antibody-coated particles agglutinate to form aggregates of diameters greater than the wavelength of the light and the latter is absorbed. There is a direct relationship between the observed absorbance value and the concentration of the antigen being measured.

Reagents and Equipment

Coagulation analyzer

Commercial microlatex reagents

Multiple adjustable pipet and tips

Normal saline

Normal and abnormal control

Procedure

1. Collect blood by clean venipuncture technique according to recommended procedures previously described.
2. Process and store the plasma samples following recommended guidelines.
3. Perform the assay according to the manufacturer's package insert.

Interpretation Since 1965, antithrombin has been considered important as a result of the description of the first known hereditary deficiency and its consequences; that is, the congenital decrease of the antithrombin level is accompanied by a high frequency of spontaneous thromboembolic disorders.

Quantitative antithrombin deficiencies are the most frequent. They are identified by both the antithrombin antigenic and activity levels being depressed. Hereditary qualitative deficiencies are less frequent and are identified by antigenic antithrombin levels being normal while antithrombin activity levels are decreased. In addition to these deficiencies, a number of acquired deficiencies have been described, including DIC, nephrotic syndrome, and liver diseases, and deficiencies resulting from oral contraceptive use, postsurgical state, and following prolonged heparin therapy.

➤ PROTEIN C ASSAYS

Protein C is a vitamin K–dependent serine protease that functions as a major regulatory protein in the control of coagulation. Activated protein C is a potent anticoagulant that acts by proteolytically inactivating factors Va and VIIIa, and also enhances fibrinolytic activity in plasma.[15] Factors Va and VIIIa are important in accelerating the activation of prothrombin and factor X.

Components of the protein C system include proteins C and S, C4b-binding protein, thrombomodulin, activated protein C inhibitor (plasminogen activator inhibitor-3), and thrombin. Protein S, also a vitamin K–dependent factor, is a necessary cofactor in the reaction in which factor Va is inactivated by protein C.

Protein C deficiency has been described as a risk factor in thromboembolic disease. Activated protein C resistance (APC-R), which is the result of a mutation in the factor V gene, has also been described.[16,17] Known as factor V Leiden, this mutation makes the factor V molecule resistant to the proteolytic activity of activated protein C, thereby negating its regulatory effect on thrombin generation and increasing the potential for the development of thromboses.

Laboratory diagnosis of a protein C deficiency is accomplished by immunologic (antigen) and functional (activity) assays.[15] Immunologic assays use Laurell rocket immunoelectrophoresis or ELISA methodology. Functional assays measure protein C by clot-based or synthetic chromogenic substrate methods. The APTT and the PT are not sensitive to decreases in protein C levels.

Protein C Immunologic Assay (Antigen)

Principle A microtiter plate coated with specific rabbit antihuman protein C antibodies captures the protein C antigen to be measured. Rabbit antiprotein C antibody coupled with peroxidase then binds to the remaining free antigenic determinants of protein C, forming a "sandwich." The bound enzyme peroxidase is then detected by its activity on the substrate orthophenylenediamine in the presence of hydrogen peroxide. The reaction is stopped with a strong acid. The intensity of the color produced is directly proportional to the protein C antigen concentration present in the plasma sample.

Reagents and Equipment

Optical density reader with 490 nm filter

Microtiter plate rocker

Vortex for mixing dilutions

Multiple adjustable pipet and tips

12×75 plastic tubes

$1\ N$ HCl

Hydrogen peroxide (H_2O_2) (30%)

Normal and abnormal controls

Procedure

1. Collect blood by clean venipuncture technique according to recommended procedures previously described.
2. Process and store the plasma samples following recommended guidelines.
3. Perform the assay according to the manufacturer's package insert.

Protein C Functional Assay (Activity)

Synthetic Substrate Assay

Principle Protein C in plasma is activated by a specific enzyme from southern copperhead snake venom. The amount of activated protein C is determined by the rate of hydrolysis of the synthetic substrate S-2366. The amount of pNA release measured at 405 nm is proportional to the protein C level.

Reagents and Equipment

Coagulation analyzer capable of reading at 405 nm

Multiple adjustable pipet and tips

Reference plasma

Normal and abnormal control

Commercial synthetic substrate kit

Procedure

1. Collect blood by clean venipuncture technique according to recommended procedures previously described.
2. Process and store the plasma samples following recommended guidelines.
3. Prepare the reference plasma according to the manufacturer's recommendations. This will be used to generate a standard curve.
4. Perform the assay according to the manufacturer's package insert. If using an automated analyzer, dilutions will be made automatically and tested according to the instrument protocol.
5. Control and patient samples are read at 405 nm and calculated from the reference curve. Results are reported as percent activity.

Comment Heparin levels up to 3.0 IU/mL do not interfere with the assay. Elevated levels of hemoglobin, bilirubin, or lipid may interfere with the assay and results from severely hemolyzed, icteric, or lipemic specimens should be interpreted accordingly.

Protein C Functional Assay (Activity)

Clot-based Assay

Principle Protein C is activated in the presence of a specific activating antigen, such as snake venom.[15] The resulting activated protein C inactivates factors Va and VIIIa, and thus prolongs the APTT compared to the baseline value.

Reagents and Equipment

APTT reagent

Commercial protein C kit containing snake venom

0.025 M CaCl$_2$

Owren-Koller buffer

Coagulation analyzer

Normal and abnormal controls

Procedure

1. Collect blood by clean venipuncture technique according to recommended procedures previously described.
2. Process and store the plasma samples following recommended guidelines.
3. Prepare the reagents according to the manufacturer's recommendations.
4. Perform a baseline APTT on normal and abnormal control plasma.
5. Add snake venom to the control plasma; repeat the APTT.
6. Repeat steps 4 and 5 for the patient plasma.
7. Protein C activity is determined based on the degree of prolongation of the APTT compared with baseline values.

Comment Heparin does not affect test results when present at a concentration less than 1.0 IU/mL. Higher levels of heparin may lead to an overestimation of the protein C level by causing an additional prolongation of the APTT.

Interpretation Low levels of protein C are observed at birth as a result of liver immaturity. In adults, the protein C level appears to be independent of age and sex. Hereditary protein C deficiency can be classified as type I or type II, according to the levels of protein C activity and antigen measured. Acquired deficiencies of protein C are observed in hepatic disorders such as hepatitis and cirrhosis, vitamin K deficiency, DIC, and oral anticoagulant therapy. In these cases, the interpretation of test results is difficult if the patient has had a history of thromboses and is receiving anticoagulant treatments.

➤ PROTEIN S ASSAYS

Protein S is a vitamin K–dependent cofactor for the anticoagulant and proteolytic effects of activated protein C. Both functional and antigenic assays for protein S have been developed. Protein S bound to C4b-binding protein (C4bBP) has little or no cofactor activity; only free protein S has functional cofactor activity.[17] In normal plasma, about 60% of protein S is complexed with the C4bBP, whereas the other 40% is in free form. It is recommended that protein S activity as well as both free protein S and total protein S antigen be determined. Total protein S can be measured by means of Laurell rocket electrophoresis or ELISA methodology. Distribution of free and bound protein S can be determined by crossed immunoelectrophoresis in which free protein S migrates faster than C4bBP-bound protein S. Semiquantitative information about protein S distribution is obtained by comparing normal plasma patterns with those in the patients.

Protein S Functional Assay (Activity)—Clotting Assay

Principle The functional protein S assay is based on the observation that activated protein C will inactivate factor Va and VIIIa in the presence of protein S. Diluted plasma is mixed with protein S–deficient plasma, which is then activated in a one-stage assay that uses factor Xa, phospholipid, and activated protein C. A linear relationship exists between the concentration of protein S and the prolonged clotting time. Normal plasma added to protein S–deficient plasma causes a prolonged clotting time proportional to the amount of normal plasma added. Functional protein S determinations are obtained by comparing the clotting time of normal plasma with that of the patient plasma. The presence of heparin and high levels of factor VIII interferes with this assay, as do oral anticoagulants.

Reagents and Equipment

Coagulation analyzer

Commercial kit

Multiple adjustable pipet and tips

Reference plasma

Normal and abnormal controls

Procedure

1. Collect blood by clean venipuncture technique according to recommended procedures previously described.
2. Process and store the plasma samples following recommended guidelines.
3. Prepare the reagents according to the manufacturer's package insert.

Comment Protein S values may be underestimated in test samples with elevated factor VIIa levels.[18] Factor VIIa may be elevated because of a clinical condition, inappropriate venipuncture, and cold activation on storage.[19] Perform additional tests when elevated factor VIIa levels are suspected by testing samples at higher dilutions using protein S–deficient plasma.

➤ SCREENING TESTS FOR THE DETECTION OF CIRCULATING ANTICOAGULANTS

Circulating anticoagulants are acquired pathologic plasma proteins that inhibit normal coagulation. Circulating anticoagulants differ from naturally occurring inhibitors such as antithrombin, α_2-macroglobulin, α_2-antitrypsin, and C1 esterase and must be differentiated from anticoagulants such as heparin and coumarin analogues. Most of these pathologic anticoagulants are inhibitors or autoantibodies of the IgG class whose inhibitory effects are directed against certain coagulation factors or demonstrate specific activity against phospholipids (such as factor VIII and the prothrombin complex).

Some of the circulating anticoagulants that have been detected thus far have been encountered in patients with the following conditions: Hemophilia A (factor VIII deficiency), Christmas disease (factor IX deficiency), DIC, pregnancy, systemic lupus erythematosus (SLE), plasma cell dyscrasias, Waldenström's macroglobulinemia, and advanced age.

The circulating anticoagulant directed against the factor VIII molecule is the most common specific factor inhibitor. It is seen in patients with hemophilia A and may be related to repeated therapeutic transfusions of antihemophilic factor (AHF), but is also seen in nonhemophiliac patients (e.g., women following childbirth or abortion, elderly individuals, and those with immunologic disorders such as rheumatoid arthritis). This is usually attributed to the elevated level of factor VIII present, which is interpreted by the immune system as being foreign. Antibodies to factor VIII may also be seen in patients known to have the severe form of von Willebrand disease.

Other specific inhibitors have been reported against factors V, IX, XI, XII, and XIII, and against inhibitors of fibrin formation.

Some patients with SLE develop an acquired circulating anticoagulant. This inhibitor is known as the lupus anticoagulant, and it demonstrates specific activity against phospholipids, thus interfering with phospholipid-dependent complexes that involve factors V and VIII.[20]

Activated Partial Thromboplastin Time (APTT)—Mixing Studies

Principle The APTT is useful as a screening test for distinguishing between factor deficiencies and circulating anticoagulants. When patient plasma is mixed with pooled normal plasma, there should be sufficient factor present to correct a prolongation caused by a factor deficiency. There is only partial or no correction in the presence of an inhibitor. Mixing studies can help determine the appropriate next steps to take to diagnose the cause of an abnormal APTT.

Reagents and Equipment

APTT reagent

CaCl$_2$ (0.025 M)
Pooled normal plasma

Procedure

1. Collect blood by clean venipuncture technique according to recommended procedures previously described.
2. Process and store the plasma samples following recommended guidelines.
3. Prepare the reagents according to the manufacturer's recommendations.
4. Perform the APTT on patient plasma according to the manufacturer's recommendations.
5. Mix the patient plasma 1:1 with pooled normal plasma.
6. Repeat the APTT on the mixture.
7. Compare the results with the patient's baseline APTT.

Note: If a time-dependent inhibitor is suspected, incubated mixing studies should also be performed.

Procedure: Incubated Mixing Studies

1. Mix patient plasma with normal control plasma in a series of six 12 × 75 test tubes as listed in Table 32–3.
2. Incubate each tube for 1 hour at 37°C.
3. Measure the APTT for each tube.

Interpretation If the APTT is corrected by normal plasma, a factor deficiency is indicated. The addition of normal plasma supplies the coagulation factor or factors that are deficient, and thus corrects the APTT. When a factor deficiency is present, there should be correction of the abnormal APTT by at least 10% to 25% normal plasma (tubes 4 and 5).

If the APTT is not corrected by the addition of normal plasma in most of the mixtures, a strong circulating anticoagulant is indicated.

A weak or time-dependent circulating anticoagulant is indicated by a prolonged APTT following incubation at 37°C for 1 hour. On incubation, a weak inhibitor progressively inactivates the coagulation factor, thus prolonging the APTT. This pattern is most typical of a factor VIII inhibitor.

Comment The circulating anticoagulant that inhibits factor VIII is most often a specific IgG antibody.[21] These antibodies are often present as weak circulating anticoagulants but are temperature- and time-dependent, thus causing only a slightly prolonged clotting time on initial testing. Mixing tests may yield APTT results intermediate between the clot-

➤ Table 32-3
DILUTION FOR APTT MIXING STUDIES

Tube No.	Patient's Plasma	Normal Control Plasma
1	0.20 mL	—
2	0.15 mL	0.05 mL
3	0.10 mL	0.10 mL
4	0.05 mL	0.15 mL
5	0.02 mL	0.18 mL
6	—	0.20 mL

ting times of patient and normal control. On incubation at 37°C, both the undiluted patient plasma and plasma mixtures show prolonged times, but the normal pooled plasma shows little or no change. Because of the nature of the factor VIII inhibitor, the mixture of patient plasma and normal pooled plasma must be incubated for a period of 60 to 120 minutes to allow for the inhibitor's progressive activity.

If a factor VIII inhibitor is present, it is important to determine the initial level of factor activity because the development of an inhibitor complicates the management of a patient with hemophilia A when therapy involves AHF concentrates. These should be monitored periodically.

Bethesda Titer

Factor VIII inhibitors may be quantified by mixing the patient plasma with a pooled plasma containing a known amount of factor VIII. The mixture is incubated at 37°C for 2 hours. The amount of inhibitor present is then calculated in Bethesda units by comparing the difference in factor activity between the patient mixture and a control mixture containing buffer. A Bethesda unit of inhibitor activity is defined as the amount of inhibitor that will inactivate half of the factor present in a mixture of equal volumes of patient plasma and pooled plasma after 2 hours' incubation at 37°C. The definition was originally defined to measure factor VIII inhibitors; however, the same method can be used to define a specific inhibitor against any factor.

If a factor VIII inhibitor is present, it is important to determine the initial level of factor activity, because the development of an inhibitor complicates the management of a patient with hemophilia A when therapy involves AHF. Evaluation of the level of inhibitor is necessary in order to make decisions regarding treatment. Therapeutic options for patients with factor VIII inhibitors include immunosuppressive drugs, plasmapheresis, or, in the event of acute bleeding episodes, infusion with porcine factor VIII.[21]

➤ SCREENING TESTS FOR THE DETECTION OF LUPUS ANTICOAGULANTS

Lupus anticoagulants (LAs) are antibodies (IgG, IgM, IgA, or a combination) directed against phospholipids, thereby prolonging in vitro phospholipid-dependent coagulation tests. First recognized in patients with SLE, LAs have been identified in a variety of disorders including malignancies, infections, and autoimmune disorders, as well as following drug therapy. The presence of an LA is usually not associated with a bleeding problem unless accompanied by thrombocytopenia, factor II deficiency, platelet dysfunction, or drug administration (e.g., aspirin). The LA, however, has been identified as a risk factor for venous and arterial thrombosis and recurrent spontaneous abortions.[22]

The laboratory diagnosis of a lupus inhibitor is critical in terms of distinguishing it from other specific factor inhibitors and to identify patients at potential risk for thrombotic problems. The Scientific and Standardization Committee (SSC) Sub-Committee for the Standardization of Lupus Anticoagulants of the International Society of Thrombosis and Hemostasis (ISTH) has defined the following criteria to make a diagnosis of a lupus anticoagulant.[23]

1. Prolongation of at least one phospholipid-dependent clotting test.

2. Evidence of inhibitory activity shown by the effect of patient plasma on pooled normal plasma.
3. Evidence that the inhibitory activity is dependent on phospholipid. This may be achieved by the addition or alteration of phospholipid, hexagonal phase phospholipid, platelets, or platelet vesicles in the test system.
4. LAs must be carefully distinguished from other coagulopathies that may give similar laboratory results or may occur concurrently with LAs. Specific factor assays and the clinical history may be helpful in differentiating LAs from these other possibilities.

Suspicion of an LA is most often aroused by an unexplained prolongation of the APTT that is not corrected by the addition of an equal volume of normal plasma. It should be noted that the time-dependent inhibition, which is usually considered an indicator of factor VIII inhibitors, has been seen with LAs, as well as factor V inhibitors. Confirmatory tests to identify an LA include those that utilize a low concentration of phospholipid in the test system, thereby increasing the LA effect such as the tissue thromboplastin inhibition test (TTIT), dilute Russell's viper venom time (dRVVT), and the kaolin clotting time (KCT), or those that increase the phospholipid, thereby neutralizing the LA effect, such as the platelet neutralization procedure. Another type of confirmatory test depends on the presence of hexagonal phase phospholipids and can also be used. It is important to note that the confirmatory test selected should correspond to the screening test that is abnormal. For example, if the APTT is abnormal, the platelet neutralization procedure would be a logical confirmatory test.

➤ CONFIRMATORY TESTS FOR LUPUS ANTICOAGULANTS

There are several confirmatory tests for the LA, including platelet neutralization procedure, anticardiolipin assay, KCT, tissue thromboplastin inhibition test, and dRVVT. The first two are described in this section.

Platelet Neutralization Procedure

Principle The platelet neutralization procedure (PNP) is based on the ability of platelets to significantly correct in vitro coagulation abnormalities.[24] The disrupted platelet membranes present in the freeze-thawed platelet suspension neutralize phospholipid antibodies present in the plasma of patients with LA. After the patient plasma is mixed with the freeze-thawed platelet suspension, the APTT will be shortened when compared with the original baseline APTT.

Interpretation A correction of the baseline APTT of a defined amount of time (i.e., 3 to 5 seconds or more) by the platelet suspension as compared with the control is indicative of the presence of an LA.

Comment Specimen collection, centrifugation, and processing are critical when testing for the presence of an LA. Coagulation assays that have a phospholipid-dependent reaction are affected by the presence of residual platelets in platelet-poor plasma. Because LAs are directed against phospholipids, the relative concentration of any platelet phospholipid contained in the sample affects the sensitivity of the assay for detection of the LA.

LAs demonstrate considerable heterogeneity and show variable differences in sensitivity and responsiveness of the reagent. This makes the selection and interpretation of an appropriate confirmatory test challenging. Despite differences in testing methodology and reagents currently available, most of these anticoagulants can be detected and identified in the routine laboratory setting.

Anticardiolipin Assay

Principle Anticardiolipin antibodies (ACAs) and LAs are antiphospholipid immunoglobulins that are IgG, IgM, IgA, or a combination. Antiphospholipid antibodies are a heterogeneous group of autoantibodies including ACA, LA, β-2 glycoprotein-1 (β2GP-1), and antiphosphatidylserine (APTS). Some patients with elevated ACAs have been reported to also have an LA. Several studies have shown that patients with the LA and the closely related ACA are prone to recurrent venous and arterial thrombosis, recurrent spontaneous abortions, and thrombocytopenia.[22] This tendency has been described as the antiphospholipid syndrome (APS).

ELISA techniques are available for measuring ACAs. The commercial kits use cardiolipin or a mixture of negatively charged phospholipids as antigens.

➤ TESTS FOR FIBRIN/FIBRINOGEN DEGRADATION PRODUCTS

Principle Plasmin proteolytically cleaves fibrin(ogen) into fragments X and Y, known as early degradation products, and fragments D and E, known as late degradation products. These FDPs share antigenic determinants with both fibrin and fibrinogen, thus allowing for detection by immunologic methods by the use of antisera to highly purified preparations of human fibrinogen fragments D and E. Measurement of FDPs provides an indirect assessment of fibrinolysis.

Thrombo-Wellcotest: Latex Agglutination Test

Principle This test is a direct latex agglutination slide test for the detection and semiquantitation of FDPs. Latex particles in glycine buffer are coated with specific antibodies to human fibrinogen fragments D and E. The presence of FDPs in either serum or urine will cause the latex particles to clump, yielding macroscopic agglutination. An approximate concentration of FDPs in the sample can be determined by testing the sample at different dilutions. Thrombin is initially added to the patient sample to ensure complete clotting and total removal of fibrinogen. The addition of proteolytic inhibitor, soybean trypsin, prevents in vitro activation of the fibrinolytic system.

Reagents and Equipment

Commercial kit

Procedure

1. Collect 2 mL of venous blood in a special FDP collection tube (provided with the test kit). Mix immediately by gentle inversion several times. Allow the blood to clot.
2. Ring the clot to allow retraction to occur. Keep the sample tube at room temperature or 37°C for 30 minutes and centrifuge to separate serum.
3. If the sample is obtained from a heparinized patient,

reptilase (Abbott Laboratories, North Chicago, IL) should be added to the blood. Reptilase and enzyme isolated from snake venom clot fibrinogen in the presence of heparin and other such antithrombins. Addition of 0.1 mL of reptilase will clot 1.0 mL of blood.
4. Label two 12 × 75 test tubes. Prepare 1:5 and 1:20 dilutions of the serum (Table 32–4). To aliquot the buffer, use the graduated dropper provided. To deliver the sample, use the disposable calibrated pipet and bulb provided in the kit. Mix well.
5. Label two rings on the glass slide provided as 1 and 2.
6. Transfer 1 drop of the dilution from test tube 2 to position 2 on the glass slide and 1 drop from test tube 1 to position 1. Deliver the dilutions in this order.
7. Thoroughly mix the latex suspension. Add 1 drop to each position on the slide.
8. Mix the latex-serum mixture. Start with position 2 on the slide, then mix position 1. When stirring the mixture, spread to fill the circles.
9. Gently rotate the slide for no longer than 2 minutes. Observe the slide for macroscopic agglutination by viewing against a dark background.

Controls

1. Label two of the rings on the glass test slide (+) and (−) for positive and negative controls.
2. Place one drop of the appropriate control and one drop of latex suspension on the slide and mix as described earlier.
3. Read the results. Failure of the controls to react as described indicates deterioration of at least one of the reagents or an improperly performed test.

Interpretation The test is sensitive to values of 2 μg of FDPs per milliliter. The presence of agglutination in position 1 indicates the presence of FDPs in a final concentration greater than 10 μg/mL. The presence of agglutination in position 2 indicates the presence of FDPs in a final concentration of greater than 40 μg/mL. For the test to be valid, if agglutination is present in position 2, it must also be present in position 1 on the slide. Agglutination in tube 1 and lack of agglutination in tube 2 indicate FDPs greater than 10 μg/mL but less than 40 μg/mL.

Lack of agglutination indicates an FDP concentration of less than 2 μg/mL. The mean normal level of serum is 4.9 ± 2.8 μg FDPs per milliliter. The normal value may be elevated during exercise and stress.

The latex agglutination assay has been documented to give false-positive results with sera from patients with rheumatoid arthritis. Trace amounts of FDPs occur in the

➤ Table 32–4
DILUTIONS FOR FDP

	Tube 1	Tube 2
Glycine buffer	0.75 mL	0.75 mL
Serum	5 drops	1 drop
Final dilution	1:5	1:20

blood of normal healthy adults and children as a result of physiologic fibrinolysis.

Comment Generally, elevated levels of FDPs are associated with thrombotic episodes such as myocardial infarction, pulmonary emboli, and deep vein thrombosis, as well as with certain complications of pregnancy.

The assay is of value in the differential diagnosis of patients with specific types of kidney diseases. Quantitation of urine FDP levels provides a useful clinical means of monitoring glomerulonephritis and kidney rejection following transplantation.

The detection of FDPs is of significant clinical value in assessing patients with DIC. A positive test result, accompanied by an elevated PT and APTT and a decrease in platelet count and possibly fibrinogen concentration, is suggestive of DIC.

D-Dimer (D-Di) Test

Principle Under the action of thrombin, fibrinogen is cleaved to give rise to fibrin monomers. These monomers form polymers, which are stabilized by factor XIII, forming covalent cross-linkages in the D domain to produce an insoluble fibrin clot. Plasmin, a potent clot-lysing enzyme, attacks fibrin clots as well as fibrinogen in the body. Unlike plasmin's action on fibrinogen, which produces FDPs, its action on the fibrin clot leads to the generation of cross-linked fibrin containing D-dimer. The latex particles provided in the D-Di test are coated with mouse anti-human D-dimer monoclonal antibodies. Test samples containing D-dimers when mixed with the latex particle suspension make the particles agglutinate. Normal D-dimer levels in plasma are less than 0.5 μg/mL. A positive D-Di test may be seen in clinical situations where active thrombosis is occurring, such as DIC, deep vein thrombosis, and pulmonary embolism.

The advantage of the D-Di test is that there is no interference from fibrinogen, so the test can be run on citrated plasma without necessitating collection in a special tube. It has limited usefulness, however, in the evaluation of primary fibrinolysis because it will only detect breakdown products from cross-linked fibrin and not those from fibrinogen. Other laboratory tests that may be useful in evaluation of the fibrinolytic system include fibrin monomers, ethanol gelation test, protamine sulfate test, and euglobulin lysis time.

➤ MARKERS OF COAGULATION ACTIVATION AND THROMBIN GENERATION

New assays have been developed that allow detection of molecular markers of thrombosis.[25] These molecular markers can provide specific and pertinent data for early diagnosis and management of coagulation disorders.

Before thrombin becomes biologically available, there is generation of biochemical markers in the blood. These markers of coagulation activation can be employed in three diagnostic applications: (1) diagnosis of spontaneous thrombosis, (2) prognosis and follow-up of thrombotic disease, and (3) monitoring of anticoagulant therapy.

Under normal conditions, all individuals produce measurable quantities of molecular markers of coagulation activation; however, significantly increased levels have been observed in persons with deep venous thrombosis, pulmonary emboli, DIC, and other thrombotic abnormalities. Because of their short half-lives, activation peptides demonstrate blood activation only as long as the thrombotic process is ongoing.

Molecular markers offer several advantages as compared with the conventional coagulation tests. Firstly, molecular markers are specific indicators of the activation of coagulation and fibrinolysis whereas conventional assays measure deficiencies of the clotting mechanism. Additionally, markers are ultrasensitive and are able to detect minute changes in the components of hemostasis.

The disadvantages of marker testing include the requirement of special anticoagulants for collection and the necessity of rapid sample processing.

Prothrombin fragment 1 + 2 (PF1+2), thrombin-antithrombin complex (TAT), soluble fibrin monomer (sFM), and thrombus precursor protein (TpP) are the markers that can be measured to determine the generation of thrombin. ELISA assays are currently available to test for these thrombotic markers.

➤ COAGULATION INSTRUMENTATION

Methods to evaluate the coagulation of blood have evolved from the manual observation of the length of time needed for whole blood to clot in a test tube to today's intricate analysis performed by highly sophisticated instruments. Interestingly, although numerous instruments, both semi- and fully automated, are available to perform coagulation testing, the manual tilt-tube method still remains as the gold standard.

General Types of Coagulation Instrumentation

Manual (Tilt-Tube) Method

In the tilt-tube method, all reagents and samples are added manually by the operator. The 37°C temperature is maintained by a water bath or heat block, which is usually monitored externally by the operator. The endpoint is determined visually by the operator by tilting the test tube at defined intervals until clot formation is observed. Timing is initiated and stopped by the operator, usually using a stopwatch. Although essentially no equipment is required (outside of a water bath or heat block, test tubes, and a stopwatch), this method is very labor-intensive and has a high coefficient of variation in results. This lead to the long-standing requirements that coagulation testing be performed in duplicate and results averaged.

Semiautomated Method

Semiautomated equipment is similar to the tilt-tube method in that it also requires that all reagents and test samples be delivered manually to the reaction cuvette. However, these instruments contain mechanisms to automatically initiate the timing device upon addition of the final reagent and an internal mechanism to detect clot formation. The equipment usually contains a device for maintaining a constant 37°C temperature, but it may not internally monitor the temperature. The advantage of semiautomated equipment is that it is relatively inexpensive and easily operated. The disadvantage is that the testing process is time-consuming and labor-intensive.

Fully Automated Method

Fully automated analyzers have only become available within the past few decades and have greatly improved coagulation testing capabilities. All reagents are automatically pipetted into the test cuvette. Timers are automatically initiated and stopped when clot formation is detected. Depending on the manufacturer and model of the analyzer, plasma samples may or may not be automatically pipetted. Fully automated analyzers contain monitoring devices and internal mechanisms to maintain and monitor a constant 37°C temperature throughout the testing process. The advantage of these systems is their improved accuracy, precision, and throughput, with reduced time required for operator intervention. The disadvantages are the cost and level of expertise needed to operate and maintain the instruments as compared with semiautomated equipment.

Methods of Endpoint Detection

Instrument methodologies used for coagulation testing are generally classified based on the principle of endpoint detection employed by the analyzer. These general classifications are:

- Mechanical
- Photo-optical
- Chromogenic
- Immunologic

Historically, coagulation instruments were only capable of providing one type of endpoint detection, such as mechanical or photo-optical. Photo-optical instruments were built to read the endpoint at a fixed wavelength of 500 to 600 nm. Later, other instruments were developed to read at a 405-nm wavelength to allow measurement of chromogenic assays. Currently, several analyzers are available that have the combined capability of reading assays using multiple detection methods within the same system, allowing laboratories to purchase and train on only one instrument instead of multiple analyzers, while still providing specialized testing capabilities on all shifts with many operators.

Mechanical Endpoint Detection

Two primary methodologies are utilized for mechanical detection of clot formation. The first is known as electromechanical detection, and incorporates a change in electrical conductivity between two metal probes immersed in a solution. During the reaction, one probe moves in and out of the solution at constant intervals. The electrical circuit between the two probes is not maintained as the moving probe rises in and out of the solution. When a clot (fibrin) is formed in the solution, the fibrin strands maintain electrical contact between the two probes when the moving probe leaves the solution, which stops the timer.[26] An example of this type of equipment is the BBL Fibrometer.

The second method of mechanical clot detection involves monitoring the movement of a steel ball within a test solution by magnetic sensors. A change in the movement of the steel ball may be detected when there is increased viscosity of the test solution, changing its range of motion, or by a break in contact with the magnetic sensors when the steel ball becomes incorporated into a fibrin clot as the cuvette rotates. These types of endpoint detection methods are utilized on the Diagnostica Stago STA[27] and the Sigma Diagnostics KC4A.[28]

Photo-Optical Endpoint Detection

Detection of clot formation measured by a change in optical density of a test sample is the basis of photo-optical instrumentation, which is also known as *turbidometric* methodology. When a light source of a specified wavelength is passed through a test solution (plasma), a certain amount of light is detected by a photo-detector or photocell located on the other side of the solution.[29] The amount of light detected is dependent on the color and clarity of the plasma sample and is considered to be the baseline light transmission value. When soluble fibrinogen begins to polymerize into a fibrin clot, formation of fibrin strands causes light to scatter, allowing less light to fall on the photo-detector (i.e., the plasma becomes more opaque, decreasing the amount of light detected).[29] When the amount of light reaching the photo-detector decreases to an exact point from the baseline value as predetermined by the instrument, this change in optical density triggers the timer to stop, indicating clot formation. This is the most common method of detection utilized on coagulation instruments at this time, such as the MDA-180 (Organon Teknika Corporation),[30] BCS (Dade Behring), and MLA Series (Medical Laboratory Automation).

Chromogenic Endpoint Detection

Chromogenic, or amidolytic, methodology is based on the use of a specific color-producing substance known as a *chromophore*. The chromophore normally used in the coagulation laboratory is para-nitroanaline (p-nitroanaline or pNA), which has an optical absorbance peak at 405 nm on a spectrophotometer. The principle of chromogenic assays is based on the attachment of pNA to a synthetic chromogenic substrate.[31] The substrate is made up of a series of amino acids, the composition of which is dependent on the structure of the enzymatic target of the coagulation protein being measured. The goal is for the coagulation protein to attack the chromogenic substrate at a specific site between a defined amino acid sequence and the pNA, thereby cleaving pNA from the substrate. Because free pNA has a yellow color, the intensity of the solution is proportional to the amount of free pNA present and is measured by a photodetector at a wavelength of 405 nm. As additional free pNA is cleaved, the amount of light absorbance is increased, leading to a greater change in optical density of the solution. The change in optical density can be either a direct or an indirect measurement of the level of the analyte being tested. This type of technology is available on a variety of instruments such as the BCS (Dade Behring),[32] MDA, STA, and AMAX (Sigma Diagnostics), and is most often seen in conjunction with the photo-optical detection methodology.

Immunologic Endpoint Detection

Immunologic assays are based on antigen-antibody reactions. Microlatex particles are coated with a specific antibody directed against the analyte (antigen) to be measured. A beam of monochromatic light is then passed through the suspension of microlatex particles. When the wavelength of light is greater than the diameter of the particles in suspension, only a small amount of light will be absorbed by the particles.[33] When the microlatex particles coated with specific antibody come in contact with the antigen present in the solution, the antigen attaches to the antibody and forms bridges between the particles, causing them to agglutinate. As the diameter of the agglutinates becomes larger and closer to the wavelength of the monochromatic light beam, the greater the amount of light that is absorbed. The increase in light absorbance is proportional to the size of the agglutinates, which, in turn, is proportional to the antigen level present in the sample, which is read from a standard curve. This technology is also incorporated into several of the instruments previously mentioned.

The introduction of new methodologies has provided the ability to perform new assays in the coagulation laboratory. Refinement of these methods has increased our ability to recognize and improve our diagnostic capabilities for determining the causes of disorders of hemostasis and thrombosis.

QUESTIONS

1. What is measured by a bleeding time?
   a. Platelet number
   b. Platelet function
   c. Intrinsic and extrinsic coagulation systems
   d. Two of the above

2. Which platelet aggregation result would be characteristic for patients with Bernard-Soulier syndrome?
   a. Incomplete aggregation with ADP
   b. Primary wave of aggregation in response to collagen
   c. Abnormal ristocetin-induced platelet aggregation
   d. Primary wave of aggregation with epinephrine

3. Which of the following tests measures the intrinsic pathway of coagulation and is used to detect factor deficiencies and hypofibrinogenemia and to monitor heparin therapy?
   a. Activated partial thromboplastin time
   b. Prothrombin time
   c. Quantitative factor assay
   d. Stypven time test (Russell's viper venom time test)

4. Which test measures the extrinsic pathway of coagulation and is used to measure factor deficiencies and monitor oral coagulation therapy?
   a. Activated partial thromboplastin time
   b. Prothrombin time
   c. Quantitative factor assay
   d. Stypven time test (Russell's viper venom time test)

5. Which test does not measure defects in intrinsic or extrinsic pathways and is affected by the levels of fibrinogen and dysfibrinogenemia, as well as the presence of circulating anticoagulants?
   a. Thrombin time
   b. Prothrombin time
   c. Reptilase time
   d. Fibrinogen

6. Which of the following conditions would show a short clotting time, indicating high fibrinogen levels?
   a. DIC
   b. Liver disease
   c. Pregnancy
   d. Fibrinolysis

7. Which condition would most likely show a decrease in factor VIII antigen?
   a. Hemophilia
   b. Female carriers of hemophilia A
   c. Myeloproliferative syndrome
   d. von Willebrand disease

8. Which APTT result would indicate the presence of a strong circulating anticoagulant?
   a. APTT not corrected by the addition of normal plasma
   b. Prolonged APTT (more than 1 hour)
   c. APTT corrected by the addition of normal plasma
   d. Any of the above results

9. Which of the following are criteria for the laboratory detection of lupus inhibitors?
   a. Abnormal APTT and/or PT
   b. Correction of APTT after platelet neutralization procedure
   c. Correction of APTT after mixing studies
   d. Two of the above

10. Using the test to measure fibrin degradation products (FDPs), which test results would be indicative of a patient having DIC? (Assume the fibrinogen concentration is indicative of DIC.)
    a. Positive FDP test result; increased PT and APTT; decreased platelet count
    b. Positive FDP test result; decreased PT and APTT; increased platelet count
    c. Negative FDP test result; increased PT, decreased APTT; decreased platelet count
    d. Negative FDP test result; decreased PT, increased APTT; increased platelet count

SUMMARY CHART

➤ The bleeding time is a screening procedure used to assess in vivo platelet function.
➤ The bleeding time is affected by platelet number and ingestion of aspirin and other drugs that inhibit platelet function.
➤ Platelet aggregation studies measure the platelets' ability to adhere to each other and release endogenous adenosine diphosphate (ADP).
➤ Platelet aggregation to ristocetin is usually abnormal in patients with von Willebrand disease.
➤ The activated partial thromboplastin time (APTT) is a screening test used to evaluate the intrinsic pathway of coagulation, which measures all the plasma coagulation factors with the exception of factors VII and XIII and platelet factor 3 (PF3).
➤ The APTT can be used to screen for inhibitors of the intrinsic pathway, such as the lupus-like anticoagulant, and to monitor heparin therapy.
➤ The prothrombin time (PT) is a valuable screening procedure used to indicate possible factor deficiencies of the extrinsic pathway.
➤ The PT test is sensitive to the vitamin K–dependent

➤ factors of the extrinsic pathway (factor VII) and common pathway (factors II and X) and is used as a means of monitoring oral anticoagulant therapy.

➤ The PT is prolonged in individuals with a factor deficiency involving a single factor (i.e., patients with a congenital deficiency) or involving multiple factors (i.e., patients with acquired deficiencies such as liver disease, oral anticoagulant therapy or patients with vitamin K deficiency).

➤ The international normalized ratio (INR) is used to standardize prothrombin time results in patients receiving oral anticoagulant therapy and should be reported along with the prothrombin time results.

➤ Nonspecific inhibitors will often have a "dilutional" effect on factor activity curves, demonstrating nonparallel curves with increasing dilutions.

➤ The thrombin time (TT) measures the conversion of fibrinogen to fibrin. It is affected by abnormal levels of fibrinogen, dysfibrinogenemia, and the presence of circulating anticoagulants (antithrombins) such as heparin and fibrin(ogen) degradation products (FDPs).

➤ The reptilase time is similar to the thrombin time in that it measures the conversion of fibrinogen to fibrin. The advantage of the reptilase time is that it is not affected by heparin.

➤ A screening test for factor XIII is clot solubility in 5 M urea or 1% monochloroacetic acid. Presence of a clot at the end of the incubation period indicates a level of greater than 1%, which is usually not associated with bleeding.

➤ Patients who present with a homozygous deficiency of factor XIII show dissolution of a fibrin clot in 5M urea or 1% monochloroacetic acid within 24 hours. This is indicative of factor XIII levels of less than 1%, which is significant as these are usually the only patients who exhibit hemorrhagic tendencies.

➤ The von Willebrand factor (vWF) molecule is composed of low-molecular-weight and high-molecular-weight portions. The low-molecular-weight portion is responsible for the procoagulant activity. The high-molecular-weight portion is the support of the von Willebrand activity or "ristocetin cofactor."

➤ It is the property of the factor VIII/vWF complex that is responsible for agglutination of platelets in the presence of ristocetin.

➤ Antithrombin (AT-III) is a naturally occurring inhibitor of blood coagulation responsible for neutralizing the activity of thrombin, factors IXa, Xa, XIa, and XIIa, and plasmin.

➤ The inhibition of thrombin by antithrombin is greatly accelerated by heparin.

➤ Functional antithrombin (activity) is measured by chromogenic assays. Immunologic antithrombin (antigen) is measured by Laurell rocket, radial immunodiffusion, or latex immunoassay techniques.

➤ A congenital decrease of antithrombin levels is accompanied by a high frequency of spontaneous thromboembolic disorders.

➤ A number of acquired antithrombin deficiencies have been described, including disseminated intravascular coagulation (DIC), nephrotic syndrome, and liver diseases; deficiencies may also occur with oral contraceptive use, postsurgically, and following prolonged heparin therapy.

➤ Protein C is a vitamin K–dependent serine protease that functions as a major regulatory protein in the control of coagulation. Activated protein C is a potent anticoagulant that acts by proteolytically inactivating factors Va and VIIIa. Protein C deficiency has been described as a risk factor in thromboembolic disease.

➤ Activated protein C resistance (APC-R), which is the result of a mutation in the factor V gene, is known as factor V Leiden. This mutation makes the factor V molecule resistant to the proteolytic activity of activated protein C, thereby negating its regulatory effect on thrombin generation and increasing the potential for the development of thromboses.

➤ Hereditary protein C deficiency can be classified as type I or type II, according to the levels of protein C activity and antigen measured. Acquired deficiencies of protein C are observed in hepatic disorders such as hepatitis and cirrhosis, vitamin K deficiency, DIC, and oral anticoagulant therapy.

➤ Protein C activity can be measured with chromogenic or clot-based assays. Protein C antigen is usually measured by enzyme-linked immunosorbent assay (ELISA) techniques.

➤ Protein S is a cofactor in the protein C pathway. It is a vitamin K–dependent factor, and is necessary in the reaction in which factors Va and VIIIa are inactivated by protein C.

➤ Protein S exists in free and bound form. Protein S bound to C4b-binding protein (C4bBP) is nonfunctional. Free protein S is the molecule active in the protein C pathway. Protein S activity is measured by clot-based assays and is extremely sensitive to poor collection technique or residual platelets in the plasma sample.

➤ Circulating anticoagulants may be detected by abnormalities in the PT or APTT, or both, and may be caused by either specific factor inhibitors such as factor VIII antibodies, or nonspecific, such as the lupus anticoagulant.

➤ The APTT is useful as a screening test to distinguish between factor deficiencies and circulating anticoagulants. When patient plasma is mixed with pooled normal plasma, sufficient factor should be present to correct a prolongation caused by a factor deficiency. There is only partial or no correction in the presence of an inhibitor.

➤ A weak or time-dependent circulating anticoagulant is indicated by a prolonged APTT following incubation at 37°C for 1 hour. On incubation, a weak inhibitor progressively inactivates the coagulation factor, thus prolonging the APTT. This pattern is most typical of a factor VIII inhibitor.

➤ Lupus anticoagulants (LAs) are antibodies (IgG, IgM, IgA, or a combination) directed against phospholipids, thereby prolonging in vitro phospholipid-dependent coagulation tests. First recognized in patients with systemic lupus erythematosus (SLE), LAs have been identified in a variety of disorders, including malignancies, infections, and autoimmune disorders, as well as following drug therapy.

➤ The presence of an LA is usually not associated with a bleeding problem unless accompanied by thrombocytopenia, factor II deficiency, platelet dysfunction, or drug administration (e.g., aspirin).

➤ The Scientific and Standardization Committee (SSC) Sub-Committee for the Standardization of Lupus Anticoagulants of the International Society of Thrombosis and Hemostasis (ISTH) has defined specific criteria to make a diagnosis of an LA.

➤ There are several confirmatory tests for LAs, including platelet neutralization procedure, anticardiolipin assay, kaolin clotting time, tissue thromboplastin inhibition test, and dilute Russell's viper venom test.

➤ Specimen collection, centrifugation, and processing are critical when testing for the presence of an LA, because the phospholipid-dependent reaction is affected by the presence of residual platelets in platelet-poor plasma.

➤ Antiphospholipid antibodies are a heterogeneous group of autoantibodies including anticardiolipin antibodies, lupus anticoagulants, beta-2 glycoprotein-1 (β2GP-1), and antiphosphatidylserine (APTS).

➤ FDPs can be measured by the Thrombo-Wellcotest or D-dimer assay. The Thrombo-Wellcotest measures both fibrin and fibrinogen breakdown products, whereas the D-dimer measures only fibrin breakdown products that have been cross-linked in a fibrin clot.

➤ Prothrombin fragment 1 + 2 (PF1+2), thrombin-antithrombin complex (TAT), soluble fibrin monomer (sFM), and thrombus precursor protein (TpP) are molecular markers that can be measured to determine the generation of thrombin.

References

1. National Committee for Clinical Laboratory Standards (NCCLS): Collection, Transport, and Processing of Blood Specimens for Coagulation Testing and General Performance of Coagulation Assays; Approved Guideline, ed 3. H21-A3, vol 18, no. 20, Wayne, PA, 1998.
2. Rodgers, RPC, and Levin, J: A critical reappraisal of the bleeding time. Semin Thromb Hemost 16:1, 1990.
3. Lind, DE: The bleeding time does not predict surgical bleeding. Blood 77:2547, 1991.
4. Kundu, SK, et al: Characterization of an in-vitro platelet function analyzer, PFA-100™. Clin Appl Thromb Hemost 2:241, 1996.
5. Hathaway, WE, and Goodnight, SH: Disorders of Hemostasis and Thrombosis. A Clinical Guide. McGraw-Hill, New York, 1993, p 43.
6. Born, GVR: Aggregation of blood platelets by adenosine diphosphate and its reversal. Nature 194:927, 1962.
7. Triplett, DA, et al: Platelet Function: Laboratory Evaluation and Clinical Application. American Society of Clinical Pathologists, Chicago, 1978.
8. Quick, AJ, et al: A study of the coagulation defect in hemophilia and jaundice. Am Med Sci 190:501, 1935.
9. Jensen R: Optimizing the INR. Clin Hem Rev 11:1:1997.
10. Hathaway, WE, and Goodnight, SH: Disorders of Hemostasis and Thrombosis. A Clinical Guide. McGraw-Hill, New York, 1993, p 176.
11. McDonagh, J: Structure and function of factor XIII. In Coleman, RW, et al (eds): Hemostasis and Thrombosis. Basic Principles and Clinical Practice, ed 3. JB Lippincott, Philadelphia, 1994, pp 301–313.
12. Ristocetin Cofactor Assay Package Insert, Helena Laboratories, Beaumont, TX, 1999.
13. Nichols, WC, et al: von Willebrand Disease. In Loscalzo, J, and Schafer, AI (eds): Thrombosis and Hemorrhage, ed 2. Williams & Wilkins, Baltimore, MD, 1998, pp 729–744.
14. Hathaway, WE, and Goodnight, SH: Hereditary von Willebrand disease. In: Disorders of Hemostasis and Thrombosis. A Clinical Guide. McGraw-Hill, New York, 1993, pp 109–116.
15. Hathaway, WE, and Goodnight, SH: Protein C deficiency. In: Disorders of Hemostasis and Thrombosis. A Clinical Guide. McGraw-Hill, New York, 1993, pp 338–340.
16. Dahlback, B, et al: Familial thrombophilia due to a previously unrecognized mechanism characterized by poor anticoagulant response to activated Protein C. Proc Natl Acad Sci USA 90:1004, 1993.
17. Comp, PC: Congenital and acquired hypercoagulable states. In Hull, R, and Pineo, GF (eds): Disorders of Thrombosis. WB Saunders, Philadelphia, 1996, pp 339–344.
18. Preda, L, et al: A prothrombin time-based functional assay of protein S. Thromb Res 60:19, 1990.
19. Ens, GE, and Newlin, F: Spurious protein S deficiency as a result of elevated factor VII levels. Clin Hemost Rev 9:18, 1995.
20. Schleider, MA, et al: A clinical study of the lupus anticoagulant. Blood 48:499, 1976.
21. Lusher, JM: Acquired inhibitors to factor VIII in non-hemophiliac patients. In Kessler, C, et al (eds): Acquired Hemophilia, ed 2. Excerpta Medica, Princeton, NJ, 1995, pp 1–8.
22. Triplett, DA: Lupus anticoagulants: Diagnostic dilemma and clinical challenge. Clin Lab Sci 10:223, 1997.
23. Brandt, JT, et al: Criteria for the diagnosis of lupus anticoagulants: An update. Thromb Haem 74:1185, 1995.
24. Bockenstedt, PL: Laboratory methods in hemostasis. In Loscalzo, J, and Schafer, AI (eds): Thrombosis and Hemorrhage, ed 2. Williams & Wilkins, Baltimore, MD, 1998, pp 517–526.
25. Jensen, R, and Ens, GE: Markers of thrombin activation. Clin Hemost Rev 8:1, 1994.
26. BBL Microbiology Systems, Division of Becton Dickinson, Cockeysville, MD.
27. STA Operator's Manual, Diagnostica Stago, Parsippany, NJ.
28. KC4A Product Information, Sigma Diagnostics Inc, St Louis, MO.
29. MLA Electra 1000 Operator's Manual, Section 3–1. Medical Laboratory Automation, Pleasantville, NY.
30. MDA 180 Operator's Manual. Organon Teknika Corporation, Durham, NC.
31. Miers, MK, et al: Cell-counting and coagulation instrumentation. In Rodak, BF (ed): Diagnostic Hematology. WB Saunders, Philadelphia, 1995, pp 626–631.
32. Blood Coagulation System (BCS) Operator's Manual. Dade Behring, Inc, Deerfield, IL.
33. Package Insert, LIATEST vWF, Diagnostica Stago, Parsippany, NJ.

33 Molecular Diagnostic Techniques in Hematopathology

Margaret L. Gulley, MD

OBJECTIVES

At the end of this chapter, the learner should be able to:

1. Describe the fundamental structure of DNA.
2. Define nucleic acid probe.
3. List the most commonly used molecular diagnostic assays and state the purpose of each assay.
4. Describe a potential clinical application of each diagnostic test.
5. Interpret a Southern blot result.

Deoxyribonucleic acid (DNA) is the inherited substance that encodes all the information needed for cell structure and function. For this information to be expressed, it must be transmitted through an intermediary substance called ribonucleic acid (RNA). DNA and RNA are collectively called *nucleic acid*. Analysis of nucleic acid in patient samples forms the foundation for a new field of laboratory medicine called *molecular diagnostics*. In no other discipline of laboratory medicine has this technology had a greater impact than in hematology, where it is used to assist in the diagnosis of certain inherited, infectious, and malignant forms of hematologic diseases.

The laboratory methods most commonly implemented in clinical settings are Southern blot analysis, polymerase chain reaction (PCR), and in situ hybridization. To understand how each of these methods is used, we must first review the structure of DNA and RNA. A glossary at the end of this textbook provides definitions of the new terms.

➤ STRUCTURE OF DNA

Human DNA is packaged into 46 chromosomes, each of which is an exceptionally large molecule formed from two very long strands of nucleotides. If all 46 chromosomes were aligned end to end, they would be 3 billion nucleotide pairs long and would stretch for over 2 meters. Inside each nucleus, the DNA strands are tightly coiled around histone proteins to form chromatin. Within these long strands of nucleotides is encoded all of the information necessary for life.[1,2]

Nucleotides are the basic building blocks of DNA, and they are composed of one of four different types of nitrogenous bases—adenine, guanine, thymine, or cytosine—attached to a deoxyribose sugar and phosphate moiety. The two strands of nucleotides that combine to form DNA are bound together by hydrogen bonds that form between the nucleotides on one strand and those on the opposite strand. According to the rules of complementary nucleotide pairing, an adenine in one strand can bond only with a thymine in the other strand, and guanine can bond only with cytosine. For this reason, the two strands of DNA are said to be complementary to each other (Fig. 33–1).

Encoded within the nucleotide sequences of DNA are functional units called *genes* that serve as templates for RNA transcription and, ultimately, protein translation. Although all nucleated cells contain a full complement of DNA constituting that person's genome, each cell ex-

5' **...GGCATCGAATGA...** 3'

3' **...CCGTAGCTTACT...** 5'

➤ **FIGURE 33–1**   DNA is composed of two strands of nucleotides that are bound to each other through hydrogen bonds (depicted as diagonal bridges). Only four types of nucleotides are present, adenine (A), thymine (T), guanine (G), and cytosine (C) Because of the characteristic biochemical structure of each nucleotide, an A on one strand can bond only to a T on the other strand, and a G can bond only to a C. Therefore, the two strands of DNA are said to be "complementary" to each other. The strands are oriented in opposite directions with respect to the sugar and phosphate groups that link adjacent nucleotides; thus each strand has a 5′ and a 3′ end. In the laboratory, the two strands of DNA may be dissociated from one another by heating them to near-boiling temperature (95°C) or treating them with an alkaline solution (high pH).

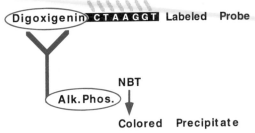

➤ **FIGURE 33–2**   A probe represents a short strand of nucleotides that can bind (or "hybridize") to its complementary target nucleotide sequence. In the example depicted here, the probe was labeled with digoxigenin so that it could be subsequently detected by a colorimetric reaction involving an antibody to digoxigenin, alkaline phosphatase and 4-nitroblue tetrazolium chloride (NBT).

presses only a fraction of the estimated 100,000 different genes, depending on its cell type and stage of differentiation. Gene expression results in the production of RNA, a molecule that resembles DNA except that it is single-stranded, contains ribose instead of deoxyribose, and substitutes uracil for thymine.

Recent advances in our understanding of the genetic basis of disease have led to the development of laboratory tests targeting DNA or RNA in patient samples. All current molecular diagnostic tests are based on our ability to identify a specific nucleotide sequence in DNA or RNA by using a "probe" that targets that sequence. A probe is simply a single-stranded segment of nucleic acid (either DNA or RNA) whose nucleotide sequence is complementary to the target sequence (either DNA or RNA). A probe binds to its target through a process called *hybridization*. Hybridization is usually accomplished by combining probe and target in a small tube (liquid phase) or on a membrane or glass slide (solid phase). In either case, the probe has usually been prelabeled so that it can be subsequently detected and used as a marker for the target sequence (Fig. 33–2).

➤ APPLICATIONS OF DNA TECHNOLOGY TO DIAGNOSTIC MEDICINE

DNA technology is potentially useful in diagnosing all diseases resulting from altered DNA. These include inherited diseases, which by definition have a genetic basis, and infectious diseases in which the identification of foreign DNA or RNA indicates that a pathogen is present. Table 33–1 provides a list of inherited and infectious diseases that commonly affect the hematopoietic system and for which probe assays have been developed.

DNA technology can also be used to help diagnose and classify various types of cancer.[12] This is because virtually all cancers harbor genetic defects that are responsible for malignant transformation. A gene whose alteration is responsible for cancer formation is called an *oncogene*. Table 33–2 lists the known oncogenes related to hematopoietic cancers. Laboratory detection of cancer-associated genetic defects not only contributes to improved diagnosis of affected patients, but in some cases may also help determine the most appropriate treatment and help monitor the efficacy of that treatment.[18,19]

Each of the previously mentioned diagnostic applications relies on prior basic and clinical research that has defined disease-specific genetic alterations and established molecular probe assays to detect those alterations. In the remainder

➤ **Table 33–1**
HEMATOLOGIC DISEASES AMENABLE TO MOLECULAR DIAGNOSIS

Inherited Diseases[3,4]

Gaucher disease

Hemoglobinopathies (sickle cell anemia, α and β thalassemias)[5]

Hemochromatosis[6]

Glucose-6-phosphate dehydrogenase deficiency

Bleeding disorders (various factor deficiencies, Bernard-Soulier syndrome, platelet storage pool deficiency, von Willebrand's disease)

Thrombotic disorders (factor V mutation, prothrombin mutation, methyltetrahydrofolate reductase mutation)[7,8]

Immunodeficiency states (deficiencies of adenosine deaminase, purine nucleoside phosphorylase, and leukocyte adhesion, DiGeorge and Wiskott-Aldrich syndromes, chronic granulomatous disease)

Porphyrias

Red cell membrane defects, including hereditary spherocytosis and elliptocytosis, and paroxysmal nocturnal hemoglobinuria

Infectious Diseases[9]

Epstein-Barr virus (EBV)[10]

Cytomegalovirus (CMV)

Human immunodeficiency virus (HIV)

Human T-lymphotropic virus type 1 (HTLV1)[11]

Malaria

Mycobacteriosis

Mycoplasmosis

Parvovirus B19

Toxoplasmosis

➤ **Table 33–2**
GENETIC ABNORMALITIES IN HEMATOPOIETIC CANCERS

Tumor Type	Karyotype	Oncogenes
Myeloid Leukemias		
Chronic myelogenous leukemia[13,14]	t(9;22)	BCR/ABL
Acute myelogenous leukemia, M2	t(8;21)	AML1/ETO
Acute myelogenous leukemia, M4eo	inv(16)	MYH11/CBFβ
Acute promyelocytic leukemia, M3[15,16]	t(15;17)	PML/RARα
B-Cell Leukemias		
Acute lymphoblastic leukemia (ALL)	t(9;22)	BCR/ABL
Pre-B ALL	t(1;19)	PBX1/E2A
Pre-B ALL	t(12;21)	TEL/AML1
ALL or mixed lineage leukemia	t(various;11)	various/MLL
B-Cell Lymphomas		
Burkitt's lymphoma	t(8;14,2 or 22)	myc/IgH, Igκ, or Igλ
Mantle cell lymphoma	t(11;14)	bc11/IgH
Follicular lymphoma[17]	t(14;18)	bc12/IgH
Diffuse large cell lymphoma	t(3;14)	bc16/IgH
Lymphoplasmacytic lymphoma	t(9;14)	PAX5/IgH
MALT lymphoma	t(11;18)	API1/MALT1
T-Cell Leukemias/Lymphomas		
Pre-T ALL	del(1p)	TAL1 deletion
Anaplastic large-cell lymphoma	t(2;5)	NPM/ALK

of this chapter, we review each of the most commonly used molecular diagnostic procedures. Readers desiring further information on the equipment, reagents, or step-by-step procedures are referred to one of several detailed protocol manuals.[20,21] Issues of quality assurance are addressed in several excellent references.[22–25] Examples of applications of these methods are found throughout this text.

➤ SAMPLE SOURCES FOR MOLECULAR PROCEDURES

DNA is a very stable molecule. For example, fragments of DNA have been recovered from fossils, skeletal remains, and bodies that were mummified thousands of years ago. Nevertheless, specimens submitted to clinical laboratories for molecular genetic assays should be handled with care to preserve intact DNA. This is particularly true for samples to be analyzed by the Southern blot technique in which prior "degradation" (i.e., nonspecific fragmentation) of the DNA invalidates the results. Intact DNA is usually well preserved in tissues that are frozen within an hour of collection, and in blood samples that are less than 2 days old.[25] One of the best tissue fixatives for preserving intact DNA is ethanol. Unfortunately, the more commonly used fixative, formalin, often interferes with molecular testing. Optimal specimen types are listed under the description of each molecular assay that follows.

Unlike DNA, RNA is unstable and is easily degraded by ubiquitous natural enzymes collectively termed *RNases*.

Therefore, special handling (described next) is required to preserve RNA in clinical samples.

➤ NUCLEIC ACID EXTRACTION

Preparation of Samples
DNA or RNA is readily extracted from blood, marrow, body fluid cells, and tissue samples.[25] In preparation for extraction of DNA from blood samples, nucleated blood cells are first separated from the more abundant red cells by centrifugation or by red cell lysis. Only nucleated cells are retained for subsequent DNA extraction, whereas the red cells and platelets are discarded because they have no nucleus and, hence, contain no chromosomes.

In contrast to blood specimens, solid tissue specimens contain relatively few red cells, so enrichment procedures are not required. Instead, frozen tissues are finely minced, whereas paraffin-embedded tissues are sliced with an instrument called a *microtome* before nucleic acid extraction.

DNA Extraction from Fresh Cells or Frozen Tissue
DNA can be separated from all of the protein and lipids that compose cells by an organic chemical extraction procedure. This procedure is based on the fact that DNA is soluble in water, whereas lipids and protein are not easily dissolved in water. First, however, the patient cells are treated with detergent and proteinase enzymes to lyse their mem-

branes and degrade their proteins. Then the organic chemical phenol is added to the cellular lysate. On centrifugation, lipids migrate to the phenol fraction at the bottom of the tube, whereas DNA remains in the aqueous fraction on top and protein byproducts collect at the interface between the two layers. The DNA that is preferentially isolated to the upper aqueous layer is simply pipetted into a fresh tube, where it is subsequently concentrated and further purified by precipitating it in a cold mixture of salt and ethanol. The DNA is then recovered by either spooling the long strands onto a stick or by centrifuging the precipitated DNA into a pellet at the bottom of the tube. Finally, the DNA is resuspended in water and stored at 4°C for up to 1 month or at −20°C indefinitely.

Commercial kits and semiautomated instruments are now available to facilitate extraction of DNA from blood and other tissues. Some kits utilize salt solutions to precipitate DNA, or they use columns to selectively bind DNA, thus avoiding exposure to hazardous organic chemicals. The purified DNA can then be quantitated (see later discussion) and analyzed by various molecular laboratory assays. Southern blot analysis requires relatively intact DNA that is free of protein contaminants, because such contaminants tend to inhibit restriction enzyme digestion. Other assays, such as PCR, can be performed on DNA that is only crudely purified or even partially degraded.

DNA Extraction from Paraffin-Embedded Tissue

First, a single 10-μm paraffin section is cut on a microtome and stuffed into a microfuge tube. Because paraffin can inhibit subsequent enzymatic reactions, some users trim excess paraffin from the block before sectioning. The resultant tissue section is typically submerged in octane to dissolve the paraffin, then washed with ethanol, dried, and incubated in a proteinase enzyme solution that degrades cellular proteins. The proteinase is subsequently heat-inactivated so that it will not interfere with future enzymatic reactions.

In nearly all cases, the DNA extracted from paraffin tissues will subsequently be used in an amplification assay such as PCR; therefore, precautions are needed to avoid contamination of the section with extraneous DNA during the histologic sectioning process. These precautions include:

1. Wear gloves. Before beginning, wipe down all work surfaces with 10% bleach to destroy any extraneous nucleic acid, then rinse with sterile water to remove residual bleach.
2. Change the microtome blade between cases so that minute amounts of tissue are not carried over to the next case.
3. Use a smooth-edged forceps to transfer the section into the microfuge tube. Between cases, wipe the forceps with 10% bleach, then rinse and dry it with clean absorbent gauze.
4. Do not allow bleach to contact the tissue to be analyzed, because it could destroy the nucleic acid.
5. Intersperse "control" blocks among the cases to evaluate for contamination by extraneous DNA.

RNA Extraction

RNA can be extracted from cells by treating them with guanidine thiocyanate, a chemical that disrupts cellular membranes and also inhibits endogenous RNase activity.

RNA is separated from cellular lipids and proteins by the same organic extraction technique described to isolate DNA. RNA is then further purified and concentrated by precipitation in isopropanol followed by centrifugation. The final product is resuspended in water and stored at −70°C pending further analysis.

Because RNase enzymes are ubiquitous, special precautions are required to prevent RNA degradation. In particular, gloves should be worn, and all solutions and plasticware should be RNase-free. Dedicated laboratory areas and reagents are recommended. Patient samples should be processed promptly upon collection.

➤ NUCLEIC ACID QUANTITATION

DNA and RNA are quantitated by spectrophotometry, which relies on the fact that nucleic acids absorb ultraviolet light of optical density (OD) 260 nm, whereas proteins absorb at OD280. Quantity is estimated using the following formulas, which are based on the concept that an OD260 of 1 corresponds to 50 μg/mL of DNA, 40 μg/mL of RNA, or 20 μg/mL of a single-stranded oligonucleotide:

Double-stranded DNA concentration (μg/μL)
= OD260 × 0.05

RNA concentration (μg/μL) = OD260 × 0.04

Single-stranded oligonucleotide concentration (μg/μL)
= OD260 × 0.02

Most commonly, a small aliquot of the unknown sample is diluted with water before spectrophotometry, so the dilution factor must be taken into account to arrive at the concentration in the original sample.

Protein contamination of a DNA sample is assessed by calculating a ratio of OD260 to OD280. The expected ratio is between 1.7 and 1.8 for DNA, and 1.9 to 2.0 for RNA. A ratio below 1.7 suggests the need for repeated organic extraction to remove impurities (usually proteins) that may interfere with restriction enzyme digestion of DNA.

Alternatively, DNA can be quantitated using either (1) a fluorometer instrument that relies on the binding of Hoechst 33258 dye or (2) electrophoresis and staining of a "yield gel," whereby lanes containing sample DNA are compared with lanes containing standard amounts of DNA. The DNA in these gels is visualized by staining with ethidium bromide, a chemical that intercalates into the DNA strands and fluoresces when exposed to ultraviolet light. Each of these techniques is suitable for quantitating very small volumes of DNA, but, unlike in the spectrophotometric method, protein contamination is not assessed.

➤ SEQUENCE-SPECIFIC FRAGMENTATION OF DNA BY RESTRICTION ENDONUCLEASES

One of the most important breakthroughs in our ability to manipulate DNA in the laboratory came with the discovery of naturally occurring enzymes that chop DNA into small fragments. An important feature of these enzymes is that they cut only at specific sequence-recognition sites. Their restricted ability to cut DNA resulted in their being named *restriction endonucleases*. These enzymes are normally produced by bacteria as a means of defending the bacteria from foreign pathogens such as bacteriophages. In diagnostic laboratories, their ability to reproducibly cleave human DNA into smaller fragments simplifies manipulation of an otherwise excessively large molecule.

In clinical laboratories, the enzymes most commonly used for sequence-specific cleavage of DNA are EcoR1, derived from *Escherichia coli* and recognizing 5'-GAATTC-3'; BamH1, derived from *Bacillus amyloliquifaciens* and recognizing 5'-GGATCC-3'; and HindIII, derived from *Haemophilus influenzae* and recognizing 5'-AAGCTT-3'. Each of these enzymes cuts human DNA into thousands of smaller fragments that can subsequently be separated by size in the Southern blot procedure or captured in vectors to produce recombinant DNA. (See Probe Production, later in the chapter.)

➤ DIAGNOSTIC PROCEDURES FOR ANALYZING DNA

Southern Blot Analysis

Purpose The purpose of Southern blot analysis is to analyze the molecular structure of DNA so that disease-specific genetic alterations can be identified.

Procedure DNA is extracted from the tissue sample, cut with restriction endonucleases to produce restriction fragments, separated by size using gel electrophoresis, and detected with probes complementary to the particular region of interest. If DNA is altered by mutation, translocation, or any other structural change, then the number or size, or both, of the resulting restriction fragments is altered accordingly (Fig. 33–3). Note that some people use the term *restriction fragment length polymorphism (RFLP)* as a synonym for the Southern blot method of detecting genetic alterations.

Sample Requirements Frozen tissue, or fresh body fluid, blood or marrow. Sufficient DNA is usually obtained from a single tube of blood (7 mL), 1 to 2 mL of marrow, or 2 mm³ of tissue or pelleted cells from a body fluid. Ethylene diaminetetraacetic acid (EDTA) anticoagulant is preferred over heparin because heparin inhibits the action of restriction endonucleases.

Assay Time Approximately 1 week.

Sensitivity Moderate (about 1 target per 20 cells, or 5%).

Specificity High.

Cost per Test Approximately $300 if only one sample is analyzed, less for batched samples.

Clinical Applications

1. To detect a disease-specific genetic abnormality that alters the size of a particular restriction fragment. Examples include certain inherited diseases, such as sickle cell anemia, and many types of cancer such as leukemia or lymphoma.[18,26] A list of cancer-related genetic defects is provided in Table 33–2. Note that B-cell tumors tend to have genetic defects involving their immunoglobulin genes, whereas T-cell tumors have defects of their T-cell receptor genes. Lymphoid tumors are thought to arise as a result of errors occurring during physiologic rearrangement of these antigen receptor genes.

2. To detect clonal rearrangement of immunoglobulin or T-cell receptor genes in lymphoid leukemias and lymphomas.[18,27,28] This helps distinguish lymphoid neoplasms from reactive lymphoid hyperplasia, and

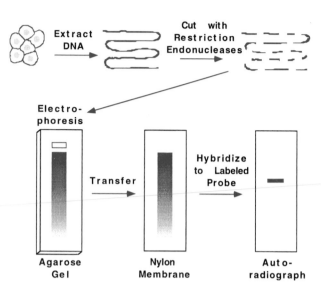

➤ **FIGURE 33–3** Southern blot analysis of DNA structure. In this procedure, DNA is extracted from cells and cut by restriction endonucleases at specific sequences. The resultant fragments are separated by size using gel electrophoresis, and then denatured into their single-stranded components by treating them with an alkaline solution. The single-stranded fragments are transferred to a nylon membrane. The membrane is soaked in a probe solution, permitting the probe to hybridize to complementary nucleotide sequences on the membrane. The probe has been labeled so that it can be localized. In the particular example shown here, radiolabeled probe binds to only one target sequence in the patient sample, thus producing a single band on the autoradiograph.

can also be used to help determine B- versus T-cell lineage of lymphoid tumors. As a rule, B-cell leukemias and lymphomas exhibit clonal rearrangement of the immunoglobulin heavy-chain gene. In most cases, they also exhibit coexistent clonal rearrangement of the kappa (κ) light-chain gene regardless of whether they express κ or lambda (λ) light-chain protein. T-cell tumors usually exhibit clonal rearrangement of the T-cell receptor beta (β) or T-cell receptor gamma (γ) genes, or both. In contrast, no clonal gene rearrangement is found in reactive lymphoid hyperplasia (Fig. 33–4).

3. To quantitate gene amplifications associated with certain tumors, such as n-*myc* gene amplification associated with neuroblastoma.

4. To detect foreign DNA associated with infectious diseases, so long as the foreign DNA is relatively abundant (at least 1 target per 20 cells).

5. To detect DNA polymorphisms in forensic or paternity assays.[29]

6. To confirm the size or origin of PCR products, or to detect disease-specific genetic alterations in those products. For example, the point mutation responsible for sickle cell anemia may be detected by a Southern blot assay or by Southern blot analysis of a PCR product.

Major Advantage Southern blot analysis is the most accurate method of detecting clonal gene rearrangement in lymphoid neoplasms.

➤ **FIGURE 33–4** *A.* Southern blot analysis can be used to identify B-cell tumors based on their characteristic clonal immunoglobulin gene rearrangements. Normally, during B-cell differentiation, the immunoglobulin kappa light-chain gene (Igκ) rearranges to produce a unique coding sequence that determines antibody specificity. This occurs through a process of splicing and deletion whereby 1 of 80 variable (V) regions is juxtaposed with 1 of 5 joining (J) regions. These rearrangements alter the size of the DNA fragments produced by the HindIII restriction endonuclease and recognized by hybridization to a probe (shown as a bar) spanning the Jκ region. Whereas each benign B cell rearranges its κ gene differently, malignant B cells contain exactly the same rearrangement that was present in the B cell from which the tumor arose. This clonal gene rearrangement alters the band pattern on a Southern blot. In addition to the 3.0-kb rearranged band that characterizes the particular rearrangement depicted here, there is also partial retention of the 5.4-kb unrearranged (germline) Igκ gene originating from residual normal cells in the sample or from the other Igκ allele in tumor cells. *B.* In the actual Southern blot autoradiograph shown here, the Jκ probe was used to detect clonal Igκ gene rearrangement in a case of chronic lymphocytic leukemia (L). In each of three different restriction endonuclease digests, the presence of two extra bands suggests that both Igκ alleles are clonally rearranged in the tumor cells or, less likely, that the tumor is biclonal. Normal control (C) tissue analyzed simultaneously identifies the position of the germline bands. A map of the Jκ region depicts the expected size of the germline bands for each restriction endonuclease.

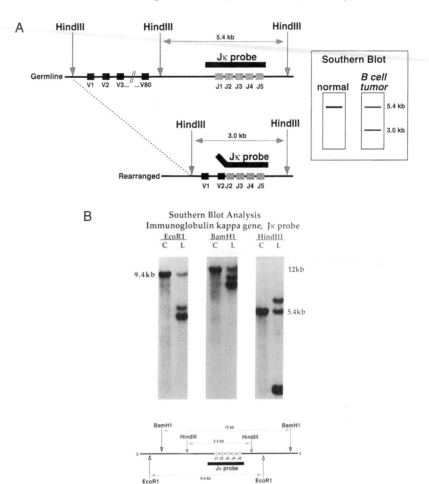

Major Disadvantages

1. Sensitivity is relatively low. For example, tumors composing less than 5% of a tissue sample are frequently undetectable. (Controls run simultaneously with patient samples can be used to evaluate the sensitivity of each Southern blot assay.)
2. Labor intensive and, therefore, costly.
3. Relatively long turn-around time.
4. Requires fresh or frozen tissue, and is not amenable to formalin-fixed tissue.

Potential Pitfalls

1. Sample DNA must be intact before beginning the Southern blot procedure. Intact DNA is characterized by very long strands of clear gel-like material that can be spooled onto a collection stick. In contrast, degraded DNA does not spool well because it is already fragmented, which confounds the ability to visualize and interpret bands on Southern blots. It should also be noted that intact DNA is difficult to pipet, whereas degraded DNA pipets easily. Pipetting of genomic DNA should be kept to a minimum because shear stresses generated by pipetting contribute to fragmentation.
2. In the next step of Southern analysis, it is essential that restriction endonuclease digestion be allowed to proceed to completion. A reasonable way to evaluate the completeness of enzymatic digestion (and the

degree of DNA degradation) is to examine the size distribution of DNA fragments in the agarose gel that is prepared during Southern analysis. These fragments may be visualized and photographed after staining them with ethidium bromide. Good-quality digestions are characterized by a graded distribution of fragment sizes, as depicted in Figure 33–3. Incomplete digestion results in an excess of large fragments, whereas degraded DNA results in an excess of small fragments.

3. Beware of "polymorphisms." Users should be aware that DNA polymorphisms can confound the proper interpretation of Southern blot results. We define polymorphisms as natural differences in nucleotide sequence that distinguish one person's DNA from another's. In fact, every person's DNA is unique, except in the case of identical twins. On average, polymorphisms occur at a rate of about 1 in every 500 nucleotide pairs. Polymorphisms can be exploited as a means of establishing identity for forensic purposes, so-called DNA fingerprinting.[29] On the other hand, polymorphisms can also interfere with molecular tests for disease-associated genetic defects. For example, a polymorphism occurring at the site where a restriction enzyme normally cleaves could result in altered band sizes on the resultant Southern blot that might mimic a disease-specific structural abnormality. To overcome this pitfall, it is prudent to confirm a low polymorphism rate at the disease locus

being examined and to design additional confirmatory tests when feasible. For example, multiple different restriction enzyme digestions are often used to establish the likelihood that an altered band pattern on a Southern blot results from a tumor-associated rearrangement as opposed to a simple base substitution at one restriction enzyme recognition site.[27] Alternatively, a tumor sample could be compared to normal tissue from the same patient to identify tumor-specific genetic defects.

Polymerase Chain Reaction

Introduction PCR is one of several methods for amplifying (i.e., copying) particular segments of DNA.[30] Because PCR was the first amplification method to be invented and the first to be introduced into clinical laboratories, it is described here in detail. A review article by Wiedbrauk describes several alternate methods of DNA amplification.[31]

Purpose The purpose of PCR is to amplify target DNA a billionfold so that it may be more easily detected or further analyzed for disease-specific genetic alterations. PCR works by enzymatically replicating one particular segment of DNA from amid all the DNA in a patient's sample. Segments as long as 40,000 base pairs (bp) have been amplified in research laboratories, but a more realistic limit in clinical samples is about 5000 bp, or even less (about 500 bp) if the DNA was extracted from fixed paraffin-embedded tissue.

Procedure DNA is isolated from the sample and mixed with (1) an enzyme called *DNA polymerase* that copies DNA by converting single-stranded into double-stranded DNA; (2) short probes that flank the target sequence and serve as primers for the initiation of DNA replication by the polymerase; and (3) the building blocks needed for generating new DNA strands (dATP, dGTP, dCTP, and dTTP). The enzymatic reaction takes place in a thermocycler instrument programmed to sequentially vary the temperature of the reaction mixture so that progressive cycles of DNA replication can occur. After about 30 cycles, which takes only a few hours, about a billion copies of the target DNA are generated (Fig. 33–5). The reaction product is easily identified as a band on gel electrophoresis. Hybridization to an internal probe is an alternative method of detecting the product and, moreover, confirming its origin. The PCR product can then be further tested for a disease-specific genetic alteration, if appropriate.

Note: The DNA polymerase used in PCR reactions is "thermostable." This means that it can sustain near-boiling temperatures and still remain active. It is this feature that allows the PCR reaction to continue through multiple heat cycles without loss of enzyme function. Thermostable polymerase is derived from bacteria such as *Thermus aquaticus* ("Taq") that have adapted to survive in geysers or hot pools.

Method Variation for Quantitative PCR In a variation of the PCR method called *real-time PCR,* amplified products are quantitated at the end of every amplification cycle, and this information is used to extrapolate how much target DNA was present in the original sample.[32] In another methodologic variation called *competitive PCR,* the patient sample is first spiked with a known amount of DNA, which then competes with target DNA during amplification. The relative proportion of PCR products generated from the target versus the spiked DNA allows calculation of the target DNA concentration in the original sample.

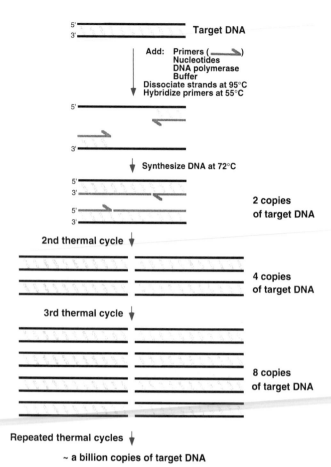

▶ **FIGURE 33–5** Polymerase chain reaction (PCR) is a method of copying a particular segment of DNA numerous times through a process of repeated cycles of heating, cooling, and DNA synthesis. To accomplish this, the target DNA is mixed with two short DNA probes called *primers* (shown as half-arrows) that are designed to span the segment of DNA to be amplified. Also added to the mixture is an enzyme called *DNA polymerase,* which converts single-stranded DNA into double-stranded DNA by incorporating nucleotides starting at the 3′ end of each primer. A thermocycler instrument is programmed to sequentially heat and cool the sample. In each heat/cool cycle, the sample is first heated to 95°C to dissociate the two strands of DNA, and then cooled to 55°C to permit binding of the primers, then warmed to 72°C for enzymatic DNA replication. After the first cycle, an exact copy of the original target DNA has been produced. Then, in subsequent cycles, the products of previous cycles can serve as templates for DNA replication, permitting an exponential accumulation of DNA copies. After 30 cycles, which takes only a few hours, approximately a billion copies of the target DNA have been synthesized.

Sample Requirements Fresh, frozen, fixed, or paraffin-embedded tissue, blood, marrow, or body fluid. Although several investigators have reported performing successful PCR reactions on single cells, most clinical assays rely on sample sizes of at least a million cells. Recommended minimum sample volumes are 1 mL of blood or body fluid, 0.5 mL of marrow, or 0.5 mm³ of tissue. Although formalin fixation results in DNA strand breakage, PCR frequently succeeds in amplifying DNA segments up to several hundred base pairs in length from formalin-fixed, paraffin-embedded tissue because only one intact target sequence is required for the reaction to proceed.

Assay Time Approximately 1 day to generate and detect the reaction product; further testing of the reaction product requires additional time.

Sensitivity High. Theoretically, one target is sufficient. In practice, amplification of one target per 10^5 cells is typically achieved.

Specificity High.

Cost per Test Approximately $100 if only one sample is analyzed, less if samples are batched, more if further testing of the PCR product is required.

Clinical Applications

1. Detect foreign nucleic acid characteristic of infectious diseases. In some cases, further molecular testing can be done to determine antibiotic resistance based on the genetic sequence of the pathogen.
2. Selectively amplify DNA that has a particular disease-associated defect, such as the point mutation characteristic of sickle cell anemia, or the *bcl2/JH* translocation characteristic of follicular lymphoma.
3. Detect minimal residual disease in cancer patients following therapy by using PCR to amplify the tumor-specific molecular defect. Such an approach has been used to predict relapse of follicular lymphoma before there is clinical or morphological evidence that residual tumor is still present.
4. Measure tumor burden so that the efficacy of anticancer therapy can be monitored.
5. Measure viral load so that the efficacy of antiviral therapy can be monitored.
6. To detect clonal immunoglobulin or T-cell receptor gene rearrangements by using primer sets that span rearranged gene segments.[33–35] Current protocols detect clonality in about 80% of lymphoid neoplasms (compared to 100% by Southern analysis).
7. To detect DNA polymorphisms for forensic or parentage tests, or to help solve dilemmas relating to misidentified samples in the clinical laboratory.[29,36]

Major Advantages

1. Extremely sensitive to low numbers of target sequences.
2. Small sample size requirements.
3. Relatively fast and inexpensive unless extensive postamplification analysis is required.
4. Permits analysis of formalin-fixed, paraffin-embedded tissue that is not suitable for Southern blot analysis.

Major Disadvantage Extreme precautions are required to avoid contamination of samples or reagents by extraneous DNA. Contamination by the abundant products generated from previous PCR reactions is a worrisome problem.

Reverse Transcriptase Polymerase Chain Reaction

Purpose The purpose of reverse transcriptase polymerase chain reaction (rtPCR) is to detect RNA in patient specimens (1) so that expression of a particular gene can be monitored, (2) so that an RNA virus can be identified, or (3) because RNA presents a better target for the detection of a particular disease-related sequence than does the DNA from which it was encoded.

Procedure RNA is extracted from tissue and converted to complementary DNA (cDNA), using the enzyme reverse

transcriptase in the presence of deoxyribonucleotides and primers. After cDNA production, conventional PCR is carried out to amplify the cDNA sequence of interest (Fig. 33–6).

The primers used in the reverse transcriptase step function to initiate enzymatic production of cDNA from an RNA template. If these primers are random hexamers, the resultant cDNA represents all of the various RNAs in the sample, whereas a longer sequence-specific primer can be used to target a particular RNA sequence of interest.

Sample Requirements Fresh blood, marrow, body fluid, or solid tissue. Because RNA is easily degraded, samples should be processed as soon as possible after collection. If RNA extraction cannot be performed immediately, the tissue or nucleated cell pellet should be stored in a sterile, sealed container at $-70°C$ until analysis. Plasma samples are often used for detection of RNA viruses. Some laboratories have reported successful rtPCR of fixed, paraffin-embedded tissue.

Assay Time Approximately 2 days.

Sensitivity High. (Theoretically, one target is sufficient.)

Specificity High.

Cost per Test Approximately $150 if only one sample is analyzed, less for batched samples.

Clinical Applications

1. Determine expression of selected genes by targeting their corresponding RNA transcripts, such as oncogenes overexpressed in tumor samples. When used to evaluate gene expression, PCR primers should be designed to flank transcript splice sites so that cDNA can be distinguished from native DNA.
2. Detect tumor-specific chromosomal translocations where chimeric RNA is transcribed across the translocation breakpoint. In many instances, breakpoint cluster regions identified at the DNA level are further clustered by the natural process of RNA splicing, thus simplifying detection of the translocation event. Examples of fusion transcripts that are amenable to rtPCR analysis include *PML/RAR*α, t(15;17); *bcr/abl*, t(9;22); *AML1/ETO*, t(8;21); *NPM/ALK*, t(2;5); *MLL/AF-4*, t(4;11); and *MYH11/CBF*β, inv16.

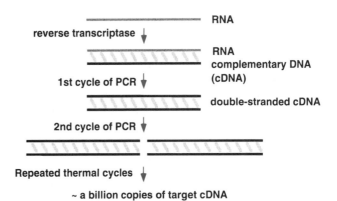

➤ **FIGURE 33–6** The reverse transcriptase polymerase chain reaction (rtPCR) procedure is a method for detecting a particular RNA transcript. First, RNA serves as a template for construction of complementary DNA (cDNA) by the enzyme reverse transcriptase. Then routine PCR is done to convert the cDNA of interest to a double-stranded sequence and to amplify that sequence so that it may be readily detected or further analyzed. This procedure is a sensitive, specific, and rapid means of amplifying disease-associated RNA in a patient sample.

3. Detect minimal residual disease in cancer patients following therapy by using rtPCR to amplify tumor-specific fusion transcripts. Such an approach has been used to predict relapse of chronic myelogenous leukemia or acute promyelocytic leukemia.[13]
4. Detect foreign organisms using probes targeting abundantly transcribed sequences or targeting viruses having RNA genomes. Examples of RNA viruses include human immunodeficiency virus (HIV), human T-lymphotropic virus type 1 (HTLV1), and hepatitis C virus (HCV).

Major Advantages

1. Sensitive to low numbers of target sequences.
2. Small sample size requirements compared to Northern blot analysis. (Northern blot analysis is an old and laborious technique for characterizing specific RNA molecules. In the Northern procedure, cellular RNA is electrophoresed, transferred to a membrane, and then hybridized to a complementary probe. This process is analogous to Southern blotting except that in the Southern blot technique, restriction enzyme digestion is not necessary because RNA is much smaller than genomic DNA. The Southern technique was first described by Dr. Edwin Southern,[37] and the term *Northern* is a pun on his name.)

Major Disadvantages

1. RNA is labile and, therefore, all RNA-based testing requires meticulous care to avoid degradation by RNases.
2. Extreme precautions are required to avoid contamination of samples or reagents by extraneous RNA, cDNA, or products of previous reactions. Physical separation of pre- and postamplification work areas is recommended.[38]

In Situ Hybridization to Cells or Tissues Immobilized on Glass Slides

Purpose The purpose of in situ hybridization is to localize DNA or RNA to particular cells in a tissue section immobilized on a glass slide.

Procedure Cells or tissue sections are immobilized on glass slides. Fresh cells or frozen sections are then fixed by immersion in 95% ethanol, whereas paraffin sections are immersed in xylene to diminish the amount of paraffin. Next, protease treatment permeabilizes cell membranes, allowing the target DNA or RNA to become accessible for hybridization. A hybridization mixture is applied that contains labeled probes (20 to 2000 bases in length) complementary to the sequence of interest. The slides are incubated for several hours at a temperature that optimizes specific hybridization of probe to target. Unbound probe is washed away, and bound probe is then detected using an appropriate signal detection method. Counterstaining permits microscopic visualization of the target nucleic acid in the context of histologic features and cytologic detail (Fig. 33–7).

Sample Requirements Fresh blood, marrow, or body fluid from which nucleated cells have been isolated; frozen tissue; or fixed paraffin-embedded tissue.

Method Variation for Flow Cytometric Analysis In a variation of this technique, fresh cells in suspension are made

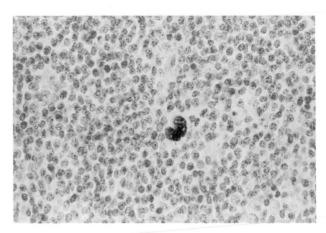

▶ **FIGURE 33–7** The in situ hybridization technique permits visualization of nucleic acid in tissue sections on glass slides. In this example, hybridization to Epstein-Barr virus EBER transcripts reveals that the viral gene product is localized to the nucleus of a Reed-Sternberg cell in a case of Hodgkin's disease. In contrast, the background lymphocytes stain only with methyl green counterstain.

permeable and then hybridized to a probe complementary to the target sequence. The probe is labeled with a fluorochrome that fluoresces in response to an input light. This signal can be detected and quantitated by flow cytometry.

Assay Time Approximately 2 days.

Sensitivity Moderate. (Theoretically, one target is sufficient, but in practice most users report difficulty detecting single-copy targets.)

Specificity High.

Cost per Test Approximately $100 if only one sample is analyzed, less for batched samples.

Clinical Applications

1. Determine the disease-related location of foreign organisms. This is especially important for pathogens that might also exist as "normal flora," such as cytomegalovirus or Epstein-Barr virus.[10]
2. Detect and localize gene expression by targeting RNA transcripts.[39]

Major Advantages

1. Permits the visualization of target nucleic acid in the context of cytologic and morphological features.
2. Sensitive to low numbers of affected cells in the sample.
3. Relatively fast results (about 2 days).

Major Disadvantage It is difficult to obtain adequate sensitivity for detecting rare targets. The assay works best for high copy number targets such as abundant RNA transcripts (e.g., EBER transcripts of Epstein-Barr virus) or abundant viral genomes (e.g., human papillomavirus in cervical carcinomas).

Fluorescence In Situ Hybridization

Purpose The purpose of fluorescence in situ hybridization (FISH) is to detect and localize specific DNA sequences in G-banded metaphase chromosomes using a probe labeled in such a way that it fluoresces in response to an input light. One option is a double hybridization in which one probe fluoresces green and another probe fluoresces red, thus allowing definitive identification of a particular translocation or deletion. Another option is hybridization to multiple probes at sites spread along the full length of a chromosome, so-called chromosome painting. Paint of a different color can be applied to each chromosome to permit evaluation of complex karyotypes.

Procedure Metaphase spreads of chromosomes are prepared on glass slides using the same methods that are employed in routine karyotyping. The chromosomal DNA is denatured and allowed to hybridize to a labeled probe complementary to the sequence of interest. Unbound probe is washed away, and the bound probe targeting the sequence of interest is visualized under a fluorescence microscope. Counterstaining with 4,6-diamidino-2-phenylindole (DAPI) permits visualization of all chromosomes (Fig. 33–8).

Sample Requirements Fresh cells capable of mitosis.

Assay Time Approximately 1 to 2 days.

Sensitivity High (1 target is sufficient).

Specificity High.

Cost per Test Approximately $100 if only one sample is analyzed, less for batched samples. This cost does not include culture, preparation of the metaphase spreads, or karyotyping.

Major Advantage FISH permits visualization of target DNA in the context of karyotypic visualization of metaphase chromosomes. This is helpful in identifying gross structural alterations that may be difficult to define by standard chromosomal G-banding techniques.[40] As an example, DiGeorge syndrome is usually characterized by small deletions of chromosome 22 that can be detected with molecular probes but are difficult to visualize on routinely prepared karyotypes.

Major Disadvantages

1. Metaphase analysis requires live cells capable of entering mitosis.
2. Visualization of fluorochromes requires input light source, and the fluorochrome fades with time.

➤ PROBE PRODUCTION

Where do DNA probes come from? Short DNA probes (less than 40 bp) can be synthesized in vitro and are readily available at reasonable prices from commercial suppliers. Longer probes are derived from cloned genomic DNA. Cloning is the process by which segments of human DNA are recombined with foreign "vector" DNA to produce "recombinant DNA." Vectors are capable of self-replicating inside bacteria. By culturing bacteria containing vector DNA hitched to a particular DNA segment of interest, one can generate millions of copies of that segment. The DNA segments can then be isolated, labeled, and dissociated into their single-stranded components to form a probe (Fig. 33–9).

An alternative process of generating short probes is by PCR amplification. In this way, multiple copies of the desired DNA sequence are generated, and these copies can be labeled and dissociated into their single-stranded components to form usable probes.

RNA probes (also known as Riboprobes) are generated from DNA templates in specialized recombinant vectors. These vectors contain transcription initiation start sites that are recognized by RNA polymerase, the enzyme that is responsible for transcribing DNA to RNA. Thousands of RNA probes can be made from a single DNA template. RNA probes are labeled during their synthesis by incorporating labeled ribonucleotides.

The optimum conditions for specific hybridization of probe to target depend on several factors, including the reaction temperature, the concentration of salt and formamide in the hybridization solution, the length of the probe and its proportion of G-C versus A-T bases, and the DNA versus RNA nature of the probe and target. For each hybridization assay, reaction conditions should be optimized so that the probe preferentially binds to its intended target rather than "cross-hybridizing" with partially matched sequences.

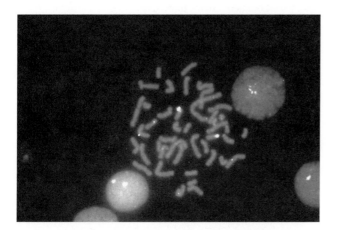

➤ **FIGURE 33–8** Fluorescence in situ hybridization (FISH) analysis helps in the diagnosis of DiGeorge syndrome, a congenital form of immunodeficiency caused by partial deletion of chromosome 22. In the example shown here, bright fluorescent signals identify the two number 22 chromosomes from among the 46 chromosomes in a cell. The DiGeorge probe and a control probe are visible on the normal chromosome 22 (*center*); however, only the control probe is seen on the other chromosome 22 (*lower right*), consistent with a deletion of DNA from the DiGeorge region. (Photomicrograph courtesy of Charleen Moore, PhD, University of Texas Health Science Center at San Antonio.)

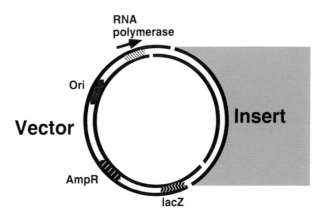

➤ **FIGURE 33–9** Vectors are vehicles for capturing and replicating specific DNA sequences. The process of using a vector to capture and manipulate a particular DNA segment is called *recombinant DNA technology*. The recombined vector/insert DNA can then be replicated inside bacterial hosts using natural cellular machinery. Specialized features built into the vector assist in tracking and controlling the vector and insert. Examples of vectors include plasmids, cosmids, and artificial chromosomes, the latter of which can hold extremely large segments of DNA (i.e., 300 kb). These vectors permit production of abundant, homogeneous probes.

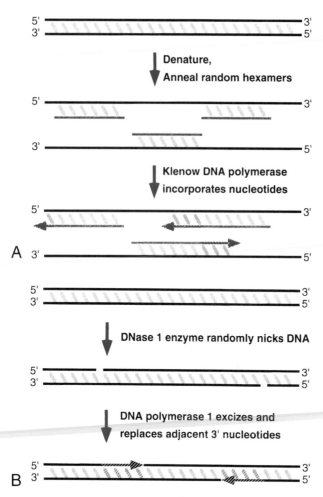

5'　3'

Denature,
Anneal random hexamers

5'　3'

3'　5'

Klenow DNA polymerase
incorporates nucleotides

5'　3'

A　3'　5'

5'　3'
3'　5'

DNase 1 enzyme randomly nicks DNA

5'　3'
3'　5'

DNA polymerase 1 excises and
replaces adjacent 3' nucleotides

5'　3'
B　3'　5'

➤ **FIGURE 33–10** DNA probes are labeled by incorporating radioisotopes or nonisotopic markers into their nucleotide strands. *A.* The random primer method capitalizes on the ability of Klenow DNA polymerase to synthesize new complementary strands of DNA starting at the free 3' ends, where "hexamers" (6 base probes of random sequence) have bound to the probe template. Addition of labeled nucleotides to the reaction mixture results in incorporation of the label into the newly synthesized DNA. *B.* The nick translation method of probe labeling relies on the ability of the enzyme DNase 1 to randomly nick the backbone of DNA. Then the enzyme DNA polymerase 1 recognizes and repairs each nick, and subsequently proceeds to replace adjacent 3' nucleotides with new ones. In this way, labeled nucleotides can be incorporated into the newly synthesized DNA.

➤ PROBE LABELS

To be useful as probes, nucleic acid fragments must be labeled in a way that is detectable following hybridization. Probes can be labeled either during their synthesis by incorporating labeled nucleotides or after their synthesis by chemically attaching labels. The labels that are most commonly used in clinical laboratories include biotin, digoxigenin, and radioisotopes.

Radioisotopes such as ^{32}P are famous for their remarkable sensitivity. They are detected by either autoradiography or a scintillation counter. Major disadvantages include their short shelf-life, high disposal costs, and the need for strict radiation safety precautions. Nevertheless, many diagnostic laboratories still use radioisotopes, particularly when sensitivity is critical to assay performance.

Biotin and digoxigenin are practical alternatives to radioisotopes. Biotin labels are recognized by avidin conjugates

in an analogous fashion to the immunochemical use of avidin-biotin conjugates. The conjugate most commonly used is alkaline phosphatase enzyme that is subsequently detected by adding a colorimetric substrate. Unlike biotin, which is a natural substance, digoxigenin is a synthetic chemical, so it is not prone to the background problems that sometimes hamper biotin reactions. Digoxigenin labels are recognized by a specific antibody carrying an alkaline phosphatase conjugate. Alkaline phosphatase catalyzes a colorimetric or chemiluminescent reaction that signals its location (see Fig. 33–2).

There are several methods for incorporating labels into probes, and commercial kits are available for each of the methods mentioned here. The most popular method of labeling a DNA probe is called *random priming.* Another is *nick translation.* Both of these procedures are suitable for labeling large DNA probes (Fig. 33–10). In contrast, short DNA probes (i.e., oligonucleotides) are efficiently labeled by a method called *end labeling,* which uses the enzyme T4 polynucleotide kinase to add labeled nucleotides to the 5' end of the probe.

➤ FUTURE PROSPECTS OF MOLECULAR ASSAYS

DNA technology is a powerful new tool for laboratory diagnosis, and tremendous advancements are expected in the coming years. Indeed, increasing numbers of probe-based kits are being approved by the Food and Drug Administration (FDA) for use in clinical laboratories. Among these are kits for evaluating tumor-specific translocations and lymphoid gene rearrangements, and kits to detect the DNA or RNA of infectious organisms.

Technological improvements will undoubtedly result in faster, less expensive, and more quantitative methods of probe analysis. At the same time, new discoveries related to the genetic basis of human disease are fostering development of even more probe tests for various disease states. It seems likely that this technology will revolutionize laboratory diagnosis of many diseases.

QUESTIONS

1. To convert double-stranded DNA into its single-stranded components, which of the following procedures may be used?
   a. Heat DNA to 95°C
   b. Expose the DNA to an alkaline pH
   c. Either of the above
   d. Neither of the above

2. Which of the following assays is most appropriate for routine clinical detection of the point mutation responsible for sickle cell anemia?
   a. In situ hybridization
   b. Fluorescence in situ hybridization
   c. Cloning
   d. Southern blot analysis

3. Which statement is true about the polymerase chain reaction (PCR)?
   a. It is a method for amplifying a particular segment of DNA.

b. The DNA polymerase that is used as a reagent in this assay cuts DNA into many fragments.

c. It is labor-intensive and expensive compared with Southern blot analysis.

d. The assay does not require any probes; therefore, you need not know anything about the sequence of the target DNA.

4. Which of the following are reasonable probe labels?
   a. Digoxigenin
   b. Biotin
   c. ^{32}P radioisotope
   d. All of the above

5. Which of the following tumor types is most likely to exhibit clonal immunoglobulin gene rearrangement?
   a. Acute myelogenous leukemia
   b. B-cell lymphoma
   c. Human T-lymphotropic virus type 1 (HTLV1)–related leukemia
   d. Chronic myelogenous leukemia

6. The following are steps in the Southern blot procedure except:
   a. Agarose gel electrophoresis
   b. Cut DNA with restriction endonuclease
   c. Synthesize DNA at 72°C
   d. DNA extraction

7. Which of the following chemicals is used to stain DNA in agarose gels?
   a. EcoR1
   b. Ethidium bromide
   c. Ethanol
   d. Formalin

8. Which of the following is true about the function of restriction endonucleases?
   a. They function to replicate DNA in the polymerase chain reaction.
   b. They incorporate labeled nucleotides in the nick translation procedure.
   c. They cut DNA at specific recognition sequences in the Southern blot procedure.
   d. They permeabilize cell membranes during in situ hybridization.

9. Which is true of the in situ hybridization procedure for analyzing paraffin tissue sections immobilized on glass slides?
   a. It localizes DNA or RNA in the context of histologic and cytologic features.
   b. It detects restriction fragment length polymorphisms.
   c. It amplifies sequences up to 5000 nucleotides in length.
   d. All of the above

10. Which of the following probes would be most appropriate for an assay in which you want to target the following DNA sequence, 5'-AAAGGGTCTCTCTTTTGGG-3'?

    a. 3'-GGGAAACTCTCTCCCCAAA-5'
    b. 5'-TTTCCCAGAGAGAAAACCC-3'
    c. 3'-TTTCCCAGAGAGAAAACCC-5'
    d. 5'-GGGAAACTCTCTCCCCAAA-3'

11. In setting up a series of PCR reactions on patient samples, it is wise to add a control tube that contains all of the reagents necessary for DNA amplification except for target DNA. What is the purpose of this control tube?
    a. To ensure that no reagent was left out of the experiment
    b. To ensure that there are no inhibitors of DNA amplification
    c. To show that PCR products can be generated under the conditions used
    d. To check for contamination of reagents by extraneous DNA

SUMMARY CHART

➤ Deoxyribonucleic acid (DNA) is a double-stranded molecule composed of long sequences of nucleotides. In the laboratory, the two strands of DNA can be denatured into single-stranded components.

➤ A DNA probe is a segment of single-stranded DNA that is complementary to the sequence of interest.

➤ All nucleated cells of the body contain the same set of genes, although any given cell expresses only a small fraction of those genes.

➤ Inherited disease results from genetic defects that are passed down from parent(s). In contrast, cancer results from acquired genetic defects that permit rampant cell growth. Molecular diagnostics tests are designed to detect these genetic defects.

➤ Each type of infectious organism has its own unique genome, and molecular diagnostic tests can be used to detect foreign pathogens in human tissues.

➤ DNA or ribonucleic acid (RNA) is the substrate for molecular diagnostic tests. DNA and RNA can be extracted from any tissue or body fluid.

➤ Southern blot analysis relies on the use of restriction enzymes to cut DNA at specific sequence-recognition sites. Restriction fragment length is altered by genetic defects, thus allowing detection of those defects using the Southern blot procedure.

➤ Polymerase chain reaction (PCR) is a method of DNA amplification that is capable of producing 1 billion copies of a particular segment of double-stranded DNA. This amplified DNA must be detected or further analyzed to generate useful data on the disease of interest.

➤ RNA can be converted to cDNA, which can then be subjected to PCR amplification.

➤ Quantitative PCR is used to measure the amount of target DNA in a patient sample. Quantitation of a particular gene sequence allows us to monitor the associated disease during therapy (e.g., measure tumor burden after treatment, or calculate viral load to evaluate the efficacy of antiviral drug regimens).

➤ In situ hybridization is a means of localizing target DNA or RNA to a particular histologic lesion that is visualized under the microscope.

➤ Fluorescence in situ hybridization enhances karyotyping by using labeled probes to visualize a particular segment of DNA within whole chromosomes.

➤ Probes are commonly labeled with biotin, digoxigenin, or ^{32}P. Labeling allows the probe to be tracked and detected following hybridization to patient nucleic acid.

ACKNOWLEDGMENTS

Polymerase chain reaction patents are owned and licensed by Roche Molecular Systems, Inc. Riboprobe is a registered trademark of the Promega Corporation.

References

1. Ross, DW: The human genome: Information content and structure. Hosp Pract 34:49, 1999.
2. Ross, DW: Introduction to Molecular Medicine, ed 3. Springer, New York, 2001.
3. Jorde, LB, et al: Medical Genetics, ed 2. Mosby, St Louis, 1999.
4. Vnencak-Jones, CL: Molecular testing for inherited diseases. Am J Clin Pathol 112(Suppl):S19, 1999.
5. Cao, A, et al: Molecular diagnosis and carrier screening for beta thalassemia. 278:1273, 1997.
6. Bacon, BR, et al: HFE genotype in patients with hemochromatosis and other liver diseases. Ann Intern Med 130:953, 1999.
7. Lutz, CT, et al: Multicenter evaluation of PCR methods for the detection of factor V Leiden (R506Q) genotypes. Clin Chem 44:1356, 1998.
8. Poort, SR, et al: A common genetic variation in the 3'-untranslated region of the prothrombin gene is associated with elevated plasma prothrombin levels and an increase in venous thrombosis. Blood 88:3698, 1996.
9. Dumler, JS, and Valsamakis, A: Molecular diagnostics for existing and emerging infections. Complementary tools for a new era of clinical microbiology. Am J Clin Pathol 112(Suppl):S33, 1999.
10. Gulley, ML: Molecular diagnosis of related diseases. J Molec Diagnostics 3:1, 2001.
11. Yamaguchi, K, et al: DNA diagnosis of HTLV-I. Intervirology 39:158, 1996.
12. Ross, DW: Introduction to Oncogenes and Molecular Cancer Medicine. Springer, New York, 1998.
13. Radich, JP, et al: Polymerase chain reaction detection of the BCR-ABL fusion transcript after allogeneic marrow transplantation for chronic myeloid leukemia: Results and implications in 346 patients. Blood 85:2632, 1995.
14. Blennerhassett, GT, et al: Clinical evaluation of a DNA probe assay for the Philadelphia (Ph1) translocation in chronic myelogenous leukemia. Leukemia 2:648, 1988.
15. Miller, WH, Jr, et al: Detection of minimal residual disease in acute promyelocytic leukemia by a reverse transcription polymerase chain reaction assay for the PML/RAR-alpha fusion mRNA. Blood 82:1689, 1993.
16. Lo Coco, F, et al: Genetic diagnosis and molecular monitoring in the management of acute promyelocytic leukemia. Blood 94:12, 1999.
17. Gribben, JG, and Schultze, JL: The detection of minimal residual disease: Implications for bone marrow transplantation. Cancer Treat Res 77:99, 1997.
18. Bagg, A, and Kallakury, BV: Molecular pathology of leukemia and lymphoma. Am J Clin Pathol 112(Suppl):S76, 1999.
19. Look, AT: Oncogenic transcription factors in the human acute leukemias. Science 278:1059, 1997.
20. Ausubel, FM: Current Protocols in Molecular Biology. Greene Publ Assoc; Wiley Interscience, New York, 1999.
21. Killeen, A: Molecular Pathology Protocols. Humana Press, Totowa, NJ, 2001.
22. Anonymous: Association for Molecular Pathology statement. Recommendations for in-house development and operation of molecular diagnostic tests. Am J Clin Pathol 111:449, 1999.
23. Farkas, DH: Molecular Biology and Pathology: A Guidebook for Quality Control. Academic Press, San Diego, CA, 1993.
24. Coleman, WB, and Tsongalis, GJ: Molecular Diagnostics for the Clinical Laboratorian. Humana Press, Totowa, NJ, 1997.
25. Farkas, DH, et al: Specimen collection and storage for diagnostic molecular pathology investigation. Arch Pathol Lab Med 120:591, 1996.
26. Saiki, RK, et al: Enzymatic amplification of beta-globin genomic sequences and restriction site analysis for diagnosis of sickle cell anemia. Science 230:1350, 1985.
27. Cossman, J, et al: Gene rearrangements in the diagnosis of lymphoma/leukemia. Guidelines for use based on a multiinstitutional study. Am J Clin Pathol 95:347, 1991.
28. Gill, JI, and Gulley, ML: Immunoglobulin and T-cell receptor gene rearrangement. Hematol Oncol Clin North Am 8:751, 1994.
29. Weedn, VW: Forensic DNA tests. Clin Lab Med 16:187, 1996.
30. Mullis, KB, and Faloona, FA: Specific synthesis of DNA in vitro via a polymerase-catalyzed chain reaction. Methods Enzymol 155:335, 1987.
31. Wiedbrauk, DL: Molecular methods for virus detection. Lab Med 23:737, 1992.
32. Kreuzer, KA, et al: LightCycler technology for the quantitation of bcr/abl fusion transcripts. Cancer Res 59:3171, 1999.
33. Segal, GH, et al: Optimal primer selection for clonality assessment by polymerase chain reaction analysis: I. Low grade B-cell lymphoproliferative disorders of nonfollicular center cell type. Hum Pathol 25:1269, 1994.
34. Segal, GH, et al: Optimal primer selection for clonality assessment by polymerase chain reaction analysis: II. Follicular lymphomas. Hum Pathol 25:1276, 1994.
35. Lombardo, JF, et al: Optimal primer selection for clonality assessment by polymerase chain reaction analysis. III. Intermediate and high-grade B-cell neoplasms. Hum Pathol 27:373, 1996.
36. Tsongalis, GJ, et al: Applications of forensic identity testing in the clinical laboratory. Am J Clin Pathol 112 (Suppl):S93, 1999.
37. Southern, EM: Detection of specific sequences among DNA fragments separated by gel electrophoresis. J Mol Biol 98:503, 1975.
38. Kwok, S, and Higuchi, R: Avoiding false positives with PCR. Nature 339:237, 1989.
39. Jin, L, and Lloyd, RV: In situ hybridization: Methods and applications. J Clin Lab Anal 11:2, 1997.
40. Fletcher, JA: DNA in situ hybridization as an adjunct in tumor diagnosis. Am J Clin Pathol 112(Suppl):S11, 1999.

Answers to Chapter Review Questions

Chapter 1
1. d
2. a
3. a
4. b
5. c
6. d
7. b
8. c
9. b
10. b
11. d
12. d

Chapter 2
1. c
2. b
3. a
4. c
5. a
6. c
7. d
8. c
9. d
10. b

Chapter 3
1. c
2. c
3. a
4. b
5. d
6. b
7. d
8. c
9. a
10. b

Chapter 4
1. c
2. b
3. a
4. d
5. c
6. c
7. d
8. a
9. c

Chapter 5
1. c
2. b
3. d
4. c
5. d
6. a
7. a
8. b
9. d
10. b
11. b
12. c
13. b
14. a

Chapter 6
1. d
2. d
3. a
4. c
5. b
6. b
7. c
8. a
9. c
10. b
11. d
12. d
13. d

Chapter 7
1. b
2. c
3. b
4. c
5. c
6. a
7. d
8. d
9. b
10. d

Chapter 8
1. a
2. c
3. d
4. b
5. d
6. a
7. c
8. d
9. a
10. b
11. c
12. b
13. c
14. c
15. b

Chapter 9
1. b
2. d
3. c
4. a
5. b
6. c
7. b
8. b
9. a

Chapter 10
1. b
2. a
3. d
4. d
5. a
6. c

Chapter 11
1. c
2. d
3. a
4. b
5. d
6. d
7. b
8. d
9. c
10. d

Chapter 12
1. b
2. c
3. a
4. d
5. d
6. c
7. b
8. a
9. b
10. c
11. b
12. a

Chapter 13
1. d
2. d
3. d
4. a
5. a
6. c
7. d
8. b
9. d
10. d
11. b
12. c
13. a
14. b
15. a
16. c
17. c

Chapter 14
1. b
2. d
3. a
4. c
5. d
6. a
7. c
8. a
9. b
10. c

Chapter 15
1. c
2. a
3. b
4. c
5. d
6. d
7. a
8. c
9. a
10. d
11. c
12. b
13. c
14. b
15. d
16. d
17. d
18. a
19. d
20. c

Chapter 16
1. b
2. a
3. d
4. c
5. d
6. b
7. c

Chapter 17
1. b
2. c
3. d
4. a
5. b
6. c
7. a
8. c
9. a
10. d
11. a
12. b
13. a
14. b
15. a
16. e
17. e
18. b
19. e

Chapter 18
1. b
2. d
3. c
4. d
5. a
6. b
7. c
8. b
9. a
10. c
11. d
12. a
13. c
14. b
15. d

Chapter 19
1. c
2. d
3. c
4. c
5. d
6. b
7. b
8. b
9. a
10. b
11. b
12. b

Chapter 20
1. d
2. a
3. b
4. c
5. a
6. d
7. c
8. b
9. c
10. a

Chapter 21	Chapter 23	Chapter 25	Chapter 28	Chapter 30	8. **a**
1. **d**	1. **a**	1. **d**	1. **b**	1. **d**	9. **d**
2. **c**	2. **d**	2. **a**	2. **c**	2. **c**	10. **d**
3. **a**	3. **c**	3. **b**	3. **d**	3. **b** and **c**	11. **c**
4. **b**	4. **b**	4. **b**	4. **d**	4. **a**	12. **d**
5. **d**	5. **a**	5. **c**	5. **b**	5. **c**	13. **c**
6. **c**	6. **c**	6. **b**	6. **a**	6. **c**	14. **d**
7. **c**	7. **a**	7. **a**	7. **a**	7. **c**	
8. **c**	8. **b**	8. **c**	8. **a**	8. **c**	Chapter 32
9. **a**	9. **d**	9. **c**	9. **d**	9. **b**	1. **d**
10. **d**	10. **b**	10. **d**	10. **a**	10. **a**	2. **c**
11. **c**	11. **d**		11. **c**	11. **c**	3. **a**
12. **d**	12. **a**	Chapter 26	12. **b**	12. **b** and **c**	4. **b**
13. **d**	13. **b**	1. **c**	13. **c**	13. **a, b**, and **d**	5. **a**
14. **c**	14. **a**	2. **d**	14. **a**	14. **b**	6. **c**
15. **d**	15. **a**	3. **d**	15. **b**	15. **d**	7. **d**
16. **b**		4. **c**		16. **b**	8. **a**
17. **d**	Chapter 24	5. **b**	Chapter 29	17. **b**	9. **d**
18. **b**	1. **b**		1. **d**	18. **a** and **d**	10. **a**
19. **d**	2. **a**	Chapter 27	2. **a**	19. **b**	
20. **c**	3. **c**	1. **b**	3. **d**	20. **b**	Chapter 33
	4. **b**	2. **b**	4. **c**	21. **a** and **c**	1. **c**
Chapter 22	5. **d**	3. **a**	5. **b**	22. **b**	2. **d**
1. **a**	6. **c**	4. **a**	6. **c**	23. **a**	3. **a**
2. **c**	7. **a**	5. **b**	7. **b**		4. **d**
3. **b**	8. **c**	6. **d**	8. **c**	Chapter 31	5. **b**
4. **d**	9. **a**		9. **c**	1. **c**	6. **c**
5. **a**	10. **b**		10. **b**	2. **a**	7. **b**
6. **b**			11. **c**	3. **b**	8. **c**
7. **b**			12. **c**	4. **c**	9. **a**
8. **b**			13. **b**	5. **c**	10. **c**
9. **c**			14. **c**	6. **d**	11. **d**
10. **d**				7. **b**	

Glossary

Abetalipoproteinemia: A disorder in which the absence of beta lipoproteins manifests itself in mental retardation and impaired food absorption. Clinical manifestations include acanthocytes, retinitis pigmentosa, and excess fat in the stool.

Abruptio placenta: Premature detachment of normally situated placenta.

Acanthocyte: An abnormal red cell that is slightly reduced in size and that possesses 3 to 12 spicules of uneven length distributed along the periphery of the cell membrane.

Achlorhydria: Absence of free hydrochloric acid in the stomach.

Acholuria: Absence of bile pigments in urine, occurring when unconjugated bilirubin does not pass through the glomerular filter.

Acrocyanosis: Bluish tinge to the extremities.

Actin: A muscle protein that, in conjunction with myosin particles, facilitates expansion and contraction.

Activated partial thromboplastin time (APTT): A test to evaluate the overall integrity of the clotting system that involves factors XII, XI, IX, VIII, X, V, II, and I. Usually a means of evaluating the intrinsic system of coagulation.

Acute-phase reactant: Plasma protein, the concentration of which increases in response to a variety of stimuli.

Adenopathy: Swelling and morbid change in lymph nodes; glandular disease.

Adenosine diphosphate (ADP): A substance used to induce platelet aggregation that may be derived from injured tissues, erythrocytes, or platelets.

Adhesion: The molecular attraction exerted between the surfaces of bodies in contact (e.g., platelets to connective tissue structures).

Afibrinogenemia: A rare blood disease characterized by the absence of fibrinogen in the plasma; may be congenital or acquired.

Agammaglobulinemia: A rare disorder in which there is a virtual absence of gamma globulins.

Agglutination: The clumping together of red blood cells or any particulate matter resulting from interaction of antibody and its corresponding antigen.

Aggregation: A clustering or clumping together (e.g., platelet aggregation, which plays a critical role in hemostasis).

Agnogenic dyspoiesis: A preleukemic disorder of unknown origin characterized by hypercellular marrow and abnormal cell maturation.

Agranulocytosis: An acute disease in which the white cell count is markedly reduced and neutropenia becomes pronounced.

Alkaline phosphatase: An enzyme that is found in a number of tissues but is chiefly used in connection with diagnosis of bone and liver disease. The granules of normal granulocytic cells contain alkaline phosphatase; patients with chronic myelogenous leukemia (CML) have decreased phosphatase activity.

Alkalosis: Excessive alkalinity of body fluids, owing to accumulation of alkalis or reduction of acids.

Allele: One of several alternate forms of a gene. In a particular person's genome, there are usually two alleles for each gene, one inherited from the mother and the other from the father. Any differences between alleles of the same gene may be referred to as *polymorphisms*.

Alloantibody: An antibody produced by an immune response that was stimulated by a foreign antigen.

Allograft: Tissue transplantation between individuals of the same species.

Alloimmunization: The process in which a patient develops antibodies to foreign or white blood cell antigen(s), or both, through transfusion or pregnancy.

Alopecia: Baldness.

Alpha (α) chain: A type of globin chain found in hemoglobin and coded for by the α gene.

Alpha methyldopa (Aldomet): A common drug used to treat hypertension; frequently the cause of a positive direct Coombs' test result.

Amaurotic: Caused by the atrophy of the optic nerve or vision centers.

Ameliorate: Moderate, improve.

Amniocentesis: Transabdominal puncture of the amniotic sac, using a needle and syringe to remove amniotic fluid. The material may then be studied to detect genetic disorders or maternal-fetal blood incompatibility.

Amphophilic: Having an affinity for acid or basic dyes, or both.

Amyloidosis: A metabolic disorder marked by extracellular deposition of amyloid (an abnormal protein) in the tissues; this usually leads to loss of function and organ enlargement.

Anamnestic (response): An accentuated antibody response following a secondary exposure to an antigen. Antibody levels from the initial exposure are not detectable in the patient's serum until the secondary exposure, when a rapid rise in antibody titer is observed.

Anaphylaxis: An allergic hypersensitivity reaction of the body to a foreign protein or drug.

Ancillary: Auxiliary, supplementary.

Androgenic: Causing masculinization.

Anemia: A condition in which there is reduced oxygen delivery to the tissues. It may result from increased destruction of red cells, excessive blood loss, or decreased production of red cells.

  Aplastic a.: A type of anemia caused by aplasia of bone marrow or its destruction by chemical agents or physical factors.

  Autoimmune hemolytic a.: An acquired disorder characterized by premature erythrocyte destruction owing to abnormalities in the individual's own immune system.

  Diamond-Blackfan a.: A congenital pure red blood cell aplasia characterized by severe chronic anemia, which manifests early in infancy and is associated with normal white cells and platelets.

  Fanconi's a.: A congenital aplastic anemia associated with genetic anomalies. Untreated patients with Fanconi's anemia usually die secondary to infections or hemorrhage.

  Hemolytic a.: A type of anemia caused by hemolysis of red blood cells resulting in reduction of normal red cell life span.

  Hypoplastic a.: A normochromic, normocytic anemia of bone marrow failure that may be idiopathic, congenital, or caused by chemical agents.

  Iron-deficiency a.: Anemia resulting from a greater demand on stored iron than can be met.

  Megaloblastic a.: Anemia in which megaloblasts are found in the blood; usually caused by a deficiency of folic acid or vitamin B_{12}.

  Microangiopathic hemolytic a.: A hemolytic process associated with thrombotic thrombocytopenic purpura (TTP), prosthetic heart valve, and burns. It is visualized in the peripheral blood smear by fragmentation of the red cells and other bizarre morphology.

  Pernicious a.: A type of megaloblastic anemia caused by a deficiency of vitamin B_{12} that is directly linked to absence of intrinsic factor (IF).

  Sickle cell a.: See **Sickle cell anemia.**

  Sideroblastic a.: A disorder in which iron is not being incorporated into heme and serum iron levels are elevated. The bone marrow is hyperplastic and contains iron-laden sideroblasts.

Aneuploidy: Having an abnormal number of chromosomes.

Angina pectoris: Severe pain and constriction about the heart caused by insufficient supply of blood to the heart.

Anisochromia: The state of being not of uniform color.

Anisocytosis: Variation in the size of erythrocytes when observed on a peripheral blood smear.

Ankyrin: A pyramid-shaped protein that is a major component of the red cell cytoskeleton.

Annealing: The process by which a probe (or oligonucleotide primer in polymerase chain reactions [PCR] reactions) binds to its complementary single-stranded target sequence.

Annexin II: An endothelial cell phospholipid that binds tissue plasminogen activator (t-PA) and plasminogen. Increased concentration is noted on leukemic promyelocytes.

Anoxia: The state of being without oxygen.

Antenatal: Occurring before birth.

Antibody: A protein substance developed in response to, and interacting specifically with, an antigen. In blood banking, it is found in serum, from either a commercial manufacturer or a patient. It is secreted by plasma cells.

> **Cross-reacting a.:** An antibody that reacts with antigens functionally similar to its specific antigen.

> **Maternal a.:** An antibody produced in the mother and transferred to the fetus in utero.

> **Naturally occurring a.:** An antibody present in a patient without known prior exposure to the corresponding red cell antigen.

Antibody screen: Testing the patient's serum with group O reagent red cells in an effort to detect atypical antibodies.

Anticoagulant: An agent that delays or prevents blood coagulation.

Antigen: A substance that is recognized by the body as being foreign and that, therefore, can elicit an immune response.

Antiglobulin test (AGT) or antihuman globulin (AHG) test: A test to ascertain the presence or absence of red cell coating by immunoglobulin (IgG) or complement, or both.

> **Direct AGT (DAT):** Used to detect in vivo cell sensitization

> **Indirect AGT (IAT):** Used to detect antigen-antibody reactions that occur in vitro.

Antihemophilic factor (AHF): A commercially prepared source of factor VIII. (See also **Hemophilia A.**)

Antihuman serum: An antibody prepared in rabbits or other suitable animals that is directed against human immunoglobulin or complement, or both. It is used to perform the antiglobulin test (AGT) or Coombs' test. The serum may be either polyspecific (anti-IgG plus anticomplement) or monospecific (anti-IgG or anticomplement).

Antiplasmin: Plasma proteins that are known to neutralize free plasmin: α_2-antiplasmin, α_2-macroglobulin.

> **α_2-a.:** The major inhibitor of plasmin.

Antipyretic: An agent that reduces fever.

Antiseptic: Preventing decay, putrefaction, or sepsis.

Antithrombin: A substance that opposes the action of thrombin and thus prevents or inhibits coagulation of blood.

Antithrombin III (AT-III): A naturally occurring inhibitor of coagulation responsible for neutralizing the activity of thrombin; factors IXa, Xa, and XIa; and plasmin. (Also known as the *heparin cofactor*.)

Anuria: Absence of urine formation.

Apheresis: A method of blood collection in which whole blood is withdrawn, a desired component separated and retained, and the remainder of the blood returned to the donor. (See also **Plateletpheresis; Plasmapheresis.**)

Aplasia: Failure of an organ or tissue to develop normally.

Apoptosis: The natural process of programmed cell death.

Ascites: The accumulation of serous fluid in the peritoneal cavity.

Asphyxia: A condition caused by insufficient intake of oxygen.

Asplenism: The state of being without a spleen.

Asthenic: Weak, caused by a muscular or cerebellar disease.

Asynchrony: The failure of events to occur in time with each other as they usually do. In hematology, nuclear and cytoplasmic development are mismatched.

Atypical lymphocyte: A benign reactive change in the morphological appearance of the lymphocyte, which is frequently secondary to a viral disease (e.g., infectious mononucleosis).

Auer rod: A rod-shaped alignment of primary granules that is present only in the cytoplasm of myeloblasts and monoblasts in leukemic states.

Autohemolysis: Hemolysis of an individual's blood corpuscles by his or her own serum.

Autoimmune: Referring to the production of antibodies directed against one's own tissues, usually in association with a disease state.

Autoimmune hemolytic anemia (AIHA): An abnormality of the immune system resulting in production of antibodies against self, which occurs because of failure of the mechanism regulating the immune response.

Autologous: Of the self.

Autosomal: Relating to any of the chromosomes other than the sex (X and Y) chromosomes.

Autosplenectomy: Formation of a fibrotic, nonfunctioning spleen caused by restrictive blood flow to the organ; often seen in sickle cell anemia.

Azotemia: The presence of increased amounts of urea in the blood.

Azurophilic granules: Primary granules.

Babesiosis: A rare, often severe and sometimes fatal disease of humans caused by the protozoan parasite of the red blood cells, *Babesia microti,* and perhaps other *Babesia* species.

Band: An immature neutrophilic granulocyte with a horseshoe- or sausage-shaped nucleus (also called a *stab*). It makes up 2% to 6% of the normal differential count.

Base pair: A nucleotide pair of A and T, or G and C, in double-stranded DNA. The length of a DNA sequence is measured in base pairs (bp), or in thousands of base pairs = kilobases (kb).

Basophil: A mature white blood cell whose cytoplasmic granules stain deep bluish-purple with basic dyes such as methylene blue. It makes up 0% to 2% of the normal differential count.

Basophilia: An absolute increase in basophils.

Basophilic normoblast: An immature red cell precursor found only in the bone marrow that is characterized by a vivid blue cytoplasm and a high nuclear-to-cytoplasmic ratio. (Synonym: **Prorubricyte.**)

Basophilic stippling: A red blood cell inclusion that consists of precipitated ribonucleoprotein and mitochondrial remnants. Stippling may be fine, coarse, or punctate and is seen in toxic states such as lead poisoning, severe bacterial infection, and drug exposure.

B cell: Named for the site of lymphopoiesis in the chicken (the bursa of Fabricius). In humans, B cells differentiate into plasma cells from lymphoid stem cells of the marrow.

Bernard-Soulier syndrome: A congenital bleeding disorder characterized by the presence of large platelets, thrombocytopenia of varying degrees, and a prolonged bleeding time.

Beta (β) chain: A type of globin chain found in hemoglobin that is coded for by the β gene.

Betke-Kleihauer technique: An acid elution test used to quantitate the amount of fetal hemoglobin present. Fetal hemoglobin is more resistant than adult hemoglobin to elution at acid pH during this procedure, and stains red.

Bilirubin: The orange or yellowish pigment in bile that is carried to the liver by the blood. It is produced from hemoglobin of red blood cells by reticuloendothelial cells in the bone marrow, spleen, and elsewhere.

> **Direct b.:** The conjugated water-soluble form of bilirubin.

> **Indirect b.:** The unconjugated water-insoluble form of bilirubin.

Bilirubinemia: A pathologic condition in which excessive destruction of red blood cells occurs, increasing the amount of bilirubin found in the blood.

Bite cells: Cells in which the removal of a portion of membrane has left a permanent indentation in the remaining cell membrane.

Blackwater fever: Hemoglobinuria following chronic falciparum malaria infection.

Bleeding time: A test used to evaluate the hemostatic role of platelets in vivo.

Bradykinin: A plasma kinin.

Buffy coat: The layer of leukocytes and platelets lying directly on top of the red cell layer seen after sedimentation or centrifugation.

Burr cells (echinocytes): Red cells with approximately 10 to 30 spicules evenly distributed over the surface of the cell.

Burst-forming unit committed to erythropoiesis (BFU-E): A primitive stem cell committed to erythropoiesis and thought to be a precursor to the colony-forming unit committed to erythropoiesis (CFU-E).

C1 esterase inhibitor: A protein in the blood that inhibits the activity of plasmin as well as the activity of C1 esterase in the complement pathway.

C3a: A biologically active fragment of the C3 molecule that demonstrates anaphylactic capabilities on liberation.

C3b: A biologically active fragment of the complement C3 molecule that is an opsonin and promotes immune adherence.

C3d: A biologically inactive fragment of the C3b complement component formed by inactivation by the C3b inactivator substance present in serum.

C4: A component of complement present in serum that participates in the classic pathway of complement activation.

C5a: A biologically active fragment of the C5 molecule that demonstrates anaphylactic capabilities as well as chemotactic properties upon liberation. This fragment has also been reported to be a potent aggregator of platelets.

Cabot's rings: A red blood cell inclusion resembling a figure 8. It is usually found in heavily stippled cells.

Cachexia: A condition that may result from chronic disease or certain malignancies whereby a state of malnutrition, weakness, and muscle wasting exists.

Calmodulin: A cytoplasmic calcium-binding protein.

Carcinoma: A neoplasm (new growth) or malignant tumor that occurs in epithelial tissue. A neoplasm can infiltrate or metastasize to any tissue or organ of the body.

Cardiac output: The amount of blood discharged from the left or right ventricle per minute.

Catecholamines: Biologically active amines, epinephrine, and norepinephrine, derived from the amino acid tyrosine. They have a marked effect on nervous and cardiovascular systems, metabolic rate, temperature, and smooth muscle.

cDNA (complementary DNA): Synthetic DNA produced from a messenger ribonucleic acid (mRNA) template by the enzyme reverse transcriptase.

Celiac: Related to the abdominal regions.

Celite: A substance that acts as a contact activator, causing the release or platelet factor 3 (PF3) and the activation of the intrinsic system.

Central venous pressure: The pressure within the superior vena cava, reflecting the pressure under which the blood is returned to the right atrium.

Centripetal: Moving toward the center.

Cerebriform: A word that is used to describe the brainlike convolutions of some nuclear chromatin material.

Chédiak-Higashi inclusions: Gigantic, fused lysosomal deposits seen in the cytoplasm of leukocytes.

Chelation: Combining of metallic ions with certain heterocyclic ring structures so that the ion is held by chemical bonds from each of the participating rings.

Chemokinesis: Increased activity of cells in the presence of a chemical attractant.

Chemotactic: Referring to the ability of white cells to move nondirectionally toward an attractant.

Chemotaxis: Describes movement toward a stimulus, particularly that displayed by phagocytic cells toward bacteria and sites of cell injury.

Cholecystectomy: Excision of a gallbladder.

Cholecystitis: Acute or chronic inflammation of the gallbladder.

Christmas factor: Plasma thromboplastin component (PTC); factor IX. It functions in the intrinsic system of coagulation.

Chromatin: A dark-staining substance located in the nucleus of the cell that contains the genetic material composed of DNA attached to a protein structure.

Chromogenic: Pigment-producing.

Circulating anticoagulants: Acquired pathologic plasma proteins that inhibit normal coagulation. The majority of these pathologic anticoagulants are inhibitors or autoantibodies of the IgG class whose inhibitory effects are directed against a specific factor or a complex of coagulation factors.

Coagulation: The process of stopping blood flow from a wound. This process involves the harmonious relationship of the blood-clotting factors, the blood vessels, and the fibrin-forming and fibrin-lysing system.

Coagulopathy: A disease affecting the blood-clotting process.

Cofactor: A factor that facilitates binding and accelerates enzymatic interaction of other coagulation factors with their target protein or substrate on an active biologic surface.

Collagen: A fibrous, insoluble protein found in the connective tissue, including skin, bone, ligaments, and cartilage; represents about 30% of the total body protein.

Colony-forming unit committed to erythropoiesis (CFU-E): A stem cell that is committed to forming cells of the red blood cell series.

Colony-forming unit–culture (CFU-C): Generation of stem cells using tissue culture methods. Current synonym is *CFU-GM,* which is a colony-forming unit committed to the production of myeloid cells (granulocytes and monocytes).

Complement: A series of proteins in the circulation that, when sequentially activated, cause disruption of bacterial and other cell membranes. Activation occurs via one of two pathways, and once activated, the components are involved in a great number of immune defense mechanisms, including anaphylaxis, chemotaxis, and phagocytosis. Red cell antibodies that activate complement may be capable of causing hemolysis.

Complement fixation (CF): An immunologic test that involves antigen combining with antibody and complement, causing inactivation of complement.

Congenital: Present at birth.

Consanguineous: Relationship by blood (i.e., being descended from a common ancestor).

Contiguous: In contact or closely associated with.

Convulsion: Involuntary muscle contraction and relaxation.

Cord cells: Fetal cells obtained from the umbilical cord at birth. They may be contaminated with Wharton's jelly.

Corticosteroid: Any of a number of hormonal steroid substances obtained from the cortex of the adrenal gland.

Coumarin drugs: Oral anticoagulants that act as vitamin K antagonists and result in depression of the concentration of prothrombin and factors VII, IX, and X; examples include warfarin (Coumadin) and dicumarol.

Counterelectrophoresis (CEP): An immunologic procedure involving electrophoretic movement of antigen and antibody, resulting in formation of a precipitin line.

Cryoglobulin: An abnormal protein in the blood that forms gels at low temperatures.

Cryoglobulinemia: An increase in the concentration of cryoglobulins in the blood.

Cryoprecipitate: A concentrated source of coagulation factor VIII that has been prepared from a single unit of donor blood. The product also contains fibrinogen, factor XIII, and von Willebrand's factor.

Cryoprotein: A protein circulating in the plasma or demonstrable in serum testing that precipitates on exposure to cold temperature.

Cryptococcosis: An infection caused by *Cryptococcus neoformans* that may affect the central nervous system with respect to the brain and meninges or the skin. It may also affect the spleen, liver, joints, and lungs.

Cyanosis: A slightly bluish or grayish discoloration of the skin caused by accumulation of reduced hemoglobin or deoxyhemoglobin in the blood as a result of oxygen deficiency or carbon dioxide buildup.

Cytochemistry: The microscopic study of the chemical constituents in cells, the purpose of which includes differentiation of cell types and assistance in the diagnosis of hematologic diseases.

Cytogenetics: The study of cytology in relation to genetics, especially the chromosomal behavior in mitosis and meiosis.

Cytokines: Growth factors, such as colony-stimulating factors and interleukins.

Cytomegalovirus (CMV): One of a group of species-specific herpesviruses.

Cytopenia: Abnormalities or deficiencies in blood cell elements.

Cytopheresis: A procedure using a machine by which one can selectively remove a particular cell type normally found in peripheral blood of a patient or donor.

Cytotoxicity: The ability to destroy.

Dacrocyte: See **Teardrop cell.**

Dactylitis: Painful swelling of the feet and hands.

Defibrinated: Deprived of fibrin (the conversion of fibrinogen into fibrin is the basis for the clotting of blood).

Delayed hemolytic transfusion reaction (DHTR): A hemolytic reaction that occurs when previously sensitized individuals have antibody levels that are undetectable and are once again exposed to the offending antigen(s). In most cases of DHTR the antibodies implicated are IgG.

Delta (δ) chain: A type of globin chain found in hemoglobin coded for by the δ gene.

Desferrioxamine: A substance obtained from certain bacteria that is used to chelate iron. This substance is used orally or parenterally in treating iron poisoning.

Diagnosis: The use of scientific and skillful methods to establish the cause and nature of a disease process.

Diapedesis: The journey of the blood cells (i.e., leukocytes) through the unruptured walls of a capillary.

Diaphoresis: Profuse sweating.

Differential: Microscopic examination of a stained blood smear to determine the relative number of each type of white blood cell; an estimate of white cell, red cell, and platelet counts; and an inspection of the morphology of red cells, white cells, and platelets.

Dimer: A compound formed by the combination of two identical molecules.

D-dimer: Degradation of cross-linked fibrin generated by plasmin.

Dimorphism: The existence of a two-cell population in the peripheral blood smear (e.g., few microcytes, few macrocytes; few hypochromic, few normochromic).

2,3-Diphosphoglycerate (2,3-DPG): An organic phosphate in red blood cells that alters the affinity of hemoglobin for oxygen. Blood cells stored in a blood bank lose 2,3-DPG, but once infused, the substance is resynthesized or reactivated.

Discocyte: See **Erythrocyte.**

Disseminated intravascular coagulation (DIC): A pathologic form of coagulation that is diffuse rather than localized, and is characterized by generalized bleeding and shock.

Diuresis: Secretion and passage of large amounts of urine.

Diuretic: An agent that increases the secretion of urine. Action is in one of two ways: by increasing glomerular filtration or by decreasing reabsorption from the tubules.

Diurnal: Occurring during the daytime.

Diverticulosis: Outpouching of the colon without inflammation or symptoms. There are many locations of diverticula, but all are saccular dilations protruding from the wall of a tubular organ.

DNA (deoxyribonucleic acid): The inherited substance that cells use to catalog, express, and propagate information. DNA is composed of two strands of nucleotides that wind around each other to form a double-stranded helix. The two nucleotide strands are held together by hydrogen bonds formed according to the following rules of complementary nucleotide pairing: G bonds with C, A bonds with T, and other combinations cannot bond. When cells divide, DNA is replicated and equally partitioned among the progeny such that each daughter cell contains a full complement of DNA known as the *genome.*

Döhle bodies: Single or multiple, round or oval, blue cytoplasmic inclusions (with Romanowsky stain) seen in neutrophils, usually associated with toxicity.

Donath-Landsteiner antibody test: A test usually performed in the blood bank to detect the presence of the Donath-Landsteiner antibody, which is a biphasic IgG antibody with anti-P specificity found in patients suffering from paroxysmal cold hemoglobinuria.

Drepanocytes: Red cells that have been transformed by hemoglobin polymerization into rigid, inflexible cells with at least one pointed projection.

Dyscrasia: An old term now used as a synonym for disease.

Dyserythropoiesis: Changes in erythroid cell nuclear chromatin pattern; some of these changes are bizarre.

Dysfibrinogenemia: A congenital disorder characterized by the synthesis of abnormal fibrinogen molecules with different functional characteristics.

Dyshematopoiesis: Abnormalities in the maturation, division, or production of blood cells.

Dyskeratosis: Any alteration in the keratinization of the epithelial cells of the epidermis.

Dysostosis: Defective ossification.

Dysplasia: Conditions or diseases characterized by developmental abnormalities or deficiencies.

Dyspnea: Labored or difficult breathing.

Dyspoiesis: Nuclear-cytoplasmic dissociation, especially in red cells.

Early degradation products: The large fragments X and Y that result from the proteolytic action of plasmin on fibrin or fibrinogen. Fragments X and Y have antithrombin activity.

Ecchymosis: A form of macula appearing in large, irregularly formed hemorrhagic areas of the skin, originally bluish-black, and changing to greenish-brown or yellow.

Echinocytes: See **Burr cells.**

Eclampsia: An acute disorder of pregnant and puerperal women, associated with convulsions and coma.

Edema: A local or generalized condition in which the body tissues contain an excessive amount of tissue fluid.

Edematous: Pertaining to swelling of body tissues.

Electrophoresis: The movement of charged particles through a medium (paper, agar, gel) in the presence of an electrical field; useful in the separation and analysis of proteins.

Elliptocyte: Pencil-shaped cells, invariably not hypochromic.

Elution: A process whereby cells that are coated with antibody are treated in such a manner as to disrupt the bonds between the antigen and the antibody. The freed antibody is collected in an inert diluent such as saline or 6% albumin. This serum can then be tested to identify its specificity using routine methods. The mechanism to free the antibody may be physical (heat, shaking) or chemical (ether, acid), and the harvested antibody-containing fluid is called an *eluate.*

Embolism: Obstruction of a blood vessel by foreign substances or by a blood clot.

Embolus: A mass of undissolved matter present in a blood or lymphatic vessel, and brought there by the blood or lymphatic circulation.

Endemic: A term used to describe disease that occurs continuously in a particular population but has a low mortality rate, such as measles; used in contrast to epidemic.

Endocarditis: Inflammation of the lining membrane of the heart. It may be caused by invasion of microorganisms or an abnormal immunologic reaction.

Endogenous: Produced or arising from within a cell or organism.

Endoplasmic reticulum: A connecting network of microcanals or tubules running through the cytoplasm of a cell that serves in intracellular transport.

Endothelium: A form of squamous epithelium consisting of flat cells that line the blood and lymphatic vessels, the heart, and various other body cavities. It is derived from the mesoderm.

Endotoxemia: The presence of endotoxin in the blood (endotoxin is present in the cells of certain bacteria, such as gram-negative organisms).

Eosinophil: A mature type of granulocyte in which cytoplasmic granules are large, round, and refractile and stain orange or red with Wright's stain. It comprises 0 to 4% of the normal differential count.

Epistaxis: Hemorrhage from the nose; nosebleed.

Epsilon (ε) chain: A type of globin chain found in embryonic hemoglobins.

Epsilon aminocaproic acid (EACA): A synthetic inhibitor of plasminogen activation.

Erythroblast: A nucleated cell from which red blood cells are developed. These cells are found in the bone marrow and seen in circulatory blood in the presence of disease.

Erythroblastosis fetalis: See **Hemolytic disease of the newborn (HDN).**

Erythrocyte: A mature red blood cell or corpuscle.

Erythrocyte sedimentation rate (ESR): The rate at which red blood cells settle per hour. It is affected by three factors: erythrocytes, plasma, and mechanical factors.

Erythrocytosis: An abnormal increase in the number of red blood cells in circulation that occurs secondary to many disorders.

Erythroid hyperplasia: As seen in the bone marrow, an increase in the number of immature red cell forms; usually a response to anemic stress.

Erythropoiesis: The production and maturation of erythrocytes.

Erythropoietin: A hormone that regulates red blood cell production.

Etiology: The study of the causes of disease.

Euglobulin: The fraction of plasma containing fibrinogen, plasminogen, and plasminogen activators with only trace amounts of antiplasmins.

Euglobulin lysis time: A coagulation procedure testing for fibrinolysins.

Exocytosis: Secretion of the contents of cytoplasmic granules.

Exogenous: Originating outside an organ or part.

Extracorporeal: Existing outside of the body.

Extramedullary hematopoiesis: Formation of blood cells in sites other than the bone marrow (i.e., liver, spleen).

Extravascular: Outside of the blood vessel.

  E. hemolysis: Hemolysis occurring within the cells of the reticuloendothelial system.

Factor assay: A coagulation procedure to assay the concentration of specific plasma coagulation factors.

Factor VIII antigen: The high-molecular-weight component of the factor VIII molecule.

Factor VIII concentrate: A commercially prepared source of coagulation factor VIII.

Favism: An inherited condition resulting from sensitivity to the fava bean, usually seen in people of Mediterranean origin who have a deficiency in the enzyme glucose-6-phosphate dehydrogenase, which may result in a severe hemolytic episode.

Femto-: A prefix used in the metric system to signify 10^{-15} of any unit. Femtoliter (fL) is used in reporting mean corpuscular volume (MCV) of erythrocytes.

Ferritin: The storage form of iron in the tissues, found principally in the reticuloendothelial cells of the liver, spleen, and bone marrow.

Fibrin: A whitish filamentous protein or clot formed by the action of thrombin on fibrinogen, converting it to fibrin.

Fibrin monomer: The altered molecule that results from thrombin splitting fibrinopeptides A and B from two of the three paired chains of the fibrinogen molecule.

Fibrinogen: A protein produced in the liver that circulates in plasma. In the presence of thrombin, an enzyme produced by the activation of the clotting mechanism, fibrinogen is cleaved into fibrin, which is an insoluble protein that is responsible for clot formation.

Fibrinogen degradation products (FDPs): The polypeptide fragments X, Y, D, and E that result from the proteolytic action of plasmin on fibrinogen or fibrin.

Fibrinolysin: The substance, also called *plasmin,* that has the ability to dissolve fibrin.

Fibrinolysis: Dissolution of fibrin by fibrinolysin, caused by the action of proteolytic enzyme system that is continually active in the body but increased greatly by various stress stimuli.

Fibrinopeptides: Peptides released when fibrinogen is converted to fibrin by thrombin. The fibrinopeptides released by thrombin are designated A and B.

  F. A: A small cleavage product released from fibrinogen by thrombin.

Fibrin-split products: Products that result from fibrin digestion.

Fibrin-stabilizing factor (FSF): Factor XIII.

Fibroblast: A flat, undifferentiated cell in connective tissue that gives rise to numerous cells that form the fibrous support tissue of the body.

Fibrosis: Excessive formation of fibrous tissue.

Fitzgerald factor: High-molecular-weight kininogen (HMWK).

Fletcher factor: Prekallikrein.

Fractures: The sudden breaking of bones.

Fragility: Liability to break, burst, or disintegrate, as erythrocytes are prone to do when exposed to varying concentrations of hypotonic salt solutions.

Fresh frozen plasma (FFP): A frozen plasma product (from a single donor) that contains all clotting factors, especially the labile factors V and VIII. It is useful for clotting factor deficiencies other than hemophilia A, von Willebrand's disease, and hypofibrinogenemia.

Friable: Easily broken or pulverized.

Gallops: Relating to cardiac rhythms, an abnormal third or fourth heart sound in a patient experiencing tachycardia. Gallops are indicative of a serious heart condition.

Gamma (γ) chain: A type of globin chain found in fetal hemoglobin. Two types exist: G-gamma ($^G\gamma$) contains glycine at position 13 of the amino acid sequence, and A-gamma ($^A\gamma$) contains alanine at the same position.

Gamma (γ) globulin: A protein found in plasma and known to be involved in immunity.

Gammopathy: Abnormalities of the immune or gamma system arising in a single disordered clone of cells that is able to synthesize immunoglobulin.

Gastrectomy: Surgical removal of part or all of the stomach.

Gastritis: Inflammation of the stomach, characterized by epigastric pain or tenderness, nausea, vomiting, and systemic electrolyte changes if vomiting persists. The mucosa may be atrophic or hypertrophic.

Gaucher's disease: A familial, lysosomal disorder caused by a deficiency in the enzyme beta-glucocerebrosidase. Three types are identified; all three have in common the triad of hepatosplenomegaly, Gaucher's cells in the bone marrow, and an increase in serum acid phosphatase.

Gene: A functional segment of DNA that serves as a template for RNA transcription and protein translation. Regulatory sequences control gene expression, so that only a small fraction of the estimated 100,000 genes are ever transcribed in any one cell. The spectrum of gene expression in a given cell depends on the cell type and stage of differentiation, and on external signals that it receives from its environment.

Gene rearrangement: A process by which segments of DNA are cut and spliced to produce new DNA sequences. The only genes known to undergo physiologic rearrangement are the immunoglobulin genes and the

T-cell receptor genes that encode antigen recognition proteins expressed by B and T lymphocytes, respectively.

Genome: The total aggregate of inherited genetic material. In humans, the genome consists of 3 billion base pairs of DNA divided among 46 chromosomes (22 pairs of autosomes and two sex chromosomes).

Genotype: The genetic constitution of a particular person. Every person's genotype is unique unless he or she has an identical twin.

Gestation: In mammals, the length of time from conception to birth.

Gigantism: Excessive development of part or all of the body.

Gla: Gamma-carboxyglutamic acid residue located on the amino-terminal end of the vitamin K–dependent coagulation proteins and plays a role in the phospholipid-dependent reactions.

Glanzmann's thrombasthenia: A congenital bleeding disorder characterized by impaired or absent clot retraction and a failure of the platelets to aggregate with most aggregating agents, particularly with ADP.

Globin: A protein constituent of hemoglobin. There are four globin chains in the hemoglobin molecule.

Glossitis: Inflammation of the tongue.

Glucose-6-phosphate dehydrogenase (G6PD): An intracellular red cell enzyme important in the hexose monophosphate pathway.

Glycolysis: Hydrolysis of sugar by an enzyme in the body.

Glycophorin: The principal integral blood cell protein, containing 60% carbohydrate and giving the red cell its negative charge. It appears on the external surface of the red cell.

Glycoprotein: A group of compounds characterized by the combination of a protein with a carbohydrate group.

Golgi apparatus: A lamellar membranous structure near the nucleus of almost all cells. The structure is best seen by electron microscopy. It contains enzymes that add terminal sugar sequences to protein moieties.

Gout: A hereditary metabolic disease that is a form of acute arthritis and is marked by inflammation of the joints. The affected joint may be at any location, but gout usually begins in the knee or foot.

GPI (glycosyl phosphatidyl inositol) anchor proteins: Proteins missing from the cell membrane in paroxysmal nocturnal hemoglobinuria, rendering cells more sensitive to lysis by complement.

Graft-versus-host (GVH) disease: A disorder in which the grafted tissue attacks the host tissue.

Granulocyte: A mature granular leukocyte; refers to band or polymorphonuclear neutrophil, eosinophil, or basophil.

Granulocytopenia: Abnormal reduction of granulocytes in the blood.

Granuloma: A granular tumor or growth usually of lymphoid and epithelial cells. It occurs in various infectious diseases such as leprosy, cutaneous leishmaniosis, yaws, and syphilis.

Granulopoiesis: The production and maturation of granulocytes.

Hageman factor: Synonym for coagulation factor XII.

Haplotypes: A term used in human leukocyte antigen (HLA) testing to denote the five genes (HLA-A, -B, -C, -D, and -DR) on the same chromosome.

Hapten: The portion of an antigen containing the grouping on which the specificity is dependent.

Haptoglobin: An α_2-glycoprotein produced in the liver, having three phenotypes with differing abilities to bind hemoglobin.

Heinz bodies: Large red blood cell inclusions that are formed as a result of denatured or precipitated hemoglobin. May be seen in the thalassemia syndromes, G6PD deficiency, or any of the unstable hemoglobin conditions.

Helmet cells: See **Bite cells.**

Hemagglutination: The clumping together of erythrocytes.

Hemangioma: A benign tumor of dilated blood vessels.

Hemarthrosis: Bloody effusion into the cavity of a joint.

Hematemesis: Vomiting of blood.

Hematocrit: The proportion of red blood cells in whole blood expressed as a percentage.

Hematoma: A swelling or mass of blood confined to an organ, tissue, or space and caused by a break in a blood vessel.

Hematopoiesis: Formation and development of blood cells, normally in the bone marrow. (Synonym: **Hemopoiesis.**)

Hematuria: Blood in the urine.

Heme: The iron-containing protoporphyrin portion of the hemoglobin wherein the iron is in the ferrous (Fe^{2+}) state.

Hemochromatosis: A disease of iron metabolism in which iron accumulates in body tissues, causing complications and tissue damage.

Hemoconcentration: An increase in the number of red cells, resulting from a decrease in the volume of plasma.

Hemodialysis: Removal of chemical substances from the blood by passing it through tubes made of semipermeable membranes. This procedure is used to cleanse the blood of patients in whom one or both kidneys are defective or absent and to remove excess accumulation of drugs or toxic chemicals in the blood.

Hemoglobin: The iron-containing pigment of the red blood cells that functions to carry oxygen from the lungs to the tissues. It consists of approximately 6% heme and 94% globin.

> **H. A:** The major portion of adult hemoglobin (95%), composed of two alpha and two beta chains.
>
> **H. A$_2$:** A small portion of adult hemoglobin (2% to 4%), composed of two alpha and two delta chains.
>
> **H. Bart's:** An abnormal hemoglobin composed of four gamma chains. Formed in alpha thalassemia major, the most severe form of thalassemia occurring in anemic, edematous stillborn infants whose hemoglobin composition is almost all hemoglobin Bart's.
>
> **H. F:** The major fetal hemoglobin, composed of two alpha and two gamma chains.
>
> **H. Gower 1:** A type of hemoglobin found in the embryo, composed of two zeta and two epsilon chains.
>
> **H. Gower 2:** A type of hemoglobin found in the embryo composed of two alpha and two epsilon chains.
>
> **H. H inclusions:** Red cell inclusions that are formed in the alpha thalassemia in which hemoglobin (four beta chains) is in high concentration.
>
> **H. Lepore:** A type of abnormal hemoglobin that is the product of a fused delta and beta gene formed by an unequal crossing-over, resulting in a hemoglobin with fused delta/beta chains; a form of thalassemia.
>
> **H. Portland:** A type of hemoglobin found in the embryo, composed of two zeta and two gamma chains.

Hemoglobinemia: Presence of hemoglobin in the blood plasma.

Hemoglobinopathies: The group of diseases caused by or associated with the presence of one of several forms of abnormal hemoglobin in the blood.

Hemoglobin-oxygen dissociation curve: The relationship between the % saturation of the hemoglobin molecule with oxygen and the environmental oxygen tension.

Hemoglobinuria: The presence of free hemoglobin in the urine.

Hemolysin: An antibody that activates complement, leading to cell lysis.

Hemolysis: The destruction of red blood cells.

> **Intravascular h.:** The disruption of the red cell membrane and release of hemoglobin into the surrounding fluid within the vasculature.
>
> **Extravascular h.:** The phagocytosis of erythrocytes by the reticuloendothelial system, primarily in the spleen and liver.

Hemolytic: Pertaining to, characterized by, or producing hemolysis.

> **H. anemia:** Anemia caused by increased destruction of erythrocytes.
>
> **H. disease of the newborn (HDN):** A disease characterized by anemia, jaundice, enlargement of the liver and spleen, and generalized edema (hydrops fetalis), and caused by maternal IgG antibodies that cross the placenta and attack fetal red cells when there is a fetomaternal

blood group incompatibility. Usually caused by ABO or Rh antibodies. (Synonym: **Erythroblastosis fetalis.**)

Hemolytic uremic syndrome (HUS): A disorder that usually affects young children and is characterized by the combination of severe hemolytic anemia and renal failure. Reticulocytosis and schistocytes are the morphological findings of this microangiopathic hemolytic anemia.

Hemopexin: A beta globulin that has the capacity to bind hemoglobin when haptoglobin has been depleted.

Hemophilia: A hereditary blood disease characterized by impaired coagulability of the blood and a strong tendency to bleed.

H. A: A sex-linked hereditary bleeding disorder characterized by greatly prolonged coagulation time, owing to a deficiency of factor VIII.

H. B: Christmas disease, a hereditary bleeding disorder caused by a deficiency of factor IX.

H. C: A hereditary bleeding disorder caused by a deficiency of factor XI.

Hemoptysis: Coughing and spitting up of blood as a result of bleeding from any part of the respiratory tract.

Hemorrhage: Abnormal internal or external bleeding. May be venous, arterial, or capillary from blood vessels into the tissues, or into or from the body.

Hemorrhagic diathesis: Predisposition to spontaneous bleeding from a trivial trauma caused by a defect in clotting or in the structure or function of blood vessels.

Hemosiderin: An iron-containing pigment derived from hemoglobin on disintegration of red cells; one method whereby iron is stored until needed for making hemoglobin.

Hemosiderinuria: The excretion of hemosiderin from disintegrated red blood cells into the urine.

Hemosiderosis: A condition in which the iron content of blood is increased.

Hemostasis: The process in which blood clots and bleeding is arrested.

Hemotherapy: Blood transfusion as a therapeutic measure.

Heparin: A sulfonated mucopolysaccharide that acts as a powerful anticoagulant at several sites in the coagulation sequence: (1) inhibition of thrombin, (2) inhibition of factor Xa, (3) inhibition of factor IXa, and (4) inhibition of factor XIIa. It is used therapeutically in the treatment of thromboembolic disease.

Hepatitis: Inflammation of the liver.

Hepatocyte: A liver cell.

Hepatomegaly: A condition characterized by enlargement of the liver.

Hepatosplenomegaly: Enlargement of the liver and the spleen.

Hereditary: Transmitted from parent to offspring.

Hereditary angioneurotic edema: A disease state in which there is no inhibition of C1 enzyme activity. There are increased levels of plasmin and complement activator.

Hereditary elliptocytosis (HE): An inherited (autosomal-dominant) intracorpuscular defect of the red cell membrane that is characterized by the presence of more than 40% elliptical red cells on the peripheral blood smear. The condition is generally asymptomatic. There is a biochemical and genetic relationship to hereditary pyropoikilocytosis (HPP).

Hereditary erythrocytic multinuclearity with a positive acid serum (HEMPAS): A type II congenital dyserythropoietic anemia (CDA), also known as Ham's test.

Hereditary hemorrhagic telangiectasia: A congenital hemorrhagic abnormality of the vascular system characterized by localized dilation and convolution of capillaries and venules, giving rise to the characteristic telangiectases.

Hereditary persistence of fetal hemoglobin (HPFH): A group of conditions characterized by the persistence of fetal hemoglobin synthesis into adult life.

Hereditary pyropoikilocytosis (HPP): A relatively rare and severe autosomal-recessive hemolytic anemia characterized by striking,

bizarre micropoikilocytosis in which the red cells bud, fragment, and form microspherocytes. In addition, the red cells are thermally unstable when heated to 45°C and strikingly fragmented in comparison to normal red cells, which fragment only at 49°C.

Hereditary spherocytosis (HS): An inherited (autosomal-dominant) intracorpuscular defect of the red cell membrane (altered spectrin) that results in the most common hereditary hemolytic anemia found in whites. The morphological hallmark of hereditary spherocytosis is the presence of spherocytes on the peripheral blood smear.

Hereditary stomatocytosis (hereditary hydrocytosis): A heterogeneous group of rare red cell membrane disorders inherited in an autosomal-dominant fashion that are characterized by the presence of stomatocytes on the peripheral blood smear and alterations in the permeability of the red cell membrane to cations.

Hereditary thrombophilia: Antithrombin-III deficiency; an autosomal-dominant disorder in which there is an increased tendency toward thrombosis.

Heterozygous: Possessing different alleles in regard to a given characteristic.

Histamine: A substance normally present in the body that is released by the mast cells and basophils. It exerts a pharmacologic action when released from injured cells.

Histiocyte: A large fixed macrophage. (See also **Macrophage.**)

Histochemistry: The science dealing with the identification of cells using chemical markers and specific chemical reactions.

Histoplasmosis: An infection caused by *Histoplasma capsulatum*, with clinical manifestations of anemia and leukopenia, enlargement of the spleen and liver, and fever.

Hodgkin's disease: A disease of unknown etiology producing enlargement of lymphoid tissue, spleen, and liver, with invasion of other tissues.

Homozygous: Possessing identical alleles in regard to a given characteristic.

Howell-Jolly bodies: Red cell inclusions that develop in periods of accelerated or abnormal erythropoiesis. They represent nuclear remnants containing DNA.

Human immunodeficiency virus (HIV): A lymphotropic (RNA) retrovirus that directly infects T helper cells (CD4 cells), causing cell lysis, loss of cellular immunity, and the acquired immunodeficiency syndrome (AIDS).

Human leukocyte antigen (HLA): Antigens found in white blood cells that are part of the major histocompatibility complex.

Humoral: Pertaining to body fluids or substances contained in them.

Hybridization: The process in which one nucleotide strand binds to its counterpart strand by forming hydrogen bonds between long stretches of complementary nucleotides.

Hybridoma: A neoplastic cell.

Hydrophilic: Having an affinity for or readily absorbing fluid.

Hydrophobic: Having an aversion to or not readily absorbing fluid.

Hydrops fetalis: Erythroblastosis fetalis. A hemolytic disease of the newborn characterized by anemia, jaundice, enlargement of liver and spleen, and generalized edema.

Hyperbilirubinemia: A condition characterized by an excessive amount of bilirubin in the blood.

Hypercoagulability: A condition in which activated coagulation factors are found intravascularly; may or may not be associated with increased incidence of thromboembolism.

Hyperkalemia: Excessive amounts of potassium in the blood.

Hyperlipidemia: A condition characterized by excessive amounts of lipids in the blood.

Hyperplasia: Excessive proliferation of normal cells in the normal tissue arrangement of an organ.

Hypersegmentation: An increase in the number of nuclear lobes or segments (more than 6) in segmented neutrophils; especially characteristic of vitamin B_{12} or folate deficiencies.

Hypersplenism: A condition arising as a result of an enlarged spleen. Red cell survival is significantly shortened.

Hypertension: Increase in blood pressure to above normal.

Hyperuricemia: Pertaining to an increased level of uric acid in the blood. Excess uric acid is converted to sodium urate crystals that precipitate in the joints and other tissues. (See **Gout.**)

Hyperuricosuria: Increased level of uric acid in the urine. Excess uric acid is converted to sodium urate crystals that precipitate in the urine.

Hyperviscosity: Excessive viscosity or exaggeration of adhesive properties seen in anemias and inflammatory disease.

Hypocalcemia: Pertaining to a deficient level of calcium in the blood.

Hypochromia: An increased area of central pallor in red cells.

Hypoferremia: Pertaining to a deficient level of iron in the blood.

Hypofibrinogenemia: A congenital disorder characterized by low levels of fibrinogen, usually without any bleeding tendencies.

Hypogammaglobulinemia: Decreased blood levels of gamma globulins seen in some disease states.

Hypogonadism: Defective internal secretion of the gonads.

Hypokalemia: Pertaining to a deficient level of potassium in the blood.

Hypopituitarism: A condition caused by deficient functioning of the hypophysis cerebri, or pituitary organ, which secretes several important hormones.

Hypoplasia: Refers to abnormal, deficient, or defective development.

Hyposplenism: Decreased or improper splenic function. A variety of conditions and splenic sizes are associated with hyposplenism; however, all have in common hematologic manifestations that suggest loss of many or all of the vital splenic functions (e.g., Howell-Jolly bodies, Pappenheimer bodies, poikilocytes, increased platelet count).

Hypotension: Decrease in blood pressure to below normal.

Hypothermia: Having a body temperature below normal.

Hypothyroidism: A condition caused by a deficiency of thyroid hormone secretion, resulting in a lowered basal metabolism.

Hypovolemia: Diminished blood volume.

Hypoxemia: A condition characterized by insufficient oxygenation of the blood.

Hypoxia: Deficiency of oxygen.

Icterus: A condition characterized by yellowish skin, eyes, mucous membranes, and body fluids owing to deposition of excess bilirubin.

Idiopathic: Pertaining to conditions without clear pathogenesis or disease without recognizable cause, as of spontaneous origin.

Idiopathic thrombocytopenia purpura (ITP): Bleeding caused by a decreased number of platelets; the etiology is unknown, with most evidence pointing to platelet autoantibodies.

Idiothrombocythemia: An increase in blood platelets with unknown etiology.

Immune response: The reaction of the body to substances that are foreign or are interpreted as being foreign. Cell-mediated or cellular immunity pertains to tissue destruction mediated by T cells, such as graft rejection and hypersensitivity reactions. Humoral immunity pertains to cell destruction caused by antibody production.

Immune serum globulin: Gamma globulin protein fraction of serum containing antibodies.

Immunoblast: A mitotically active T or B cell.

Immunodeficiency: A decrease in the normal concentration of immunoglobulins in serum.

Immunogenicity: The ability of an antigen to stimulate an antibody response.

Immunoglobulin (Ig): One of a family of closely related, yet not identical, proteins that are capable of acting as antibodies: IgA, IgD, IgE, IgG, and IgM. The principal immunoglobulin in exocrine secretions such as saliva and tears is IgA. IgD may play a role in antigen recognition and the initiation of antibody synthesis. IgE is produced by the cells lining the intestinal and respiratory tracts and is important in forming reagin. The main immunoglobulin in human serum is IgG. A globulin formed in almost every immune response during the early period of the reaction is IgM.

Immunologic memory: The development of T and B memory cells that have been sensitized by exposure to an antigen and respond rapidly under subsequent encounters with the antigen.

Immunologic unresponsiveness: Development of a tolerance to certain antigens that would otherwise evoke an immune response.

Immunoprecipitin: An antigen-antibody reaction that results in precipitation.

Inflammation: Tissue reaction to injury. The succession of changes that occurs in living tissue when it is injured.

Inhibitor: A chemical substance that stops enzyme activity.

Insidious: Without warning.

In situ hybridization: Detection of DNA or RNA within native cells by hybridization to a complementary probe. This permits microscopic visualization of the target sequence in the context of cytologic or morphological features of the tissue on glass slides. In a variation of this procedure called fluorescence in situ hybridization (FISH), the target is usually a karyotypic preparation of chromosomes, and the probe is labeled in such a way that it fluoresces in response to an input light signal.

Insomnia: Inability to sleep, or sleep prematurely ended or interrupted by periods of wakefulness.

Interferon: A protein or proteins formed when cells are exposed to viruses. Noninfected cells exposed to interferon are protected against viral infection.

Interleukin (IL): A family of polypeptide products (proteins) produced by many cell types that are involved in lymphocyte recruitment, lymphocyte proliferation, and cellular responses in immunology.

Intravascular hemolysis: Hemolysis occurring within the blood vessels. (See **Hemolysis.**)

Intrinsic factor (IF): A protein secreted by the parietal cells of the stomach that is necessary for vitamin B_{12} absorption.

Intrinsic system: Initiation of blood clotting that occurs through a surface-mediated pathway.

In utero: Within the uterus.

In vitro: In glass, as in a test tube.

In vivo: In the living body or organism.

Ischemia: Local and temporary deficiency of blood supply to the tissues.

Isoagglutinins: A term used to denote the ABO antibodies anti-A, anti-B, and anti-A, B.

Isoimmune: An antibody produced against a foreign antigen in the same species.

Jaundice: A condition characterized by yellowing of the skin and the whites of the eyes. One cause is excess hemolysis, which results in increased circulating bilirubin. Another cause is liver damage caused by hepatitis.

Juvenile: A common-usage term that is a synonym for neutrophilic metamyelocyte.

Kaolin: A surface-activated substance.

Karyorrhexis: A necrotic stage with fragmentation of the nucleus, whereby chromatin is distributed irregularly throughout the cytoplasm.

Karyotype: A photomicrograph of a single cell in the metaphase stage of mitosis that is arranged to show the chromosomes in descending order of size.

Keratocytes: Synonymous with **Burr cells.**

Kernicterus: A form of icterus neonatorum occurring in infants. It develops at 2 to 8 days of age, and the prognosis is poor if untreated.

Ketosis: The accumulation in the body of the ketone bodies: acetone, beta-hydroxybutyric acid, and acetoacetic acid.

Kinin: A general term for a group of polypeptides that have considerable biologic activity (e.g., vasoactivity).

Koilonychia: A disorder of the nails, which are abnormally thin and concave from side to side, with the edges turned up.

Late degradation products: The terminal fragments D and E that result from the proteolytic action of plasmin on fibrin or fibrinogen. Fragments D and E are known to inhibit fibrin polymerization.

Lepore: See **Hemoglobin Lepore.**

Leptocyte: Synonymous with **Target cell.**

Lethargic: Sluggish; having a lack of energy.

Leukemia: A chronic or acute disease of unknown etiologic factors characterized by unrestrained growth of leukocytes and their precursors in the tissues.

Leukemic hiatus: A phase of leukemia in which the normal maturation series of white cells is not seen because blast cells crowd out normal cells.

Leukemoid reaction: A moderate or advanced degree of leukocytes in the blood that is not a result of a leukemic disease. These reactions are frequently observed as a feature of infectious disease, drug and chemical intoxication, or secondary to nonhematopoietic carcinoma.

Leukoagglutinins: Antibodies to white blood cells.

Leukocyte: A colorless cell in blood, lymph, and tissue; important to immune system functioning.

Leukocytosis: An increase in number of leukocytes (more than 10,000 cells per cubic millimeter) in the blood.

Leukoerythroblastosis: The presence of immature white cells and nucleated red cells on the blood smear; frequently denotes a malignant or myeloproliferative process.

Leukopenia: An abnormal decrease in the number of leukocytes in the blood.

Leukopheresis: Withdrawal of leukocytes from the circulation. It may be used to obtain leukocytes for administration to patients with severe granulocytopenia.

Linkage analysis: The process of following the inheritance pattern of a particular gene in a family based on its tendency to be inherited together with another locus on the same chromosome.

Littoral cells: Cells located in the walls of blood sinuses or lymph, characterized by their flattened appearance.

Locus: A specific position along the DNA sequence composing a particular chromosome, analogous to a street address.

Lymphadenitis: Inflammation of the lymph nodes.

Lymphadenopathy: Disease of the lymph nodes.

Lymphocyte: A white blood cell formed in lymphoid tissue throughout the body, generally described as nongranular and including small and large varieties. It makes up approximately 20% to 45% of the total leukocyte count.

Lymphocytosis: An increase in lymphocytes within the blood.

Lymphoma: Asymmetric enlargement of a group of lymph nodes, which destroys the normal histologic lymph node architecture.

Lymphopoiesis: Refers to the growth or development of lymphocytes.

Lysosomes: Part of an intracellular digestive system that exists as separate particles in the cell. Even though their importance in health and disease is certain, all the precise ways in which lysosomes effect changes are not understood.

Lysozyme (muramidase): A hydrolytic enzyme destructive to cell walls of certain bacteria. It is present in body fluids and found in high concentration within granulocytes.

Macrocephaly: Enlargement of the head.

Macrocyte: A red cell 9 μm in diameter or larger.

Macrocytosis: Refers to a condition in which erythrocytes are abnormally large.

Macroglobulin: A protease inhibitor present in the blood that inhibits the activity of plasmin.

Macroglobulinemia: Abnormal presence of high-molecular-weight immunoglobulins (IgM) in the blood.

Macro-ovalocytes: Refers to a condition in which ovalocytes are abnormally large.

Macrophage: A cell of the reticuloendothelial system having the ability to phagocytose particulate substances and to store vital dyes and other colloidal substances; found in loose connective tissues and various organs of the body.

Major histocompatibility complex (MHC): Present in all mammalian and ovarian species (analogous to human HLA complex); HLA antigens are within the MHC at a locus on chromosome 6.

Malabsorption syndrome: Disordered or inadequate absorption of nutrients from the intestinal tract. It may be caused by a disease that affects the intestinal mucosa, such as infections, tropical sprue, gluten enteropathy, or pancreatic insufficiency, or by antibiotic therapy.

Malaria: An acute and sometimes chronic infectious disease caused by the presence of protozoan plasmodium parasites within red blood cells.

Mast cell: A tissue basophil. (See **Basophil.**)

Mastocytosis: An increase in the number of mast cells.

Mastoiditis: Inflammation of the air cells of the mastoid process.

May-Hegglin anomaly: Inclusions found in the hereditary leukocyte and platelet disorder; similar, but not identical to, Döhle bodies.

Mean corpuscular hemoglobin (MCH): A measure of hemoglobin content of red corpuscles. It is reported in picograms.

$$MCH = \frac{\text{Hemoglobin in g/100 mL} \times 10}{\text{RBC count, millions of cells/}\mu L}$$

Mean corpuscular hemoglobin concentration (MCHC): A measure of concentration of hemoglobin in the average red cell.

$$MCHC = \frac{\text{Hemoglobin in g/100 mL} \times 100}{\text{Hematocrit, \%}}$$

Mean corpuscular volume (MCV): A measure of the volume of red corpuscles expressed in cubic micrometers or femtoliters.

$$MCV = \frac{\text{Hematocrit, \%} \times 10}{\text{RBC count, millions of cells/}\mu L}$$

Mediastinal: Related to the mediastinum.

Mediastinum: A septum or cavity between two principal portions of an organ.

Medullary: Concerning marrow or medulla.

Megakaryocyte: The intermediate platelet precursor cell in the bone marrow, not normally present in peripheral blood. It is a large cell, usually having a multilobed nucleus, that gives rise to blood platelets owing to a pinching off of the cytoplasm.

Megakaryopoiesis: The development of megakaryocytes in the blood.

Megaloblast: A large, nucleated, abnormal red cell precursor, 11 to 20 μm in diameter, oval and slightly irregular, resulting from a nuclear-cytoplasmic maturation asynchrony characteristic of vitamin B_{12} or folate deficiency.

Megaloblastoid: A term used to describe changes in the bone marrow that are morphologically similar to, yet etiologically different from, megaloblastic change.

Meiosis: A type of cell division of germ cells in which two successive divisions of the nucleus produce cells that contain half the number of chromosomes present in somatic cells.

Melena: Black tarry feces caused by the action of intestinal juices on free blood.

Melanocyte: A pigment-producing cell.

Menorrhagia: Menstrual bleeding that is excessive in number of days or amount of blood, or both.

Menstruation: The periodic discharge of a bloody fluid from the uterus, occurring at more or less regular intervals during the life of a woman from puberty to menopause.

Metamyelocyte: An immature neutrophilic granulocyte with a kidney bean–shaped nucleus or an indent, with the presence of specific granules (neutrophilic, eosinophilic, or basophilic) in the cytoplasm (such as neutrophilic metamyelocyte, eosinophilic metamyelocyte, basophilic metamyelocyte).

Metaphyseal dysostosis: Defective bone formation in the metaphysis (the portion of a developing long bone between the diaphysis, or shaft, and the epiphysis).

Metaplasia: Conversion of one kind of tissue into a form that is not normal for that tissue.

Metarubricyte: Synonymous with **Orthochromic (orthochromatophilic) normoblast.**

Metastasis: Movement of bacteria or body cell, especially cancer cells, from one part of the body to another. Change in location of a disease or of its manifestations or transfer from one organ or part to another not directly connected. Spread is by the lymphatic system or bloodstream.

Metastatic: Pertaining to metastasis. (See above.)

Methemoglobin: A form of hemoglobin wherein the ferrous ion (Fe^{2+}) has been oxidized to ferric ion (Fe^{3+}), possibly owing to toxic substances such as aniline dyes, potassium chlorate, or nitrate-contaminated water.

Microaggregates: Aggregates of platelets and leukocytes that accumulate in stored blood.

Microcephaly: Abnormal smallness of the head, often seen in mental retardation. This condition is congenital.

Microcyte: An abnormally small red cell with a diameter of less than 6 μm.

Microcytosis: Refers to a condition in which the erythrocytes are abnormally small.

Microspherocytes: Small, sphere-shaped red blood cells seen in certain kinds of anemia.

Mitochondria: Slender microscopic filaments or rods 0.5 μm in diameter that can be seen in cells by using phase-contrast microscopy or electron microscopy. They are a source of energy in the cell and are involved in protein synthesis and lipid metabolism.

Mitosis: Type of cell division in which each daughter cell contains the same number of chromosomes as the parent cell. All cells except sex cells undergo mitosis.

Mixed field: A type of agglutination pattern in which there are numerous small clumps of cells amid a sea of free cells.

Mixed lymphocyte culture (MLC): A technique for typing cells in which lymphocytes of different individuals are co-cultured.

Mixed lymphocyte reaction (MLR): A method of tissue typing that exploits the fact that T lymphocytes are stimulated to grow in the presence of cells carrying foreign histocompatibility class II antigens.

Monoclonal: An antibody derived from a single ancestral antibody-producing parent cell.

Monocyte: A white blood cell that normally constitutes 2% to 10% of the total leukocyte differential count. This cell is 9 to 12 μm in diameter and has an indented nucleus and an abundant pale bluish-gray cytoplasm containing many fine red-staining granules.

Mononuclear phagocyte system: Formerly called the *reticuloendothelial system;* a system of mononuclear phagocytic cells scattered throughout the body. It includes monocytes and macrophages in the blood and bone marrow, histiocytes of loose connective tissue, reticular cells of lymphatic organs, Kupffer cells of the liver, cells lining blood sinuses of the spleen, and others.

Morbidity: The number of sick persons or cases of disease in relationship to a specific population.

Mortality: The death rate; ratio of number of deaths to a given population.

Mucopolysaccharidoses: A group of hexosamine-containing polysaccharides that are the major constituent of mucous.

Multiparous: Having borne more than one child.

Multiple myeloma: A neoplastic proliferation of plasma cells, characterized by very high immunoglobulin levels of monoclonal origin.

Mutant: A variation of genetic structure.

Mutation: A change in a gene potentially capable of being transmitted to offspring.

> **Frameshift m.:** A change in which a message is read incorrectly because either a base is missing or an extra base is added. This results in an entirely new polypeptide because the triplet sequence has been shifted one base.

> **Point m.:** A change in a base in DNA that can lead to a change in the amino acid incorporated into the polypeptide. The change is identifiable by analyzing the amino acid sequences of the original protein and its mutant offspring.

Myalgia: Muscle pain.

Myeloblast: The first recognizable "mother cell" (precursor) of the granulocytic cell line.

Myelocyte: An immature granulocyte characterized by an eccentrically located round nucleus and specific granules (neutrophilic, eosinophilic, or basophilic) in the cytoplasm (such as neutrophilic myelocyte, eosinophilic myelocyte, or basophilic myelocyte).

Myelodysplasia: Abnormal division; maturation and production of erythrocytes, granulocytes, monocytes, and platelets.

Myelodysplastic syndrome (MDS): A group of primary hematologic disorders associated with abnormal division, maturation, and production of erythrocytes, granulocytes, monocytes, and platelets; also referred to as *preleukemic myelodysplastic syndrome.*

Myelofibrosis: Replacement of the bone marrow by fibrous tissue.

Myeloid-to-erythroid (M:E) ratio: A differential count of bone marrow obtained by dividing the number of granulocytes and their precursor cells by the number of nucleated red cells.

Myelokathexis: A moderate neutropenia related to defective release of mature granulocytes into peripheral circulation.

Myeloperoxidase: An enzyme that is present in the primary (azurophilic) granules of polymorphonuclear neutrophils, eosinophils, and monocytes-macrophages.

Myelophthisic: The process that occurs primarily in the bone marrow as a result of the crowding out of normal elements by malignant cells. A consequential reduction in normal marrow cells and release of immature hematopoietic cells (especially nucleated red cells) into the blood occurs.

Myelopoiesis: The growth or development of myeloid cells in the bone marrow.

Myeloproliferative: Referring to a group of disorders characterized by autonomous proliferation of one or more hematopoietic elements in the bone marrow. In many cases, the liver and spleen are enlarged.

Myoglobin: Muscle hemoglobin.

Necrosis: The pathologic death of one or more cells of a portion of tissue or organ.

Neonatal: Pertaining to the first 6 weeks after birth.

Neoplasm: A new and abnormal formation of tissue such as a tumor or growth.

Neuraminidase: An enzyme that cleaves sialic acid from the red cell membrane.

Neutralization: Inactivation of an antibody by reacting it with an antigen against which it is directed.

Neutropenia: The presence of abnormally small numbers of neutrophils in the circulating blood.

Neutrophil: A medium-sized mature leukocyte with a three- to five-lobed nucleus and cytoplasm containing small lilac-staining granules. Neutrophils normally constitute 50% to 70% of leukocytes in the blood.

Neutrophilia: An abnormal increase in neutrophil leukocytes.

Niemann-Pick disease: An infant disease characterized by a deficiency of sphingomyelinase, fatal within the first 2 years of life. It is characterized by anemia, enlargement of the liver and spleen, and leukocytosis.

Nondisjunction: Failure of a pair of chromosomes to separate during meiosis.

Nonresponder: An individual whose immune system does not respond well in antibody formation to antigenic stimulation.

Normocyte: Having a normal erythrocyte.

Normovolemic: Having a normal blood volume.

Nuclear-to-cytoplasmic (N:C) ratio: The proportion of nucleus to cytoplasm found in nucleated cells; often used in identification of cell maturity.

Nucleotide: The basic building block of DNA, composed of a nitrogenous base (A = adenine, T = thymine, G = guanine, or C = cytosine) attached to a sugar (deoxyribose) and a triphosphate moiety. RNA is similarly composed except that the sugar is ribose and T is replaced by U = uracil.

Obstetric: Referring to the branch of medicine that concerns itself with the management of women during pregnancy, childbirth, and puerperium.

Oculocutaneous: Relating to the eyes and the skin.

Oliguria: Diminished amount of urine formation.

Oncogene: A gene that contributes to the development of cancer. Most oncogenes are altered forms of normal genes (called proto-oncogenes) that function in key biochemical pathways related to cell growth or differentiation.

Opisthotonos: Extreme arching of the spine.

Opsonin: A substance in the blood serum that acts on microorganisms and other cells, facilitating phagocytosis.

Organomegaly: Enlargement of any of the specific organs of the body.

Orthochromic (orthochromatophilic) normoblast: An immature red cell precursor characterized by pink cytoplasm and a small, round, pyknotic nucleus. This stage of maturation is normally found only in the bone marrow.

Orthodontic: Referring to the branch of dentistry that deals with the prevention and correction of irregularities of the teeth.

Orthostatic hypotension: Decreased blood pressure when the body is in an erect position.

Osmolality: The osmotic concentration of a solution determined by the ionic concentration of dissolved substances per unit of solvent.

Osmotic fragility: The ability of the red cells to withstand different salt concentration; this is dependent on the volume, surface area, and functional state of the red blood cell membrane.

Osteoblast: An immature bone marrow cell responsible for the formation of osteocytes.

Osteoclast: A giant multinuclear cell formed in the bone marrow of growing bones.

Osteomyelitis: Inflammation of the bone, especially the marrow, caused by a pathogenic organism.

Osteoporosis: Increased porosity of the bone, seen most often in elderly women.

Osteosclerosis: An abnormal increase in the density of bone tissue, resulting from some abnormality affecting osteoclasts.

Ovalocyte: An abnormal red cell that is egg-shaped or elliptical. (Synonym: **Elliptocyte.**)

Oxyhemoglobin: The combined form of hemoglobin and oxygen.

P$_{50}$: The partial pressure of oxygen or oxygen tension at which the hemoglobin molecule is 50% saturated with oxygen under standard in-vitro conditions of temperature and pH.

Pagophagia: The craving to eat ice.

Pallor: Paleness; lack of color.

Panagglutinin: An antibody capable of agglutinating all red blood cells tested, including the patient's own cells.

Pancytopenia: A depression of each of the normal bone marrow elements: white cells, red cells, and platelets in the peripheral blood.

Panel: A large number of group 0 reagent red cells that are of known antigenic characterization and are used for antibody identification.

Panhyperplasia: An abnormal increase in all affected cells.

Panmyelosis: Increase in all the elements of the bone marrow.

Papilledema: Edema and inflammation of the optic nerve at its point of entrance into the eyeball.

Pappenheimer bodies: Basophilic inclusions in the red blood cell that are cluster-like. They are believed to be iron particles; confirmation is made by Prussian blue stain.

Parachromatin: The portions of the nuclear chromatin that are non-stained or lightly stained.

Paracoagulants: A variety of substances capable of converting soluble fibrin monomer complexes into insoluble fibrin. These include protamine sulfate, ethanol, and material from staphylococci.

Paracoagulation tests: Coagulation procedures used to indicate the presence of soluble fibrin monomer complexes, which is indirect evidence of the action of thrombin on fibrinogen.

Paraproteinemia: A general term for abnormalities of the immunoglobulins, associated with one of several disease states.

Parenchymal: Relating to parenchyma, the essential parts of an organ that are concerned with its function in contradistinction to its framework.

Parenteral: Entry into the body through the intravenous (IV) or intramuscular (IM) route rather than the alimentary route.

Paresis: Partial or incomplete paralysis.

Paresthesia: Numbness.

Paroxysm: A sudden, periodic attack or recurrence of symptoms of a disease.

Paroxysmal cold hemoglobinuria (PCH): A type of cold autoimmune hemolytic anemia usually found in children suffering from viral infections in which a biphasic IgG antibody can be demonstrated with anti-P specificity. (See also **Donath-Landsteiner antibody test.**)

Paroxysmal nocturnal hemoglobinuria (PNH): An uncommon acquired form of hemolysis caused by an intrinsic defect in the red blood cell membrane, rendering it more susceptible to hemolysins in an acid environment, and characterized by hemoglobin in the urine following periods of sleep.

Pathogenesis: Origination and development of a disease.

Pathognomonic: Specifically distinctive or characteristic of a disease or pathologic condition.

Perfusion: Supplying an organ or tissue with nutrients and oxygen by passing blood or other suitable fluid through it.

Perioral paresthesia: Tingling around the mouth, occasionally experienced by apheresis donors, resulting from the rapid return of citrated plasma that contains citrate-bound calcium and free citrate.

Peroxidase: An enzyme that hastens the transfer of oxygen from peroxide to a tissue that requires oxygen; essential to intracellular respiration.

Petechiae: Pinpoint hemorrhages from arterioles or venules.

Phagocyte: A cells that ingests foreign particles, microorganisms, or other cells.

Phagocytosis: Ingestion and digestion of bacteria and particles by phagocytes.

Pharmacologic: Relating to the study of drugs and their origin, natural properties, and effects on living organisms.

Phlebotomy: Surgical opening of a vein to withdraw blood.

Phosphoglyceromutase (PGM): A red cell enzyme involved in the glycolytic pathway.

Phospholipid: A lipid containing phosphorus groups, found in the RBC membrane.

Photodermatitis: Lesion development on exposure to sunlight.

Phototherapy: Exposure to sunlight or artificial light for therapeutic purposes.

Phox: Phagocyte oxidase subunits whose interaction results in the formation of active oxygen metabolites during the respiratory burst.

Pica: A perversion of appetite associated with ingestion of material not fit for food, such as starch, clay, ashes, or plaster; it is associated with severe iron-deficiency anemia.

Pico-: A prefix used in the metric system to signify 10^{-12}. A picogram is used in reporting the mean corpuscular hemoglobin.

Pinguecula: A yellowish discoloration near the corneal-scleral junction of the eye.

Pinocytosis: The process by which cells absorb or ingest nutrients and fluid.

PIVKA: Proteins induced by vitamin K absence or antagonist; it is seen in patients receiving long-term warfarin treatment.

Plaques: Small, flat growths.

Plasma: The liquid portion of whole blood containing water, electrolytes, glucose, fats, proteins, and gases. Contains all the clotting factors necessary for coagulation but in an inactive form. Once coagulation occurs, the fluid is converted to serum.

Plasma cell: A B lymphocyte–derived cell that secretes immunoglobulins or antibodies.

Plasmacyte: A plasma cell.

Plasmacytosis: The presence of plasma cells in blood.

Plasma protein fraction (PPF): Also known as Plasmanate. Sterile pooled plasma stored as a fluid or freeze-dried. It is used for volume replacement.

Plasma thromboplastin antecedent (PTA): Factor XI involved in the intrinsic coagulation pathway.

Plasmacytomas: Localized or generalized tumor masses of plasma cells.

Plasmapheresis: Removal of blood, separation of plasma by centrifugation, and reinjection of the cells into the body. Used as a means of obtaining plasma and in the treatment of certain pathologic conditions.

Plasmin: A fibrinolytic enzyme derived from its precursor, plasminogen.

Plasminogen: A protein found in many tissues and body fluids. It is important in preventing fibrin clot formation.

    P. activators: Endothelial cell–derived plasma proteins, which convert plasminogen to plasmin.

    P. activator inhibitors: Endothelial cell proteins, which bind to tissue plasminogen activator (t-PA) and urokinase to inhibit their actions.

Plasmodium: See **Malaria.**

Platelet: A round or oval disc, 2 to 4 μm in diameter, derived from the cytoplasm of the megakaryocyte, a large cell in the bone marrow. Plays an important role in blood coagulation, hemostasis, and blood thrombus formation.

Platelet adhesion: The interaction of platelet surface glycoproteins with connective tissue elements of the subendothelium, requiring von Willebrand's factor as a plasma cofactor.

Platelet aggregation: Platelet-to-platelet interaction, dependent on calcium.

Platelet concentrate: Platelets prepared from a single unit of whole blood or plasma and suspended in a specific volume of the original plasma. Also known as *random donor platelets.*

Platelet-derived growth factor (PDGF): A hematopoietic growth factor that stimulates fibroblasts to divide and secrete collagen.

Platelet factor 3 (PF3): A phospholipid found within the platelet membrane required for coagulation. PF3 assays are used to evaluate platelet disorders.

Platelet plug: Platelets that function to arrest bleeding by "plugging" any damage in the vessel wall and providing phospholipids essential for blood coagulation. The development of a hemostatic platelet plug depends on adhesion, aggregation, and consolidation.

Plateletpheresis: A procedure using a machine by which one can selectively remove platelets from a donor or patient.

Platelet-rich plasma (PRP): Plasma that is derived from a citrated blood sample spun at 1500 rpm for 5 minutes.

Platelin: A substance that acts in vitro similar to platelet factor 3.

Plethoric Congestion causing distension of the blood vessels.

Pleural effusion: Fluid in the pleural space.

Pluripotential stem cells: A generalized parent cell that gives rise to a common lymphoid stem cell, which differentiates into T- or B-cell ontogeny or a colony-forming unit (CFU).

Pneumonitis: Inflammation of the lung.

Poikilocytosis: Variation in shape of red cells.

Polyacrylamide gel: A type of matrix used in electrophoresis upon which substances are separated.

Polyagglutination: A state in which an individual's red cells are agglutinated by all sera regardless of blood type.

Polychromasia: Describes the bluish-gray color of some younger red cells in evaluation of red blood cell morphology. Increased polychromasia is a sign of a very active bone marrow.

Polychromatophilic normoblast: An immature red cell precursor characterized by bluish-gray cytoplasm and a round, eccentrically located nucleus with a distinct chromatin/parachromatin pattern of staining, and normally only found in the bone marrow. (Synonym: **Rubricyte.**)

Polyclonal: Antibodies derived from more than one antibody-producing parent cell.

Polycythemia: An excess of red blood cells in the peripheral blood.

    P. vera: A chronic life-shortening myeloproliferative disorder involving all bone marrow elements, characterized by an increase in red blood cell mass and hemoglobin concentration.

Polymerase chain reaction (PCR): A procedure for copying a specific DNA sequence a billionfold. To accomplish this, short DNA probes are designed to flank the target sequence. These probes serve as primers to initiate synthesis of new complementary nucleotide strands by the enzyme DNA polymerase. The whole process takes place in a thermocycler, an instrument that sequentially varies the reaction temperature to optimize probe binding, DNA synthesis, and denaturation. Thirty such cycles of DNA synthesis generate about a billion copies of the target sequence extending up to several thousand base pairs in length. The final product is removed from the thermocycler and subjected to further analysis by methods such as gel electrophoresis, ELISA plate detection, or DNA sequencing. In a variation called *real-time PCR,* the products are automatically quantitated at the end of each cycle to facilitate their detection and extrapolate the original target DNA concentration.

Polymorphism: A genetic system that possesses numerous allelic forms, such as a blood group system.

Polymorphonuclear neutrophil (PMN): A mature granulocyte with neutrophilic granules and a segmented nucleus (also called *segmented neutrophil*). (See **Neutrophil.**)

Polyspecific Coombs' sera: A reagent that contains anti-human globulin sera against IgG and C3d.

Porphobilinogen: A precursor of porphobilin that is a dark-pigmented nonporphyrin.

Porphyrias: A group of inherited disorders caused by excessive production of porphyrins in the bone marrow or the liver. Two types are recognized: erythropoietic and hepatic.

Portal hypertension: Increased pressure in the portal vein as a result of obstruction of the flow of blood through the liver.

Postpartum: Occurring after childbirth.

Precipitation: The formation of a visible complex (precipitate) in a medium containing soluble antigen (precipitinogen) and the corresponding antibody (precipitin).

Precipitin: An antibody formed in the blood serum of an animal by the presence of a soluble antigen, usually a protein. When added to a solution of the antigen, it brings about precipitation. The injected protein is called the *antigen* and the antibody produced is the *precipitin.*

Preleukemia (myelodysplastic syndrome): A clinical syndrome in which the bone marrow shows marked hypocellularity with clusters of immature cells that in many cases evolve into true nonlymphocytic leukemia.

Priapism: Abnormal, painful, and continued erection of the penis caused by disease, accompanied by loss of sexual desire.

Primary fibrinolysis: Activation of the fibrinolytic system that is not secondary to coagulation.

Primary hemostasis: The interaction of platelets and the vascular endothelium to stop bleeding following vascular injury.

Proaccelerin: Factor V; it functions in the common pathway of coagulation as a cofactor.

Proband: The initial subject presenting with a mental or physical disorder; the heredity of this individual is studied to determine if other members of the family have had the same disease or carry it. (Synonym: **Propositus/proposita.**)

Probe: A tool for identifying a particular nucleotide sequence. A probe is a strand of nucleotides whose sequence is complementary to the target sequence and is thus capable of hybridizing to it. Probes are usually labeled in a way that permits their detection, so that the probe serves as a marker for the target sequence. Probes and their targets may be composed of either deoxyribonucleotides (DNA) or ribonucleotides (RNA). For probe binding to be effective, both the probe and target must be single stranded. Double-stranded nucleic acid can be converted to its single-stranded components by the application of heat or a strong alkaline solution.

Proconvertin: Factor VII; it functions in the extrinsic system of coagulation.

Prodrome: A symptom indicative of an approaching disease.

Progranulocyte: An immature white blood cell precursor found only in the bone marrow that is the characteristic stage of maturation at which azurophilic nonspecific granules first appear in the cytoplasm of the granulocytic cell line.

Pronormoblast: The first recognizable "mother cell" (precursor) of the erythrocytic cell line. (Synonym: **Rubriblast.**)

Prophylaxis: Any agent or regimen that contributes to the prevention of infection and disease.

Propositus/Proposita: The initial individual whose condition led to investigation of a hereditary disorder or to a serologic evaluation of family members. (Synonym: **Proband.**)

Proprioception: The awareness of posture movement and change in equilibrium and the knowledge of position, weight, and resistance of objects in relation to the body.

Prorubricyte: See **Basophilic normoblast.**

Prostaglandins: A group of fatty acid derivatives present in many tissues, including prostate gland, menstrual fluid, brain, lung, kidney, thymus, seminal fluid, and pancreas.

Prosthesis: Replacement of a missing part by an artificial substitute, such as an artificial extremity.

Prostration: Absolute exhaustion.

Protamine sulfate: A substance used to detect the presence of soluble fibrin monomer complexes. It is also used to neutralize the effects of heparin. (See also **Paracoagulants.**)

Prothrombin: Factor II; it functions in the common pathway of coagulation.

Prothrombin complex: A commercially prepared concentrate of the vitamin K–dependent factors, prothrombin, and factors VII, IX, and X in lypholized form. Preparations of prothrombin complex are used therapeutically to treat acquired and congenital hemorrhagic disorders.

Prothrombin consumption test (PCT): A test that measures prothrombin activity in serum after coagulation has taken place.

Prothrombin time (PT): A test to evaluate the overall integrity of the clotting system that involves factors VII, X, V, II, and I. Commonly referred to as a means of evaluating the extrinsic system of coagulation.

Protoporphyrin: A porphyrin whose iron complex forms the heme of hemoglobin and the prosthetic groups of myoglobin and certain respiratory pigments.

Pruritus: The symptom of itching.

Aquagenic p.: Itching that occurs after exposure to warm water.

Pulmonary artery wedge pressure: Pressure measured in the pulmonary artery at its capillary end.

Pulse pressure: The difference between the systolic and the diastolic blood pressures.

Punctate: Having pinpoint punctures or depressions on the surface; marked with dots.

Purpura: A condition with various manifestations and diverse causes characterized by hemorrhages into the skin, mucous membranes, internal organs, and other tissues.

Pyelogram: A radiograph of the ureter and renal pelvis.

Pyknosis (pyknotic): Condensation and shrinkage of cells through degeneration.

Pyoderma: Any acute inflammatory skin disease of unknown origin. Bacteria may be cultured from the lesions, but there are normal resident flora.

Pyogenic: Producing pus (e.g., pyogenic infection).

Pyropoikilocytosis: See **Hereditary pyropoikilocytosis.**

Pyroprotein: A serum protein that precipitates on exposure to hot temperatures.

Pyruvate kinase deficiency: An enzymatic disorder in the Embden-Meyerhof pathway caused by a deficiency in pyruvate kinase. Hemolysis and anemia persist after splenectomy. The trait is autosomal recessive.

Quaternary complex: An inhibitory configuration involving VIIa, Xa, tissue factor, and tissue factor pathway inhibitor.

***RAS* gene:** The gene that plays a central role in relaying signals from the outside of the cell to the nucleus, thereby aiding in the proliferation and differentiation of hematopoietic precursor cells.

_R._ mutation: Mutation in the *RAS* gene that leads to cellular dysplasia.

Raynaud's disease: A peripheral vascular disorder characterized by abnormal vasoconstriction of the extremities on exposure to cold or during emotional stress. A history of symptoms for at least 2 years is necessary for diagnosis.

Recessive: In genetics, incapable of expression unless carried by both members of a set of homologous chromosomes; not dominant.

Recipient: A patient who is receiving a transfusion of blood or a blood product.

Recombinant human erythropoietin (rHuEpo): A genetically engineered erythropoietin.

Red cell distribution width (RDW): This measurement is included on some instrumentation as part of the complete blood count. It measures the distribution of red blood cell volume and is equivalent to anisocytosis on the peripheral blood smear. It is calculated as the coefficient of variation of the red cell volume and is expressed as a percentage (normal is 11.5% to 14.5%).

Refractory: Not responsive to therapy.

Reniform–kidney bean shape: The characteristic shape of the nucleus of metamyelocytes; often used to distinguish metamyelocytes from myelocytes and neutrophilic bands; may also be used to characterize the appearance of reactive lymphocytes.

Replication: The process by which DNA is copied during cell division. Replication is carried out by the enzyme DNA polymerase, which recognizes single-stranded DNA and fills in the appropriate complementary nucleotides to produce double-stranded DNA. Synthesis usually begins at a junction where double-stranded DNA lies next to single-stranded DNA, and synthesis proceeds in a 5' to 3' direction. In the laboratory, replication of specific DNA sequences can be artificially induced. This permits us to produce and label DNA probes, determine the sequence of target DNA, and amplify DNA sequences as exploited by polymerase chain reaction.

Reptilase: An enzyme, thrombin-like in nature, derived from the venom of *Bothrops atrox*. It predominantly hydrolyzes fibrinopeptide A from the fibrinogen molecule, in contrast to thrombin, which hydrolyzes fibrinopeptides A and B.

R. time: A coagulation procedure similar to the thrombin time except that clotting is initiated with the snake venom enzyme reptilase.

Respiratory distress syndrome (RDS): A condition, formerly known as *hyaline membrane disease,* accounting for more than 25,000 infant deaths per year in the United States. Clinical signs, including delayed onset of respiration and low Apgar score, are usually present at birth.

Respiratory syncytial virus (RSV): A common viral cause of acquired neutropenia in children.

Restriction endonuclease: An enzyme that cleaves double-stranded DNA at a specific nucleotide sequence. For example, EcoR1 cleaves DNA only where the sequence 5′-GAATTC-3′ is present. A variety of other endonucleases have different sequence recognition sites. The ability to reproducibly cleave DNA into smaller fragments simplifies molecular analysis of an otherwise quite long molecule. (Human chromosomes exceed 10^7 nucleotides in length.)

Reticular dysgenesis: A disorder characterized by a combined deficiency of antibody production and cellular immunity; reported to be a selective failure of stem cells committed to the myeloid and lymphoid cell lines. Death occurs shortly after birth.

Reticulin: A substance found in the connective fibers of reticular tissue; bone marrow.

Reticulocyte: A red blood cell containing a network of granules or filaments representing an immature stage in development. It normally comprises about 1% of circulating red blood cells.

Reticulocytopenia: A condition characterized by decreased erythrocytes.

Reticuloendothelial system (RES): A term applied to those cells scattered throughout the body that have the power to ingest particulate matter. It includes histiocytes of loose connective tissue; reticular cells of lymphatic organs; Kupffer cells of the liver; cells lining blood sinuses of the spleen, bone marrow, adrenal cortex, and hypophysis; and other cells.

Retinopathy: Any disorder of the retina.

Rh immune globulin (RhIg): A passive form of anti-D given within 72 hours of delivery to all Rh-negative mothers delivering an Rh-positive fetus.

Ribonucleic acid (RNA): A nucleic acid that controls protein synthesis in all living cells. There are three different types, and all are derived from the information encoded in the DNA of the cell. Messenger RNA (mRNA) carries the code for specific amino acid sequences from the DNA to the cytoplasm for protein synthesis. Transfer RNA (tRNA) carries the amino acid groups to the ribosome for protein synthesis. Ribosomal RNA (rRNA) exists within the ribosomes and is thought to assist in protein synthesis.

Ribosome: A cellular organelle that contains ribonucleoprotein and functions to synthesize protein. Ribosomes may be single units or clusters called *polyribosomes* or *polysomes.*

Rickettsia: Any of the microorganisms belonging to the genus *Rickettsia.*

Ristocetin: Drug used in platelet aggregation studies.

Rouleaux: A group of red blood corpuscles arranged like a roll of coins, owing to an abnormal protein coating on the cells' surfaces; seen in multiple myeloma and Waldenström's macroglobulinemia.

Rubriblast: See **Pronormoblast.**

Rubricyte: See **Polychromatophilic normoblast.**

Russell's viper venom (Stypven): Snake venom with thromboplastic activity.

Sarcoidosis: A disease of unknown etiology characterized by widespread granulomatous lesions that may affect any organ or tissue of the body.

Sarcoma: Cancer arising from connective tissue such as muscle or bone. It may affect the bones, bladder, kidneys, liver, lungs, parotids, and spleen.

Schistocyte: An abnormal red cell that is formed when pieces of the red cell membrane become fragmented. Whole pieces of the red cell membrane appear to be missing, causing bizarre-looking red cells.

Sclera: A tough, white fibrous tissue that covers the so-called white of the eye. It extends from the optic nerve to the cornea.

Scleroderma: A chronic disease of unknown etiology that causes sclerosis of the skin and certain organs, including the gastrointestinal tract, lungs, heart, and kidneys. The skin feels tough and leathery, may itch, and later becomes hyperpigmented.

Screening cells: Group O reagent red cells that are used in antibody detection or screening tests.

Scurvy: A deficiency of vitamin C characterized by hemorrhagic manifestations and abnormal formation of bones and teeth.

Secondary fibrinolysis: Indirect activation of the fibrinolytic system by thrombin stimulation of endothelial cells to release tissue plasminogen activator (t-PA) and urokinase.

Senescence: The aging process of the red cells.

Sensitization: A condition of being made sensitive to a specific substance (such as an antigen) after the initial exposure to that substance. Results in the development of immunologic memory that evokes an accentuated immune response with subsequent exposure to the substance.

Sepsis: A pathologic state, usually febrile, resulting from the presence of microorganisms or their poisonous products in the bloodstream.

Septicemia: Presence of bacteria in the blood. The microorganisms may multiply and cause overwhelming infection and death.

Sequestration: An increase in the quantity of blood within the blood vessels, occurring physiologically or produced artificially.

Serine protease inhibitors: Plasma proteins such as antithrombin-III. The activity of the various enzymes (serine proteases) involved in the coagulation sequence is controlled to a variable extent primarily by plasma proteins generally known as inhibitors.

Serine proteases: A family of proteolytic enzymes with the amino acid serine at the active site.

Serositis: Inflamed condition of a serous membrane.

Serotonin: A chemical present in platelets that is a potent vasoconstrictor.

Serum: The fluid that remains after plasma has clotted.

Sex linkage: A genetic characteristic located on the X or Y chromosome.

Sézary syndrome: Skin disease characterized by infiltration with atypical Sézary cells. The exfoliative dermatitis is considered a variant form of mycosis fungoides.

Shift to the left: An abnormal cell maturation situation that occurs when increased bands, less mature neutrophils, and a smaller average number of lobes are found in segmented cells; it may be caused by infection, hematologic disorders, or physiologic factors.

Shift to the right: An abnormal cell maturation situation that occurs when more than one hypersegmented cell is seen; it is indicative of vitamin B_{12} or folate deficiency.

Shock: A clinical syndrome in which the peripheral blood flow is inadequate to return sufficient blood to the heart for normal function, particularly transport of oxygen to all organs and tissues.

Sickle cell: An abnormal red cell seen in patients who possess high quantities of hemoglobin S, an abnormal hemoglobin. The red cell is crescent or sickle shaped.

Sickle cell anemia: A hereditary, chronic anemia in which abnormal sickle- or crescent-shaped erythrocytes are present. It is caused by the presence of hemoglobin S in the red blood cells. The gene that causes this disease occurs with high frequency in African and Mediterranean populations.

Sickle trait: Blood that is heterozygous for the gene coding for the abnormal hemoglobin of sickle cell anemia.

Sideroblast: A ferritin-containing normoblast in the bone marrow. It makes up from 20% to 90% of normoblasts in the marrow.

Siderocyte: A nonnucleated red blood cell containing iron in a form other than hematin and confirmed by a specific iron stain such as the Prussian blue reaction.

Siderosis: A form of pneumoconiosis resulting from inhalation of dust or fumes containing iron particles.

Sodium dodecyl sulfate (SDS): An anionic detergent that renders a net negative charge to substances it solubilizes.

Somatic: Pertaining to nonreproductive cells or tissues.

Southern blot: A procedure to evaluate the structure of DNA, named after its inventor, Dr. Edwin Southern. First, DNA is cleaved at specific nucleotide sequences by the action of restriction endonucleases. The resulting DNA fragments are separated by size using agarose gel electrophoresis, and then denatured using a strongly basic solution that converts double-stranded DNA into its single-stranded components. The fragments are transferred to a membrane where they are immobilized and then hybridized to a complementary labeled probe. Detection of the probe label permits identification of the DNA fragments containing the sequence of interest. Genetic defects often result in alteration of the size or number of the target fragments, or both.

Specificity: The affinity of an antibody and the antigen against which it is directed.

Spectrin: A large molecule, found on the inner surface of red blood cell membrane, that is responsible for the biconcave shape of the red cell as well as for its deformability.

Spectrophotometer: Device for measuring amount of color in a solution by comparison with the spectrum.

Spherocyte: An abnormal red blood cell shape. Spherocytes are smaller than normal red cells, have a concentrated hemoglobin content, and have a decreased surface-to-volume ratio.

Spherocytosis: See **Hereditary spherocytosis.**

Splenomegaly: Enlargement of the spleen seen in several blood disorders.

Sprue: A disease endemic in many tropical regions and occurring sporadically in temperate countries, characterized by weakness, loss of weight, steatorrhea, and various digestive disorders.

Spurious: Not true or genuine; adulterated; false.

Stab: See **Band.**

Staphylococcal clumping test: A coagulation procedure used to detect the presence of fibrin-fibrinogen degradation products. The test uses a strain of staphylococcus that clumps in the presence of fibrinogen, fibrin monomers, or X and Y fragments.

Steatorrhea: Increased secretion of sebaceous glands; fatty stools.

Stenosis: Constriction or narrowing of a passage or orifice.

Steroid hormones: Hormones of the adrenal cortex and the sex hormones.

Stertorous: Pertaining to laborious breathing.

Stomatocyte: An abnormal red cell shape; this shape appears as having a slitlike area of central pallor.

Strabismus: A disorder of the eye in which optic axes cannot be directed to same object. Strabismus can result from reduced visual activity, unequal ocular muscle tone, or an oculomotor nerve lesion.

Streptokinase: A product of beta-hemolytic streptococci capable of liquefying fibrin.

Stroma: The red cell membrane that is left after hemolysis.

Stuart-Prower factor: Factor X; it functions in the common pathway of coagulation.

Stypven time test: A coagulation procedure used to distinguish between a deficiency of factor VIII and a deficiency of factor X.

Supernatant: Floating on the surface, as oil on water.

Supervention: The development of an additional condition as a complication to an existing disease.

Syncytial: Of the nature of a syncytium, which is a group of cells in which the protoplasm of one cell is continuous with that of adjoining cells, such as the mesenchyme cells of the embryo.

Systemic: Pertaining to a whole body rather than to one of its parts.

Systemic lupus erythematosus (SLE): A disseminated autoimmune disease characterized by anemia, thrombocytopenia, increased IgG levels, and the presence of four IgG antibodies: antinuclear antibody, antinucleoprotein antibody, anti-DNA antibody, and antihistone antibody. It is believed to be caused by suppressor T-cell dysfunction.

Systolic pressure: The maximum blood pressure that occurs at ventricular concentration; the upper value of a blood pressure reading.

Tachycardia: Abnormal rapidity of heart action, usually defined as a heart rate greater than 100 beats per minute.

Tachypnea: Abnormal rapidity of respiration.

Tanned red cell hemagglutination inhibition immunoassay (TRCHII): A test that is the reference method for the assay of fibrinogen degradation products.

Target cell: This abnormal red cell looks like a "bull's eye," with hemoglobin concentrated in the center and on the rim of the cell.

Tay-Sachs disease: Originally termed *amaurotic infantile idiocy,* this disorder is an autosomal-recessive gangliosidosis caused by a deficiency of the enzyme hexosaminidase A. Its incidence in the Ashkenazi Jewish population is 100 times greater than that in the non-Jewish population.

T cell: One of the cells derived from lymphoid stem cells.

Teardrop cell: An abnormal red cell, shaped like a tear, seen frequently in the myeloproliferative disorders. (Synonym: **Dacrocyte.**)

Telangiectasia: The presence of small, red focal lesions, usually in the skin or mucous membrane, caused by dilation of capillaries, arterioles, or venules.

Template bleeding time: The elapsed time it takes for a uniform incision made by a template and blade to stop bleeding; a test of platelet function in vivo, assuming a normal platelet count.

Tertian malaria: Malaria in which sporulation occurs every 48 hours. Symptoms are more common during the day; paroxysms are divided into chill, fever, and sweating stages. Benign tertian malaria is caused by *Plasmodium vivax,* malignant tertian malaria by *Plasmodium falciparum.*

Tetany: A nervous affection characterized by intermittent spasms of the muscles of the extremities.

Thalassemia: A group of hereditary anemias produced by either a defective production rate of alpha- or beta-hemoglobin polypeptide. This disorder is inherited in homozygous or heterozygous state.

   T. major: The homozygous form of deficient beta chain synthesis, which is very severe and presents itself during childhood. Prognosis varies; however; the younger the child when the disease appears, the more unfavorable the outcome.

Thermal amplitude: The range of temperature over which an antibody demonstrates serologic or in vitro activity, or both.

Thrombin: An enzyme that converts fibrinogen to fibrin so that a soluble clot can be formed.

Thrombin time (TT): A coagulation procedure that measures the time required for thrombin to convert fibrinogen to an insoluble fibrin clot.

Thrombocythemia: A condition marked by increased platelets in the blood.

Thrombocytopathies: Inherited disorders of platelets.

Thrombocytopenia: Decreased numbers of platelets.

Thrombocytosis: Increased numbers of platelets.

Thromboembolism: An embolism; the blocking of a blood vessel by a thrombus (blood clot) that has become detached from the site of formation.

Thrombophilia: An acquired or inherited coagulation disorder in which the person is hypercoagulable, or prone to clotting, usually caused by a deficiency in one or more of the naturally occurring inhibitors.

Thrombopoiesis: The formation of platelets.

Thrombosis: The formation or development of a blood clot or thrombus.

Thrombotic thrombocytopenic purpura (TTP): A severe condition characterized by thrombocytopenia, microangiopathic hemolytic anemia, renal dysfunction, neurologic abnormalities, and fever.

Thymidine: An essential ingredient used in DNA synthesis and incorporated by T lymphocytes undergoing blast transformation in response to foreign HLA-D antigens in the mixed lymphocyte culture test.

Thymoma: A disorder of the thymus marked by anemia as a result of selective hypoplasia of red blood cell precursors in bone marrow.

Thyromegaly: Enlargement of the thyroid gland.

Tinnitus: Buzzing in the ears.

Tissue factor: An endothelial cell phospholipid that forms a complex with factor VIIa to activate factor X.

    T. factor pathway inhibitor: A plasma protein that inhibits tissue factor–factor VIIa complex in the extrinsic clotting cascade.

Tissue plasminogen activator (t-PA): A clotting factor produced by vascular endothelial cells that selectively bind to fibrin as it activates fibrin-bound plasminogen.

Tissue thromboplastin: Factor III; it functions in the extrinsic system of coagulation.

Titer score: A method used to evaluate more precisely than simple dilution by comparing the titers of an antibody. Agglutination at each higher dilution is graded on a continuous scale; the total is the titer score.

Total iron-binding capacity (TIBC): The amount of iron that transferrin can bind; normal range is 250 to 360 μg/dL. TIBC = unsaturated iron-binding capacity (UIBC) or amount of additional iron that transferrin can bind above that which is already complexed + serum Fe.

Toxic granulation: Medium to large metachromatic granules that are evenly distributed throughout the cytoplasm. May be seen in severe bacterial infections, severe burns, and other conditions.

Trabeculae: Bands or bundles of connective tissue.

Trait: A characteristic that is inherited.

Transcription: The process of RNA production from DNA, which requires the enzyme RNA polymerase.

Transferase: An enzyme that catalyzes the transfer of atoms or groups of atoms from one chemical compound to another.

Transferrin: A glycoprotein synthesized in the liver, with the primary function of iron transport.

Transforming growth factor-beta (TGF-β): The most important growth factor, secreted by megakaryocytes and monocytes, involved in the pathogenesis of bone marrow fibrosis. TGF-3 promotes secretion of collagen from fibroblasts.

Transfuse: To perform a transfusion.

Transfusion: The injection of blood, a blood component, saline, or other fluids into the bloodstream.

    T. reaction: An adverse response to a transfusion.

Translation: The production of protein from the interactions of the RNAs.

Translocation: The transfer of a portion of one chromosome to its allele.

Transplacental: Through the placenta.

Transposition: The location of two genes on opposite chromosomes of a homologous pair.

Ubiquitous: Existing everywhere at the same time.

Uremia: The presence of urine or urine components in the blood.

Urokinase: A trypsin-like protease, found in the urine and synthesized by the kidney, that activates plasminogen by proteolytic cleavage. Differs from tissue plasminogen activators in that urokinase reacts with plasminogen in the fluid phase of blood.

Urticaria: A vascular reaction of the skin similar to hives.

Vaccine: A suspension of infectious organisms or components of them that is given as a form of passive immunization to establish resistance to the infectious disease caused by the same organism.

Vacuolization: The presence of cavity in a cell's protoplasm.

Valvular: Relating to or having a valve.

Variable region: The portion of the immunoglobulin light and heavy chains in which amino acid sequences vary tremendously. These amino acid variations permit the different immunoglobulin molecules to recognize different antigenic determinants. In other words, the variable region determines the antigen against which the antibody will react, thus providing each antibody molecule with its unique specificity. The variable region is located at the amino terminal region of the molecule.

Vascular: Pertaining to or composed of blood vessels.

Vasculitis: Inflammation of a blood or lymph vessel.

Vasoconstriction: Constriction of blood vessels.

Vasodilation: Dilation of blood vessels, especially small arteries and arterioles.

Vaso-occlusive: Obstruction of the vasculature by some pathologic process that seriously impedes blood flow.

Vasovagal syncope: Syncope resulting from hypotension caused by emotional stress, pain, acute blood loss, fear, or rapidly rising from a recumbent position.

Venipuncture: Puncture of a vein for any purpose.

Venom: A poison excreted by some animals such as insects or snakes and transmitted by bites or stings.

Venule: A tiny vein continuous with a capillary.

Verrucous: Wartlike, with raised portions.

Vertigo: Dizziness.

Viremia: Refers to the presence of a virus in the blood.

Viscosity: Having sticky or glutinous attributes.

Vitamin K: A fat-soluble vitamin required for maintenance of normal blood levels of the vitamin K–dependent factors: prothrombin and factors VII, IX, and X. Vitamin K is necessary for carboxylation of specific glutamic acid residues in the postprotein synthesis of the vitamin K–dependent factors.

von Willebrand's disease (vWD): A congenital bleeding disorder inherited as an autosomal-dominant trait and characterized by a decreased level of factor VIII:C and a prolonged bleeding time.

von Willebrand's factor (vWF): A component of the factor VIII molecule that mediates platelet interaction with subendothelium.

WAIHA: Warm autoimmune hemolytic anemia.

Whole blood clotting time: A test that evaluates the overall activity of the intrinsic system of coagulation.

Wiskott-Aldrich syndrome: A congenital platelet storage pool defect characterized by immunologic alteration, recurrent pyogenic infections, and eczema.

Xerocyte: A dehydrated red blood cell having a peculiar morphological appearance (i.e., hemoglobin concentration at one pole of the red cell).

Zeta (ζ) chain: A type of globin chain found in embryonic hemoglobin.

Zymogen: A substance that, when paired with its zymase, becomes an enzyme.

Bibliography

Chapter 2

Foucar, K: Bone marrow examination, techniques, morphologic review and decision making process. In: Bone Marrow Pathology. American Society of Clinical Pathologists, Chicago, 1995, pp 21–57.

Hanson, CA: Bone marrow examination in clinical laboratory medicine. In McClatchey, KD (ed): Clinical Laboratory Medicine. Williams & Wilkins, Baltimore, MD, 1994, pp 848–851.

Weitberg, AB: Study of bone marrow. In Handin, RI, et al (eds): Blood, Principles and Practice of Hematology. JB Lippincott, Philadelphia, 1995, pp 61–79.

Chapter 7

Affronti, J, and Baillie, J: Gastroscopic follow-up of pernicious anemia patients. Gastrointest Endosc 40:129, 1994.

Allen, RH, et al: Metabolic abnormalities in cobalamin (vitamin B_{12}) and folate deficiency. FASEB J 7:1344, 1993.

Curtis, D, et al: Elevated of serum homocysteine as a predictor for vitamin B_{12} or folate deficiency. Eur J Haematol 52:227, 1994.

Elia, M: Oral and parental therapy for B_{12} deficiency. Lancet 352:1721, 1998.

Flippo, TS, and Holder, WD: Neurologic degeneration associated with vitamin B_{12} deficiency. Arch Surg 128:1391, 1993.

Gross, S, and Roath, S: Hematology. A Problem Oriented Approach. Williams & Wilkins, Baltimore, MD, 1996, pp 25–30.

Hoffbrand, AV, and Jackson, BF: Correction of the DNA synthesis defect in vitamin B_{12} deficiency by tetrahydrofolate: Evidence in favor of the methyl-folate trap hypothesis as the cause of megaloblastic anemia in vitamin B_{12} deficiency. Br J Haematol 83:643, 1993.

Hsing, AW, et al: Pernicious anemia and subsequent cancer. A population-based cohort study. Cancer 71:745, 1993.

Jacob, RA, et al: Homocysteine increases as folate decreases in plasma of healthy men during short-term dietary folate and methyl group restriction. J Nutr 124:1072, 1994.

Lotspeich-Steininger, CA, et al: Clinical Hematology. Principles, Procedures, Correlations. JB Lippincott, Philadelphia, 1998, p 163.

Michie, CA, et al: Folate deficiency, neural tube defects, and cardiac disease in UK, Indians and Pakistanis. Lancet 351:1105, 1998.

Norman, EJ, and Morrison, JA: Screening elderly populations for cobalamin (vitamin B_{12}) deficiency using the urinary methylmalonic acid assay by gas chromatography mass spectrometry. Am J Med 94:589, 1993.

Otega, RM, et al: Nutritional assessment of folate and cyanocobalamin status in a Spanish elderly group. Int J Vitam Nutr Res 63:17, 1993.

Robinson, SH, and Reich, PR: Hematology, Pathophysiologic Basis for Clinical Practice, ed 3. Little, Brown, Boston, 1993, pp 75–103.

Span, J, et al: A reversible case of pernicious anemia. Am J Gastroenterol 88:1277, 1993.

Stern, SC, et al: Management of megaloblastic anemia. Lancet 349:135, 1997.

Tungtrongchitr, R, et al: Vitamin B_{12}, folic acid and haematological status of 132 Thai vegetarians. Int J Vitam Nutr Res 63:202, 1993.

Turgeon, ML: Clinical Hematology. Theory and Procedures. Philadelphia, Lippincott Williams & Wilkins, 1999, pp 125–127.

Waters, HM, et al: High incidence of type II autoantibodies in pernicious anemia. J Clin Pathol 46:45, 1993.

Wickramasinghe, SN, and Fida, S: Correlations between holo-transcobalamin II, holo-haptocorrin, and total B_{12} in serum samples from healthy subjects and patients. J Clin Pathol 46:537, 1993.

Wild, J, et al: Investigation of folate intake and metabolism in women who have had two pregnancies complicated by neural tube defects. Br J Obstet Gynaecol 101:197, 1994.

Wood, ME, and Bunn, PA: Hematology/Oncology Secrets. Hanley & Belfus, Philadelphia, 1994, pp 34–38.

Young, SN: The use of diet and dietary components in the study of factors controlling affect in humans: a review. J Psychiatry Neurosci 18:235, 1993.

Chapter 8

Alter, BP, and Young, NS: The bone marrow failure syndromes. In Nathan, PG, and Orkin, SH (eds): Hematology of Infancy and Childhood, ed 5. WB Saunders, Philadelphia, 1998, p 237.

Jandl, JH: Aplastic anemia. In Blood: Textbook of Hematology, ed 2. Little, Brown, Boston, 1996, p 201.

Shadduck, RK: Aplastic anemia. In Buetler, E, et al (eds): Williams Hematology, ed 5. McGraw-Hill, New York, 1995, p 238.

Williams, DM: Pancytopenia, aplastic anemia, and pure red cell aplasia. In Lee, GR, et al (eds): Wintrobe's Clinical Hematology, ed 10. Williams & Wilkins, Baltimore, MD, 1998, p 1449.

Chapter 12

Bunn, HF, and Forget, BG: Hemoglobin: Molecular, Genetic and Clinical Aspects. WB Saunders, Philadelphia, 1986.

Fosburg, MT, and Nathan, DG: Treatment of Cooley's anemia. Blood 76:435, 1990.

Higgs, DR, and Weatherall, DJ (eds): Baillere's Clinical Haematology, vol 6. WB Saunders, London, 1993.

Higgs, DR, et al: A review of the molecular genetics of the human α-globin gene cluster. Blood 73:1018, 1989.

Kazazian, HH: The thalassemia syndromes: Molecular basis and prenatal diagnosis in 1990. Semin Hematol 27:209, 1990.

Modell, B, and Berdoukas, V: The Clinical Approach to Thalassemia. Grune & Stratton, New York, 1984.

Stamatoyannopoulos, G, et al (eds): The Molecular Basis of Blood Diseases. WB Saunders, Philadelphia, 1994.

Steinberg, MH: Review: Thalassemia: Molecular pathology and management. Am J Med Sci 296:308, 1988.

Weatherall, DJ (ed): The Thalassemias. Methods in Hematology. Churchill-Livingstone, New York, 1983.

Weatherall, DJ, and Clegg, JB: The Thalassemia Syndromes. Blackwell Scientific Publications, Boston, 1981.

Weatherall, DJ, et al: The hemoglobinopathies. In Scriver, CR, et al (eds): The Metabolic Basis of Inherited Diseases. McGraw-Hill, New York, 1989, p 2281.

WHO Working Group: Community Control of Hereditary Anemias: Memorandum from a WHO meeting. Bull WHO 61:63, 1983.

WHO Working Group: Hereditary Anemias: Genetic Basis, Clinical Features, Diagnosis and Treatment. Bull WHO 60:643, 1982.

Chapter 14

Chisholm, M: Haematologic disorders in liver disease. In Wright, R, et al (eds): Liver and Biliary Disease, Pathophysiology, Diagnosis, Management. WB Saunders, Philadelphia, 1992.

Erslev, AJ: Anemia of endocrine disorders. In Williams, WJ, et al (ed): Hematology, ed 6. McGraw-Hill, New York, 2000.

Jandl, JH: Blood. Lippincott, Williams & Wilkins, Philadelphia, 1996.

Means, RT: The anemia of chronic disorders. In Lee, GR, et al (eds): Wintrobe's Clinical Hematology, ed 10. Williams & Wilkins, Baltimore, MD, 1998.

Rapaport, SI: Introduction to Hematology, ed 2. JB Lippincott, Philadelphia, 1987.

Wiggins, RC, et al: Mechanisms of vascular injury. In Tisher, CC, and Brenner, BM (eds): Renal Pathology with Clinical and Functional Correlations, ed 2. Lippincott, Williams & Wilkins, Philadelphia, 1993.

Chapter 18

Adams, JA, et al: Primary polycythemia, essential thrombocythemia and myelofibrosis three facets of a single disease process? Acta Haematol (Basel) 79:33, 1988.

Babior, BM, and Stossed, TP: Hematology: A Pathophysiological Approach, ed 3. Churchill Livingstone, New York, 1994.

Baron, BW, et al: Combined plateletpheresis and cytotoxic chemotherapy for symptomatic thrombocytosis in myeloproliferative disorders. Cancer 72:1209, 1993.

Barosi, G, et al: A prognostic classification of myeloid metaplasia. Br J Haematol 70:400, 1988.

Berk, PD, et al: Therapeutic recommendations in polycythemia vera based on Polycythemia Vera Study Group Protocols. Semin Hematol 23:132, 1986.

Bick, RL, et al: Hematology, Clinical and Laboratory Practice, vol 2. Mosby-Year Book, St Louis, MO, 1993, pp 533–542, 1239–1257.

Canize, D, et al: The value of cell cultures for the diagnosis of mixed myelodysplastic/myeloproliferative disorders. Haematologica 83:3, 1998.

Chaiter, Y, et al: High incidence of myeloproliferative disorders in Ashkenazi Jews in northern Israel. Leuk Lymphoma 6:252, 1992.

Chintagumpala, MM, et al: Treatment of thrombocythemia with anagrelide. J Pediatr 127:495, 1995.

Dalla, KP, et al: α-Interferon in myelofibrosis: A case report. Br J Haematol 86:654, 1994.

Dickstein, JI, and Vardiman, JW: Issues in the pathology and diagnosis of the chronic myeloproliferative disorders and the myelodysplastic syndromes [review]. Am J Clin Pathol 99:515,519, 1993.

Dutcher, TF: Hematologic Morphology for Teachers and Learners. ASCP National Meeting. ASCP Press, Chicago, 1994.

Gaidano, G, et al: Molecular mechanism of tumor progression in chronic myeloproliferative disorders. Leukemia 8(Suppl 1):S27, 1994.

Garcia, S, et al: Idiopathic myelofibrosis terminating in erythroleukemia. Am J Hematol 32:70, 1989.

Gersuk, GM, et al: Quantitative and functional studies of impaired natural killer (NK) cells in patients with myelofibrosis, essential thrombocythemia, and polycythemia vera. I. A potential role for platelet-derived growth factor in defective NK cytotoxicity. Nat Immun 12:136, 1993.

Greenberg, BR, and Wilson, FD: Cytogenetics of fibroblastic colonies in Ph'-positive chronic myelogenous leukemia. Blood 51:1039, 1978.

Gruppo Italiano Studio Politemia: Polycythemia vera: The natural history of 1213 patients followed for 20 years. Ann Intern Med 123:656, 1995.

Handin, RI, et al: Blood: Principles and Practices of Hematology. JB Lippincott, Philadelphia, 1995.

Hoogstraten, B, and Duiant, JR: Hematologic Malignancies. International Union Against Cancer, Current Treatment of Cancer. Springer-Verlag, Berlin/Heidelberg, 1986.

Jandl, JH: Blood: Textbook of Hematology, ed. 2. Little, Brown, Boston, 1996.

Jowitt, SN, et al: Case report: Pleural effusion secondary to extramedullary haemopoiesis in a patient with idiopathic myelofibrosis responding to pleurodesis and hydroxyurea. Clin Lab Haematol 19:283, 1997.

Joy, G, and Logan, PM: Residents' corner. Answer to case of the month #55. Intrathoracic intramedullary hematopoiesis secondary to idiopathic myelofibrosis. Can Assoc Radiol J 49:200, 1998.

Kikawa, Y, et al: Successful treatment of essential thrombocythemia evolving into agnogenic myeloid metaplasia with interferon-α. J Pediatr Hematol Oncol 20:463, 1998.

Kung, C, et al: Polycythemia: Primary or secondary: The differential diagnostic value of stem cell cultures. Schweiz Med Wochenschr 123:53, 1993.

Landolfi, R, et al: Bleeding and thrombosis in myeloproliferative disorders: Mechanisms and treatment. Crit Rev Oncol Hematol 20:203, 1995.

Lee, GR, et al (eds): Wintrobe's Clinical Hematology, ed 10. Williams & Wilkins, Baltimore, MD, 1999.

Leoni, P, et al: Antibodies against terminal galactosyl alpha (1–3) galactose epitopes in patients with idiopathic myelofibrosis. Br J Haematol 85:313, 1993.

Manoharan, A, et al: Effect of chemotherapy on tear drop poikilocytes and other peripheral blood findings in myelofibrosis. Pathology 20:7, 1988.

Martyre, MC, et al: Elevated levels of basic fibroblast growth factor in megakaryocytes and platelets from patients with idiopathic myelofibrosis. Br J Haematol 97:441, 1997.

McKenzie, SB: Textbook of Hematology, ed 2. Williams & Wilkins, Baltimore, MD, 1996.

Perez-Encinas, M, et al: Familial myeloproliferative syndrome. Am J Hematol 46:225, 1994.

Michiels, JJ, and Ten Kate, FJ: Erythromelalgia in thrombocythemia of various myeloproliferative disorders. Am J Hematol 39:131, 1992.

Murphy, S: Therapeutic dilemmas: Balancing the risks of thrombosis, and leukemic transformation in myeloproliferative disorders: FK Schattauer Verlagsgesellschaft mfH (Stuttgart) 78:622, 1997.

Petrini, M, et al: Cytogenetic remission induced by interferon-α in a myeloproliferative disorder with trisomy 8. Br J Haematol 92:941, 1996.

Pizzo, PA, and Poplack, DG: Principles of Pediatric Oncology, ed. 3. Lippincott-Raven, Philadelphia, 1997.

Radaelli, F, et al: Treatment of myeloproliferative syndrome with hydroxyurea. Ann Hematol 73:205, 1996.

Randi, ML, et al: Which tests are most useful in distinguishing between reactive thrombocytosis and the thrombocytosis of myeloproliferative disease? Clin Lab Haematol 14:267, 1992.

Rogers, BA: Want to live with polycythemia vera for a few hours? Lab World 12:33, 1981.

Rosenthal, DS: Clinical aspects of chronic myeloproliferative diseases [review]. Am J Med Sci 304:109, 1992.

Rosenthal, N, and Sessen, FA: Course of polycythemia. Arch Intern Med 62:903, 1938.

Sacci, S: The role of α-interferon in essential thrombocythemia, polycythaemia vera and myelofibrosis with myeloid metaplasia (MMM): A concise update. Leuk Lymphoma 19:13, 1995.

Schofield, JR, and Robinson, WA: A new myeloproliferative syndrome. Am J Hematol 48:186, 1995.

Schwartz, CL, and Cohen, HJ: Myeloproliferative and myelodysplastic syndromes. In Pixxo, PA, and Poplack, DG (eds): Principles and Practice of Pediatric Oncology. Lippincott-Raven, Philadelphia, 1997.

Silverstein, MN: Agnogenic Myeloid Metaplasia. Publishing Science, Boston, 1975.

Spivak, JL, and Eichner, ER: The Fundamentals of Clinical Hematology, ed 3. Johns Hopkins University Press, Baltimore, MD, 1993.

Stein-Martin, EA, et al: Clinical Hematology Principles, Procedures, Correlations, ed 2. Lippincott-Raven, Philadelphia, 1998.

Sterkers, BY, et al: Acute myeloid leukemia and myelodysplastic syndromes following essential thrombocythemia treated with hydroxyurea: High proportion of cases with 17p deletion. Blood 91:616, 1998.

Takimoto, Y, and Kimura, A: Basic and clinical study of platelet-derived growth factor gene expression. Rinsho Ketsueki 35:364, 1994.

Tefferi, A, and Hoagland, HC: Issues in the diagnosis and management of essential thrombocythemia. Mayo Clin Proc 69:651, 1994.

Turk, W: Beitrage zur Kenntnis des Symptomenbildes Polycythamie mit Milztumor und Zyanose. Wein Klin Wochenschr 17:153, 1904.

Van Genderen, PJ, and Michiels, JJ: Primary thrombocythemia: Diagnosis, clinical manifestations and management. Ann Hematol 67:57, 1993.

Von Haller: Elementa physiologiae corporis humani. (Lausanne) 2:34, 1757.

Wasserman, LR: Polycythemia Vera Study Group: A historical perspective. Semin Hematol 23:183, 1986.

Westwood, N, et al: Primary polycythaemia: Diagnosis by non-conventional positive criteria. Eur J Haematol 51:228, 1993.

Chapter 19

Begemen, H, and Rastetter, J: Atlas of Clinical Hematology. Springer-Verlag, Berlin, 1989.

Foucar, K: Bone Marrow Pathology. ASCP Press, Chicago, 1995.

Handin, RI, et al: Blood, Principles and Practice of Hematology. JB Lippincott, Philadelphia, 1995.

Hoffman, R, et al: Hematology: Basic Principles and Practice, ed 3. Churchill Livingstone, Philadelphia, PA, 2000.

Knowles, DM (ed): Neoplastic Hematopathology. Williams & Wilkins, Baltimore, MD, 1992.

Mufti, GJ, et al: An Atlas of Malignant Haematology, Cytology, Histology and Cytogenetics. Lippincott-Raven, Philadelphia, 1996.

Richard, LG, et al (eds): Wintrobe's Clinical Hematology, ed 10, vols I and II. Lea & Febiger, Philadelphia, 1998.

Chapter 23

Alper, CA: The plasma proteins. In Williams WJ, et al (eds): Hematology, ed 6. McGraw-Hill, New York, 2000.

Alving, BM, and Griffin, JH: Venous thrombosis: How to make the best use of the laboratory to guide therapy. Consultant January:64, 1995.

Antithrombin Hereditary Deficiency Case Study: Consultation reports and discharge summary. Fairfax Hospital-INOVA Health System, 1993–1996.

Bajaj, SP: Interaction and Regulation of Tissue Factor Induced Coagulation. Hemostasis and Thrombosis: Update. St Louis University Seminar, pp 1–13.

Bauer, K: Activation of the factor VII–tissue factor pathway. Thromb Haemost 78:108, 1997.

Bennett, JS, and Shattil, SJ: Platelet function. In Williams, WJ, et al (eds): Hematology, ed 6. McGraw-Hill, New York, 2000.

Bick, RL: Hypercoagulability and thrombosis. In Bick, RL (ed): Hematology: Clinical and Laboratory Practice. CV Mosby, St Louis, MO, 1992, pp 1463–1493.

Bick, RL, and Murano, G: Physiology of hemostasis. In Bick, RL (ed): Hematology: Clinical and Laboratory Practice. CV Mosby, St Louis, MO, 1992, pp 1285–1309.

Bloom, AL: Physiology of blood coagulation. Haemostasis 20(Suppl 1):14, 1990.

Bombeli, T, et al: Anticoagulant properties of the endothelium. Thromb Haemost 77:408, 1997.

Broze, GL, Jr: Tissue factor pathway inhibitor. Hamostaseologie 17:82/73–86/77, 1997.

Clemetson, KJ: Primary hemostasis: Sticky fingers cement the relationship. Curr Biol 9:R110, 1999.

Comp, PC: Control of coagulation reactions. In Williams, WJ, et al (eds): Hematology, ed 6. McGraw-Hill, New York, 2000.

Cox, D: Methods for monitoring platelet function. Am Heart J 1998, 135(5Pt 280)S:170, 1998.

Dahlback, B, et al: Familial thrombophilia due to a previously unrecognized mechanism characterized by poor anticoagulant response to activated protein C: Prediction of a cofactor to activated protein C. Proc Natl Acad Sci USA 90:1004, 1993.

Edgington, T, et al: The structural basis of function of the tissue factor VII, a complex in the cellular initiation of coagulation. Thromb Haemost 78:401, 1997.

Fass, D: The Hemostatic Mechanism. Bleeding and Thrombosing Diseases: The Basics and Beyond. Mayo Clinic Seminar, 1997, pp 1–5.

Gastineau, DA: Screening Tests of Hemostasis. Mayo Clinic Seminar, 1997, pp 1–5.

Griffin, JH, et al: Diagnosis and treatment of hypercoagulable states. Education Program, American Society of Hematology, 1996, pp 106–111.

Hathaway, WE, and Goodnight, SH, Jr: Disorders of Hemostasis and Thrombosis: A Clinical Guide. McGraw-Hill, New York, 1993, pp 15–19, 50–56, 339–340, 347–352.

Hawiger, J: Formation and regulation of platelet and fibrin hemostatic plug. Hum Pathol 18:111, 1987.

Hirsh, J, et al: Approach to the thrombophilic patient. In Colman, RW, et al (eds): Hemostasis and Thrombosis: Basic Principles and Clinical Practice, ed 3. JB Lippincott, Philadelphia, 1994, pp 1543–1561.

Holmson, H: Composition of platelets. In Williams, WJ, et al (eds): Hematology, ed 6. McGraw-Hill, New York, 2000.

Hursting, MJ: An enzyme-linked immunosorbent assay for prothrombin fragment 1.2 [F1.2]. Am Clin Lab 32, 1992.

Jaffe, EA: The role of blood vessels in hemostasis. In Williams, WJ, et al (eds): Hematology, ed 6. McGraw-Hill, New York, 2000.

Jensen, R: Naturally occurring anticoagulants—Part I. Clin Hemost Rev September:1, 1996.

Jensen, R: Naturally occurring anticoagulants—Part II. Clin Hemost Rev October: 1, 1996.

Kaczor, DA, et al: Evaluation of different mixing study reagents and dilution effect in lupus anticoagulant testing. Am J Clin Pathol 95:408, 1991.

Kjeldsburg, CR, (ed): Practical Diagnosis of Hematologic Disorders, ed 2. ASCP Press, Chicago, 1995, pp 627–631.

Lazarchick, J, and Kizer, J: Interaction of the fibrinolytic, coagulation, and kinin systems and related pathology. In Harmening, DM (ed): Clinical Hematology and Fundamentals of Hemostasis, ed 2. FA Davis, Philadelphia, 1992, pp 486–497.

Mammen, EF: Congenital coagulation protein disorders. In Bick, RL (ed): Hematology: Clinical and Laboratory Practice. CV Mosby, St Louis, MO, 1992, pp 1391–1414.

Michelson, AD, et al: The effects of aspirin and hypothermia on platelet function in vivo. Br J Haematol 104:64, 1999

Morrisey, J, et al: Factor VIIa–tissue factor: Functional importance of protein membrane interactions. Thromb Haemost 78:112, 1997.

Packham, MA: Role of platelets in thrombosis and hemostasis. Can J Physiol Pharmacol 72:278, 1994.

Rick, ME: Grand rounds at the clinical center of the National Institutes of Health. Protein C and Protein S: Vitamin K–dependent inhibitors of blood coagulation. JAMA 263:701, 1990.

Roth, GJ, and Caverley, DC: Aspirin, platelets and thrombosis: Theory and practice. Blood 83(4):885–898, 1994.

Ruggeri, ZM: New insights into the mechanisms of platelet adhesion and aggregation. Semin Hematol 31:229, 1994.

Saito, H: Normal hemostatic mechanisms. In Ratnoff, O, and Forbes, C (eds): Disorders of Hemostasis, ed 3, vol 2. WB Saunders, Philadelphia, 1996, pp 23–46.

Schmaier, A: Contact activation: A revision. Thromb Haemost 78:108, 1997.

Sherry, S: Fibrinolysis, Thrombosis and Hemostasis: Concepts, Perspectives and Clinical Applications. Lea & Febiger, Malvern, PA, 1992, pp 71–87.

Sixma, JS, and Wester, J: The hemostatic plug. Semin Hematol 14:265, 1997.

Smith, WL, and Lands, WE: Stimulation and blockade of prostaglandin biosynthesis. J Biol Chem 246(21):6700, 1971.

Thompson, A, and Harker, L: Manual of Hemostasis and Thrombosis, ed 3. FA Davis, Philadelphia, 1998, pp 21–33.

Triplett, DA: The Diagnosis and Management of Thrombophilia. Hemostasis and Thrombosis Symposium, Hershey, PA, May 2, 1997.

Triplett, DA: Hemostasis: A Case Oriented Approach. Igaku-Shoin, New York, 1995, pp 1–60.

Wiltsie, JC: The Hemostatic History—The Most Important Test. Mayo Clinic Seminar, 1997, pp 1–7.

Zimmerman, TS, and Ruggeri, ZM: Laboratory diagnosis of von Willebrand disease. In Bick, RL (ed): Hematology: Clinical and Laboratory Practice. CV Mosby, St Louis, MO, 1992, pp 1441–1445.

Chapter 27

Greaves, M: Antiphospholipid antibodies and thrombosis. Lancet 353:1348, 1999.

Roubey, RAS: Immunology of the antiphospholipid syndrome: Antibodies, antigens and autoimmune response. Thromb Haemost 82:656, 1999.

Triplett, DA: Antiphospholipid-protein antibodies: Laboratory detection and clinical relevance. Thromb Res 78:1, 1995.

Vermylen, J, et al: Antibody-mediated thrombosis. Thromb Haemostas 78:420, 1997.

Warkentin, TE, et al: Heparin-induced thrombocytopenia: Towards consensus. Thromb Haemost 79:1, 1998.

Chapter 29

ADVIA® 120 Hematology System Operator's Guide: V1.03.01,1997–1999, Bayer Corporation, Diagnostics Division, Tarrytown, NY.

Bessman, JD, et al: Improved classification of anemias by MCV and RDW. Am J Clin Pathol 80:322, 1983.

Brown, BA: Hematology Principles and Procedures, ed 6. Lea & Febiger, Philadelphia, 1993, pp 373–374.

Burns, ER, and Wenz, HG: Quantitative evaluation of the hematopoietic system. In Tilton, RC, et al (eds): Clinical Laboratory Medicine. Mosby-Year Book, St Louis, MO, 1992, p 859.

CELL-DYN® 3200 and 3500 Operator's Manuals 9140181B and 9140285A, November 1997. Abbott Laboratories, Abbott Park, IL.

Coulter® Hematology Education Series: Significant Advances in Hematology. Coulter Electronics, Hialeah, FL, 1983.

Coulter® Hematology Education Series: Significant Advances in Hematology. Coulter Electronics, Hialeah, FL, 1989.

Dotson, M: Automation in hematology. In Schoeff, LE, and Williams, RH (eds): Principles of Laboratory Instruments. CV Mosby, St Louis, MO, 1993, p 361.

Sysmex Reagents America, Inc: Sysmex SE-Series Hematology Analyzers, Los Alamitos, CA.

Turgeon, ML: Clinical Hematology: Theory and Procedures, ed 2. Little, Brown, Boston, 1993, p 313.

Watson, JS, and Dotson, M: Multiparameter hematology instruments. In Lotspeich-Steininger, CA, et al (eds): Clinical Hematology: Principles, Procedures and Correlations. JB Lippincott, Philadelphia, 1992, p 496.

Chapter 31

Abramson, JS, and Wheeler, JG: The Neutrophil. Oxford Press, Oxford, England, 1993.

Archer, RK, and Broome, J: Studies on the peroxidase reaction of living eosinophils and other leukocytes. Acta Haematol 29:47, 1963.

Bell, A, et al: Use of cytochemical and FAB classification in leukemias and other pathologic stages. Am J Med Technol 47:6, 1981.

Brownnman, GP, et al: The contribution of cytochemistry and immunophenotyping to the reproducibility of the FAB classification in acute leukemia. Blood 68:134, 1986.

Carson, F: Histotechnology: A Self-Instructional Text, ed 2. ASCP Press, Chicago, 1993.

Catovsky, D, and Foa, R: The Lymphoid Leukaemias. Butterworths, London, England, 1990.

Dacie, JV, and Lewis, SM: Practical Hematology, ed 6. Churchill Livingstone, New York, 1984.

Elghetany, M, et al: The use of cytochemical procedures in the diagnosis of acute and chronic myeloid leukemia. Clin Lab Med 4:90, 1990.

Ellas, JM: A rapid sensitive myeloperoxidase stain using 4-chlor-1-naphthol. Brief scientific reports. Am J Clin Pathol 73:797, 1980.

Handin, RI, et al: Blood: Principles and Practice of Hematology. JB Lippincott, Philadelphia, 1995.

Heckner, F, et al: Practical Microscopic Hematology, ed 4. Lea & Febiger, Philadelphia, 1994.

Janckila, AJ, et al: The cytochemistry of tartrate-resistant acid phosphatase. Am J Clin Pathol 70:45, 1978.

Kaplow, LS: Substitute for benzidine in myeloperoxidase stains. Am J Clin Pathol 63:451, 1974.

Kass, L: Esterase activity in erythroleukemia. Am J Clin Pathol 67:368, 1977.

Kass, L, and Peters, CL: Esterase in acute leukemias. Am J Clin Pathol 69:273, 1978.

Katayama, I, and Yang, JPS: Reassessment of a cytochemical test for differential diagnosis of leukemic reticuloendotheliosis. Am J Clin Pathol 68:268, 1977.

Kjedsberg, C, et al: Practical Diagnosis of Hematologic Disorders. ASCP Press, Chicago, 1989.

Kung, PC, et al: Terminal deoxynucleotidyl transferase in the diagnosis of leukemia and malignant lymphoma. Am J Med 64:788, 1978.

Lee, EJ, et al: Minimally differentiated acute nonlymphocytic leukemia. A distinct entity. Blood 5:1400, 1987.

Li, CY, et al: Acid phosphatase isoenzyme in human leukocytes in normal and pathologic conditions. J Histochem Cytochem 18:473, 1970.

Li, CY, et al: Esterase in human leukocytes. J. Histochem Cytochem 21(1):1–12, 1973.

Li, CY, et al: Modern Modalities for the Diagnosis of Hematologic Neoplasms: Color Atlas/Text. Igaku-Shoin, New York, 1996.

Lotspeich-Steininger, CA, et al: Clinical Hematology: Principles, Procedures and Correlations. JB Lippincott, Philadelphia, 1992.

Melvin, L: Comparison of techniques for detecting T-cell acute lymphocytic leukemia. Blood 54:1, 1979.

Miale, JB: Laboratory Medicine: Hematology, ed 6. CV Mosby, St Louis, MO, 1982.

Nadjii, M, and Morales, AR: Immunoperoxidase: II. Practical applications. Lab Med 15:33, 1984.

Naeim, F, et al: Recent advances in diagnosis and classification of leukemias and lymphomas. Dis Markers 8:231, 1990.

Nathan, DG, and Oski, FA: Hematology of Infancy and Childhood. WB Saunders, Philadelphia, 1993.

Rodak, BF: Diagnostic Hematology. WB Saunders, Philadelphia, 1995.

Rozenszajn, L, et al: The esterase activity in megaloblasts, leukaemic and normal haemotopoietic cells. Br J Haematol 14:605, 1968.

Rutenberg, AM, et al: An improved histochemical method for the demonstration of leukocyte alkaline phosphatase activity: Clinical application. J Clin Lab Med 65, 1965.

Seo, IS, et al: Myelodysplastic syndrome. Diagnostic implications of cytochemical and immunocytochemical studies. Mayo Clin Proc 68:47, 1998.

Sheehan, HL, and Storey, GW: An improved method of staining leukocyte granules with Sudan black B. J Pathogen Bacteriol 59:336, 1947.

Sun, T, et al: Atlas of Cytochemistry & Immunochemistry of Hematologic Neoplasms. ASCP Press, Chicago, 1985.

William, WJ, et al (eds): Hematology, ed 5. McGraw-Hill, New York, 1995.

Wislocki, GB, et al: The occurrence of the periodic acid-Schiff reaction in various normal cells of blood and connective tissue. Blood 4:562, 1949.

Yam, LT, et al: Cytochemical identification of monocytes and granulocytes. Am J Clin Pathol 55:283, 1971.

Chapter 32

Ambruso, DR, et al: Antithrombin III deficiency: Decreased synthesis of a biochemically normal molecule. Blood 60:1, 1982.

Automated APTT (package insert). Organon Teknika Corporation, Durham, NC.

Bauer, JD: Clinical Laboratory Methods, ed 9. CV Mosby, St Louis, MO, 1982.

Bertina, RM, et al: Mutation in blood coagulation factor V associated with resistance to activated protein C. Nature 359:64, 1994.

Biggs, R, and Rizza, CR: Human Blood Coagulation: Hemostasis and Thrombosis, ed 3. Blackwell Scientific, Boston, 1984.

Bloom, AL: The von Willebrand syndrome. Semin Hematol 27:4, 1980.

Bockenstedt, PL: Laboratory methods in hemostasis. Thromb Hemorrhage 26:455, 1994.

Comp, PC: Laboratory evaluation of protein S status. Semin Thromb Hemost 16:177, 1990.

Comp, PC, et al: An abnormal plasma distribution of protein S occurs in functional protein S deficiency. Blood 67:504, 1986.

Comp, PC, et al: Determination of functional protein C, and antithrombotic protein, using thrombin thrombomodulin complex. Blood 63:15, 1984.

Dahlback, B, and Hildebrand, B: Inherited resistance to activated protein C is corrected by anticoagulation cofactor activity found to be a property of factor V. Proc Natl Acad Sci USA 91:1396, 1994.

Dahlback, B, et al: Familial thrombophilia due to a previously unrecognized mechanism characterized by poor anticoagulant response to activated protein C: Prediction of a cofactor to activated protein C. Proc Natl Acad Sci USA 90:1004, 1993.

Data-Fi Fibrinogen Determination Kit (package insert). Dade Behring, Inc, Deerfield, IL.

de Ronde, H, and Bertina, RM: Laboratory diagnosis of APC-resistance: A critical evaluation of the test and the development of diagnostic criteria. Thromb Haemost 72:880, 1994.

Ebert, R: PTs, PRs, ISIs, and INRs: A primer on prothrombin time reporting. Part II: Limitations of INR reporting. Clin Hemost Rev 7:1, 1993.

Eliman, L, et al: The Thrombo-Wellcotest as a screening test for disseminated intravascular coagulation. N Engl J Med 288:633, 1973.

Ens, G: Disorders leading to thrombosis. Clin Hematol 56:639, 1992.

Ens, G, and Jensen, R: Coagulation instrumentation review. Clin Hemost Rev 7;1, 1993.

Ens, G, and Jensen, R: Diagnosis and management of acquired bleeding disorders. Clin Hemost Rev 7:1, 1993.

Epstein, DJ, et al: Radioimmunoassay for protein C and factor X. Am J Clin Pathol 82:573, 1983.

Ewing, NP, and Kasper, CK: In vitro detection of mild inhibitors to factor VII in hemophilia. Am J Clin Pathol 77:6, 1982.

Exner, T, et al: Comparison of test methods for the lupus anticoagulant: International survey on lupus anticoagulants-I (ISLA-1). Thromb Haemost 64:478, 1990.

Francis, RB, and Thomas, W: Behavior of protein C inhibitor in intravascular coagulation and liver disease. Thromb Haemost 52P:71, 1984.

Guglielmone, HA, and Vides, MA: A novel functional assay of protein C in human plasma and its comparison with amidolytic and anticoagulant assays. Thromb Haemost 67:46, 1992.

Harker, L, and Thompson, AR: Manual of Hemostasis and Thrombosis, ed 3. FA Davis, Philadelphia, 1983.

Hemostasis Committee of the "Société Française De Biologie Clinique": Laboratory heterogeneity of the lupus anticoagulant: A multicentre study using different clotting assays on a panel of 78 samples. Thromb Res 66:349, 1992.

Henry, JB: Clinical Diagnosis and Management by Laboratory Methods, ed 17. WB Saunders, Philadelphia, 1984.

Hoyer, LW: The factor VIII complex: Structure and function. Blood 58:1, 1981.

Jensen, R: Activated protein C resistance. Clin Hemost Rev 9:1, 1995.

Jensen, R: Optimizing the INR. Clin Hemost Rev 11:1, 1997.

Jensen, R, and Ens, G: Advances in the diagnosis of lupus anticoagulant. Clin Hemost Rev 7;1, 1993.

Jensen, R, and Ens, G: Components of the protein C anticoagulant system Part I. Clin Hemost Rev 6:1, 1992.

Jensen, R, and Ens, G: Components of the protein C anticoagulant system Part II. Clin Hemost Rev 6:1, 1992.

Jensen, R, and Ens, G: ELISA application in hemostasis. Clin Hemost Rev 7:1, 1993.

Jensen, R, and Ens, G: Serine protease inhibitors. Clin Hemost Rev 7:1, 1993.

Laroche, P, et al: Rapid quantitative latex immunoassays for diagnosis of thrombotic disorders. Thromb Haemost 62:379, 1989.

Latallo, ZS, and Teisseyre, E: Evaluation of reptilase-R and thrombin clotting time in the presence of fibrinogen degradation products and heparin. Scand J Haematol 4:261, 1971.

Laurell, CB: Electroimmunoassay. Scand J Clin Lab Invest 124:21, 1972.

Laurell, CB: Quantitative estimation of proteins by electrophoresis in agarose gel containing antibodies. Ann Biochem 15:45, 1966.

Lee, RL, and White, PD: A clinical study of the coagulation time of blood. Am J Med Sci 145:495, 1913.

Lenahan, JG, and Smith, K: Hemostasis, ed 16. General Diagnostic Division of Warner-Lambert Company, Morris Plains, NJ, 1982.

Macfarlane, RG: A simple method for measuring clot retraction. Lancet 1:1199, 1939.

Mammen, EF: Congenital abnormalities of the fibrinogen molecule. Semin Thromb Hemost 1:184, 1974.

Mannucci, PM, et al: Familial dysfunction of protein S. Thromb Haemost 62:763, 1989.

Martinoli, JL, and Stocker, K: Fast functional protein C assay using Protac, a novel protein C activator. Thromb Res 43:253, 1986.

McGann, MA, and Triplett, DA: Interpretation of antithrombin III activity. Lab Med 13:12, 1982.

Miale, JB: Laboratory Medicine: Hematology, ed 6. CV Mosby, St Louis, MO, 1982.

Mielke, CH, et al: The standardized normal ivy bleeding time and its prolongation by aspirin. Blood 34:204, 1969.

Murano, G, and Bick, RL: Basic Concepts of Hemostasis and Thrombosis. CRC Press, Boca Raton, FL, 1980.

Nor-Partien Fibrinogen Kit (package insert). Behring Diagnostics, La Jolla, CA, 1988.

Olson, JD, et al: Evaluation of ristocetin-Willebrand's factor assay and ristocetin-induced platelet aggregation. Am J Clin Pathol 63:210, 1975.

Palkuti, H, and Jackson, MP: International Normalized Ratio (INR)—Clinical Significance and Applications. Bio/Data Corporation, 1995.

Patterson, BB: Clot observation—A review of an important but neglected coagulation test. Lab Med 7;12, 1976.

Platelet Neutralization Procedure. Department of Air Force, Lackland AFB, TX, 1980.

Preda, L, et al: A prothrombin time-based functional assay of protein S. Thromb Res 60:19, 1990.

Protein C Antigen Rocket EID Method (package insert). Helena Laboratories, Beaumont, TX, 1989.

Protopath Proteolytic Enzyme Detection System: Antithrombin III Synthetic Substrate Assay for Determination of AT-III Activity in Plasma (package insert). American Dade, Division of American Hospital Supply Corp, Miami, FL, 1986.

Ramsey, R, and Evatt, BL: Rapid assay for von Willebrand's factor activity using formalin-fixed platelets and microtitration technique. Am J Clin Pathol 72:996, 1979.

Reptilase-R (package insert). Abbott Laboratories, Diagnostics Division, IL, 93-4260, 1974.

Russell's Viper Venom Reagent for Factor X Assays (package insert). General Diagnostics, Morris Plains, NJ, 1976.

Sadler, JE: A revised classification of von Willebrand disease: For the Subcommittee on von Willebrand Factor of the Scientific and Standardization Committee of the International Society on Thrombosis and Haemostasis. Thromb Haemost 71:520, 1994.

Sahud, MA: Laboratory diagnosis of inhibitors. Semin Thromb Hemost 26:195, 2000.

Sala, N, et al: A functional assay of protein C in human plasma. Blood 63:671, 1984.

Shitamoto, BS, et al: Postpartum hemophilia. Am J Clin Pathol 78:5, 1982.

Sirridge, MS, and Shannon, R: Laboratory Evaluation of Hemostasis and Thrombosis, ed 3. Lea & Febiger, Philadelphia, 1983.

Spero, JA, et al: Disseminated intravascular coagulation: Findings in 346 patients. Thromb Haemost 43:28, 1980.

Stenflo, J, and Jonsson, M: Protein S, a new vitamin K–dependent protein from bovine plasma. FEBS Lett 101:37, 1979.

Sukhu, K, et al: Evaluation of the von Willebrand factor antigen assay using an immuno-turbidimetric method (STA Liatest vwF) automated on the MDA 180 coagulometer. Clin Lab Haematol 22:29, 2000.

Sussman, LN: The clotting time—an enigma. Am J Clin Pathol 60:5, 1973.

Thrombo-Wellcotest (package insert). Wellcome Research Laboratories, Brekenham, England, 1974.

Triplett, DA: The laboratory diagnosis of lupus anticoagulants. Presented at the Fifth International Symposium of Antiphospholipid Antibodies. San Antonio, TX, September, 1992.

Triplett, DA, and Harms, CS: Procedures for the Coagulation Laboratory. American Society of Clinical Pathologists, Chicago, 1981.

Triplett, DA, et al: Platelet Function: Laboratory Evaluation and Clinical Application. American Society of Clinical Pathologists, Chicago, 1978.

Vinazzer, H, et al: Protein C: Comparison of different assays in normal and abnormal plasma samples. Thromb Res 46:1, 1987.

von Kaulla, F, and von Kaulla, N: Deficiency of antithrombin III activity associated with hereditary thrombosis tendency. J. Med 3;349, 1972.

Walker, FJ: Regulation of activated protein C by a new protein—A possible function for bovine protein S. J Biol Chem 255:5521, 1980.

INDEX

Note: Page reference in italics indicates a figure; page reference followed by "t" indicates a table.